RETURN OF THE TRAILBLAZER

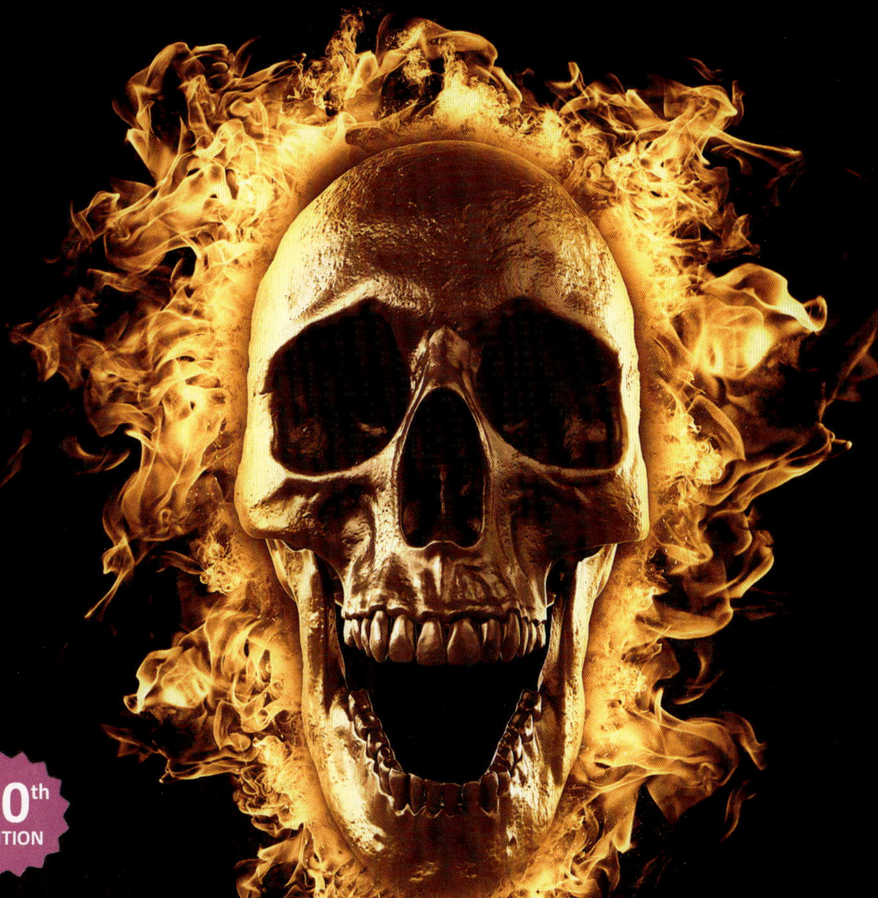

20th EDITION

FREE SUPPLEMENT

Textbook of Forensic Medicine & Toxicology

V V Pillay

Important Sections of New Indian Criminal Laws – 2024

Free Supplement with

V V Pillay – Textbook of Forensic Medicine & Toxicology (20th Edition)

Important Sections of New Indian Criminal Laws that have Replaced Older Statutes

- **Bharatiya Nyaya Sanhita 2023 (BNS)** replaces **Indian Penal Code 1860 (IPC).**
  - BNS has 358 sections (instead of 511 sections of IPC).
  - 20 new crimes have been added.
  - Imprisonment sentence has been increased for 33 crimes.
  - Amount of fine has been increased in 83 crimes.
  - Mandatory minimum punishment has been introduced for 23 crimes.
- **Bharatiya Nagarik Suraksha Sanhita 2023 (BNSS)** replaces **Criminal Procedure Code 1973 (CrPC).**
  - BNSS has 531 sections (instead of 484 sections of CrPC).
  - 177 provisions have been changed.
  - 9 new sections and 39 new sub-sections have been added.
  - 44 new provisions and clarifications have been added.
  - Timelines have been added to 35 sections and audio-video provision has been added at 35 places.
- **Bharatiya Sakshya Adhiniyam 2023 (BSA)** replaces **Indian Evidence Act 1872 (IEA).**
  - BSA has 170 provisions (instead of 167 provisions of IEA).
  - 24 provisions have been changed.

All the above have received the assent of the President of India on 25th Dec 2023.

IMPORTANT CHANGES*

Bharatiya Nyaya Sanhita 2023 (BNS) (*previously,* Indian Penal Code)

I. **Additions**:

The following Section has been **added** to the **Bharatiya Nyaya Sanhita 2023 (BNS)** (*previously*, **Indian Penal Code**):

226 BNS – Criminalises any attempt to commit suicide in order to compel or restrain exercise of lawful power by a public servant, punishable with imprisonment up to 1 year or fine or both, or community service.

II. **Deletions**:

The following Sections have been **deleted** from the erstwhile Indian Penal Code, and therefore do not figure in the **Bharatiya Nyaya Sanhita 2023 (BNS)**:

1. **124-A IPC** (sedition)
2. **309 IPC** (attempt to commit suicide)
3. **377 IPC** (punishment for unnatural sexual offences)
4. **497 IPC** (adultery)

III. **Substitutions**:

- **2(6) BNS** replaces **46 IPC** – **Definition of death** (no change)
- **2(11) BNS** replaces **52 IPC** – **Definition of good faith** (no change)
- **2(14) BNS** replaces **44 IPC** – **Definition of injury** (*the word "denotes" is replaced with "means"*): "Injury" means any harm whatever illegally caused to any person, in body, mind, reputation or property.
- **2(23) BNS** replaces **51 IPC** – **Definition of oath** (no change)
- **2(24) BNS** replaces **40 IPC** – **Definition of offence** (*Except in the Chapters and Sections mentioned in sub-clauses (a) and (b), the word "offence" means a thing made punishable by this Sanhita*).
- **20 BNS** replaces **82 IPC** – **Criminal responsibility of child under 7 years** (no change)
- **21 BNS** replaces **83 IPC** – **Criminal responsibility of child 7-12 years** (no change)
- **22 BNS** replaces **84 IPC** – **Criminal responsibility of person with unsound mind – McNaughten Rule** (no change)
- **23 BNS** replaces **85 IPC** – **Criminal responsibility of person with involuntary intoxication** – (no change)
- **24 BNS** replaces **86 IPC** – **Criminal responsibility of person with voluntary intoxication** – (no change)
- **25 BNS** replaces **87 IPC** – **Act not intended/known to cause death or grievous hurt done with consent** (no change)

**Those which are underlined are MOST important!*

- **26 BNS** replaces **88 IPC** – **Act done in good faith for benefit of person with consent, not intended to cause death** (no change)
- **27 BNS** replaces **89 IPC** – **Act done in good faith for benefit of minor/person of unsound mind with consent of guardian** (*the words "insane person" are replaced with "person of unsound mind"*).
- **28 BNS** replaces **90 IPC** – **Consent given under fear or misconception is invalid** (no change)
- **30 BNS** replaces **92 IPC** – **Act done in good faith for benefit of person without consent** (no change).
- **63 BNS** replaces **375 IPC** – **Defines rape** (*Age of consent: 15 years is replaced by 18 years in BNS. Exception 2 of Section 63 states that "sexual intercourse or acts by a man with his wife, the wife not being under 18 years of age, is not rape"*).
- **64 BNS** replaces
  376(1) IPC – **Punishment for rape** (no change)
  376(2) IPC – **Punishment for custodial rape** (no change).
- **65(1) BNS** replaces **376(3) IPC** – **Punishment for raping girl under 16 years** (no change).
- **65(2) BNS** replaces **376AB IPC** – **Punishment for raping girl under 12 years** (no change).
- **66 BNS** replaces **376A IPC** – **Punishment for causing death or persistent vegetative state of rape victim** (no change).
- **67 BNS** replaces **376B IPC** – **Punishment for sexual intercourse by man with his own wife, who is living separately** (no change).
- **68 BNS** replaces **376C IPC** – **Punishment for sexual intercourse by forcibly inducing/enticing a female to have sexual intercourse, by a man using his authority** (no change).
- **70(1) BNS** replaces **376D IPC** – **Punishment for gang rape** (no change).
- **70(2) BNS** replaces
  - **376DA IPC** – Punishment for gang rape of victim under 16 years
    and
  - **376DB IPC** Punishment for gang rape of victim under 12 years

  (*Death sentence was provided under section 376DB of IPC for gang rape of woman under 12 years of age. No death penalty was provided for gang rape of woman aged below 16 but above 12 in section 376DA.* ***Now, section 70(2) of BNS provides death penalty for gang rape of any woman under 18 years of age***).
- **71 BNS** replaces **376E IPC** – **Punishment for repeat offenders of rape** (no change).
- **72 BNS** replaces **228A(1)/(2) IPC** – **Punishment for disclosure of identity of victim of certain offences such as rape** (*the word "minor" is replaced by "child"*).
- **73 BNS** replaces **228A(3) IPC** – **Punishment for printing or publishing any matter relating to court proceedings without permission**.
  - *Punishment for both – imprisonment up to 2 years and fine.*
- **74 BNS** replaces **354 IPC** – **Punishment for assault or use of criminal force to woman with intent to outrage her modesty** – **indecent assault** (no change).
- **75 BNS** replaces **354A IPC** – **Punishment for sexual harassment** (no change).
- **76 BNS** replaces **354B IPC** – **Punishment for intent to disrobe a woman** (*the words "Any man who" is replaced by "Whoever"*).
- **77 BNS** replaces **354C IPC** – Deals with **voyeurism** (no change).
- **78 BNS** replaces **354D IPC** – Deals with **stalking** (no change).
- **79 BNS** replaces **509 IPC** – **Punishment for word, gesture or act intended to insult the modesty of a woman** (no change).
- **80 BNS** replaces **304B IPC** – **Punishment for dowry death** (no change).
- **84 BNS** replaces **498 IPC** – **Punishment for enticing/taking away/detaining married woman with criminal intent** (no change).
- **85 BNS** replaces **498A IPC** – **Punishment for husband or his relative for subjecting wife to cruelty** (no change).
- **87 BNS** replaces **366 IPC** – **Kidnapping or abducting a woman to compel her for marriage, etc** (no change).
- **88 BNS** replaces **312 IPC** – **Punishment for causing miscarriage** (no change).
- **89 BNS** replaces **313 IPC** – **Punishment for causing miscarriage without woman's consent** (no change).
- **90 BNS** replaces **314 IPC** – **Punishment for causing death by an act done with intent to cause miscarriage** (no change).
- **91 BNS** replaces **315 IPC** – **Punishment for any act done with intent to prevent a child from being born alive, or to cause it to die after its birth** (no change).
- **92 BNS** replaces **316 IPC** – **Punishment for causing death of quick, unborn child by an act amounting to culpable homicide** (no change).
- **93 BNS** replaces **317 IPC** – **Punishment for exposure and abandonment of child <12 years by parent or guardian** (no change).
- **94 BNS** replaces **318 IPC** – **Punishment for concealment of birth by secret disposal of dead body** (no change).

- **96 BNS** replaces **366A IPC** – **Procuration of child for illicit intercourse** (*the words "minor girl under the age of 18 years" are replaced by the word "child" and made gender neutral*).
- **100 BNS** replaces **299 IPC** – **Definition of culpable homicide not amounting to murder** (no change).
- **101 BNS** replaces **300 IPC** – **Definition of culpable homicide amounting to murder** (no change).
- **103(1) BNS** replaces **302 IPC** – **Punishment for murder** (no change).
- **103(2) BNS** is a **new sub-section** – "*When a group of five or more persons acting in concert commits murder on the ground of race, caste or community, sex, place of birth, language, personal belief or any other similar ground, each member shall be punished with death or with imprisonment for life, and shall also be liable to fine*".
- **104 BNS** replaces **303 IPC** – **Punishment for murder by person already undergoing life imprisonment** (*BNS gives an alternate punishment for the life-convict murderer as death 'or with imprisonment for life, which shall mean the remainder of that person's natural life', whereas in IPC, the only punishment mentioned is death sentence for murder by a life convict*).
- **105 BNS** replaces **304 IPC** – **Punishment for culpable homicide not amounting to murder** (*Minimum imprisonment for five years is added, and fine is made mandatory*).
- **106 BNS** replaces **304A IPC** – **Punishment for causing death by rash or negligent act**.
  - ***Sub-section 1*** – up to 5 years imprisonment and fine. (if doctor is involved in negligent death of patient – up to 2 years and fine)
  - ***Sub-section 2*** – if it is a hit and run traffic death, up to 10 years imprisonment and fine.
- **107 BNS** replaces **305 IPC** – **Abetment of suicide of child or person of unsound mind** (*punishment enhanced from 10 years to life imprisonment or death*).
- **108 BNS** replaces **306 IPC** – **Abetment of suicide by person not being a child or of unsound mind** (no change).
- **109 BNS** replaces **307 IPC** – **Attempt to commit murder** (no change).
- **110 BNS** replaces **308 IPC** – **Attempt to commit culpable homicide** (no change).
- **114 BNS** replaces **319 IPC** – **Defines hurt** (no change).
- **115 BNS** replaces **323 IPC** – **Punishment for voluntarily causing hurt** (*fine increased from 1000 to 10,000*; rest is the same).
- **116 BNS** replaces **320 IPC** – **Definition of grievous hurt**. (*Clause 8 of 320 IPC has been changed in Sub-section h of 116 BNS as follows: "Any hurt which causes the sufferer to be during the space of 15 days in severe bodily pain, or unable to follow his ordinary pursuits is considered grievous hurt". In 320 IPC, it was 20 days*).
- **117 BNS** replaces **322** and **325 IPC** – **Punishment for causing grievous hurt**.
  - **117(3)**: "*Whoever commits an offence in the course of which causes that person to be in permanent disability or in persistent vegetative state, shall be punished with rigorous imprisonment for a term which shall not be less than ten years but which may extend to imprisonment for life, which shall mean imprisonment for the remainder of that person's natural life*".
- **118(1)** and **(2) BNS** replace **324** and **326 IPC** – **Punishment for voluntarily causing grievous hurt by dangerous weapons or means**
  - *Fine is increased to 20,000 rupees under 118(1)*
  - *Mandatory imprisonment is added, i.e., 1 year, under 118(2)*
- **123 BNS** replaces **328 IPC** – **Punishment for causing hurt by means of poison with intent to commit an offence** (no change).
- **124(1) BNS** replaces **326A IPC** – **Punishment for voluntarily causing grievous hurt by acid, or causes a person to be in persistent vegetative state** (*10 years to life imprisonment, and fine paid to victim*). Neither is required to be irreversible.
- **124(2) BNS** replaces **326B IPC** – **Punishment for voluntarily throwing, or attempting to throw acid** (*5–7 years imprisonment and fine*).
- **125(a) BNS** replaces **337 IPC** – **Causing hurt by rash and negligent act endangering life or personal safety of others** (*fine increased from Rs 500 to Rs 5000;* rest is the same).
- **125(b) BNS** replaces **338 IPC** – **Causing grievous hurt by rash and negligent act endangering life or personal safety of others** (*punishment increased from 2 years to 3 years imprisonment, with/without fine increased from Rs 1000 to Rs 10,000*).
- **130 BNS** replaces **351 IPC** – **Defines assault** (no change).
- **131 BNS** replaces **352 IPC** – **Punishment for assault** (*Fine is increased from Rs 500 to Rs 1000*).
- **137(1) BNS** replaces **361 IPC** – **Defines kidnapping** (no change).
- **137(2) BNS** replaces **363 IPC** – **Punishment for kidnapping** (no change).
- **138 BNS** replaces **362 IPC** – **Defines abduction** (no change).
- **140(1) BNS** replaces **364 IPC** – **Kidnapping or abducting in order to murder** (no change).
- **140(2) BNS** replaces **364A IPC** – **Kidnapping for ransom**, etc (no change).

- 141 BNS replaces 366B IPC – **Importation of boy (*<18 years*) or girl (*<21 years*) from foreign country for illicit intercourse**.
- 143 BNS replaces 370 IPC – **Trafficking of person** (*the word "minor" is replaced by "child"*)
- 144 BNS replaces 370A IPC – **Exploitation of trafficked person** (*enhancement of maximum punishment to 10 years*)
- 200 BNS replaces 166B IPC – **Punishment for non-treatment of victim** (no change).
- 208 BNS replaces 174 IPC – **Non-attendance to summons** (*imprisonment same, i.e., 6 months, but fine enhanced to Rs 10,000*).
- 211 BNS replaces 176 IPC –
  - **Omission to give notice or information to public servant by person legally bound to give it** — *shall be punished with simple imprisonment for a term which may extend to 1 month, or with fine up to Rs 5000, or with both;*
  - **Where the notice or information required to be given respects the commission of an offence** - *simple imprisonment for a term which may extend to 6 months, or with fine up to Rs 10,000, or with both;*
- 212 BNS replaces 177 IPC – **Punishment for**
  - **Furnishing false information** (*imprisonment up to 6 months, with/without fine up to Rs 5000*).
  - **Furnishing false information related to commission of an offence** (*imprisonment up to 2 years, with/without fine*).
- 227 BNS replaces 191 IPC – **Giving false evidence, i.e., perjury** (no change).
- 228 BNS replaces 192 IPC – **Fabricating false evidence** (no change).
- 229 BNS replaces 193 IPC – **Punishment for perjury** (no change).
- 234 BNS replaces 197 IPC – **Punishment for issuing or signing false certificate** (no change).
- 238 BNS replaces 201 IPC – **Causing disappearance of evidence, or giving false information to screen offender** (no change).
- 239 BNS replaces 202 IPC – **Intentional omission to give information of offence by person bound to inform** (no change).
- 241 BNS replaces 204 IPC – **Destruction of document or electronic record to prevent its production as evidence** (*punishment enhanced from 2 years to 3 years, with/without fine*).
- 286 BNS replaces 284 IPC – **Punishment for negligent conduct with respect to poison** (*up to 6 months imprisonment, with/without fine which has been enhanced from Rs 1000 to Rs 5000*).
- 292 BNS replaces 290 IPC – **Punishment for public nuisance in any case not otherwise punishable** (*fine raised from Rs 100 to Rs 1000*).
- 296 BNS replaces 294 IPC – **Punishment for obscene acts and songs, including exhibitionism** (no change).
- 301 BNS replaces 297 IPC – **Punishment for committing trespass in any place of worship, or a burial site, or offers any indignity to a human corpse, including necrophilia** (no change).
- 355 BNS replaces 510 IPC – **Punishment for misconduct in public by drunken person** (*Fine Rs 1000, or community service*).

Bharatiya Nagarik Suraksha Sanhita 2023 (BNNS) (*previously,* Criminal Procedure Code)

- 2(1)(g) BNSS replaces 2(C) CrPC – **Cognizable offence** (no change).
- 33 BNSS replaces 39 CrPC – **Public to provide information of certain offences under BNS** (no change).
- 51(1) BNSS replaces 53(1) CrPC –
  - *When a person is arrested on a charge of committing an offence of such a nature that there are reasonable grounds for believing that an examination of his person will afford evidence as to the commission of the offence, it shall be lawful for a registered medical practitioner, acting at the request of any police officer, to make such an examination as is reasonably necessary, and to use such force as is reasonably necessary for that purpose.*
- 51(2) BNSS replaces 53(2) CrPC –
  - *Whenever the person of a female is to be examined under this section, the examination shall be made only by, or under the supervision of, a female registered medical practitioner.*

    Explanation — "Examination" shall include the examination of blood, blood stains, semen, swabs in case of sexual offences, sputum and sweat, hair samples and finger nail clippings by the use of modern and scientific techniques including DNA profiling.
- 52 BNSS replaces 53A CrPC – **Examination of rape accused by medical practitioner** (*the words "police officer not below the rank of Sub-Inspector" are replaced by "any police officer"*).
- 53 BNSS replaces 54 CrPC – **Examination of arrested person by medical officer** (*When any person is arrested, he shall be examined by a medical officer in the service of the Central Government or a State Government, and in case such medical officer is not available, by any registered medical practitioner soon after the arrest is made*).

- 58 BNSS replaces 57 CrPC – **Person arrested not to be detained for more than 24 hours.** (no change)
- 63-71 BNSS replace 61-69 CrPC – Deal with **Summons** (*The following clause is added: "Summons can be in the form of electronic communication and shall bear the image of the seal of the Court or digital signature. Service of summons through electronic communication shall be considered duly served, and a copy of such summons shall be attested and kept as proof of service of summons"*).
- 184 BNSS replaces 164A CrPC – **Medical examination of rape victim** (*"Without delay" is replaced by "Within a period of 7 days" for medical practitioner to forward the report to Investigating officer*).
- 194 BNSS replaces 174 CrPC –
  - **Police inquest** (*The report shall be signed by such police officer and other persons, and shall be forwarded to the District Magistrate or the Sub-divisional Magistrate within 24 hours*).
  - Mandatory autopsy of woman who dies within 7 years of marriage.
- 196 BNSS replaces 176 CrPC – **Magistrate's inquest** (*"Judicial Magistrate" is replaced by "Magistrate", and Metropolitan Magistrate is removed*).
- 326 BNSS replaces 291 CrPC – **Deposition of medical witness** (no change).
- 366 BNSS replaces 327 CrPC – **Examination of a survivor of sexual assault must be conducted *in camera*** (no change).
- 389 BNSS replaces 350 CrPC – **Summary procedure for punishment for non-attendance by a witness in spite of summons having been received** (*Fine increased from Rs 100 to Rs 500*).
- 397 BNSS replaces 357C CrPC – **Information to the police about rape, and free treatment of rape victim** (*BNS sections replace corresponding IPC sections. "under sections 4, 6, 8 or section 10 of the Protection of Children from Sexual Offences Act, 2012" is added*).
- 456 BNSS replaces 416 CrPC – **Compulsory commutation of death sentence of a pregnant woman to life imprisonment** (*earlier, death sentence was postponed until after delivery, but not necessarily commuted*).

Bharatiya Sakshya Adhiniyam 2023 (BSA) (*previously,* Indian Evidence Act)

- 2(1)(e) BSA replaces 3 IEA – **Evidence** (*the following have been added - "including statements given electronically"*).
- 26 BSA replaces 32 IEA – **Cases in which statement of relevant fact by person who is dead or cannot be found, etc., is relevant. Includes dying declaration** (no change).
- 39(1) BSA replaces 45 IEA – **Opinion of experts** (*The following words "or any other field" are added. Thus, scope is expanded greatly.*).
- 110 BSA replaces 107 IEA – **Presumption of being alive** – burden of proving death of person known to have been alive within 30 years (no change).
- 111 BSA replaces 108 IEA – **Presumption of death** – burden of proving that person is alive who has not been heard of for 7 years (no change).
- 120 BSA replaces 114A IEA – **Presumption as to absence of consent in certain cases of rape** (no change).
- 142 BSA replaces 137 IEA – **Procedures in examining witness in a court of law** (no change).
- 143 BSA replaces 138 IEA – **Order of examining witness in a court of law** (no change).
- 146(1) BSA replaces 141 IEA – **Leading question** (no change).
- 146(2) & (3) BSA replace 142 IEA – **When leading questions cannot be asked** (no change).
- 146(4) BSA replaces 143 IEA – **When leading questions may be asked** (no change).
- 149 BSA replaces 146 IEA – **Questions lawful in cross examination** (no change).
- 151 BSA replaces 148 IEA – **Court to decide when a witness can be compelled to answer** (no change).
- 154 BSA replaces 151 IEA – **Indecent and scandalous questions** (no change).
- 157 BSA replaces 154 IEA – **Question by party to his own witness – hostile witness** (no change).
- 162 BSA replaces 159 IEA – **Refreshing memory by witness** (no change).
- 165 BSA replaces 162 IEA – **Production of documents in court** (no change).

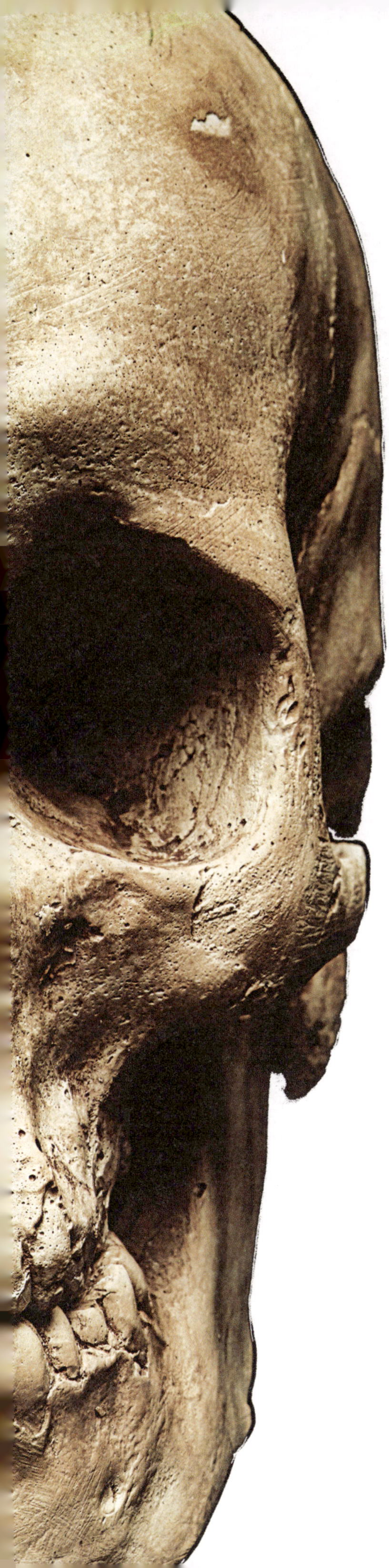

Textbook of Forensic Medicine & Toxicology

V V Pillay, MD, DCL

Chief, Poison Control Centre
Head, Analytical Toxicology
Professor and Head, Forensic Medicine & Toxicology
Amrita School of Medicine
Amrita Vishwa Vidyapeetham (Deemed-to-be-University)
Cochin, Kerala, India

20th Edition

*Prepared **exactly** as per the new MBBS curriculum (Competency Based Undergraduate Curriculum for the Indian Medical Graduate or CBME-2018) along with subsequent amendments.*

Completely revised, profusely illustrated, and embellished with landmark case histories, shocking true stories, fascinating anecdotes, and mnemonics for an enlightening and fulfilling read.

Paras Medical Publisher®
Hyderabad ▪ New Delhi, India

DEDICATION

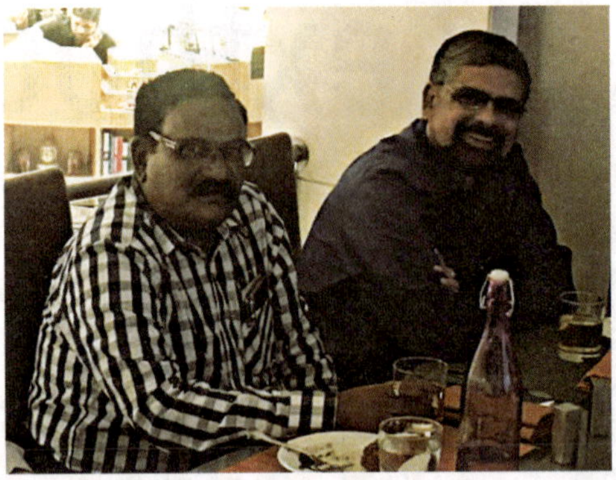

Dedicated to the memory of one of my closest friends from medical school days, **Dr Raphael Ranjan**; within a month after a reunion party with a few other friends, as we relived our wild and carefree days, planning some more parties for the next year, this terrible news came like a bolt out of the blue: Ranjan had suddenly passed away due to a massive heart attack. The image posted above is from that 'last supper' (*Ranjan is at the left*). The following is an apt eulogy to a chum that I will never forget (the lyrics have been tweaked a little from the original song "Seasons in the Sun" by Terry Jacks):

Goodbye my friend, it's hard to die
When all the birds are singing in the sky
We had joy, we had fun
We had seasons in the sun
But the wine and the song
Like the seasons, have all gone
Goodbye Ranjan, my favourite friend
You gave me love and helped me find the sun
And every time that I was down
You would always come around
And get my feet back on the ground
Goodbye Ranjan, it's hard to die
When all the birds are singing in the sky
Now that the spring is in the air
With the flowers everywhere
I wish that we could both be there.......

TEXTBOOK OF FORENSIC MEDICINE & TOXICOLOGY

PARAS®

Explore the New Possibilities

Paras Medical Publisher
5-1-475, First Floor, Putlibowli
Hyderabad – 500095, Telangana, India

Branch Office:
2/25, Ground Floor, Arun House
Daryaganj, Ansari Road
New Delhi – 110002, India

1/ed 1965, 11/ed 1999, 12/ed 2001, 13/ed 2003, 14/ed 2004, 15/ed 2010, 16/ed 2011, 17/ed 2016, 18/ed 2017 19/ed 2019, 20/ed 2023

ISBN: 978-81-8191-560-3

FAN PAGE

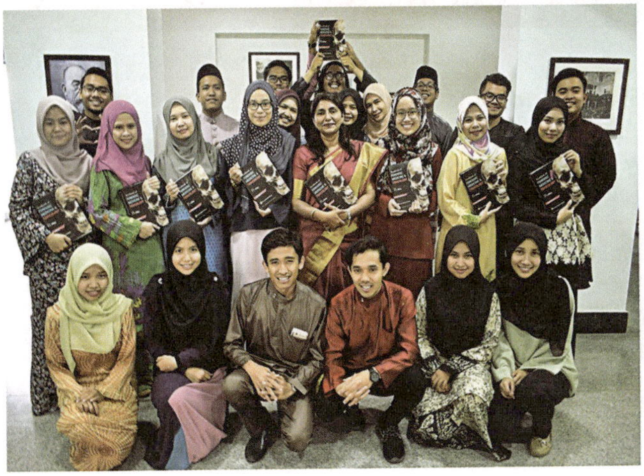

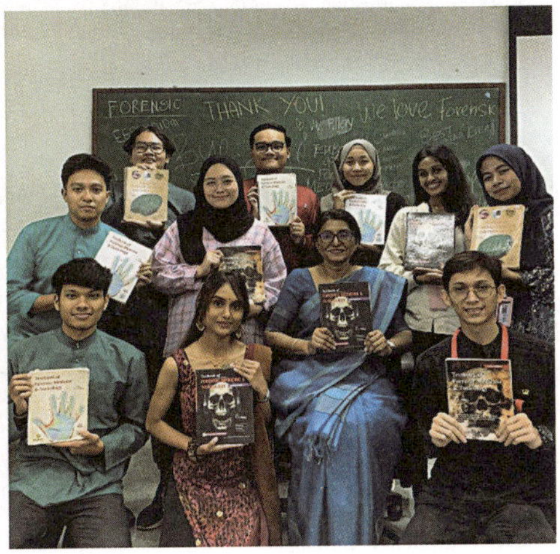

Talking about Pillay Sir's textbook,
You are bound to have a second look!
A feast to the eyes,
That will surely make you more wiser.
A concoction of pulsating cases, in Boxes
Newspaper clippings of familiar faces and hoaxes.
Apt anecdotes, which are thrilling
Oh such information, is truly fulfilling!
Interesting illustrations, exciting references to movies and pictures that are perfect,
Tables, figures, glossy pages and the hard bound cover, all add on to that special effect.
Kudos to the editor for all the hard work he took
It's good to see the maestro's smiling face in the book!

Dr Ajee Kuruvilla with Students
Dept of Forensic Medicine & Toxicology
International Medical School (MSU), Ramaiah Campus, Bangalore

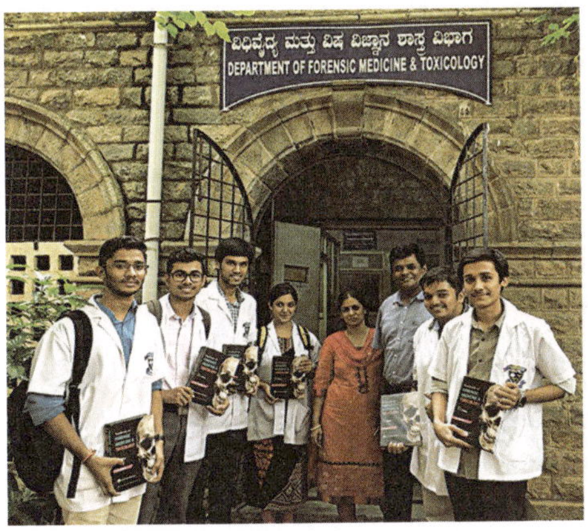

Dr S Venkata Raghava and Dr CN Sumangala with Students
Dept of Forensic Medicine & Toxicology
Bangalore Medical College & Research Institute (BMCRI), Bangalore

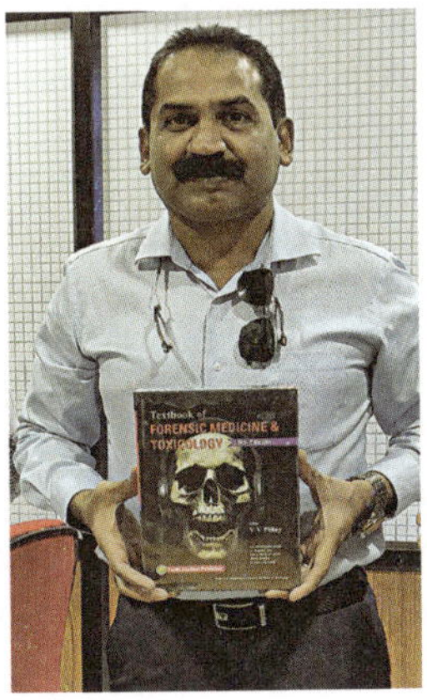

Dr Jayaprakash (JP)
Renowned Expert
and PG Entrance
Exam Coach

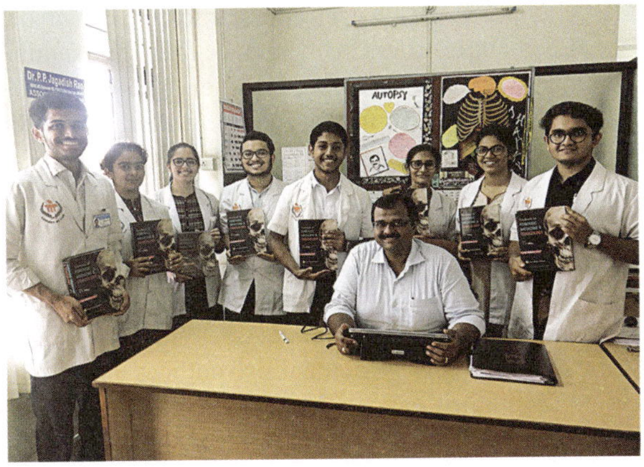

Dr Jagadish Rao PP and Students
Dept of Forensic Medicine & Toxicology
Kasturba Medical College
Mangalore

How to Read the Book!

Why Red, Green and Black Text?

The 20th edition of the trailblazing "*Textbook of Forensic Medicine & Toxicology*" has been prepared **exactly** as per the Competency Based Undergraduate Curriculum (2018) along with its amendments, of the National Medical Commission.

The entire textual matter is **Colour Coded** as per the nature of information being discussed:
- **Red** print matter – *Necessary to Know* (essential information!)
- **Black** print matter – *Need to Know* (required information)
- **Green** print matter – *Nice to Know* (optional information)

This translates as
- **Red** = Pass
- **Red** + **Black** = First Class
- **Red** + **Black** + **Green** = Distinction

It is advisable to **read** the red, black and green matter at the start of the course, and later exercise your choice as you approach the examination, depending on the time available or your inclination (pass, first class or distinction!).

ADDITIONAL POINTS OF IMPORTANCE!

- This is a compact book covering all the information as per the new CBME curriculum of the NMC.
- It is the Editor's genuine belief that anything that is not mentioned in this book is **outside the scope** of the new curriculum, which means that it is **outside the syllabus**.
- There are no Chapters, only **Topics**. This is how it is mentioned in the new curriculum. The concept of Chapters is outdated.
- Every **Topic** will have one or more **Competencies (Outcomes)**. The number of Competencies will depend upon the extent of information to be covered, and has been explicitly laid out in the new curriculum.
- Each **Topic** is designated by the alphabets **FM** (which stand for Forensic Medicine) followed by a **number**, while the **Competency** is designated as a **running number** following a full stop after the Topic number.
  - For example, the first Topic in the book is designated as Topic 1, while each Competency under it is mentioned as running numbers following a full stop.
  - Since Topic 1 has 11 Competencies, they will be discussed in serial order as follows: FM1.1, FM1.2,.....until FM1.11.
- Each **Topic** differs in importance from the examination point of view. There are two main categories:
  - **Core Topic** designated by the alphabet **Y** (Must Achieve)
  - **Non-Core Topic** designated by the alphabet **N** (Desirable)
- **Core Topics** can be assessed in **Formative Assessment** (Internal Assessments and Day-to-Day Assessment) as well as **Summative Assessment** (University examination), while **Non-Core Topics** are not to be assessed in University examination, but can be assessed in Internal Assessments and Day-to-Day Assessment.
  - In short, Core Topics are essential to pass the University examination, while Non-Core Topics are useful to clear the Internal Assessment which is necessary to be eligible to take the University examination.
  - Please note that Internal Assessment marks cannot be added to University examination marks.
- While the new curriculum also outlines the **Learning Domains** for each **Competency** (Knowledge, Skill, Attitude and Communication), as also the expected **Level of Achievement** (Knows, Knows How, Shows How, Performs), these are more important for teachers than the students, so this book will not trouble you with unnecessary details.

In **Summary**, remember the following when reading the book:
- **Colour Coding** of print matter – **Red** (essential), **Black** (required) **or Green** (optional).
- Nature of Topic –
  - **Core** (Day-to-Day Assessment, Internal Assessment and University exam)
  - **Non-Core** (Internal Assessment and Day-to-Day Assessment only)

HAPPY READING!

Acknowledgements

Grateful acknowledgements are due to:

- My colleagues who have contributed to this edition (information, photographs, drawings). All such material has been explicitly credited to the respective contributor wherever it has been incorporated.
- The following distinguished persons from Amrita Institute of Medical Sciences & Research, Cochin for their constant support and encouragement: **Dr Prem Nair**, **Dr Gireesh Kumar KP**.
- Sub-editors and major contributors of previous editions: **Dr BK Bastia**, **Dr Joseph T John**, **Dr Ch Lakshmi Kumar**, **Dr P Sampath Kumar**, **Dr Ajee Kuruvilla**, **Dr Rohan Monis**, **Dr Jagadeesh N**, **Dr Prateek Rastogi**, **Dr Jagadish Rao PP**, **Dr Vina Vaswani**, **Dr Walter Vaz**.
- My wife **Dr Minnie** who has always stood by me; our dear daughter **Dr Roshni**, who has had the rare good fortune of having been taught the subject of Anatomy by her own dedicated mother, and Forensic Medicine & Toxicology by her unconventional father; and our dynamic son-in-law **Dr Balram Rathish**, who was also our own student.
- Mr Divyesh Kothari of Paras Medical Publisher for ensuring excellence in the presentation of textual matter, illustrations, and images, and the over-all get-up of the book.

And above all to:

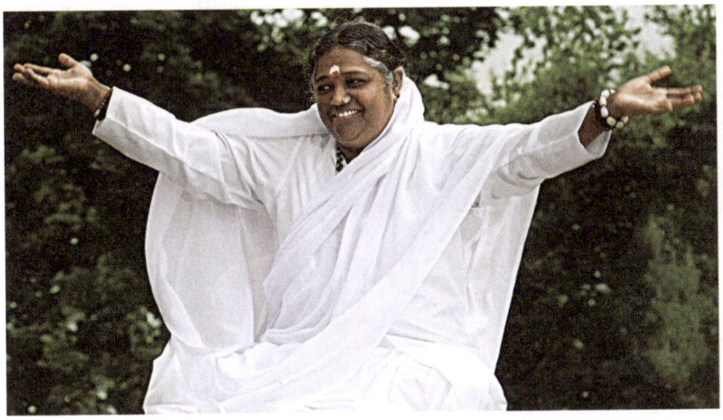

Her Holiness **Sri Mata Amritanandamayi Devi**
for unwavering divine inspiration leading to my own sense of fulfillment and accomplishment.

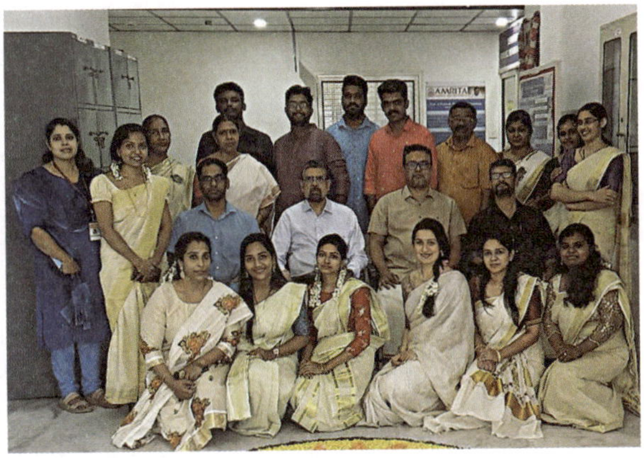

Faculty and Staff
Dept of Forensic Medicine & Toxicology
Amrita Institute of Medical Sciences
for flawless dedication and cooperation

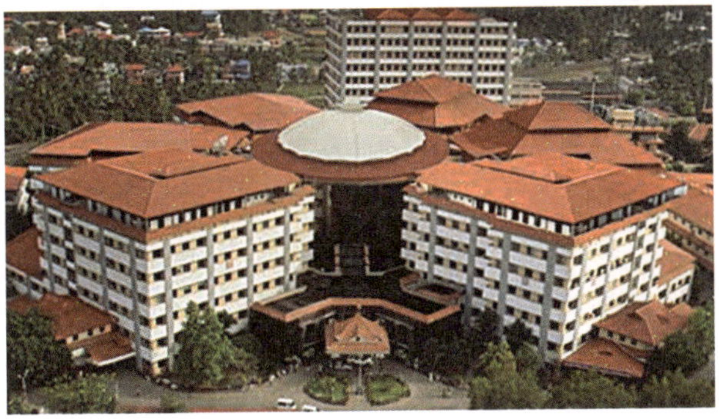

Amrita Institute of Medical Sciences & Research Centre
Cochin, Kerala

Table of Contents

SECTION 1 — FORENSIC MEDICINE

Topic 1 : General Information

Competencies: 11 (1.1 to 1.11)

Topic 2 : Forensic Pathology

Competencies: 35 (2.1 to 2.35)

Topic 3 : Clinical Forensic Medicine

Competencies: 33 (3.1 to 3.33)

Topic 4 : Medical Jurisprudence (Medical Law and Ethics)

Competencies: 30 (4.1 to 4.30)

Topic 5 : Forensic Psychiatry

Competencies: 6 (5.1 to 5.6)

Topic 6 : Forensic Laboratory Investigations in Medicolegal Practice

Competencies: 3 (6.1 to 6.3)

Topic 7 : Emerging Technologies in Forensic Medicine

Competencies: 1 (7.1)

SECTION 2 — TOXICOLOGY

Topic 8 : General Toxicology

Competencies: 10 (8.1 to 8.10)

Topic 9 : Chemical Toxicology

Competencies: 6 (9.1 to 9.6)

Topic 10 : Pharmaceutical Toxicology

Competencies: 1 (10.1)

Topic 11 : Biotoxicology

Competencies: 1 (11.1)

Topic 12 : Sociomedical Toxicology

Competencies: 1 (12.1)

Topic 13 : Environmental Toxicology

Competencies: 2 (13.1 to 13.2)

Annexures

Section 1

FORENSIC MEDICINE

Topic 1

GENERAL INFORMATION

Number of Competencies – 11 (FM 1.1 to 1.11)

FM 1.1: Non-Core – Written/Viva Voce
- Demonstrate knowledge of basics of Forensic Medicine in the form of definitions of
  - Forensic Medicine
  - Clinical Forensic Medicine
  - Forensic Pathology
  - State Medicine
  - Legal Medicine
  - Medical Jurisprudence

DEFINITIONS

Forensic Medicine (Legal Medicine)

The term *forensic* is derived from the Latin word 'forensis' pertaining to forum. Forum is a term that refers to a market place in ancient Rome, where civil and legal matters were discussed, and justice was dispensed.

- **Forensic Medicine (or Legal Medicine) is a branch of Medicine, which deals with the application of medical knowledge in the administration of law and justice.**
- A medical practitioner may have to, on some occasion, give evidence as an expert witness in a court of law to prove the innocence or guilt of an accused, or to authenticate or disprove a criminal charge of assault, rape or murder brought against an individual. He should be aware of the laws relating to the practice of medicine. A knowledge about legal procedures and some sections of the **Indian Penal Code** (IPC), **Criminal Procedure Code** (CrPC) and **Indian Evidence Act** (IEA), related to various offences, is desirable.

Clinical Forensic Medicine

- **Clinical Forensic Medicine deals with the medicolegal aspects of patient care (diagnosis and management). It also includes the examination of victims and perpetrators of criminal assault, rape, child abuse, etc.**
- Apart from these, there are some special categories under the term "Clinical Forensic Medicine" such as:
  - **Traffic medicine** (e.g., examination of injured vehicle drivers, occupants and pedestrians).
  - **Age estimation** in persons having no personal documents.
  - Examination to determine **criminal responsibility of a mentally unsound person**.

Forensic Pathology

- **Forensic Pathology deals with the investigation of intentional (homicidal and suicidal) and unintentional (accidental) death and also deaths from natural causes which are unclear.***
- The primary role of the forensic pathologist is to determine the **cause of death** based on a detailed autopsy. In addition to the examination of the dead victim, the forensic pathologist may also be involved in the examination of the accused/suspect, the scene of crime and the collection of evidentiary material. He has to attend courts of law as an expert witness, provide opinion on the cases he has examined and help in the administration of justice.

State Medicine

- **State Medicine refers to administration and control by the government, of medical and hospital services provided to a population, and paid for out of funds raised by taxation.**

Medical Jurisprudence

('*Juris*' = law and '*Prudence*' = knowledge)

- **Medical Jurisprudence deals with the legal aspects of medicine such as the legal rights, privileges, duties and obligations of a medical practitioner.**
- Medical practitioners must be aware of legal implications of their medical practice. They should be familiar with the various statutes, rules and regulations that are in force, as well as possess a working knowledge of the functioning of statutory bodies and Medical Councils.

FM 1.2: Non-Core – Written/Viva Voce
- Describe the history of Forensic Medicine.

HISTORY OF FORENSIC MEDICINE

A. **Outside India**:

- **3000 to 2000 BCE****:
  - **Imhotep** (2667-2600 BCE) (**Fig. 1.1**), the Grand Vizier to the Pharaoh Djoser of Egypt is considered to be the world's **first physician**. The oldest known written manual of surgery and trauma, describing 48 cases of wounds, fractures, dislocations and tumours, is attributed to Imhotep. **Sir Sydney Smith**, Regius Professor of Forensic Medicine, University of Edinburgh in an article in *BMJ*, in 1950, described Imhotep as the **first medicolegal expert**.***

***Source**: *Kanchan T, Krishan K. Encyclopedia of Forensic Sciences, 2nd ed; 2013.*

****BCE** *stands for "**Before Common Era**". It was formerly referred to as BC (Before Christ).*

*****Source**: *Smith S. The history and development of Forensic Medicine. Br Med J. 1951;1:599–607.*

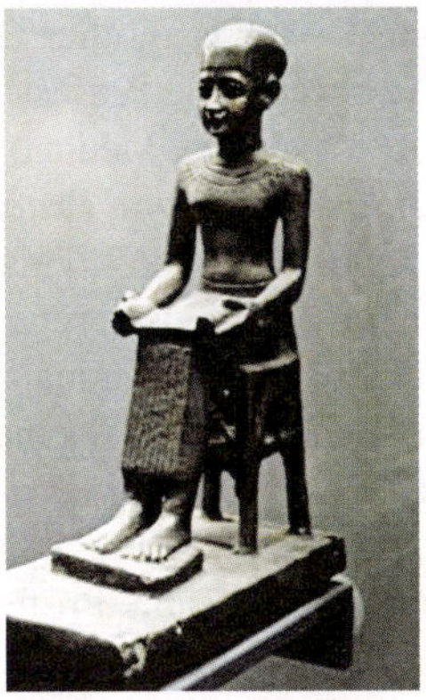

Fig. 1.1 Imhotep

- **2000 to 1000 BCE**:
  - **Hammurabi code** – It is the **oldest written code of law** by the King of Babylon in 1755-1750 BCE, enumerating the responsibilities of a doctor while treating patients.
- **1000 to 50 BCE**:
  - **Hippocrates of Kos** (460-370 BCE) (**Fig. 1.2**) – He is generally acknowledged as the **Father of Medicine**. His teachings included medicolegal aspects of wounds and medical ethics.

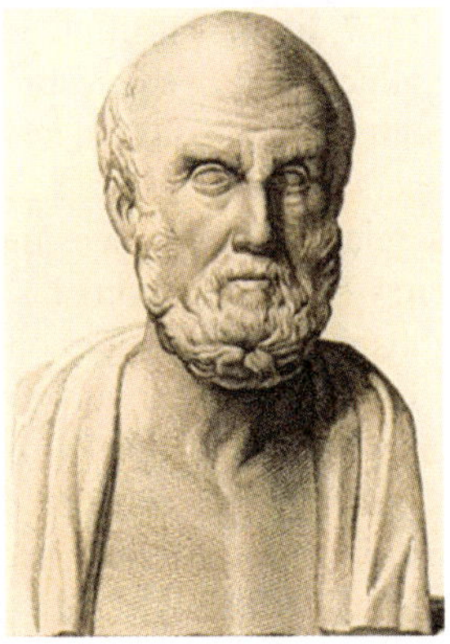

Fig. 1.2 Hippocrates

  - In Rome, **Julius Caesar** (100–44 BCE) is said to have been delivered by a surgical operation practiced to save the life of newborn babies, which later came to be called ***Caesarean section***.
  - **Antistius** – The first recorded autopsy was performed in **44 BCE** by **Antistius** (a Roman physician) on Julius Caesar's body after his assassination, during which he determined that of the 23 stab wounds, one wound to the chest that ruptured Caesar's aorta was the fatal one. **This was the first ever medicolegal autopsy report.**
  - According to ***Jewish law*** of the olden days, a person who attempted suicide was said to be possessed by evil spirits, and hence deserved punishment. Similar ideology was shared by people in Rome and Greece during this period.
- **001 to 100 CE***:
  - **Pliny the Elder** (23-79 CE) first made a mention about suspended animation, and sudden & natural deaths in his treatise, leading to the evolution of forensic literature from as early as 2nd and 3rd centuries.
- **500 to 1000 CE**:
  - ***Justinian Code*** (529 CE) prescribed regulations for medical practice and imposition of penalties for malpractice.
  - ***Visigothic Code*** (***Lex Visigothorum***) is a set of laws outlined by king Chindasuinth of the Visigothic Kingdom in his 2nd year of rule (642-643 CE).
  - The ***Bavarian Code*** (around 741 CE) prescribed punishment for administering abortifacients to cause criminal abortion.
  - The ***Lex Alamannorum*** (7–8th century) gave detailed descriptions of wounds on body and made mention of compulsory medicolegal examination of injuries by competent medical experts.
- **1100 to 1200 CE**:
  - **Frederick II** (1194–1250) who was one of the most powerful emperors of the Middle Ages, made it compulsory that in order for a person to practice medicine, he must fulfill the following criteria:
    - Born legitimately.
    - Aged 21 years.
    - Studied philosophy for 3 years.
    - Studied medicine for 5 years according to the teaching of Hippocrates, Galen and Avicenna.
    - Served 1 year apprenticeship.
    - Taken oath to help the poor and needy after taking the final examination.

    This was how **State Medicine** was born, which is even now reflected in the code of medical ethics that regulates the conduct of registered medical practitioners.
- **1200 to 1500 CE**:
  - In 1249, **Hugo De Lucca**, a surgeon, was appointed as "Medicolegal expert" in Italy.
  - In China, **Hsi Yuan Lu** (1250) was published, which was a handbook containing descriptions of postmortem examinations.
  - In 1374, the Pope sanctioned autopsy examinations.
- **1500 to 1700 CE**:
  - Emperor Charles V created a code called ***Constitutio Criminalis Carolina*** (around 1530 CE) which recognized the essentiality of medical testimony in deaths due to homicide, poisoning, abortion or infanticide.
  - **Ambroise Pare** (1510–1590) (**Fig. 1.3**), a French surgeon, wrote a treatise on different medicolegal problems and how to differentiate antemortem injuries from postmortem injuries. He is generally considered as the **Father of Forensic Pathology**.
  - **Paulo Zacchia** (1584–1659) (**Fig. 1.4**), an Italian physician, published ***Quaestiones Medico-legales***. He is

CE stands for "Common Era**". It was formerly referred to as AD ("in the year of our Lord").*

considered as the **Father of Forensic Psychiatry** and the **Father of Legal Medicine**.

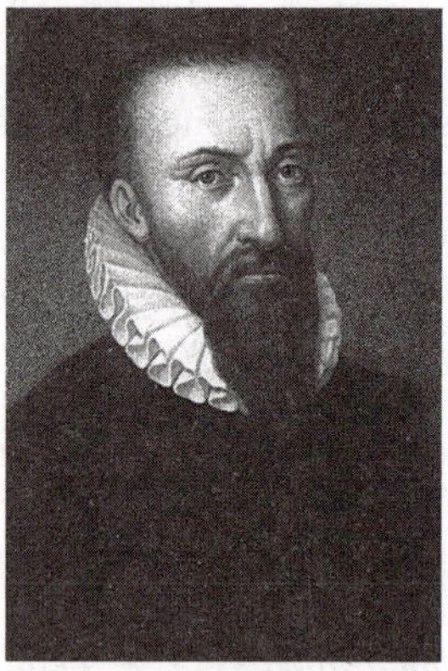

Fig. 1.3 Ambroise Pare

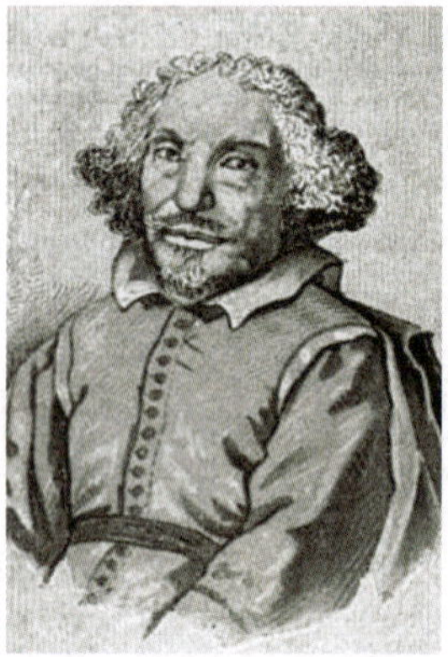

Fig. 1.4 Paulo Zacchia

- **18th century**:
  - In 1701, **Valentini** published ***Pandectae medico-legalese*** which was a work challenging that of Paulo Zacchia.
  - **Andrew Duncan** (1773–1832) became the first Professor of Medical Jurisprudence at Edinburgh in 1807.
- **19th century**:
  - **Mathieu Orfila** (1787–1853) (**Fig. 1.5**), a Spanish toxicologist and chemist, founded the science of toxicology. He is generally considered to be the **Father of Toxicology**.

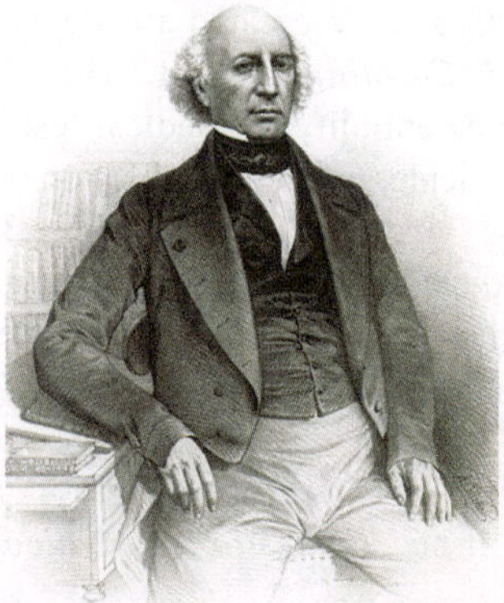

Fig. 1.5 Mathieu Orfila

  - **Alfred Swaine Taylor** is another famous name during this period. He became the Professor of Medical Jurisprudence at Guy's Hospital Medical School in 1834. His first edition of ***Principles and Practice of Medical Jurisprudence*** appeared in 1865. This book has stood the test of time, and is still revised regularly.
  - For mentally compromised criminals, the ***McNaughten's Rules*** were framed in **1843**. This marked the beginning of modern day **Forensic Psychiatry**.
  - **Sir Robert Christison** (1797–1882), a Scottish physician and toxicologist became Professor of Medical Jurisprudence at the age of 25 years in 1822, and was involved as medicolegal expert in the infamous case of *Burke and Hare*.
  - **Alphonse Bertillon** (1853–1914) was a French police officer and Biometrics researcher who applied the anthropological technique of Anthropometry to law enforcement creating an identification system based on physical measurements. **Anthropometry** was the first scientific system used by police to identify criminals. Before that time, criminals could only be identified by name or photograph. The method was however eventually supplanted by the Fingerprint system.
  - In 1858, **Sir William Herschel** initiated fingerprinting in India. In 1877, he first instituted the use of fingerprints on contracts and deeds to prevent the repudiation of signatures in Kolkata, and he registered government pensioners' fingerprints to prevent the collection of money by relatives after a pensioner's death.
  - In 1880, **Henry Faulds**, a Scottish surgeon in a Tokyo hospital, published his first paper on the usefulness of fingerprints for identification and proposed a method to record them with printing ink. Returning to Great Britain, in 1886, he offered the concept to the Metropolitan Police in London, but it was dismissed at that time.
  - **Sir Francis Galton** (1822–1911) (**Fig. 1.6**) published a detailed statistical model of fingerprint analysis and identification in his 1892 book "**Finger Prints**". He had calculated that the chance of a "false positive" (two different individuals having the same fingerprints) was about 1 in 64 billion.

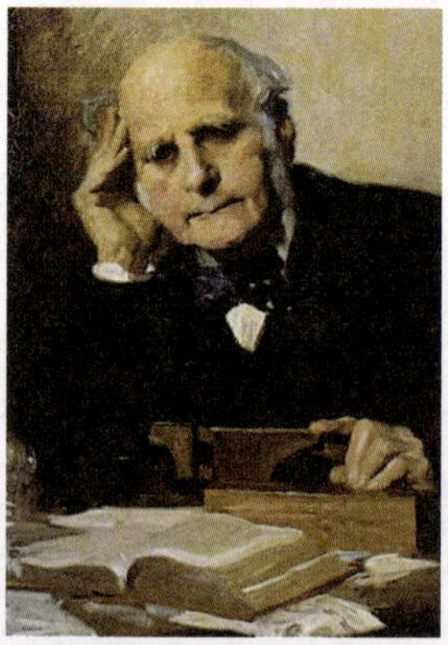

Fig. 1.6 Sir Francis Galton

- In 1892, **Juan Vucetich**, an Argentine chief police officer, created the first method of recording the fingerprints of individuals on file.
    - In that same year, Francisca Rojas was found in a house with neck injuries, while her two sons were found dead with their throats cut. Rojas accused a neighbour, but despite brutal interrogation that neighbour would not confess to the crimes. Inspector Álvarez, a colleague of Vucetich, went to the scene and found a bloody thumb mark on a door. When it was compared with Rojas' prints, it was found to be identical with her right thumb. She then confessed to the murder of her sons. **This was the first known murder case to be solved using fingerprint analysis**.
- In Kolkata, the first ever **Fingerprint Bureau** was established in **1897**, after the Council of the Governor General approved a committee report that fingerprints should be used for the classification of criminal records. The bureau employees **Azizul Haque** (a police officer) and **Hem Chandra Bose** developed a fingerprint classification system eventually named after their supervisor, **Edward Henry**.
- The study of insects infesting a decaying corpse to find out the time since death (**Forensic Entomology**) began with the pioneering work of French entomologist **Jean Pierre Megnin** during 1887–1894.

- **20th century and beyond**:
    - In 1909, **Archibald Reiss** founded the first ever **Forensic Science University** (Institut de Police Scientifique) in Lausanne, Switzerland.
    - **Dr Edmond Locard** (1877–1966) (**Fig. 1.7**), a French criminologist, who became known as the "Sherlock Holmes of France" formulated the basic principle of forensic science: "Every contact leaves a trace". This became known as "**Locard's exchange principle**."
        - In 1910, Dr Locard established the first ever **Criminal Laboratory (Forensic Science Laboratory)** in the world.

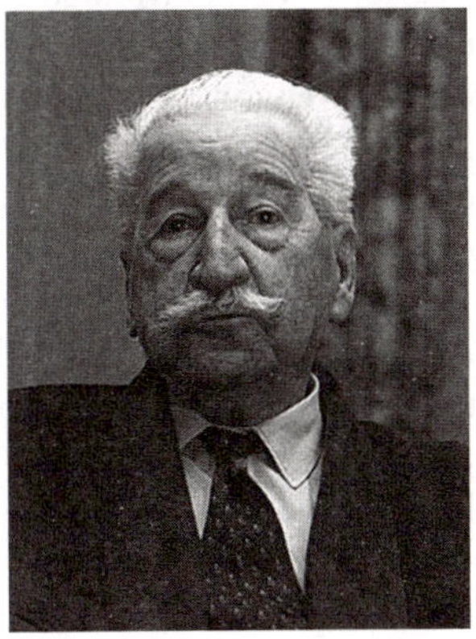

Fig. 1.7 Dr Edmund Locard

- **Forensic Medicine (Forensic Pathology)** evolved quickly as a specialty in the 20th century with the help of notable experts such as **Dr Bernard Spilsbury, Dr Sydney Smith, Dr Keith Simpson** and **Dr Milton Helpern**.
    - Dr Keith Simpson published "**Forty Years of Murder – An Autobiography**" in 1978, which recounted some of his most famous cases. It is considered a forensic classic.
- In 1984, **Sir Alec Jeffreys** (**Fig. 1.8**), a British geneticist working in University of Leicester, first developed the technique called **DNA Fingerprinting** (now referred to as DNA Profiling or DNA Typing), which is today considered to be the most revolutionary technique in the world for identification purposes. He is commonly referred to as the **Father of Forensic DNA Analysis**.

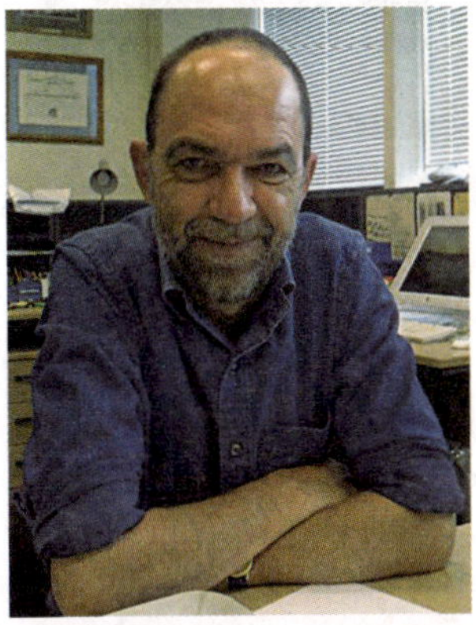

Fig. 1.8 Sir Alec Jeffreys

B. In India:

Forensic Medicine in India has attained its present state of development by passing through several phases of evolution amidst superstition, religion and magic through the centuries, and subsequently imbibing Western concepts under the British regime. In ancient times, no person was safe from attacks to himself or his property: a tooth for a tooth, an eye for an eye and a life for a life was the rule of law.

- **Manu** (3102 BCE) in his famous treatise ***Manu Smriti*** prescribed various rules relating to minimum age of marriage, punishment for offences (sexual) and as to how a disease or intoxication could render one incapable of making a contract or depose in court.
- During the Vedic Age (2000 to 1000 BCE), ***Rig Veda*** was written, which mentioned about how physicians successfully cured patients literally on the verge of death. Similarly, other Vedas mentioned crimes such as adultery, incest, abortion, murder and prescribe punishments for the same. In ***Atharva Veda*** (1500 BCE), there is mention of cures from arrows, stab wounds, snake bites, etc.
- Criminal abortion (*Brunahatya*) and suicide (*Atmahatya*) were specially mentioned as punishable under law in the Vedas. Even the nature of poison was attempted to be detected from the nature of flame and the sound of fire when

the stomach or heart of the deceased (dead due to poisoning) was put in the fire.

- **Post-Vedic Period**:
  - *Sushruta Samhita* compiled by **Sushruta (Father of Indian Surgery)** (approx. 800–700 BCE) (**Fig. 1.9**) dealt not only with the management of surgical cases, but also detailed the good qualities of an ideal physician.

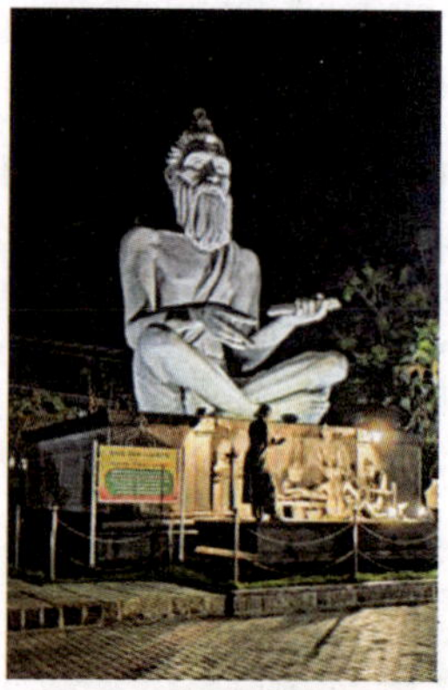

Fig. 1.9 Sculpture of Sushruta at AIMS, Cochin

  - *Kautilya's Arthasastra* was written during this period. It is said to be the best treatise ever written in India on **medicolegal investigation of crimes**, and administration of law and justice. **Kautilya** (or **Chanakya** – 375-283 BCE) advised medical examination in case of deaths due to assaults, poisoning and asphyxia, similar to the postmortem examinations conducted today.
  - *Charaka Samhita* mentioned about training and duties for physicians. Also, poisons were classified, as well as treatment measures for poisoning.
  - **Charaka (Physician Hippocrates of India)** (1st century CE to 2nd century CE) also laid down guidelines as to how a student should be trained to become a physician. Hence, he is also known as the **Father of Indian Medicine**. The physicians of those days were held in high esteem, both by the King and the general public.
  - **1000 to 1600 CE**:
    - This period witnessed the invasion of India by foreign powers such as the Turks, Pathans and Moghuls. Their law was based mainly on the Hadith. Judiciary was based on ***Sharia rules***, which included harsh punishments like cutting of body parts, throwing to wild animals, etc.
    - ***Unani*** system of medicine was introduced during this period.
  - **17th to 19th centuries**:
    - The Portuguese, Dutch and French invaded and ruled the country. Later, the *English East India Company* was established, and the British conquered the country, introducing a whole new system of medicine and legal procedures.
    - **Dr Buckley (Bulkley)** carried out the **first postmortem examination in India** at Madras, in **1693** on a suspected case of arsenic poisoning.
    - The **first medical college** in the country was started in **1835** at **Calcutta**. Similar colleges were later set up in Madras and Mumbai.
    - ***Coroner's system*** was introduced in Kolkata and Mumbai by the **Coroner's Act 1871**. But, rest of the country followed the *Police system*.
    - **Dr CTO Woodford** served as the **first Professor of Medical Jurisprudence** in the country, in **1845**.
    - ***Indian Penal Code*** was published in **1860**, codifying various crimes and punishments. It was drafted under the presidentship of Lord Macaulay.
    - ***Criminal Procedure Code*** was first published in **1882**, which streamlined the criminal procedures in the country.
    - ***Indian Evidence Act*** of **1872** codified laws with respect to evidence.
  - **The Present Day**:
    - After 1947, amendments were made to the above mentioned Acts. Medical Jurisprudence changed its nomenclature to Forensic Medicine. **Dr Jaising P Modi** (1875–1954) (**Fig. 1.10**) became the **first Indian physician to handle cases of medicolegal nature**.

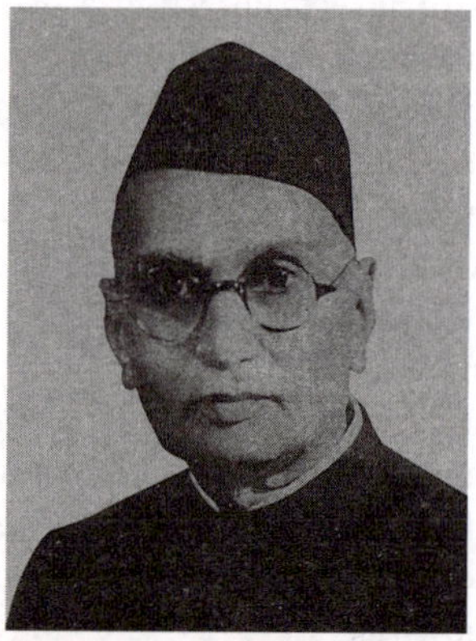

Fig. 1.10 Dr Jaising P Modi

    - Among the early forensic medical experts of India, two professors who contributed extensively to the growth of the specialty include **Prof Bhooshana Rao** and **Prof ATS Iyengar**.
    - Forensic Medicine together with Toxicology is now a part of the medical curriculum in all universities throughout the country, and has been greatly strengthened in the new MBBS curriculum (Graduate Medical Education or GME-2018).
    - The first DNA Fingerprinting Laboratory in India was set up in 1995 by **Dr Lalji Singh** – Centre for DNA Fingerprinting and Diagnostics (CDFD) at Hyderabad.
      - Dr Lalji Singh (1947–2017) (**Fig. 1.11**) is popularly known as the **"Father of Indian DNA Fingerprinting"**.

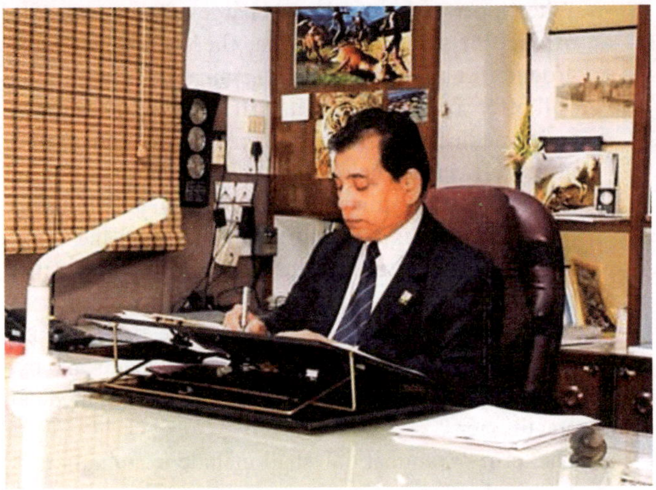

Fig. 1.11 Dr Lalji Singh

- The field of Medical Toxicology has received a boost with the establishment of **Poison Control Centres**, one of which set up by the Editor of this book in 2003 in Amrita Institute of Medical Sciences (AIMS) in Cochin, Kerala is the most full-fledged centre with state-of-the-art poison information and analytical services.
- For an overview of the historical evolution of the specialities of Forensic Medicine and Toxicology in a pictorial manner, comprising images of stalwarts who helped shape these two fascinating branches of medicine, arranged in chronological order, every reader of this book is invited to visit the **Dept of Forensic Medicine & Toxicology (FMT)** of **AIMS Cochin**. The two walls of the department corridor are lined by the famous forensic and toxicology experts (**Wall of Fame**) and infamous criminals caught with the help of forensic science (**Wall of Shame**) (**Fig. 1.12**).

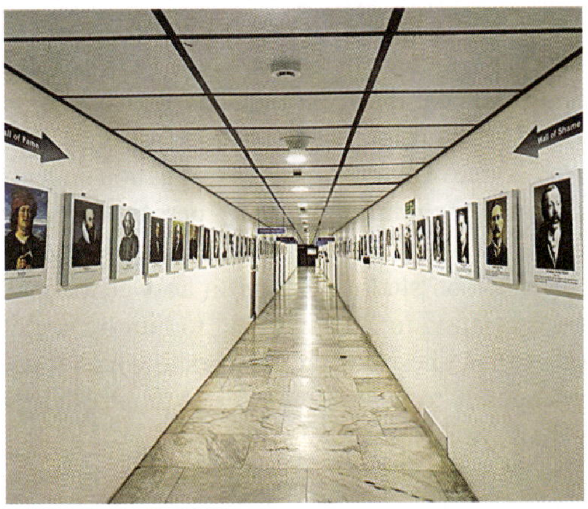

Fig. 1.12 The Corridor of the FMT Dept in AIMS, Cochin

FM 1.3: Non-Core – Written/Viva Voce
- **Describe legal procedures including**
  - Criminal Procedure Code
  - Indian Penal Code
  - Indian Evidence Act
  - Civil and Criminal Cases
  - Inquest (Police Inquest and Magistrate's Inquest)
  - Cognizable and Non-cognizable Offences

LEGAL PROCEDURE

Some Important Sections of The Indian Penal Code

Section	*Offence*
166B	Punishment to a doctor for refusal to provide medicolegal examination and treatment of a sexual assault victim (imprisonment for up to 1 year).
299	Culpable homicide not amounting to murder.
300	Culpable homicide amounting to murder.
302	Punishment for culpable homicide amounting to murder.
303	Murder by a person already undergoing life imprisonment.
304	Punishment for culpable homicide not amounting to murder.
304A	Causing death by rash and negligent act.
304B	Dowry death.
306	Abetment of suicide.
309	Attempt to commit suicide: Although section 309 is still in effect, the **Mental Healthcare Act, 2017 (enacted July 2018) has restricted its application**. The relevant provision of the new act states: *Notwithstanding anything contained in section 309 of the Indian Penal Code, any person who attempts to commit suicide shall be presumed, unless proved otherwise, to have severe stress and* ***shall not be tried and punished*** *under the said Code.*
312	Causing miscarriage, if woman is quick with child.
313	Causing miscarriage without woman's consent.
314	Death caused by an act done with intent to cause miscarriage (without woman's consent).
315	Act done with intent to prevent a child from being born alive, or to cause it to die after its birth.
316	Causing death of a quick unborn child by an act amounting to culpable homicide.
317	Exposure of a child under 12 years, by parent or guardian with intention of abandoning it.
318	Concealment of birth by secret disposal of dead body.
323	Voluntarily causing hurt.
324	Voluntarily causing hurt by dangerous weapons or means.
325	Voluntarily causing grievous hurt.
326	Voluntarily causing grievous hurt by dangerous weapons or means.
326A	Punishment for acid throwing (vitriolage).

326B	Punishment for attempted acid throwing.
328	Administering stupefying drug or poison with intent to cause hurt, etc.
352	Assault or use of criminal force.
354	Assault or use of criminal force to a woman with intent to outrage her modesty.
354A	Sexual harassment.
354B	Act with intent to disrobe a woman.
354C	Voyeurism
354D	Stalking
363	Kidnapping
364	Kidnapping or abducting in order to murder.
364A	Kidnapping for ransom, etc.
366	Kidnapping or abducting a woman to compel her for marriage, etc.
366A	Procuration of minor girl.
375	Rape
376	Punishment for rape.
376A	Punishment for whoever commits rape in the course of which an injury is inflicted which causes the death of the woman, or causes the woman to be in a persistent vegetative state.
376B	Punishment for sexual intercourse with one's own wife, who is living separately, whether under a decree of separation or otherwise, without her consent.
376C	Punishment for intercourse by superintendent of jail, remand home, etc., or by anyone on the management of a hospital or being on the staff of a hospital, etc.
376D	Punishment for rape by one or more persons constituting a group or acting in furtherance of a common intention ('gang rape').
376E	Punishment for rape by someone who has been previously convicted of an offence punishable under section 376 or any of its sub-sections.
377	Unnatural sexual offences. On 6 Sept 2018, the Supreme Court of India **decriminalised Section 377 in relation to homosexuality** (consensual homosexual sex between adults), but allowed Section 377 to remain in force relating to sex with minors, non-consensual sexual acts, and bestiality.
497	Adultery. On 27 Sept 2018, the Supreme Court of India revoked Section 497, and therefore **adultery is no longer a crime** in India. However, it can be a reason for civil issues such as divorce.
498	Enticing or taking away, or detaining, with criminal intent, a married woman.
498A	Punishment for subjecting a married woman to cruelty.

Some Important Sections of Criminal Procedure Code (CrPC)

- **Section 53**: Examination of accused by medical practitioner at the request of a police officer:
  - When a person arrested on a charge of committing an offence of such a nature that there are reasonable grounds for believing that an examination of his person will offer some evidence, it shall be lawful for a registered medical practitioner, acting at the request of a police officer not below the rank of sub inspector, to make such an examination of the person arrested as is reasonably necessary in order to ascertain the facts, and to use such force as reasonably necessary for that purpose.
  - Whenever the person of a female is to be examined under this section, the examination shall be made only by, or under the supervision, of a female registered medical practitioner.
  - The term "examination" shall include examination of blood, blood stain, semen, swabs in case of sexual offences, sputum and sweat, hair samples and finger nail clippings by the use of scientific techniques including DNA profiling, and such other tests which the registered medical practitioner thinks necessary in a particular case.
- **Section 53A: Examination of person accused of rape, by a medical practitioner**:
  - When a person is arrested on a charge of committing an offence of rape, and there are reasonable grounds for believing that an examination of his person will afford evidence as to the commission of such offence, it shall be lawful for a registered medical practitioner acting at the request of a police officer not below the rank of a sub inspector, to make such an examination of the arrested person, and to use such force as is reasonably necessary for that purpose.
  - The registered medical practitioner conducting such examination, shall without delay, examine such person and prepare a report of his examination, and forward the report to the investigating officer, who shall forward it to the Magistrate.
- **Section 61: Summons to witness**:
  - Every summons issued by a court shall be in writing, in duplicate, signed by the presiding officer of such court and shall bear the seal of the court.
- **Section 161: Examination of witness by police**:
  - Any police offer making an investigation under this section may examine orally any person supposed to be acquainted with the facts and circumstances of the case.
  - Such person shall be bound to answer truly all questions relating to such case put to him by such officer, other than questions the answers to which would have a tendency to expose him to a criminal charge or to a penalty or forfeiture.
  - The police officer may reduce into writing any statement made to him in the course of an examination under this section; and if he does so, he shall make a separate and true record of the statement of each such person whose statement he records.

- **Section 174: Inquiry by Police Officer into cause of death**:
  - When the officer in charge of a police station receives information that a person has committed suicide, or committed an offence resulting in death of another person, he shall immediately give intimation thereof to the nearest Executive Magistrate, and shall proceed to the place of death, and there, in the presence of two or more respectable inhabitants of the neighbourhood, make an investigation, and draw up a report of the apparent cause of death, describing such wounds as may be found on the body, and stating in what manner, or by what weapon or instrument, such wounds appear to have been inflicted.
  - The report will be signed by such police officer and other persons, and shall be forwarded to the District Magistrate or the Sub Divisional Magistrate.
  - When –
    - The case involves suicide by a woman within 7 years of her marriage; or
    - The case relates to the death of a woman within 7 years of her marriage under any circumstance that raises a reasonable suspicion that some other person instigated or compelled her to do so; or
    - The case relates to the death of a woman within 7 years of her marriage and any relative of the woman has made a request in this behalf; or
    - There is any doubt regarding the cause of death; or
    - The police officer for any other reason considers it expedient so to do;

    He shall submit to such rules as the State Government may prescribe in this behalf, and forward the body with a view to its being examined, to the nearest Civil Surgeon, or any other qualified medical man.
- **Section 176: Inquiry by Magistrate into cause of death**:
  - When the case is of the nature referred to in sub-sections 1–3 of **Section 174**, the nearest Magistrate empowered to hold inquests shall hold an enquiry mentioned into the cause of death, either instead of, or in addition to, the investigation held by the police officer.
  - Where –
    - Any person dies or disappears while he is in the custody of the police
    - or in any other custody authorised by the Magistrate or the Court
    - or rape is alleged to have been committed on any woman, while such person or woman is in the custody of the police, either instead of, or in addition to the inquiry or investigation held by the police, an inquiry shall be held by the Judicial Magistrate, within whose local jurisdiction the offence has been committed.
  - The Magistrate holding such an inquiry shall record the evidence taken by him in connection therewith in any manner hereinafter prescribed according to the circumstances of the case.
  - Whenever such Magistrate considers it expedient to make an examination of the dead body of any person who has been already buried, in order to discover the cause of his death, the Magistrate may cause the body to be exhumed and examined.
  - The Judicial Magistrate or the Executive Magistrate or police officer holding an inquiry or investigation, as the case may be shall, within 24 hours of the death of a person, forward the body with a view to its being examined to the nearest Civil Surgeon or other qualified medical man appointed in this behalf by the State Government, unless it is not possible to do so for reasons to be recorded in writing.
- **Section 244: Evidence for prosecution**
  - When, in any warrant case instituted other than on a police report, the accused appears before a Magistrate, he shall proceed to hear the prosecution and take all evidences as may be produced in support of the prosecution.
  - The Magistrate may, on the application of the prosecution, issue summons to any of its witnesses directing him to attend, or to produce any document or other thing.
- **Section 327** (*Amended as per Code of Criminal Procedure [Amendment] Act, 2008*):
  - The court examination of a survivor of sexual assault must be conducted ***in camera*** – which means that there will be **no general public** present in the court. The only people allowed will be the Judge, public prosecutor, defence lawyer and the staff of the court.
- **Section 357C** (*Criminal Law Amendment Act 2013*):
  - Hospitals (both public and private) are required to provide free treatment to survivors of sexual assault. This cannot be denied for the want of a police requisition.

Some Important Sections of the Indian Evidence Act (IEA)

- **Section 45: Opinion of experts**:
  - When the court has to form an opinion upon a point of foreign law, or science or art, the opinion upon that point of persons specially skilled in such foreign law, science or art, are relevant facts. Such persons are called **experts**.
- **Section 113 A: Presumption as to abetment of suicide by a married woman**:
  - When the question is whether the commission of suicide by a woman had been abetted by her husband or any relative of her husband, and it is shown that she had committed suicide within a period of 7 years from the date of her marriage, and that her husband or such relative of her husband had subjected her to cruelty, the court may presume that such suicide had been abetted by her husband, or by such relative of her husband.
- **Section 113 B: Presumption as to dowry death**:
  - When the question is whether a person has committed dowry death of a woman, and it is shown that soon

before her death, she had been subjected to cruelty or harassment for, or in connection with, a demand of dowry, the court shall presume that such person had caused the death.

- **Section 114 A: Presumption as to absence of consent in certain prosecutions for rape:**
  - In a prosecution for rape under clause (a) or clause (b) or clause (d) or clause (e) or clause (g), or subsection (2), of section 376 of the Indian Penal Code, where sexual intercourse by the accused is proved, and the question is whether it was without consent of the woman alleged to have been raped, and she states in her evidence before the court that she did not consent, the Court shall presume that she did not consent.
- **Section 137: Procedures in examining witness in a court of law**:
  - Examination-in-chief – The examination of a witness by the party who calls him shall be called his examination-in-chief.
  - Cross-examination – The examination of witness by the adverse party shall be called cross examination.
  - Re-examination – The examination of a witness by the party who called him, subsequent to the cross examination, shall be called re-examination.
- **Section 138: Order of examinations**:
  - Witnesses shall be first examined-in-chief, then (if the adverse party so desires) cross-examined, then (if the party calling him so desires) re-examined.
  - The chief examination and cross-examination must relate to relevant facts, but the cross-examination need not be confined to the facts to which the witness testified on his examination-in-chief.
  - Direction of re-examination – The re-examination shall be directed to the explanation of matters referred to in cross-examination; and, if new matter is, by permission of the Court, introduced in re-examination, the adverse party may further cross-examine upon that matter.
- **Section 141: Leading questions**:
  - Any question suggesting the answer which the person putting it wishes or expects to receive, is called a leading question.
- **Section 142: When leading questions must not be asked**:
  - Leading questions must not, if objected to by the adverse party, be asked in an examination-in-chief.
- **Section 143: When leading questions may be asked**:
  - Leading questions may be asked in cross-examination.
- **Section 146: Questions lawful in cross-examination**: When a witness is cross-examined, he may, in addition to the questions herein before referred to, be asked any questions which tend
  - to test his veracity
  - to discover who he is, and what is his position in life, or
  - to shake his credibility, although the answer to such question might tend directly or indirectly to incriminate him, or might expose him to a penalty or forfeiture:
    - Provided that in prosecution for rape or attempt to commit rape, it shall not be permissible to put questions in the cross-examination of the prosecutrix as to her general moral character.
- **Section 148: Court to decide when a witness is compelled to answer**:
  - If any such question relates to a matter not relevant to the suit or proceeding, except in so far as it affects the credibility of the witness by injuring his character, the court shall decide whether or not the witness shall be compelled to answer it, and may, if it thinks fit, warn the witness he is not obliged to answer it.
- **Section 151: Indecent and scandalous questions**:
  - The court may forbid any questions or inquiries which are regarded as indecent or scandalous, although such questions or inquiries may have some bearing on the questions before the court, unless they relate to a fact in issue, or to matters necessary to be known, in order to determine whether or not the fact in issue existed.
- **Section 159**: **Refreshing memory**:
  - A witness, while under examination, can refresh his memory when he is questioned, or so soon afterwards that the Court considers it likely that the transaction was at that time fresh in his memory.
  - The witness may also refer to any such writing made by another person, and read by witness within the time aforesaid, if when he read it he knew it to be correct.
  - When witness may use copy of document to refresh memory – Whenever a witness may refresh his memory by reference to any document, he may, with the permission of the Court, refer to a copy of such document, provided the court is satisfied that there is sufficient reason for the non-production of the original.
  - An expert may refresh his memory by reference to professional treatises.

CIVIL AND CRIMINAL CASES

- **Case**: An action, cause of action, matter of dispute or law suit.
  - There are basically four types of court cases:
    - **Warrant case** – A case relating to an offence punishable with death, imprisonment for life, or imprisonment for a term exceeding two years.
    - **Summons case** – A case relating to an offence which is not punishable by a term of imprisonment exceeding 2 years.
    - **Civil case** – It is a dispute between two private parties relating to wealth, property, etc.
    - **Criminal case** – It is a case between the Government (represented by the police) and a private party (suspect/accused) concerning matters of public interest and safety, e.g., assault, robbery, murder and rape.

INQUEST

- **An inquest is a legal inquiry into the circumstances and cause of death, in a case of sudden, suspicious or unnatural death.**
  - Types of Inquest:
    - Police Inquest
    - Magistrate's Inquest
    - Coroner's Inquest
    - Medical Examiner's System

Police Inquest

- Conducted by an officer in charge of a police station.
- On receipt of information of an unnatural death, the police officer informs the nearest Magistrate, and proceeds to the place of death.
- He then conducts an inquest in the presence of two or more respectable inhabitants of the neighbourhood (**panchas**).
- After the necessary investigation, a report is drawn up on the apparent cause of death as judged by the state of the body, the injuries present on the body, hearsay evidence, circumstantial evidence, etc. This document is called **panchanama** or **inquest report** (**Box 1.1**). This is signed by the police officer and the persons present at the inquest.
- If any foul play or unnatural death is suspected, the police officer forwards the body for postmortem examination to the nearest medical officer, along with a written request and a copy of the panchanama, to help him find out the probable cause of death. If the autopsy report confirms that the death is due to an unnatural cause, further enquiry and trial of the case is carried out in the usual manner by the magistrate concerned, to whom the entire records of the case are transferred by the police officer.

Coroner's Inquest

- Conducted by a **Coroner** who is either a medical professional with legal qualifications, or a graduate in law.
- Until recently, the Coroner's Inquest existed in the city of Mumbai, from where it has now been abolished. Previously, it was also conducted in various other cities such as Kolkata. **Today, the Coroner system of inquest does not exist anywhere in India**. It is however the prevalent method of inquiry in the UK (England, Wales & Northern Ireland),* Canada, Hong Kong, Australia, New Zealand, Sri Lanka and some states of the USA.
- A coroner holds an inquest on receipt of information of any unnatural, obscure, sudden or suspicious death. He also investigates deaths of convicts in jail, deaths of persons in police custody and deaths of patients in mental hospitals.
- The Coroner's Court is a **court of enquiry**, and not of trial. He is empowered to summon witnesses and record their

Box 1.1—Inquest Report (Panchanama)

Report of investigation under section 174 Cr.P.C. on the body of a person found dead at .... AM/PM .... on the .... day of ....(month) .... (year)

- Name, occupation and residence of persons composing the panchayat:
- Name of the deceased, sex, age, occupation, father's name and residence:
- By whom first found dead, when, and where?:
- By whom last seen alive, where and when, and in whose company, and whether he carried any valuable property with him:
- Height, colour and descriptive marks:
- Married or single:
- State of corpse, its posture and exact state of limbs, eyes, mouth, etc.:
- If any wounds, particulars thereof, and list of all property found in the corpse:
- Minute description of exact spot:
- Where corpse was found & if in water, depth thereof:
- When body is found in a well, information on the following points should be given:
  - Is the well a public or private property?
  - If the latter, to whom does it belong?
  - Is it near a public road or pathway?
  - Does it have a parapet wall and float?
- By which relative, body is recognized, and their statement given in short (blood relatives, such as parents, brothers, sisters always to be examined, if there are any)
- Abstract of evidence of other persons examined:
- Apparent cause of death:
- If by violence, apparently, by what weapon:
- If any person is suspected, who and why?
- Was the deceased insured in any company?
- If corpse is not sent for medical examination, why?
- If corpse is sent, for what purpose and by whose order, and No. of Constable who went with it. (the date and hour when the body is sent should also be given here)
- By whose order, corpse was buried or burnt?
- Opinion of the panchas as to cause and manner of death:
- Signatures of such of the panchas who concur with the above opinion:
- Station house officer's signature:
- If name and residence of deceased is unknown, state what steps have been taken to:
  - Ascertain the same, and secure identification.
  - Have fingerprints of the deceased been taken and sent to the Finger Print Bureau concerned?
- Was the body warm or cold when first found?
- Any reason to suspect foul play?
- Duration of investigation:
- Investigation commenced at .... Investigation closed at ....

Signatures of witnesses ....

Signature of the Investigating Officer.....................

**Scotland does not have Coroner system; inquest is conducted by an officer called "Procurator Fiscal".*

evidence on oath. He can order for postmortem examination and exhumation whenever required.

Magistrate's Inquest

- A magistrate (usually an **executive magistrate**) conducts inquest in the following circumstances*:
    - **D**owry death
    - **P**rison death
    - **P**olice custody death
    - **P**olice firing death
    - **P**sychiatric hospital death
    - **E**xhumation
- Magistrate's inquest is done all over India (in the situations described above).

Medical Examiner's System

- Medical Examiner's System is a type of inquest which is **prevalent in most of the states of USA**.
- All sudden, unexpected, or unnatural deaths are analysed by a Medical Examiner who is a forensic pathologist.
- This type of inquest is considered **superior to all other types of inquest**, because it is conducted by a forensic pathologist with medical, scientific and legal knowledge.

COGNIZABLE AND NON-COGNIZABLE OFFENCES

Cognizable Offence

- A **cognizable offence** means an offence in which a police officer has the authority to make an arrest without a warrant and to start an investigation with or without the permission of a court.
- The police can file a First Information Report (FIR) only for cognizable offences.
- In cognizable cases, the police can conduct an investigation without prior permission of a Magistrate.
- Cognizable cases are more serious than non-cognizable cases. Normally, serious offences are defined as cognisable and usually carry a sentence of 3 years or more.
- They are usually **non-bailable offences.**
    - Examples: Rape, murder, theft, kidnapping, etc.

Non-Cognizable Offence

- A **non-cognizable offence** means an offence in which a police officer cannot make an arrest without a warrant, and cannot start an investigation without the permission of a court.
- In this type of crime, a criminal complaint is lodged with the metropolitan magistrate who should order the concerned police station to initiate an investigation. The police officer is expected to file the charge sheet with the court which is followed by a trial.
- After the trial, if the accused is found guilty, the court passes the order to issue a warrant to arrest the accused.
- They are usually **bailable offences**.
    - Examples: Forgery, cheating, defamation, public nuisance, etc.

FM 1.4: Non-Core – Written/Viva Voce

- Describe the Courts in India and their powers:
    - Supreme Court
    - High Court
    - Sessions Court
    - Magistrate's Court
    - Labour Court
    - Family Court
    - Executive Magistrate Court
    - Juvenile Justice Board

COURTS

- Members of the medical profession may be required to attend court to give evidence in medico-legal cases. Therefore, it is desirable that all medical practitioners possess some basic knowledge about criminal courts and court procedures.

Types of Courts

A. *Supreme Court*

- The Supreme Court of India came into being on 28 January 1950.
- It is the supreme judicial body of India and the **highest court of India** under the constitution. It is the most senior constitutional court, and has the power of judicial review.
- The Chief Justice of India is the head and chief judge of the Supreme Court, and the court consists of a maximum of 34 judges.
- It has extensive powers in the form of original, appellate and advisory jurisdictions.
- As the constitutional court of the country, it takes up appeals primarily against verdicts of the High Courts of various states of the Union, and other courts and tribunals. It safeguards fundamental rights of citizens and settles disputes between various government authorities as well as the central government vs state governments, or state governments versus another state government in the country.
- As an advisory court, it hears matters which may specifically be referred to it under the Constitution by the President of India.
- The law declared by the Supreme Court becomes binding on all courts within India.

B. *High Court*

- The High Courts of India are the courts with **highest powers in each state and union territory** of the country.
- They can try any offence and pass any sentence authorized by law.
- However, the work of most High Courts primarily consists of appeals from lower courts and writ petitions.
- Judges in a High Court are appointed by the President of India in consultation with the Chief Justice of India and the Governor of the state. High courts are headed by a Chief Justice.

*Mnemonic (to help remember the 6 indications): ***D 4P E***.

Table 1.1 High Courts of India – An Overview

State/UT	Court	Principal Seat	Bench(es)
Andaman and Nicobar Islands	Calcutta High Court	—	Port Blair
Arunachal Pradesh	Gauhati High Court	—	Itanagar
Andhra Pradesh	Andhra Pradesh High Court	Amaravati	—
Assam	Gauhati High Court	Guwahati	—
Bihar	Patna High Court	Patna	—
Chandigarh	Punjab and Haryana High Court	Chandigarh	—
Chhattisgarh	Chhattisgarh High Court	Bilaspur	—
Dadra and Nagar Haveli and Daman and Diu	Bombay High Court	Mumbai	—
National Capital Territory of Delhi	Delhi High Court	New Delhi	—
Goa	Bombay High Court	—	Panaji
Gujarat	Gujarat High Court	Ahmedabad	—
Haryana	Punjab and Haryana High Court	Chandigarh	—
Himachal Pradesh	Himachal Pradesh High Court	Shimla	—
Jammu and Kashmir	Jammu and Kashmir High Court	Srinagar/Jammu	—
Jharkhand	Jharkhand High Court	Ranchi	—
Karnataka	Karnataka High Court	Bangalore	Dharwad and Gulbarga
Kerala	Kerala High Court	Kochi	—
Ladakh	Jammu and Kashmir High Court	Srinagar/Jammu	—
Lakshadweep	Kerala High Court	Kochi	—
Madhya Pradesh	Madhya Pradesh High Court	Jabalpur	Gwalior and Indore
Maharashtra	Bombay High Court	Mumbai	Aurangabad and Nagpur
Manipur	Manipur High Court	Imphal	—
Meghalaya	Meghalaya High Court	Shillong	—
Mizoram	Gauhati High Court	—	Aizawl
Nagaland	Gauhati High Court	—	Kohima
Odisha	Orissa High Court	Cuttack	—
Pondicherry (Puducherry)	Madras High Court	Chennai	—
Punjab	Punjab and Haryana High Court	Chandigarh	—
Rajasthan	Rajasthan High Court	Jodhpur	Jaipur
Sikkim	Sikkim High Court	Gangtok	—
Tamil Nadu	Madras High Court	Chennai	Madurai
Telangana	Telangana High Court	Hyderabad	—
Tripura	Tripura High Court	Agartala	—
Uttar Pradesh	Allahabad High Court	Prayagraj	Lucknow
Uttarakhand	Uttarakhand High Court	Nainital	—
West Bengal	Calcutta High Court	Kolkata	Jalpaiguri

- The Calcutta High Court is the oldest High Court in the country, established on 2 July 1862.

***Some interesting questions relating to High Courts*:**

1. **How many High Courts are there in India?**
   There are 25 High Courts in India at present.
2. **Which of the states in India share a common High Court?**
   The states of Punjab and Haryana have a common High Court in Chandigarh. Also, the North-Eastern states (Assam, Mizoram, Nagaland, Arunachal Pradesh) share the same High Court in Guwahati.
3. **Which are the High Courts having jurisdiction over more than one State or Union Territory?**
   a. Bombay High Court has jurisdiction over Maharashtra, Dadar and Nagar Haveli, Daman, Diu and Goa.
   b. Kolkata High Court has jurisdiction over West Bengal and Andaman & Nicobar Islands.
   c. Madras High Court has jurisdiction over Tamil Nadu and Pondicherry.
   d. Guwahati High Court has jurisdiction over Assam, Nagaland, Mizoram and Arunachal Pradesh.
   e. Kerala High Court has jurisdiction over Kerala and Lakshadweep.
   f. Punjab & Haryana High Court has jurisdiction over Punjab, Haryana and Chandigarh.

C. *Sessions (District) Court*

- A District court is referred to as Sessions Court when it exercises its jurisdiction on criminal matters under the Code of Criminal Procedure (CrPc).
- A Sessions Court is the **highest criminal court in a district** and the court of first instance for trying serious offences, i.e., those carrying punishment of imprisonment of more than seven years, life imprisonment or death.
- The court is presided over by a Judge, appointed by the High Court of that particular state. The High Court may also appoint Additional Sessions Judges and Assistant Sessions Judges in this court.
- Sessions Court has the power to impose the full range of penalties for criminal acts, including the death penalty, but the latter has to be confirmed by the respective High Court before it can be carried out.

D. *Magistrates Courts*

- There are six categories of magistrates in the Judiciary of India*:
  - Chief Judicial Magistrate
  - Sub-Divisional Judicial Magistrate
  - Judicial Magistrate First Class
  - Judicial Magistrate Second Class
  - Metropolitan Magistrate
  - Executive Magistrates (including District Magistrate, Additional District Magistrate, Sub Divisional District Magistrate, etc.)
- The Chief Judicial Magistrate [CJM] (incl. Additional Chief Judicial Magistrate) can hear all types of criminal cases.
- All magistrates' courts are controlled by the CJM. But though the CJM looks over the work of judicial magistrates, he cannot take any action against them. The CJM can only report the misbehaviour of judicial magistrates to the High Court.
- The Chief Judicial Magistrate can sentence a person to jail up to 7 years and impose fines of up to any amount.
- There is a Sub-Divisional Judicial Magistrate (SDJM) in every subdivision. They hear cases related to the Dowry Act, Essential Commodities Act, and other criminal cases.
  - The SDJM can sentence a person to imprisonment for up to 3 years and impose fine up to Rs. 10,000.
- A Judicial Magistrate First Class can also sentence a person to jail for up to 3 years and impose a fine of up to Rs. 10,000.
- A Judicial Magistrate Second Class can sentence a person to jail for up to one year and impose a fine of up to Rs. 5000.
- According to Section 16 of the CrPc, in every metropolitan area, there shall be established as many courts of Metropolitan Magistrates, as the State Government may, after consultation with the High Court, specify.
  - Metropolitan Courts are to be established at such places in every metropolitan area having population of 10 lakhs or more. It has jurisdiction throughout such metropolitan area.
  - A Metropolitan Magistrate is a first class magistrate under the general control of the District & Sessions Judge and is subordinate to the Chief Metropolitan Magistrate.
  - A Metropolitan Magistrate may pass a sentence of imprisonment for a term not exceeding 3 years, or a fine not exceeding 10,000 rupees.
- An Executive Magistrate is an officer of the Executive branch (as opposed to the Judicial branch) who is invested with specific powers under both the CrPC and the IPC.
- Normally, the Collector of the district is appointed as the District Magistrate. Similarly, the Sub-Collectors are appointed as the Sub-Divisional District Magistrates (SDMs). Tahsildars and Deputy/Additional Tahsildars are appointed as ordinary Executive Magistrates.
- These officers cannot try any accused nor pass verdicts.
- A person arrested on the orders of a court located outside the local jurisdiction should be produced before an Executive Magistrate who can also set the bail amount for the arrested individual to avoid police custody, depending on the terms of the warrant.
- The Executive Magistrate also can pass orders restraining persons from committing a particular act or preventing persons from entering an area (Section 144 CrPC). The Executive Magistrates alone are authorised to use force against

**As per Criminal Procedure Code, 1973 (CrPC).*

people. In plain language, they alone can disperse an "unlawful assembly".

- Technically, the police are to assist the Executive Magistrate. Executive Magistrates can dictate to the police the manner of force (baton or lathi charge/tear gas/blank fire/actual firing) and also, how much force should be used. They can also seek the assistance of the Armed Forces to quell a riot.

E. ***Labour Court***

- The term "labour court" is used in reference to a judicial forum to resolve disputes between employers and workmen. It has two-fold jurisdiction, viz civil as well as criminal, and is not subordinate to the High Court.
- Labour Courts deal with all types of disputes between employers and employees under the provisions of Industrial Disputes Act and other labour laws. The courts are presided over by judicial officers of the cadre of District Judges.
- Labour Courts deal mainly with recovery of wages and other employment benefits provided to employees under the Employment Act 1955, such as overtime pay, maternity allowance, termination benefits, etc.
- The "Labour Court" is not a statutory tribunal like the "Industrial Court" but refers to the hearing conducted by a Labour Officer of the Labour Department into complaints by employees. Cases handled can come under various other Acts also:
  - Workmen's Compensation Act, 1923
  - Industrial Disputes Act, 1947
  - Employees State Insurance Act, 1948
  - Factories Act, 1948
- In the Constitution of India, articles 14-16, 19(1)(c), 23-24, and 39(d) directly concern labour rights.
  - Article 14 specifies that everyone should be equal before the law.
  - Article 15 specifically says the state should not discriminate against citizens.
  - Article 16 extends a right of "equality of opportunity" for employment or appointment under the state.
  - Article 19(1)(c) gives everyone a specific right "to form associations or unions".
  - Article 23 prohibits all trafficking and forced labour.
  - Article 24 prohibits child labour under 14 years of age in a factory, mine or "any other hazardous employment".
  - Bonded Labour System (Abolition) Act 1976, abolishes bonded labour.
  - Article 39(d) of the Constitution provides that men and women should receive equal pay for equal work. The Equal Remuneration Act 1976 serves to implement this principle as legislation.
- Health and safety issues are an important component of labour law, and are covered by:
  - The Workmen's Compensation Act 1923, which requires compensation to be paid, if workers are injured in the course of employment for injuries, or benefits to dependants.
  - Occupational Safety, Health and Working Conditions Code, 2020, which provides for a safe working environment at the work place.
  - Sexual Harassment of Women at Workplace (Prevention, Prohibition & Redressal) Act, 2013, which seeks to protect and provide a mechanism for women to report incidents of sexual harassment at their place of work.

F. ***Family Court***

- Family courts hear all cases that relate to familial and domestic relationships. Each state and each country has a different system utilized to address family law cases, including decisions regarding divorce. In India, **The Family Courts Act, 1984** was enacted to provide for establishment of family courts with a view to promoting conciliation in, and secure speedy settlement of disputes relating to marriage and family affairs.
- The matters which are dealt in a Family Court in India are matrimonial reliefs which include:
  - nullity of marriage
  - judicial separation
  - divorce
  - restitution of conjugal rights
  - declaration as to the validity of marriage and matrimonial status of the person
  - property of the spouses
  - declaration as to the legitimacy of any person, guardianship of a person or custody of any minor
  - maintenance issues.
- It is the duty of the family court to resolve all matters through conciliation and settlement.
- Family courts have jurisdiction to give the custody of a child to a proper person.
- Procedure to be followed by the Family Court:
  - Family courts have the power to make their own procedure.
  - They are not required to record the oral statement of any witness at length.
  - The Family Court can receive any document or statement even if it is not admissible under Indian Evidence Act.
  - The Court can take assistance of medical and welfare experts as well as counsellors.
  - ***In camera*** proceedings can be ordered, if the parties desire.*
- Appeal against a decision of a Family Court can be made directly to the High Court within 30 days of passing the order or the judgement. Such appeal can be on both question of law and question of fact.

*"***In camera***" *means that the general public is not allowed to watch the proceedings.*

G. *Juvenile Justice Board*

- **The Juvenile Justice (Care and Protection of Children) Act, 2015** (*hereinafter referred to as* ***JJ Act, 2015***) is a new legislation which repeals the Juvenile Justice Act, 2000. One of the primary reasons for the introduction of this act was to address the commission of heinous offences by juveniles aged 16–18. This development comes after the infamous Nirbhaya Case of Delhi in 2012.
- The primary focus of this Act is on the procedural aspect, with regard to pendency in cases, accountability of the functionaries, etc. It has also highlighted the categories of '**child in conflict with law**' under Section 2(13) and '**child in need of care and protection**' under Section 2(14) of the Act. The Indian Constitution envisages a welfare state, where the children would be free from abuse and exploitation.
- The Juvenile Justice Board is an institutional body constituted under Section 4 of the JJ Act, 2015. At least one Juvenile Justice Board is established by the State Government for each district. The Board exercises its powers and discharges functions relating to the 'child in conflict with law' as has been defined under Section 2(13) of this Act.
- The **constitution of the Board** is as follows:
  - Metropolitan Magistrate or Judicial Magistrate First Class (referred to as Principal Magistrate)
  - Two social workers (one being a woman)
- **Powers granted to Juvenile Justice Board**:
  - The Bench shall have all the powers conferred by the Code of Criminal Procedure (CrPC) on a Metropolitan Magistrate or a Judicial Magistrate First Class.
  - The Placement of Persons under the JJ Act, 2015 has been divided into two categories.
    - *Category 1*: **A person who ceases to be a child during an inquiry** – If an inquiry has been initiated in respect of any child under the Act and during such course of the inquiry, if the child completes the age of 18 years, then the inquiry can be continued and orders can be passed as if such person was a child.
    - *Category 2*: **A person who was below the age of 18 years when the offence was committed** – Any person who has completed 18 years of age, and is arrested for the commission of an offence when he/she was below 18 years, then such person shall be treated like a child during the process of inquiry.
- When an alleged child in conflict with law is produced before the Board, it shall exercise its power to hold an inquiry according to the provisions of this Act and may pass orders as it deems fit.
- The Board is also empowered to inquire into heinous offences under Section 15 of the Act. Such preliminary assessment has to be disposed of within a period of 3 months from the date of first production of the child before the Board.
- **Functions of Juvenile Justice Board**:
  - Ensuring participation of the child and the parent throughout the process.
  - Ensuring protection of the child's rights throughout the process of arresting the child, inquiry, aftercare and rehabilitation.
  - Ensuring the availability of legal aid for the child through various legal services institutions.
  - Providing a qualified interpreter or translator to the child, if he/she fails to understand the language during the course of proceedings.
  - Directing Probation Officer/Child Welfare Officer/Social Worker to undertake a social investigation into the case, and directing them to submit the report within 15 days.
  - Adjudicating and disposing of cases pertaining to children in conflict with the law according to the process mentioned in Section 14.
  - Conducting inspection every month of residential facilities for children in conflict with the law and recommending various measures for improvement in the quality of services provided.
  - Ordering the police for registration of FIR if any offence is committed against any child in conflict with the law.
  - Conducting a regular inspection of jails meant for adults, to check, if any child is lodged in such jails.
  - Taking immediate measures for the transfer of a child found in jails for adults, to an observation home. Any child who is in conflict with law cannot be kept in police lock-up or jail under any circumstances.

FM 1.5: Non-Core – Written/Viva Voce
- Describe Court procedures including
  - Issue of Summons
  - Conduct money
  - Types of witnesses
  - Recording of evidence: oath, solemn affirmation, examination in chief, cross-examination, re-examination and court questions
  - Conduct of doctor in witness box

COURT PROCEDURES

Summons (Subpoena)

- **Subpoena or Summons is a document commanding the attendance of a witness in a court of law, under a penalty** (*sub* – under, *poena* – penalty).
- A summons is issued by the court, in writing, signed by the presiding officer and is served on the witness by a police officer or an officer of the court, or any other person specifically authorised for the purpose (**Box 1.2**).
- It is issued in duplicate, one of which is to be returned after signing, while the other is retained by the witness.
- A summons must be implicitly obeyed, unless there are valid and urgent reasons. A witness who willfully avoids to appear before a court after having been duly served a summons, is guilty of **contempt of court**. The penalty for non-compliance of summons is a **warrant of arrest** and a compulsory appearance before the court.

- In the matter of attending a court in response to a summons, it must be borne in mind that a witness must give **priority to a criminal case over a civil case**, if he is summoned to two courts at the same time, because criminal cases have priority over civil matters. Similarly, if he is summoned by two criminal courts on the same day, he is to give preference to the **higher court which takes precedence over a lower court**.

Conduct Money

- In civil cases, the medical officer is usually paid money to meet his travelling expenses from his place of residence to the court, and back. This is called **conduct money**. This is paid to him at the time the summons is served on him. If this amount is not paid to him, he may ignore the summons, if he so desires. If he feels the sum is inadequate, he can inform the court accordingly and get it enhanced.
- In criminal cases, however, no such fee is given usually, and it is the bounden duty of every citizen to attend the court whenever summoned.

Box 1.2—Proforma of a Subpoena (Summons to a Witness) (Cr.P.C Sections 61 & 244)

To Dr. ....
Whereas complaint has been made before me that Mr..................... of .... has committed, or is suspected to have committed the offence U/S ..... IPC on .... at ...., and it appears to me that you are likely to give material evidence, or to produce any document or other thing for the prosecution, You are hereby summoned to appear before this Court on .... at ...., to produce such document or thing to testify what you know concerning the matter of the said complaint, and not to depart thence without leave of court; and you are hereby warned that, if you neglect or refuse to appear on the said date, without just excuse, a warrant will be issued to compel your attendance.
Dated..............
(Seal of the Court) Signature ....

(The Summons is issued in duplicate. The witness has to acknowledge the receipt of the summons by signing on the reverse side of the original. The signed original has to be returned to the court. The copy is to be retained with the witness.)

WITNESSES

- Witnesses are of two kinds, namely, **common witness** and **expert witness**.
  - A **common** or **ordinary witness**, is one who testifies only to the facts observed by him. His evidence requires only common intelligence and knowledge. He is not capable of forming opinion or drawing conclusions from the facts observed by him.
  - An **expert witness** on the other hand, is one who is skilled in scientific, technical or professional matters, and who on account of his professional training, experience and ability, is capable of forming opinions, or drawing inferences, e.g., a doctor who conducts an autopsy.
  - Sometimes, a witness deliberately conceals the truth or gives false evidence. After making a particular statement in court, he contradicts this subsequently. He is therefore presumed to have an interest or motive for concealing the truth, or giving false evidence. The court therefore declares him to be **hostile**. It is possible that a common witness or expert witness may turn hostile. When a **hostile witness** is being examined, leading questions are permissible even during examination-in-chief.

Procedure in Court*

1. **Oath**
   a. Once the Medical Officer who is summoned makes his appearance in court, his evidence is recorded after administration of the oath.
   b. An **oath** is a declaration required by the law, to be made before the court by the witness. The oath is as follows: "*I swear in the name of God, that the evidence I shall give to the court shall be the truth, the whole truth, and nothing but the truth. So help me God.*"
   c. If the witness is an atheist, he makes a **solemn affirmation** as follows: "*I solemnly affirm that the evidence I shall give to the court shall be the truth, the whole truth, and nothing but the truth.*"
   d. Once a witness has been sworn, he is liable to be prosecuted for **perjury** (willful utterance of falsehood), if he does not speak the truth, or willfully conceals the truth (punishable under **sec 193 IPC**).
2. **Examination-in-Chief**
   a. Examination-in-chief is the examination of the witness by the counsel (advocate) of the party which has called him. In government prosecution cases, the **public prosecutor** commences the examination-in-chief, the purpose of which is to apprise the court of all the facts of the case.
   b. Leading questions are not allowed in examination-in-chief, except when a hostile witness is being examined. A **leading question** is one which itself suggests the answer.
      i. For e.g., "*Doctor, was not the injury caused by a sharp weapon?*" is a leading question. Normally, the question should be phrased in this manner – "*Doctor, by what weapon has this injury been caused?*"
3. **Cross-Examination**
   a. Cross-examination follows examination-in-chief. It is the examination of the witness by the counsel (advocate) of the opposite party, namely counsel for the accused (**defense counsel**).
   b. The purpose of cross-examination is to highlight inaccuracies and contradictions in the statements of the

**Trial by Jury was abolished in India in the 1960s, following a recommendation by the Law Commission in 1958.*

witness, and thereby to prove to the court that this evidence is not valid.

c. **Leading questions** are allowed during cross-examination. The witness must therefore be very careful in answering the questions. He may be asked questions to test his truthfulness, skill and character. A medical witness must not feel insulted, must avoid losing his temper, and must answer the questions with dignity and poise. He may sometimes be stumped for an answer, when asked an absurd question (**Box 1.3**). After all, even lawyers are human!

4. **Re-Examination**
   a. Cross-examination is followed by re-examination. It is conducted by the counsel who has conducted the examination-in-chief.
   b. The purpose of re-examination is to clear any doubts that may have arisen during cross-examination.
   c. Leading questions are not allowed.
   d. No new matter may be introduced without the permission of the judge and the consent of the counsel of the opposing party. In the event of a new topic being introduced, the opposing party has the right to cross-examine on the new matter.

Court Questions: These are questions put forward by the presiding officer of the court. These questions are posed to clear doubts, if any, and can be asked at any stage of the trial proceedings.

Box 1.3—Some Wise Court Questions

The following are questions actually asked of witnesses by attorneys during trials:
- "Now doctor, isn't it true that when a person dies in his sleep, he doesn't know about it until the next morning?"
- "The youngest son, the twenty-year old, how old is he?"
- "Were you present when your picture was taken?"
- "Were you alone or by yourself?"
- "Was it you or your younger brother who was killed in the war?"
- "Did he kill you?"
- "How far apart were the vehicles at the time of the collision?"
- "You were there until the time you left, is that true?"
- "How many times have you committed suicide?"
- "Doctor, which human species do these skeletal remains belong to?"

Source: All except the 10th entry are from the *Massachusetts Bar Association Lawyers Journal* (as mentioned in *Anil Aggrawal's Page of Forensic Jokes, Puns & Tidbits*: *http://aniljokes.tripod.com/forensicjoke001.html*).

Last entry: Question asked to the Editor of this book (*VV Pillay*) by the Defence Counsel in a Sessions Case at Mangalore, Karnataka.

Conduct of a Doctor in the Court

1. Go to court well prepared with the details of the case. Take care to have answers ready for anticipated questions.
2. Be in possession of all relevant certificates, documents and notes.
3. Do not attempt to memorise anything, since you are allowed to refresh your memory by consulting your report or notes.
4. Be well dressed and modest.
5. Speak audibly and clearly.
6. Use simple language, and avoid technical terms as far as possible.
7. Do not exaggerate anything. Avoid the use of superlatives, e.g., "*It was the* ***biggest wound*** *I have ever seen........*".
8. Do not fumble while referring to any case notes or records.
9. Do not discuss the case with anybody except the lawyer who has called you.
10. Address the Judge respectfully – "*Sir*" or "*Madam*" or "*Your Honour*". When entering the room, bow to him/her before taking your seat.
11. Avoid discrepancies between your earlier statements and your testimony to the court.
12. Do not evade any question. If a question is unclear, ask for it to be repeated or rephrased.
13. If you do not know the answer to a particular question, be frank and admit it.
14. Do not lose your temper. Always remain calm, composed and courteous.
15. Do not argue. Disagree firmly with anything you are not convinced about. But do not give the impression of being dogmatic.
16. Do not give rambling, long-winded answers. Try to be brief and precise.
17. As far as possible do not volunteer any statement on your own. However, if you feel that by not making some statement, injustice may result, do mention it.
18. Express opinions only on the basis of your own knowledge and experience. You can however utilise published opinion on scientific facts by qualified writers.
19. Be honest. If you have made some mistake, admit it. Do not attempt to cover up any lapses or errors.
20. Be absolutely impartial. Even though you may have been called by the prosecutor, present your facts objectively without taking sides.
    a. Remember the following quotation made by **Dr PCH Brouardel**, a 19th century French medico-legalist: "***If the law has made you a witness, remain a man of science. You have no victim to avenge, no guilty man to convict, and no innocent man to save. You must bear testimony within the limits of science.***"*

**Kulich RJ, Driscoll J, Prescott Jr JC, Pelletier NJ, Driscoll S, Cooke W, Correa L, Mehta NR. The Daubert Standard, a primer for pain specialists. Pain Med. 2003;4:75–80.*
Some textbooks incorrectly ***mention*** *the name of the author of this famous quote. The correct name is* ***Dr PCH Brouardel.***

FM 1.6: Non-Core – Written/Viva Voce
- Describe Offences in Court including
  - Perjury
  - Court strictures vis-a-vis Medical Officer

OFFENCES IN COURT

Perjury

- Once a witness has been sworn in a court of law, he is liable to be prosecuted for **perjury** (willful utterance of falsehood), if he does not speak the truth, or willfully conceals the truth (punishable under **Sec 193 IPC**).

Court Strictures vis-a-vis Medical Officer

- The term "**court stricture**" or more correctly "**judicial stricture**" means that the court has expressed disapproval of some aspect of the conduct of a lawyer or a witness in a court of law, in the form of critical remarks made by the presiding judge.
- A stricture is the signature of disapproval. It is not a sentence of punishment, but a scathing comment that can be deeply humiliating to the person concerned. When it goes into the records of a case, it can be highly stigmatizing to the recipient of such a stricture. If the latter is an expert witness such as a doctor, his reputation can be significantly affected not only in relation to the case in question, but also sometimes in future court appearances as well. Every medical witness must be alert to this possibility when tendering evidence.
- All witnesses, whether common or expert, are expected to adhere to some norms of behaviour, besides being completely factual in their testimony. In the case of a doctor as an expert witness, all efforts must be taken to demonstrate to the court that due diligence had gone into the preparation and deposition of evidence, and that there was no glaring negligence in coming to conclusions or framing an opinion.

PLEASE NOTE, STUDENTS AND TEACHERS!

Incredible though it may seem, as per the CBME curriculum for FMT (2018), all the above Competencies (FM 1.1 to 1.6) are Non-Core! Which means, they are actually desirable to know (nice to know) only, and not really essential to know (must know)!

FM 1.7: Core – Written/Viva Voce
- Describe
  - Dying Declaration
  - Dying Deposition

DYING DECLARATION

- **A dying declaration is a statement, written or oral, made by a person who is on the verge of dying as a result of unnatural causes.**
  - The statement should relate to the cause of his imminent death, or any of the circumstances of the transaction resulting in his present condition.
  - Such a declaration is **admissible in court**, when the cause of that person's death is the subject of enquiry. It may provide useful information and help to obtain justice.
  - A person who is accused of a crime cannot make a dying declaration, but only a person who is the victim of a crime.
  - Statements unconnected with the actual crime are not admissible in a dying declaration.
- It is believed that a person who is about to die will speak only the truth. A dying declaration has the same measure of worth, as that of a statement made on oath, in the court.
- A dying declaration is valid even if the declarant lives for some days after making the declaration, but in that case, it may be relied on only as corroborative evidence.
- As soon as a doctor knows that the victim of a crime who is in danger of dying, has something of importance to say to the court, he must send for a magistrate.
  - If the doctor feels that the declarant may die before the arrival of the magistrate, he can record the declaration himself.
  - It is desirable (but not mandatory) to certify that the declarant was in a state of sound mind (***compos mentis***) at the time of making the declaration.
- Although no oath is administered, a dying declaration is admissible in court as if this had been done, provided it is recorded as per the guidelines laid down for the purpose.
- The declaration must be recorded in the presence of two witnesses.
- It is to be recorded verbatim, in the language in which the victim prefers to speak.
- No information must be elicited by asking leading questions. No prompting or suggestions should be made to the declarant, and undue influence must not be imposed on the declarant.
- **The investigating police officer should not be present when the declaration is being made**.
- If the dying person is unable to speak, but is able to make gestures in answer to questions, it can be recorded after deciphering the gestures. The medical officer recording the declaration should only mention the precise nature of the gestures so made, and not interpret them himself. Interpretation is done subsequently by the court.
- After the complete declaration has been recorded, it must be read over to the declarant, and must if possible, be signed by him. It must then be attested by the writer and the witnesses.
  - If the declarant dies or becomes unconscious while the declaration is being made, the medical officer writing it must record as much information as he has obtained and sign it.
- The declaration must be **forwarded to the magistrate in a sealed envelope**.
- If a dying declaration is recorded by a magistrate, and in the presence of the accused who is given an opportunity

to cross examine the declarant, it is called a **dying deposition**.

- A dying deposition has greater value than dying declaration in court, for the reason that it is recorded by a Magistrate, in the presence of the accused who is permitted to cross examine the declarant.
  Note: This is however NOT prevalent in India.

DYING DEPOSITION*

- Dying deposition is also a form of dying declaration. The main difference being that it is recorded by a magistrate in the presence of the accused or his/her lawyer.
- The magistrate records the evidence after administering oath in the presence of the accused or his/her lawyer.
- Legally, **a dying deposition has more value than a dying declaration** as the accused has the opportunity to challenge and cross-examine the victim who is making the statement.
- The medical officer's presence is not essential, but he/she may have to certify the mental fitness of the victim.
  Note: Currently this is not in practice in India, as there is no provision of dying deposition in the Indian Evidence Act.

> **FM 1.8: Core – Written/Viva Voce**
> - Describe the latest decisions/notifications/resolutions/circulars/standing orders related to medico-legal practice issued by Courts/Government authorities, etc.

Some of the latest decisions/notifications/resolutions/circulars/standing orders related to medicolegal practice issued by Courts/Government authorities, etc., include the following:

A. **The Criminal Law (Amendment) Act, 2013**

The Criminal Law (Amendment) Act, 2013 inserted new sections 326A, 326B, 354A, 354B, 354C, and 354D in the Indian Penal Code (IPC).

Some Highlights:

1. **Sec 326A of IPC** deals with cases of **acid attacks** and specifies punishment for such a crime. It states that: *Whoever causes permanent or partial damage or deformity to, or burns or maims or disfigures or disables, any part or parts of the body of a person, or causes grievous hurt by throwing acid on, or by using any other means with the intention of causing or with the knowledge that he is likely to cause such injury or hurt, shall be punished with* ***imprisonment of 10 years, but which may extend to imprisonment for life, and with fine***. *Provided further that any fine imposed under this section shall be paid to the victim.*
2. **Sec 326B of IPC** specifies the punishment for **attempted acid throwing**. It states that: *Whoever throws or attempts to throw acid on any person or attempts to administer acid to any person, or attempts to use any other means, with the intention of causing permanent or partial damage or deformity or maiming or disfigurement or disability or grievous hurt to that person, shall be punished with imprisonment for* ***5 years, but which may extent to 7 years and also be liable to fine***.
   Explanation: For the purposes of Section 326A and this section, "acid" includes any substance which has acidic or corrosive character or burning nature, that is capable of causing bodily injury leading to scars or disfigurement or temporary or permanent disability.
3. **Sec 354A of IPC: Sexual harassment**: Provides for rigorous imprisonment up to 3 years, or with fine, or with both in case of offence described in clauses (i), (ii) or (iii); imprisonment up to 1 year, or with fine, or with both in other cases.
   Only protects women.
   Clauses:
   i. physical contact and advances involving unwelcome and explicit sexual overtures
   ii. a demand or request for sexual favours
   iii. forcibly showing pornography
   iv. making sexually coloured remark
   v. any other unwelcome physical, verbal or non-verbal conduct of sexual nature.
4. **Sec 354B of IPC: Intent to disrobe a woman**: Imprisonment not less than 3 years but which may extend to 7 years and with fine. Only protects women against anyone who "*assaults, or uses criminal force to any woman, or abets such act, with the intention of disrobing or compelling her to be naked.*"
5. **Sec 354C of IPC**: Defines '**Voyeurism**' as any man who watches, or captures the image of, a woman engaging in a private act in circumstances where she would usually have the expectation of not being observed either by the perpetrator or by any other person. It carries a punishment of 1 year in prison, extendable to 3 years, and shall also be liable to fine. A second or subsequent conviction will entail imprisonment for a term which shall not be less than 3 years, but which may extend to 7 years, and shall also be liable to fine. **Explanation**: For the purpose of this section, 'private act' includes an act of watching a woman, in a place that would reasonably be expected to provide privacy, whose genitals, posterior or breasts are exposed, or covered only in underwear; or the victim is using a lavatory; or the victim is doing a sexual act that is not of a kind ordinarily done in public.
6. **Sec 354D of IPC**: Defines '**Stalking**' as any man who—
   - follows a woman and contacts, or attempts to contact such woman to foster personal interaction repeatedly, despite a clear indication of disinterest by the woman; or

---

**It is strange that this ('dying deposition') should feature in the new curriculum, as it is not practiced in India. Teachers must refrain from setting questions on such obsolete content.*

- monitors the use by a woman of the internet, email or any other form of electronic communication.

Whoever commits the offence of stalking shall be punished on first conviction with imprisonment of 3 years in prison, and shall also be liable to fine; and be punished on a second or subsequent conviction, with imprisonment for a term which may extend to 5 years, and shall also be liable to fine.

7. **Section 370 of IPC** has been substituted with new sections, **370** and **370A** which deal with **trafficking of person for exploitation**. If a person recruits, transports, harbours or receives a person, by using threats, or force, or coercion, or by abuse of power, for exploitation including prostitution, slavery, forced organ removal, etc. will be punished with imprisonment ranging from at least 7 years to life.
8. **Section 375 of IPC**: The term '**rape**' is extended to include acts in addition to vaginal penetration. The definition is broadly worded with acts like penetration of penis into the vagina, urethra, anus or mouth; or any object or any part of body to any extent, into the vagina, urethra or anus of a woman, or making another person do so; to apply mouth or touching private parts. Except in certain aggravated situations, the punishment will be imprisonment not less than 7 years, but which may extend to imprisonment for life, and shall also be liable to fine. In aggravated situations, punishment will be rigorous imprisonment for a term which shall not be less than 10 years but which may extend to imprisonment for life, and shall also be liable to fine.
9. **Sec 376A of IPC**: Has been added which states that if a person committing the offence of **sexual assault**, "*inflicts an injury which causes the death of the person or causes the person to be in a* ***persistent vegetative state****, shall be punished with rigorous imprisonment for a term which shall not be less than 20 years, but which may extend to imprisonment for life, or with death.*"
   a. In case of "**gang rape**", persons involved regardless of their gender shall be punished with rigorous imprisonment for a term which shall not be less than 20 years, but which may extend to life, and shall pay compensation to the victim which shall be reasonable to meet the medical expenses and rehabilitation of the victim.
   b. The age of consent in India has been increased to 18 years, which means any sexual activity irrespective of presence of consent with a woman below the age of 18 will constitute **statutory rape**.
10. Certain changes have been introduced in the **Criminal Procedure Code** and **Indian Evidence Act**, like the process of recording the statement of the victim has been made more victim friendly and easy.

    The two critical changes are:
    a. the '**character of the victim**' is now rendered totally irrelevant,
    b. there is now a presumption of '**no consent**' in a case where sexual intercourse is proved and the victim states in the court that she did not consent.

B. **The Protection of Children from Sexual Offences Act or POCSO (2012)**: This was enacted to provide a robust legal framework for the protection of children from offences of sexual assault, sexual harassment and pornography, while safeguarding the interest of the child at every stage of the judicial process. The framing of the Act seeks to put children first by making it easy to use by including mechanisms for child-friendly reporting, recording of evidence, investigation and speedy trial of offences through designated Special Courts. The new Act provides for a variety of offences under which an accused can be punished.

Offences under the act include:

- ***Penetrative Sexual Assault***: Insertion of penis/object/ another body part in child's vagina/urethra/anus/mouth, or asking the child to do so with them or some other person.
- ***Sexual Assault***: When a person touches the child, or makes the child touch them or someone else.
- ***Sexual Harassment***: Passing sexually coloured remark, sexual gesture/noise, repeatedly following, flashing, etc.
- ***Child Pornography***
- ***Aggravated Penetrative Sexual Assault/Aggravated Sexual Assault***

The act is **gender-neutral** for both children and for the accused.

With respect to pornography, the Act criminalises even watching, or collecting pornographic content involving children.

The Act also makes abetment of child sexual abuse an offence.

C. **Unnatural Offences (Sodomy) – Section 377 IPC**: On **06 Sept 2018**, the Supreme Court ruled that **Section 377 of the Indian Penal Code (IPC) is unconstitutional** "*in so far as it criminalises consensual sexual conduct between adults of the same sex*".

Homosexuality thus has been de-criminalized in India (with certain conditions).

D. **Attempt to Commit Suicide – Section 309 IPC**: Section 309 of Indian Penal Code (IPC) deals with unsuccessful suicides, whereby attempting to commit suicide was punishable with imprisonment up to 1 year. Considering longstanding demand and recommendations of the Law Commission of India, which has repeatedly endorsed the repeal of this section, the Govt of India in Dec 2014 decided to decriminalise attempts to commit suicide by dropping Section 309 of the IPC from the statute book. Even though that has not officially been done, in 2017, the new Mental Healthcare Act of India was signed. **Section 115(1)** of the act effectively **decriminalizes suicide**, saying "*any person who attempts to commit suicide shall be presumed to have severe stress and shall not be tried and punished under the said Code.*"

E. **Adultery – Section 497 IPC**: Section 497 of the Indian Penal Code (IPC) has been criticized on the one hand for allegedly treating woman as the private property of her husband, and on the other hand for giving women complete protection against punishment for adultery. This section was unanimously struck down on 27 Sept 2018 by the Supreme Court as being unconstitutional and demeaning to the dignity of women.

   Adultery continues to be grounds for seeking divorce in a Civil Court, but is no longer a criminal offence in India.

F. **Guidelines for Medical Examination of Arrested Persons**: As per **Section 57 of Criminal Procedure Code (CrPC)**, a person arrested should not be detained more than 24 hrs, and Section 54 (1), (2) & (3) mandates statutory medical examination of arrested persons before producing him/her before the magistrate.

   The following guidelines have recently been issued in this regard:
   - After arresting the accused and before producing him/her before the magistrate concerned within the statutory time limit, the mandatory medical examination prescribed under Section 54 CrPC should be carried out. When such an arrested person is brought for mandatory medical examination, the doctor concerned shall complete the medical examination without delay.
   - After remanding the accused person in judicial custody or police custody, the Police Officer concerned shall, as early as possible give a request to the Medical Officer to carry out detailed examination as per proforma prescribed by National Human Rights Commission. Such a request should mention whether he/she is in judicial custody or police custody.
   - The remanded person shall be taken before the Medical Officer as far as possible, to take blood and sputum samples. If these facilities are not available, then the medical officer concerned should inform the same to the police, and he may be referred to another hospital having these facilities for taking blood and other fluids as required for examination.
   - Since testing for HIV has to be done after counselling the persons concerned as per the existing norms, the remanded person suspected of having HIV or Hepatitis may be referred to ICTC (Integrated Testing and Counselling Centre) after their admission in prisons. The prison officers concerned will send them to ICTC with police escort as per the Prison Act.
   - The test results of blood and other fluids may be made available to the prison authorities or police authorities as the case may be, by the medical officers concerned within 24 hours of the examination, so that persons with communicable diseases may be quarantined and treated accordingly.
   - The prison authority should take all efforts to keep the remanded person separately till complete result of medical examination is available.
   - In the case of police custody, the police concerned shall ensure that the remanded person is not in physical contact with other arrested persons till the completion of medical examination.

G. **Amendment to Section 114B Indian Evidence Act: Presumption of custodial death or injury**: In a prosecution of a police officer for an offence constituted by an act alleged to have caused death or bodily injury to a person, if there is evidence that the death or injury was caused during a period when that person was in the custody of the Police, the court may presume that the death or injury was caused by the Police Officer having custody of that person during that period.

FM 1.9: Core – Written/Viva Voce
- Describe the importance of documentation in medical practice in regard to medicolegal examinations, medical certificates, and medicolegal reports, especially
  - Maintenance of patient case records, discharge summary, prescribed registers to be maintained in health centres
  - Maintenance of medicolegal register like accident register
  - Documents of issuance of wound certificate
  - Documents of issuance of drunkenness certificate
  - Documents of issuance of sickness and fitness certificate
  - Documents for issuance of death certificate
  - Documents of medical certification of cause of death-form numbers 4 and 4A
  - Documents for estimation of age by physical, dental and radiological examination and issuance of certificate.

DOCUMENTATION IN MEDICAL PRACTICE

Proper documentation of cases of patient management and preservation of such documents are important aspects of medical and medicolegal practice. Every doctor is expected to be aware of the legalities involved in such documentation, which may subsequently become crucial evidence in certain kinds of litigation in the form of "documentary evidence".

Documentary Evidence

- This comprises documents produced before the court, and include:
  - Medical certificate
  - Medicolegal report
  - Dying declaration

Medical Certificates

- These are certificates which pertain to sickness, fitness, insanity, death, etc.
- They are issued only by a registered medical practitioner and are admissible in court.
- It is however, an offence to issue a false certificate. When a medical practitioner is not sure of the cause of death or

when he suspects foul play, he must refuse to issue a death certificate and must inform the police.

Sickness and Fitness Certificates*

- Only a registered medical practitioner can issue sickness and/or fitness certificates.
- Sickness certificate is issued for the expected duration of an illness and is required to be produced by employees of various organizations (whether private or government), various educational institutes, and also for the purpose of receiving insurance claims.
- **Sickness certificate** is issued when the person is still sick and undergoing treatment.
- **Fitness certificate** is issued at the time of resuming duties once the patient is cured of the illness and is fit to rejoin work. Hence, a fitness certificate is only issued at the end of the medical treatment.
- These certificates should preferably be issued on letter-heads bearing the name, qualifications, registration number and address of the RMP, and it should be in the prescribed format.
- The certificate is to be issued to the patient himself or to the guardian who has already given consent for examination and treatment for the illness of the patient.
- The physician must ensure that any statements made in these certificates are to the best of his or her knowledge, accurate, and based upon current clinical information. No part of the certificate should be untrue, misleading or improper in any way.
- A physician must never state that a patient has been under his or her care unless that is actually the case. The duration of the care should be clearly indicated. The duration of illness mentioned in the certificate should be limited to the period during which the patient was actually under care and observation of the practitioner.
- The certificate must be accompanied by a brief resume of the case giving the nature of the illness, its symptoms, causes and duration.
- The practitioner should preserve with him a duplicate copy of the certificate issued, and retain it at least for 2 years. Otherwise, he should maintain a register with details of all certificates issued with serial number and the signature of the patient to whom a particular certificate was issued. If more than one copy of a certificate is required to be given to the patient, it is to be marked as duplicate.
- Medical practitioners can demand fees for issuing such certificates, unless they are issued from hospitals providing free service.
- The practitioner should sign the certificate legibly at the end along with the registration number and also the signature/left thumb impression of the patient, attested by him.
- If during the course of treatment of such illness, the practitioner comes across any other disease or ailment, which he has actually not treated (e.g., colour blindness noticed in a patient being treated for malaria) then that information should not be included in the sickness/fitness certificate without the expressed written consent of the patient. In such cases, the rules that are applicable for professional secrecy and privileged communication should be followed.

Guidelines for preparing a Sickness Certificate

- The certificate should have legible handwriting.
- Two identification marks should be mentioned in detail. The marks should be preferably from exposed parts of the body. The exact description of the marks as regards the location, site, size, colour, etc., should be mentioned.
- The name of the RMP should be mentioned in full. The RMP who has examined the patient should only issue the certificate.
- Name of the patient is to be written in full along with the age, sex and address.
- The exact nature of illness should be mentioned. Any use of short forms or abbreviations should be avoided.
- The expected duration of the illness (in number of days) must be mentioned in the sickness certificate. If the RMP is of the opinion that any further increase in duration of treatment is anticipated, then such a comment can be added.
- The signature of the medical practitioner along with the name in legible handwriting, registration number, date, time and place of examination should be mentioned.
- Signature/Left thumb impression of the patient must be obtained in the presence of the RMP himself.
- If the patient informs the doctor that he was ill for the last 3 days, which information the doctor is not in a position to verify, then he should mention such a fact as follows: 'as per the information provided by the patient, he was ill since (date)'. However, the duration of illness in the sickness certificate must be from the date on which the patient visited the doctor.
- If preprinted stationery is used, the practitioner shall delete words which are irrelevant.

Guidelines for preparing a Fitness Certificate

- The certificate should have legible handwriting.
- Two identification marks should be mentioned in detail. The marks should be preferably from exposed parts of the body. The exact description of the marks as regards the location, site, size, colour etc should be mentioned.
- The name of the RMP should be mentioned in full. The RMP who has examined the patient should only issue the certificate.
- Name of the patient is to be written in full along with the age, sex and address.
- The exact nature of illness should be mentioned. Any use of short forms or abbreviations should be avoided. The nature of illness should mention the ailment for which the

Source: Parts of this section have been adapted from the format used by Department of Forensic Medicine, Rural Medical College, Loni (Maharashtra), with the kind courtesy of the Medicolegal Association of Maharashtra (MLAM).

patient approached the RMP and which was being treated by him.

- The exact duration (in number of days) of illness suffered by the patient must be mentioned in the fitness certificate.
- The date from which the RMP considers the patient to be fit to resume his duties should be clearly mentioned.
- The signature of the medical practitioner along with the name in legible handwriting, registration number, date, time and place of examination should be mentioned.
- Signature/Left thumb impression of the patient must be obtained in the presence of the RMP himself.
- If preprinted stationery is used, the practitioner shall delete words which are irrelevant.

***Liabilities for issuing false or misleading medical certificates*:**

- Issuing of a false certificate is not only ethically wrong but also attracts the provisions of Indian Penal Code.
  - **Sec 197 of the IPC** states that "*Whoever issues or signs any certificate relating to any fact knowing or believing that such certificate is false in any material point, shall be punished in the same manner as if, he gave 'false evidence'*".
- Issuing of a false certificate is considered as "**Professional Misconduct**" and can lead to penal erasure of the name of the practitioner from the medical register.

Box 1.4—Format of Sickness Certificate

This is to certify that I .... have personally examined Mr/Ms ....s/ w/ d/ o ...., aged about ...... years, sex (male/female/other),occupation .... resident of .... (whose signature/left thumb impression is verified as under).
He/she is suffering from (disease) .... and I have advised him/her...
I do consider that absence of ....days with effect from ...., i.e., from .... to .... is absolutely necessary for restoration of his/ her good health.

Identification marks of patient:
1.......................
2.......................

Signature ....
Name, Qualification,
Regn Number, Designation
(Rubber stamped)

....
Verified signature
Or
Left thumb impression of patient

Date:

- A physician may be required to testify in proceedings involving disputes between an employer and the employee (i.e., the physician's patient) based on the sickness/fitness certificate provided. Physicians can be summoned as witnesses in legal proceedings under oath, and their clinical notes may be examined and cross-examined by legal counsel. Carelessness in preparation of these forms can have serious medicolegal implications.
- If the patient suffers any damage due to mention of any untrue, incorrect or misleading information in the sickness/fitness certificate issued by an RMP, he/she has the right to avail legal remedy by filing a civil suit.

Box 1.5—Format of Fitness Certificate

This is to certify that I .... have personally examined Mr/Ms .... s/ w/ d/ o ...., aged about .... years, sex (male/female/other), occupation.. resident of .... (whose signature/left thumb impression is verified as under), and found that he/she has completely recovered from his/her illness and is now fit to resume duties with effect from.............
I also certify that before arriving at this decision, I have examined the original medical certificate and statement of the case on which leave was granted or extended, and have taken them into consideration in arriving at my decision.

Identification marks of patient:
1......................
2......................

Signature ....
Name, Qualification,
Regn Number, Designation
(Rubber stamped)

....
Verified signature
Or
Left thumb impression of patient

Date:

*Death Certificate**

- **Death certificate** is
  - a legal document issued by a medical practitioner which states when a person died, or
  - a document issued by a government civil registration office that declares the date, location and cause of a person's death, as entered in an official register of deaths.
- An official death certificate is usually required to be provided when applying for probate or administration of a deceased's estate.
- The government registration office would usually be required to provide details of deaths, without production of

**Source: Some parts of this section have been taken from the article "Medical certification of cause of death" by Dr PC Srivastava, Dr Shikha Saxena & Professor MKB Sahai – IJMU. 2009;4(1).*

a death certificate, to enable government agencies to update their records, such as electoral registers, government benefits paid, passport records, etc.

- The Registration of Births and Deaths under Municipal Acts stipulates that notice must compulsorily be given by a doctor in attendance, at the time of the birth or death of an individual.
- Proper death certification begins with a fundamental understanding of the cause and manner of death. During the process of medical certification of the cause of death, it is incorrect to write "heart failure," "cardiac failure," "cardiopulmonary arrest", "respiratory arrest" and "brain death" without mentioning the underlying pathological cause. It should be remembered that every death which occurs due to one or the other cause ends in cardio-respiratory failure. Cardiac failure or respiratory failure means simply the cessation of circulation or respiration leading to somatic and cellular death.
- The data on cause of death contained in the certificate serves many purposes, such as assessing the effectiveness of public health programmes, providing a feedback for future policy and implementation, better health planning, etc. Medical certification of the cause of death by a registered medical practitioner is thus very important and must be as accurate as possible. He should have the knowledge of the underlying cause of death of his patient which initiated the train of morbid events leading directly to death; and certification of cause of death.
- The cause of death must be properly determined before lawful disposal of the dead body. In cases where the cause of death is unknown, the body should be subjected to medicolegal (forensic) or pathological (clinical) autopsy to ascertain the cause of death depending upon the circumstances. This will fulfil the requirements of International Classification of Diseases (ICD-11) developed by WHO when death certificates are issued.
- **Cause of death** is a disease, abnormality, injury or poisoning that contributes directly or indirectly to death. A death often results from the combined effects of two or more conditions. These conditions may be completely unrelated, arising independently of each other; or causally related to each other.
  - The **underlying cause**, i.e., the disease or injury which has initiated the sequence of events should get selected for the purpose of tabulation.
  - Those morbid conditions or injuries consequent to the underlying cause relating to death are termed as **antecedent** and **immediate cause**.
- According to the legal provisions made in the Registration of Births and Deaths Act, 1969, the certification of the cause of death by a medical practitioner who has attended the deceased during the latter's last illness is mandatory.
- The medical practitioner shall, after the death of that person, forthwith issue to the person required under this Act to give information concerning the death, a certificate in the prescribed form stating to the best of his knowledge and belief the causes of death; and the certificate shall be received and delivered by such person to the Registrar at the time of giving information concerning the death as required by this Act.
- The registered medical practitioner's primary responsibility is to complete the medical part of the certificate regarding all diseases, morbid conditions or injuries which either resulted in or contributed to death.
- In the case of unnatural deaths and other medicolegal cases in which medicolegal autopsy is indicated, the last attending medical practitioner should **not** issue the "death certificate". The case should be informed to the police and the dead body should be kept in safe custody till it is forwarded for medicolegal autopsy after an inquest.
- The medical practitioner is not entitled to charge any fee for issuing a death certificate. He should not refuse, nor cause unnecessary delay in issuing a death certificate.
- The recommended format of death certificate is mentioned in **Box 1.6**.
  - Form No. 4 is for institutional (hospital) deaths, while Form No. 4A is for non-institutional deaths.
- It is the legal responsibility of the person in charge of a Medical Institution to report all births and deaths occurring therein to the Registrar of Births & Deaths in the prescribed form **within 21 days** under the **Registration of Births & Deaths (RBD) Act, 1969**.

Medicolegal Reports

- **Medicolegal reports** are documents prepared by medical officers in compliance with a written requisition issued by a magistrate or police officer.
- A medicolegal report may pertain to **injury (wound), sexual offence, death**, etc. It contains facts observed by the medical officer, and his opinion drawn therefrom. His opinion must be based upon the observations made by him, and not on hearsay evidence.

Documentation procedure and other related information pertaining to **wound certificate, drunkenness certificate** and **age certificate** have been discussed under relevant sections (*consult Index*).

Dying Declaration

Discussed under FM 1.7 *(page no. 19)*.

> **FM 1.10: Core – Written/Viva Voce**
> - Select appropriate cause of death in a particular scenario by referring ICD-10 code

FM 1.11: Core – Written/Viva Voce
- Write a correct cause of death certificate as per ICD-10 document*

Medical Certification of Cause of Death

- As per **ICD-10** (now **ICD-11**)**, two separate formats, one for **perinatal deaths** and another for **all other deaths**, exist for medical certification of cause of death.
- The one to be used in **non-perinatal deaths** has two variants:
  - for **hospital deaths** and
  - **non-hospital deaths**.
- The difference between the two is minimal. The most important portion is the portion where cause of death is mentioned.
- The preliminary portion of the form gives the available information about the personal particulars of the deceased including date and time of death.
  - Since the medical officer cannot declare a person dead without attending and examining him, this entry will be of the time when he has first seen the individual dead, irrespective of when the death has occurred.
    - For example, if an old man has died during his sleep at night and the medical officer examines him at 06:00 hours the next morning, the individual is declared to have died at 06:00 hours.
  - However, all such cases of deaths, unattended by a medical officer, are to be reported as medicolegal deaths. The actual time of death will then be decided during the inquest and postmortem examination along with the cause of death. Since the medical certificate of cause of death is filled after the postmortem examination, the legal time of death will be registered as that decided after the inquest.
  - Similarly, dilemma may arise in situations of prolonged attempts to revive a person thought to be in suspended animation. The time of death then is when revival measures are considered futile and stopped.
- If the identity of the deceased is not known, then the name will be entered as "Unknown" in all the documents including the medical certificate of cause of death, and will be replaced by the correct information when available.
- In 1967, the 20th World Health Assembly defined the causes of death to be entered on the medical certificate of cause of death as "all those diseases, morbid conditions or injuries which either resulted in or contributed to death, and the circumstances of the accident or violence which produced any such injuries". In a given situation more than one of the above conditions may be present, which may be completely unrelated to each other or they may be causally related to each other, i.e., one leading to the other, thus establishing a sequence.
- In Part I of the Cause of Death certificate, the disease or circumstances of accident/violence, which started the chain, is listed as the Underlying Cause of Death and the subsequent events in the chain are called as Antecedent Cause of Death and Immediate Cause of Death. The entire sequence gives the complete picture of the cause of death.
  - Example: In a patient with diabetes mellitus, who died of septicaemia due to gangrene of a limb:
    - Immediate Cause: Septicaemia
    - Antecedent Cause: Gangrene of limb
    - Underlying Cause: Diabetes mellitus
- If the individual was suffering from any other disease which is not related to the underlying cause and hence cannot be part of the sequence, but, in the opinion of the certifier, has contributed to death, such a condition too is to be recorded in Part II of the certificate. However, if the co-existing disease has not contributed to death, it has no place in the medical certificate of cause of death. Thus the certificate, unlike his medical records, is not a list of all diseases which the individual was suffering from at the time of death.
- The underlying cause of death which started the sequence should be the last entry under I. Consequently, if there is no chain of events and underlying cause is the only event, it should be entered under (a) as it is both the immediate & underlying cause. Evidently, line (a) must always have an entry. Due thought should be given to the last entry under I as it is picked up for statistical purposes as underlying cause of death.
- After entering the conditions sequentially, the duration of existence of each one of them is to be reflected under the heading "Interval between onset and death". This entry will give the chronology of events and thus ensure the correctness of the sequence.
- Having provided all the available information to the best of his knowledge, the certifier signs the certificate giving his name, qualifications, designation and registration number. The date and time of signature will be the same as that of death mentioned in the beginning of the certificate, except in cases where the cause of death has been certified after an autopsy.
- The bottom portion of the medical certificate of cause of death is to be filled up by the certifier, detached and handed over to the relatives. This document enables them to get the municipal permission for cremation/burial, as well as

---

**Source*: *Some parts of this section have been taken from the article "Medical certification of cause of death" by RB Kotabagi, RK Chaturvedi, A Banerjee – Med J Armed Forces India. 2004;60(3):261–72.*

***The ICD-11 is the eleventh revision of the International Classification of Diseases (ICD), and replaces the ICD-10 as the global standard for recording health information and causes of death. It was released on 18 June 2018, and officially endorsed by all WHO members during the 72nd World Health Assembly on 25 May 2019.*

Box 1.6—Formats of Death Certificate

Form No 4

MEDICAL CERTIFICATE OF CAUSE OF DEATH

(Hospital In-patients. Not to be used for stillbirths)
To be sent to Registrar along with Form No.2 (Death Report)

Name of the Hospital……………………………………………………………………………………

I hereby certify that the person whose particulars are given below died in the hospital, in Ward No…… on…………at…………..AM/PM.

<table>
<tr><td colspan="5">NAME OF DECEASED:</td><td>For Use of Statistical Office</td></tr>
<tr><td>Sex</td><td colspan="4">Age at death</td><td rowspan="3"></td></tr>
<tr><td rowspan="2">Male
Female
Other</td><td>If 1 year or more, age in years</td><td>If less than 1 year, age in months</td><td>If less than 1 month, age in days</td><td>If less than 1 day, age in hours</td></tr>
<tr><td></td><td></td><td></td><td></td></tr>
<tr><td colspan="4">CAUSE OF DEATH</td><td></td><td></td></tr>
<tr><td colspan="3">I
Immediate Cause
State the disease, injury or complication which caused death, not the mode of dying such as heart failure, asthenia, etc</td><td>(a) ……………………………
due to (or as a consequence of)</td><td rowspan="3">Interval between onset and death
(approx)</td><td rowspan="3"></td></tr>
<tr><td colspan="3">Antecedent Cause
Morbid conditions, if any, giving rise to the above cause, stating underlying conditions last</td><td>(b)……………………………
due to (or as a consequence of)</td></tr>
<tr><td colspan="3">II
Contributory Cause
Other significant conditions contributing to the death, but not related to the disease or condition causing it</td><td>(c) ……………………………
……………………………
……………………………</td></tr>
</table>

Manner of Death
(How did the injury occur)

1. Natural 2. Accident 3. Suicide 4. Homicide 5. Pending Investigation

If deceased was a female, was the death associated with pregnancy? 1. Yes 2. No
If yes, was there a delivery? 1. Yes 2. No

Name and Signature of the Medical Attendant
(certifying the cause of death)

Date of Verification

(to be filled and handed over to the relative of the deceased)

Certified that Shri/Smt/Kum……………………………………………………….S/W/D of Shri……………………………
R/O……………………………………………………………………………………was admitted to this hospital on..………...
and expired on…………………………………………

Doctor……………………………………………..
(Medical Suptdt)
Name of Hospital……………………………….

Form No 4A

MEDICAL CERTIFICATE OF CAUSE OF DEATH

(For non-institutional deaths. Not to be used for stillbirths)
To be sent to Registrar along with Form No.2 (Death Report)

I hereby certify that the person Shri/Smt/Kum..son/wife/daughter of.................
resident of..was under my treatment from..............to ....
and he/she died on ....at.............AM/PM.

<table>
<tr><td colspan="5">NAME OF DECEASED:</td><td>For Use of Statistical Office</td></tr>
<tr><td>Sex</td><td colspan="4">Age at death</td><td rowspan="3"></td></tr>
<tr><td rowspan="2">Male
Female
Other</td><td>If 1 year or more, age in years</td><td>If less than 1 year, age in months</td><td>If less than 1 month, age in days</td><td>If less than 1 day, age in hours</td></tr>
<tr><td></td><td></td><td></td><td></td></tr>
<tr><td colspan="4">CAUSE OF DEATH</td><td></td><td></td></tr>
<tr><td colspan="3">I
Immediate Cause
State the disease, injury or complication which caused death, not the mode of dying such as heart failure, asthenia, etc</td><td>(a) ....
due to (or as a consequence of)</td><td rowspan="3">Interval between onset and death
(approx)</td><td rowspan="3"></td></tr>
<tr><td colspan="3">Antecedent Cause
Morbid conditions, if any, giving rise to the above cause, stating underlying conditions last</td><td>(b)..............................
due to (or as a consequence of)</td></tr>
<tr><td colspan="3">II
Contributory Cause
Other significant conditions contributing to the death, but not related to the disease or condition causing it</td><td>(c) ....
....
..............................</td></tr>
</table>

Manner of Death
(How did the injury occur)

1. Natural 2. Accident 3. Suicide 4. Homicide 5. Pending Investigation

If deceased was a female, was the death associated with pregnancy? 1. Yes 2. No
If yes, was there a delivery? 1. Yes 2. No

Name and Signature of the Medical Attendant
(certifying the cause of death)

Date of Verification

(to be filled and handed over to the relative of the deceased)

Certified that Shri/Smt/Kum..S/W/D of Shri................................
R/O..was under my treatment from...........to.............
and expired on......................at.....................AM/PM

Doctor..
(Medical Suptdt)
Name of Hospital...................................

acts as a reference to obtain the extract of the death register (Death Certificate) from the registering authority.

- It may be noted that this portion, handed over to the relatives does not mention the medical cause of death. Even the Death Certificate issued by the registering authority does not mention the medical cause of death. This procedure is adopted to maintain confidentiality of information of the cause of death in accordance with the Registration of Births & Deaths Act of 1969. Hence, the certifier should send the medical certificate of cause of death along with death report forms to the registering authority directly. Thus, the medical cause of death is entered and available only in the Death Register maintained by the registering authority.

ADDENDUM — 1

*(Some of the following information is not mentioned specifically in the new curriculum as '**Competency**', but is important all the same.)*

MEDICAL EVIDENCE

- The term "**Evidence**" means all information which the court permits, which is helpful in relation to matters of fact under enquiry. It may be **documentary** or **oral** or **circumstantial**.
  - Evidence produced in the form of documents is called **documentary evidence**.
  - Evidence which is stated orally is called **oral evidence**.
  - Evidence obtained from the circumstances surrounding a case is called **circumstantial evidence**.

Documentary Evidence*

- This comprises documents produced before the court, and include:
  - Medical certificate
  - Medicolegal report
  - Dying declaration

Oral Evidence

- **Oral evidence refers to evidence which is tendered verbally.**
- Oral evidence, as far as possible, must be **direct**, i.e., if it refers to a fact which can be seen, heard or perceived, then it must be the evidence of a person who says he saw, heard or perceived it. In other words, it must be the evidence of the actual witness.
- However, it is not always necessary that oral evidence must be direct. Exceptions to direct oral evidence include:
  - Dying declaration.
  - Expert opinion expressed in a treatise, when the author is dead, or cannot be found, or is otherwise incapable of giving evidence.
  - Deposition of medical witness in a lower court.
  - Chemical examiner's report.
- **Oral evidence is superior to documentary evidence**, because it can be subjected to cross-examination.
- **Hearsay Evidence**: Hearsay evidence is the evidence of one who has no personal knowledge of the facts of the case, but just repeats what he has heard others say.
  - For example, if Mr A has seen Mr B shooting Mr X with a revolver, and if Mr A testifies that he has witnessed this incident, then it is **direct evidence**. But, if Mr A has got information from Mr Z that Mr B shot Mr X, then it is **hearsay evidence**, and it is not permissible in court, as the witness cannot be cross-examined.

Circumstantial Evidence

- It is the **evidence obtained from suspicious circumstances.**
  - For example, the sudden disappearance of a person who is suspected to be the criminal. In some cases, circumstantial evidence is more reliable than eye witness accounts.

ADDENDUM — 2

*(Most items in the following glossary are not mentioned specifically in the new curriculum as '**Competencies**', but they are important to know.)*

Box 1.7—Glossary of Common Legal Terms

Accused: One who is accused of/alleged to have committed a crime, but which has not yet been proved in a court of law.
Acquittal: It means the accused has been absolved, i.e., he is not guilty, and therefore can be set free. Once an accused has been acquitted, he cannot be tried again for the same offence by the same court.
Affidavit: Voluntary, written statement of facts made under oath before an officer of the court or before a notary public.
Appeal: It is a complaint made to a superior court of an injustice done, or error committed by an inferior one, whose judgement or decision is requested to be corrected or reversed.
Appellant: The person who files an appeal.
Arrest: Apprehension of a person (usually an accused) by judicial authorities, resulting in deprivation of his liberty.
- **Warrant of arrest** – It is a written order, which is signed, sealed, and issued by a magistrate, and addressed to a police officer or some other person specially named, commanding him to arrest the person named in it.

Assailant: One who has committed an assault.
Bail: It is defined as the security on behalf of an accused person, on giving which, he is released from custody, pending investigation or court trial.
- **Anticipatory bail** – It is a direction granted by the Sessions or High Court to release a person on bail issued even before the person is arrested.

Case: An action, cause of action, matter of dispute or law suit.

contd.

*Already discussed in preceding sections. This is specifically mentioned in the new curriculum and must be read thoroughly by every student.

- **Warrant case** – A case relating to an offence punishable with death, imprisonment for life or imprisonment for a term exceeding 2 years.
- **Summons case** – A case relating to an offence which is not punishable by a term of imprisonment exceeding 2 years.
- **Civil case** – It is a dispute between two private parties relating to wealth, property, etc.
- **Criminal case** – It is a case between the Government (represented by the police) and a private party concerning matters of public interest and safety, e.g., assault, robbery, murder, rape, etc.

Case law: Legal principles derived from judicial decisions. It is different from statutory law which is enacted by the legislature.

Cause of action: A set of facts which gives a person a right to file a proceeding in a civil court.

Charge: A formal accusation in writing against a person that he has committed an offence.

Charge sheet: It is a report alleging the commission of a crime by an accused person submitted to a magistrate by the police on completion of an investigation.

Common law: Judge-made law as opposed to codified law.

Complaint: A legal document that is the initial pleading on the part of the plaintiff in a civil suit. The purpose of this document is to give the defendant notice of the alleged facts. The complaint is usually attached to the summons.

Contempt of court: It means intentional insult or interruption to a court in any stage of a judicial proceeding.

Conviction: It means that an accused has been proved in a court of law, to be guilty of the crime alleged to have been committed by him. The "accused" is now termed a "convict."

Court of justice: It denotes a Judge who is empowered by law to act judicially alone, or a body of Judges which is empowered by law to act judicially as a body.

Culpability: Being at fault, deserving punishment or reproach, for some act or cause of action.

Damage: Injury suffered by a party as a result of the action of another.

Damages: Compensation (usually monetary) that is payable to a victim, as decided by the court.

Decree: The document under the seal of the court setting out the relief granted to a party or parties.

Defendant: The party against whom a complaint has been filed. He is the same as an "accused."

Defence counsel: The legal practitioner who acts on behalf of the accused, and challenges the evidence of the prosecution. In other words, he defends the defendant.

Deposition: The evidence given under oath by a person (usually a witness) in a court of law.

Document: It describes any matter expressed or inscribed upon any substance by means of letters, figures, or marks, intended to be used, or which may be used as an evidence of that matter.

Evidence: It means anything by which any alleged matter of fact is either established or disproved.

- **Demonstrative or Real evidence** – The use of an article or object, rather than the statement of a witness to prove a fact in question.
- **Material evidence** – Proof of facts that directly affect an element of the cause of action.
- **Prima facie evidence** – A level of proof which is sufficient to establish the fact, and if not rebutted, becomes conclusive of the fact.

Exhibit: Any document or object produced for inspection before the court.

Good faith: Nothing is said to be done or believed in good faith, which is done or believed without due care and attention.

Inquiry: A procedure that is conducted by a magistrate or court as per the Criminal Procedure Code, which does not amount to a trial.

Investigation: It is a procedure carried out by a police officer or other person (other than a magistrate) as per the Criminal Procedure Code, for the collection of evidence.

Judge: It is a term that denotes not only those persons officially designated as a judge in a court of law, but also every person who is empowered by the law to give, in any judicial proceeding, civil or criminal, a definite judgement. It includes for instance, collectors of districts and executive magistrates.

Jury: A sworn body of people convened to render an impartial verdict officially submitted to them by a court, or to set a penalty or judgment. In criminal cases there are usually 12 members (jurors). Trial by jury does not exist in India.

Offence: It is any act or omission made punishable by law.

- **Cognizable offence** – It is an offence for which a police officer may arrest a person without a warrant, e.g., theft, rape, murder, etc.
- **Non-cognizable offence** – It is an offence for which a police officer cannot arrest a person without a warrant, e.g., forgery, cheating, etc.

Offender: One who has committed an offence.

Public Prosecutor: A lawyer appointed by the Government for conducting prosecutions on behalf of the state in judicial proceedings of the High Court, Sessions Court or Magistrate's Court.

Search warrant: It is a written authority given to a police officer or any person by a competent magistrate or court for the search of any general or specified thing or document.

Statute: The law passed by the legislature.

Statute of limitation: The time period up to which a plaintiff may file a lawsuit.

Suit: A civil proceeding in a court of law.

Trial: It is a legal process in accordance with the law whereby the question of guilt or innocence of any person accused of an offence is determined.

- **Court trial** – A trial without a jury, where a judge determines the facts as well as the law.

Verdict: The formal decision or finding made by a judge or jury at the end of a trial. The verdict may be in favour of either the plaintiff or defendant.

Topic 2

FORENSIC PATHOLOGY

Number of Competencies – 35 (FM 2.1 to 2.35)

FM 2.1: Core – Written/Viva Voce

- **Define, describe and discuss death and its types including**
  - Somatic/Clinical/Cellular Death
  - Molecular Death
  - Brain Death
    - Cortical Death
    - Brainstem Death

DEATH

- **Thanatology is a branch of science that deals with the study of death**. The term 'thanatology' is derived from '*Thanatos*', the Greek God of Death, and the suffix '*-ology*' is derived from the Greek suffix '*-logia*' meaning 'study of'.
- Death is an inevitable reality and in the past was considered to be a simple and straightforward phenomenon. The doctor would declare a person dead once he was convinced that there was cessation of life in the patient. This meant that the patient had stopped breathing, his heart had stopped beating, there was unresponsiveness and his body had turned cold.
- Though cessation of heartbeat was enough to consider a person as dead in the past, it is no longer an evidence of death today, since the heart is now able to be substituted with that of a 'just deceased donor' or a mechanical one. Moreover, modern biomedical innovations like the resuscitator and cardiac pacemaker have made it imperative to establish a set criteria by which the moment of death could be identified.
- The basic concept is that death is the irreversible loss of the capacity for consciousness and capacity to breathe. Since both the functions reside in the brainstem, the modern concept of diagnosing death is to identify whether a person's brainstem is alive or not.

Somatic/Clinical Death

- **Somatic death (Clinical death)** refers to the complete and irreversible cessation of the function of the brain, followed by the cessation of the functions of the heart and the lungs.
- Although the heart may have stopped, the respiration has ceased and the brainstem is functionless, tissues retain the 'vital principle of life' for some time. The body is dead as a whole, but the biological properties of the component parts may still be demonstrable. The muscles contract to mechanical or electric stimulus. The pupils respond to appropriate pharmacological stimuli.

Molecular Death

- The time during which the properties (described above) persist, soon runs out. Over a period of time, these individual tissues and cells die.
- **Molecular death (Cell death)** refers to the cessation of functions of individual tissues and cells of the body.
- The whole body is now dead. In this way, a person dies in bits and pieces. Therefore, death is a process, not an event.

Brain Death

- **Brain death** is the complete loss of brain function (including involuntary activity necessary to sustain life).
- It differs from
  - **Persistent vegetative state**, in which the person is alive and some autonomic functions remain.
  - **Coma**, whether caused by injury and/or illness, even if it is very deep, as long as some brain and bodily activity and functions remain.
  - **Locked-in syndrome**.
- Brain death is used as an indicator of legal death in many countries, and patients classified as brain-dead can have their organs surgically removed for organ donation. But it is defined inconsistently and often confused by the public. Various parts of the brain may keep functioning when others do not anymore, and the term "brain death" has been used to refer to various combinations.
  - For example, although one major medical dictionary considers "**brain death**" to be synonymous with "**cerebral death**" (death of the cerebrum), the US National Library of Medicine Medical Subject Headings (MeSH) system defines brain death as including the brainstem. The distinctions are medically significant because, for example, in someone with a dead cerebrum but a living brainstem, spontaneous breathing may continue unaided, whereas in whole-brain death (which includes brainstem death), only life support equipment would maintain ventilation.

Cortical Death

- In **cortical brain death**, the cortex is destroyed. Often the brainstem is still intact, e.g., **persistent vegetative state**, i.e., the patient can survive indefinitely if sufficient nutrition is available.
- Absence of cerebral cortical function can be determined by
  - Testing for electrical activity with an EEG (electroencephalogram).
  - Lack of verbal response.

- Lack of spontaneous or coordinated eye movements.
- Absence of cerebral circulation.

Brainstem Death

- The brainstem is the posterior part of the brain, adjoining and structurally continuous with the spinal cord. It provides the main motor and sensory innervation to the face and neck via the cranial nerves. Though small, this is an extremely important part of the brain as the nerve connections of the motor and sensory systems from the main part of the brain to the rest of the body pass through the brain stem. This includes:
  - Corticospinal tract (motor)
  - Posterior column-medial lemniscus pathway (fine touch, vibration sensation and proprioception)
  - Spinothalamic tract (pain, temperature, itch and crude touch).
- The brainstem also plays an important role in the regulation of cardiac and respiratory function. It also regulates the central nervous system, and is pivotal in maintaining consciousness and regulating the sleep cycle.
- The term "**brainstem**" includes the following: **medulla oblongata, pons** and **midbrain** (**Fig. 2.1**). If this small area is dead, the person becomes irreversibly unconscious and irreversibly apnoeic.

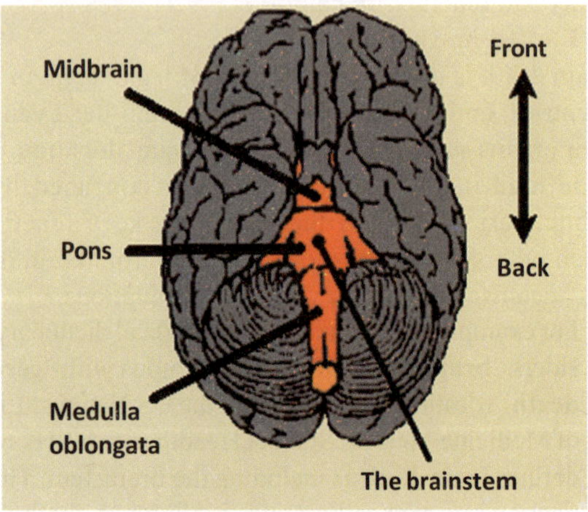

Fig. 2.1 Brainstem

Diagnosis of Brainstem Death

The diagnosis of brainstem death involves **three steps**:

1. The patient must be comatose and unable to breathe spontaneously, and therefore unconscious and on a ventilator. The cause of coma must be 'irremediable structural brain damage.'
2. Exclusion of the cause of coma as due to drugs, hypothermia or profound metabolic disturbance, which may reversibly impair brainstem function.
3. Establishing that all the brainstem reflexes are absent and that the patient fails to breathe, even when taken off the respirator, after performing the ***apnoea test***.

British Code (Harvard Criteria) for Diagnosing Brainstem Death

- Criteria:
  - Unreceptivity
  - Unresponsiveness
  - No movements or breathing
  - No reflexes with further delineation of brainstem reflexes, and
  - Flat electroencephalogram or EEG (repeated after 24 hours with no change).
- Preconditions:
  - Comatose patient on a ventilator
  - Positive diagnosis of cause of coma (irremediable structural damage)
- Exclusions:
  - Primary hypothermia
  - Drugs
  - Severe metabolic or endocrine disturbances
- Tests:
  - Absent brainstem reflexes
  - Apnoea

Testing the **Brainstem Reflexes** (**Fig. 2.2**):

- ***Pupillary response*** to light (***Light reflex***) (afferent 2nd and efferent 3rd cranial nerve) – Making the pupil constrict.
- ***Corneal reflex*** (***Blink reflex***) (afferent 5th and efferent 7th cranial nerve) – Blinking response to corneal stimulation.
- ***Oculovestibular reflex*** (afferent 8th and efferent 3rd & 6th cranial nerves) – Doll's eye movement in response to irrigation of the tympanic membranes of the ears with ice-cold water.
- ***Grimacing reflex*** (afferent 5th and efferent 7th cranial nerve) – In response to painful stimulus over face, and
- ***Gag or cough reflex*** (afferent 9th and efferent 10th cranial nerve) – In response to intubation.

  If all the above-mentioned reflexes are tested properly and are found to be absent, it means that one is examining the brainstem slice by slice, in a series of tests whose results reinforce one another in confirming the fact that the brainstem is dead.
- ***Apnoea Test***
  - The apnoea test aims at proving that the patient is incapable of breathing. In doing this test, one disconnects the patient from the ventilator, and allows the carbon dioxide to build up to a point, where it would trigger off respiration, if there were any cells still alive in the respiratory centre of the brainstem.
  - The ventilator is disconnected for a period of 10 minutes, but to prevent anoxia developing, one must preoxygenate the patient thoroughly before the test. This is done by administering 100% oxygen for 10 minutes, then making the subject breathe a mixture of 95% oxygen and 5% carbon dioxide, which ensures that one starts with high oxygen and reasonably high carbon dioxide. At the end of the disconnection period, one

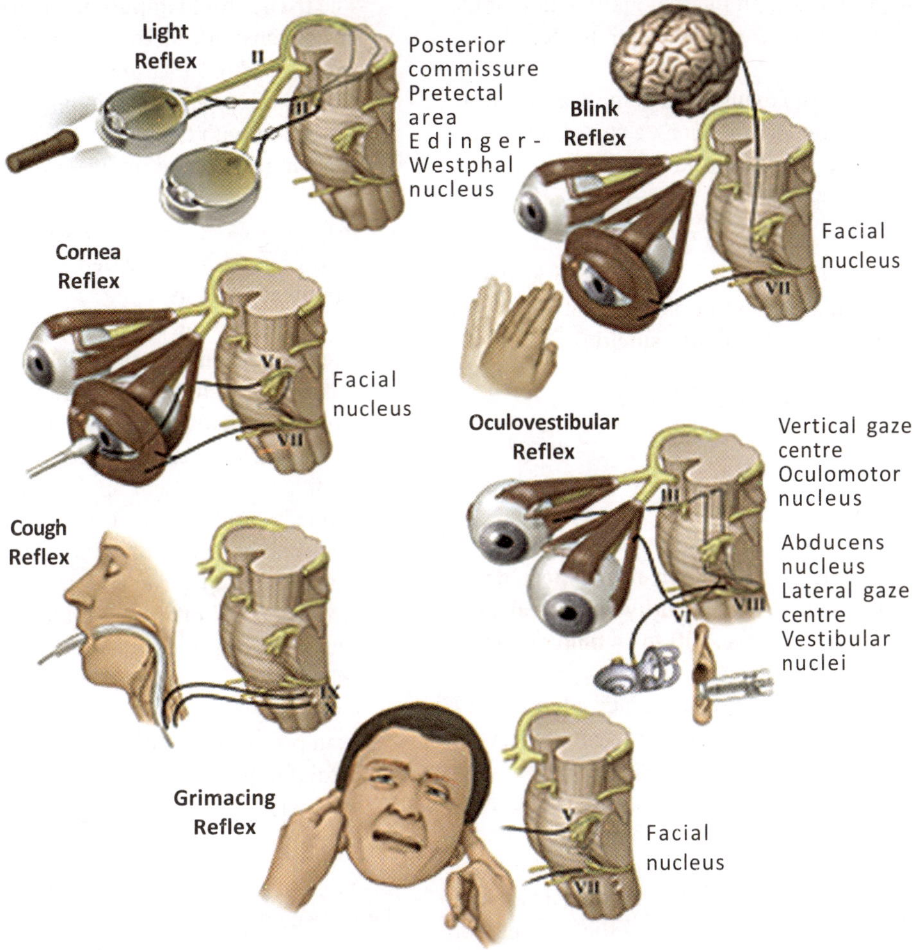

Fig. 2.2 Brainstem reflexes

should estimate the carbon dioxide in the arterial blood to ensure it has reached a level of 50 mm Hg.

- The time of death is the time at which brainstem death is established, and not some later time when the ventilator is switched off, or the heartbeat ceases. Clinicians should emphasize this when explaining the situation to the relatives and they should make it clear that ventilation is not being withdrawn to let the patient die, but because continued ventilation is immaterial for a patient who is already dead. The only justification for maintaining ventilation for a short time is to preserve the condition of the organs, when it has been agreed that they are to be made available for transplantation.

Board of Medical Experts to Certify Brainstem Death

- The **registered medical practitioner** treating the patient whose brainstem death has occurred.
- The **medical administrator** in charge of the hospital in which brainstem death has occurred.
- **Neurologist/Neurosurgeon** nominated from the panel of names approved by an appropriate authority and
- An **independent medical specialist** nominated from the panel of names approved by the appropriate authority.

> **FM 2.2: Core – Written/Viva Voce**
> - **Describe and discuss**
>   - Natural death
>   - Unnatural death

CAUSE & MANNER OF DEATH

- A distinction is often made between the **cause of death**, which is a specific disease or injury, versus **manner of death**, which is primarily a legal determination.
- **Cause of death** refers to the actual reason for a person's death, e.g., an illness or infection, stab injury of heart, gunshot injury, etc.
- **Manner of death** refers to the legality of the cause of death, i.e., whether it is **natural** or **unnatural**, and if it is the latter, whether it is an **accident**, **suicide** or **homicide**.

Natural Death

- The expression '**natural death**' means that the death was caused entirely by natural disease, and that it was not caused by trauma or poisoning.

- It results from an illness or an internal malfunction of the body not directly caused by external forces, other than infectious disease.
  - For example, a person dying from complications from influenza or pneumonia (infection), a stroke, a heart attack or sudden heart failure would be listed as having died from natural causes.

Unnatural Death

- The expression '**unnatural death**' means that the death was not the result of natural disease or old age, but by trauma or poisoning in the form of **homicide**, **suicide** or **accident**.

> **FM 2.3: Core – Written/Viva Voce**
> - Describe and discuss issues related to sudden natural deaths

SUDDEN NATURAL DEATH

- **Sudden death** is defined as **the sudden or unexpected termination of life of an apparently healthy individual, usually from some natural disease, within 24 hours of onset of symptoms**.
- It is usually taken to mean that death occurred unexpectedly, and within 24 hours after the onset of symptoms, with or without known pre-existing conditions. The emphasis is on the unexpected character, rather than the suddenness of the death. In fact, sometimes the individual may linger on for a few hours or days after the abrupt onset of illness.
- The expression '**natural death**' means that the death was caused entirely by natural disease, and that it was not caused by trauma or poisoning.
- The purpose of a medicolegal autopsy in sudden deaths is to determine whether violence or poisoning has been in any way responsible for the death. Absence of external evidence of injury does not preclude death from physical violence. The age of the deceased, authentic information as to past health status and the presence or absence of witnesses at the time of death are all helpful in deciding the necessity for an autopsy.
- Sudden deaths are more frequent in older individuals, and they usually take place under circumstances which arouse no suspicion. It is the sudden death of younger individuals that invariably arouses suspicion. Medical officers must never issue death certificate in a case of sudden death, and instead must suggest that an autopsy be done.
- When there is no apparent cause of death as revealed by the police inquest, and on external examination of the body, death due to natural causes should be suspected. In that case, a detailed examination of all the systems should be conducted. Each organ has to be weighed and the naked eye observations have to be recorded. Bits of tissues should be taken from all the organs. If there is difficulty in interpreting the morbid anatomical changes in any of the organs, that organ as a whole can be preserved and despatched to the forensic pathologist for expert opinion.
  - The **tissues** for **histopathological examination** have to be collected in wide-mouthed glass bottles. The preservative used is **10% formalin**. If bits of tissues are sent for examination, gross findings should be provided to the expert with the history of the case.
  - A **peripheral blood smear** should be taken for examination.
  - In all such cases, relevant **viscera and body fluids** must be preserved in **saturated saline** and despatched for **chemical analysis**.
  - Samples of **blood** must be collected for **biochemical**, **haematological** and **microbiological examinations** also. Sterile bottles have to be used for the collection of materials for microbiological examinations. If diseases like leukaemia are suspected, bone marrow should be taken.
  - If injuries are present on the body, they should be examined and details recorded. Effort must be made to find out the cause of injuries found on the body by examination of the scene, interrogation of witnesses, etc. If, on the other hand, the natural cause of death was a result of the injury, the relation has to be established. Injuries can either precipitate or hasten death of a person who is already suffering from a disease. For example, trivial injuries may precipitate death by myocardial infarction in a person having coronary arteriosclerosis.

Causes of Sudden Natural Death

- Diseases of the cardiovascular system account for about 45% of sudden deaths, diseases of the respiratory system 25%, diseases of the nervous system about 20% and the rest occur due to diseases of other organs.
- The most common causes appear to be:
  - Coronary artery disease with **myocardial infarction**.
  - Non-atherosclerotic coronary artery disease, **cardiomyopathy, myocarditis**.
  - Cerebrovascular accident (**cerebral stroke**).
  - Subarachnoid haemorrhage due to **rupture of berry aneurysm**.
  - Sudden rupture of a diseased blood vessel with fatal bleeding, such as the **rupture of an aortic aneurysm**.
  - Massive **pulmonary embolism**.
  - Acquired respiratory distress syndrome (ARDS) due to any cause.
  - Perforation of peptic ulcer.
  - Fulminating infectious disease without any recognizable symptoms until death, e.g., **lobar pneumonia, bacterial endocarditis**, etc.
  - A shift in the position of a viscus, causing sudden shock as in **volvulus, strangulated hernia, twisted ovarian cyst**, etc.
  - **Anaphylactic shock** due to any cause.
  - Sudden infant death syndrome.

> **FM 2.4: Core – Written/Viva Voce**
> - Describe the salient features of Organ Transplantation and The Human Organ Transplant (Amendment) Act 2011
> - Discuss the ethical issues regarding organ donation

ORGAN TRANSPLANTATION

- Organ transplantation is a medical procedure in which an organ is removed from one body and placed in the body of a recipient, to replace a damaged or missing organ.
- The donor and recipient may be at the same location, or organs may be transported from a donor site to another location.
- Organs and/or tissues that are transplanted within the same person's body are called **autografts**.
- Transplants that are performed between two subjects of the same species are called **allografts**. Allografts can either be from a **living person** or a **cadaver**.
- **Organs** that are commonly transplanted include:
  - Heart, kidneys, liver, lungs, pancreas, intestine, thymus and uterus.
    - Kidneys are the most commonly transplanted organs, followed by the liver and the heart.
- **Tissues** that are commonly transplanted include:
  - Bones, tendons (both referred to as musculoskeletal grafts), cornea, skin, heart valves, nerves and veins.
    - Cornea and musculoskeletal grafts are the most commonly transplanted tissues; these in fact outnumber organ transplants by more than tenfold.
- Organ donors may be living, brain dead or dead via circulatory death. Tissue may be recovered from donors who die of circulatory death, as well as of brain death – up to 24 hours past the cessation of heartbeat. Unlike organs, most tissues (with the exception of cornea) can be preserved and stored for up to 5 years, meaning they can be "banked".
- Transplantation raises a number of bioethical issues, including the definition of death, when and how consent should be given for an organ to be transplanted, and payment for organs for transplantation. A particular problem is organ trafficking.
- **Transplantation medicine** is one of the most challenging and complex areas of modern medicine. Some of the key areas for medical management are the problems of transplant rejection, during which the body has an immune response to the transplanted organ, possibly leading to transplant failure and the need to immediately remove the organ from the recipient. When possible, transplant rejection can be reduced through serotyping to determine the most appropriate donor–recipient match and through the use of immunosuppressant drugs.
- **Types of Donor**:
  - ***Living Donor***: In living donors, the donor remains alive and donates a renewable tissue, cell or fluid (e.g., blood, skin), or donates an organ or part of an organ in which the remaining organ can regenerate or take on the workload of the rest of the organ (e.g., single kidney, partial liver, lung lobe, small bowel, etc.).
  - ***Deceased Donor (Cadaveric Donor; Beating Heart Donor)***: Deceased donors are people who have been declared brain dead and whose organs are kept viable by ventilators or other mechanical mechanisms until they can be excised for transplantation. Such a beating heart cadaver is a body that is pronounced dead in all medical and legal definitions, connected to a ventilator and retains cardio-pulmonary functions. This keeps the organs of the body, including the heart, functioning and alive. As a result, the period of time in which the organs may be used for transplantation is extended.

The Human Organ Transplant (Amendment) Act 2011

- **The Transplantation of Human Organs Act (THOA), 1994** was enacted in the year 1994 and was adopted in all States except erstwhile State of J&K and Andhra Pradesh which have their own legislation in this regard. The main purpose of the Act is to regulate the removal, storage and transplantation of human organs for therapeutic purposes and for the prevention of commercial dealings in human organs.
- The Act was amended in 2011 and the **Transplantation of Human Organs (Amendment) Act 2011**, came into force on 10-1-2014 in the States of Goa, Himachal Pradesh, West Bengal and Union Territories. Several other states have adopted the amendment Act subsequently, including Rajasthan, Jharkhand, Kerala, Orissa, Punjab, Maharashtra, Assam, Haryana, Gujarat, Bihar, Uttar Pradesh, etc.
- The amended Act is now named **Transplantation of Human Organs and Tissues Act (THOTA), 1994 (Amended 2011)**.
- Brainstem death is recognized as 'legal death' in India under the THOTA, since 1994, like many other countries, and has revolutionized the concept of organ donation after death. After natural cardiac death only a few organs/tissues can be donated (like cornea, bone, skin and blood vessels), whereas after brain stem death almost 37 different organs and tissues can be donated including vital organs such as kidneys, heart, liver and lungs.
- The amended Act and revised Rules have many provisions for promotion of organ donations from cadavers.

Important **amendments** include the following:

- Tissues have been included along with 'Organs'.
- 'Near relative' definition has been expanded to include spouse, son, daughter, father, mother, brother, sister, grandfather, grandmother, grandson and granddaughter.
- Provision of 'Retrieval Centres' and their registration for retrieval of organs from deceased donors. Tissue Banks must also be registered.
- Provision of **Swap Donation** included:
  - Also called '**Paired Exchange Programme**'. Sometimes, a loved one may want to donate a kidney, but their blood type is incompatible. Transplant centres can help such incompatible recipient/donor through a process called paired exchange, which involves two living donors and

two recipients. If the recipient from one pair is compatible with the donor from the other pair, and vice versa – the transplant centre can arrange for a "swap" – for two simultaneous transplants to take place. This allows two transplant candidates to receive organs and two donors to give organs, though the original recipient/donor pairs were unable to do so with each other.

- There is provision of mandatory inquiry from the attendants of potential donors admitted in ICU and informing them about the option to donate – if they consent to donate, inform retrieval centre.
- Provision of mandatory '**Transplant Coordinator**' in all hospitals registered under the Act.
- To protect vulnerable and poor, there is provision of higher penalties for trading in organs.
- Constitution of Brain Death Certification Board has been simplified – wherever neurophysician or neurosurgeon is not available, an anaesthetist or intensivist can be a member of board in his place, subject to the condition that he is not a member of the transplant team.
- National Human Organs and Tissues Removal and Storage Network and National Registry for Transplant to be established.
- There is provision of **Advisory Committee** to aid and advise Appropriate Authority:
  - **Role of Authorization Committee (AC)** – The purpose of this body is to regulate the process of authorization to approve or reject transplants between the recipient and donors other than a first relative. The primary duty of the committee is to ensure that the donor is not being exploited for monetary consideration to donate their organ. The joint application made by the recipient and donor is scrutinized and a personal interview is essential to satisfy to the AC the genuine motive of donation and to ensure that the donor understands the potential risks of the surgery.
  - **Role of Appropriate Authority (AA)** – The purpose of this body is to regulate the removal, storage and transplantation of human organs. A hospital is permitted to perform such activities only after being licensed by the authority. The removal of eyes from a dead body of a donor is not governed by such an authority and can be done at other premises and does not require any licensing procedure. The powers of the AA include inspecting and granting registration to the hospitals for transplant surgery, enforcing the required standards for hospitals, conducting regular inspections of the hospitals to examine the quality of transplantation and follow-up medical care of donors and recipients, suspending or cancelling the registrations of erring hospitals, and conducting investigations into complaints for breach of any provisions of the Act. The AA issues a license to a hospital for a period of 5 years at a time and can renew the license after that period. Each organ requires a separate license.
- Enucleation of corneas has been permitted to be done by a trained technician.
- The Act has made provision of greater caution in case of minors and foreign nationals, and prohibition of organ donation from mentally challenged persons.
- Source of Organs for Transplant: Source may be Living or Deceased Donor:
  - **Living Donor Transplant**:
    - Near relative donor (mother, father, son, daughter, brother, sister, spouse).
    - Other than near relative donor: Such a donor can donate only for reasons of affection and attachment, or for any other special reason and that too with the approval of the authorisation committee.
  - **Deceased Donor Transplant**:
    - ***Donor after Brainstem death***: Organ donation is practically possible in the situation of brainstem death, e.g., a victim of road traffic accident, etc., where the brainstem is dead and person cannot breathe on his own but can be maintained through ventilator, oxygen, fluids, etc., to keep the heart and other organs working and functional.
    - ***Donor after Cardiac death (DCD)***: Practically, in Indian scenario only tissues are donated after cardiac death. But, a few centres like PGI Chandigarh has started DCD.

Ethical Issues Regarding Organ Donation

- The presence of a growing middle class, the lack of a national health insurance scheme, the growing disparity between the rich and the poor, and to some extent the presence of technology in the country makes the process of commodification of organs a simple, quick and attractive business proposition for some and a solution for others. In many affordable middle class or upper class families, even when there are relatives in good health who can donate, the general argument that is often presented is "why donate and take any risks when you can buy a kidney?" Organ trade in India like other problems such as child labour and prostitution has a societal issue to it. It relates to the exploitation of the poverty-stricken people by alluring them with financial gains that at times can be large and can meet their immediate short-term financial needs. But, unlike other similar exploitative social situations, organ donation requires an invasive surgical procedure that has both physical and psychological implications.
- In India, where the deceased donation rate is abysmally small, there is a serious need to curb commerce in organs. There are currently over 150 transplant centres in India performing thousands of kidney transplants annually. Out of these transplant centres, a few centres undertake a few hundred liver transplants annually, while some of these centres also do an occasional heart transplant.
- Kidney donation is steadily rising in India, and unrelated living donations are being reported in the media, including a few deaths. Although kidney donation is a relatively safe

surgery, the rising incidence of diabetes and hypertension in India makes the young donors potentially risk their health in the long-term. In some of the studies, it has been noted that when the motive of donation has been purely commercial, donors in the post-operative period have been more prone to ill-health. Whereas, when the donation was purely altruistic, there was the feel-good factor and the psychological recovery was much better.

- In one field study, it was found that more than 90% of participants sold their kidneys to pay off debts. The average family income declined by one-third after removal of the kidney, and the number of participants living below the poverty line increased. A total of three-fourths of the participants were still in debt at the time of the survey. A significant proportion of participants reported deterioration in their health status after nephrectomy.
- Another study found that most of the donors were women who were deeply in debt, and most of the money was squandered by their husbands in gambling and liquor, and the promise of a better future was never realized. In this study, it was found that there is a one-way trade in some of the "kidney belt regions" of southern India, the trade route extending from organ sellers – usually poor rural women – to hospitals and recipients – often wealthy people from the Gulf States.
- Giving in to market forces and making organs a commodity is fraught with dangers, and erodes social, moral and ethical values. It is not an alternative that can be acceptable to overcome the problem of organ shortage in a civilized society. By their very nature, such markets are indiscriminate, promiscuous and inclined to reduce everything, including human beings, their labour and even their reproductive capacity to the status of commodities, to things that can be bought, sold, traded and sometimes even stolen.
- The Bellagio Task Force (Dept of Anthropology, University of California), conducted an ethnographic research in some sites in Brazil, India and South Africa between 1997 and 1998. Their findings were as follows:
  - Strong and persistent race, class and gender inequalities and injustices exist in the acquisition, harvesting and distribution of organs.
  - Violation of national laws that prohibit the sale of organs.
  - The collapse of cultural and religious sanctions against body dismemberment and commercial use exist in the face of the enormous market pressures in the transplant industry.
  - Persistent and flagrant human rights violations of cadavers in public morgues exist, with organs and tissues removed without any consent for international sale.
- Since clinical demand far outstrips organ donation rate, clearly defined allocation criteria are required. Criteria should follow the principles of human rights and should not be based on a recipient's gender, race, religion or economic condition.
- The high demand and poor supply of kidneys in rich countries like the United States has widened over the years. This has resulted in many patients travelling abroad for transplant surgery. Some of the countries that have weak regulatory mechanisms have given in to the market forces and include India, Iran, China, Pakistan, Philippines, Brazil, etc.
- The total number of road accidents exceeds 1 lakh per annum in India, and many of these end in fatalities. Most of the time, the cause of death is head injury, making such cases potential organ donors. Even if 5–10% of such deceased patients became organ donors, it would mean that there would be no requirement for a living person to donate an organ. Promoting the deceased donation programme would not only help kidney transplants, but also liver, heart, pancreas and lung transplants to thrive in the country.
- Understanding the ethics of organ donation is important, if we are to tackle challenges that are emerging with cutting edge regenerative medicine such as stem cells transplants, cloning and tissue re-engineering. The ethical principles of organ donation is an acid test that will help us in evolving and resolving many of the future moral issues that we are likely to encounter.

FM 2.5: Core – Written/Viva Voce

- Discuss moment of death, modes of death – coma, asphyxia and syncope

MOMENT OF DEATH

- Death is a process, not an event, and therefore there is no real '**moment of death**'. The entire body does not die at the same time; different organ systems and tissues die at different times.
- However, in order to legally declare a person as dead, the current concept is to define death as the irreversible loss of the capacity for consciousness and capacity to breathe. Since both the functions reside in the brainstem, the modern concept of diagnosing death is to identify whether a person's brainstem is alive or not. (*Brainstem death is discussed in earlier sections of this topic – refer Index.*)

MODES OF DEATH

- The expression '**Mode of Death**' is an **outdated and obsolete** one, and it is strange that it finds mention in the new curriculum. It is a term that is not recommended to be used any more, and must not be taught to students. It is being described here only to condemn it.
- Formerly, it was said that there are three 'modes of death', depending on which organ system was primarily affected:
  1. Asphyxia: Death due to respiratory failure.
  2. Syncope: Death due to cardiovascular collapse.
  3. Coma: Death due to cessation of brain function.

Today, we know that these are erroneous concepts and must never be used in scientific discourses on death.

FM 2.6: Core – Written/Viva Voce

- Discuss
  - Presumption of death
  - Presumption of survivorship

- Presumption of survivorship and death are guided by **Sections 107** and **108** of the **Indian Evidence Act**. These sections deal with the burden of proving the death of a person known to have been alive for 30 years, and proving a person is alive who is missing since 7 years, respectively.
- **Section 107 IEA (Presumption of survivorship)**: Burden of proving death of person considered to have been alive for the last 30 years – When the question is whether a man is alive or dead, and it is shown that he was alive for the last 30 years, the burden of proving that he is actually dead is on the person who affirms it.
  - To prove the death of a person known to be alive for 30 years, it is mandatory to prove when he died, which day he died and how he died.
  - The burden of proving the details of the death lies upon the person claiming the death of that person, and if he successfully proves the death of the person considered alive for the last 30 years, then the court will declare the death of the concerned person.
- **Section 108 IEA (Presumption of death)**: Burden of proving that a person is still alive who has not been heard of for 7 years – Provided that when the question is whether a man is alive or dead, and it is proved that he has not been heard of for 7 years by those who would naturally have heard of him, if he had been alive, the burden of proving that he is still alive is shifted to the person who affirms it.
  - The Court will consider a person dead, if he has been missing for 7 years or more, unless it is proved that the concerned person is alive.

FM 2.7: Core – Written/Viva Voce

- Describe and discuss suspended animation

SUSPENDED ANIMATION

- **Suspended animation is a state where the metabolic needs of the body are at such low ebb that the person appears apparently dead.**
- His pulse is not palpable, heart sounds are not audible, respiratory movements are not visually perceptible and reflexes are either absent or not possible to elicit.
- The person is not actually dead, and he can be revived in most cases by resuscitation.
- Recognizing this condition is important in order to prevent premature certification of death.
- Causes*:
  - **S**edative overdose
  - **H**ypothermia
  - **E**lectrocution
  - **N**ewborn baby
  - **D**rowning
- Some 'sanyasis' (Hindu ascetics) are supposed to have the power to induce in themselves a state of 'suspended animation' voluntarily.
- Some practitioners of yoga are also said to have the capacity to induce in themselves a state resembling suspended animation (*Samadhi*).

FM 2.8: Core – Written/Viva Voce/OSPE (Objective Structured Practical Examination)

- Describe and discuss postmortem changes including
  - Signs of death
  - Cooling of body
  - Postmortem lividity
  - Rigor mortis
  - Cadaveric spasm
  - Cold stiffening
  - Heat stiffening

POSTMORTEM CHANGES

For convenience, **postmortem changes** are being described under the following headings:

- **Immediate changes**, which result in:
  - Complete and irreversible cessation of the functions of the brain, heart and the lungs
  - Muscles of the body become flaccid
  - Corneal reflexes are abolished
- **Early changes**, which take place within the first 12–24 hours. They comprise:
  - Changes in the skin
  - Changes in the eye
  - Algor mortis (postmortem cooling)
  - Livor mortis (postmortem staining)
  - Rigor mortis (postmortem stiffening)
- **Late changes** include:
  - Putrefaction and its modifications:
    - Adipocere
    - Mummification
  - Skeletonization

Early Changes after Death

I. *Changes in the Skin*

- Elasticity of the skin is lost soon after death.
- Skin that was translucent in life becomes pale.

II. *Changes in the Eye*

- The cornea loses its lustre with the passage of time, and becomes dull, hazy, and finally opaque and wrinkled.
- Desiccation of the conjunctiva makes it discoloured, which is referred to as "**tache noire**".**

**Mnemonic: SHEND.*

***Pronounced "tosh nwar".*

- Full form – **Tache noire de la sclerotique**, which is French for "*black spot of the sclera*" is one of the ocular signs of death in which a reddish-brown discolouration occurs transversely across the sclera. It occurs when the eyes are not completely closed so that the sclera is exposed to air (**Fig. 2.3**).

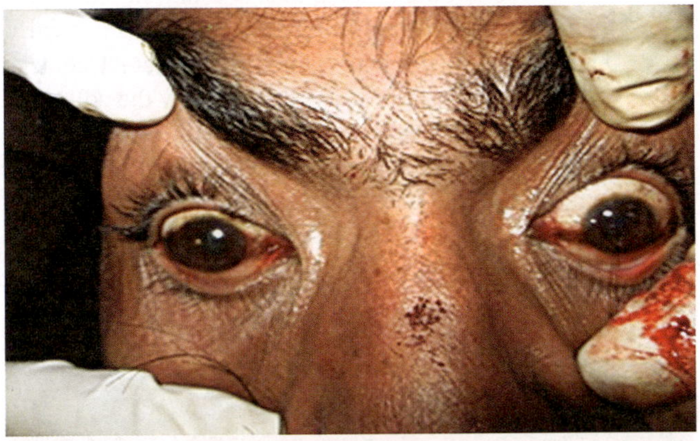

Fig. 2.3 Tache noire

- Intraocular tension falls so rapidly that by 2 hours after death, the tension is nearly zero and the eyeball appears sunken.
- If the retina could be viewed through an ophthalmoscope, the columns of blood in the vessels may be seen to be broken up into segments, which is referred to as '**trucking**.'

III. *Algor Mortis (Postmortem Cooling; Chill of Death)*

- There is a constant balance between heat production and heat loss during life. After death, heat production is lost and hence the body starts cooling. Dead body loses its heat by conduction, convection and radiation.
- Measurement of the rate of cooling helps in estimating the time since death. When the rate of cooling is plotted on a graph, the pattern of the curve assumes a **sigmoid shape** (**Fig. 2.4**).
- The body surface starts losing heat rapidly, but the core body temperature does not alter until a gradient is established between the core body temperature and the surface. As there is no significant change in the core body temperature for sometime which may be up to 2–3 hours after death, an initial plateau is seen. When once the gradient is established between the core body temperature and the surface, the rate of cooling is approximately proportional to the difference in temperature between the body and the surface.
- This aspect is in accordance with the Newton's law of cooling, which means that after the initial plateau, the curve dips down progressively before it becomes nearly flat at the bottom. The curve may even rise before becoming flat due to heat produced by putrefactive changes.

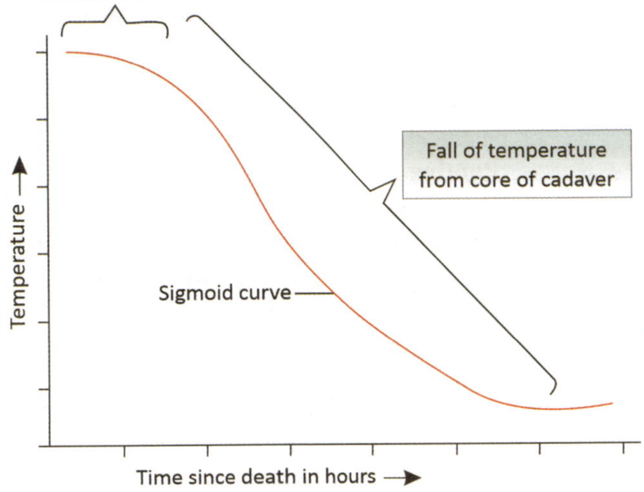

Fig. 2.4 Sigmoid curve of postmortem cooling

- The preferred site for measuring the inner core body temperature is either the **rectum**, or the **axilla**, or the **abdominal cavity**.
  - The usual method is to use a rectal thermometer, which is introduced deep inside the rectum (several centimetres), or alternatively, the thermometer may be kept in contact with the under-surface of the liver through a slit made in the anterior abdominal wall in the right hypochondrium.
  - At the same time, the environmental temperature is also measured.
  - The time since death is then calculated (after taking two readings at an interval of 1 hour), by the following formula:

$$\frac{\text{Normal body temperature} - \text{Temperature of cadaver}}{\text{Rate of fall of temperature/hour}} = \text{Time since death}$$

- ***A rule of thumb states that there is a decrease of 1.5°F every hour.***
- ***The Glaister Equation* estimates the hours elapsed since death as follows***:

$$\frac{98.7°\text{F} - \text{Rectal temperature (in Fahrenheit)}}{1.5°\text{F/ hr}}$$

**Carly Berdan: Improving Methods to Estimate Time of Death from Body Temperature – A Thesis. Submitted to the Faculty of New Jersey Institute of Technology and Rutgers, The State of University of New Jersey – Newark, Federated Biological Sciences Department; August 2018.*

- However, there are a number of variables which need to be taken into account:
  - The body temperature at the time of death is presumed to be normal. This may not be the case. In fact in some cases, there is a slight rise in the temperature of the body after death. This is known as **postmortem caloricity**, and may be seen in:
    - **Pontine haemorrhage**
    - Bodies which at the time of death had suffered violent muscular contractions (**exertion**)
    - Asphyxial deaths such as **strangulation**
    - Death due to **septicaemia**
    - **Strychnine** poisoning

    (***Mnemonic***: *PESSS*)
  - If the environmental temperature is extremely cold, the process of cooling of the body is hastened, while in very hot climates the body may not cool at all.
  - Obesity lessens the heat loss, as fat is a bad conductor of heat.
  - Ratio between the body surface and the body mass: children and old people cool more rapidly.
  - Presence of thick clothing at the time of death slows the rate of heat loss.
- In addition to the commonly employed sites for measuring the body temperature mentioned above, other sites have been proposed by various investigators, including the axilla, nasal cavity, trachea, middle ear cavity, etc.
- Electronic thermometer and thermocouple have been employed in the place of chemical thermometer by some investigators.
- **Henssge's nomogram** is said to be the most accurate method of measuring the time of death by means of temperature measurement. It is a method to determine the postmortem interval using temperature, but unlike the Glaister Equation, it also takes into consideration some other important factors. In order to use this nomogram, body temperature, ambient temperature, body weight, clothing and whether the body was in air or water, etc., are all factored into the equation.

IV. *Livor Mortis (Postmortem Lividity; Postmortem Staining; Hypostasis; Suggillation)*

- With the stoppage of functions of the heart after death, active circulation of blood in the body ceases. The blood which is fluid in nature, gradually settles down in the toneless capillaries of the dependent parts of the body, seen externally as patches of purplish discolouration through the skin (**livor mortis, postmortem lividity, postmortem staining, hypostasis, suggillation**) (**Fig. 2.5**).
- This settling of blood in the dependent parts is in accordance with the law of gravity.
  - Thus, if the body is in supine position, the postmortem lividity will be seen on the back.
  - In deaths due to hanging, lividity is seen on the hands, feet and the lower parts of the face above the ligature.
  - In drowning, where the body usually floats with the back facing up and the limbs hanging down, the lividity is seen over the limbs, abdomen and the face.

  Distribution of the lividity, thus is useful in indicating the **position of the body** after death.
- Those parts of the body which are in actual contact with the surface they lie on, do not show the colour as the toneless capillaries are pressed by the weight of the body. Such areas are known as areas of **contact flattening**. Thus, in the body which is lying supine, postmortem lividity is not seen over the shoulder blades, buttocks, calves, etc.

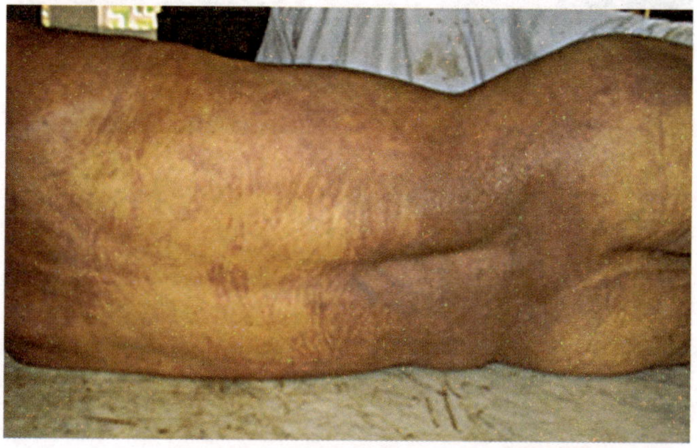

Fig. 2.5 Postmortem lividity (with pale areas of contact flattening) (*Courtesy*: *Dr RV Bardale*)

- If the deceased was wearing a tight collared shirt, a band of pale area may be seen around the neck, where lividity does not develop, and this could be confused with a strangulation mark by an inexperienced person. Proper interpretation of such findings is important.
- Postmortem lividity begins as mottled patches ranging from 1 to 2 cm in diameter. These patches gradually increase in size with the passage of time and coalesce with each other till they become one uniform area of staining.
- Though the time of the appearance of these patches is variable, they are generally seen 2–3 hours after death. If the position of the body is altered, these patches gradually disappear, & appear in new dependent parts.
- If the body is left undisturbed for some time (usually 6–8 hours), lividity becomes well developed and **fixed**, and does not alter in position even with subsequent alteration in the position of the body.
  - This was till recently thought to be due to clotting of blood in the blood vessels. In fact, the word '**fixation**' itself is erroneous. If the position of the body is altered after 'fixation' and left in the new position for some more time, the intensity of the lividity gradu

ally fades, even though some colour, due to haemolysis staining the tissues, may remain in the primary position.
  - Blood is usually found fluid in capillaries and venules, and this blood is responsible for postmortem lividity. Thus, clotting of blood is not entirely responsible for the fixation.
- 'Fixation' is an apparent phenomenon. If pressure is applied over the area of lividity in the early stages, it blanches (**Fig 2.6**). Once fixation occurs, the area of lividity will not blanch.

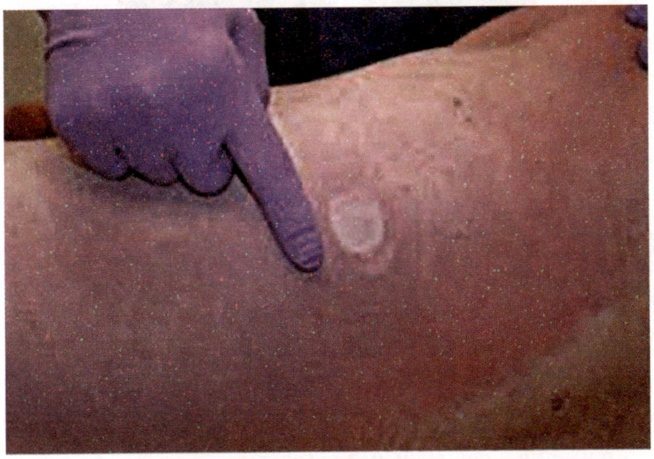

Fig. 2.6 Postmortem lividity which is not yet fixed (blanching on pressure by a finger)

- **Colour of the lividity** in certain cases helps in arriving at the cause of death. For example, it is:
  - Cherry red or pink in carbon monoxide poisoning
  - Bright (brick) red in cyanide poisoning
  - Dark blue in aniline dye poisoning
  - Greenish blue in hydrogen sulphide poisoning
  - Brown shades:
    - Brownish in phosphorus poisoning
    - Reddish brown in poisoning with nitrates
    - Chocolate brown in poisoning with chlorates
  - *Some books mention that opium (or opiate) poisoning gives rise to blackish lividity which is WRONG.*
- Patches of lividity may sometimes be seen over non-dependent areas. The possible mechanism for this is the squeezing of column of blood in the deeper veins against gravity, towards the skin surface, by the muscles developing rigor mortis. Such patches could be mistaken for contusions.
  - This confusion is easily resolved by making an incision over the discoloured area.
  - If it is contusion, staining of the tissue is seen which cannot be washed off.
  - If it is lividity, the blood oozes out from the freshly cut blood vessels, and the fresh stain can be easily washed off with water.
  - If still doubt persists, microscopic examination of tissue from the suspected area clinches the diagnosis.
- As the process of formation of postmortem lividity is purely a physical phenomenon, it is seen in the dependent parts of the internal organs also. It is important to bear this in mind, lest the appearance of it in the organs may be mistaken for some significant condition of medicolegal bearing.
- Significance of lividity in postmortem clocking is not very reliable. However, scientists have tried instruments utilizing light, to measure PM lividity and its application to establish the time since death, with some significant correlation between them.
- Evaluation of PM lividity using colorimeter-measuring system has also been tried with some success in postmortem clocking.
- **Note**:
  - PM lividity disperses with the onset of putrefaction.
  - PM lividity may not develop at all, if the body is tossed and turned continuously as seen in fast flowing waters of rivers or the sea.
  - PM lividity cannot be appreciated well in dark coloured subjects.
  - PM lividity may not be appreciable even in fair skinned bodies, if they have bled profusely or were severely anaemic.

V. *Rigor Mortis (Postmortem Stiffening)*

- During life, muscles are supple and in a slightly contracted state. After passing through a phase of **primary flaccidity** soon after death during which they are totally relaxed, the muscles over a period of time, gradually stiffen. This stiffening is known as **rigor mortis**.
- Rigor mortis affects all the muscles in the body, both skeletal and smooth.
- Rigor mortis is a physico-chemical phenomenon. Recalling one's memory of the elementary structure of the muscle is necessary to understand the mechanism of its formation.
  - A muscle mass is made up of a number of bundles of long fibres.
  - Each muscle fibre in the bundle consists of densely packed myofibrils, which are the contractile elements.
  - These myofibrils are made up of two protein filaments, actin and myosin.
  - Separation of actin and myosin is responsible for extensibility and softness of the muscles.
  - Coming together of these actin and myosin filaments, which results in contraction is dependent on the energy provided by adenosine triphosphate (ATP). Constant supply of ATP is maintained in life.
  - Failure of resynthesis of ATP after death results in the muscles becoming hard and rigid. However, some amount of ATP is still available after death till the glycogen reserve lasts. When once this glycogen reserve is depleted, there is no more ATP available,

and the contractile elements are converted into dehydrated, stiff, gel-like mass resulting in the muscles themselves becoming hard andrigid (rigor mortis).

- Rigor mortis becomes noticeable first in the eye lids, then the muscles of the face, jaw and neck. Then it is seen to affect the upper limbs (**Fig. 2.7**), thorax, abdomen and the lower limbs. Though rigor mortis is basically due to chemical changes, the physical aspect is responsible for this apparent proximo-distal progression, viz., smaller muscles having less glycogen reserves than the larger muscles are first to be affected.

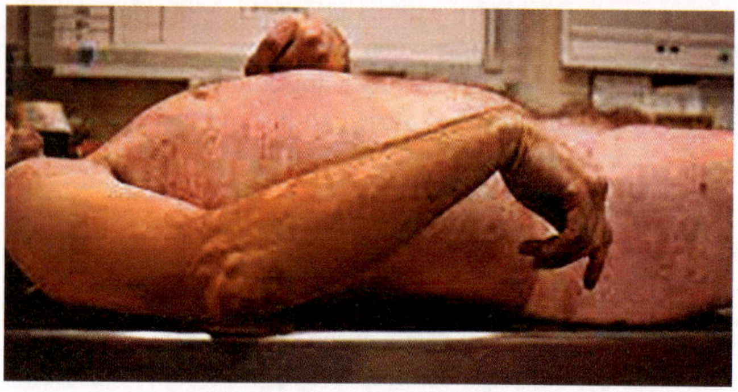

Fig. 2.7 Rigor mortis of upper limb

- It is generally considered that by the first 12 hours after death, rigor affects the whole body. It is retained for another 12 hours, and passes off in the next 12 hours with the onset of putrefaction. This **rule of 12**, also known as the **march of rigor**, is only a generalization of the time since death. In some locations in India (e.g., Kerala), it has been shown that rigor mortis may actually follow the **rule of 6**, i.e., it sets in, remains, and disappears from the body in 6 hours respectively.
- Rigor passes off in the same order in which it made its proximo-distal progression.
- With the passing away of the rigor, the muscles once again become softened. This is the phase of **secondary flaccidity**.

Cadaveric Spasm

- Another condition, rarely seen but commonly talked about, is **cadaveric spasm** or **instantaneous rigor**, where instead of primary flaccidity after death, the muscles usually belonging to small groups go into a sudden state of stiffening.
- This condition, though of unknown cause, when seen, is usually associated with violent deaths coupled with emotional disturbance at the time of death, as in
  - Drowning (where grass or weeds may be clutched in the hands) (**Fig. 2.8**).
  - Suicide by shooting (where the weapon may be tightly grasped in the hand), etc.

Other conditions that result in the body becoming stiff after death include:

- Thermal deaths (**pugilistic attitude**): The stiffening of the body in death due to burns (**heat stiffening**) is due to coagulation of muscle proteins,

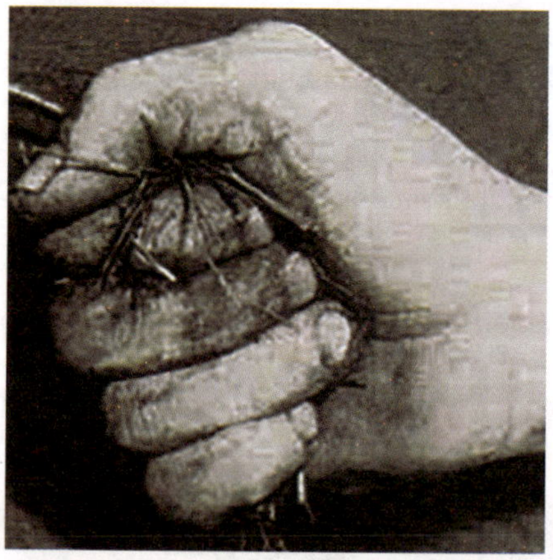

Fig. 2.8 Cadaveric spasm of the hand (weeds clutched in the hand of a victim of drowning)

- While in exposure to severe cold (**cold stiffening**), the body becomes stiff due to freezing of the subcutaneous fat and the water content in the body, forming icicles.
- Putrefaction: Gases evolved during the putrefactive process also stiffen the body (**gas stiffening**), but poses no problem in distinguishing it from rigor mortis.

Note:

- Application of force results in breaking of rigor, which does not set in again when once broken.
- As rigor is a chemical phenomenon, any condition that depletes ATP fast, will hasten its early development. For example, violent muscular contractions at the time of death due to epilepsy, strychnine poisoning, tetanus, electrocution, etc.
- In robust, healthy young individuals, it appears late because of good glycogen reserve in the muscle mass.
- As rigor mortis is not functionally related to the nervous system, it can develop in paralysed limbs also.
- As rigor is also not dependent on blood supply, it develops even in amputated limbs.
- If a body is frozen soon after death, and such a body is brought back to normal environmental temperature, rigor mortis which had been arrested till then, will appear subsequently. Estimation of time since death from such thawed bodies becomes erroneous.
- Apart from postmortem clocking, rigor mortis helps in identifying any alteration in the position of the body, if the position in which the body has undergone rigor is incompatible with the position in which it was discovered at the scene.

FM 2.9: Core – Written/Viva Voce/OSPE (Objective Structured Practical Examination)

- Describe
  - Putrefaction
  - Mummification
  - Adipocere
  - Maceration

LATE CHANGES AFTER DEATH

Putrefaction*

- Onset of putrefaction initiates the breakdown of complex organic constituents of the body into simpler inorganic substances. Such breakdown of complex structure is facilitated by **autolysis** and **bacterial action**, while the destruction of the body tissues by various fauna expedites the process of disintegration.
  - **Autolysis**: The digestive action of various enzymes released by the cells after death leads to softening and liquefaction of tissues. Soft tissues like the brain, lungs, pancreas, gall bladder and stomach are affected earliest. Architectural patterns of the organs are lost. The process of autolysis is independent of any bacterial action. It is an aseptic chemical process.
    - **Maceration** of the dead foetus inside the uterus is a classical example of autolytic putrefaction.
  - **Bacterial action**: Any condition conducive for rapid bacterial growth results in early onset of putrefaction. Bacteria disseminate and multiply fast after death, as stagnant blood offers an excellent medium for their growth. Apart from the normally inhabiting bacteria of the body, bacteria from outside also may enter the body through open wounds. These bacteria generally comprise *Streptococcus* sp, *Staphylococcus* sp, *Escherichia coli*, *Proteus* sp and *Clostridium welchii*.
    - While autolysis produces limited gross change, bacterial action is the major component of putrefaction.

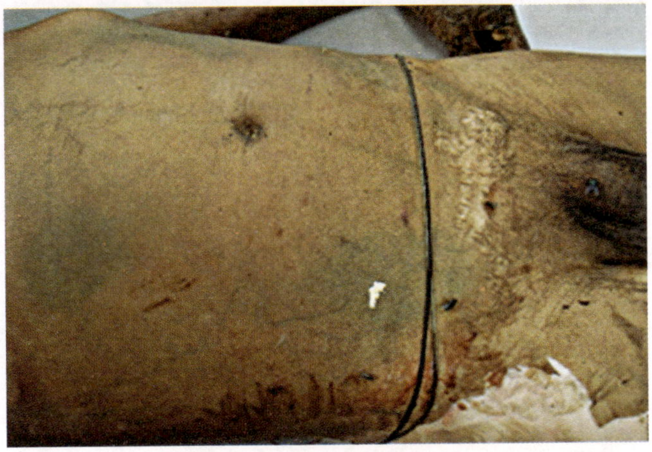

Fig. 2.9 Greenish discolouration of Rt iliac fossa (*Courtesy*: *Dr Rajesh V Bardale*)

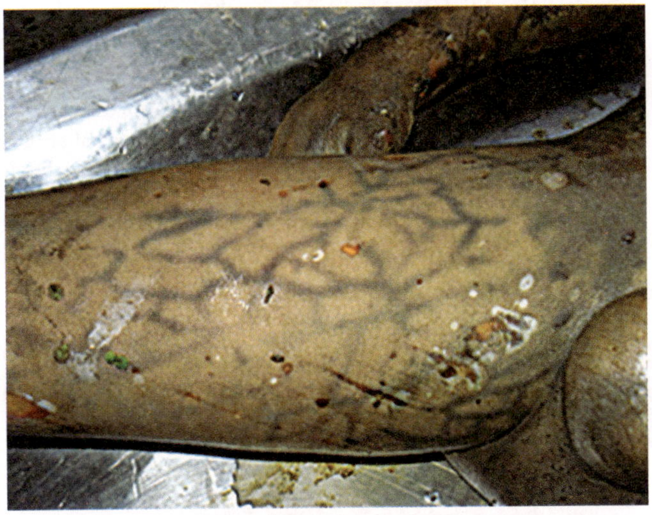

Fig. 2.10 Marbling over thigh (*Courtesy*: *Dr Rajesh V Bardale*)

Changes Occurring due to Putrefaction

- **Greenish discolouration in the right iliac fossa is the earliest external manifestation of the onset of putrefaction, which occurs around 12–24 hours after death** (**Fig. 2.9**). This is the area where the caecum lies, the contents of which are more fluid and rich in bacteria. Hydrogen sulphide produced by the bacteria acts on the haemoglobin (that has now become extracellular due to haemolysis), to produce sulphaemoglobin. This imparts the greenish hue. With the passage of time this greenish discolouration, which is very obvious in fair skinned bodies, subsequently spreads to the abdomen, and also makes its appearance in the chest, face and the limbs. Coalescence of these coloured areas results in the entire body becoming greenish or greenish-black.
- Later, in about **36–48 hours**, a network of veins becomes visible in the form of a characteristic mosaic-like pattern (**marbling**), over various parts of the body like the root of the neck, shoulder, etc. (**Fig. 2.10**). This results from staining of the vessel walls due to diffusion of haemoglobin.
- By the time the colour changes become visible externally, **evolution of gases** would have started internally. These gases possess very unpleasant smell. They include hydrogen sulphide, ammonia, carbon dioxide, carbon monoxide, methane, etc. These gases by themselves are not of any medicolegal significance, but the pressure effects they produce when they accumulate in sufficient quantity are so much as to bring about gross changes in the appearance of the body. Evolution of gases results in **ballooning effects** and **dispersion of postmortem lividity**.
  - **Ballooning effects**:
    - Gases easily collect in the hollow viscera resulting in their voluminous expansion.
    - The stomach and the intestines which balloon out, increase the intra-abdominal pressure resulting in distension of abdomen, and pushing of the diaphragm upwards.
    - Lungs are squeezed by this pressure, and froth oozes from the mouth and nostrils.
    - The gases not only accumulate in the hollow viscera, but also penetrate into every tissue and organ.

__Note__: Some books refer to this incorrectly as Putrification. The correct term is Putrefaction.

Soft tissues of the body like the breast, scrotum, periorbital tissues, etc., increase in their size enormously.

- Eyeballs protrude out of the sockets, the cheeks puff out and so also the lips.
- The tongue protrudes through the mouth, and on exposure to air becomes dark in colour.
- The facial features alter so much that even the resemblance to a normal human face is lost. At this stage, identification by external features becomes extremely difficult even to the closest relatives (**Fig. 2.11**).
- Percolation of putrefactive gases into the undersurface of the skin results in the epidermal layer ballooning out, which resembles blisters caused by scalding (**Fig. 2.12**). In contrast to protein-rich fluid present in the blisters caused by scalding, **putrefactive blisters** contain only air.
- The epidermal layer from the hands and feet slip off like gloves and stockings. It is important to retain and preserve this part of the skin, as it can yield a full set of fingerprints that may help in establishing identity.
- Increased pressure inside the abdomen may result in the expulsion of foetus in the case of a pregnant deceased (**postmortem delivery**).
- Uterus and rectum may protrude out due to pressure.
- Though the evolution of gases may commence as early as 18 hours after death, a full-blown picture to develop may take 48–72 hours.

- **Dispersion of postmortem lividity**:
  - Evolution of gases moves the blood in the blood vessels. If the blood is clotted, it now liquefies, and haemolysis takes place. Movement of this blood results in dispersion of postmortem lividity in any direction.
  - Therefore, assessment of the position of the body at the time of death based on lividity at this stage, becomes difficult.

- **Colliquative putrefaction**: In 3–5 days after death, the nails and the hair become loose and can be pulled off with ease. The teeth become loose and can be pulled out from their sockets. The abdomen and the thorax may burst open. The sutures on the skull get loosened (**Fig. 2.13**), the liquefied brain matter oozing out through these deficiencies. With further progression of putrefaction, from 5 to 10 days, **colliquative putrefaction** ensues, resulting in the tissues and organs being converted into a soft, thick, black, pultaceous mass, totally losing their architecture. However, even at this stage, organs such as the **prostate** and non-gravid **uterus** can be identified, as they resist putrefaction, thus helping in the identification of the sex.

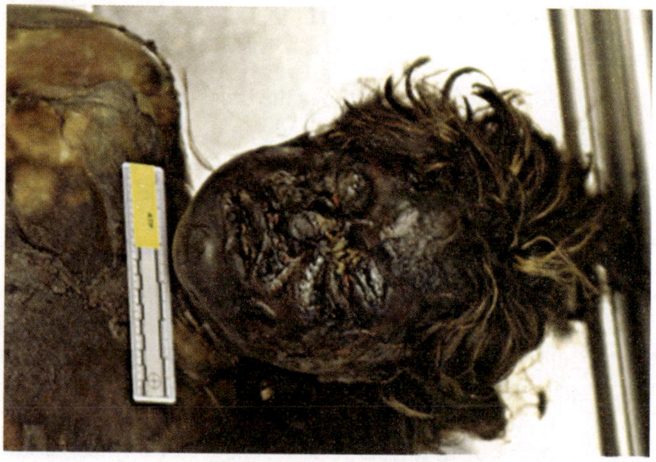

Fig. 2.11 Advanced putrefaction distorting facial features (*Courtesy*: *Dr Abraham Philip*)

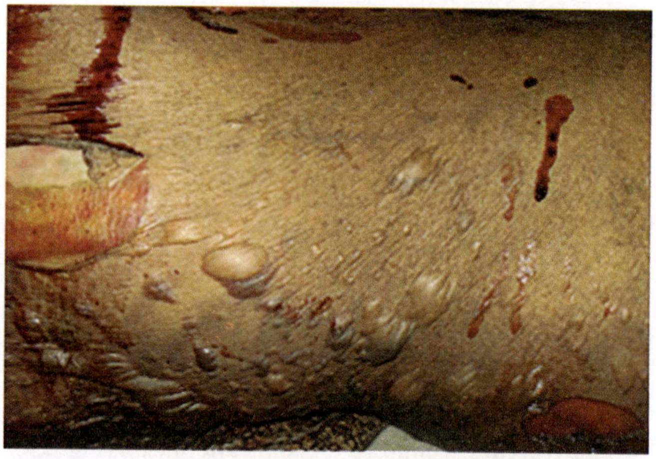

Fig. 2.12 Putrefactive blisters (*Courtesy*: *Dr Rajesh V Bardale*)

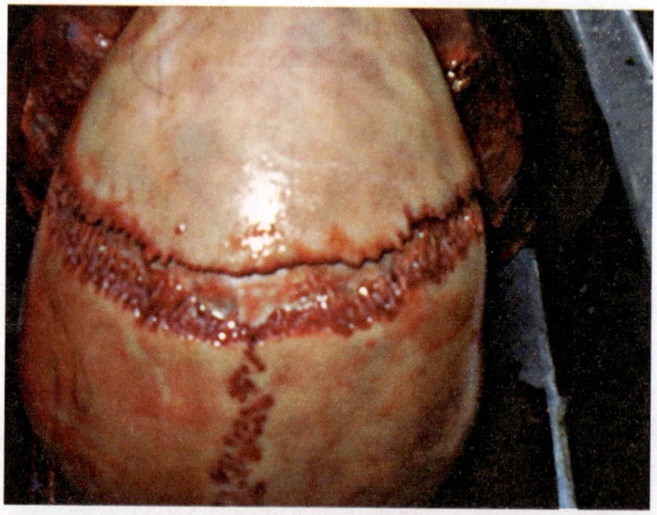

Fig. 2.13 Postmortem separation of skull sutures (*Courtesy*: *Dr Rajesh V Bardale*)

- This liquefied unrecognizable pultaceous mass gradually falls off from the bony attachments leaving the skeleton exposed. If a dead body is lying in the open, it may take 1–3 months for complete **skeletonisation**. If the body is buried, skeletonisation may take place in two to six months. If the body is encased in a coffin, more time is required for skeletonisation.
- **Odour mortis**: This refers to the "odour signatures" unique to the decomposition of human remains with potential ramifications on cadaver dog training procedures, and in the development of field-portable analytical instruments which can be used to locate human remains in shallow burial sites.
- Sometimes the environmental conditions may arrest the progression of putrefaction and may deviate it to either **adipocere** formation or **mummification**.
  - **Adipocere** (**Saponification; Grave Wax**): This arrests the further progression of putrefaction.
    - Adipocerous change is due to hydrogenation and hydrolysis of body fat.
    - The prerequisites for adipocerous change of the body fats include:
      - abundant body fat
      - humid climate
      - still air
      - warm temperature
      - bacteria producing fat-splitting enzymes, like *Clostridium welchii*.
    - Thus a body lying on damp soil, in a shady place, with optimum environmental temperature, and no free air current blowing over it, undergoes adipocerous change.
    - Adipocere is yellowish in colour and has the appearance of rancid butter (**Fig. 2.14**), giving off a sweetish but disagreeable smell.
    - Transformation of the body fat into adipocere is usually seen over areas such as cheeks, breasts, buttocks, or limbs, though rarely the whole body is affected.
    - It takes generally about 3 weeks for adipocere to develop fully.
    - As the progression of putrefaction is arrested, the facial features are recognizable, which helps in identification of the deceased by friends or relatives.
    - Similarly, as the wounds are also preserved without much alteration, the weapons used (and to a certain extent the cause of death), can be identified.
    - The approximate time since death can also be estimated.
  - **Mummification**:
    - In hot and dry climate, where there are warm air currents freely flowing over the body, putrefactive process becomes arrested and the body becomes mummified due to dehydration and desiccation of the tissues and the organs.

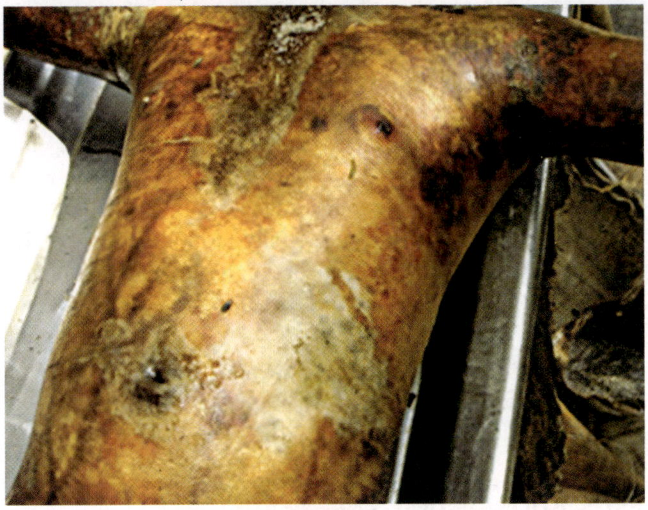

Fig. 2.14 Adipocere involving almost the entire body (*Courtesy*: *Dr Rajesh V Bardale*)

    - The skin is dark and tightly adherent to the skeletal frame.
    - Mummification usually requires 3–6 months.
    - A mummified body does not emanate any foul smell.
    - Mummification helps in identification, as the general facial features are preserved.
    - It also helps in recognizing the presence of wounds.
    - Estimation of the approximate time of death and place of death is possible.

Note:
- Rate of putrefaction varies depending on whether the body is in an open place, buried or in water. It is generally presumed that if the rate of putrefaction is considered as 1 unit of time on open ground, it is 2 units in water and 8 units in deeply buried bodies. This is known as **Casper's dictum**.
- Putrefaction occurs rapidly at temperatures between 20°C

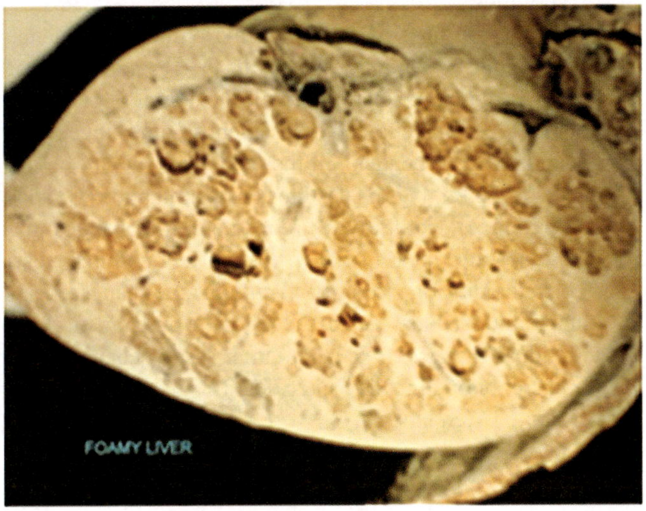

Fig. 2.15 Foamy liver (*Courtesy*: *Dr Shashidhar C Mestri*)

and 40°C. Therefore, bodies exposed to the sun, especially in summer, decompose faster. Putrefaction will be arrested below 0°C. A dead body can be kept in a cold chamber, or covered with ice and salt to slow down decomposition. If the body has to be preserved for weeks, it has to be embalmed.

- Evolution of gases in solid organs like liver leads to an alteration in the architecture visible to the naked eye. In such cases, the liver on cut section has a honeycomb appearance (**foamy liver**) (**Fig 2.15**).

> **FM 2.10: Core – Written/Viva Voce/OSPE (Objective Structured Practical Examination)**
> - Discuss the estimation of time since death

ESTIMATION OF TIME SINCE DEATH

The time since death or *postmortem interval* is the period that has elapsed between death and the actual time of the postmortem examination.

- Though the exact time of death can rarely be estimated on the basis of autopsy findings, an approximate range can usually be deduced by interpretation of the various changes that take place after death.
- Estimation of the time since death within a narrow range is possible only in the early period. Once putrefaction sets in, this range becomes wider. However, entomological study can help in narrowing the range considerably.
- Evidence for estimating the time since death generally falls under the following three categories:
  - **Corporal evidence** – that which is present in the dead body.
  - **Environmental evidence** – that which is present in the vicinity and general surroundings of the deceased.
  - **Anamnestic evidence** – that which is based on the deceased's ordinary habits, movements and day-to-day activities.
- Assessing the time of death by environmental evidence and anamnestic evidence is mostly the responsibility of the investigating officer, in India. The doctor is generally not involved. The doctor's assessment of time since death is exclusively dependent on the evidence that can be deduced by the findings on postmortem examination (**Corporal evidence**). Naturally, he relies upon the changes that take place after death such as postmortem cooling, postmortem lividity, rigor mortis and putrefactive changes, bearing in mind all those factors that alter the outcome of these individual changes. **Box 2.1** summarises the changes useful in computing the time since death.
- **Additional Methods**
  - ***Gastric emptying time***: If the time of the last meal is known, presence or absence of food and the state of digestion in the stomach helps to a certain extent in estimating the time since death. But, the rate of emptying of the stomach depends on many variables including the type of food eaten, the emotional state of the person, any surgical procedure done on the stomach such as gastrojejunostomy, etc. Therefore, this method must be used only as corroborative evidence.
  - ***Bladder content***: It is usual to empty the bladder before going to bed. On the morning of the death, if the body is found to be warm and supple and the bladder is full, it means that the person has died in the early hours of the morning, and hence the time since death is very short, probably within the last 1 or 2 hours. On the other hand, if the body has developed a certain amount of rigor and is cold to touch, and the bladder is full, it means that the person must have died the previous night, probably before going to bed. This is fairly good corroborative evidence.
  - ***Biochemical changes***: Though a lot of research work has been undertaken to estimate the time since death based on biochemical changes such as changes in the potassium content of the vitreous humour, pericardial fluid enzymes, level of lactic acid and non-protein nitrogen of CSF and a plethora of other chemical parameters, they are mostly only of academic interest. As the antemortem values of these chemicals vary substantially, they are of limited practical value.
  - ***Circumstantial evidence***:
    - If the body is found in an open place, the state of grass underneath the body helps in the estimation of time since death. As the grass becomes deprived of sunlight for photosynthesis, they gradually turn yellow, due to conversion of chlorophyll to xanthophyll. The usual time required for such a change in colour is 3–5 days.
    - Uncollected mail or newspapers, recent purchases of household materials with dated bills, condition of the food in the kitchen, etc., are other factors which can be taken into consideration in assessing the time since death.
  - ***Entomology of the Cadaver***: Foul-smelling gases that emanate due to putrefaction attract various insects.
    - The study of the life cycle of these insects which infest dead bodies, in order to know the time of death and some other useful information, is known as **Forensic Entomology**.
      - There are eight successive waves of invasion from the beginning of putrefaction right up to skeletonization.
      - Initially, two-winged flies predominate, but later there will be involvement of several other kinds of insects including beetles.
      - Two-winged flies such as blue bottles, flesh flies, house flies, etc., lay their **eggs** in about 18–36 hours (sometimes as early as 6–10 hours).

- Mostly these eggs are laid in the mucocutaneous junctions such as lips, nostrils, anus, vagina or even in open wounds.
- The eggs hatch into larvae (***maggots***) within 12–24 hours (**Fig. 2.16**). These larvae are voracious eaters and they grow in size up to 4–5 days, during which time they devour the tissues and hasten the process of disintegration of the body.
- The maggots then enclose themselves inside shell-like structures (***pupae***), which in another 4–5 days break open to release young flies (***nymphs***).
- The role of the doctor while doing autopsies on such maggot-infested bodies is only to pick up these maggots, preserve them properly and send them to a qualified entomologist for species identification. Maggots immersed in boiling absolute alcohol die instantly in extended position, which facilitates measurement of their length.
- Calculation of time since death is done as follows:

  Time since death = A + B x (cd)

  where **A** is the stage of invasion (in hours, days, weeks or months), **B** is the stage of life cycle (in hours or days) and **cd** represents climatic factor correction.
- Study of insect's life cycle is the job of an entomologist. The doctor should not guess the postmortem interval from his very limited knowledge of entomology.

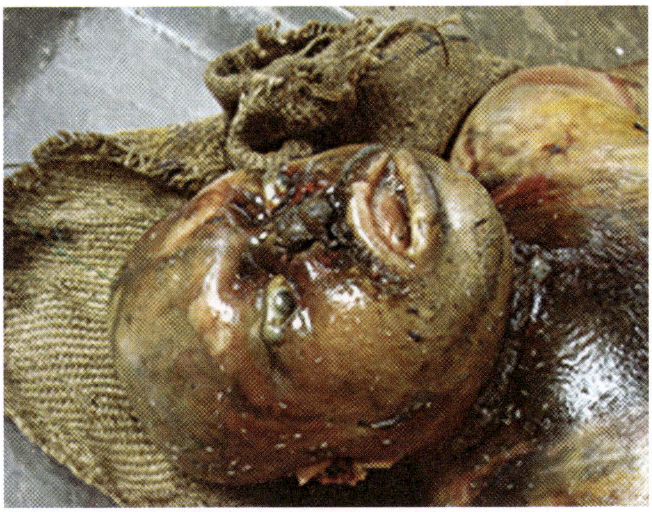

Fig. 2.16 Maggots crawling over the face (*Courtesy*: *Dr Rajesh V Bardale*)

- Usefulness of **chemical analysis of maggots for poisons**, which are not destroyed by the putrefying process, should be kept in mind. This type of study has come to be called **Forensic Entomotoxicology**.

Box 2.1—Postmortem Changes and Postmortem Interval

Condition of the body	Time since death
Warm supple body, transparent cornea, no patches of postmortem lividity	*Within 1 hr*
Patches of lividity on the dependent parts, rigor mortis appreciable in the muscles of the face	*2–3 hrs*
PM lividity well developed and 'fixed', rigor mortis at least in the upper part of the body, body surface cold	*6–8 hrs*
Rigor mortis all over the body, with or without greenish discolouration over the right iliac fossa, body cold	*Around 12 hrs*
Body cold and stiff, greenish discolouration over the right iliac fossa, eggs of flies	*12–24 hrs*
Body is cold, rigor has receded, greenish discolouration over the abdomen and chest, distension of the abdomen with evolution of gases	*24–36 hrs*
Marbling, distended abdomen and thorax, presence of maggots, post-mortem blisters	*36–48 hrs*
Whole body bloated, face unrecognisable, nails and hairs easily pulled off, grown maggots or pupae all over the body	*3–5 days*
Colliquative putrefaction where the internal organs are reduced to black unrecognisable pultaceous mass	*1 week (5–10 days)*
Most of the soft tissues gone, organs that putrefy late like prostate and non-gravid uterus recognizable	*2 weeks*
Skeletonization (exposed body)	*1–3 months*

FM 2.11: Core – Written/Viva Voce/OSPE (Objective Structured Practical Examination)

- Describe and discuss autopsy procedures including
  - Postmortem examination
  - Different types of autopsies
  - Aims and objectives of postmortem examination.

AUTOPSY PROCEDURES

- Though **necropsy** is the most accurate term for the investigative dissection of a dead body, the term **autopsy** is used more commonly. **Postmortem examination** is an alternative expression, but it unfortunately suffers from a lack of precision about the extent of examination, for in some countries many bodies are disposed of after external examination without dissection.

Types of Autopsy

1. **Medicolegal Autopsy**
   a. Performed only on the instructions of a legal authority responsible for the investigation of sudden, suspicious, obscure, unnatural or criminal deaths.
   b. In India, such legal authority may be represented by a police officer or a magistrate. The information so obtained is invaluable in the administration of justice, in convicting criminals, and in protecting innocent suspects.
   c. Consent of the next of kin (closest relative) is not necessary for conducting the autopsy, but an official requisition from police or magistrate is essential.
   d. The main objectives include identity fixation (if the identity is unknown or uncertain), cause of death, manner of death, time of death, etc.
2. **Clinical or Pathological Autopsy**
   a. Performed in death due to natural causes, in order to ascertain the exact cause, if the diagnosis made by the treating physician is to be confirmed or refuted, or if diagnosis could not be arrived at all while the patient had been alive.
   b. The consent of the next of kin is essential.
   c. There is no need for a requisition from the police or the magistrate.
3. **Psychological Autopsy**
   a. This is not really an autopsy at all, but instead refers to the perusal of medical and personal history, and other background information of a deceased person who had committed suicide, in order to arrive at the motive for the act.
4. **Endoscopic Autopsy**
   a. It has been suggested that if a conventional autopsy is difficult or impossible to undertake for any reason, a postmortem endoscopic examination can be performed with the help of a trocar and telescopic device coupled to a video camera. This is referred to as endoscopic autopsy.
   b. But, there are serious limitations to this technique, and hence is not generally recommended.
5. **Virtual Autopsy (Virtopsy)**
   a. Of late, some forensic pathologists in Western countries are beginning to consider modern cross-sectional imaging techniques to supplement and even partially replace traditional autopsy. Computed tomography (CT) is the imaging modality of choice for two- and three-dimensional documentation and analysis of autopsy findings including fracture systems, pathologic gas collections (e.g., air embolism, subcutaneous emphysema after trauma, hyperbaric trauma, decomposition effects) and gross tissue injury.
   b. Various post-processing techniques can provide strong forensic evidence for use in legal proceedings. Magnetic resonance (MR) imaging has had a greater impact in demonstrating soft-tissue injury, organ trauma and non-traumatic conditions. However, the differences in morphologic features and signal intensity characteristics seen at antemortem versus postmortem MR imaging have not yet been studied systematically.
   c. The documentation and analysis of postmortem findings with CT and MR imaging and post-processing techniques is claimed to be investigator-independent, objective and noninvasive, and will lead to qualitative improvements in forensic pathologic investigation.
   d. Future applications of this approach include the assessment of morbidity and mortality in the general population and, perhaps, routine screening of bodies prior to burial.

Aims and Objectives of A Medicolegal Autopsy

1. To identify the **cause** and **manner of death**.
2. To **identify the deceased**, if unknown.
3. To determine the **time of death** and **injury**.
4. To document the injuries, if any.
5. To deduce how the injuries occurred.
6. To document any natural disease present.
7. To determine any contributory or causative factors to the death.
8. To provide expert testimony, if the case goes to trial.
9. In a case of infanticide, to decide whether the infant was **born alive**.

FM 2.12: Core – Written/Viva Voce/OSPE (Objective Structured Practical Examination)

- Describe the
  - Legal requirements to conduct postmortem examination and
  - Procedures to conduct medicolegal postmortem examination

RULES (LEGAL REQUIREMENTS) OF A MEDICOLEGAL AUTOPSY

- Every registered medical practitioner who is called upon to undertake a medicolegal autopsy is legally obliged to do so at the earliest possible time.
- No fees must be charged for conducting a medicolegal autopsy.
- **Permission** or **authorization**:
  - In India, a police officer or a magistrate can give authorization for a medicolegal autopsy. Without such permission, a medicolegal autopsy must not be performed.
  - There is no need to take permission or consent from the relatives of the deceased.
- Whenever a body is sent for autopsy, it must always be accompanied by a **dead body challan** and an **inquest report**.
- A **dead body challan** is the formal requisition submitted to the medical officer by the investigating police officer for performing a medicolegal autopsy.
  - It contains the name, address, age, sex, religion, etc., of the deceased.
  - It also contains information about the time, and location from where the body was recovered, distance from the site to the mortuary, and name and address of the police official and the relatives accompanying the corpse.
  - The medical officer has to fill in the column indicating the time of receipt of the case at the mortuary, and the time of commencement of the postmortem examination.
- An **inquest report** or **panchanama** is the preliminary investigation report of the investigating police officer. It contains:
  - The available history of the case,
  - The details of the belongings of the dead body and
  - A provisional opinion of the police officer, as well as two respectable inhabitants of the locality (panchas).
- **Place**: Ideally, an autopsy should be performed in a well-equipped mortuary. But depending upon the circumstances, it can well be performed at the site itself without undue delay, as in the case of exhumation and mass disasters. But this should be done only on requisition by a magistrate.
- **Treatment** or **hospital records**: These should accompany the inquest report and the dead body challan. If they are not supplied, the medical officer can ask the investigating officer to procure them. By studying the treatment history, a doctor can avoid unnecessary investigations, e.g., a fruitless search for a broken piece of weapon which has already been removed surgically, can be avoided. Availability of these records will also serve as a check against future manipulations or tampering of treatment records, especially in deaths due to alleged negligence.
- Before beginning the autopsy, the body must be properly identified by the police officer concerned. In case of unidentified bodies, photographs and fingerprints should be taken by the police.
- The medical officer should always ascertain the circumstances surrounding the case before beginning the autopsy. Inquest reports and hospital records must be scrutinized thoroughly.
- The medical officer should try to limit the number of those present in the autopsy hall to the barest minimum. Not only is there a greater risk of loss of confidentiality, but sheer numbers can make the mortuary overcrowded. This will hamper movement, cause distraction, and add to the risk of infection and contamination. No one should be present merely as a casual observer, not even senior police officers (unless they are directly involved in the investigation).
  - When the deceased has been under medical care before death, it is acceptable practice to allow and encourage the physician concerned to be present at the autopsy, as he is in possession of relevant (and sometimes vital) medical history.
  - All persons present at an autopsy should be listed and named by the medical officer in a separate register, or in the autopsy report.
- Autopsies are best done in daylight, otherwise colour changes relating to bruises, jaundice, etc., are likely to be missed.*
- Detailed notes must always be made at the time of autopsy.
  - It is better to dictate the notes to an assistant while the autopsy is in progress. Subsequently, the medical officer must verify the notes and sign it. All corrections should be initialled. Nothing should be erased.
  - If no assistant is available, the doctor should prepare the report immediately after completion of the autopsy. A tape recorder may be used.
  - Sketches should be made of all major injuries and lesions.
- **Verification of injuries noted in the inquest report**: All injuries mentioned in the inquest report must be verified as being present or absent while doing an autopsy. A mismatch is not infrequent, mainly due to wrong interpretation of lesions by the police. For example, a postmortem abrasion in the neck may have been interpreted by the investigating officer as an antemortem injury due to assault. Conversely, a delayed bruise or "come-out bruise" may not be recorded at all by the police. So, if a doctor fails to find the injuries recorded in the inquest report, he should mention that the injuries are either absent, or were misinterpreted, or merely comprise postmortem artefacts.

**Actually this is a contentious issue, and many forensic pathologists today say that good quality artificial light (that simulates day light as far as possible) is quite sufficient to undertake medicolegal autopsies. In fact, the vast majority of autopsy rooms in the West are located in the basement of the hospital, where the question of daylight does not arise at all. Increasingly, this approach is being adopted in India also.*

- **Number of doctors required**: In most cases, a single registered medical practitioner empowered by the state government is all that is required to perform a medicolegal autopsy. But, if requested by the magistrate, as in dowry death cases and custodial deaths, a team of two doctors may be required to perform an autopsy.
- **Video recording**: As per the recommendations of the National Human Rights Commission, all autopsies in the case of death occurring in police custody or prison have to be videotaped. So, if arrangements have not been made by the police, the doctor must insist on it, in order to avoid possible controversy in future.
- **Visit to the scene of crime**: If a visit to the scene of crime is possible, it should be undertaken without delay, especially in cases such as murder, poisoning, traffic accidents, sex crimes and firearm injuries. Examination of the scene can provide certain important clues to the nature and circumstances of the crime, and can help in the reconstruction of the sequence of events.
- The body should never be embalmed before autopsy, as it will alter the toxicological evidence completely.
- Every medicolegal autopsy must be thorough, meticulous and complete. A partial autopsy should never be done. Useful information can be obtained through careful observation, even in grossly decomposed bodies.
- The information obtained during an autopsy is not privileged. The question of professional secrecy does not arise when an autopsy is done under legal obligation. Hence, a doctor conducting an autopsy has to divulge all the relevant information to the investigating authorities.
- The postmortem report should ideally be submitted within 24 hours of completion of autopsy.

INFRASTRUCTURAL REQUIREMENTS OF A MEDICOLEGAL AUTOPSY

Minimum requirements of a mortuary for performing medicolegal autopsies include the following:

- **Autopsy table** – Stainless steel or masonry type, with adequate running water and drainage facility.
- **Instruments (Fig. 2.17; Table 2.1)**:
  - Scalpels
  - Cartilage knives
  - Dissecting knives
  - Amputation knife
  - Enterotome
  - Large and small dissecting scissors
  - Forceps (toothed and serrated)
  - Large clamps
  - Bone saw
  - Chisel
  - Hammer
- **Other requirements**:
  - Almirahs with locking facility
  - Aprons
  - Surgical and heavy duty gloves

Instruments & Accessories for Autopsy

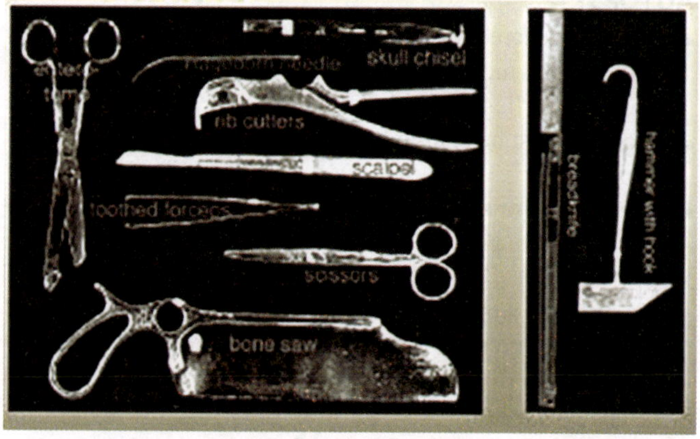

Fig. 2.17 Autopsy instrument set

  - Sponges
  - Swabs
  - Microscope slides
  - Syringes and needles
  - Glassware
  - Wide-mouthed glass bottles (1 L and 500 mL capacity), with screw caps
- **Chemicals**:
  - Rectified spirit
  - Common salt (powder)
  - Formalin
  - Sodium fluoride

PROCEDURE OF A MEDICOLEGAL AUTOPSY

External Examination

- External examination is a vital part of autopsy. Often, it provides more information than internal examination, but it is always desirable to observe both external and internal appearances closely, and attempt to correlate all the findings to get a cohesive picture.
- External examination of the body is traditionally done in three steps:
  - Identification of the body
  - Estimation of the time of death
  - Determination of the cause of death.

Identification

- A general and brief description of the body with regard to sex, age, weight, height, complexion, general condition of the body, nutritional status, gross deformities and description of hair regarding colour, nature, length and distribution are essential in every medicolegal autopsy, irrespective of whether the identity is known or not.
- If the body is that of an unknown person, in addition to the above descriptions, details must be given of the clothing, identification features such as moles and old scars, and the police must be requested to record fingerprints, and take photographs of the body.

Table 2.1 Autopsy Equipment and Instruments

Instrument	Uses
Dissection scissors	To cut open body tissues
Rubber gloves	Disposable gloves are used to prevent contamination of evidence and to keep the wearer safe
Goggles	To protect foreign objects from getting in the eyes
Jackets, aprons, etc.	To protect against infection
Autopsy saw	To cut tough structures like bones
Scalpels and blades	Used during autopsy to cut bodily tissues
Hammer and chisel	To break the skull
Bone saw/Bone cutting forceps	For cutting bones
Sternal saw	For cutting into the chest of the body by cutting the sternum
Toothed forceps	For tearing or holding structures
Skull key	A T-shaped chisel used as a lever while removing skull cap
Brain knife	To cleanly cut the brain
Rib shears	To cut through the ribs while opening the chest
Dissecting scissors	For sharp cutting
Speculum	For vaginal and rectal examinations
Non-absorbable sutures	Usually nylon to close the body cavities
Postmortem needles	Large thick needles for suturing the skin after an autopsy to return the body to a natural looking state
Medical syringes	For fluid aspiration
Foley catheter	For evacuation or irrigation of the bladder to collect a urine sample
Swabs	Collecting smears
Double-ended probe	Used for probing
Formaldehyde	Primary preservative for histopathology
Saturated common salt solution/Rectified spirit	Primary preservative for viscera for chemical analysis

Estimation of Time of Death

- The various methods that help in deducing the time of death have been described in earlier sections. If the exact time of death is known, or hospital records are available, a general description of the body in relation to the condition of the eyes, postmortem lividity, and rigor mortis (or features of decomposition), is sufficient.
- As per the recommendations of the National Human Rights Commission in relation to custodial deaths, rectal temperature must also be recorded (by means of a chemical thermometer).
- If the body was preserved in cold storage or refrigerated, estimation of time since death is obviously going to be difficult. So this fact must be recorded in the postmortem report, along with a brief description of the body.

- Entomological evidence is important in decomposing bodies, and the medical officer must be familiar with the procedures relating to collection of specimens, preservation and despatch.

Determination of Cause of Death

- **Examination of wrappings**: The body may be brought to the mortuary enclosed in plastic or cloth wrapping. It should be examined carefully for trace evidence which may have been dislodged from the body.
- **Hospital dressings**: These should be described in detail, with particular mention of their nature and position. Any application of ointment, medication, etc., should be noted, as also the position of catheters and drainage tubes.
- **Clothing**:
  - These should be examined in situ for evidence of any tear, loss of buttons or general disarray.
  - Cuts and tears, if present, have to be correlated with the external injuries on the body.
  - In the case of firearm injuries, burns or blackening of the clothing must be described and correlated with the external body injuries. The area of blackening must be measured, which could give an idea about the range of fire.
  - Stains in clothing due to blood, semen, saliva, vomit, poison, vitriolage, faeces, mud, grass, etc., must all be recorded meticulously. If it is decided to take photographs, two photographs are essential: one of long range to indicate the exact location of the stain, and another of close range to record the details of the stain itself.
  - In the case of death due to poisoning or burns, an attempt must be made to detect characteristic odours.
  - All clothing should be carefully removed by unbuttoning or unzipping. Special care must be taken to ensure that the clothing retains its evidentiary value, right up to the time of the trial. In all cases, it must be air dried, preserved, sealed and handed over to the investigating police officer.
- **Examination of the body**:
  - The entire body surface from head to toe must be examined thoroughly before washing the body.
  - Traces of blood, semen, saliva or any foreign material, if present, should be collected by swabbing or scraping as required.
  - Any characteristic odour emanating from the body must be noted. In the case of immolation by fire, smelling the scalp hair may help in finding out whether an accelerant such as petrol or kerosene was used.
  - After completing the survey of the body surface, the cadaver is washed thoroughly using running water, so that the wounds obscured by stains will be rendered more prominent.
  - Any deformity in the normal body structure has to be described in detail. Fractures must be ruled out by handling suspected regions manually. Confirmation can be done by incising the area.
  - Signs of disease such as oedema, ascites, icterus, anaemia, eczema, etc., must be looked for. Special note must be made of cyanosis, congestion or pallor, if present.
  - The status of natural orifices (mouth, nose, ear, urethra, vagina, anus) is to be carefully observed, and any abnormality or discharge if present, must be recorded. The mouth in particular must be examined closely for evidence of salivary dribble, discolouration due to poisoning, peculiar odour, foreign bodies, etc. In a suspected drug-related death, the nasal orifices must be examined for evidence of "snorting," i.e., intake of drug by insufflation.
  - ***Documentation of injuries***:
    - Great care must be taken to examine and record injuries. Sometimes, a tiny puncture in the skin may be the only sign of the cause of death, e.g., snakebite. Such inconspicuous injuries may be even more difficult to appreciate in dark skinned people. Similarly, injuries of the scalp may be difficult to appreciate as the scalp hair frequently obscures them. Suspect regions must be shaved cautiously, and the injuries noted both by inspection and palpation. A hand lens is sometimes needed to differentiate an incised wound from a split laceration.
    - In a case of hanging or strangulation, the ligature used must be described properly before removing it and documenting the ligature mark.
    - In the case of stab and firearm injuries, the exact location of the wound as measured from the heel must be recorded.
    - All external injuries must be described as to their nature, dimensions, exact location and direction, whenever possible. While taking measurements, a flexible measuring tape is to be preferred for accurate recording of dimensions in regions with undulating surface. Injuries must be described as far as possible in centimetres or millimetres, and not in inches or feet, although the police appear to be more familiar with the inch/foot system than the metric system.
    - Description of old scars and lesions is also important. An old scar on the inner aspect of the wrist may indicate a previous attempt at suicide. Similarly, scars over the back of the hand or in the bend of the elbow may indicate intravenous drug abuse.
    - Written descriptions of external wounds should ideally be supplemented by suitable sketches and photographs.

Internal Examination

The three major body cavities must always be examined in detail. However, the spinal column need not be opened, if there is no specific indication. In case of suspected poisoning, certain viscera and body fluids must be preserved for chemical analysis. In general, it is better to begin by examining that part or cavity suspected to be affected most. However, before dissecting the neck, it is ideal to drain away the blood by opening the cranium and other body cavities, in order to avoid artefacts.

Incisions

For the Trunk

- ***I-shaped incision***: The usual incision is a straight line from the chin to the pubis (symphysis menti to symphysis pubis), with a deviation at the umbilicus in order to avoid cutting through it. The skin over the neck and trunk can thus be reflected laterally on either side.
- ***Y-shaped incision***: Begins at a point close to the acromial process and extends down below the breast, and then medially across to the xiphoid process. A similar incision is made on the opposite side of the body. From the xiphoid process, the joint incision is carried downwards in a straight line to the pubis.
- ***Modified Y-shaped incision***: This incision begins behind each ear from the mastoid, extends down to the mid-point of the clavicle and then progresses medially to the sternal notch from where it continues downwards to the symphysis pubis. Such an incision is preferred in strangulation, hanging and any other condition, where the larynx has been traumatised, as the skin of the neck can be dissected upwards up to the mandible, and raised clear to provide an excellent view of the neck structures. However, this incision should not be made until the skull cap and brain have been removed, to avoid artificial haemorrhages in neck structures which can be confused with true antemortem trauma.
- A fourth type of incision has been suggested (***cosmetic autopsy incision***) (**Fig. 2.19**), mainly to avoid disfigurement of the body by the anterior-type incision employed in the three conventional incisions, which can be distressing to the relatives and friends when the body is displayed for viewing after the autopsy.*
  - In this incision technique, the body is first placed prone, and the scalp is incised in the usual manner (coronally, mastoid to mastoid), following which the skin is cut down to the posterior aspect of acromion bilaterally.
  - A curved incision is then made bilaterally from the tip of the acromion up to the mid-axillary line, and then extended down to the iliac crest.
  - The posterior flap of the scalp is reflected back up to the occiput, and the anterior flap up to the frontal ridge.
  - The posterior flap is then reflected back all down the trunk up to the superior border of the sacrum.
  - The whole of the back of the neck, chest and abdomen is thus laid bare.
  - The body is now turned over (supine), and a curved incision is made from the acromion to the mid-axillary line bilaterally, as in the case of the posterior incision.
  - Another incision is now made from the mid-axillary line on the iliac crest bilaterally, over the inguinal ligament, to meet at the symphysis pubis.
  - To open the abdominal cavity, a para-medial incision is made on the rectus near the symphysis pubis which is extended upward up to the xiphoid process.
  - The thorax is opened by removing the sternum after cutting through the costo-chondral junctions, and separating the sternoclavicular joints.
  - The whole of the chest and abdomen are now open for inspection.

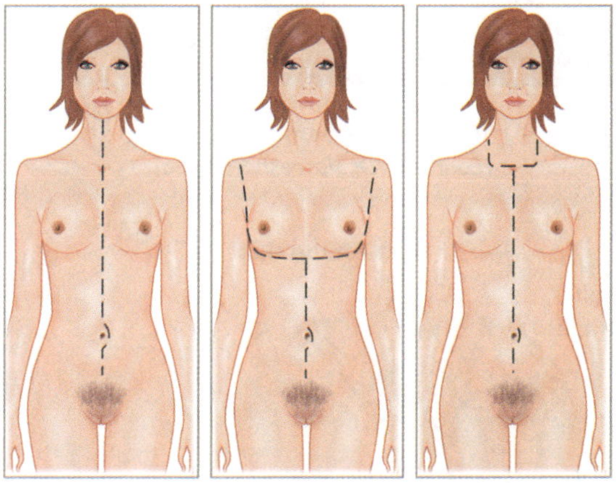

Fig. 2.18 Trunk incisions for autopsy

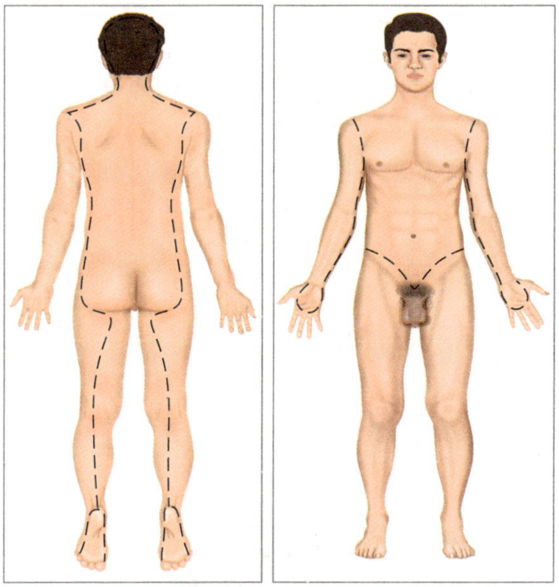

Fig. 2.19 Cosmetic autopsy incision

*Source: Patowary A. The fourth incision. Am J Forensic Med Pathol. 2010;31:37–41.

For the Scalp

- *Coronal incision* (**Fig. 2.20**): The incision for access to the skull begins from behind each ear, and extends upwards on either side to meet over the crown of the head.

Opening the Body Cavities

- The skin, subcutaneous tissue and fat are flayed laterally from the main incision, taking care not to extend beyond the lateral edge of the neck, or the outer third of the clavicles.
- Over the thorax, the tissues (including the pectoral muscles) are flayed to the mid-axillary line in the upper part, and in the lower part, even further posteriorly towards the costal margins.
- The anterior abdominal wall is similarly separated, stripping back the skin and fat to expose the muscles – or the full thickness of skin, fat and muscle can be reflected together. Muscles must be cut from the costal margins, and if thick fat overlies, a few transverse relieving incisions can be made on the peritoneal surface of the lower abdominal wall.

Thorax

- The thorax is opened by first disarticulating both sterno-clavicular joints. The ribs are cut through (lateral to the costochondral junctions) from a point on the lower costal margin, up to the sterno-clavicular joints.
- When the sternum and medial ends of ribs are free, the sternum is lifted and dissected away from the mediastinum, keeping the blade of the knife close to the bone, in order to avoid cutting the pericardium.
- The sternum is examined for fractures or other lesions, before it is put aside.
- The whole of the thorax and abdomen is now open for inspection. The degree of inflation of the lungs should be assessed, noting complete or partial collapse, emphysema and over-distension.
- If pneumothorax has been suspected beforehand, a postmortem radiograph is the best confirmation. Alternatively, the chest wall can be punctured in the mid-axillary line, after filling the pocket between the ribcage and reflected skin, with water. If bubbles escape into the water, it is indicative of pneumothorax. The test cannot succeed, if there is a patent communication between pleural cavity and the bronchial tree. The pleural cavities are examined for adhesions, effusions, pus, blood, fibrin and even for extravasated gastric contents.

Abdomen

- The abdomen is inspected for evidence of ascites, faeculent fluid, pus or blood.
- The omentum may show inflammation or fat necrosis, or it may be totally devoid of fat (as in starvation deaths).
- The coils and loops of bowel are examined for any abnormalities, e.g., infarction, peritonitis, distension, etc. Beware of mistaking postmortem hypostasis for necrosis or mesenteric haemorrhages (**Fig. 2.21**) or strangulated bowel. Though the dark colour may be similar, hypostasis has irregular segments when the gut is stretched out, whereas in infarction, the discolouration occupies one continuous section. When well established, the bowel wall will be lustreless and friable.
- Finally, the bowel is gently moved aside to look at the posterior part of abdomen: a retro-peritoneal haemorrhage from a ruptured aorta may be present.

Removal of the Viscera

There are a number of methods of removal of viscera from the body, once the major cavities have been opened up:

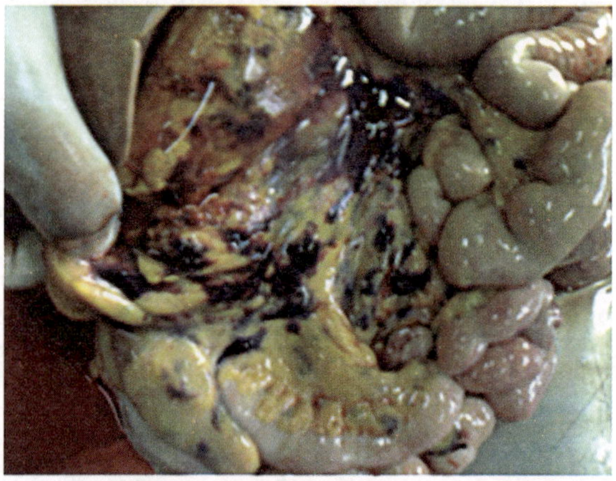

Fig. 2.21 Mesenteric haemorrhage (*Courtesy*: *Dr Hareesh S Gouda*)

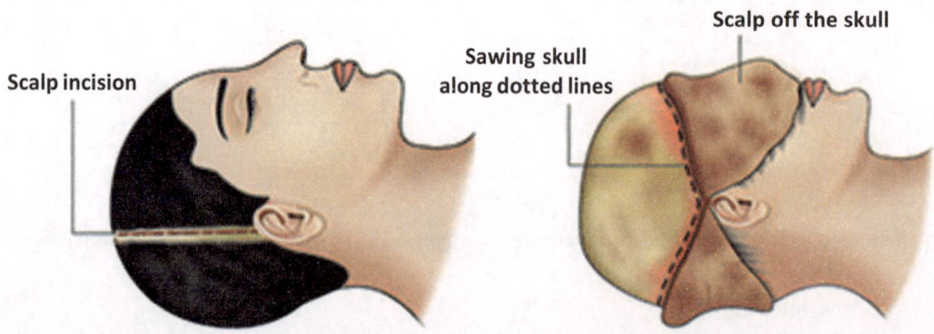

Fig. 2.20 Scalp autopsy incision and sawing of skull

1. **Technique of R Virchow**: In this technique, after opening the body cavities, the organs are removed one by one. This method is widely employed, with some modifications.
2. **Technique of C Rokitansky**: This technique is characterised by in situ dissection and removal of organs as required.
3. **Technique of A Ghon**: The thoracic and cervical structures, the abdominal organs and the urogenital systems are all removed as organ blocks (***en-bloc removal***).
4. **Technique of M Letulle**: The thoracic, cervical, abdominal and pelvic organs are removed as one block (***en-masse removal***), and subsequently dissected into organ blocks. It is widely practiced in the mortuaries of most medical colleges in India, with some modification.

Procedure

- First, the intestines are removed. The greater omentum is lifted upwards to expose the coils of small intestine. The uppermost part of the jejunum is identified, where it passes retroperitoneally to join the terminal duodenum. Here, the mesentery is perforated with a knife, and the gut is cut through between double ligatures. The mesentery is then stripped off the entire intestinal length until the ileo-caecal valve is reached.
- The caecum is then mobilised medially using traction, with minimum use of the knife (to avoid puncturing it). When the hepatic flexure is reached, the omentum is pulled downwards to draw the transverse colon tense against the mesocolon, which is cut through taking care not to open the adjacent stomach. The splenic flexure is then pulled medially and downwards, and the descending and sigmoid colon are separated from the posterior abdominal wall. The upper rectum is cut between double ligatures.
- **Removal of Neck Structures**
  - To make the removal of neck structures easier, a wooden block (10–15 cm high) should be placed under the shoulders of the cadaver which allows the head to fall back, and thus extends the neck. This must be done gently to avoid the well-known **undertaker's fracture**, which is a subluxation of the lower cervical spine, due to tearing of inter-vertebral disc between C6 and C7. There is danger of misinterpreting this as an antemortem injury.
  - The neck structures are now freed by passing a knife under the skin of the upper neck, until it enters the floor of the mouth. The knife is then run around the inside of the mandible to free the tongue. The tissues at the back and sides of the pharynx are divided, and the tonsilar area is cut through.
  - The fingers of one hand are passed up behind the mandibular symphysis to grasp the tongue, which is then drawn down, the remaining tissues behind the larynx being divided to release the neck structures. This should be done as far laterally as possible, so that the carotids can be removed along with the laryngeal structures.

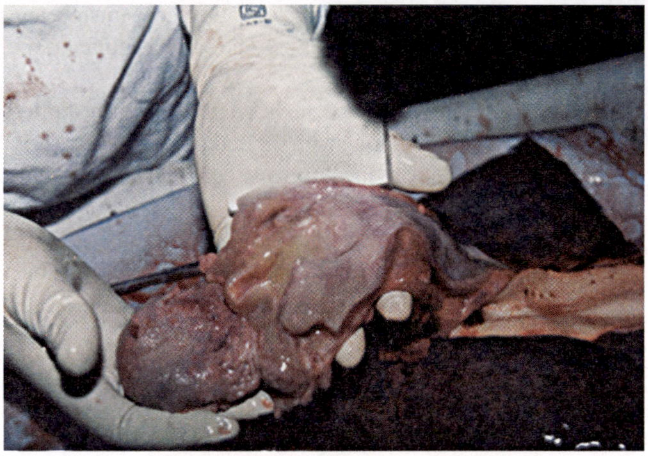

Fig. 2.22 Glottic oedema (*Courtesy*: *Dr Geetha O*)

  - The pharynx and glottis should be examined at this stage to look for any obstruction, bleeding or any other abnormality of the upper airway (**Fig. 2.22**).
- **Removal of Thoracic Contents**
  - The subclavian bundles of vessels and nerves are divided by passing the knife from the inside of the thorax (around the medial ends of the clavicles and first ribs), to release the trachea and oesophagus.
  - With gentle traction, the neck structures are held up and pulled caudally, while carefully clearing all attachments to the thoracic spine with the knife. Traction should be minimal and, as soon as the thorax is entered, the hand should move from the neck structures to place two fingers under the upper lobes of the lungs, lifting them and the mediastinum, as the knife clears the midline structures down to the diaphragm.
  - If the neck structures are pulled too hard to drag out the thoracic viscera, they may get ripped off. In addition, the descending aorta may suffer transverse intimal tears from traction, which can resemble the genuine "ladder tears" seen in many traffic accidents.
  - Pleural adhesions may prevent clean removal of the lungs. If these are minimal, they can be cut through. If the whole pleural cavity is obliterated by adhesions, the lungs may be pulled away by making a cleavage plane with the hand, thereby stripping off the adhesions.
- **Removal of Abdominal Contents**
  - When the chest organs have been cleared, they are laid back in the thoracic cavity, and the diaphragm is incised. The left leaf of the diaphragm is stretched, while the knife cuts through it laterally, near the costal margin. The cut should curve posteriorly under the organs to reach the spine, where it must pass through the cruciate ligaments, and then progress caudally behind the kidney which is mobilised forwards.

- The knife cut then curves up over the psoas muscle and ends at the brim of the pelvis. The same is done on the opposite side.
- The thoracic organs are now lifted and gently pulled free of the cavity along with the abdominal viscera. Any resistance is due to incompletely cut cruciate ligaments which must be severed.
- The iliac vessels and ureters are cut through, and the whole bulk of viscera is removed to the dissecting table, where running water and adequate illumination must be available.

- **Removal of Pelvic Contents**
  - The bladder is cut open, and the mucosa and trigone inspected, before the prostate is incised for examination.
  - The testis on each side is pushed upwards through the inguinal canal, which is widened with the knife.
  - In a female dead body, the ovaries are incised and the fallopian tubes are examined, before the uterus is sliced in the midline from fundus to cervix.
- **Removal of Cranial Contents**
  - After incising the scalp across the posterior vertex, from the mastoid process of one side to the corresponding mastoid process on the other side, the tissues are reflected forwards to the lower forehead, and backwards to the occiput.
  - If head injury is present or suspected, the scalp should be reflected right back to the nape of the neck, paying attention to the tissues behind and below each ear to avoid damaging the vertebral and basilar arteries.
  - The skull is sawn through, using either hand-saw or power tools. The sawing should preferably be angled, with a horizontal cut from the forehead to a point behind the ears, joined by a second cut passing diagonally upwards over the occipito-parietal area (**Fig. 2.20**). This will prevent the skull cap slipping out of position, after it has been replaced and the scalp has been sutured, at the conclusion of the autopsy.
  - The calvarium (skull cap) is removed by leverage after cutting through completely. Hammer and chisel should not be used in forensic autopsies, even to ensure that the dura remains intact. The risk of extending an existing fracture or even causing new fractures because of hammering, is too high merely to justify an unmarked dural membrane. A cut dura is easily recognised as such by a pathologist. What is more important is to inspect the surface of the exposed dura and brain for evidence of oedema, bleeding or inflammatory conditions. The skull cap is carefully inspected for fractures, and the dura is peeled off from its inner aspect to study the inner surface.
  - To remove the brain, the superior sagittal sinus is first incised with fine scissors or scalpel, and then examined for thrombosis.
  - The dura is cut all along the line of cleavage of the skull and folded back. Look for subdural or subarachnoid haemorrhage. Subdural haemorrhage can be easily washed away, whereas subarachnoid haemorrhage cannot be washed off. Examine the leptomeninges for inflammatory changes.
  - Free the falx-cerebri from the cribriform plate and fold it backwards. Lift the frontal lobe of the brain by inserting the fingers of one hand under it. The optic chiasma and the cranial nerves are now identified and cut one by one, as far away from the brain as possible.
  - Cut the tentorium on either side, and pass a narrow pointed knife through the foramen magnum, to cut the cervical cord well below the medulla.
  - Remove the brain gently with both hands. Strip away the remaining dura from the base of the skull and inspect for fractures (**Fig. 2.23**). The brain is weighed before dissection.

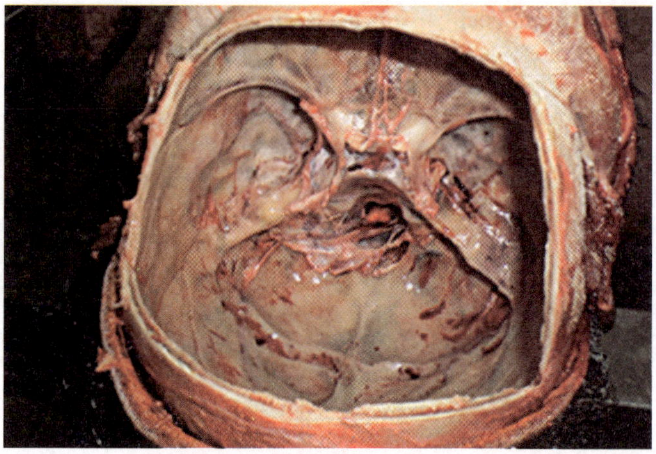

Fig. 2.23 Base of skull (after stripping off the dura) (*Courtesy*: *Dr Prateek Rastogi*)

- **Removal of Spinal Cord**
  - This is not normally done. It is undertaken only if there are specific indications.
  - The posterior approach is usually preferred in an adult. The body is placed in the prone position and a midline incision is made from the occipital protuberance to about the 4th lumbar vertebra.
  - The skin and underlying tissues are dissected away on either side of the vertebral spines, and the laminae are exposed. These are divided as close as possible to the transverse processes by means of an adjustable double-blade saw.
  - A transverse incision is made at the lower end of the midline exposure to enable the dissector to grasp the lumbar end of the freed spinous processes with the bone forceps. The spinous processes can be lifted upwards in one piece.
  - The spinal cord enveloped by the dura mater is now exposed and inspected. The dura is gripped with for-

ceps and drawn aside gently to expose the extradural nerves, which are divided on either side.

- The dura is picked up with the forceps so as to raise the cord gently, allowing the dissector to cut the remaining connections. The spinal cord and dura mater are now divided as near the foramen magnum as possible and removed.

Dissection of Viscera

Brain

- Examine the brain surface for evidence of injury, infection or bleeding. Identify and scrutinise the **Circle of Willis** (**Fig. 2.24**).
  - **Circle of Willis (Circulus arteriosus cerebri)**
    - An arterial anastomosis that unites the internal carotid and vertebro-basilar systems.
    - It lies in the subarachnoid space within the basal cisterns that surround the optic chiasma and infundibulum.
    - The anterior cerebral arteries are derived from the internal carotid artery and are linked by a small, but functionally important, anterior communicating artery.
    - Posteriorly, the two posterior cerebral arteries formed by the division of the basilar artery, are joined to the ipsilateral internal carotid artery by a posterior communicating artery.

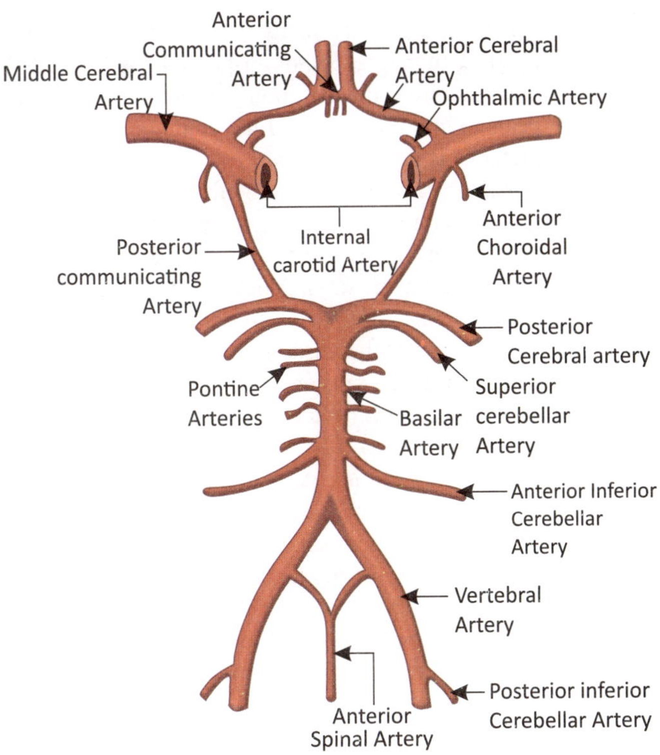

Fig. 2.24 Circle of Willis

- The brain is now placed on a flat board with the convexity in view, and the frontal pole away from the dissector.
- The hemispheres are separated with the left hand. A brain knife is placed in the longitudinal sulcus, and horizontal sections are made on either side just above the level of corpus callosum.
- The white matter of the brain is examined with particular reference to petechial haemorrhages, often seen in death from fat embolism.
- The lateral ventricles are now opened by incising the white matter with a scalpel. Inspect the choroid plexus and locate the interventricular foramen. The fornices and corpus callosum are cut and bent backwards. Examine the thalamus and caudate nucleus.
- The third ventricle is now exposed. Look for any abnormalities. Pass a probe through the aqueduct of Sylvius. Expose the fourth ventricle by cutting along the vermin in the midline.
- With a long knife make parallel horizontal incisions, a little below the incision already made on the cerebral hemisphere. The internal and external capsule, as well as the basal ganglia are now exposed and examined.
- The cerebellum and brainstem are removed. Each cerebellar hemisphere is incised to expose the dentate nucleus.
- Serial sections are made through the pons, medulla and the remaining cord.
- If the brain is oedematous, the gyri appear flattened and the sulci get narrowed.
- Tentorial herniation produces a groove (**Kernohan's notch**) on the surface of mid brain.
- Foraminal herniation produces indentations of medulla and cerebellum.

Spinal Cord

- The spinal cord along with its coverings is stretched out on the dissecting board.
- The dura is opened by scissors and forceps in the midline, the cord being exposed and its membranes and outer surface inspected.
- The cord is sectioned by a series of transverse incisions about half an inch apart and the cut surfaces inspected. It is advisable to dip the knife in water before commencing this dissection, as the cord will otherwise stick to the blade.

Other Viscera

- The thoracic and abdominal viscera are laid on a cutting bench under good illumination.
- Wash the viscera with ample water to flush the tissues as the dissection proceeds. Some pathologists maintain that this should not be done, as water can affect the quality of histological sections, a view which is debatable. In any case, the gross appearance of organs is usually far more important than microscopic findings, in most forensic autopsies.

- **Structures of the mouth and neck**:
    - The tongue is examined for disease or injuries.
    - It should be sliced to detect deep haemorrhages (seen in strangulation), mostly at the sides and centre of the mid-part of the tongue.
    - Gross congestion, which may be due to either pressure on the neck or other congestive modes of death, is sometimes evident in the posterior part of the tongue.
    - The tonsils and pharyngeal walls are inspected.
    - The glottis is examined for mechanical or infective obstruction, and the hyoid and thyroid horns are palpated for fractures.
    - The oesophagus is opened up to the cardiac end of the stomach, and any suspicious material present such as capsules, tablets, etc., are retained for analysis.
    - The carotid artery on each side is slit-opened, and if thrombosis is suspected, the intracranial part should be examined in the cavernous sinus.
    - The thyroid gland should be sliced and inspected.
    - The trachea and main bronchi should be examined for disease or obstruction. Gastric contents are often found as a postmortem artefact; it should not be assumed that antemortem aspiration has occurred merely due to the presence of gastric contents in the air passages.
- **Lungs**:
    - The lungs are removed, and carefully examined for evidence of patchy collapse, emphysema or petechiae (especially around the hilum and in the interlobar fissures) (**Fig. 2.25**).
    - Both lungs are weighed.
    - Then, each lung is laid on the dissecting board with the hilum facing down. Each lung is grasped by the left hand and cut across in the sagittal plane from apex to base, with a large brain knife wielded parallel to the board. This produces an antero-posterior slice, the lower medial part carrying the hilum. The two halves can now be opened like a book, and the surfaces examined for oedema, tumour, pneumonic consolidation, infarction, trauma, abscess, etc.
    - The smaller bronchi must be examined for mucosal thickening, infection or blockage.
    - The smaller pulmonary arteries may reveal thrombosis or embolism that was not visible in the larger vessels (**Fig. 2.26**).

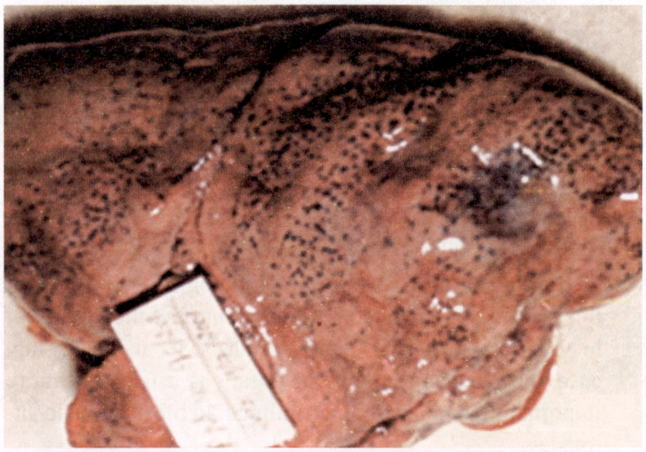

Fig. 2.25 Lung – Multiple petechiae on surface (*Courtesy*: *Dr Shashidhar C Mestri*)

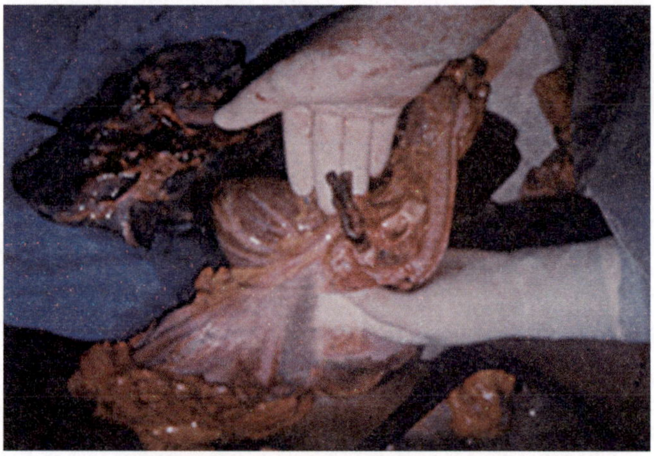

Fig. 2.26 Antemortem thrombus – Pulmonary vasculature (*Courtesy*: *Dr Geetha O*)

- **Heart**:
    - There are almost as many ways of examining the heart as there are pathologists, and each operator must therefore decide upon the method which appeals to him most. One of the commonly followed methods is described here.
    - A pair of scissors is used to cut open the common iliac artery and extended right up to the aortic arch, and further beyond up to a few centimetres above the aortic valve, staying outside the reflection of pericardium.
    - The interior of the aorta is studied for evidence of atheroma, aneurysms or trauma.
    - The inferior vena cava is opened from its lower end upwards.
    - The pericardium is examined through a small nick for the presence of fluid or blood (**Fig. 2.27**), then opened widely with scissors.
    - The heart is delivered through the incision and inspected externally for adhesions, discolouration, pallor or aneurysmal dilatation.
    - In a child, the thymus is examined and dissected out at this stage.
    - The presence of air embolism can be tested by filling the pericardial sac with water and puncturing the right ventricular wall (under water) with a scalpel. Escaping air in the form of bubbles is indicative of air embolism, provided the body is not putrefied.

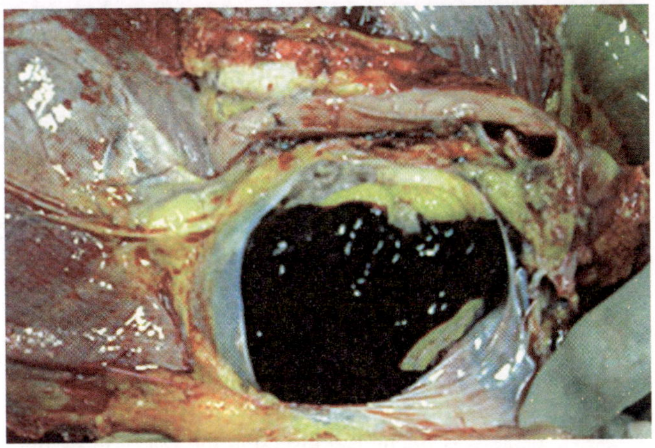

Fig. 2.27 Antemortem clot in the pericardial cavity (*Courtesy*: *Dr Hareesh S Gouda*)

Gases of putrefaction will give a false-positive result. To differentiate between the two, the following method has been suggested:

- Aspirate the right ventricle with a syringe filled with 4 mL of 2% pyrogallol solution which has been alkalinized by adding 0.5 mL of 0.5 N sodium hydroxide. The solution will turn brown in air embolism, while putrefactive gases will not produce such a change in colour.

- The heart is removed by holding it up with the left hand, so that its attachment is tensed against the neighbouring structures. A long knife is passed horizontally across the reflection of the pericardium cutting through the roots of aorta and other great vessels.
- The detached heart is washed and placed in the anatomical position on the dissecting board, with the apex facing the operator and the anterior surface upwards (**Fig. 2.28**). It should not be weighed until all blood contained in the chambers has been removed.

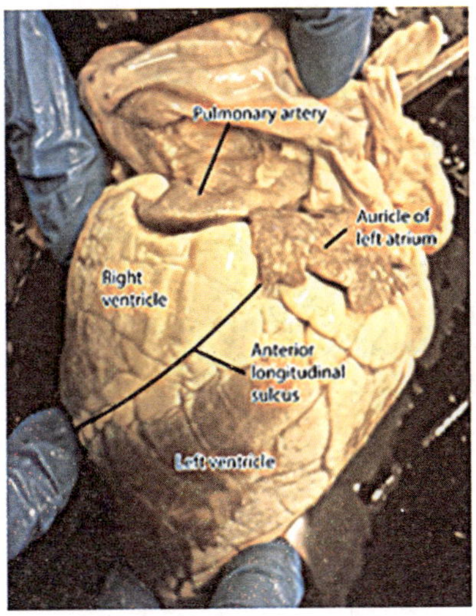

Fig. 2.28 Anterior surface of heart

- The general size and shape should be noted. Any dilatation or thickening of the pulmonary conus should be noted as an index of right ventricular hypertrophy, especially if striae of transverse muscle fibres are present.
- The right atrium is then opened. The interior of the atrium, as well as the septum and tricuspid valve are examined.
- The interventricular septum is identified externally, and a cut is made about 1.5 cm to the right of and parallel to the septum over the right ventricle, which should be deep enough to enter the chamber. The cut must run up through the pulmonary conus and into the pulmonary artery. It is also extended downwards to the apex of the ventricle.
- A pair of fine scissors is now used to pass and cut into the tricuspid valve from the opened atrium. The whole of the right side of the heart can now be opened and displayed (**Fig. 2.29**). It should be washed out, and the endocardium examined for lesions (**Fig. 2.30**). The patency of the valve is tested under running water.

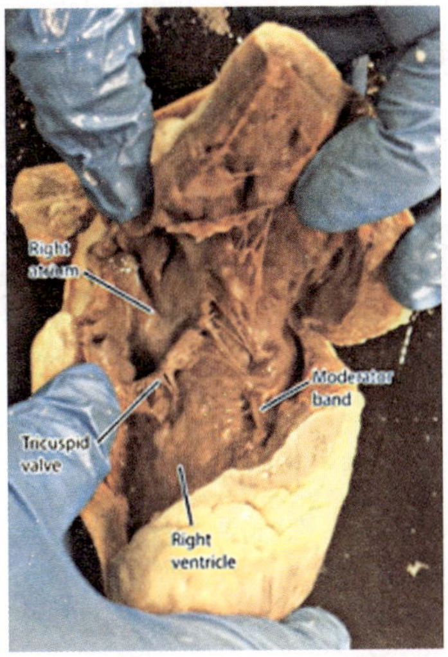

Fig. 2.29 Right side of heart opened

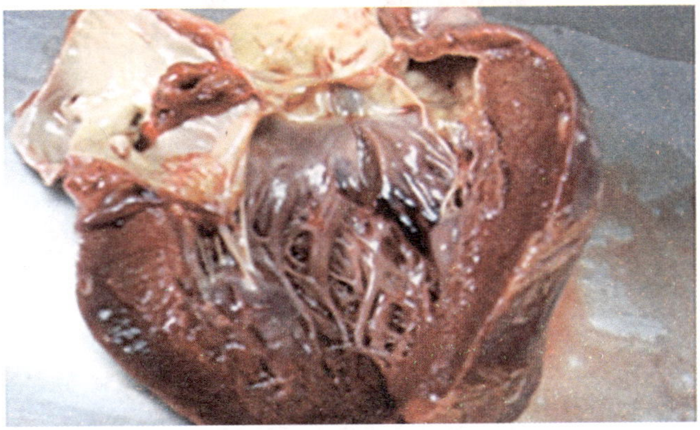

Fig. 2.30 Sub-endocardial haemorrhages (*Courtesy*: *Dr Prateek Rastogi*)

- A similar procedure is followed on the left side. The scissors is introduced into a pulmonary vein and passed horizontally across to an opposite vein, thus opening the left atrium. Two fingers are introduced into the mitral valve to estimate its size and detect any stenosis.
- The heart is restored to the anatomical position and a cut is made parallel to the septum on the left side, going deep as the left ventricle is thicker. Guided by the fingers still in the mitral valve, the cut is extended upwards through that valve and out from the top of the atrium.
- Observe whether there is any hypertrophy of the ventricular walls. Various estimates of the normal weight exist for the human heart, but there is considerable variation depending on the sex and body weight. As a rule of thumb however, we can accept up to 380 g as normal in an adult man of average build.
- After weighing the heart, the endocardium and valves are examined in more detail.

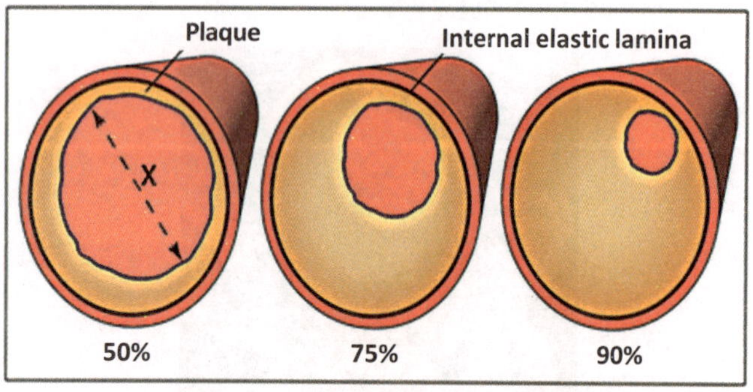

Fig. 2.31 Coronary artery segments with different degrees of atherosclerotic stenosis. The diagrams demonstrate a 50% area stenosis, 75% stenosis and 90% stenosis; diameter x is usually less than 2 mm in the left main stem and less than 1 mm in other major coronary arteries

- The coronary arteries must be scrutinised with reference to narrowing of lumen or stenosis (**Fig. 2.31**). The ostia are examined for congenital variations (which are frequent), and for obstruction (**Fig. 2.32**). Serial cuts are then made at intervals of not more than 3 mm, first into the left coronary artery, followed by the circumflex branch laterally, until the vessel becomes too small, as it dips down from the epicardium to become intra-muscular. The anterior descending branch is then followed down the front of the septum almost to the apex.
- The right coronary artery is dealt with in the same way, beginning from the point where the right ventricle was opened, transecting the artery in its mid part. Serial cuts are made back to the aorta, and then the distal segment is followed laterally until it becomes the posterior descending branch. During this process, the dominance of right versus left vessels is noted.
- Difficulty arises when severe calcification exists in the coronary arteries. The only solution then is to decalcify the vessels. Postmortem angiography is the other alternative, but if the autopsy case-load is high, this can be difficult to accomplish.
- Observe the surface as well as the cut sections of the heart to look for evidence of old or recent myocardial infarction (**Fig. 2.33**).

- **Abdominal and pelvic organs**:
  - The stomach is washed externally in a stream of water and a small cut is made in the greater curvature, which is then opened widely with scissors.
  - The contents are collected into a container and the gastric mucosa is examined for signs of inflammation, erosion, ulceration, etc.
  - The contents are examined with reference to the nature, quantity, state of digestion, presence of foreign matter, smell, etc.
  - The liver is dissected out, weighed and scrutinized. Serial sections are made (**Fig 2.34**), and the cut sur-

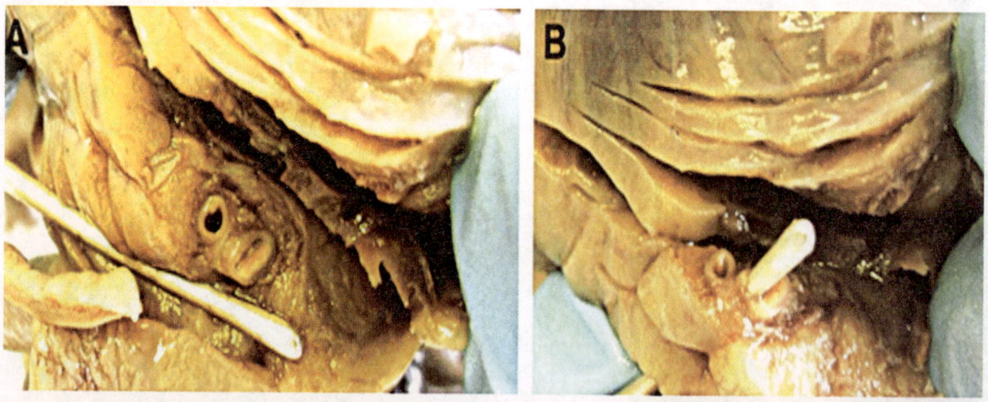

Fig. 2.32 **(A)** The left anterior descending (LAD) coronary artery with a diagonal branch. The LAD contains eccentric atheroma and collapse of the lumen with a slit-like space. **(B)** A 2-mm probe which has opened up the lumen of the LAD indicating non-significant stenosis

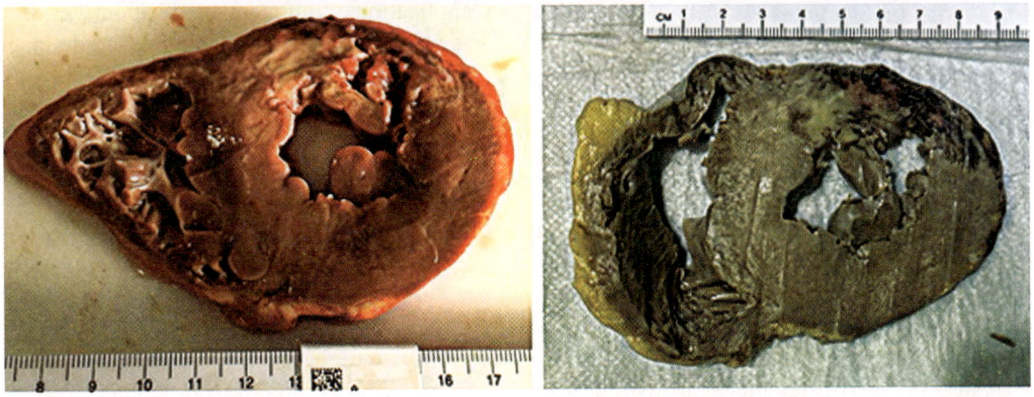

Fig. 2.33 One-week-old myocardial infarction of posterior left ventricle, with focal rupture, in fresh state (left) and after formalin fixation (right). Infarcted area is pale, whereas the rupture is haemorrhagic (dark red)

faces are examined for evidence of congestion, fatty change, cirrhosis, abscesses, haematoma, etc.

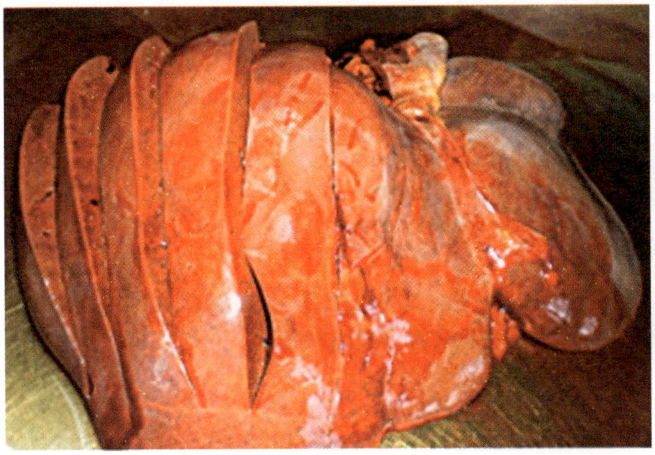

Fig. 2.34 Dissected liver
(*Courtesy*: *Dr Prateek Rastogi*)

- The pancreas is not ordinarily examined in detail, unless there is a specific reason. In relevant cases, look for calculi in the duct system or acini, evidence of fat necrosis, etc.
- The adrenals are examined next, the right one being located on top of the right kidney, while the left is situated on the medial side of the left kidney. The amount of cortical fat and presence of bleeding or other abnormality is noted in each gland.
- The kidneys are exposed by incising their capsules. They can usually be peeled out of their capsules unless these are adherent. The renal vessels can be examined when the aorta is opened. The kidneys are detached at their hilum and weighed, then cut lengthwise to examine the interior (**Fig. 2.35**). The width of the cortex is about 1 cm in a healthy subject. The granularity of the surface and the clarity of the cortico-medullary junction is assessed, as well as the size of the renal pelvis.

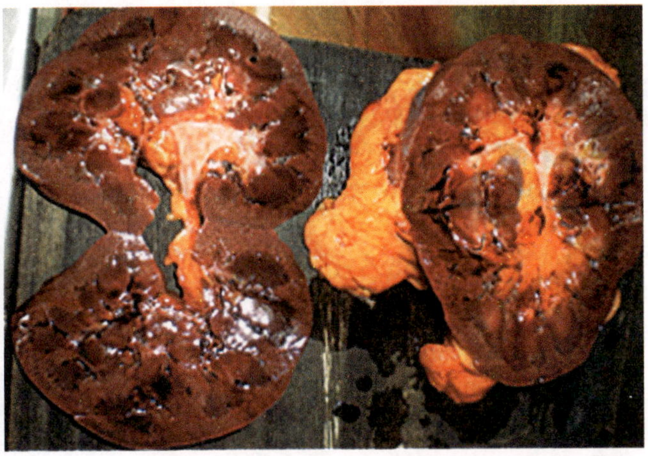

Fig. 2.35 Dissected kidney
(*Courtesy*: *Dr Prateek Rastogi*)

- The spleen is removed by cutting through its pedicle, and is sliced after weighing.
- The small intestine can be examined now. However, it is not customary to open the entire length of the small bowel, unless there is some specific indication.
- In a female dead body, it is important to examine the uterus after removing it along with the fallopian tubes, ovaries and a portion of the vagina.
- The cervix is scrutinised for evidence of ulceration, erosion, laceration, mucosal plug, etc. The uterine cavity is examined for products of conception, blood clots and foreign bodies. Both the ovaries must be incised to look for corpus luteum, congestion, cysts, etc.
- In a male dead body, the prostate may have to be examined, though this is not usually done. Testes must be examined in sudden, unexpected deaths, especially if the victim had died in the course of a brawl or assault. The scrotum should not be incised; instead an internal approach can be made via the inner aspect of the inguinal canal.

FM 2.13: Core – Written/Viva Voce
- Describe and discuss obscure autopsy

NEGATIVE OR OBSCURE AUTOPSY

- When at the conclusion of a complete and thorough post-mortem examination, inclusive of all relevant investigations such as histopathological, toxicological and biochemical investigations, no cause can be attributed to the death, it is termed as a **negative autopsy** or **obscure autopsy**.
- Approximately, 2–5% of all autopsies are negative in nature.
- Some investigators prefer to differentiate the two, and state that:
  - An **obscure autopsy** is one where the cause of death is difficult to determine even though a complete and meticulous examination was performed (external and internal), while
  - A **negative autopsy** is one where in addition to a meticulous examination, all investigations (histopathology, toxicology, etc.) are also inconclusive.

Causes of Obscure Autopsy

- Inadequate history.
- Advanced putrefaction.
- Death due to certain kinds of poisons, e.g., narcotic drugs.
- Death due to anaphylaxis.
- Death due to concealed puncture wounds.
- Electrocution deaths.

Causes of Negative Autopsy

- Death due to cardiac arrhythmias.
- Death due to vagal inhibition.
- Death due to cerebral concussion.

FM 2.14: Core – Written/Viva Voce/OSPE
(Objective Structured Practical Examination)
- Describe and discuss
  - Examination of clothing
  - Preservation of viscera on postmortem examination for chemical analysis and other medicolegal purposes
  - Postmortem artefacts

POSTMORTEM EXAMINATION – EXAMINATION OF CLOTHING

- **Examination of wrappings**: A dead body may be brought to the mortuary enclosed in plastic or cloth wrapping. It should be examined carefully for trace evidence which may have been dislodged from the body.
- **Hospital dressings**: These should be described in detail, with particular mention of their nature and position. Any application of ointment, medication, etc., should be noted, as also the position of catheters and drainage tubes.
- **Clothing**:
  - These should be examined in situ for evidence of any tear, loss of buttons or general disarray.
  - Cuts and tears, if present, have to be correlated with the external injuries on the body.
  - In the case of firearm injuries, burns or blackening of the clothing must be described and correlated with the external body injuries. The area of blackening must be measured, which could give an idea about the range of fire.
  - Stains in clothing due to blood, semen, saliva, vomit, poison, vitriolage, faeces, mud, grass, etc., must all be recorded meticulously. If it is decided to take photographs, two photographs are essential: one of long range to indicate the exact location of the stain, and another of close range to record the details of the stain itself.
  - In the case of death due to poisoning or burns, an attempt must be made to detect characteristic odours.
  - All clothing should be carefully removed by unbuttoning or unzipping. Special care must be taken to ensure that the clothing retains its evidentiary value, right up to the time of the trial. In all cases, it must be air dried, preserved, sealed and handed over to the investigating police officer.

POSTMORTEM EXAMINATION – PRESERVATION OF VISCERA FOR CHEMICAL ANALYSIS

- In every case of death due to poisoning, an attempt must be made to demonstrate the presence of poison by standardised analytical methods. For this purpose, the pathologist conducting the autopsy must collect certain of the viscera and body fluids, and despatch them through the police to the nearest forensic science laboratory.
- While submitting the samples for analysis, it must be ensured that the correct quantity has been preserved in appropriate preservative in suitable, sealed containers.
- Viscera to be collected are mentioned in **Table 2.2**, while recommended preservatives are listed in **Table 2.3**.
- In reality, all that is required for toxicological analysis is 5–10 mL of blood and 25–50 mL of urine stored and transported in cold condition, without any preservative. A bit of liver or kidney may be required in addition in a few cases. The practice of sending large quantities of viscera and body fluids for analysis to the forensic science lab in every suspected poisoning case as is done in India is quite outdated and needs to be avoided.

POSTMORTEM ARTEFACTS*

There are several inherent pitfalls that must be avoided in the course of medicolegal autopsies which can lead to erroneous

*__Note__: *Incorrectly spelt as* ***'Artifact'*** *in many textbooks, which actually refers to a man-made object, such as a piece of art or tool, that is of particular cultural, historical or archaeological interest.*

or fallacious conclusions. Every forensic pathologist must familiarise himself with these **postmortem artefacts** that are liable to misinterpretation (**Figs. 2.36 & 2.37**). While an exhaustive discussion on this matter is unfortunately beyond the scope of this book, some of the more commonly encountered artefacts have been mentioned in **Box 2.2**.

Table 2.2 Viscera and Body Fluids to be Preserved in Suspected Poisoning

1. **Routine Viscera & Body Fluids** (*to be preserved routinely for analysis, in every case of poisoning*)

SPECIMEN	QUANTITY
1. Stomach	Entire
2. Stomach contents	Entire (preferably)
3. Small intestine (jejunum)	30 cm (entire length in infants)
4. Small intestinal contents	Up to 100 g
5. Liver (portion containing gall bladder)	500 g (entire liver in infants)
6. Kidney	One half of each kidney (both kidneys in infants)
7. Urine	30–50 mL
8. Blood	10–20 mL

2. **Special Viscera** (*all or any of these should be preserved in addition to routine viscera, in certain specific cases of poisoning*)

SPECIMEN	QUANTITY	POISON
1. Cerebrospinal fluid	As much as can be withdrawn	Alcohol
2. Brain	Half (one hemisphere)	Alcohol, anaesthetics, barbiturates, carbon monoxide, cyanide, opiates, strychnine
3. Spinal cord	Entire length	Gelsemine, strychnine
4. Lung	One	Inhaled poisons
5. Skin (with underlying tissues)	Affected portion	Corrosives, injected poisons
6. Long bone (preferably femur)	10 cm length	Heavy metals
7. Scalp hair (plucked)	15–20 strands	Heavy metals

Table 2.3 Preservatives for Viscera and Body Fluids

SPECIMEN	PRESERVATIVE
1. Viscera	Rectified spirit* or Saturated saline
2. Blood	For every 10 mL, use 30 mg potassium oxalate** and 100 mg sodium fluoride***
3. Urine	100 mg sodium fluoride for every 10 mL

**Not to be used in poisoning due to alcohol, phosphorus, acetic acid, phenol and paraldehyde.*
***In cases of oxalic acid and ethylene glycol poisoning, do not preserve blood in potassium oxalate*
****For carbon monoxide and other gaseous/volatile poisons, use glass or plastic tube and ensure that there is very little headspace after filling.*

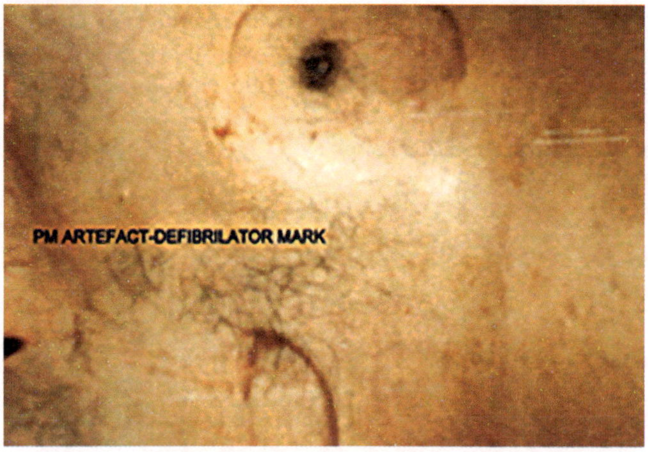

Fig. 2.36 Defibrillator injury
(*Courtesy*: *Dr Shashidhar C Mestri*)

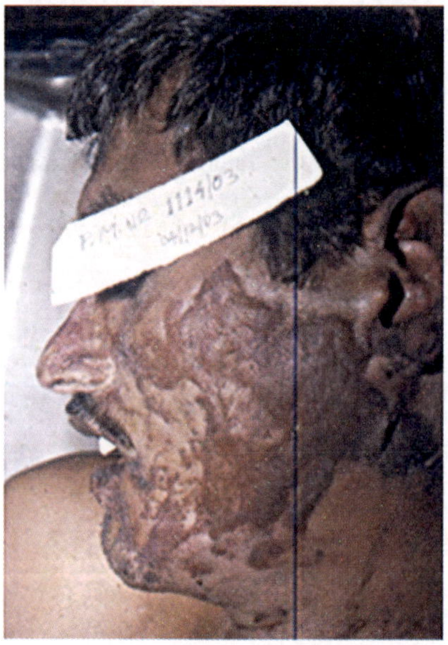

Fig. 2.37 Postmortem ant bite erosions
(*Courtesy*: *Dr EJ Rodrigues*)

Box 2.2—Postmortem Artefacts

- Aspiration of gastric contents may occur as an agonal terminal event, or due to resuscitation, or handling of the body after death. This should not be confused with death due to choking.
- **Prinsloo-Gordon haemorrhage**: Misinterpretation of extravasation of blood into the soft tissues of the neck, entirely due to dissection, as a mimic of bruising related to trauma. Essentially, handling (blunt dissection) and incising congested blood vessels (sharp dissection) can cause blood to track between and within the strap muscles. These haemorrhages may be only localized to the upper posterior pharynx or may extend along the posterior pharyngeal wall and spread into the posterior mediastinum. The main pitfall with the Prinsloo-Gordon haemorrhage has been to confuse this artefact with haemorrhages that may occur with **strangulation**.
  - By dissecting the neck after vascular decompression, such "haemorrhages" could be avoided. Thus, the layered dissection of the neck was introduced to medicolegal autopsy work in the 1950s.
- Defibrillator used as a part of resuscitative procedure may produce contusions over chest. Similar is the case with external cardiac massage which may even cause ribs to be fractured.
- Positive pressure breathing done through a respirator may cause emphysematous condition of the lungs.
- Fractures of skull, cervical spine (*undertaker's fracture*), ribs or extremities may result from rough handling of a dead body.
  - **Undertaker's fracture** is an artefact related to poor handling of a corpse characterized by subluxation of lower cervical spine (tearing of the intervertebral disc) at C6-C7 vertebral level.
- Abrasions may result from a recently dead victim being dragged on a rough surface.
- Rough handling can break rigor mortis leading to wrong conclusions about the time of death.
- Bodies placed in cold storage immediately after death can develop pink colouration of postmortem lividity, which may be mistaken for carbon monoxide poisoning.
- Postmortem lividity in internal organs such as the heart, stomach, intestines, etc., may be mistaken for congestion, inflammation or disease.
- Tight clothes can produce marks resembling ligature mark (neck) or bruising (trunk).
- In a burnt body, fractures of skull or limb bones can occur due to heat, and must not be confused with traumatic fractures.
- Insect or animal bites on a dead body may be mistaken for antemortem injuries.
- Decomposition can cause a number of changes that may be mistaken to be due to antemortem violence, e.g., oozing of blood stained fluid from mouth and nose.

FM 2.15: Core – Written/Viva Voce/OSPE (Objective Structured Practical Examination)

- Describe special protocols for the conduct of medicolegal autopsies in cases of death in custody or following violation of human rights as per National Human Rights Commission Guidelines.

NATIONAL HUMAN RIGHTS COMMISSION (NHRC) PROTOCOL FOR MEDICOLEGAL AUTOPSIES IN POLICE CUSTODIAL DEATHS

The **National Human Rights Commission (NHRC)** issued guidelines for the conduct of medicolegal autopsies in **1993**, which were subsequently amended in **2001**. As per these guidelines (protocol), the following salient points must be followed:

1. Information relating to any custodial death must be intimated to the NHRC (*henceforth referred to as 'Commission'*) within 24 hours of its occurrence.
2. Magistrate's inquest is mandatory in all custodial deaths.
3. In order to help in proper assessment of 'time since death', determination of rectal temperature and study of rigor mortis at the time of the first examination at the scene is essential by a medical officer or a trained police officer.
4. A medicolegal autopsy (postmortem examination) is mandatory, and must be videographed to facilitate an independent review of the examination at a later stage, if required. At the time of the video recording, the voice of the doctor should be recorded, and he must narrate his prima facie observations while conducting the postmortem examination.
5. The postmortem examination must be done by a board of at least three doctors preferably from three different institutions. Moreover, doctors conducting the postmortem must hold a postgraduate degree in forensic medicine. They must have at least 5 years experience of conducting the postmortem examination.
6. The postmortem examination must be performed strictly as per the proforma designed by the Commission.
   Precautions to be taken:
   i. Both the hands of the deceased should be wrapped in white paper bags, and the body should be covered in special body bags having zip pouches for proper transportation.
   ii. Clothing should not be removed by the police or any other person as it must be examined, preserved and sealed by the doctor conducting the autopsy. It should be sent for further examination at the FSL; a detailed note regarding examination of the clothing is to be incorporated in the postmortem examination by the concerned doctor.
   iii. In case of alleged firearm death, the body should be subjected to radiological examination (X-ray/CT scan) prior to autopsy.
   iv. While describing the injuries, the distance from heel, as also from the midline, must be taken in respect of each injury which will help later in reconstruction of events.
   v. Photographs: A total of 20–25 colour photographs of the whole body should be taken, and some photographs should be taken before removing the clothes. The postmortem number, date of examination and scale for dimensions must be incorporated in the frame of the photograph itself.
7. The postmortem report must be typed or computer generated, and must not be hand written.
8. Fingerprints of the deceased must be taken on separate sheet and attached by the doctor to the main postmortem report.
9. All reports must reach the Commission within 2 months of the incident (magistrate's inquest report, postmortem report, video cassette).
10. If any viscera/body fluids have been set aside for histopathological or toxicological or forensic examination of any kind, such reports must be sent to the Commission as soon as the results are obtained. However, the postmortem report must be sent within the deadline stipulated (with or without the other reports).

FM 2.16: Core – Written/Viva Voce/OSPE (Objective Structured Practical Examination)

- Describe and discuss examination of mutilated bodies or fragments, charred bones and bundle of bones

EXAMINATION OF MUTILATED BODIES/FRAGMENTS/ CHARRED BONES/BUNDLE OF BONES

- Mutilated bodies or fragments, charred bones and bundle of bones sent for examination to a Forensic Expert are usually either those recovered after exhumation, or those recovered from burial sites, cremation sites, burnt buildings, deserted areas, dustbins, ditches, forests, etc. The examination of such **skeletal** or **body remains** should be undertaken with great care, in order to provide information which may be vital to the investigation (**Fig. 2.38**). The following facts should be elucidated:
  - **Human or not**: Can be determined by noting morphological features. It is difficult when only small body parts or bone fragments are available. Precipitin test will be helpful in such cases.
  - **Male or female**: Mutilated or fragmented body parts may offer clues as to the sex of the individual, depending on which parts are available for examination. With regard to skeletal remains, in post-pubertal bones, sex

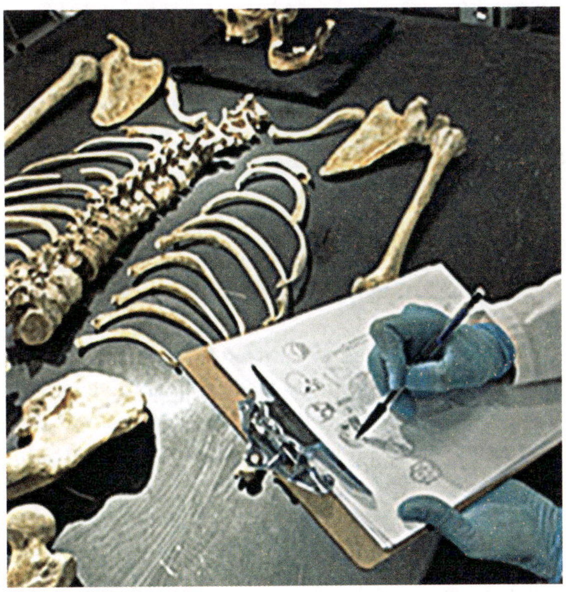

Fig. 2.38 Systematic examination of skeletal remains

differences can be determined from an examination of pelvis, skull, sacrum, etc.

- **One or more individuals**: This can be ascertained by sorting and assigning the individual body parts or bones to their anatomical positions. If there are no disproportionate or duplicated body parts or bones, and the age and sex of all the parts or bones are same, it can be safely concluded that all the body parts or bones belong to the same individual.
- **Probable stature**: Can be assessed by measuring limb parts in the case of dismembered or fragmented body remains, or long bones in the case of skeletal remains, and applying appropriate formulae.
- **Age of the individual**: Can be determined by the examination of skin or hair, if available (in the case of body parts); and teeth, ossification status and suture closure (in the case of skeletal remains).
- **Identity**: The superimposition technique can be employed for establishing identity in the case of the skull. If soft tissues or tooth pulp or bone marrow are available, DNA fingerprinting can be done.
- **Time of death**: It is difficult to tell precisely the time of death. But, an intelligent guess may be made from the condition of the soft parts, ligaments and bones. Skeletonisation generally takes place within 3–6 months after burial, and sooner if the body is exposed to inclemental conditions.
- **Cause of death**: It is usually impossible to find out the cause of death from an examination of body parts or bones, unless there is evidence of serious injury to vital body parts, or major fractures in the vital parts of the skeleton (e.g., skull). However, it is often difficult to distinguish between an antemortem fracture and a postmortem artefact. Presence of vital reaction, blood clots or evidence of reparative processes indicate antemortem nature.

FM 2.17: Core – Written/Viva Voce

- Describe and discuss exhumation

EXHUMATION

- The term **'Exhumation'** refers to the retrieval of a previously buried body for postmortem examination.
  - This term should be restricted to the removal of a body interred in a legitimate fashion in a graveyard (interment = burial), rather than the recovery of an uncoffined, clandestinely buried victim of a suspicious death. The latter is actually a "scene of crime," and the pathologist should treat it as such.

Indications

- Where some civil legal matter needs to be investigated, such as personal injuries for insurance purpose, or civil litigation relating to negligence – usually after road traffic, industrial or other accidents.
- Where new information, or substantiated allegations arise to suggest that a death was due to unnatural causes, criminal abortion, or some form of injury or poison that was not elucidated prior to burial.
- Where a second autopsy needs to be done because the first autopsy report is being challenged as to its veracity, or because it is ambiguous.
- In ancient or historical circumstances, to study either the individual, or a series of individuals, for academic interest.

Procedure

- The body is exhumed only on written order from an executive or judicial magistrate. Under Section 176(3) of the Criminal Procedure Code, an order for exhumation can be given by the District Collector, Additional District Magistrate, Sub Collector, RDO, Tahsildar or Deputy Tahsildar. They are all Executive Magistrates.
- There is no time limit for ordering an exhumation in India.
- It is done under the direct supervision of the medical officer and in the presence of a police officer.
- It is advisable to conduct an exhumation early in the morning, as exposure to strong sunlight will accelerate putrefactive processes.
- Before beginning to dig, the grave should be positively identified by examining the plan of the graveyard, or by questioning the persons who had accomplished the burial (**Fig. 2.39**).
- The grave is then carefully dug out. The soil must be carefully screened for small objects like teeth, bullet(s), hyoid bone, thyroid cartilage, etc.
- In a case of suspected poisoning, about 500 g of earth in actual contact with the body from the top, bottom, sides, above and below, should be collected and sent for chemical analysis as a control sample, to rule out contamination of the body by a poison present in the soil itself.
  - Eight jars may be used for soil samples: for soil from top, bottom, front, back, left and right sides of the casket, as well as two jars containing soil from about 25 yards away from the grave.
- In coffined bodies, the coffin must be identified by the person who had made it. The coffin or the body is lifted out, and the body is identified by as many persons as possible who had been present at the time of burial. Any debris in the coffin must be sent for chemical analysis.
- Exhumation of a recently buried body can be unpleasant, and sometimes hazardous.
- Disinfectants should not be sprinkled on the body.
- The examiner should wear masks and thick rubber gloves, and stand away from the direction of the wind.
- Once the body has been lifted out, postmortem examination is done in the usual way.
- Viscera should be preserved for chemical analysis. If viscera are not distinguishable, masses obtained from the areas of these organs should be preserved. If viscera/masses are not present, then hair, nails, teeth, bones and skin should be preserved.

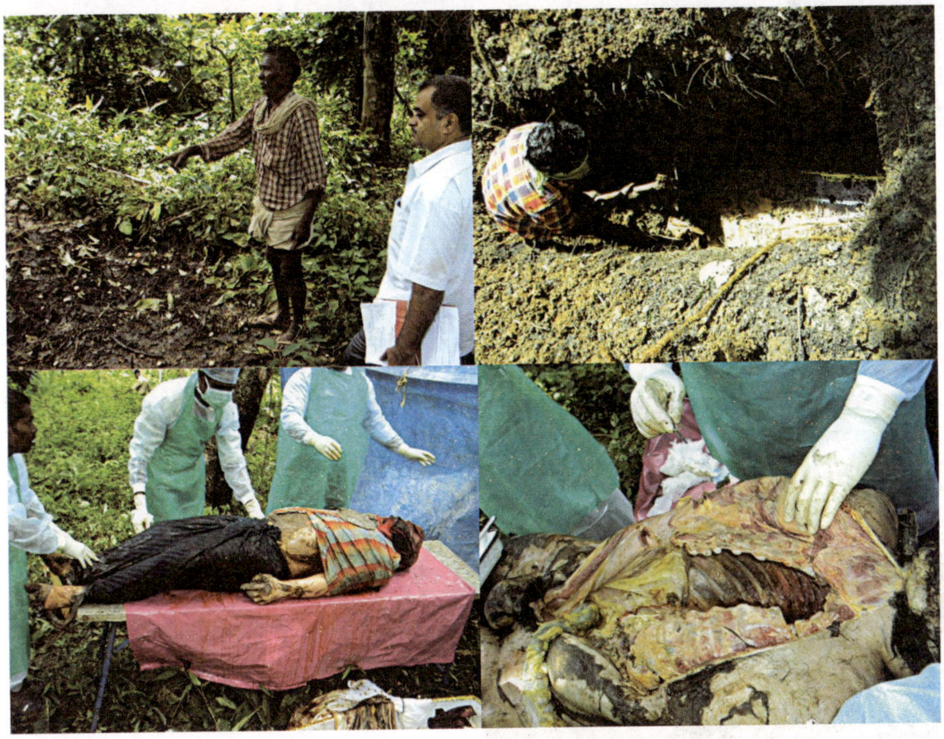

Fig. 2.39 Exhumation in progress (*Courtesy*: *Dr PS Sanjay*)

- If skeletonisation has taken place, ascertain the age, sex, height and cause of death. Even negative information gained, such as absence of alleged or suspected fractures may be of considerable value.
- If only bones are recovered during exhumation (as in very old graves), the bones must be boiled before examination. Maceration by this process may reveal diagnosis not available otherwise by ordinary examination. Maceration by this process is recommended not only in medicolegal autopsies, but also in historical material.

> **FM 2.18: Core – Written/Viva Voce**
> - Crime Scene Investigation:
>   - Describe and discuss the objectives of crime scene visit
>   - Duties & responsibilities of doctors at crime scene
>   - Reconstruction of sequence of events after crime scene investigation

CRIME SCENE INVESTIGATION

One of the most important aspects of crime investigation, with which all doctors (especially forensic experts) must be familiar, is a detailed study of the crime scene.

- Meaning of the term "**Crime Scene**": In a broad sense, the crime scene includes more than the actual location where the crime was committed. It also includes other locations, where evidence has been generated. For example, a person may have been murdered in one place, the body dumped in another place and the car used to transport it may have been abandoned in yet another location. All these are part of the crime scene and can contain important evidence.
- **Approach to Crime Scene Investigation**: This section deals with the investigation of a homicide crime scene from a forensic expert's viewpoint. The analysis of a crime scene and subsequent collection of physical evidence requires skill, knowledge and aptitude. The manner in which a crime scene was studied would have an important, sometimes crucial, bearing on the eventual success of the investigation. A systematic approach is necessary to ensure:
  - Harmonious coordination between crime scene officers and investigating officers.
  - Thorough and effective crime scene analysis.
  - Orderly collection of evidence.
  - Correct interpretation and deductions.
- **Assessment of Crime Scene (Fig. 2.40)**: Every attempt must be made to answer the following questions during the course of crime scene investigation:
  - **Who?**
    - Who is the victim?
    - Who reported the crime?
    - Who saw or heard anything?
  - **What?**
    - What happened?
    - What is the nature of the crime?
    - What were the actions of the victim?
    - What do the witnesses say?
    - What clothing and personal property are present on the deceased?

    - What injuries or marks are present on the body?
    - What is the time of death?
    - What type of weapon was used?
    - What could be the cause and manner of death?
- **When?**
    - When was the body discovered?
    - When was the victim last seen alive?
    - When was the crime reported?
- **How?**
    - How did the victim sustain the injuries?
    - How much time has passed between injury and death?

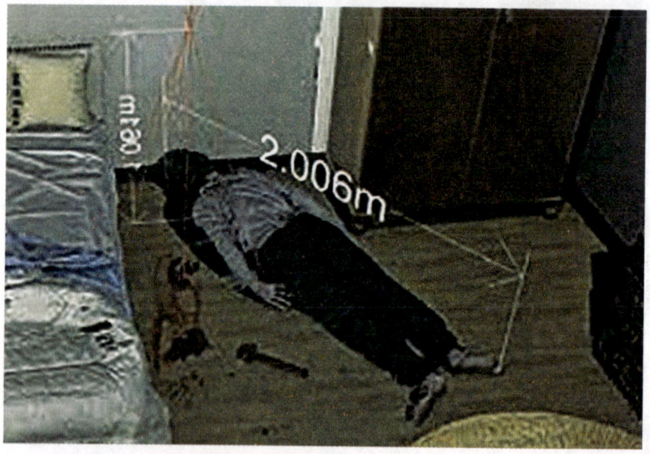

Fig. 2.40 Documenting a crime scene

- **Where?**
    - Where is the body located?
    - Where did the death occur?
    - Where was the victim last seen?
    - Where did the injuries occur?
    - Where were the witnesses during the incident?
- **Why?**
    - Why was the victim at this location?
    - Why was the crime committed?
    - Why was this type of weapon used?
    - Why was the deceased found at this particular time?

■ **Scene Security**:
- It is important to ensure proper security of the crime scene, and to keep curious onlookers at bay. Though this is mainly the responsibility of the investigating officer, the forensic expert must do his bit to see that no tampering or destruction of evidence occurs at the scene. The perimeter of the crime scene is taped off with **barricade tape** (**Fig. 2.41**) in order to keep only those necessary on site.
    - Barricade tape is a brightly coloured tape (often incorporating a two-tone pattern of alternating yellow-black or red-white stripes or the words "Caution" or "Danger" in prominent lettering). It is also known as **barrier tape**, **caution tape**, **warning tape** or **danger tape**.
- The main objectives of securing a crime scene include:
    - Prevention of destruction or contamination of evidence.
    - Prevention of leakage of vital information to the general public which could hinder investigation.
    - Ensuring chain of custody.
    - Ensuring proper recovery of evidence and recording of the same.
    - Removal of all unauthorized persons from the scene.

■ **Sequential Approach to Crime Scene Search**: It is important to conduct a search of the crime scene in a scientifically based sequential manner, so that best results are obtained and no evidence is lost or rendered useless. The following is an example of such a sequential approach:
- Identifiable evidence should be collected from an area before it is dusted for fingerprints.
- Bloodstains and other forensic evidence should be collected before dusting for fingerprints.
- Polished floors need to be examined with oblique lighting to locate latent foot/shoe prints.
- Visible hairs, fibres, etc., should be collected from an area before tape lifts, sweeping or vacuuming.
- Tape lift areas of interest before removing the dead body.

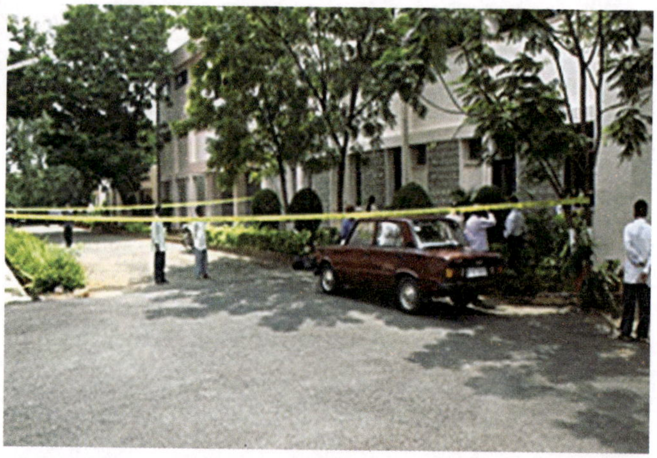

Fig. 2.41 Barricade tape at a crime scene

■ **Specific Duties of Forensic Pathologist at the Crime Scene**: The main role of a forensic pathologist at the crime scene is to help find out the:
- Fact that the victim is really dead: Search for pulse, heartbeat, evidence of breathing, etc. Use stethoscope!
- Identity of the deceased: Observe and record distinctive physical characteristics of the victim. Details can be recorded at the time of the autopsy.
- Time of death: The following methods may help: study of livor mortis, rigor mortis, temperature of the body (use chemical thermometer and determine rectal or core body temperature), signs of decomposition, etc.
- Cause and manner of death: An initial assessment can be attempted at the crime scene, which can be later verified at autopsy.

- Age of the victim: A rough estimate suffices at the crime scene.
- Evidence of any sexual assault: Look for disturbance or disarray of clothing, injuries around private parts, evidence of seminal emission, etc. Ensure that swabbing of stains is done.
- Nature of injuries: At the crime scene, it is enough to deduce whether the injuries have resulted from the use of a blunt or sharp weapon, firearm, etc. Details can be worked out later at autopsy.
- Whether it is a case of poisoning: Look for evidence of odour, frothing from the mouth, poison or drug containers lying around, etc.
- The best method of recording and preserving evidence relating to the death: Careful instructions should be given to the photographer, police artist, etc., as to how best to record important findings on the body of the deceased.

Collection, Packing & Despatch of Evidentiary Material

Collection

The principal methods of collection of trace material from a crime scene include:

- **Handpicking**: Gross and macroscopic items large enough to be seen visually should be recovered by hand or by the use of tweezers. As far as possible, gloves must be worn.
- **Tape lifting**: This is an effective method of collecting material such as hairs and fibres from a variety of surfaces, especially garments (**Fig. 2.42**) and motor vehicle seats. Transparent adhesive tape of no more than 7.5 cm length is applied to the surface and then placed over a clean piece of glass or rigid plastic, which is then put inside a clean, labeled plastic bag. Care should be taken not to tape too much material on a single tape piece. Fingerprints can also be tape-lifted from surfaces.
- **Swabbing**: Dry swabs are used to collect minute particles, while swabs moistened with distilled or injection water can be used to collect body fluids.
- **Sweeping**: This method is particularly useful for collecting material from inaccessible sites, or where there is a mass of material to be collected. The best implement for sweeping is a paintbrush approximately 2.5 cm wide. It is imperative that a clean brush is used each time.
- **Vacuuming**:
  - Collection of microscopic material from garments, motor vehicles and other large objects is best facilitated by vacuuming.
  - Specialized nozzles (custom-made from stainless steel) must be employed.
  - Ordinary vacuum cleaners must not be used.
  - Material is collected on to a clean filter paper or cotton material resting on the perforated plate located in the central compartment.
  - When not in use, the nozzle should be cleaned and stored in a sealed plastic bag.

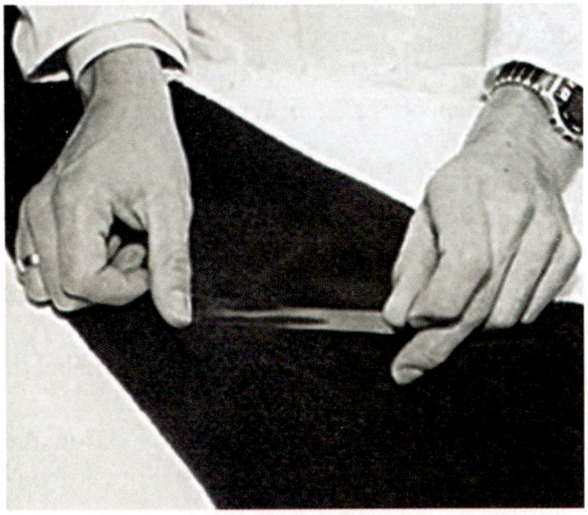

Fig. 2.42 Recovering fibres from a garment using clear adhesive tape

Packing and Despatching

Procedures for packing and despatching are the same as for any specimen in medicolegal cases. A summary is given below:

- **Blood**:
  - On absorbent material:
    - Cut material, air dry and pack separately.
    - Include control sample. Pack large items in paper, while small samples can be placed in plastic vials.
  - On non-absorbent material:
    - *Wet*: Suck up with pipette, or soak small piece of cotton.
    - *Dry*: Use scalpel to scrape off the stain, or rub with moistened cotton. Include controls. Pack in plastic or glass vials.
- **Saliva**:
  - *Wet*: Collect on clean white gauze. Air dry and pack.
  - *Dry*: Use moistened swab. Pack in plastic container.
- **Semen**:
  - Stains can be photographed.
  - Items bearing seminal stains must be collected, air dried and packed. Pack in paper bags.
- **Paint**:
  - If possible, collect the item (tool, clothing or vehicle) containing the evidence.
  - Collect paint chips separately. Pack in folded paper inserted inside envelope, plastic bag or plastic container.
- **Hairs and Fibres**:
  - If hairs or fibres are present on a movable item, collect the item.
  - If it is a fixed object, use plastic tweezers or adhesive tape to collect the hairs or fibres.
  - Pack in folded paper inserted inside envelope, plastic bag or plastic container.

- **Clothing (Figs. 2.43 & 2.44)**:
  - Photograph, note and describe.
  - Remove clothing from body over clean white paper, air dry and pack.
  - Pack trace material from clothing separately.
  - Pack in paper bags. Each item must be placed in a separate bag.
- **Ammunition**:
  - Projectiles, cartridges, shot or wads, must be wrapped in tissue paper or small plastic bags.
  - Each item is placed in a separate plastic or cardboard container.
  - It is advisable not to mark ammunition. Label the container instead.
  - Wash projectiles and air dry, if removed from the body. Pack each item separately in plastic or cardboard container.
- **Cigarette butts**:
  - Collect with plastic tweezers, air dry and pack.
  - Look for trace evidence: lipstick, fingerprints, etc.
  - Pack each butt separately in plastic or glass vials.

All packed evidentiary items must be labelled and sealed.

Recording Evidence at Crime Scene

This can be done by:

- **Photography**: Must be done preferably by a police photographer. There are specialized techniques for effective indoor and outdoor photography (**Fig. 2.45A** & **B**).
- **Videography**: Not always required.
- **Sketching**: Must always be undertaken. The forensic expert at the scene can himself draw the scene, taking care to label the various components of the crime scene in relation to nearby landmarks (**Fig. 2.46**).

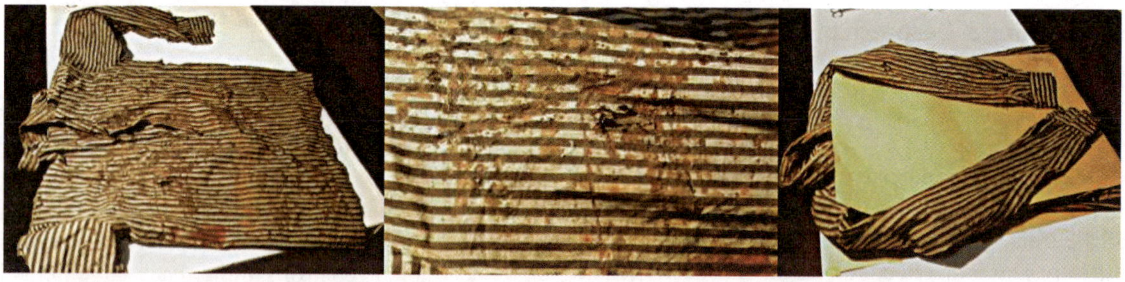

Fig. 2.43 Protecting a cut on the shirt, and method of packing (*Courtesy*: *Dr MB Rao*)

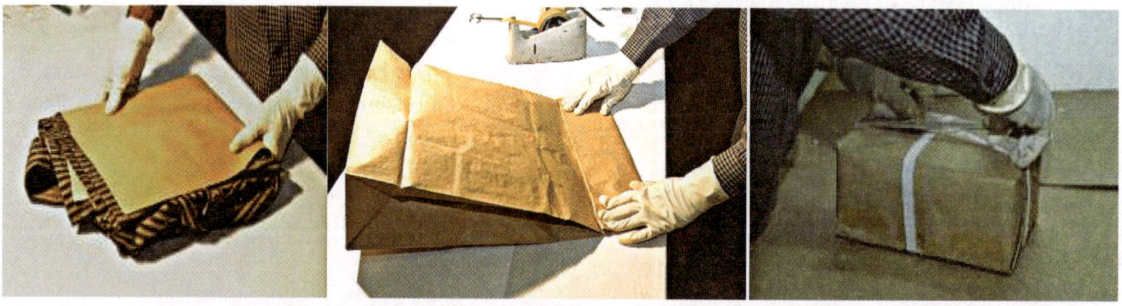

Fig. 2.44 Packing and sealing blood stained clothing (*Courtesy*: *Dr MB Rao*)

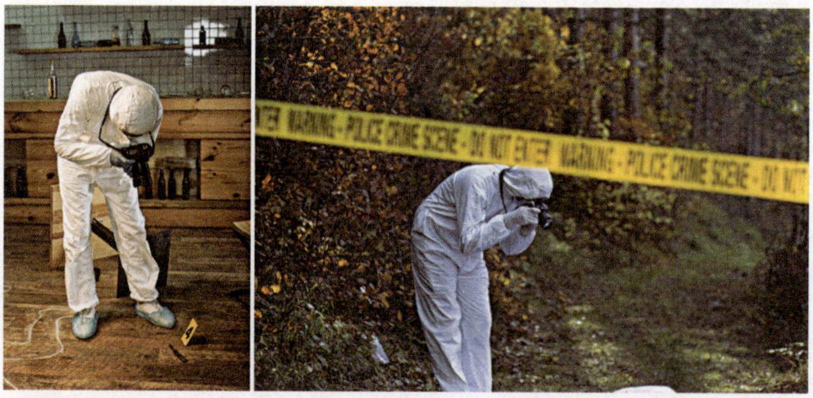

Fig. 2.45 Crime scene photography: **(A)** Indoor; **(B)** Outdoor

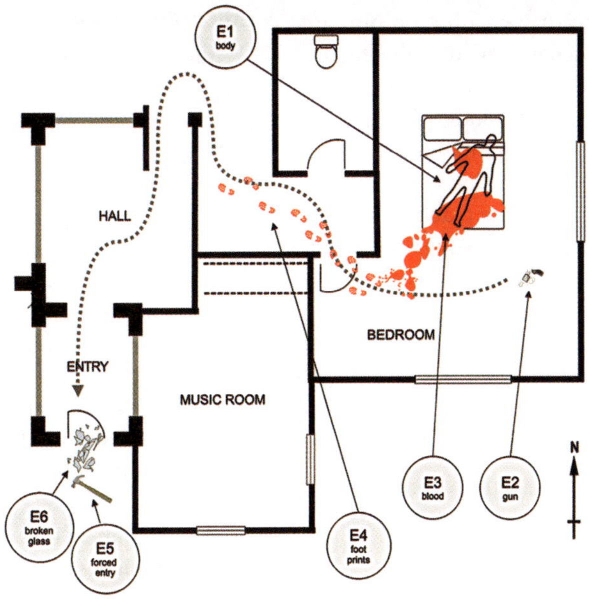

Fig. 2.46 An example of a crime scene sketch

> **FM 2.19: Core – Written/Viva Voce**
> - Investigation of anaesthetic, operative deaths:
>   - Describe and discuss special protocols for conduct of autopsy and for
>   - Collection, preservation and dispatch of related material evidence

SURGICAL AND ANAESTHETIC DEATHS

Causes of Surgical and Anaesthetic Deaths

A. **Those Directly Caused by the Disease or Injury for which the Operation or Anaesthetic was Necessitated**

a. In the advanced stage of some diseases, a heroic effort may have to be taken to save the life of the patient, and if such intervention leads to the death of the patient, the disease from which he was suffering is cited as the cause of death, and the intervening procedure is not taken into account. But in cases where the patient had been relatively well, when he was wheeled into the operation theatre and is subsequently brought out dead, the suspicion of the relatives may be aroused, and such death might lead to an investigation.

b. The American Society of Anesthesiologists (ASA) has classified deaths during surgical procedures as follows:

i. ASA Risk I: Normal healthy patient.
ii. ASA Risk II: Mild systemic disease.
iii. ASA Risk III: Severe systemic disease limiting activity but not incapacitating.
iv. ASA Risk IV: Incapacitating systemic disease that is a constant threat to life.
v. ASA Risk V: Moribund patient not expected to survive 24 hours without an operation.
vi. E: Emergency operation.

Categories I, II and III require full medicolegal investigation, as death is unexpected in these cases. It is important to note that in those cases, where surgical operation was done in a victim of trauma, it may be impossible to separate the relative contribution of each to death.

B. **Those Caused by a Disease or Abnormality Other than that for which the Procedure was being Carried out**

a. In case death was caused by a disease other than that for which the procedure was carried out, and its existence was known beforehand, the pathologist must evaluate the need for the operation.

b. However, if the disease had not been suspected by the clinicians, or if specialised diagnostic procedures were not available, the death can be excused.

c. But the presence of common conditions such as hypertension, ischaemic heart disease, lung disease, etc., can lead to medicolegal problems, if proper care had not been taken in their diagnosis or treatment.

C. **Surgical or Diagnostic Procedure Mishap**

a. Failure of a surgical technique might be inadvertent as happens in some unusually difficult operative circumstances, or anatomical abnormalities, or it may be accidental due to failure of the equipment, or it might be a result of error or incompetence on the part of the surgeon, in which case he can be sued for negligence.

D. **Mishap or Complication of Anaesthetic Administration**

a. Overdosage of Anaesthetic Agent:

i. True anaesthetic deaths arising out of overdosage of the anaesthetic agent are very rare, and if at all they do occur, it is due to ill-advised polypharmacy.

ii. Though data regarding the blood levels of various anaesthetic agents at different grades of anaesthesia are available in the literature, they are of limited use in practice. The current trend is to achieve a light plane of unconsciousness with a barbiturate or some other hypnotic, accompanied by the inhalation of nitrous oxide and oxygen, along with small quantities of a liquid agent like halothane. Muscular relaxation is achieved by the use of relaxants.

iii. Anaesthetic gases are known to cause dependence (physical or psychological), among anaesthesiologists, dentists and paramedical personnel to whom they are readily available.
   - Etheromania is the dependence caused by ether, and is characterized by rapid onset and sudden abatement. Etheromania is of two types – acute and subacute.
     - In the acute variety, the person becomes delirious, and suffers from hypomania and convulsions leading to death.
     - In the subacute type, the person becomes aggressive and psychotic. It is usually difficult to determine whether the death was due to accidental overdosage or due to suicidal ingestion in such cases.

iv. Muscular relaxation is achieved by the use of relaxants such as gallamine, pancuronium bromide, tubocurarine, etc., which compete with acetylcholine at the motor end plate, or with agents such as succinylcholine, decamethonium iodide, etc., which depolarize the motor end plate rendering it inexcitable to acetylcholine. Whatever be the mode of action, the end result is the same – paralysis – the only difference being the former are long acting agents, while the latter are short acting. Overdose with tubocurarine and pancuronium bromide can be treated with neostigmine, while prolonged mechanical ventilation is the only solution to overdosage with succinylcholine and similar agents.

b. Anaesthetic Misadventure: An anaesthetic misadventure or a critical incident as it is called, is a human error or equipment failure that could have led (if not discovered or corrected in time), or did lead to an undesirable outcome, ranging from increased length of hospital stay to death. Most cases of anaesthetic morbidity and mortality occur from one of the following causes:

i. Complications of anaesthetic procedure.

ii. Human error: A variety of factors associated with human error have been reported: emergency case, lack of experience with technique or equipment, failure to perform a normal check, lack of skilled assistance, restricted access to patient and inadequate supervision of the patient due to distraction, fatigue, inattention, boredom or anxiety.

iii. Equipment failure: Equipment failure is a relatively minor cause of anaesthetic mishaps.

Medicolegal Issues

- While most surgical procedures carry with them an element of risk, there is an increased risk of serious morbidity, and even mortality in the case of complicated procedures, infants, aged patients and persons with pre-existing diseases, especially diabetes, hypertension, endocrine diseases, immunological disorders, etc. Also, emergency surgical procedures generally are associated with greater risk than elective procedures for obvious reasons.
- Lack of empathy and failure of proper communication with the patient and his relatives are the main precipitating factors of negligence suits.
- Anaesthetists and surgeons should ensure the following in order to minimise the possibility of malpractice actions:
  - Always establish a proper physician–patient relationship.
  - Establishment of identity is important in surgery, which also includes the type of surgery to be performed, the side (in bilateral structures), self-identification, i.e., the patient must feel the presence of the doctor during surgery, and lastly re-identification, so that the patient sees the familiar face of doctor on awakening.
  - Informed consent of the patient (or that of a relative) with particular regard to the physical status of the patient, and associated disabilities must be obtained. Legally, separate consent for anaesthesia apart from surgery has to be taken.
  - Documentation regarding pre-anaesthetic evaluation and assessment of the patient, and pre-operative record of events is of vital importance. Automated anaesthesia records systems similar to the 'black-box' in aviation are available, which are clearer and more complete than handwritten records, reduce the workload of the anaesthetist, and can prove to be a valuable tool for retrospective analysis of anaesthetic mishaps.
  - Detailed, written records of the actual anaesthetic administered, the dose, route, etc., must also be ensured. The anaesthetic chart should contain details of premedication given, methods of induction and the periodic recording of the vital parameters at regular intervals as the surgery proceeds. Details of the recovery phase are also to be recorded.
  - A written record must not be modified, once it has been made. If any alteration is done because of a genuine error, it must be done without delay and initialled by the surgeon or anaesthetist in charge, with date and time, stating reasons for such alteration.
  - Regarding any new instrumentation/technology, it is imperative to ascertain whether the anaesthetist had acquired the necessary skill to operate it, by formal training or by the demonstration of a salesperson, as also the rate of success of the procedure in his hands.
  - During the postoperative period (which is usually taken as up to 30 days following a surgical procedure), intensive care is very important, and the patient must be

managed in a specialized intensive care unit with necessary facilities, equipment and trained staff. Prophylaxis against cardiac deaths and deep vein thrombosis (DVT) may be required. For instance, administration of anticoagulants, use of calf pumps and thromboembolic deterrent (TED) stockings are helpful in preventing DVT and pulmonary thromboembolism, two of the commonest postoperative complications.

- All unexpected deaths occurring during the course of anaesthesia, surgery or childbirth or within a short time thereafter should be reported to the police, as they come under the definition of unnatural death. It is always desirable to request for an autopsy to ascertain the cause of the unexpected death. An open approach such as this will enable the doctor to defend himself effectively against possible litigation.
- Apportioning responsibility between the anaesthetist and the surgeon may be difficult in actual practice. Both have contractual obligations to the patient to exercise reasonable skill and care. Each one is responsible only for his own negligent act.
    - The surgeon may be held vicariously responsible for negligence committed by his assistants and nurses, but not any member of the anaesthetic team.
    - The anaesthetist is an independent contractor, and is solely liable for his acts of omission and commission, and vicariously responsible for mistakes committed by his assistants.

Autopsy in a Case of Surgical or Anaesthetic Death*

Role of the Autopsy

- When death occurs following surgery, the role of the autopsy is to determine the cause of death and the impact, if any that the surgery had on the cause of death.
- People who die during or following surgery may die from a wide variety of causes, which can be broadly classified as follows:
    - **Death due to the natural disease for which the operation was performed**, for example, death during an emergency aortic aneurysm repair as a result of a retroperitoneal haemorrhage due to a ruptured abdominal aortic aneurysm.
    - **Death due to a complication of surgery**, for example, death as a result of haemorrhage, wound infection or bone cement implantation syndrome shortly after the instillation of bone cement during a cemented hemiarthroplasty for a fractured osteoporotic femoral neck.
    - **Death due to late complications of surgery**, for example, death as a result of small bowel infarction due to peritoneal adhesions following a right hemicolectomy.
    - **Death due to an anaesthetic complication**, for example, death as a result of malignant hyperpyrexia or allergic reaction to drugs provided.
    - **Death due to metabolic complications**, for example, diabetic ketoacidosis, paralytic ileus or salt–water imbalance.
    - **Death due to an operative or anaesthetic error**, for example, death as a result of peritonitis caused by inadvertent perforation of the transverse colon during a laparoscopic cholecystectomy or incorrect size prosthesis being implanted or death as a result of asphyxia caused by premature removal of an endotracheal tube.
    - **Death due to an unrelated cause**, for example, death resulting from an ischaemic stroke, 3 days after a radical prostatectomy for adenocarcinoma of the prostate, in the absence of disseminated disease.

Pathology Encountered at Autopsy

- The pathologies encountered during an autopsy investigating a postoperative death will depend on the nature of the operation performed, the age of the patient (and the presence or absence of comorbidities) and the interval between surgery and death.
- Common causes of death:
    - Bacterial sepsis (including pneumonia, urinary tract infection, wound infection, peritonitis).
    - Pulmonary thromboembolism.
    - Anastomotic breakdown, particularly bowel.
    - Haemorrhage, potentially at any site.
- Common causes that are less often the direct cause of death:
    - Ischaemic heart disease.
    - Hypertensive heart disease.
    - Intracranial haemorrhage.
    - Chronic obstructive pulmonary disease exacerbation following abdominal surgery.
- Less common causes of death:
    - Malignant hyperpyrexia.
    - Halothane hepatitis.
    - Drug-induced hepatitis (e.g. antibiotic induced).
    - Anaphylaxis.

Clinical Information Relevant to the Autopsy

Autopsies investigating postoperative deaths ideally should only be undertaken once the clinical history has been reviewed. This allows the autopsy pathologist to plan the autopsy examination and to identify questions that the autopsy should seek to answer. If there are areas of concern, discussion with the surgical, anaesthetic and nursing team may be relevant. When reviewing the clinical history the following components should receive particular attention:

- Pre-admission/Admission clerking (past medical history, diagnosis, drug history, allergies)
- Consent form
- Operation note
- Anaesthetic chart
- Drug cards
- Postoperative care (medical and nursing)

***Source**: *Royal College of Pathologists. Guidelines on Autopsy Practice: Postoperative Deaths; May 2019. London, UK.*

- Any ante-mortem histopathology, clinical chemistry, haematology and/or microbiology results.

Autopsy Procedure

External Examination

- Following a postoperative death, the external examination often determines the approach to the internal structures and any devices that exist. Consequently, careful inspection of the body to identify all surgical wounds/scars, cannulae and sites of prior placement of lines, catheters, drains, fixators, etc., is important. These should be recorded in terms of size, if appropriate, with additional commentary on features of infection, poor healing or other pathology, if present.
- The general status of the body should be considered in terms of nutrition, jaundice, oedema, tissue swelling and/or ulceration (often decubitus).
- Evidence of a sepsis-related process in terms of marbling and disseminated intravascular coagulation should be considered and photography may be of particular assistance. If sepsis is likely, appropriate samples for microbiology should be collected before the body is opened.

Evisceration

- Evisceration of the body tissues should be performed by the pathologist undertaking the autopsy, or at least by the anatomical pathology technician in concert with the pathologist, to avoid missing vital pathology.
- The body cavities will need to be opened sequentially, depending on the issues of the case. Thus, incisions may be made outside standard protocols to inspect the under surface of the skin and subcutaneous tissues with regard to drainage lines and other devices.
- The body cavities may be opened likewise in a non-standard fashion to test for issues with the devices implanted. The position of the device and its status (e.g. haemorrhage, infection, misplacement) is often best appreciated at the start of evisceration rather than after organs and tissues have been removed.
- Photography of any pathology is of benefit, as the case progresses.
- The evisceration should include:
  - Opening the body cavities (exploring the surgical wound in the process).
  - Inspection of the contents of body cavities in situ before evisceration.
  - Noting the placement of devices and the presence or absence of any local complications.
  - Removal of pacemakers, defibrillator units, nerve stimulators and other devices.
  - Inspection of surgical anastomoses for evidence of dehiscence.
  - Photography of the organs and devices in situ.
  - Evisceration as usual, taking care to work towards anastomoses so as not to place tension on them/cause artefactual dehiscence.
- Additional samples, beyond those taken in the standard autopsy, are recommended. Where death has occurred during surgery, blood should be sampled for immunology (mast cell tryptase) and lung tissue should be sampled for frozen section histopathological lung examination with an Oil Red O stain to identify fat emboli. Where death occurs after the immediate operative period, deep tissue samples should be collected from the operative site for microbiological culture.
- Medical devices: There are two broad groups of medical devices that can be considered. Firstly, those that are structural and, secondly, those which have direct tissue interaction/functionality.
  - The first group includes metal prostheses associated with joint surgery (hip repair, intramedullary nail, joint spacers, etc.) and the well-recognised intrauterine device for contraception. Of increasing importance are mesh devices used for abdominal and sometimes perineal reconstruction. Close attention to possible sepsis and pronounced sclerosis around these items should be made.
  - The more interactive types of device include classic forms of permanent pacemakers (single lead, dual lead), although defibrillator pacemakers are increasingly seen as standard medical therapy. Likewise, central nervous systems stimulators for epilepsy, auditory loops and bladder stimulators (for cases of spinal cord disease) are to be considered as part of the standard autopsy if they are present. Such implanted electronic devices must be deactivated before the autopsy examination and should be handled in accordance with relevant guidelines.
- Organ retention: In general, whole organ retention is not required, particularly if photography is available. Retention of the heart to permit detailed examination by a cardiac pathologist following complex cardiac surgery may be required.
  - Histological examination: Gross observation alone may miss infections, ischaemia and embolic phenomena. Histological examination of the major organs, generally the heart, lungs, liver and kidneys, is always recommended. Samples of the heart may include one or more pieces of native/graft vasculature, which can usually be mounted in the same block but often also require decalcification for full analysis. The number of blocks from cardiac tissues for analysis can be a matter of one or two blocks but could potentially include multiple samples from the mid-ventricular level tissues and/or samples of the cardiac conduction tissues (pacemaker cases).
  - With the exception of samples retained for frozen section, tissue samples should be fixed in a 10% solution of buffered formalin. Thereafter, routine processing to paraffin is appropriate.

Toxicological Evaluation

- If the clinical history raises concerns that death may have been due to a drug overdose or metabolic derangement (such as ketoacidosis), samples should be collected for toxicological analysis.
- The pathologist should determine whether blood samples obtained in life still exist, as these typically are the most useful for testing. This should be done as a matter of urgency, if the samples are to be retained before they are discarded by the laboratory.
- At autopsy, samples of blood, urine, vitreous humour and gastric contents should be collected.

Microbiology Investigations

- Where the clinical history suggests that death may be due to sepsis, blood from the neck veins or heart should be obtained for culture, ideally before the body is opened.
- Additional samples will depend on whether the history and macroscopic findings suggest a focus of infection. Where a focus is evident, bacteriological samples should be obtained for microscopy, culture and sensitivity.
- It is not necessary to retain samples for virology in every autopsy. Where there is suspicion that death may have been caused or contributed to by a viral infection, samples should be collected for virology. Where no focus of infection is evident, a nasal swab or bronchial swab, and solid fragments of lung tissue, myocardium and brain are required. Samples of cerebrospinal fluid or other fluid collections may be relevant and should be retained for analysis.

Immunological Investigations

- It is not necessary to retain samples for immunology in every postoperative death autopsy. Blood should be retained for immunology, if the clinical history raises the possibility of anaphylaxis as a cause death (for mast cell tryptase analysis).
- If the clinical history raises the possibility of hepatitis, blood should be retained for serology and an autoantibody screening.

Imaging

- Imaging of the body has been available for many decades. Traditionally, plain X-rays have been used, although increasingly postmortem computed tomography and, to a lesser extent, postmortem magnetic resonance imaging are available.
- Any autopsy case with imaging assessment should always have an external review, but can proceed to radiological review promptly, unless the mortuary has a policy of scanning all cases. This is particularly useful in cases of multiple trauma, where assessment of bony structures and body compartments can be readily appreciated in transverse section or reconstructed format. The possibility to combine this with injection of dye into vessels or other hollow structures may assist in understanding the role of any leakage, thrombosis or obstructions.
- Imaging-based postmortem examination should never be undertaken without an appropriate and thorough external examination of the body having been performed by a medical practitioner with appropriate expertise/qualifications.

Arriving at Final Opinion

- The final opinion should set out the pathological sequence logically. The clinicians and relatives are going to study the autopsy report very closely, as may lawyers, and indeed the general public/press.
- Explain the cause of death in lay terms.
- Consider whether death occurred despite surgery or because of surgery.
- Consider whether the autopsy reveals evidence of surgical or anaesthetic error.
- Consult a more experienced pathologist to review the case, autopsy photographs and histology, if the pathology and cause of death are not clear.
- The autopsy alone may not resolve the cause of death in all perioperative and postoperative deaths and a multidisciplinary approach with input from surgeons, anaesthetists and clinical pathologists may assist the forensic pathologist in identifying the most probable/reasonable cause of death.

> **FM 2.20: Core – Written/Viva Voce/OSPE (Objective Structured Practical Examination)**
> - Mechanical Asphyxia:
>   - Define, classify and describe asphyxia
>   - Medicolegal interpretation of postmortem findings in asphyxial deaths

DEFINITION OF ASPHYXIA

- Literally, the term **asphyxia** denotes absence of pulsation (*pulselessness*), though its usage in Forensic Medicine has generally come to mean a lack of oxygen.
- Actually, **asphyxia is best described as an interference with respiration due to any cause – mechanical, environmental or toxic**.
- The term **anoxia refers to a lack of oxygen**.

In this section, we shall focus mainly on the mechanical causes of asphyxia, and not the toxic or environmental causes, which will be discussed under the section on **Toxicology**.

CAUSES OF ASPHYXIA

- Closure of external respiratory orifices: **Smothering**.
- Occlusion of air passage by pressure on the neck: **Hanging, strangulation** or **throttling**.
- Occlusion of air passage from within: **Choking**.
- Lack of oxygen in the atmosphere, or inhalation of irrespirable gases: **Suffocation**.
- Restriction of respiratory movements of the chest or abdomen: **Traumatic asphyxia**.
- Prevention of gas exchange in the lung by fluids: **Drowning**.

- Inability to utilize oxygen by peripheral tissues: **Poisoning** (e.g., cyanide).

Mechanical Asphyxia

The main types of mechanical asphyxia include the following (*mnemonic – HSSD*)

- **H**anging
- **S**trangulation
- **S**uffocation: **G**agging, **O**verlying, **S**mothering, **C**hoking, Traumatic **A**sphyxia, **B**urking (*mnemonic – GOSCAB*)
- **D**rowning

Postmortem Findings or Signs of Asphyxia

1. ***Classical Signs***

- **Oedema and congestion of organs**: When the neck is compressed (as in hanging or strangulation), the venous return gets obstructed. This leads to congestion, i.e., the face, lips and tongue become swollen and red. Sometimes, there is darkening due to cyanosis (*vide infra*). Congestion is associated with tissue swelling, if there is continued venous obstruction. When circulation stops completely with ensuing anoxia, the walls of capillaries become permeable resulting in exudation of fluid from the capillaries into neighbouring tissues, leading to oedema.
- **Petechial haemorrhages**: Due to the impaired integrity of capillary walls, red blood cells escape through, producing small bleeding points, varying from pinpoint to pinhead size. These are known as petechial haemorrhages or **petechiae** or **Tardieu spots** (**Fig. 2.47**). They are also attributed to rupture of venules, and are most commonly seen in the sclera, conjunctiva or over serous membranes such as pleura and pericardium. If the bleeding spots are larger than 2 mm, they are called **ecchymoses**.
- **Cyanosis**: The colour of oxygenated blood is normally scarlet red. When haemoglobin is not fully saturated with oxygen, i.e., it is reduced, the blood assumes a bluish colour. This is known as **cyanosis** (**Fig. 2.48**). For this to happen, there should be at least 5 g of reduced haemoglobin per 100 mL of blood. Cyanosis is especially marked in traumatic asphyxia.

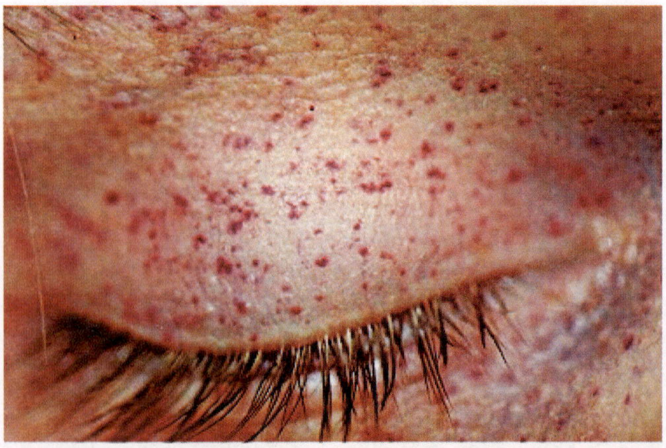

Fig. 2.47 Tardieu spots

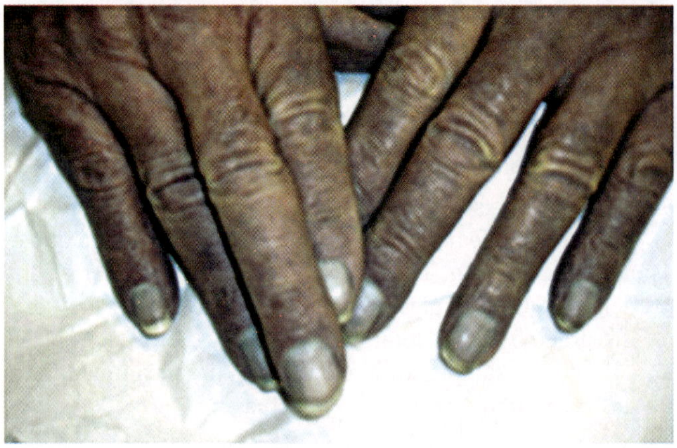

Fig. 2.48 Cyanosis of fingertips

2. ***Non-specific Signs***

- Abnormal fluidity of the blood.
- Dilatation of right chambers of the heart, and great veins.

3. ***Specific Signs***

Signs on the body which indicate the exact way in which the fatal chain of events was initiated, as well as changes which clearly indicate the type of asphyxial death, are referred to as **specific signs**. These include:

- Ligature mark on the neck in hanging.
- Fingernail abrasions on the neck in manual strangulation.
- Fluid medium in the air passages and stomach in drowning.
- Foreign body in the larynx in choking, gagging, etc.

DEFINITION OF ANOXIA/HYPOXIA

Asphyxia from any cause results in **anoxia**, which refers to lack of oxygen; or **hypoxia**, which refers to diminution of oxygen.

CAUSES OF ANOXIA/HYPOXIA

The different types of anoxia/hypoxia (based on the cause) are as follows:

1. **Anoxic Anoxia**

   This is due to **defective oxygenation of blood** in the lungs (hypoxic hypoxia) or a total failure in oxygenation (anoxic anoxia). In vitiated atmosphere such as the bottom of an unused well, or the interior of a granary, silo, or underground sewer, inhalation of inert or toxic gases results in decreased saturation of oxygen in the blood. This can also be due to mechanical interference of the passage of air into or down the respiratory tract caused by smothering, choking, throttling, strangulation and hanging, or by external compression of the chest and abdominal walls as in traumatic asphyxia, or primary cessation of respiratory movements through paralysis of respiratory centre as in the case of electrical injury and certain kinds of poisoning.

2. **Anaemic Anoxia**

   Death initiated by a **reduced oxygen carrying capacity of the blood** is called anaemic anoxia, which may be seen in massive haemorrhage or carbon monoxide poisoning.

3. **Stagnant Anoxia**
   This occurs due to **impaired circulation** resulting in reduction of oxygen delivery, which can be seen in death from shock.
4. **Histotoxic Anoxia**
   Death initiated by **depression of oxidative process in the tissues** is called histotoxic hypoxia or histotoxic anoxia, which can be seen in death due to acute cyanide poisoning.

> **FM 2.21: Core – Written/Viva Voce/OSPE (Objective Structured Practical Examination)**
> - Mechanical Asphyxia:
>   - Describe and discuss different types of Hanging
>   - Describe and discuss different types of Strangulation
>   - Including clinical findings, causes of death, postmortem findings and
>   - Medicolegal aspects of death due to Hanging and Strangulation, including examination, preservation and dispatch of ligature material.

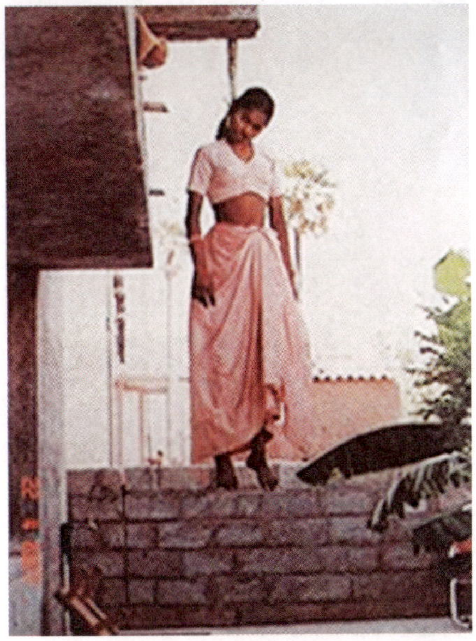

Fig. 2.49 Complete hanging (*Courtesy*: *Dr BM Balaraj*)

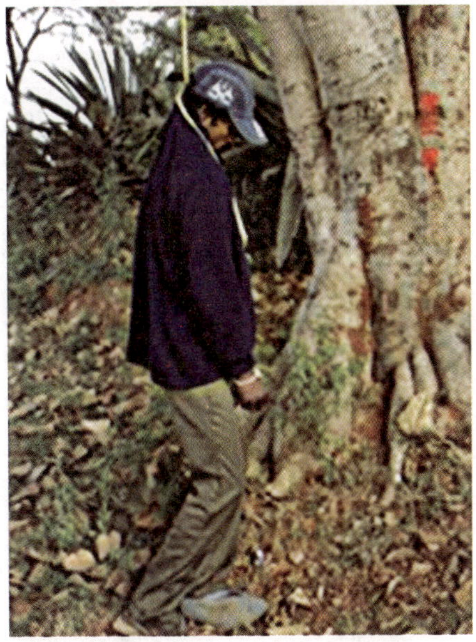

Fig. 2.50 Partial hanging (*Courtesy*: *Dr MD Nithin*)

HANGING

Definition

- **Hanging results from constriction of the neck as a result of suspension of the body by a ligature, where the constricting force is the weight of the body or a part of the body.**
- Hanging should always raise the presumption of suicide, while strangulation (*vide infra*) must always be considered homicidal, unless proved otherwise.

Types of Hanging

- When the feet do not touch the ground and the body is completely suspended by the ligature, it is called **complete hanging** (**Fig. 2.49**). If the body is in a reclining or sitting or kneeling position, or if the feet touch the ground, it is called **partial (or incomplete) hanging** (**Fig. 2.50**).
- When the body is suspended by a ligature running upwards from either side of thyroid cartilage, and the **point of suspension is at the nape of the neck (near occiput)**, it is called **typical hanging** (**Fig. 2.51**).
- When the point of suspension is elsewhere such as **the right or left side of the neck**, or even the **front of the neck**, it is called **atypical hanging** (**Figs. 2.52 & 2.53**).
- Hanging is invariably **suicidal**.
- **Accidental** and **homicidal** hangings are rare.
- **Lynching**: It is a form of homicidal hanging, where a person suspected to be involved in dacoity, murder or rape, is overpowered by a mob, and hanged forcibly from a tree or lamp post.
  - The term "lynching" is derived from the name **Charles Lynch** (1736–1796), a justice of the peace who administered rough and instant justice in Virginia (USA). Lynching was originally a system of punishment used by Whites against African American slaves (Blacks) (**Fig. 2.54**). Today the meaning has been extended to include any act of violence (not just homicidal hanging) inflicted by a mob upon the body of another person which results in death of that person.
- **Judicial hanging**: In some countries (including India), hanging is the mode of legal execution of death sentence (*page no. 82*).
- **Postmortem hanging**: Occasionally, after a victim has been murdered, the body may be suspended to simulate hanging, in order to mislead the police into believing it to be a case of suicide. Findings of asphyxia will not be prominent in such a case.
- **Auto-erotic hanging**: This is also known as sexual asphyxia, and is a rare type of hanging seen mostly in white males in

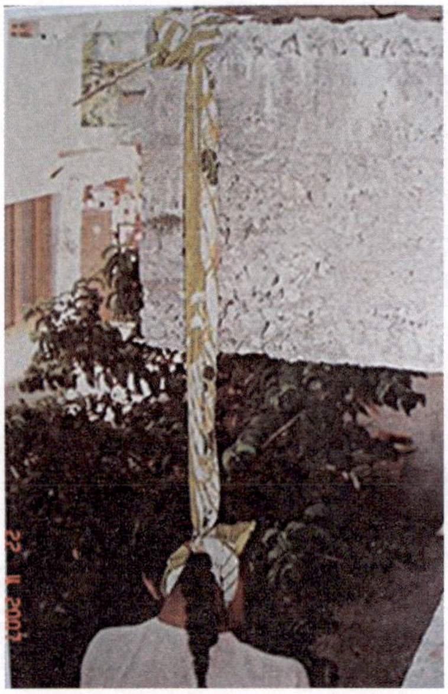

Fig. 2.51 Typical hanging
(*Courtesy*: *Dr BM Balaraj & Dr MD Nithin*)

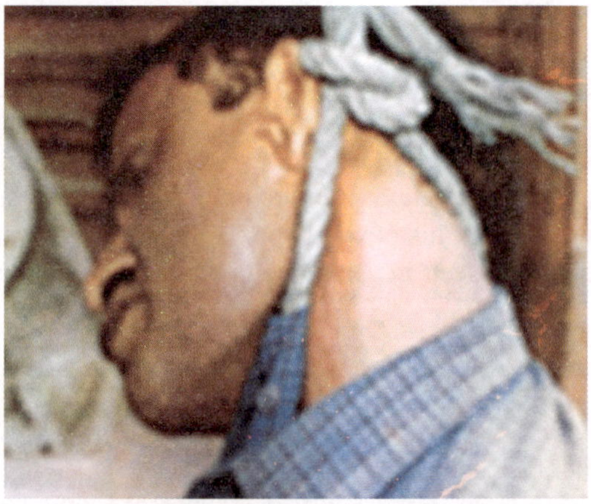

Fig. 2.52 Atypical hanging (knot on left side)
(*Courtesy*: *Dr Shashidhar C Mestri*)

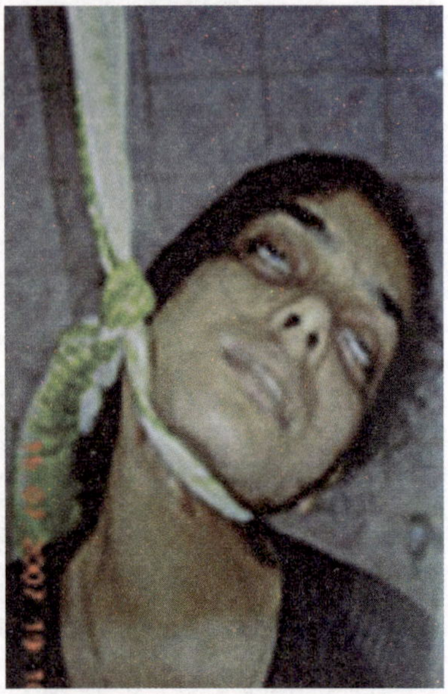

Fig. 2.53 Atypical hanging (knot on right side)
(*Courtesy*: *Dr BM Balaraj & Dr MD Nithin*)

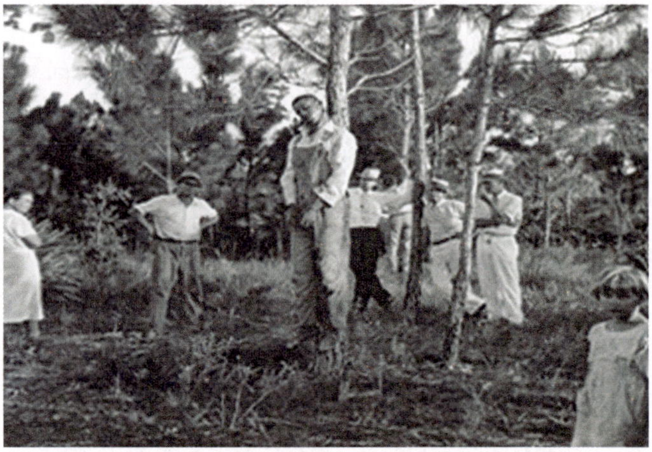

Fig. 2.54 Lynching of a Black male by White community (somewhere in the US in the 1860s)

Western countries. It is one form of sexual paraphilia. The individual partially asphyxiates himself with a ligature. The resulting partial anoxia is believed to enhance sexual pleasure by masturbation.

Clinical Signs & Symptoms

A victim of hanging experiences the following:

- Ringing in the ears (tinnitus)
- Blurring of vision
- Mental confusion
- Loss of power of thought
- Loss of consciousness
- Convulsions, leading to death.

Causes of Death

Immediate Causes

- Prevention of entry of oxygen into respiratory passages (**airway occlusion**).
- Vascular congestion from compression of large veins, subsequently interfering with blood supply to the brain leading to anoxia (**cerebral apoplexy**).
- **Combination of the above**.
- Compression of arteries of the neck with direct anoxic consequences on the brain (**cerebral anaemia**).
- Sudden cardiac arrest due to **reflex vagal inhibition**.

Delayed Causes

- Infection.
- Sequelae of hypoxia to the brain.
- Oedema of the organs, especially the lungs.

Mechanism of Death

- A constricting pressure of just 2 kg is sufficient to compress the jugular venous system leading to intracranial venous congestion. The victim loses consciousness gradually and the inexorable build up of venous engorgement produces cerebral oedema, anoxia and eventually death.
- A constricting pressure of 5 kg obliterates both carotid arteries. The victim loses consciousness rapidly, and the abrupt cessation of blood to the brain results in cerebral anoxia.
- These mechanisms explain why suicide victims may succumb even in cases of partial hanging, where the body does not hang free of the ground. In cases of complete hanging, where the entire body weight is suspended on the ligature and no part of the body touches the ground, there is immediate occlusion of air passage along with obliteration of great vessels in the neck.
- Airway occlusion can be the result of direct compression of the larynx or trachea, or alternatively, the ligature may force the base of the tongue upward and backward against the posterior pharyngeal wall, pushing the soft palate upward and depressing the epiglottis over the laryngeal opening. The pressure needed to occlude the trachea is 15 kg.
- Pressure on the baroreceptors situated in the carotid sinus, the carotid sheaths and the carotid body can result in slowing of the heart or cardiac arrest. The impulses travel to the 10th cranial nerve nucleus through the glossopharyngeal nerve, and return via the vagus nerve to inhibit the heart.

Autopsy Findings

- In every case of hanging, the scene of the incident should be inspected with reference to the type of platform, evidence of stains, signs of struggle, presence of suicide note, or pornographic material (in auto-erotic sexual asphyxia).
- The body should be examined for injuries, type of clothing and the nature of ligature mark.
- **Ligature Mark**
  - The **ligature material** used could be anything from a bed sheet to a leather belt, wire, rope (**Fig. 2.55**), sheet or even a handkerchief, as in most cases there is little premeditation. The length, width and pattern of the material should be noted. The most important point is matching of ligature material with the ligature mark.
  - The ligature material should always be cut away from the knot, and preserved for later laboratory examination (**Fig. 2.56**).
  - An important point relating to the mode of application of ligature is that, a ligature knotted firmly following the first turn, and then knotted after the second turn is unlikely to be a suicide.
  - The position of the knot in suicidal hanging is commonly over the back of the neck, around the occiput (**typical hanging**) or on either sides of the neck (**atypical hanging**).

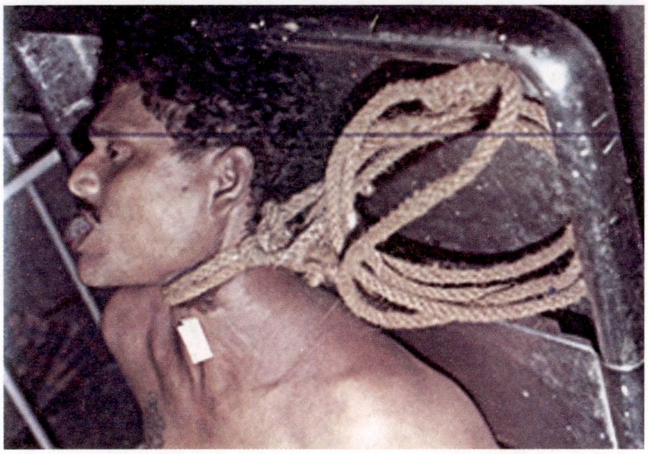

Fig. 2.55 Ligature material – Coir rope (*Courtesy*: *Dr EJ Rodrigues*)

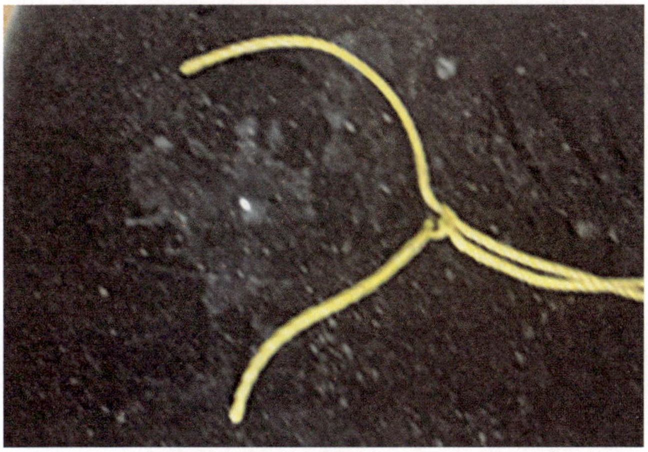

Fig. 2.56 Cutting ligature away from the knot (*Courtesy*: *Dr Prateek Rastogi*)

    - The most common position is on the right side of the neck.
  - The point of suspension chosen by a suicide normally will be one that is within reach, with or without the aid of some platform.
  - The ligature leaves a distinct furrow of its own width and pattern on the skin surface. The bed of the furrow may be pale, and the edges reddish-brown due to abrasion caused by the constriction. Sometimes the entire mark appears reddish-brown. Ecchymosis and congestion of adjacent skin may be seen.
  - Grooving of the ligature mark is due to congestion and associated oedema. These are generally more marked near the upper border of the mark. The ligature groove will be deepest on the opposite side of the knot when the noose is tied with a fixed knot.
  - In general, the thinner and tougher the material used, the more pronounced is the ligature mark (**Fig. 2.57**). Similarly, the softer and broader the material, the less distinct is the ligature mark.

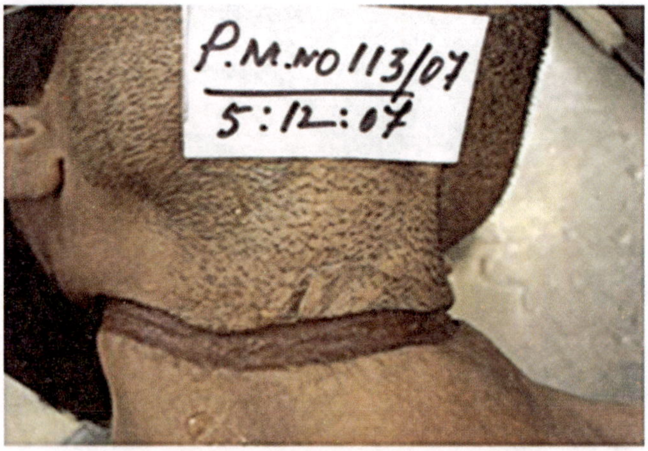

Fig. 2.57 Deep and prominent ligature mark (*Courtesy*: *Dr BM Balaraj & Dr MD Nithin*)

- The skin in the region of the ligature mark is generally dry and hard.
- The pattern of the ligature used often gets imprinted on the skin as a **pressure abrasion**.
- Ligature mark is usually situated above the level of the hyoid bone, and is oblique, passing backwards and upwards symmetrically on either side to the point of suspension. The mark is not seen at the point of suspension, and also in those regions where there is intervening hair or clothing.
- When hanging is from a low point of suspension, the mark may be horizontal and could resemble strangulation, although in hanging it is invariably above the level of the thyroid cartilage.
- There may be more than one ligature mark when the material has been wound around the neck more than once. In such cases, the skin between the ligature marks will appear bruised due to pinching.
- Microscopically, the ligature mark displays the usual characteristics of an abrasion, showing desquamation and flattening of cells of the epidermis. If death has occurred quickly, vital reaction may be quite difficult to demonstrate.
- Hanging can be accomplished even without the use of a noose. For example, suspension could occur from a steering wheel in the case of a vehicular accident, or from the rungs of a ladder when the person who is using it slips while climbing.

■ **The Knot**
- In most cases of suicide by right-handed victims, the knot is situated on the right side because tying of the knot is easier.
- It may be a slip knot as is usual in suicidal hanging, or a binding knot.
  - A **slip knot** (or **running knot**) (**Fig. 2.58**) is generally created by attaching a rope to itself, creating a loop which can be tightened. In other words, the 'tail' of the rope is passed through a small loop on the end of that same rope. This gives rise to a progressively constricting, larger, second loop which is termed '**running noose**'.*
  - A **binding knot** (**Fig. 2.59**) is a knot that uses a rope which passes at least once around the neck, and is held in place by the two ends of the rope being knotted together. This gives rise to a '**fixed noose**'.
- A third type of knot used in professional executions by hanging is the **hangman's knot** (**Fig. 2.60**). This is actually a slip knot having multiple turns in the knot.

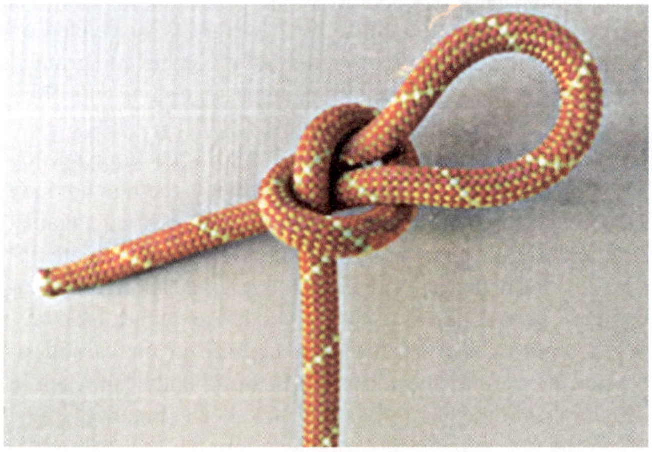

Fig. 2.58 Slip knot

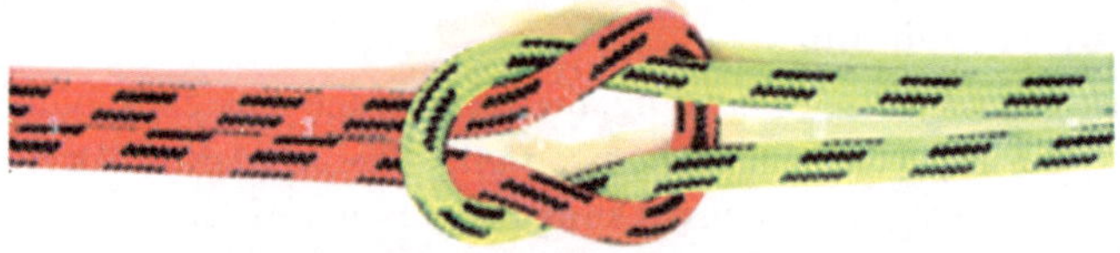

Fig. 2.59 Binding knot

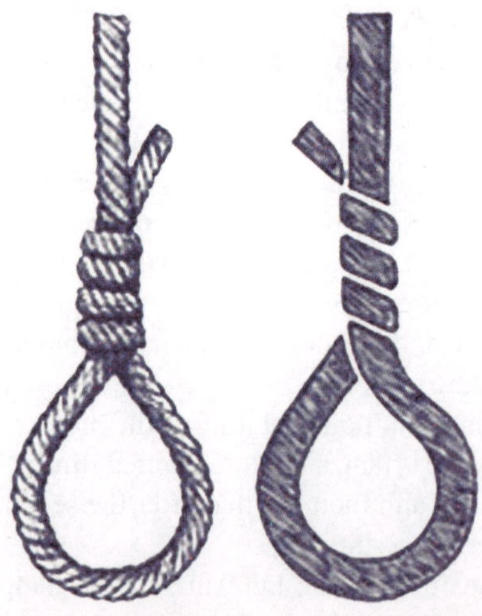

Fig. 2.60 Hangman's knot

**Note*: *Not 'running nose'*!

- The common sites for the knot include the right or left side of the neck, and the occiput. Cases of suspension where the knot is below the chin, are rare.
- The groove is deepest opposite the position of the knot.

■ **Other External Features**
- The face may be congested, puffed up and bluish.
- Bloody froth may be seen in the region of the mouth.
- Postmortem lividity is seen in the distal parts of upper and lower limbs (**Fig. 2.61**), which gets fixed after 6–8 hours. This is because the hands and feet constitute the dependent parts of the body, in the suspended state. If the body remains suspended for a long time, petechial haemorrhages are seen on the lower limbs.
- The head is tilted away from the knot.
- The ligature may press on the salivary glands causing increased salivary secretion, which causes **dribbling of saliva** from the angle of the mouth (**Fig. 2.62**). If the body is viewed later, dried up salivary stains running down from the angle of the mouth on to the front of the chest may be seen. This conclusively suggests the **antemortem nature of hanging**.
- The tongue is protruded and may have been bitten.
- If the knot presses on the cervical sympathetic ganglia, the eye on that side remains open and the pupil is dilated. This is also a vital antemortem feature, and is often referred to as **le facie sympathique** (**Fig. 2.63**).

■ **Neck Dissection**
- Blood often extravasates into the subcutaneous tissues of the neck, beneath the ligature mark.
- Contusion of sternocleidomastoid and platysma may be present.
- The intima of the carotids may be ruptured transversely.
- Occasionally, the **hyoid bone is fractured**. If such is the case, it is more common in the case of a deceased above 40 years of age, in whom the greater cornua have fused with the body.
- As the **hyoid bone** is pressed backwards against the vertebrae, it results in an **anteroposterior compression** or **outward compression fracture** (**Fig. 2.71**, *page no. 87*). This is also called **abduction fracture**. The greater cornua therefore diverge outwards. The broken fragments of the bone also have an outward angulation and can be freely moved only outwards, but cannot be manipulated inwards. The periosteum is torn on the inner aspect of the fracture.

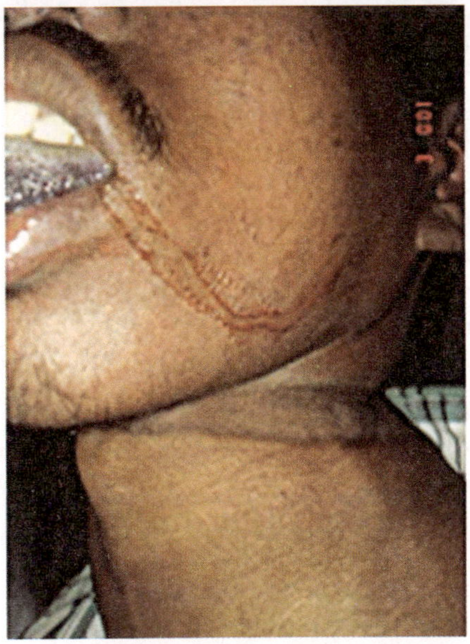

Fig. 2.62 Hanging – Salivary dribbling (*Courtesy*: *Dr BM Balaraj & Dr MD Nithin*)

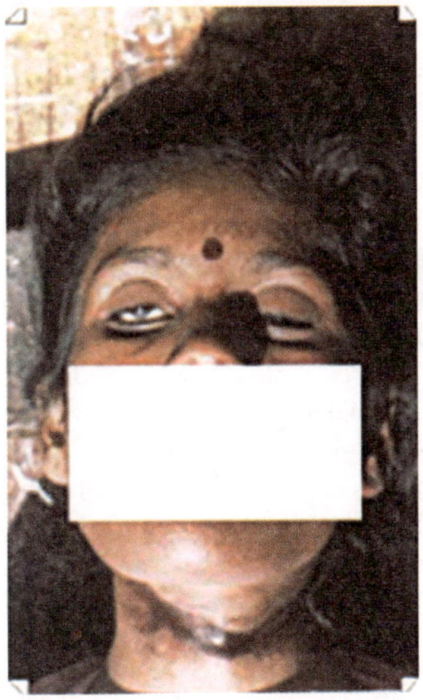

Fig. 2.63 Hanging: Le facie sympathique (*Courtesy*: *Dr Pratik Patel*)

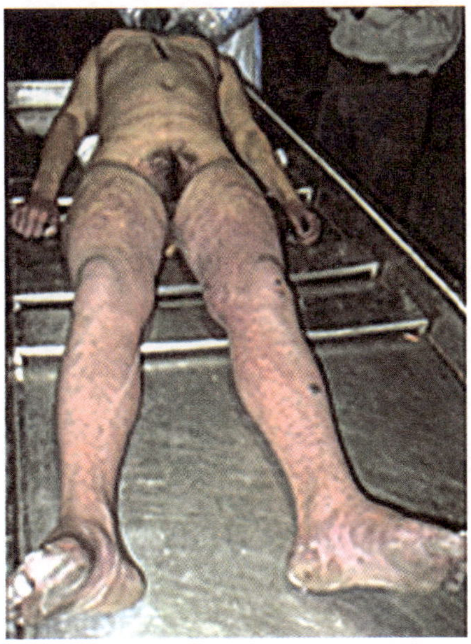

Fig. 2.61 Hanging – PM lividity on dependent parts of limbs

- Superior horn of thyroid cartilage may be found fractured in some cases.
- The lymph nodes of the neck above and below the ligature mark show evidence of congestion, stasis & haemorrhage. This is never seen in postmortem hanging.
- In hanging associated with a long drop, destruction of larynx and fracture-dislocation of cervical vertebrae are common. Punctate haemorrhages may be present in the laryngeal mucous membrane.

- **Internal Features**
  - All the usual signs of asphyxia are generally seen (*76 p*).

Medicolegal Aspects

Hanging is invariably suicidal. Accidental and homicidal hangings are rare.

- **Suicidal hanging**:
  - Any material that is immediately available may be used as ligature material.
  - A foot stool may be found at the scene of death, wherein the person attempting suicide ties one end of the ligature material to the beam or ceiling fan, stands on the stool, adjusts the noose around his neck and steps off the stool.
  - When the feet do not touch the ground and the body is completely suspended by the ligature, it is called **complete hanging**. If the body is in a reclining or sitting position, or if the feet touch the ground, it is called **partial (incomplete) hanging**.
  - When the body is suspended by a ligature which runs upwards from either side of the thyroid cartilage, and the point of suspension is above the occiput, it is called **typical hanging**. When the point of suspension is elsewhere such as the right or left side of the neck, it is called **atypical hanging**.
- **Accidental hanging**:
  - Tragic cases have been recorded of accidental hanging in children who play dangerous games that include simulation of hanging (e.g., cops and robbers). Some have luckily survived.
  - Although by definition hanging is defined as suspension of the body by a ligature, it may occur without the use of a ligature, e.g., being suspended from the rung of a ladder, if one slips while climbing.
- **Homicidal hanging**:
  - This is difficult to accomplish unless the victim is a child, or a weak and feeble individual, or one who is weakened by alcohol or drugs.
  - **Lynching**: It is a form of homicidal hanging where a person suspected to be involved in dacoity, murder or rape, is overpowered by a mob, and hanged forcibly from a tree or lamp post.
- **Judicial hanging**:
  - In some countries, hanging is the mode of legal execution of death sentence. Countries which use this method of execution include India, Pakistan, Bangladesh, Singapore, Malaysia, South Korea, Iran, Iraq, Egypt, Jordan, Lebanon, Kuwait and Syria, besides many countries in Africa and the Caribbean. Two states in the USA offer hanging as an option to the usual method (lethal injection: Washington and Delaware).
  - There are four forms of judicial hanging:
    - **Short drop hanging**: The condemned person drops just a few inches, and his suspended body weight and physical struggling cause the noose to tighten, resulting in death by strangulation or reflex vagal inhibition.
    - **Suspension hanging**: The condemned person is lifted into the air using a crane, and death results in the same manner as for short drop hanging.
    - **Standard drop hanging**: Where the condemned person drops from a pre-determined height, usually 4–5 feet, which may or may not break the neck.
    - **Measured or long drop hanging**: As practised currently in India, where the distance the person falls when the trapdoors open is calculated according to his weight, height and physique, and is designed to break his neck. This method is supposed to be the most humane form of judicial hanging.*
  - The condemned man is first led to the gallows, and his face is covered with a black mask. The noose is adjusted around his neck.
  - He is then made to stand on a platform, which by means of a lever is pulled back, so that he drops down to 5–9 feet usually.
  - When he comes to the end of the rope, there is a violent jerk which causes a fracture dislocation of upper cervical vertebrae. This disrupts the brainstem resulting in instantaneous death.
  - It is to be noted that the **Indian armed forces** (army, navy and air force) also allow judicial execution of somebody who is sentenced to death, by means of **firing squad** (as an alternative to hanging). Section 166 of the Army Act 1950, Section 163 of Air Force Act 1950, and Section 147 of Navy Act 1957 all deal with the way an execution of death sentence is to be carried out and states, "*In awarding a sentence of death, a court-martial shall, in its discretion, direct that the offender shall suffer death by being hanged by the neck until he be dead, or shall suffer death by being shot to death*".
- **Postmortem hanging**:
  - Occasionally, after a victim has been murdered, the body may be suspended to simulate hanging, in order to mislead the police into believing it to be a case of suicide. Findings of asphyxia will not be prominent in such a case.
  - **Table 2.4** mentions the important differentiating points between antemortem and postmortem hanging.

This does not seem to be true as the Supreme Court of India is currently debating its subsitution by alternative (more humane) methods such as* ***lethal injection**, in response to a petition filed in 2017. In May 2023 the Central Govt finally agreed to constitute an expert panel to study the issue.*

Table 2.4 Differences between Antemortem and Postmortem Hanging

	Antemortem Hanging	Postmortem Hanging
Ligature mark	Prominent, reddish (turning brownish and parchment-like with time)	Not prominent
Salivary dribble	Present at angle of mouth (stains may be present over front of chest)	Absent
Le facie sympathique	Present occasionally	Absent
Drag marks on body	Absent	May be present
Rope fibres	May be seen on hands of victim	Absent
General asphyxial signs	Often present	Absent

- **Auto-erotic hanging**:
  - This is also known as **sexual asphyxia**, **asphyxiophilia**, **hypoxiphilia** or **Kotzwainism** (named after the 18th century Czech musician – Frantisek Kotzwara – who indulged in this activity).
  - It is a rare type of hanging seen mostly in White males in Western countries. It is one form of sexual paraphilia. Of late, cases are being reported from India also.
  - The individual (often dressed in female attire) partially asphyxiates himself with a ligature (**Fig. 2.64**). The resulting partial anoxia is believed to enhance sexual pleasure by masturbation.
  - The neck is usually protected by a soft cloth, so that the ligature mark is not seen.
  - Some element of bondage (tying) is also seen in such auto-erotic hanging cases.
  - Pornographic literature may be seen scattered around.
  - These cases invariably occur in secluded or private spots.
  - Death can occur sometimes, since the margin between constriction of neck to enhance sexual pleasure, and that which can lead to fatal asphyxia is very narrow.

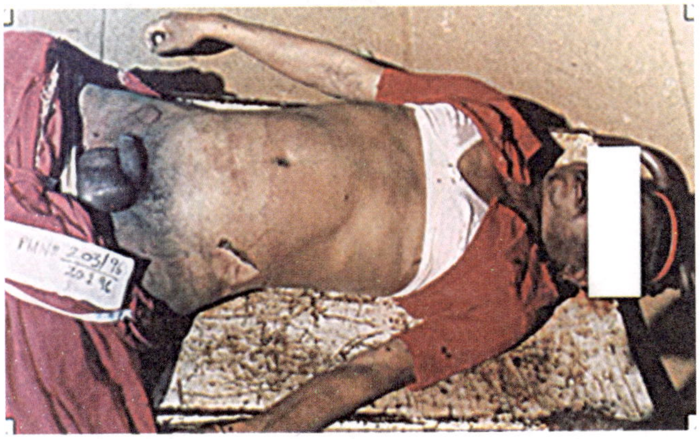

Fig. 2.64 Auto-erotic asphyxial death (*Courtesy*: *Dr Pratik Patel*)

STRANGULATION

Definition

- Strangulation refers to the application of external pressure on the neck either by bare hands, or by a ligature, or by any other material. **It is a form of asphyxia caused by constriction of the neck without suspending the body**.
- Strangulation that is effected by a ligature is called **ligature strangulation**, while that which is accomplished by bare hands is called **manual strangulation**, or **throttling**.

Manual Strangulation (Throttling)

- When the hands are used to squeeze or compress the neck, the resulting asphyxia is called manual strangulation or throttling.
- Occasionally, compression of carotid structures (e.g., carotid sinus), may result in reflex cardiac arrest (**Fig. 2.65**).
- **It is always homicidal**. Rarely, a playful tweak on the neck has resulted in death from vagal inhibition.

Autopsy Findings

- Signs of asphyxia are seen. In addition, the following specific findings may be present:

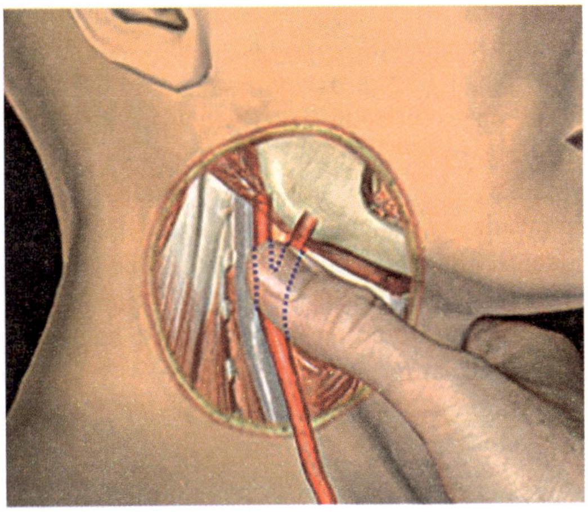

Fig. 2.65 Pressure on carotid sinus during strangulation

- Bruising of the neck: Bruising occurs due to the assailant's fingers grasping the neck. The bruises are usually circular, dark red or purple in colour, and are 1–2 cm in size (formerly called '***six penny bruises***').* If the fingers slide over the skin, elongated marks may be seen.
- Abrasions on the neck: Scratches may be caused by the fingernails of either the assailant or the victim. They may be curved or linear. During autopsy, scrapings from under the fingernails of the deceased may be taken for DNA fingerprinting and compared with that of the suspect, because the victim may have scratched the assailant in an attempt to ward off the attack.
- Internal appearances: The tissues of the neck are often markedly contused. Bleeding may be seen in the strap muscles or platysma. If excessive force has been applied, bleeding from larynx may have occurred.

Ligature Strangulation

- Material used for ligature strangulation can be anything from flexible rubber tubing to cloth, or sticks, wooden planks, belt, wire, rope, etc. (**Fig. 2.66**).

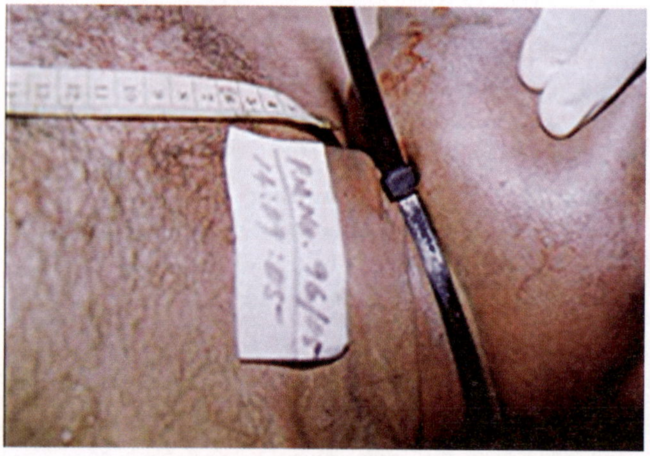

Fig. 2.66 Ligature strangulation (*Courtesy*: *Dr BM Balaraj & Dr MD Nithin*)

- The ligature is usually wound transversely around the neck, sometimes with several turns, and is often below the level of the thyroid cartilage.
- Intense congestion of the face, bleeding from nose, mouth and even ears are characteristic features.
- Involuntary passage of urine, defaecation, etc., are more common than in hanging.
- In infants, homicidal strangulation may be brought about by winding the umbilical cord around the neck.
- Variations of ligature strangulation include **bansdola, mugging** and **garroting**.
  - **Bansdola**: In this form of strangulation, a wooden pole or rod is placed over the front of, and another behind the neck. One end of these rods is fastened together by a rope. The other ends when forcefully brought together squeeze the neck to cause death.
  - **Mugging**: It is brought about by squeezing the neck of the victim in the crook of the elbow, or the bend of the knee.
  - **Garroting**:
    - This was a method of judicial execution in some countries. The victim is made to wear a neck collar of metal. Death is brought about by tightening the collar.
    - Garroting may also be effected by an assailant who comes up behind a seated victim, throws a ligature around his neck and pulls it tight. This was popular among the Mafia gangs of the USA, who employed it to execute their enemies (**Fig. 2.67**). Since there is an upward pull, the resulting ligature mark may resemble that of hanging. The ligature that is used in such cases is called a **garrote**, which consists of two wooden handles attached to a length of flexible wire (**Fig. 2.68**); the wire is looped over the victim's head and pulled taut in one motion.

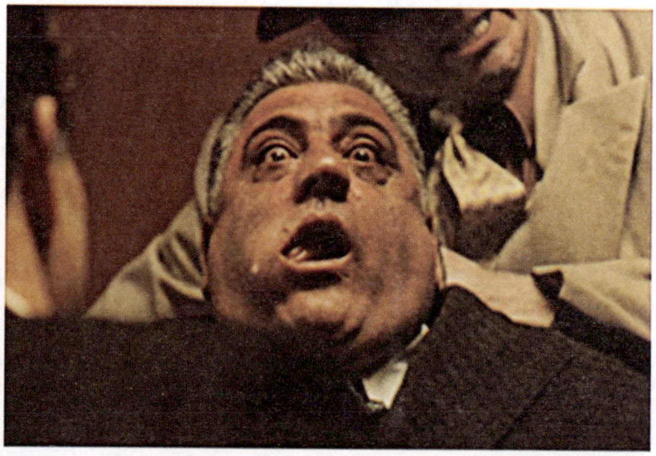

Fig. 2.67 A scene depicting a man (Luca Brasi) being garroted in the film 'The Godfather'

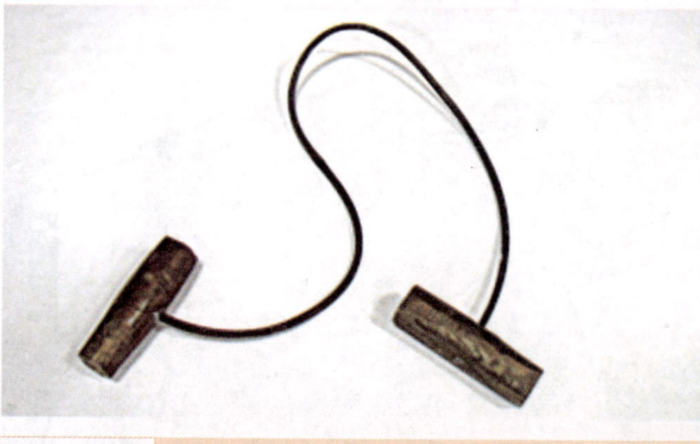

Fig. 2.68 Garrote

**Why should we call these 'six penny bruises'? Has anybody in India seen a six penny coin?? In fact, even in Britain where these coins were minted, stopped their circulation from 1980 onwards.*

Autopsy Findings

- Classical and non-specific signs of asphyxia are prominent.
- Tongue is often protruded.
- Bleeding from the ears or the nose may be seen.
- The **ligature mark** is usually seen as a depression around the neck because of the oedema of the tissues above and below it (**Fig. 2.69**).
  - The skin over the mark is invariably dry and hard. The base of the mark appears pale, while the edges may show small abrasions.
  - The width of the mark depends on the ligature used. The pattern of the ligature may get imprinted on the skin as a **pressure abrasion**. The mark is usually situated around the middle of the neck at the level of the thyroid cartilage, in contrast to the higher location in hanging.
  - In most cases, it runs horizontally, contrasting with the oblique direction in hanging. Sometimes, several turns may have been effected with the ligature, which is then secured with one or more knots.
  - The ligature mark completely encircles the neck in strangulation, while in hanging it is absent near the point of suspension.
  - The position of the knot is indicated by a wider impression on the skin. The type of knot is generally a binding knot.
  - The occurrence of a narrow zone of engorgement or bruising immediately above and below the groove, confirms that the victim was alive at the time when the ligature was applied. In addition, abrasions may be present. Fingernail marks, sometimes linear and vertical may also be present, suggesting efforts on the part of the victim to ease the pressure of the ligature.
  - Even if putrefaction has set in, the ligature mark usually remains distinct.
- Asphyxial component is always more pronounced in strangulation, as compared to hanging.
- Carotid arteries often show transverse intimal tears.
- **Fracture** of left or right superior horn of **thyroid cartilage** is a common feature. If more force is applied, there may also be fracture of cricoid cartilage and tracheal rings.

Medicolegal Aspects

- Strangulation is usually homicidal.
- Suicidal strangulation is rare, because once anoxia sets in, the pressure over the neck gets relaxed. In very rare cases, suicide may be effected successfully by strangulation when the victim manages to keep the ligature tight by knotting it, or twisting it, sometimes employing a stick as a lever.
- Accidental strangulation is rare, but it may occur when an article of clothing such as a dupatta, neck band or cord gets tightly drawn around the neck, in an abrupt manner.
- **Pseudostrangulation**: In the neck of a dead (obese) person or infant, the skin folds may sometimes mimic ligature marks, which may be confused with strangulation marks. However, dissection will reveal the absence of bruising or abrasions.
- The important differentiating points between hanging and strangulation are mentioned in **Table 2.5**.

FRACTURES OF HYOID & THYROID

- The locations of hyoid bone and thyroid cartilage in the neck are depicted in **Fig. 2.70**.
- The hyoid bone calcifies, i.e., it becomes a single bone, by the age of 40–45 years. In younger individuals, it is usually cartilaginous and hence fractures are uncommon.
- The thyroid horns are especially vulnerable to pressure on the neck.
- Antemortem fractures of the thyroid and hyoid are diagnosed by evidence of haemorrhage around the fracture site, with blood spots under the periosteum.
- The broken region may be slightly crepitant.
- Microscopically, there may be extravasation of RBCs.

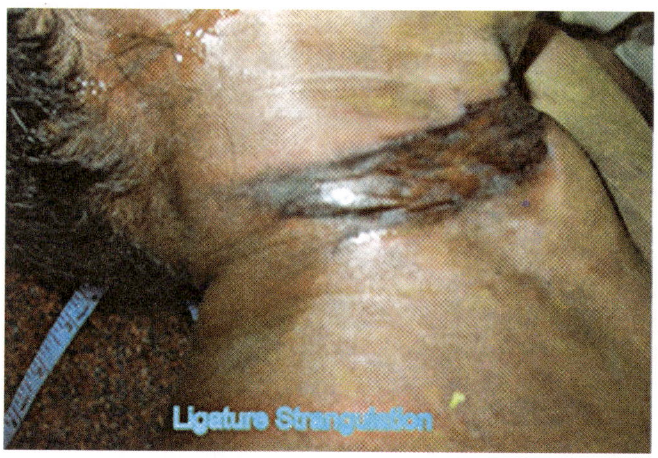

Fig. 2.69 Strangulation – deep furrow in the neck (*Courtesy: Dr Shashidhar C Mestri*)

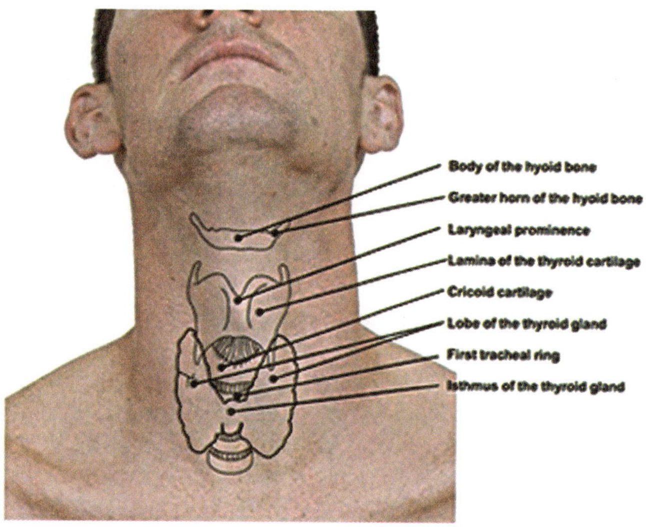

Fig. 2.70 Location of hyoid bone and thyroid cartilage in the neck

Table 2.5 Differences between Hanging and Strangulation

	Hanging	Strangulation
Ligature mark	▪ Oblique, above the level of thyroid cartilage. ▪ Not encircling the neck completely. ▪ Base is pale, hard and parchment-like.	▪ Transverse, at or below the level of thyroid cartilage ▪ Completely encircling the neck with crossing of the ligature mark. ▪ Base is soft and reddish.
Neck injury	▪ Neck may appear stretched or elongated. ▪ Under the ligature, on reflection of skin, tissues look pale. ▪ Bruising of neck muscles is less common.	▪ Neck is not overstretched. ▪ Under the ligature, on reflection of skin, tissues are reddish. ▪ Bruising of neck muscles is more common.
Hyoid bone	Fracture may occur.	Fracture is uncommon.
Thyroid cartilage	Fracture is less common.	Fracture is more common.
Larynx and trachea	Damage is rare.	Damage is more common.
Carotid arteries	May be damaged.	Intact
Signs of asphyxia	Less prominent.	More prominent.
Face	Pale, petechiae uncommon.	Congested, livid & marked with petechiae.
Tongue	Swelling and protrusion less marked.	Swollen and protruded markedly.
Bleeding	From ears, nose and mouth is less common.	From external orifices is more common.
Involuntary discharge of urine, faeces	Uncommon	Common
Saliva	Dribbling often present.	Absent
Seminal emission	Can occur.	Absent

- There are three types of hyoid bone fractures:
  - **Antero-posterior** or **Outward compression type (Abduction fracture)** – Most often seen in cases of **hanging**, where the hyoid bone is forced backwards due to which the divergence of the greater horns is increased, resulting in a fracture with outward displacement of the fractured fragment. The periosteum is disrupted on the inner side alone and the fragment can be easily moved outwards, but inward movement is restricted.
  - **Inward compression type (Adduction fracture)** – Seen in **throttling**, where the greater horns are squeezed towards each other by the constricting hand as a result of which the bone gets fractured with inward displacement of fractured fragment. The periosteum is therefore disrupted on the outer side alone, and the fragment can be easily moved inwards, but outward movement is restricted.
  - Rarely, a third type of hyoid bone fracture occurs called **avulsion**, **traction** or **tug fracture**, which results from muscular overactivity. It is an indirect type of fracture without direct injury to the hyoid.

FM 2.22: Core – Written/Viva Voce/OSPE (Objective Structured Practical Examination)

- **Mechanical Asphyxia:**
  - Describe and discuss pathophysiology, clinical features, postmortem findings and medicolegal aspects of traumatic asphyxia
  - Describe and discuss obstruction of nose & mouth, suffocation and sexual asphyxia

*This Competency is to do with **suffocation** as a form of **mechanical asphyxia**, and will be discussed as such.*

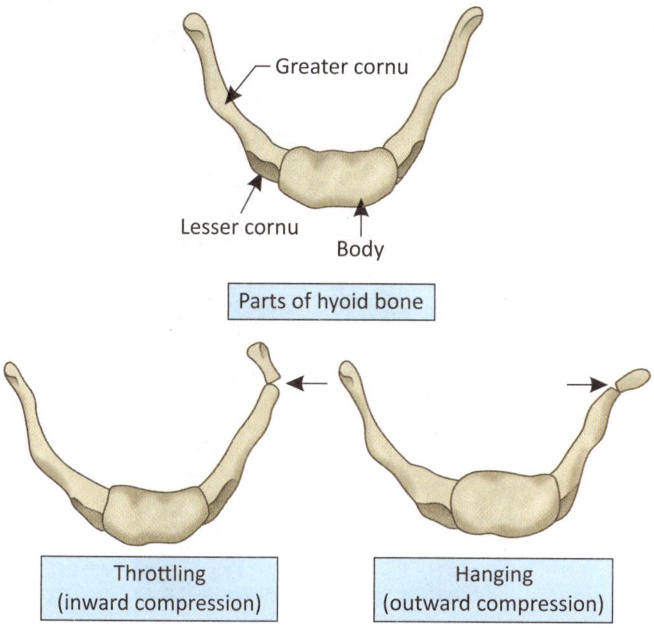

Fig. 2.71 Hyoid bone fracture types

SUFFOCATION

Definition

- **Suffocation is a type of mechanical asphyxia caused by obstruction of the passage of air into the lungs (excluding constriction of the neck and drowning).**

Causes/Types

Suffocation may be produced by:

- **External means**: By closure of mouth and nostrils, e.g., **smothering**, **overlying** (also referred to as **overlaying**), or by pressure over the chest or abdomen, e.g., **traumatic asphyxia**.
  - A combination of **smothering** and **traumatic asphyxia** is called **burking**.
- **Internal means**: Closure of glottis or mouth by insertion of soft cloth, paper, etc., e.g., **gagging**, or impaction of a bolus of food or foreign body deep into the airways, e.g., **choking**.
- **Environmental causes**: This refers to death caused by reduction of oxygen in the atmosphere. This may occur in a wide variety of situations such as **decompression**, **high altitude**, **vitiated atmosphere**, etc.

To summarise, **suffocation** includes gagging, overlying, smothering, choking, traumatic asphyxia (crush asphyxia), burking and inhalation of irrespirable gases.*

Smothering

- Here, death is due to **mechanical occlusion of the mouth and nose**, for instance by pressing a pillow or any other soft material over the mouth and nose, or by manually closing these orifices (**Fig. 2.72**).

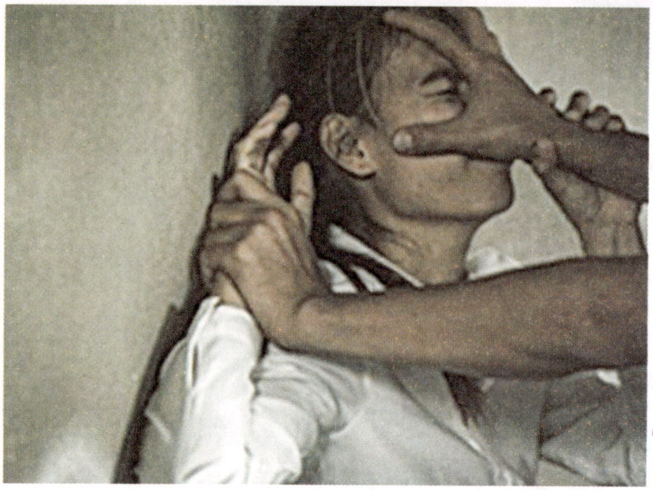

Fig. 2.72 Manual smothering

- Infants and elderly individuals are the usual victims of smothering.
- A circular pale area around the mouth and nose is often seen.
- Discolouration, congestion, petechiae, etc., may be seen over the face and in the eyes (**Fig. 2.73**).
- Scratches and nail marks on the face of the victim are also frequently present.
- Lips, gums and tongue may show bruising and lacerations.
- Internally, intra-thoracic petechiae are common.
- **Plastic Bag Suffocation**: This is encountered in children who put their heads in plastic bags for fun. Such accidental deaths have also resulted in sexually deviant adults due to covering of the head with polythene sheet or other impermeable material, during auto-erotic sexual acts (*page 83*). Plastic bags may be used to homicidally smother a victim whose hands are tied, or is unconscious (**Fig. 2.74**).
- **Glue Sniffing/Volatile Substance Abuse**:
  - This is a form of drug abuse indulged in mostly by street urchins of major cities in Western countries, and is being increasingly reported from India also.
  - It involves the inhalation of volatile agents such as paint removers, adhesives, shoe polish, cigarette-lighter fluid, etc. Gasoline or petrol inhalation is also sometimes encountered.
  - In some cases, volatile substances are poured into a plastic bag and inhaled.
  - Volatile substances usually produce euphoria followed by disorientation and unconsciousness, especially when inhalation is through container. On becoming unconscious, the mouth and nose remain firmly fixed on the container. Hypoxia and hypercapnia exacerbate the toxic effects of the substance.
  - Death may result from cardiac arrhythmias.

Choking

- **Choking refers to blockage of the trachea or larynx by a foreign body**, e.g., coins, dentures, fish bones, food particles, seeds, aspiration of vomitus, etc. (**Fig. 2.75**).

*Mnemonic: **GOSCABI***

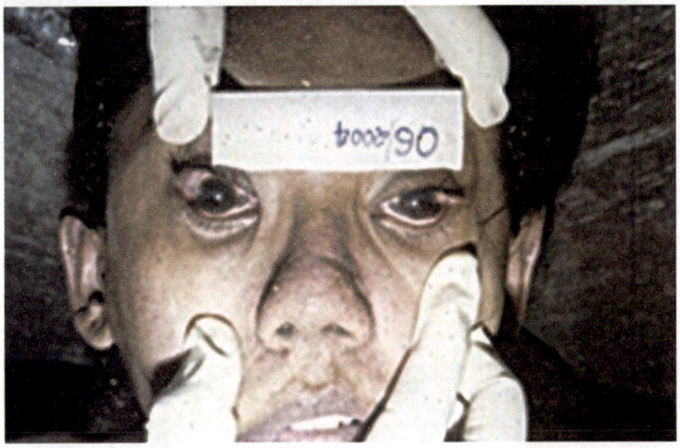

Fig. 2.73 Homicidal smothering (*Courtesy: Dr EJ Rodrigues*)

- Death may result from neurogenic cardiac arrest or hypoxia. If death is due to the latter, all the usual signs such as congestion, cyanosis and petechiae may be present at autopsy.
- Another example of choking is the entry of blood into the airways in a case of cut-throat injury.
- It is important to remember that in order to effectively occlude an air passage, the object need not always be as large as the lumen of the air passage. Even an object smaller in size than the lumen can cause a complete block because of reflex spasm of the respiratory passage.
- **Cafe Coronary**:
  - Although by and large, choking is simple mechanical obstruction, entry of foreign material may in some cases cause death due to vagal inhibition.
  - A person under the influence of alcohol may sometimes choke over a large piece of meat or bone, due to depressed gag reflex.
  - The foreign body in the larynx or trachea causes parasympathetic stimulation from laryngeal nerve endings, which results in cardiac arrest and death.

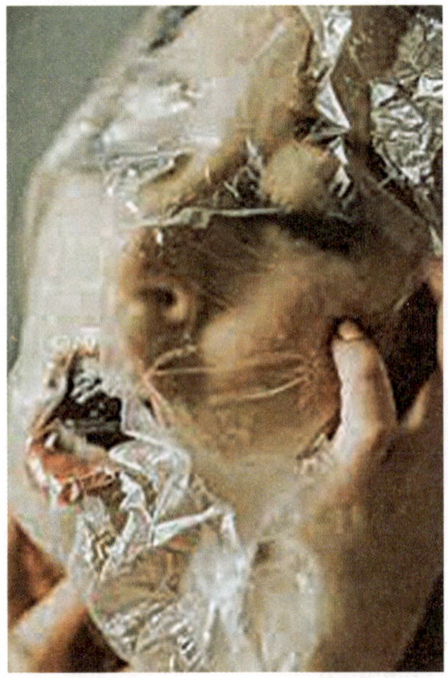

Fig. 2.74 Homicidal plastic bag suffocation

  - This term is actually a misnomer, and was the result of such cases being earlier attributed (mistakenly) to myocardial infarction.
  - When a person chokes on food or any object, a bystander who is present at the scene must apply the **Heimlich manoeuvre (maneuver)** (**Fig. 2.76**):
    - This involves the rescuer standing behind the patient and using his hands with fingers interlinked to exert pressure in the region of the pit of the stomach (just below the xiphoid). This compresses the lungs and exerts pressure on any object lodged in the trachea, hopefully expelling it. It amounts to stimulating an artificial, explosive cough. Due to the forceful nature of the procedure, even when done correctly it can injure the person on whom it is performed. Bruising to the abdomen is highly likely, and if care

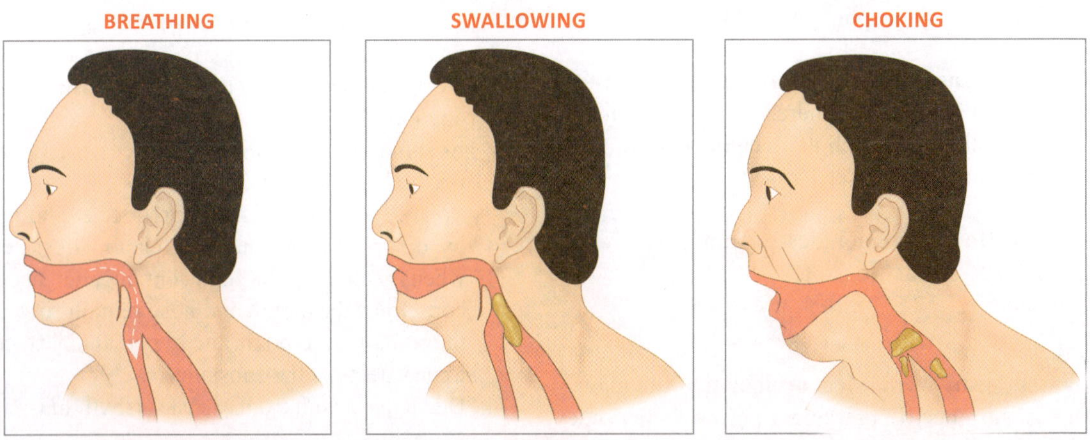

Fig. 2.75 Choking: Food entering the larynx

is not taken, more serious injuries can occur, including fracture of the xiphoid process or ribs.

- The Red Cross recommends a "**Five-and-Five**" (**Fig. 2.77**) approach to delivering first aid:
  - Give 5 back blows: First, deliver five back blows between the person's shoulder blades with the heel of the hand.
  - Give 5 abdominal thrusts: Perform five abdominal thrusts (Heimlich manoeuvre).
  - Alternate between 5 blows and 5 thrusts until the blockage is dislodged.

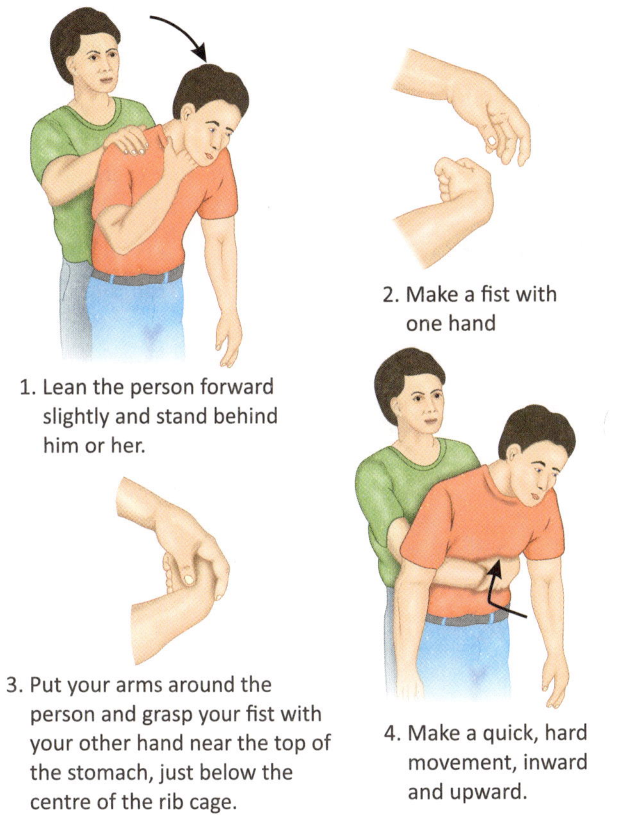

Fig. 2.76 Heimlich manoeuvre

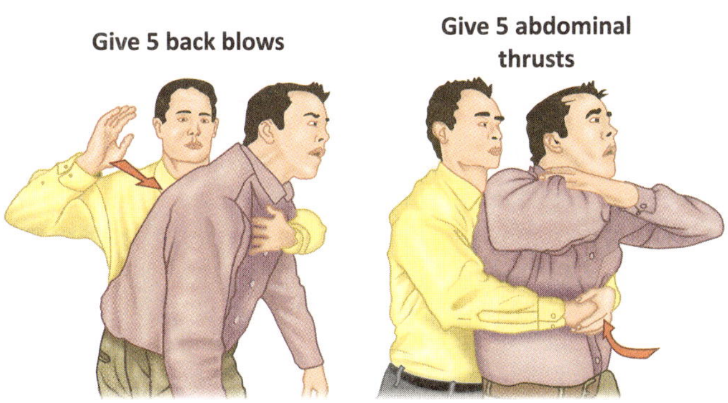

Fig. 2.77 Five-and-Five approach

Gagging

- This is strictly speaking, a form of choking. The usual situation arises from a **soft cloth being thrust into the mouth of a person to render him incapable of shouting**.
- Even if the cloth happens to be small in size, it partially blocks the air passage, soaks up saliva and swells. Due to constant foreign body irritation, there is pooling of saliva, and death subsequently occurs due to obstruction of air passages.
- As is evident from above, it may be accidental when done to render a person speechless in the course of the commission of a crime. It may however be homicidal in infants.

Traumatic Asphyxia (Crush Asphyxia, Compression Asphyxia)

- In this case, death results from **pressure and fixation of the chest and/or abdomen**. Thus, if a person is crushed under a vehicle or in a house collapse, or an earthquake, or in a stampede, the result is traumatic asphyxia. The steering wheel of a motor car violently impinging on the driver's chest in a car accident, is also an example of traumatic asphyxia. Because of the pressure on the chest, the victim is unable to breathe and dies of asphyxia.
- As would be evident from the foregoing, traumatic asphyxia is mostly an accidental phenomenon.
- **Autopsy findings**:
  - Gross congestion, cyanosis and petechiae of the face, neck and shoulders are the most remarkable findings (**Fig. 2.78**).
  - There is often a very dark discolouration of the body above the level of constriction.
  - Instead of petechiae, haemorrhages are frequently seen in the conjunctivae.
  - Copious bleeding may occur through the ears and nostrils.
  - There may be injuries resulting from the heavy object pinning the chest.
  - Internally
    - Subpleural haemorrhages and Tardieu's spots are observed.
    - The right heart and all the veins above the atria are markedly distended. The blood is forced back into the great veins due to pressure on the chest. As the venous valves in the subclavian vessels prevent displacement into arms, the extra volume is forced up the valveless jugular system to cause congestion of the head and the neck. All the appearances of asphyxia (external and internal), are intensely pronounced.
    - Injuries to the chest, including fractures of the ribs and lacerations of the lungs and heart may be seen. If ribs are fractured, they are usually bilateral, multiple and involve the angles of the ribs.

- In a steering wheel impact, there may be a transverse fracture of the sternum at the junction of the manubrium with the body (***buckled sternum***).

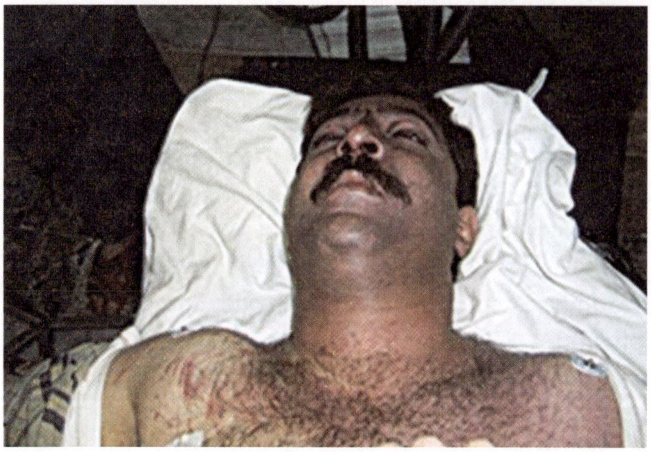

Fig. 2.78 Traumatic asphyxia – Intense congestion of face and upper chest

Overlying (Overlaying)

- This occurs when a parent or some other adult shares the same bed with an infant. **During sleep, he/she may inadvertently roll over the infant, asphyxiating it**.
- Along with petechial haemorrhages, there may be evidence of flattening of the nose and face.
- A clear pattern of the object (fabric) involved in compression, is sometimes seen on the infant's cheek or body.
- There may be bloodstained froth at the mouth and nose.

Burking

- This term is derived from the notorious criminal **William Burke**, who with his accomplice **William Hare**, killed old people (mostly beggars and tramps) by a **combination of smothering and traumatic asphyxia**, and sold the bodies to the medical school in Edinburgh (**Fig. 2.79**).
  - The **Burke and Hare murders** were a series of 16 killings committed over a period of about 10 months in 1828 in Edinburgh, Scotland.
  - The infamous duo would select victims who had no relations or friends (so that police complaints could be avoided), invite them to their derelict apartment and ply them with alcohol.

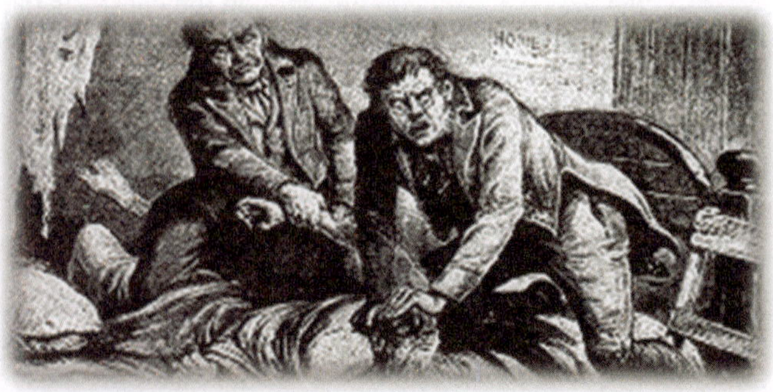

Fig. 2.79 Burking

- As soon as their guest was drunk enough, Hare would wrestle him to the floor and close his mouth and nostrils with his hands, while Burke would sit on the poor victim's chest. Thus, an effective combination of intoxication and asphyxia (involving **smothering** and **traumatic asphyxia**), would result in a quick, non-messy death.
- The dead body would then be delivered to the Anatomy Department of Edinburgh Medical School (which had a perpetual shortage of cadavers for dissection), and invariably received by Professor Robert Knox, who paid handsomely for each corpse!
- Both Burke and Hare were arrested, but as the latter turned approver, only Burke was convicted. He was hanged shortly afterwards, and his body was dissected in the very same medical school, where he used to deliver his macabre goods! Burke's skeleton is preserved to this day in the Anatomy Department of Edinburgh Medical School.

SEXUAL ASPHYXIA

Discussed on page 83 (under Auto-erotic Hanging).

> **FM 2.23: Core – Written/Viva Voce/OSPE (Objective Structured Practical Examination)**
> - **Mechanical Asphyxia:**
>   - Describe and discuss types, pathophysiology, clinical features, postmortem findings and medicolegal aspects of drowning.
>   - Diatom test and Gettler test.

DROWNING

Definition

- **It is a form of asphyxial death which results from complete or partial submersion of a person in a liquid medium.**
  - Death occurs due to entry of fluid into the respiratory passages, or due to the effects of severe water and electrolyte imbalance.

Mechanism

In order to understand the mechanism as well as the autopsy findings, it is necessary to appreciate what happens when a person (who cannot swim) falls into water.

- Initially, he sinks to a depth directly proportional to the momentum of the fall. The inherent buoyancy however tends to make the person float rather than sink. Additionally, his struggling movements, and the air trapped in the clothes help him to rise to the surface.
- In his desperate attempts at inhaling air, large gulps of water enter the throat, and may be partly inhaled and partly swallowed. The water which inadvertently enters the respiratory passages acts as a foreign irritant, and excites a strong reflex. Consequently, a large volume of air is driven out of the lungs.

- There is therefore a greater need for air, and the vicious cycle of drowning continues till a large quantity of water enters the lungs.
- Asphyxia consequently occurs, which leads to insensibility, and the victim finally succumbs.
- The barotrauma to the middle ear results in haemorrhages which causes vestibular disturbance, and this makes the victim lose his sense of direction under water.
- During the struggle for life under water, the victim may grasp anything within his reach. This accounts for objects such as weeds or mud occasionally found grasped in the hand of the victim, as a manifestation of **cadaveric spasm**.

Types of Drowning

A. ***Wet Drowning***:

- In this type of drowning (the commonest type), water is completely inhaled into the lungs.
- **Freshwater Drowning**:
  i. Drowning in fresh water causes dilution of the blood up to 70%, within a couple of minutes.
  ii. This causes **haemodilution** resulting in lysis of RBCs, which in turn leads to hyperkalaemia and hyponatraemia.
  iii. The circulation becomes overloaded.
  iv. Fresh water also denatures surfactant, which causes decreased lung compliance.
  v. There is a fall in systolic blood pressure.
  vi. Myocardial anoxia occurs, and death results from ventricular fibrillation.
- **Seawater Drowning**:
  i. Seawater constitutes a hypertonic medium.
  ii. Due to **haemoconcentration**, as much as 40% of water from circulating blood is withdrawn into the lungs and massive pulmonary oedema is produced.
  iii. There is increased serum sodium concentration (hypernatraemia).
  iv. Pulmonary oedema and myocardial anoxia cause death.

  Death in freshwater takes 2–3 minutes, whereas it is delayed up to 4–5 minutes in seawater (**Table 2.6**).

B. ***Dry Drowning***:

- The water enters the larynx, but is prevented from entering the lungs due to immediate and severe laryngeal spasm.

C. ***Secondary Drowning (Post-immersion Syndrome)***:

- Death occurs due to secondary effects of drowning, after a gap of half an hour to a few days following resuscitation.
- Death is due to cerebral anoxia and irreversible brain damage, associated with electrolyte disturbances and metabolic acidosis. Bronchopneumonia is also common.

D. ***Hydrocution (Immersion Syndrome)***:

- Death results from cardiac arrest due to vagal inhibition, as a result of cold-water stimulation of the nerve endings on the surface of the body, the epigastrium and the ear and nasal passages.

Causes of Death in Drowning

- Asphyxia
- Ventricular fibrillation
- Myocardial anoxia
- Laryngeal spasm
- Vagal inhibition
- Exhaustion
- Head injuries (from striking against objects during a fall into river, well, etc.).

Autopsy Findings

External Appearances

- The clothing is wet.
- The skin is wet, cold and clammy. It appears pale due to contraction of superficial blood vessels.
- Body temperature falls to the temperature of the water in a few hours.
- Postmortem lividity is seen in the head, neck and front of chest. It is usually bright pink in colour due to the imbibi-

Table 2.6 Differences between Freshwater and Seawater Drowning

	Freshwater	Seawater
Time required for fatality	2–3 min	4–5 min
Changes in the blood	Haemodilution Hyponatraemia Hyperkalaemia	Haemoconcentration Hypernatraemia
Changes in the lungs	Ballooned out and lighter Pinkish Emphysematous Crepitant Less froth Retains shape after removal from body	Ballooned out and heavier Purplish/Bluish Soft and jelly-like No crepitus Copious froth Flattens out on removal from body

tion of oxygen through water, but it may be dusky and cyanotic, if the body had been floating face down, buttocks up, and hands and feet dangling down. This is in fact the usual position of a body floating in water after putrefactive gases begin to form. However, if the water is turbulent and constantly turns the body, postmortem staining may not be seen at all.

- **Cutis anserina (goose fleshing)** occurs due to contraction of erector pilorum muscles (**Fig. 2.80**). There is a puckered appearance of skin with hairs standing on end.

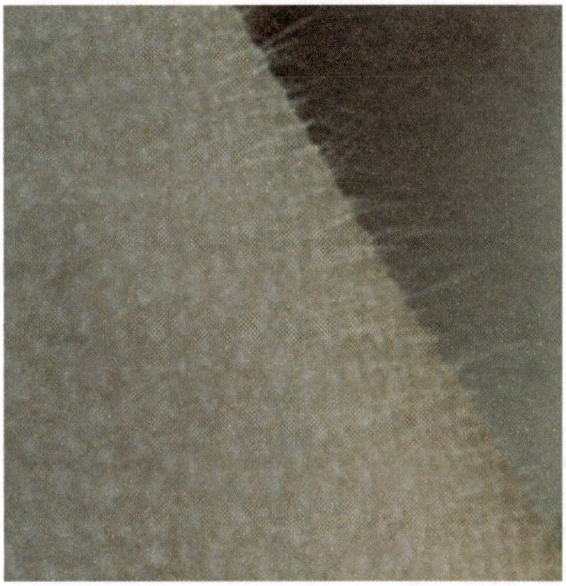

Fig. 2.80 Cutis anserina

- Rigor mortis sets in and passes off early, due to exhaustion resulting from the person's struggle under water.
- Conjunctivae are often congested; subconjunctival ecchymoses may be present.
- Hands affected by **cadaveric spasm** may contain various objects grasped while struggling in the water, such as seaweed, sand, straw, etc.
- After 48–72 hours or more, the skin of the palms and the soles becomes bleached, wrinkled and soddened (**Fig. 2.81**). This is called "**washerwoman's hands and feet**".*
- Putrefaction leads to accumulation of gases, and the body rises to the surface of water to float (**floater**).
- **Froth**:
  - A fine, white, tenacious, persistent, frothy foam in the shape of a balloon, or mushroom, or horn, is invariably seen at the nose and mouth (**Fig. 2.82**).
  - This is formed by the water inhaled into the lungs, which acts as an irritant prompting the secretion of mucus. Water, air, desquammated epithelium and mucus, are all churned up to form froth by violent respiratory efforts.
  - Sometimes, the froth is tinged pink due to blood from ruptured capillaries. This froth is pathognomonic of drowning.

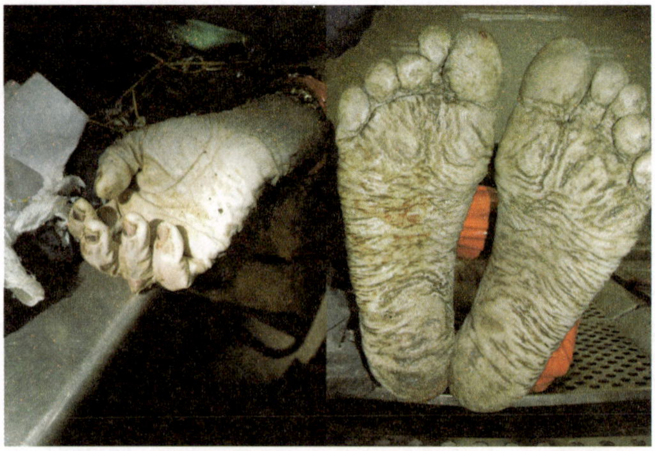

Fig. 2.81 Washerwoman's hands and feet

  - Copious froth exudes out when pressure is exerted on the chest. Froth may also be seen in cases of poisoning due to opium, organophosphates and snakebite, but it is never as copious as in drowning.
  - However, in dry drowning, froth may not be present at all.

Internal Appearances

- Airways contain stiff foam or frothy fluid or grit, gravel, mud, etc.
- Water in the air passages and stomach, especially dirty marshy water which is not potable, is an important finding to confirm death due to drowning.
- **Lungs**:
  - Large subpleural haemorrhages may be produced due to rupture of interalveolar partitions beneath the pleura. These are called **Paltauf's haemorrhages**. They are more prominent over the lower lobes and the interlobar surfaces.
  - The lungs appear ballooned, oedematous, and have a heavy and boggy feel. They are doughy and spongy, water-logged, and pit on pressure. This is referred to as **emphysema aquosum**. The condition develops only when the conscious victim of drowning struggles for survival, whereas a related condition called **oedema aquosum** develops when a body is passively immersed in water, or when the victim is unconscious. It is a mere flooding of the lungs.
  - Because of water-logging, rib marks are often seen on the lung surfaces.
  - On cut section, watery, frothy fluid exudes out of the lungs.
  - In deaths due to laryngeal spasm (**dry drowning**), these changes in the lungs and in the respiratory tree are not seen.

**Note*: *May be called "washerman's hands and feet" as well.*

- In saltwater drowning, the lungs appear purple, and are much more oedematous than in freshwater drowning. Further, in the latter case, lungs appear pinkish, and crepitus is heard on applying pressure.

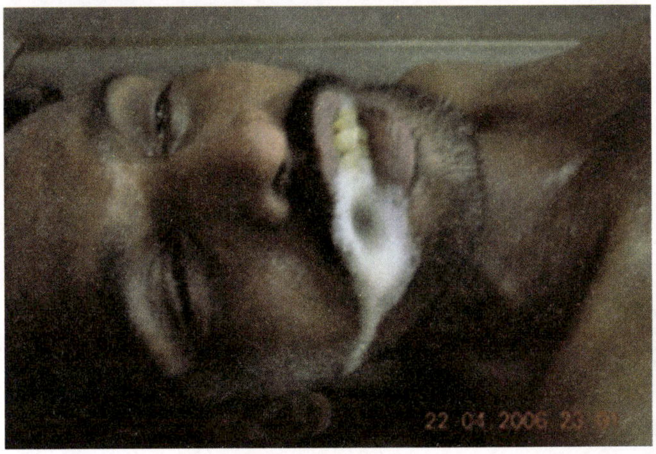

Fig. 2.82 Drowning – Froth (*Courtesy*: *Dr Prateek Rastogi*)

- The blood is likely to remain in a fluid state, free from clots, due to prevention of coagulation resulting from the release of plasminogen activator from damaged endothelium of pulmonary capillaries.
- Water may be detected in the middle ear, resulting from violent respiratory excursions, which force the water into the ear. This never happens in **postmortem submersion**, i.e., submersion of the body after death, which is sometimes resorted to deliberately, for the purpose of misleading criminal investigation.
- Haemorrhages may occur in the middle ear and mastoid air cells, due to barotrauma produced by the pressure exerted by the surrounding water.

Main differences between **antemortem drowning** and **postmortem submersion** have been listed in **Table 2.7**.

Diatom Test

- Most samples of water contain microscopic, unicellular algae or plankton called **diatoms**, which possess silicaceous cell membranes, and vary in size from 10 to 80 μm (**Fig. 2.83**). As a result of the hard cell wall, these microorganisms are resistant to heat and acids.
- In wet drowning, diatoms get aspirated into the lungs along with inhaled water, and then pass into the venous circulation through ruptured pulmonary capillaries or alveolar walls.
- They get distributed to various organs of the body and the bone marrow.

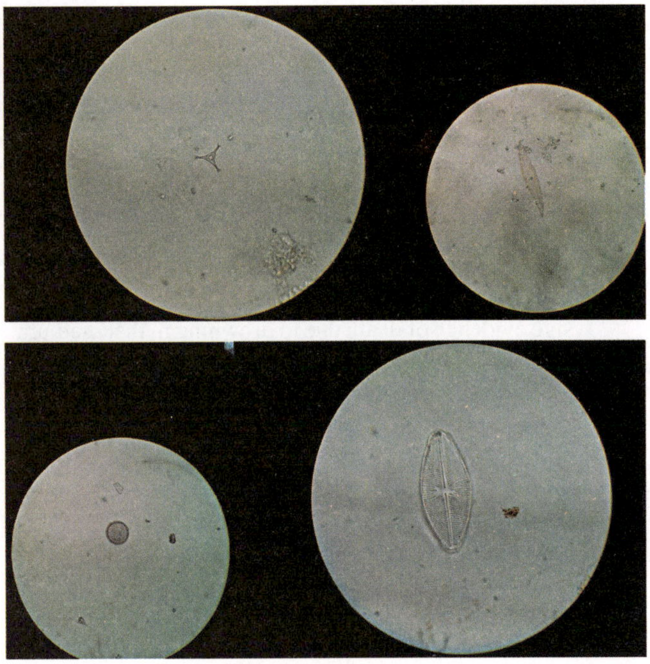

Fig. 2.83 Diatoms – Various shapes and sizes (*Courtesy*: *Dr Anu Sasidharan*)

Table 2.7 Differences between Antemortem Drowning and Postmortem Submersion

	Antemortem Drowning	Postmortem Submersion
Froth	Fine, persistent froth at the mouth and nose, which increases by pressure on chest.	No froth
Cadaveric spasm	May be seen rarely, with the victim clutching weeds, etc.	Absent
Water in stomach/ small intestine	May be present, which suggests active peristalsis	Absent
Sand particles	May be present till secondary bronchioles	Absent
Haemorrhage in mastoid air cells of middle ear	Present, though difficult to demonstrate	Absent

Note: The absence of any of the above features does not conclusively rule out antemortem drowning.

- These diatoms are demonstrable histologically, and their presence in the blood, viscera or bone marrow along with their presence in control samples of water from where the body was fished out, is pathognomonic of drowning.
- A simple test can be performed on the sternal bone marrow to demonstrate these diatoms:
  - The marrow is subjected to acid digestion, centrifuged and the sediment examined under the microscope. A sample of bone marrow (minimum 5 g) can be taken from the sternum or long bones, and digested with nitric acid for 1–2 hours. Then, the fluid is centrifuged, and the deposit is examined microscopically. Through acid digestion, all organic matter will be dissolved except diatoms which resist it because of their silicaceous covering.
  - A sample of the drowning medium (water in which the body was submerged) should also be subjected to microscopic examination. A few drops of tincture iodine/Lugol's iodine is added to the water sample and allowed to stand for 24 hours. Then, it is centrifuged at 3000 rpm. The supernatant fluid is discarded. The deposit is examined microscopically. If both the medium and the marrow contain the same type of diatoms, it is conclusive evidence of death due to drowning in that medium. Tissues like lungs, kidney, brain, etc., can also be subjected to this test.
  - A great advantage of this test is that diatoms resist putrefaction and are present even in highly decomposed bodies.
  - A negative diatom test however does not rule out the possibility of drowning, since it could be a case of dry drowning.
- Indian studies corroborate a number of Western studies, which indicate that the biggest drawback of the diatom test is that diatoms can be demonstrated even in non-drowning death. Hence, extreme caution should be exercised while opining on the cause of death in a medicolegal case, on the basis of a positive diatom test alone.
- Today, most experts agree that the **Diatom test**, like the **Gettler test** (*vide infra*) has too many flaws and must **NOT** be undertaken to conclusively diagnose death by drowning. At best, it can be considered as a supplementary laboratory test.

Gettler Test

- The **Gettler test** or **Chloride test** is done by withdrawing 10 mL of blood from each ventricle of the heart and subjecting it to estimation of chlorides.
- Normal value of chloride is 600 mg% in both chambers.
- In seawater drowning, there is said to be 30–40% increase of the chloride level in the blood in left ventricle, while in freshwater drowning, the chlorides get reduced by 50%.
- This change is of course not evident in dry drowning.
- **Actually, the Gettler test is only of historical interest, and has no practical relevance.**

Medicolegal Aspects of Drowning

- Before deciding the manner of death (accidental, suicidal or homicidal), it must first be established with certainty that it is a case of antemortem drowning, and not postmortem submersion. The points in favour of **antemortem drowning** are as follows:
  - Copious fine, lathery,* tenacious froth exuding from mouth and nose.
  - Material such as weeds, sand, etc., gripped in the hands.
  - Petechiae in the face; congestion of eyes.
  - Paltauff's haemorrhages on the surface of lungs (subpleural).
  - Ballooned out, crepitant lungs full of frothy fluid that oozes out on cut section.
  - Sand or mud particles within bronchi and bronchioles.
  - Water (especially, muddy or otherwise non-drinkable) in the stomach and intestines.
  - Water in the middle ear: Water can be aspirated from the middle ear and mastoid air cells in antemortem drowning.
  - Positive diatom test (in wet drowning).
- Most cases of drowning are either accidental or suicidal in nature. The former are more common in young children, elderly individuals and non-swimmers, while the latter are more common in women.
- Homicidal cases are very rare. But, cases do get reported from time to time.
- Death occurring in shallow water should be considered as homicide, unless otherwise proved. Tying of limbs or attaching a weight to the body is not always indicative of homicide. A person who is determined to drown himself may resort to this, especially if he is a swimmer.
- If injuries are found, they should be carefully evaluated with regard to the location, nature, etc. An examination of the scene is necessary to find out whether the injuries could have been sustained during the act of drowning.
- It is important to remember that bodies in water may be attacked by fish and various types of postmortem injuries can occur. These will however have irregular margins, and will be devoid of vital reaction.

> **FM 2.24: Core – Written/Viva Voce**
> - **Thermal deaths:**
>   - Describe the clinical features, postmortem findings and medicolegal aspects of injuries due to physical agents like
>   - Heat (heat hyperpyrexia, heat stroke, sun stroke, heat exhaustion/prostration, heat cramps) and
>   - Cold (systemic and localized hypothermia, frostbite, trench foot, immersion foot).

**Note*: *Not leathery, as mentioned in some textbooks! 'Lathery' is derived from 'lather', the kind of foam that one gets when washing briskly with soap and water.*

EFFECTS OF HIGH ENVIRONMENTAL TEMPERATURE*

When the human body is exposed to high environmental temperature for a prolonged time, the following effects are seen:

- Heat cramps
- Heat exhaustion
- Heat stroke

Heat Cramps

- These occur in persons who are working in a hot atmosphere, and perspire profusely, for instance, manual labourers, firemen, miners and stokers (hence, the synonyms **fireman's** or **miner's** or **stoker's cramps**).
  - They are characterised by painful cramps of the voluntary muscles.
  - Profuse perspiration results in substantial loss of water and sodium chloride from the system, which accounts for the cramps.
  - Treatment consists of restoring fluid and salt intake.

Heat Exhaustion

- This occurs in persons who physically exert themselves for a long period in a hot and humid atmosphere. It results from dehydration and salt depletion.
  - Heat exhaustion (also referred to as **heat collapse**, **heat prostration** or **heat syncope**), is characterised by headache, pallor, profuse perspiration, vomiting, subnormal temperature, muscular weakness and circulatory collapse. Urine becomes scanty.
  - Treatment consists of administering fluids of glucose-saline with sodium bicarbonate.
  - The condition is rarely fatal.

Heat Stroke

- This results from hyperpyrexia following exposure to excessive heat (**sunstroke**, **heat hyperpyrexia**, **thermic fever**).
  - There is a disturbance in the normal physiology of the heat-regulating centre in the hypothalamus.
  - The victim first experiences headache, visual disturbances, nausea, vomiting and dizziness, and then suddenly becomes unconscious. The body is flushed and hot, with dry skin. The body temperature may go as high as 43°C. The pulse is feeble and rapid, and the respiration stertorous.
  - Treatment involves removal of the patient's clothing, and immersion of the person (up to his neck) in a tap-water bath till the temperature comes down to 38°C.
  - This condition is often fatal, if not treated in time.
- **Autopsy Findings**:
  - Most of the victims die from disseminated intravascular coagulation.
  - The most striking autopsy findings are large areas of pulmonary haemorrhage.
  - The brain is congested and oedematous, with petechial haemorrhages in the white matter. Such haemorrhages are also found elsewhere in other organs of the body.
  - Microscopically, there are micro-thrombi in small blood vessels of many organs with small foci of necrosis of parenchymal cells.
  - Hepatic failure at times contributes to the death.
  - Skeletal muscles may demonstrate rhabdomyolysis.

Differences between heat exhaustion and heat stroke are mentioned in Table 2.8.

Table 2.8 Differences between Heat exhaustion and Heat stroke

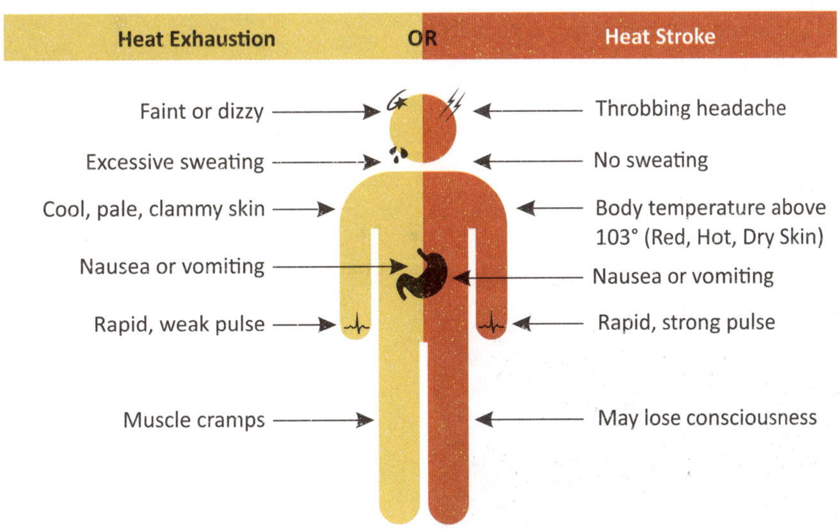

*__Note__: *Remember the confusing synonyms for each of these conditions!*
Heat cramps = Fireman's cramps or Miner's cramps or Stoker's cramps.
Heat exhaustion = Heat collapse or Heat prostration or Heat syncope.
Heat stroke = Sunstroke or Heat hyperpyrexia or Thermic fever.

EFFECTS OF LOW ENVIRONMENTAL TEMPERATURE

Hypothermia

- This is usually defined as a condition in which the body's core temperature falls below 35°C.
- Exposure to cold, exhaustion, fatigue, lack of food, disease, injuries, drugs or alcoholic intoxication are usually major causative or aggravating factors of such a condition.
- There is a progressive decrease in the metabolic processes in all the organs, a lowered oxygen dissociation from oxyhaemoglobin and oxymyoglobin and a diminished blood flow through organs and tissues. The mechanism for temperature regulation becomes progressively inoperative.
- However, hypothermia protects the central nervous system from the effects of ischaemia, and is an important cause of "apparent death" (**suspended animation**). The heart rate slows down, and the cardiac output falls. Cardiac fibrillation occurs at temperatures below 28°C.
- Treatment involves administration of pre-warmed glucose by intragastric drip, and antibiotic prophylaxis.
- If death is imminent, a peculiar feature sometimes occurs called **paradoxical undressing**, wherein the person appears to actually feel warm instead of experiencing cold, and therefore removes all his clothes. Hence, in some cases of death due to hypothermia, the victim may be found naked (**Fig. 2.84**).
    - One explanation for the effect is a cold-induced malfunction of the hypothalamus, the part of the brain that regulates body temperature.
    - Another explanation is that the muscles contracting peripheral blood vessels become exhausted (loss of vasomotor tone) and relax, leading to a sudden surge of blood (and heat) to the extremities, fooling the person into feeling overheated.
- Another feature that is sometimes encountered, especially in slowly developing hypothermia is **terminal burrowing** or **hide-and-die syndrome**. The afflicted will enter small, enclosed spaces, such as underneath beds or behind wardrobes (**Fig. 2.85**). It is often associated with paradoxical undressing.
    - Researchers claim this is "an autonomous process of the brain stem, which is triggered in the final state of hypothermia and produces a primitive and burrowing-like behaviour of protection, as seen in hibernating animals."

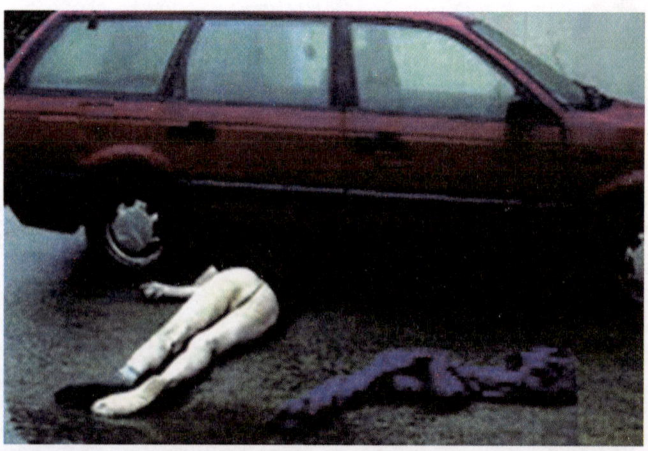

Fig. 2.84 Paradoxical undressing in a case of hypothermic death

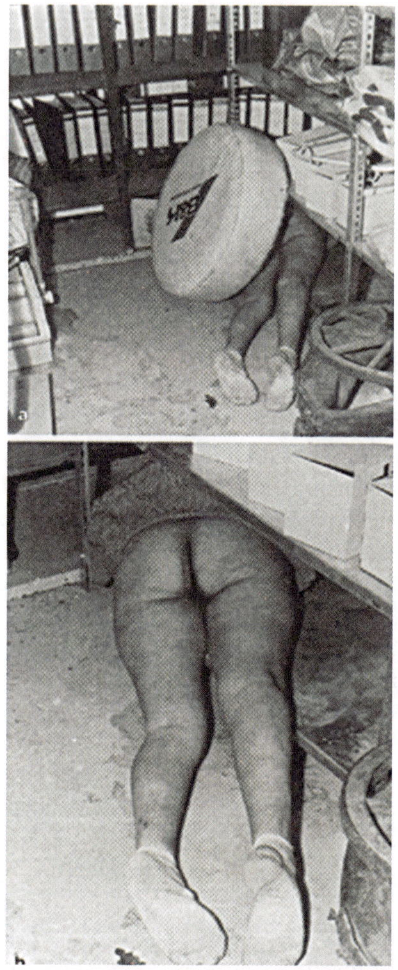

Fig. 2.85 Hide and die syndrome (Terminal burrowing)

- Local effects of hypothermia produce frostbite and immersion foot (trench foot).
    - **Frostbite** (**Fig. 2.86**) occurs at temperatures ranging from 5°C to 8°C. If this is continued for several hours, gangrene occurs. There is localized damage to skin and other tissues due to the extreme cold. Frostbite is most likely to happen in body parts farthest from the heart, and those with large exposed areas. Commonest site is the hand (especially the tips of the fingers). Frostbitten areas will turn discoloured, purplish at first and soon turn black. After a while, nerve damage becomes so great that feeling is lost in the frostbitten areas. Blisters will also occur. If feeling is lost in the damaged area, checking it for cuts and breaks in the skin is vital. Infected

open skin can lead to gangrene and amputation may be needed.

- **Trench foot** (**Fig. 2.87**) is a condition caused by prolonged exposure of the feet to damp, unsanitary and cold conditions. Immersion foot occurs when feet are cold and damp while wearing constricting footwear. Unlike frostbite, trench foot/immersion foot does not require freezing temperatures, and can occur in temperatures up to 60°Fahrenheit (about 16°Celsius). Affected feet become numb, and then turn red or blue. As the condition worsens, they may swell. Blisters and open sores form, which lead to fungal infections; this is sometimes called **tropical ulcer** (**jungle rot**). If left untreated, it usually results in gangrene, which requires amputation. If trench foot/immersion foot is treated properly, complete recovery is normal, though it is marked by severe, short-term pain when feeling returns.

- **Autopsy Findings** (hypothermic death): A distinctive **bright-pink** colour of the blood and tissues is said to be characteristic of non-dissociation of oxygen from haemoglobin (**Fig. 2.88**). There may also be prominent patches of purple discolouration of the limbs.

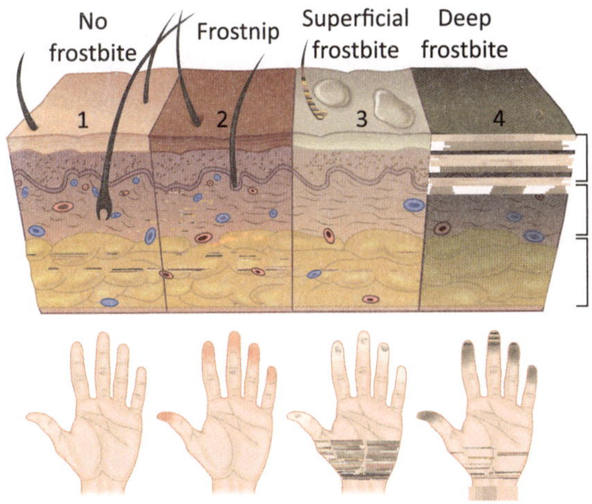

Fig. 2.86 Frostbite – Stages (degrees) of severity

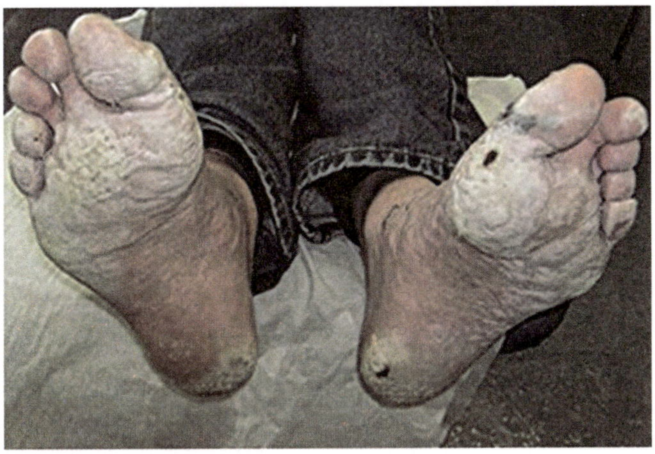

Fig. 2.87 Trench foot

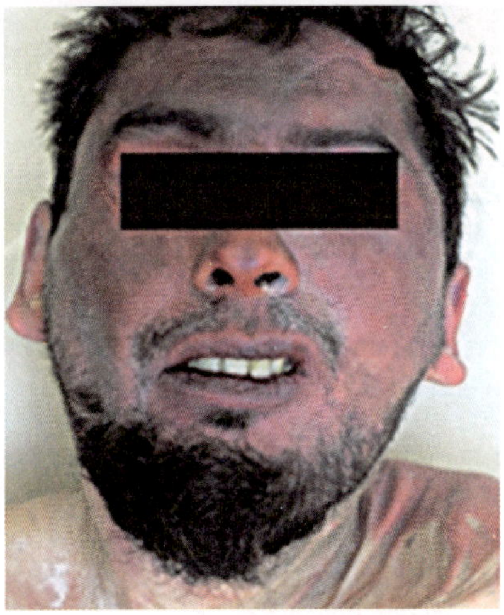

Fig. 2.88 Pink colour of skin – hypothermic death

> **FM 2.25: Core – Written/Viva Voce**
> - **Thermal deaths:**
>   - Describe types of injuries, clinical features, pathophysiology, postmortem findings and medicolegal aspects in cases of
>   - Burns
>   - Scalds
>   - Lightning
>   - Electrocution
>   - Radiation

EFFECTS OF HEAT ON THE BODY

Heat is a form of energy which when transferred to the body produces thermal injury in the form of **scalds** or **burns**, the former resulting from moist heat, and the latter from dry heat.

Thermal injuries can result from the application of:

- Flame
- Hot liquids
- Hot gases
- Solid heated substances like metal or glass
- Lightning
- Electricity
- Ultraviolet or infrared rays
- X-ray
- Corrosive chemical substances

Scald

- **Scalds** are produced due to application of moist heat to the body in the form of **boiling liquid** or **steam**.
  - Boiling liquids that can scald include water, milk, oil, etc.
- Corrosive liquids (acids and alkalis) do not cause scalds; they cause burns.
- Depending on the **severity**, scalds are classified into first, second and third degrees:
  - **First degree**: Reddening of the skin.
  - **Second degree**: Blister formation (**Fig. 2.89**).
  - **Third degree**: Drying and desiccation of deeper tissues.

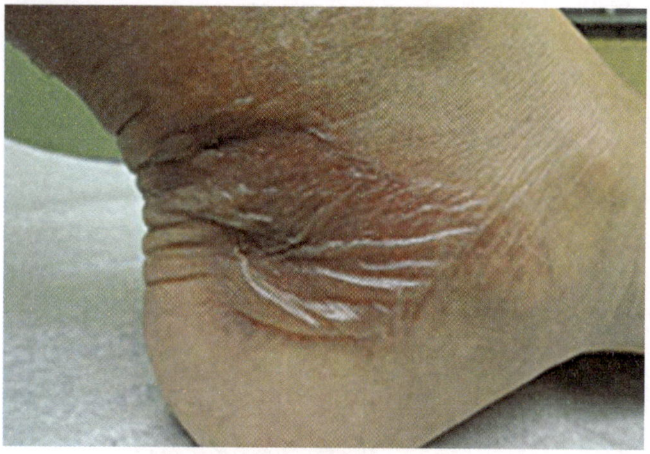

Fig. 2.89 Scald blister

- When external heat is applied to the human body, the extent of damage depends on the applied temperature, the time for which it is applied, and the ability of the body to conduct excess heat. Temperatures as low as 44°C can cause damage, if there is prolonged period of contact.
- Scalds do not show evidence of blackening or charring, unlike burns (**Fig. 2.90**).
- However, there may be evidence of splashing of the boiling liquid on the body, as well as trickle marks.
- Scalds usually heal without significant scarring or contracture formation.
- Death is rare, unless the body is extensively scalded by boiling liquid.

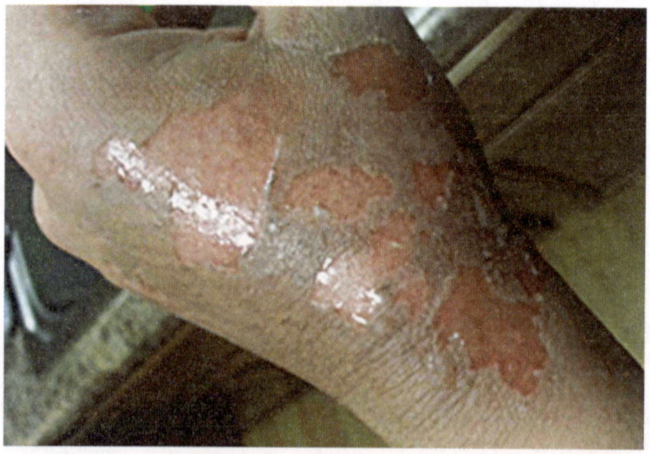

Fig. 2.90 Extensive scald injury – no evidence of blackening or charring

Burn Injury

Classification

A. Based on Depth:

1. **Dupuytren's Classification**: Dupuytren classified burns into six degrees depending on the severity of the burns.
    - First Degree: Erythema (reddening of the skin), followed by desquammation of superficial layer of epidermis.
    - Second Degree: Blister formation.
    - Third Degree: Destruction of the epidermis.
    - Fourth Degree: Destruction of the whole thickness of skin.
    - Fifth Degree: Destruction of muscles.
    - Sixth Degree: Destruction of bone, nerve trunks, etc.
2. **Hebra's Classification**: Hebra classified burns into three degrees, merging every two degrees of Dupuytren into one.
3. **Wilson's Classification** (**Fig. 2.91**): Wilson put forth a simpler and clearer classification (*vide infra*). On naked eye examination, the depth of the burn is difficult to make out, and hence he considered Dupuytren's classification to be of limited value in the practical situation.
    - **First Degree: Epidermal burns**
        - In this type of burn injury, the lesion is confined to the epidermis. There may be blistering without loss of epidermis. If the blister bursts, a reddened base is seen.
        - There is capillary dilatation and transudation of fluid into the tissues, causing swelling.
        - First-degree burns heal without scarring.
    - **Second Degree: Dermo-epidermal burns**
        - There is destruction of full thickness of skin.
        - The epidermis is coagulated or charred.
        - There is a central zone of necrotic tissue surrounded by first-degree burns or hyperaemia. The central necrosis sloughs off and the epidermis grows in from the margins.
        - Scarring is inevitable, and due to formation of contractures, there is disfiguration.
    - **Third Degree: Deep burns**
        - There is destruction of deeper tissues below the skin surface.
        - The skin is totally destroyed, though in some deep burns, islands of intact dermis may be found.
        - Damage to subcutaneous fat, and loss of muscle, bone, etc., is seen.

B. Based on Surface Area

1. **The Rule of Nines**
    - This is employed for the assessment of percentage of burns (used when burns are superficial in nature) (**Fig. 2.92**).
    - **Table 2.8** summarises the calculation of surface area involved, on the basis of the rule of nines.
    - It is important to remember that the calculation is slightly different in children < 5 years old. Since the head is proportionately larger in a child relative to the rest of the body as compared to that of an adult, the percentage allotted for the head and neck is 18% and not 9%. Since the lower limbs are proportionately smaller, the percentage allotment is 13.5% for each lower limb, i.e., 27% for both put together, instead of 36%.
    - Today, however, it is recommended to use the **Lund and Browder Chart** for accurate estimation of the surface area involved (**Fig. 2.93**). The rule of nines is only a rule

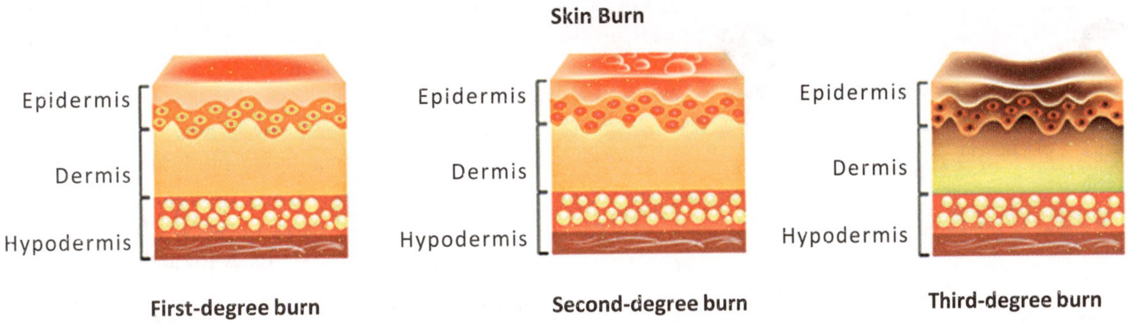

Fig. 2.91 Wilson's classification of degree of burn injury

Table 2.8 Rule of Nines

Body Part Affected	Percentage of Burns
Head & Neck	9
Right upper extremity	9
Left upper extremity	9
Right lower extremity	18
Left lower extremity	18
Front of trunk	18
Back of trunk	18
Genitals	1

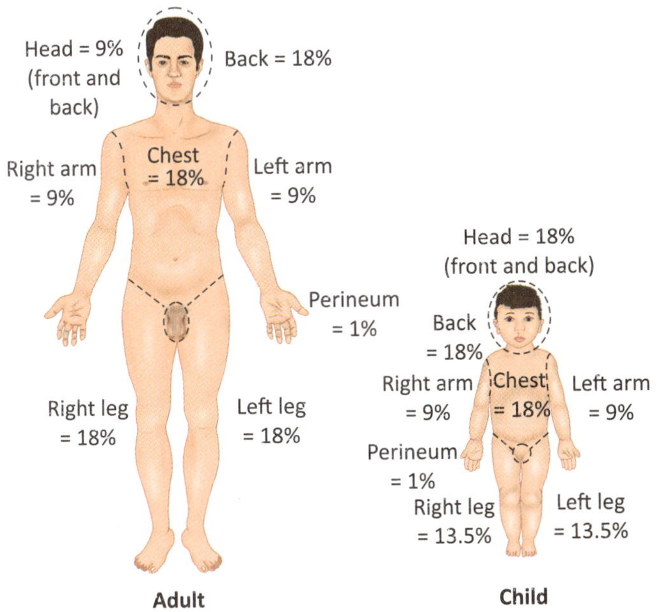

Fig. 2.92 Rule of Nines

of thumb, but it is adequate for autopsy purposes in deceased individuals.

General Features of Burns

- A burn injury will be more severe, if the heat applied is of great intensity. However, if the body is exposed to heat for a long time, it will show severe burn even if the intensity is less.
- The severity of burn also depends on the area involved. Burns affecting the face, genitals or lower part of the abdomen are more dangerous than burns in other parts of the body.
- Infants and elderly individuals are more susceptible to complications of burns.
- **Heat Haematoma**:
  - A haematoma may form in the extradural space between the skull and the dura mater when the cranium is exposed to tremendous heat.
  - It resembles a traumatic extradural haematoma, and may originate from venous sinuses, or from emissary veins in the diploe of the skull.
  - It can be differentiated from traumatic extradural haemorrhage by the presence of charring of the skull.
  - The clot itself is soft and friable with honeycomb appearance, and follows the distribution of charring of the outer table of the skull.
- **Heat Ruptures**:
  - Heated skin contracts and splits (**Fig. 2.94**). Such defects may appear to the inexperienced observer as antemortem wounds.
  - They are usually seen on the elbows, knees and over the extensor surfaces of other joints, as well as on the head.
- **Heat Rigor**:
  - Heat rigor is observed mainly in the muscles. This phenomenon is seen particularly in cases with extensive burn injury. It is due to coagulation and denaturation of proteins.
  - The posture of the body in such cases will demonstrate generalised flexion of the trunk, arms and legs. The upper limbs are held out with the fingers curled inwards, akin to the characteristic attitude of a pugilist (boxer) who is ready for a bout. Hence, this is sometimes referred to as the **pugilistic (boxer's or fencer's) attitude** (**Fig. 2.95**).

- It is important to note that the pugilistic attitude does not necessarily indicate that the burns are antemortem in nature. This is seen even if a dead body is burnt.

- **Heat Fractures**
  - Due to intense heat, bones may get fractured, especially the cranial vault and the limb bones. Such fractures are characteristically fissured in nature.
  - In severe and extensive burns, the body may become charred (carbonized) (**Fig. 2.96**) and even fragmented.

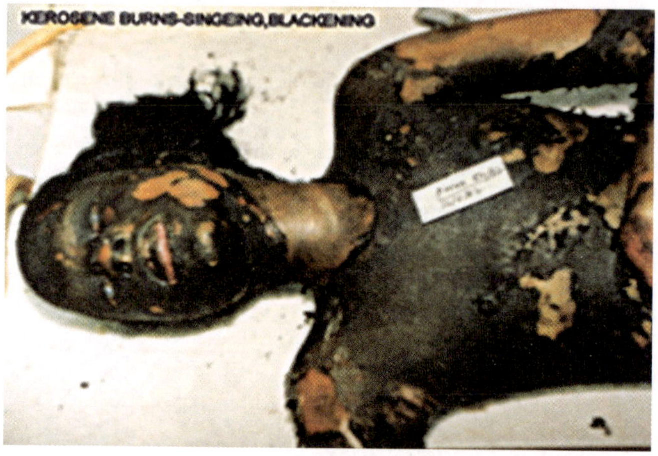

Fig. 2.96 Extensive burns with charring (*Courtesy*: *Dr Shashidhar C Mestri*)

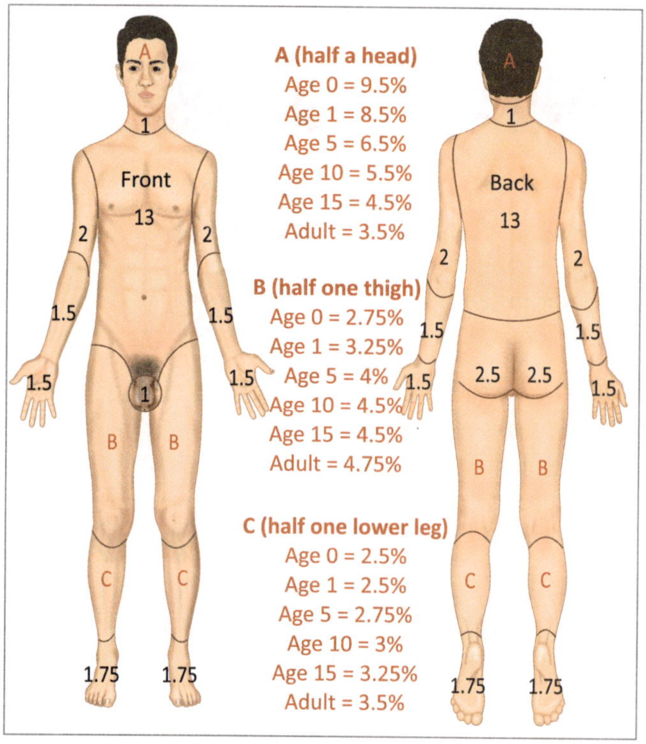

Fig. 2.93 Lund and Browder Chart

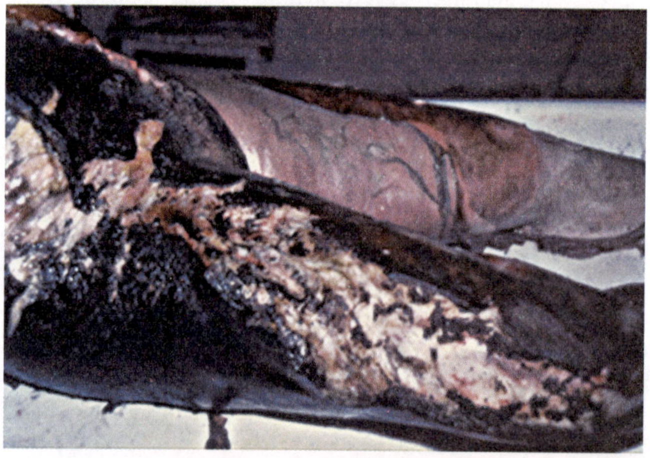

Fig. 2.94 Heat rupture – Lower limb (*Courtesy*: *Dr Geetha O*)

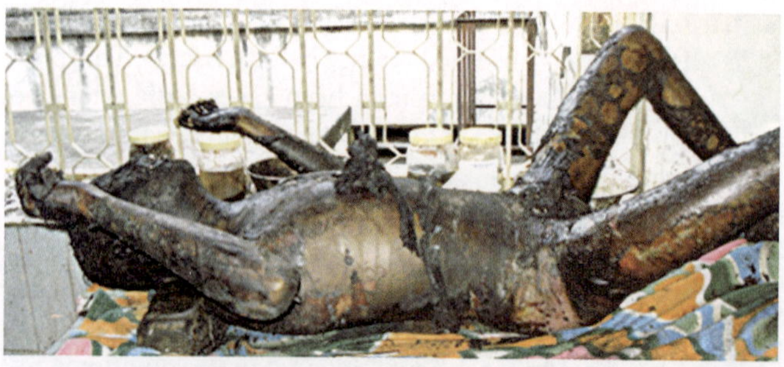

Fig. 2.95 Pugilistic attitude (*Courtesy*: *Dr Rajesh Bardale*)

Clinical Management of Scalds and Burns

Mild or Moderately Severe

1. First Aid
   a. Cool the area with running water for 20 minutes.
   b. Cold water compresses are useful for analgesia for localised burns.
   c. Do not apply ice.
   d. For chemical and eye burns, irrigate with copious volumes of water.
   e. Plastic (cling) wrap useful after cooling (limits evaporation and heat loss).
2. Pain Relief
   a. Paracetamol and codeine (PO) – 20–30 mg/kg paracetamol, 0.5–1 mg/kg codeine.
   b. Morphine (IV) – 0.1 mg/kg given in titrated boluses.
   c. Morphine (IM) – 0.2 mg/kg
3. Airway and Breathing
   a. Assess for the presence of stridor, hoarseness, black sputum or respiratory distress, singed nasal hairs or facial swelling.
   b. Oropharyngeal burns and significant neck burns usually require immediate intubation even if the airway is not yet compromised.
4. Circulation
   a. Early hypovolaemia is rarely related to the burn injury and other sources of bleeding should be sought.

b. For circumferential burns, check for signs of circulatory obstruction and the need for an escharotomy; elevate the limb.
c. For electrical burns, monitor ECG continuously. If high-voltage limb burn, early fasciotomy might be required.

Severe

1. Airway and Breathing
   a. For signs of airway burn or lung injury, arrange intubation as soon as possible and before airway swelling occurs.
2. Circulation
   a. If >10% of body surface involved, commence burns fluid resuscitation, and calculate fluid requirements from the time of injury. Preferably insert IV line through uninvolved skin.
   b. Insert urinary catheter, if burn > 15% SA, or if significant perineal burn.
   c. If >10% deep partial thickness or full thickness burns, start feeding within 6–18 hours.
3. Investigations
   a. Hb, Hct, electrolytes, blood glucose, blood group, etc.
   b. COHb and cyanide levels (if fire in confined space).
4. Eye Care
   a. Burns to the eyes require early copious irrigation with normal saline or water and ophthalmologic opinion.
5. Document the Following
   a. Time of burn
   b. Extent – Consult charts
   c. Depth
   d. First aid
   e. Tetanus status
6. Other Measures
   a. Analgesia should be adequate; children may require morphine initially before assessment and initial dressings.
   b. Immobilisation with sling and splinting is suggested for upper limb burns.
   c. Closed dressings are recommended for partial thickness burns.
   d. Blisters have a protective function, and reduce pain, if they are left intact for a few days.
   e. If blisters are small, not near a joint and not obstructing the dressing, leave alone.
   f. Large blisters and those overlying a joint should be de-roofed.
   g. Opaque blister fluid occurring after a few days suggests infection. The blister should then be de-roofed and dressed.

Causes of Death in Burns

- Death due to burns may be the result of
  - **Neurogenic shock** due to pain
  - **Hypovolaemic shock** due to loss of fluid
  - **Toxaemia** as a result of absorption of toxic material from the burnt site or
  - **Septicaemic shock** due to infection.
- Death occurring within 24 hours is usually due to neurogenic shock, hypovolaemia or toxaemia.
- Delayed deaths, which occur after 72–96 hours, are usually the result of infection, or renal damage, or haemorrhage from erosions (**Curling's ulcers**) of gastrointestinal tract (**Table 2.9**).
- Death can also occur from smoke inhalation (carbon monoxide poisoning), or mechanical trauma due to falling masonry, if a building is on fire with occupants trapped inside.

Autopsy Findings

1. **External**
   a. The body may demonstrate "**pugilistic attitude**" (which is however seen in both antemortem and postmortem

Table 2.9 Death due to Burns (Causes, Fatal Period and Autopsy Features)

Cause	Fatal Period	Autopsy Features
Shock 1. Neurogenic 2. Hypovolaemic 3. Endotoxic 4. Septicaemic	 Instantaneous Within 24–48 hours 24 hours later 48 hours later	 No specific features Pallor, organs may be pale Focus of infection Acute tubular necrosis Adrenal haemorrhage possible
Suffocation Inhalation of smoke, noxious gases, e.g., carbon monoxide	Immediate to first few hours	Look for soot particles in the trachea. May be absent, if time gap prolonged.
Injuries, Accidents Occur while attempting to escape from the fire, e.g., jumping off a high rise building.	Depends on the nature and severity of the injury	Despite the obvious burns, look for signs of injury and record meticulously. The presence of injuries may complicate autopsy features of burns.

burns). **Table 2.10** outlines the salient differences between antemortem and postmortem burns.

b. Antemortem burns appear reddened and blistered. Hair is singed or burnt. Even pubic hair, eyelashes and eyebrows may be involved.

c. Blisters may be seen (**Fig. 2.97A**), but they occur also in postmortem burns, and even in a putrefying body (**Fig. 2.97B**); the medical officer must therefore be careful while interpreting the cause of such dermal blisters.

d. Often, there may be signs of gross infection of burns on a dead body with discolouration and pus formation (**Fig. 2.98**). This is of course clinching evidence of the antemortem nature of burns.

e. In case of scalding, the body and clothes may be wet. If the scalding fluid has trickled down, the scald effect diminishes along its track, being maximum at the site of initial contact with skin.

f. Burning of clothes, singeing of hair, charring of the body, etc., are not seen in scalds.

g. Heat ruptures may be evident, which must not be confused with antemortem incised wounds.

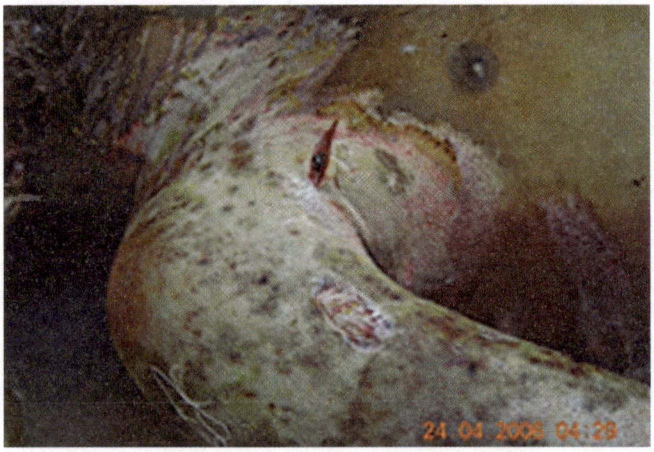

Fig. 2.98 Infected burns

2. **Internal**

a. Blood may be **cherry red** in colour, due to the presence of carboxyhaemoglobin.

b. Extradural heat haematoma may be seen.

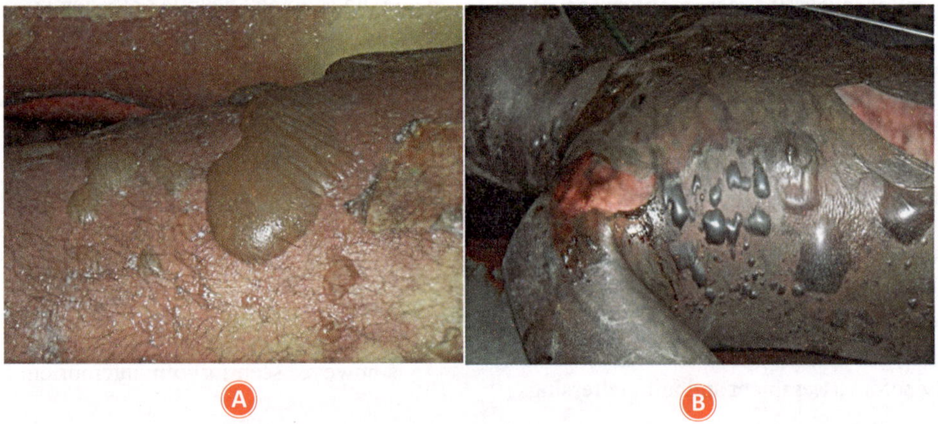

Fig. 2.97 **(A)** Blisters in antemortem burns; **(B)** Blisters in putrefying body (*Courtesy*: *Dr Prateek Rastogi*)

Table 2.10 Differences between antemortem and postmortem burns

Feature	Antemortem Burns	Postmortem Burns
1. **Line of redness**	Present around the burned part.	Absent
2. **Blisters**	Contain serous fluid with proteins and chlorides. Base is red.	Contain fluid and air. No proteins and chlorides. Base is dry and hard.
3. **Vital reaction**	Present	Absent
4. **Enzymatic activity** (*by histochemistry*)	Present (time related): Tissue cathepsin – immediate Serotonin – 10 mts Histamine – 20 mts. Esterase and ATPase – 1 hr Acid phosphatase – 3 hrs Alkaline phosphatase – 4 hrs	Absent

c. The brain is congested, and may demonstrate a "cooked" appearance.
d. **Soot particles** or carbonaceous material may be seen in the respiratory passages due to smoke inhalation. However, carbon monoxide intoxication can occur without visible soot in the airways.
e. **Curling's ulcers** may be seen in the stomach and duodenum.
f. Serous pleural effusions are common. Lungs are congested and appear "cooked."
g. Spleen and adrenals may be enlarged, congested and softened.

Medicolegal Aspects of Burns

- First, determine whether the burns are antemortem or postmortem in nature:
  - **Features of antemortem burns**:
    - Line of redness around the burn.
    - Blisters contain serous fluid rich in proteins and chlorides.
    - Soot in airways.
    - Cherry red colour of blood and tissues.
    - Evidence of infection.
- Next, determine the manner of burning: accidental, suicidal or homicidal:
  - **Accidental**:
    - It is the commonest cause of burns.
    - Examples: Dress catching fire while cooking, careless disposal of lighted matches/cigarettes, firecracker mishaps, automobile or aircraft accident, etc.
  - **Suicidal**:
    - Mostly in women. May be related to dowry harassment. Some fire accelerant (usually kerosene) is often used in such cases.
    - **Self-immolation**: An act of killing oneself as a sacrifice, usually by setting oneself on fire. Self-immolation is sanctioned by some elements of Mahayana Buddhism and Hinduism, and it has been practiced for many centuries, especially in India, for various reasons, including jauhar, sati, political protest, devotion and renouncement. Certain warrior cultures, such as those of the Charans and Rajputs, also practiced self-immolation. The practice continues in India even today with hundreds of self-immolations reported every year.
  - **Homicidal**
    - Rare, but cases are reported from time to time.
    - **Incendiary warfare**: Incendiary warfare involves the technique of 'firebombing' which is designed to damage a target, generally an urban area, through the use of fire, caused by incendiary devices, rather than from the blast effect of large bombs.
  - **Preternatural combustion**: Can a body go up in flames on its own? Incredible as it may seem, cases are on record where this has apparently happened. However, closer examination usually reveals a more plausible explanation, e.g., drinking alcohol (which is flammable) and smoking at the same time in bed or on a couch while alone, and then falling asleep with a smouldering cigarette in hand that may come in contact with the alcohol.

Lightning*

- When there is discharge of electricity between clouds, **lightning** occurs.
  - When the charge jumps between the cloud and the earth, it is called **lightning strike** (**Fig. 2.99**). Lightning chooses the easiest path (not the shortest), and hence it often takes a wandering, zigzag path.
- When lightning strikes a person, a potential of 1000 million Volts causes a 20,000-Ampere current to pass through the body of the victim (***direct effect***). This induces lethal electrocution. The current may then disperse over an area close to where the victim is standing (***indirect effect***).
- When the lightning flash strikes a nearby metallic object, it may give rise to induced voltage.
- The atmospheric gases become heated to 20,000°C, and this heating of gases in the path of lightning causes an explosive expansion. Although the duration of explosion is for a fraction of a second, the blast effect can be devastating. Objects may be fragmented and flung away from the site of lightning.
- Lightning can incapacitate humans in four different ways:
  - **Direct strike**: The electrical charge strikes the victim first. If the victim's skin resistance is high enough, much of the current will ***flash*** around the skin or clothing to the ground, resulting in a surprisingly benign outcome. Metallic objects in contact with the skin may concen-

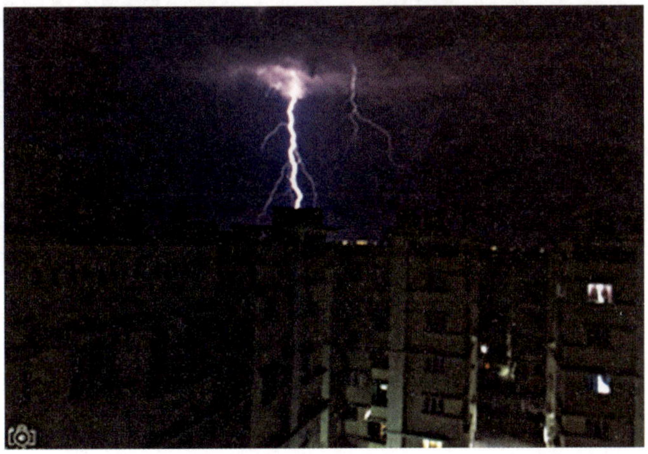

Fig. 2.99 Lightning strike (thunder bolt) (*Courtesy*: Dr Vivek Kumar)

****Note***: *Not 'Lightening', which refers to lighten something that is dark coloured!*

trate the lightning strike, preventing the flashover effect and resulting in more serious injuries.
- '**Splash**': ***Splash*** hits occur when lightning prefers a victim (with lower resistance) over a nearby object that has more resistance, and strikes the victim on its way to the ground.
- **Ground strike**: ***Ground strikes***, in which the bolt lands near the victim and is conducted through the victim and his or her connection to the ground (such as through the feet, due to the voltage gradient in the earth), can cause great damage.
- **EMP or electromagnetic pulse**: Results from close strikes, especially during positive lightning discharges.

- **Autopsy Findings**:
  - **External lesions** mostly take the form of burns:
    - ***Linear burns***: They vary from 6 to 25 mm in width. They are linear in shape, and are found more commonly on moist surfaces of the skin, because moist skin offers less resistance than dry skin.
    - ***Arborescent burns***: There is formation of superficial, thin, irregular, tortuous markings on the skin. They resemble the branching pattern of a tree, hence the name. Sometimes, the pattern resembles a fern leaf (**filigree burns** or **keraunographic markings** or **Lichtenberg figures**) (**Fig. 2.100**). These marks are formed when capillaries beneath the skin rupture due to the electrical discharge, and they usually appear within hours of the strike though they tend to disappear within a few days. They generally occur on the upper body.
    - ***Surface burns***: These burns occur due to heating up of metallic objects worn or carried by the person. Sometimes the object becomes **magnetised**. This can be ascertained with the help of a pocket compass.

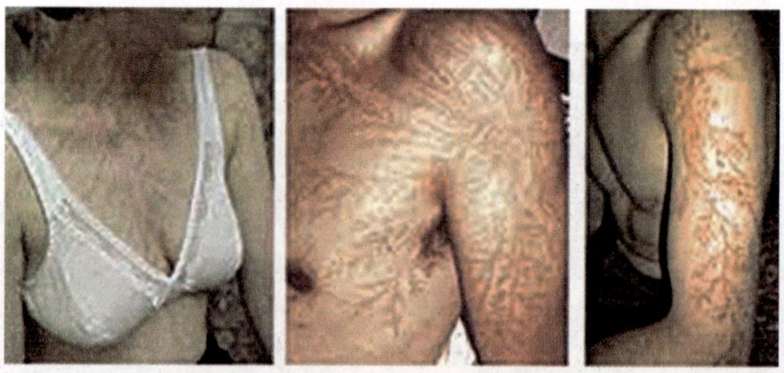

Fig. 2.100 Arborescent burns on various parts of the body of lightning-struck victims

- **Other Effects**:
  - Clothes may be torn.
  - Shoes may burst open.
  - Rupture of tympanic membrane is often seen.
  - Injuries from the skin may extend to involve subcutaneous tissue, muscle and bone.
  - Bony injuries may show periosteal elevation and destruction of superficial layers of the bone, or fractures.
  - Petechial haemorrhages may be seen in the brain and the spinal cord. Chromatolysis and fragmentation of axons are common.
  - Congestion of all organs, and pulmonary oedema are also common.

Electrocution

Injuries caused by electrocution respect all the known laws of physics and thus are predictable in their manifestations, under different physical conditions.

- Electrical current is of two types: **direct current** and **alternating current** (**DC** and **AC**). All modern homes and electrical appliances run on alternating current. **AC is more dangerous to the human body than DC**. AC can be fatal at 4–6 times lower strength than DC. This is because when alternating current comes in contact with muscles, it produces tetanic stimulation, which induces muscle spasm and does not allow the person to release contact with the source of current. An alternating current of 70–80 mA (milliAmperes) can be fatal, whereas direct current (DC) of 200–250 mA can be tolerated without much damage.
- The resistance of the skin varies greatly, according to dryness. Wet skin may have a thousand fold reduction in resistance compared to dry skin.
- The point at which the electric current enters the body is called the point of entry. The point of exit denotes the point from where the electric current leaves the body. Burns may be seen both at the point of entry as well as the point of exit.
  - The electrical burn at the **point of entry** is called **Joule burn** or **endogenous burn** (**Fig. 2.101**): It resembles the size and shape of the object causing it. Generally, it appears as a round or oval, shallow crater, surrounded by a ridge of skin, 2–4 mm high. The floor is composed of pale, flattened skin with a surrounding hyperaemic zone.
- The effects of electrocution vary depending on the point of entry and exit.

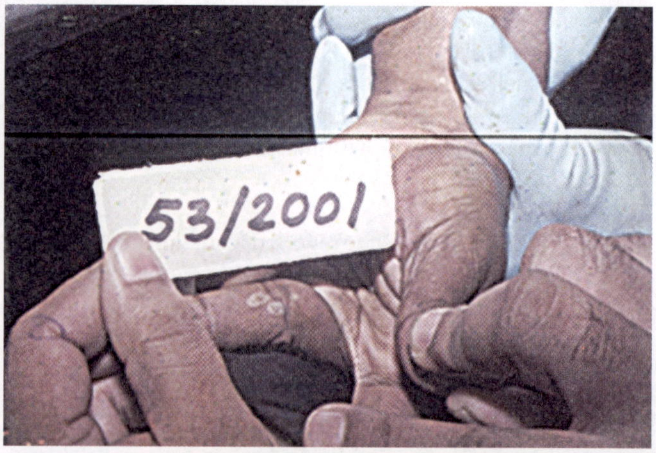

Fig. 2.101 Joule burn (*Courtesy*: *Dr EJ Rodrigues*)

- If the point of entry is in one upper limb, and the earthing point is in the opposite foot, the current will pass across the chest in a diagonal direction and be most likely to produce myocardial fibrillation.
- Electrical current passing through the lower parts of the body may not produce fibrillation at all.
- Current passing through the head may not affect the heart, but can cause brainstem damage with central respiratory paralysis.
- Sometimes, the entry and exit points of the current are spread over such wide areas that no focal lesions are present on the body, more so when the skin is wet or the body is immersed in water.

- Death lurks in bathrooms where electrocution is common due to wet floors, wet skin or metal plumbing that acts as a good conductor. Added to this, the presence of faulty earthing, current leakage and downright carelessness in handling electrical appliances make the bathroom a veritable graveyard for the unsuspecting, especially young children and frail, old people.
- Other types of burns:
  - **Spark burn** is produced by intermittent contact with a live object, and is due to arcing of current from the conductor to the skin. A yellowish parchment-like skin surrounded by a pale area is seen. Sometimes thermal burns are seen over large surface areas of the body. While working with high-tension wire, etc., a person may be thrown off to a distance, yet may show different types of burns. This is also due to arcing. Occasionally, there is actual charring of the skin with carbonisation.
  - At times, there is confluence of spark burns resulting in a **crocodile skin** effect (**Fig. 2.102**).
- **Causes of Death in Electrocution**:
  - Ventricular fibrillation.
  - Respiratory failure due to spasm of respiratory muscles.
  - Cerebral anoxia.
  - Delayed death due to complications of burns.

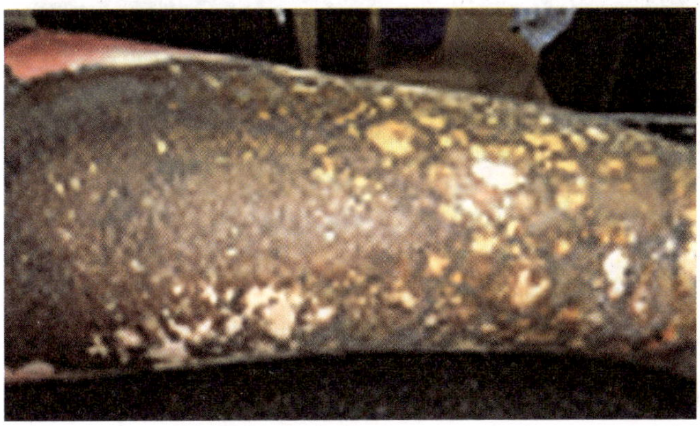

Fig. 2.102 Crocodile burns (high voltage) (*Courtesy: Dr Hareesh S Gouda*)

- **Autopsy Findings & Medicolegal Significance**:
  - Burns may be seen at the point of entry and exit. At the point of entry, the burn (Joule burn) may resemble the shape of the object causing electrocution. The skin may be ruptured at the point of exit.
  - All the organs are congested. Petechial haemorrhages are seen on serous surfaces. There may be pulmonary oedema.
  - Electrocution is by and large accidental. However, there are cases of electrocution due to suicidal and homicidal intentions.
  - **Judicial electrocution** is practiced in some states of the USA.
    - Judicial electrocution is presently practised in the following states of the USA: Alabama, Arkansas, Connecticut, Florida, Georgia, Indiana, Kentucky, Nebraska, Ohio, South Carolina, Tennessee, Vermont and Virginia. But in most of these states, the condemned prisoner is first given the option of lethal injection as a substitute method of execution, if he prefers that. Some of these states have in fact abolished the electric chair totally.
    - The actual protocol and voltage varies from state to state. The scalp and the left calf of the condemned person are shaved. One hour prior to the execution, sponges soaked in brine are applied to these areas, to enhance the conductivity of the skin. The condemned man is made to sit in a wooden chair and straps are applied to secure his hands, legs and chest. Metal electrodes are applied and an alternate current of 2400 Volts (7.5 amps) is applied for 7 seconds, followed by 600 Volts for 17 seconds, the whole being repeated twice. After 5 minutes, a physician confirms death, or otherwise the procedure is repeated till life becomes extinct.

Radiation Injury

- Radiation injury is caused by exposure to ionizing radiation, which can be particulate radiation caused by protons, neutrons, alpha rays and beta rays, or electromagnetic radiation due to X-rays. Gamma rays with short wavelength are also included in the latter.
- The radioactive elements, on entering the body, act on cells causing death. This occurs in two ways: chromosomal breaks (double stranded DNA) and production of free radicals.
- Radiation injury has its most pronounced effect on cells in the mitotic phase of cell division. Epithelial cells of the GI tract and lymphoid tissue are especially susceptible.
- A single large dose of irradiation can lead to death (as observed in victims of the Hiroshima and Nagasaki bombings at the end of World War II).

- At doses greater than 100 Gy (10,000 rad), death occurs within 24–48 hours.* This is known as **acute radiation syndrome**.
  - Acute radiation syndrome (ARS), also known as radiation sickness or radiation poisoning, is a collection of signs and symptoms that are caused by being exposed to high amounts of ionizing radiation, in a short period of time (**Fig. 2.103**). The symptoms of ARS can start within an hour of exposure, and can last for several months. Within the first few days the symptoms are usually nausea, vomiting and loss of appetite. Later, leukopenia occurs with weakness and fatigue, alopecia, hypotension, dizziness, high fever, shock, infections and death in a few days to weeks.
    - It is generally divided into three types: **bone marrow, gastrointestinal and neurovascular syndrome**, with bone marrow syndrome occurring at 0.7–10 Gy, and neurovascular syndrome occurring at doses that exceed 50 Gy.
  - Treatment of ARS is generally supportive care. This may include blood transfusions, antibiotics, colony-stimulating factors or stem cell transplant.
  - A sensational case of political assassination accomplished through acute radiation syndrome concerned the Russian defector **Alexander Litvinenko** who was poisoned by KGB agents with radioactive polonium-210 in Nov 2006 in London (**Box 2.3**).

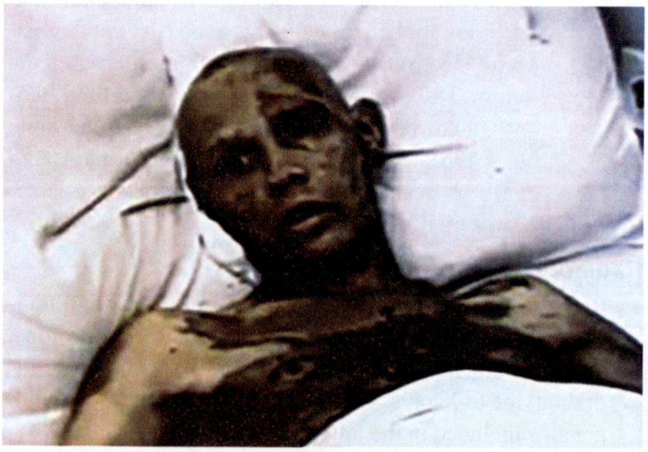

Fig. 2.103 Victim of acute radiation syndrome

- ARS differs from chronic radiation syndrome (CRS), which occurs following prolonged exposures to relatively low doses of radiation. At sub-lethal doses, delayed effects result in somatic changes such as sterility, premature abortions and foetal abnormalities. Increased incidence of malignancies (both haematological and solid organ) have been observed.
- In the case of a **nuclear explosion** like the one that **Japan** suffered in **World War II**, generation of thermal radiation consisting of ultraviolet rays, infra-red and light rays, creates a tremendous amount of heat, comparable to the interior of the sun in a volume of space a few inches in diameter. Because the reaction is completed in microseconds, a violent explosion results. Near the hypocentre, the temperature of 6000°C incinerates the body, blisters tile surfaces and instantly ignites flammable objects. At distances of about 3 km, the skin is charred, but at distances closer to the hypocentre, internal tissues are injured as if they are roasted, and death is instantaneous. As thermal radiation and the penetrating nuclear radiation of gamma rays and neutrons act upon the body simultaneously, the combined effects would be lethal for those out in the open within 1500 m of the hypocentre, even for those who are not injured by the trauma.

Box 2.3—Assassination by Radiation – The Alexander Litvinenko Case (2006)

Alexander Litvinenko was a former officer of the Russian KGB, who escaped prosecution in Russia and received political asylum in Great Britain. He authored two books in which he accused the Russian secret services of staging Russian apartment bombings and other terrorism acts to bring Vladimir Putin to power.

On 1st Nov 2006, Litvinenko suddenly fell ill and was hospitalized. Earlier that day, he had met two former KGB officers, Andrei Lugovoi and Dmitri Kovtun. Lugovoi was a former bodyguard of Russian ex-Prime Minister Yegor Gaidar (also reportedly poisoned in Nov 2006). Litvinenko also had lunch at a sushi restaurant on Piccadilly in London, with an Italian acquaintance, Mario Scaramella. The latter attached to a Commission investigating KGB penetration of Italian politics, claimed to have information on the death of Anna Politkovskaya, 48 years, a journalist who was killed at her Moscow apartment in Oct 2006. He passed Litvinenko papers supposedly concerning her fate. On 20th Nov, it was reported that Scaramella had gone into hiding and feared for his life. Litvinenko died on 23rd Nov.

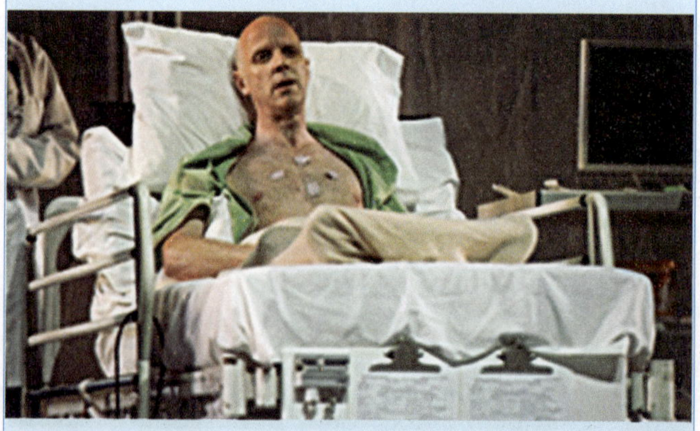

Alexander Litvinenko in his hospital bed

contd

**Note*: *Gy stands for Gray, which is a unit of ionizing radiation dose in the International System of Units (SI). Rad is a unit of absorbed dose of ionizing radiation.*

Shortly after his death, the UK's Health Protection Agency (HPA) stated, tests had established that Litvinenko had significant amounts of the radionuclide Polonium-210 (^{210}Po) in his body. British and US Government sources both said the use of ^{210}Po as a poison had never been documented before, and this was probably the first time a person had been tested for its presence in his or her body. The poison was in Litvinenko's tea cup.

Polonium could be identified only after Litvinenko's death; it was not detected earlier because it does not emit gamma rays, which are encountered with most radioactive isotopes. Polonium-210 emits only alpha particles that do not penetrate even a sheet of paper, or the epidermis of human skin, thus being invisible to normal radiation detectors. Hospitals only have equipment to detect gamma rays. However, both gamma rays and alpha particles are classified as ionizing radiation which can cause radiation damage. An alpha-emitting substance can cause significant damage only if ingested or inhaled, acting on living cells like a short-range weapon. Litvinenko was tested for alpha-emitters using special equipment.

Litvinenko's autopsy took place on 1st Dec. According to doctors, his body had five times the level of polonium-210 that would be considered lethal.

FM 2.26: Core – Written/Viva Voce

- Describe and discuss clinical features, postmortem findings and medicolegal aspects of death due to starvation and neglect.

STARVATION

Starvation results from the deprivation of a regular and constant supply of food, which is necessary for the maintenance of the nutritional balance of the body.

- The term "**starvation**" includes both
  - **sub-nutrition** (intake of insufficient **quantity** of food), as well as
  - **malnutrition** (intake of insufficient **quality** of food).
    - Malnutrition can and does occur as a separate entity, while sub-nutrition must always include some degree of malnutrition.
- **Starvation** is regarded as ***acute***, when the necessary quantity of food and water are suddenly and completely withheld, and ***chronic***, when there is a gradual deficiency in the supply of food.
- In India, starvation deaths due to **famine** are not an unknown occurrence, though it is not so common today.
- **Inanition** refers to the symptoms and effects of starvation, while **cachexia** refers to acute loss of body weight.
- **Neglect** and **starvation** are not synonymous, but are often so closely associated that the two conditions are usually considered together. Death can occur from deliberate or negligent lack of provision of proper care and nutrition of children. In general, though there are many exceptions, nutritional neglect and physical battering tend to be mutually exclusive. The abused child is usually well nourished, while the emaciated child is usually uninjured.

Causes of Starvation

- Famine
- Fasting
- Malnutrition
- Overpopulation
- Poverty
- War
- Anorexia nervosa
- Bulimia nervosa
- Depression
- Coma
- Diabetes mellitus
- Digestive disease

General Features of Starvation

- A minimum of 1900 calories of food per day is the average dietary requirement for an adult, below which the effects of starvation will begin to manifest (**Fig. 2.104**).
- There is danger to life when more than 40% of the original body weight has been lost, though the speed of loss is relevant.
- Total lack of food is likely to cause death in about 50–60 days, if adequate water is available, while if it is not, death is greatly accelerated.
- Total deprivation of water results in death in about 10 days.
- The rapidity of death also depends on the weather, temperature of the environment and the original fitness (or fatness!) of the individual.

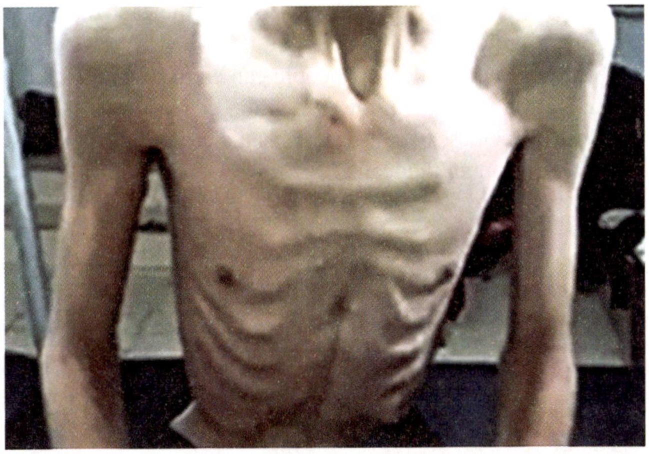

Fig. 2.104 Victim of starvation

Signs and Symptoms of Starvation

- An acute feeling of hunger lasts for the first 2 days.
- Loss of fat and emaciation make their appearance in about 4 days.
- There is progressive loss of body weight.
- The skin becomes dry, shriveled, thin, parchment-like, fissured and drawn tight over bony prominences.

- The cheeks become hollowed out, and lips are dry and cracked.
- The abdomen becomes scaphoid, i.e., sunken inwards (**Fig. 2.105**).
- The person feels weak, and may look pale and cadaverous. Pallor is due to anaemia resulting from inadequate intake of iron, proteins, vitamins and other required elements.
- Pupils get dilated.
- Tongue is dry and coated. The breath turns offensive.
- Hair becomes dry, lustreless and brittle. Nails become brittle and ridged.
- Pulse is feeble, and blood pressure is low because of cardiac atrophy.
- There may be oedema of the feet due to decrease in blood proteins (hypoproteinaemic oedema).
- The temperature is subnormal.
- There is constipation at first, but later diarrhoea sets in.
- Urine is scanty and dark coloured.
- The mind usually remains clear till the end. The person may become delirious just before death.
- In contrast to the generalized drying up of tissues in most cases of starvation as listed above, some individuals may develop ***wet starvation***: oedema of face, trunk and extremities, in association with pleural effusion and ascites.

Factors Modifying the Effects of Starvation

1. **Age**: Old people generally withstand the effects of starvation better than young adults because of their lower food requirements. Similarly, a mature adult can withstand starvation better than a growing child.
2. **Sex**: Women can usually combat starvation better than men for the same reason as above, as also the fact that they generally possess more body fat.
3. **State of health**: Healthy people can endure the effects of starvation better than the sick.
4. **Body fat**: Obese people can withstand the effects of starvation better than the lean.
5. **Cold**: Exposure to cold aggravates the effects of starvation, because it accelerates the basal metabolic rate.

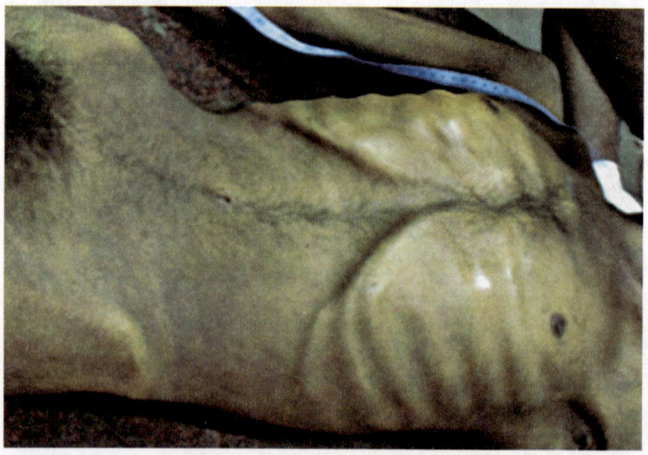

Fig. 2.105 Starvation – Scaphoid abdomen (*Courtesy*: *Dr Shashidhar C Mestri*)

Treatment

- Rest and warmth must be provided and maintained.
- Solid food must not be given straight away.
- Small sips of warm water mixed with glucose or fruit juice can be given at frequent intervals.
- Later solid food can be given in gradually increasing quantities. Administration of protein hydrolysate helps to raise the level of blood proteins and thus combat oedema.
- If treatment is hurried with immediate institution of normal feeding, there is a potential risk of precipitating the "**refeeding syndrome**," which can be fatal.
  - **Refeeding syndrome**:
    - Usually occurs within 4 days of starting to feed.
    - Patients can develop fluid and electrolyte disorders, especially hypophosphataemia, along with neurologic, pulmonary, cardiac, neuromuscular and haematologic complications. Most effects result from a sudden shift from fat to carbohydrate metabolism, and a sudden increase in insulin levels after refeeding, which leads to increased cellular uptake of phosphate.
    - Intracellular movement of electrolytes occurs, along with a fall in the serum electrolytes including phosphate, potassium, magnesium, glucose and thiamine.
    - Refeeding syndrome can cause confusion, coma, convulsions and death.

Postmortem Findings

- **External**
  - ***Emaciation***: The degree of loss of weight is an indication of the duration of starvation.
  - Pupils: Dilated.
  - Skin: Dry, shrivelled, thin, parchment-like, fissured and drawn tight over bony prominences (**Fig. 2.106**). Trophic ulcers may be present.
  - Hair: Dry, lustreless and brittle.
  - Nails: Brittle and ridged.
  - Lips: Dry and cracked.
  - Tongue: Dry and coated.
  - There may be oedema of the feet.
- **Internal**
  - Loss of body fat (**Fig. 2.107**) and atrophy of muscles.
  - Stomach and small intestine: Small and contracted.
  - **Gall bladder**: Distended with bile.
  - Omentum and mesentery: Devoid of fat.
  - Large intestine: Contains hard faecal matter. There may be generalized ulceration of colonic mucosa.
  - All organs except brain, shrunken and reduced in size (**Fig. 2.108**). Brain is often oedematous.
  - Bones: Demineralized.

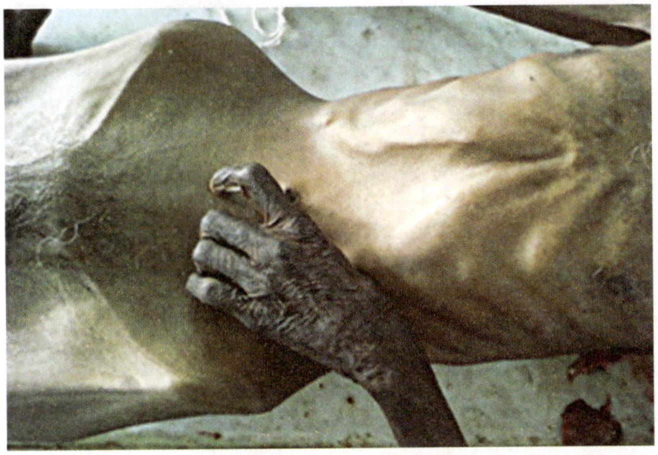

Fig. 2.106 Emaciation with parchment-like skin drawn tight over bony prominences (*Courtesy: Dr Nilesh Tumram*)

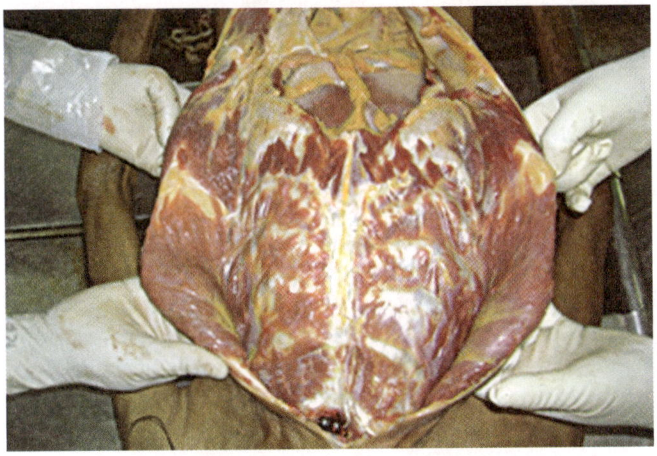

Fig. 2.107 Starvation – Depleted subcutaneous fat (*Courtesy: Dr Pannag S Kumar*)

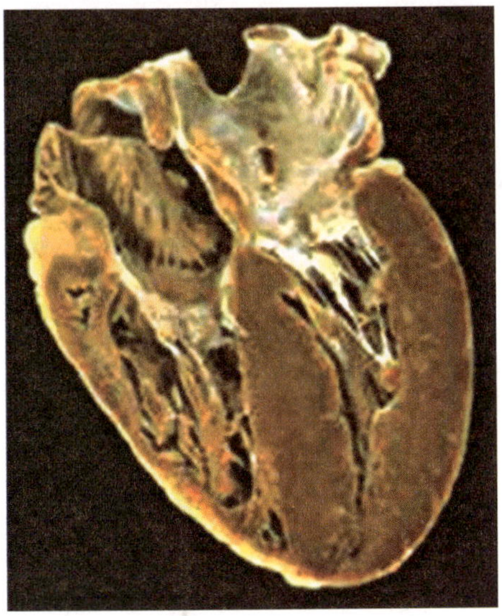

Fig. 2.108 Brown atrophy of heart

Cause of Death

- In acute starvation, death occurs from inanition and circulatory failure.
- In partial/chronic starvation, the vitality of the individual is reduced, and death may result from intercurrent disease. Multiple organ failure with ventricular fibrillation as the terminal event is the usual end result.

Medicolegal Importance

Starvation may be **accidental**, **suicidal** or **homicidal**.

- In cases of **accidental starvation**, the circumstances are self-explanatory, such as famine, ship-wreck, entombment in mines or diseases such as stricture of the oesophagus.
  - The right to food is not just a basic human right, but also a basic human need. It is the state's responsibility to ensure that its people do not starve and die due to hunger and starvation. Under the Indian Constitution, there is no fundamental right to food, but the issue can be brought under Article 21, which guarantees the "Right to life and liberty" to all the citizens. The Supreme Court has directed that the Chief Secretary of a state would be held responsible for all starvation deaths in that state, if such deaths are reported and proved to have occurred.
- **Suicidal starvation** is rare, though it may be seen among mentally disturbed individuals, and occasionally among prisoners who go on a **hunger strike** as a form of protest. Voluntary starvation for religious or political reasons is well known.
- In **homicidal cases**, the victim is usually an infant who has been deliberately and wilfully deprived of food. Successful prosecution in cases of fatal infant starvation depends on establishing the fact that the death resulted from failure to offer the child sufficient food. This deficiency must be coupled with evidence that the mother was aware of the gravity of the child's condition, and that she did nothing to ameliorate the situation in spite of availability of resources.
  - Starvation has historically been used as a death sentence. From the beginning of civilization through to the Middle Ages people were immured, or starved to death.
    - **Immurement** is a form of execution, where a person is walled up within a building and left to die from starvation or dehydration.
    - Anarkali was a legendary woman said to be loved by the 16th-century Mughal Prince Salim, who later became Emperor Jahangir (**Fig. 2.109**). When this illicit relationship became known to his father, Mughal Emperor Akbar, the latter had her executed by immurement. Anarkali is depicted in the 1960 Bollywood film Mughal-e-Azam in which she is portrayed by Madhubala (**Fig. 2.110**).
  - Mass **homicide** is sometimes inflicted on an enemy population during a war, the most horrific example of which is the **Holocaust** perpetrated by Nazi Germans during World War II (1939–1945). Many deaths from starvation

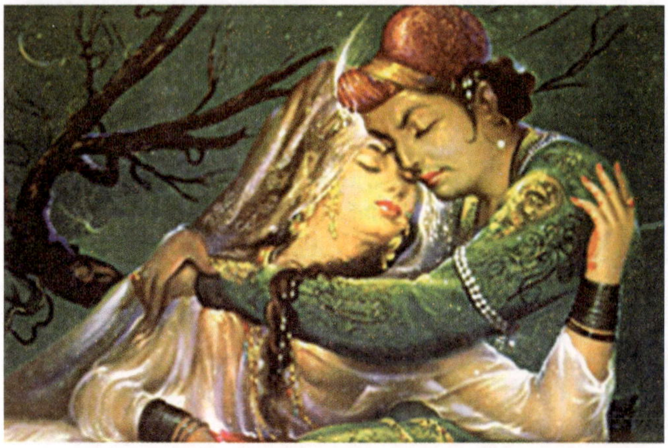

Fig. 2.109 Anarkali and Salim

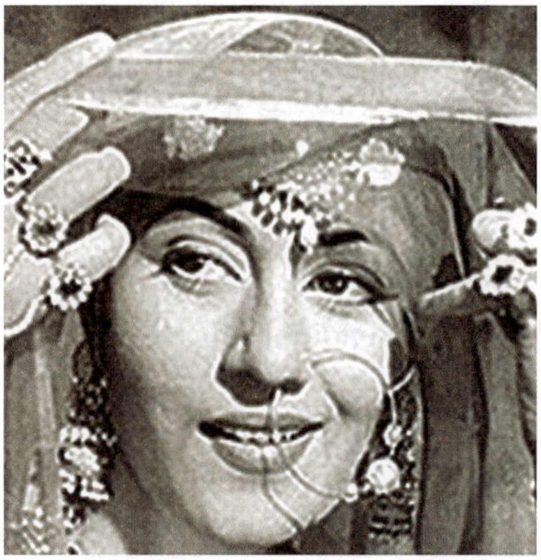

Fig. 2.110 Madhubala as Anarkali

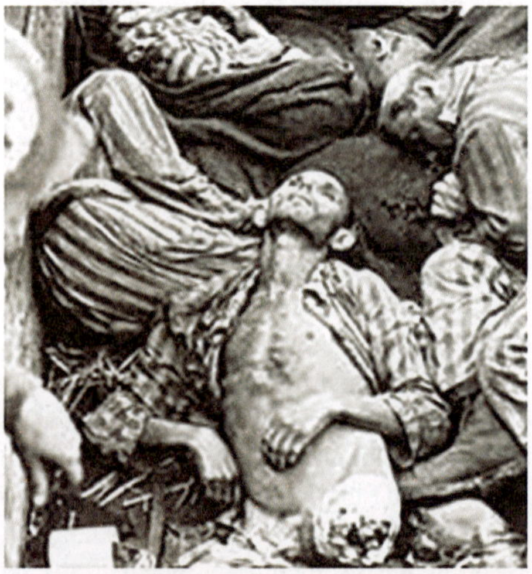

Fig. 2.111 Victims of starvation – Belsen concentration camp

took place in Nazi concentration camps in Belsen and other places in Germany during that time (**Fig. 2.111**).

FM 2.27: Core- Written/Viva Voce

- Define and discuss
    - Infanticide
    - Foeticide
    - Stillbirth.

INFANTICIDE

- Though the legal definition and implications of infanticide vary from country to country, the medical concept is more or less universally accepted. **Infanticide refers to the deliberate killing of a child below the age of 1 year**.
    - In England, Germany and the UK, there is a clear-cut distinction between homicide and infanticide, and a charge of infanticide is less serious than a charge of murder, if committed by the mother due to stress factors surrounding birth and lactation.
    - In India, no such distinction exists, and the mother is punished under Section 302 (IPC), the same as for murder.

FOETICIDE

- **Killing of a foetus prior to birth**.
- Prenatal sex determination followed by selective abortion of female foetuses is the main cause for the declining sex ratio at birth in India. Women most clearly at risk are those who already have one or two female children. Based on conservative assumptions, the practice accounts for more than a million missing female births yearly, translating over the past 2 decades into the abortion of several million female foetuses, and the skewed male-to-female ratio.

NEONATICIDE

- **Killing of a newborn infant**.
- The perpetrator is invariably the mother, and the cause of death is usually either asphyxia or abandonment.

STILLBIRTH

- **Birth of a baby after 28 weeks of gestation, which did not at any time after being completely expelled from its mother, breathe or show any other signs of life**.

FM 2.28: Core– Written/Viva Voce/OSPE (Objective Structured Practical Examination)

- Describe and discuss
    - Signs of intrauterine death
    - Signs of live birth
    - Viability of foetus
    - Age determination of foetus
    - DOAP session of ossification centres
    - Hydrostatic test
    - Sudden Infant Death Syndrome
    - Munchausen's Syndrome by Proxy

INTRAUTERINE DEATH OF FOETUS

Dead Birth

- **A dead born child is one which has died in utero, and shows any one of the following signs after it is completely born**:
  - **Maceration**:
    - This is a process of **aseptic autolysis** (**Fig. 2.112**). Unlike putrefaction which is due to bacteria, there is no bacterial action in maceration.
    - The cells break down due to enzymatic action (autolysis), and the body becomes soft and flaccid.
    - The skin appears purplish brown and peels easily.
    - After the foetus dies in utero, the cerebral hemispheres shrink in size. As a result, the bones of the cranial vault loosen and begin to override each other. This overriding of the cranial bones seen on X-ray is called **Spalding sign*** (**Fig. 2.113**).
    - Signs of maceration become evident only about 24 hours after the death of the foetus. However, skin slippage can occur as early as 6–12 hours, and constitutes the earliest sign of maceration.

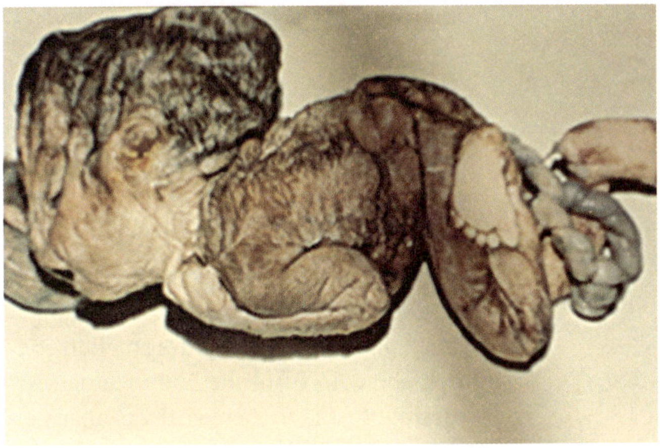

Fig. 2.112 Macerated foetus (*Courtesy*: *Dr Shashidhar C Mestri*)

  - **Putrefaction** – If there is rupture of the membranes, air entry is facilitated and putrefaction sets in.
  - **Mummification** – When liquor amnii is scanty, the foetus becomes dry and shrivelled.
  - **Rigor mortis** – In the early stages after intra-uterine death, if the foetus has developed to nearly full term, rigor mortis may set in. The delivery of such a foetus may be difficult.

VIABILITY

- **The ability of a foetus to lead a separate existence after birth, by virtue of a certain degree of development, is called viability**.
- Although in some cases, infants have reportedly survived even though the gestation period was only 180 days, for practical purposes, the minimum duration required to make a foetus viable is taken as **210 days (seven 30-day months)**.

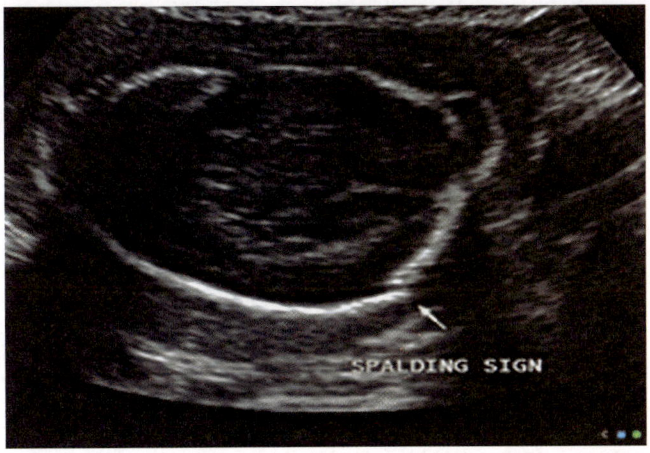

Fig. 2.113 Spalding sign on ultrasound

- Some factors which help in assessing the viability include weight, crown–heel length and appearance of ossification centres. At 7 months, the average weight is 1.3 kg, and the crown–heel length is 35 cm.
- **Rule of Haase**** – It is a rough method of determining the gestational age of a foetus after delivery. The square root of the crown–heel length (cm) gives the gestational age (months), up to 5 months intrauterine life. For example, a length of 16 cm indicates the age of the foetus to be 4 months. Beyond the 5th month, the length of the foetus (cm) when divided by 5, provides its age in months. For example, a length of 30 cm divided by 5 shows the age to be 6 months.
- **Ossification centres** – By 28th week, the centre for the proximal end of the tibia, as well as the centres for cuneate, capitate and cuboid bones appear. The centre for the proximal end of the tibia is the most reliable, that of the cuneate and capitate least reliable, and that of the cuboid is of intermediate value.

LIVE BIRTH

- The term **live birth** is used when a **child has shown signs of life, even if only a part of the child was out of the womb, though the child may not have breathed or been born completely**.
- Causing the death of such a child is treated in the same manner as homicide.

Signs of Live Birth

- In India, the law presumes that every child that was discovered in a dead condition was born dead, unless the contrary can be proved. In civil cases, any sign of life such as a cry, movement of the body, or hand or foot, after birth is likely to be accepted as proof of live birth. Sometimes, a child may cry even while it is still in the uterus or vagina

**Note*: *Alfred Baker Spalding, an American gynaecologist, first pointed this out (in 1922).*

***Carl Friedrich Haase (1788–1865) was a German Obstetrician.*

(after the membranes have ruptured). This is called **vagitus uterinus** and **vagitus vaginalis**, respectively. And yet when the child is actually born, i.e., has come to the exterior, it may be found to be without signs of life.

- Hence, in criminal cases, the cry of the child alone is not proof enough of live birth. Such proof that is acceptable to the court can only be furnished after **postmortem examination**:
  - **Umbilical cord**:
    - If the cord has separated, it indicates that birth took place several days earlier.
    - Generally, in the first 12–24 hours after birth, the umbilical cord becomes dry and shriveled.
    - On the 2nd day, a zone of redness is seen at the attachment of the cord to the umbilicus.
    - It is also important to consider as to whether the cord was cut or torn. In the case of a torn cord, the edges appear ragged and ripped.
  - **Presence of vernix**:
    - This merely indicates that the child was not washed. It does not indicate live birth.
    - **Vernix** (also known as **vernix caseosa**) (**Fig. 2.114**) is the waxy or cheese-like white substance found coating the skin of newborn humans. It is secreted by the foetus's sebaceous glands in utero, and is hypothesized to have antibacterial properties.
    - It is different from **lanugo**, which is soft, fine hair covering the foetus while inside the uterus. It is usually shed shortly after birth.

Lanugo

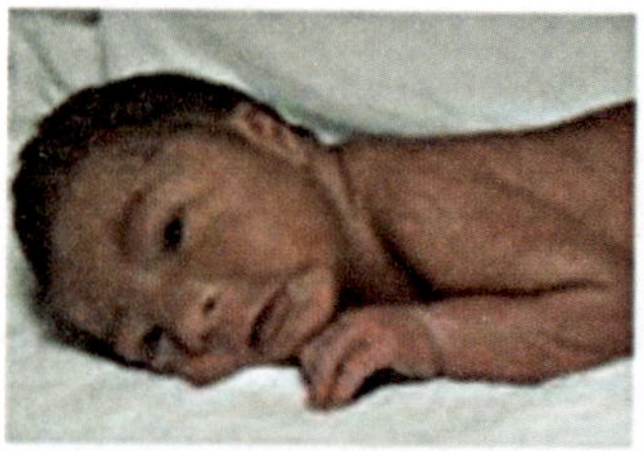

Vernix caseosa

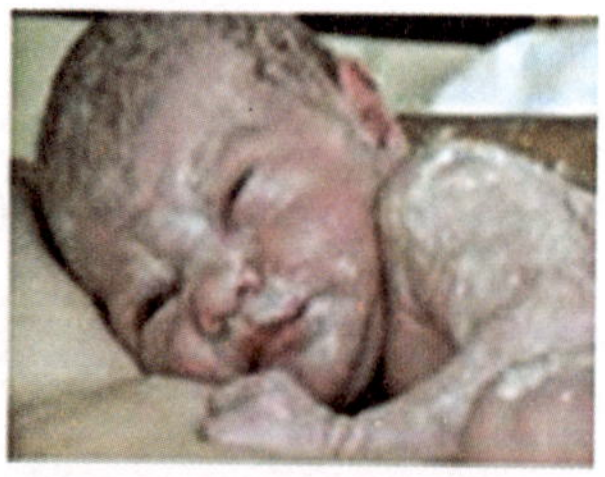

Fig. 2.114 Lanugo hair and Vernix caseosa

  - **Food in the stomach**: Presence of milk or food in the stomach is a conclusive sign of live birth.
  - **Proof of breathing**: The following points are relevant:
    - The shape of the chest is flat before respiration, after which it becomes drum shaped.
    - The diaphragm is at the level of the 6th or 7th rib after respiration has taken place. Otherwise, it is at the level of the 3rd or 4th rib.
    - The lungs are voluminous, with the medial edges overlapping the mediastinum. The margins become rounded after respiration is established. Before respiration the lungs are firm in consistency, but respired lungs are spongy, elastic and crepitant, due to being distended with air.

- **Hydrostatic test**: The hydrostatic test is based on the principle that if the infant has breathed, the lungs will float in water. Each lung is cut into pieces and tested for floatation in water. A piece of liver can serve as control. If the liver bit floats, the test has no meaning, because it is clear that putrefaction has set in. If all the pieces of lung float, they are crushed under a weight and tested again.
  - ***Inference***: Floatation is positive when the baby has respired. But, if the pieces sink after pressure, no respiration has taken place. If some pieces float while others sink, it means feeble respiration has taken place.
  - ***Drawbacks***: Expanded lungs may sink due to oedema, pneumonia, atelectasis and obstruction by alveolar duct membrane. On the other hand, unexpanded lungs may float due to putrefaction or artificial respiration.
  - The hydrostatic test is superfluous (i.e., not necessary), if the foetus is:
    - below 180 days of gestation
    - macerated
    - grossly deformed
    - showing milk in the stomach.
- The hydrostatic test is of limited value. It can only be used as a suggestive pointer to live birth, but it is not conclusive.
- **Other indicators**:
  - The lungs of a stillborn are dark, small and heavy (like liver).
  - Before respiration, the lungs are smaller, constituting about 1/70th of the body weight. After respiration, due to increased vascular volume it becomes 1/35th of the body weight (this is also sometimes called the **Ploucquet's test**).
  - The texture of the unrespired lung is rubbery and firm with sharp margins. On slicing, the interior is uniform in colour and texture. On rubbing a small piece between the fingers, close to the ears, no sound is heard. In the case of a respired lung, crepitation can be made out.
  - Histological appearance: In a respired lung, alveoli appear expanded with flattened epithelium.
  - Presence of air in the stomach and intestine (which float in water if double-ligated). This is referred to as **Breslau's second life test** or **Stomach-bowel test**.
  - The disappearance of gelatinous tissue from the middle ear after respiration is established,

may point to maturity of the infant (**Wredin's test**).
- Foetal haemoglobin, which is 80% at birth, decreases to 7–8% in 3 months.

CAUSES OF INFANT DEATH

Death of a foetus may be due to natural or unnatural causes.

- **Natural causes** include immaturity, foetal malformations and birth trauma.
- **Unnatural causes** may be accidental or criminal.
  - **Accidental causes** may be due to prolonged labour, cord twisting around the neck or cord prolapse. Sometimes, a foetus is born with the membranes covering the head (**caul**) which if not incised soon after birth, may lead to asphyxia (**Fig. 2.115**).
    - **Precipitate labour**:
      - Precipitate labour is said to occur when all the stages of labour merge with each other, and the birth takes place in an abnormally short time.
      - The mother may experience mild pain which she may attribute to a distended rectum, and therefore she may attempt to defaecate, as a result of which the child may be born into the lavatory pan. The child may sustain skull fractures or bleed from the torn end of the umbilicus. It may inhale faecal matter which may be demonstrable in the lungs.

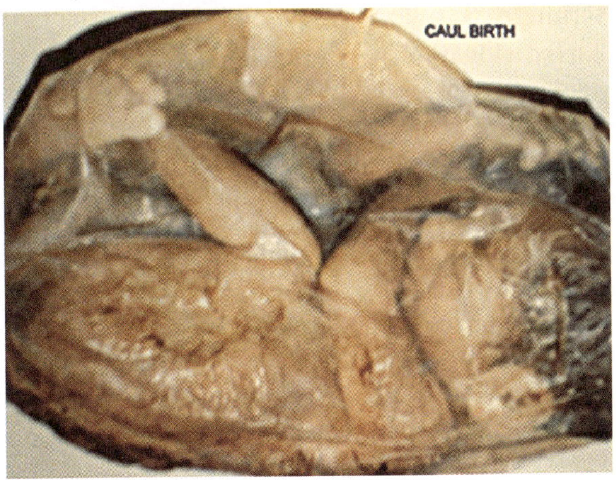

Fig. 2.115 Caul birth (*Courtesy: Dr Shashidhar C Mestri*)

      - Precipitate labour occurs when the pelvis is very roomy and the foetus is very small. In such cases, **caput succedaneum** or **cephalhaematoma** which are pointers to obstructed labour, **are absent**.
        - **Caput succedaneum** is a soft swelling on the presenting part of the scalp formed during delivery and contains blood and serous fluid. The swelling does not cross over the midline, as it is limited by the attachment of pericranium to the bones of the vault. In breech delivery, it may be seen on the buttocks. Caput resolves in 1–7 days.
        - **Cephalhaematoma** is due to accumulation of blood deep to the scalp. It is limited to suture lines. It takes about one to three months to resolve and shows colour changes similar to a bruise.
  - **Criminal causes** of infant death constitute the offence of **infanticide**. These may be the result of acts of omission or acts of commission.
    - **Acts of omission** (or neglect):
      - Failure to protect the child from heat or cold
      - Failure to provide assistance during labour
      - Failure to clear the air passages of mucus
      - Failure to cut the umbilical cord
      - Failure to feed the child.
    - **Acts of commission**: The following constitute some common examples:
      - Smothering, e.g., by blocking the air passage by a pillow or soft cloth.
      - Strangulation, e.g., by ligature, sash of the baby's frock or even the umbilical cord.
      - Manual strangulation or throttling.
      - Banging the head of the child against a wall.
      - Burning
      - Drowning
      - **Concealed puncture wounds**, e.g., in the axilla, inner canthus of the eye, vagina, rectum, through a fontanelle, etc., usually accomplished by the insertion of a stout needle or fine-bladed knife.
      - Poisoning.

CONCEALMENT OF BIRTH

- **Section 318** of the **Indian Penal Code** recognizes intentional concealment of birth and/or secret burial or disposal of a dead child as a crime punishable with fine or imprisonment up to 2 years, irrespective of whether the child dies during, before or after birth.

ABANDONING OF INFANTS

- If the parent or guardian of a child below 12 years, or anyone entrusted with the care of such a child, leaves it in any place with the intention of abandonment, he/she is punishable up to 7 years imprisonment (**317 IPC**).

SUDDEN INFANT DEATH SYNDROME or SIDS (COT DEATH, CRIB DEATH)

Definition

- SIDS is defined as the **sudden death of an infant which remains unexplained, even after a thorough case investigation, including performance of a complete autopsy, examination of the death scene and review of the clinical history**.
- The incidence of SIDS is 2–3/1000 live births, with a slight male preponderance.
- Most cases involve infants between the ages of **2 weeks to 2 years**, with maximum incidence between 3 and 7 months.
- Occur commonly at night or in the wee hours of the morning.
- Twins are at greater risk.
- In many cases, there is a prior history of running nose or coryza (common cold).

Possible Causes

- Overlaying of the infant by drunken parents.
- Prone sleeping position.
- Inadvertent smothering by soft cloth or pillow.
- Sleep apnoea, which causes hypoxia and respiratory depression.
- Hypotonic babies, whose neck posture reduces the airway lumen.
- Dust mite allergy.
- Cow's milk allergy.
- Calcium or selenium deficiency.
- Viraemia.
- Hyperthermia or hypothermia.
- Anaphylactic shock.

Autopsy Findings

The following may be seen:

- Blood-stained froth in the mouth.
- Evidence of laryngitis, tracheitis, tracheobronchitis or congenital heart disease may be seen in some cases.
- Multiple petechial haemorrhages are often noticed in the heart, lungs and thymus.

Preventive Measures (Fig. 2.116)

- The parent/caregiver of an infant must not sleep along with the baby, as far as possible. A **separate, properly designed crib** must be used for the baby.
- Ensure that the infant always **sleeps on its back**. Never allow it to sleep prone (face down).
- Use only a **firm mattress** and avoid soft bedding.
- Ensure that the room in which the baby is sleeping is **well ventilated** at all times.
- The baby must be **breast fed** as far as possible. Discourage bottle feeding in the early months after delivery.
- **Do not allow anyone to smoke** in the vicinity of a sleeping baby.
- **Do not medicate an infant** without consulting a paediatrician.

Follow the

ABCs

of **Safe Sleep**

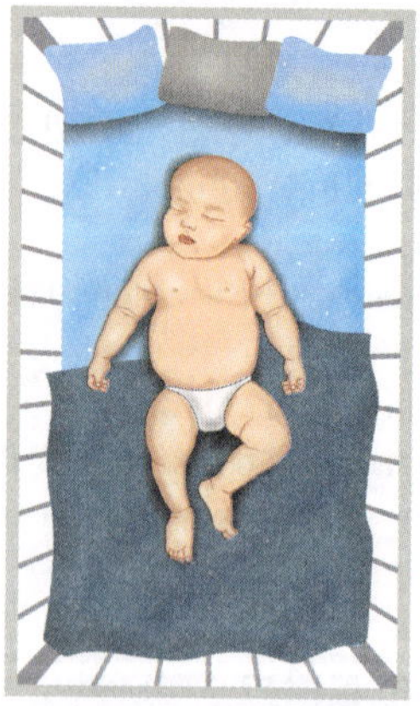

A **Alone**
Baby should sleep **Alone**

B **Back**
Put baby on its **Back**

C **Crib**
Put baby on safe **Crib**

Fig. 2.116 Prevention of SIDS

MÜNCHAUSEN SYNDROME BY PROXY

Synonyms

MSbP, Factitious Disorder by Proxy

Description

- **An individual – usually a mother – deliberately makes another person (usually her own child) sick, or convinces others that the person is sick**.
- The parent or caregiver misleads others into thinking that the child has medical problems by lying and reporting fictitious episodes. He or she may exaggerate, fabricate or induce symptoms.
- As a result, doctors usually order tests, try different types of medications, and may even hospitalize the child, or perform surgery to determine the cause.
- Because the parent or caregiver appears to be so caring and attentive, often no one suspects any wrongdoing. It is not unusual for medical personnel to overlook the possibility of MSbP because it goes against the belief that a parent or caregiver would never deliberately hurt his or her child.
- Children who are subject to MSbP are typically of preschool age, although there have been reported cases in children up to 16 years old. There are equal numbers of boys and girls; however, 98% of the perpetrators are female.

Diagnosis of MSbP

Clues:

- Child who has multiple medical problems that do not respond to treatment.

- Physical or laboratory findings that are highly unusual, do not correspond with the child's medical history, or are physically or clinically impossible.
- Short-term symptoms that tend to stop when the perpetrator is not around.
- Parent who is not reassured by "good news" when test results find no medical problems, but continues to believe that the child is ill.
- Parent/Caregiver who appears to be medically knowledgeable or fascinated with medical details or appears to enjoy hospital environment.
- Parent or caregiver who is unusually calm in the face of serious difficulties with the child's health.

Child Sexual Abuse

This is related to paedophilia, and is discussed in detail in the section on "Sexual Offences and Paraphilias." *(page no. 270)*

FM 2.29: Core – Role Play

- Demonstrate respect to the directions of courts, while appearing as witness for recording of evidence under oath or affirmation, examination in chief, cross examination, re-examination and court questions, recording of evidence.

Theoretical aspects have been discussed in Topic 1 under the following Competency: FM 1.5: **Non-Core**: Describe Court procedures *(page no. 16)*.

FM 2.30: Core – Written/Viva Voce

- Have knowledge/awareness of latest decisions/notifications/resolutions/circulars/standing orders related to medico-legal practice issued by Courts/Government authorities, etc.

These have been discussed under various Topics interspersed throughout the book.

FM 2.31: Core – Written/Viva Voce

- Demonstrate ability to work in a team for conduction of medico-legal autopsies in cases of death following alleged negligence, medical dowry death, death in custody or following violation of human rights as per National Human Rights Commission Guidelines on exhumation.

Discussed under the following Competency of Topic 2 *(page no. 64)*:

FM 2.15: Core – Written/Viva Voce/OSPE (Objective Structured Practical Examination)

- Describe special protocols for the conduct of medicolegal autopsies in cases of death in custody or following violation of human rights as per National Human Rights Commission Guidelines.

FM 2.32: Core – Written/Viva Voce

- Demonstrate ability to exchange information by verbal, or nonverbal communication to the peers, family members, law enforcing agency and judiciary.

COMMUNICATING WITH PATIENTS

- Good communication skills have been considered extremely important for medical practitioners in the Western world since decades. Its significance is now being acknowledged in our country and many educators have expressed the view that it is "the need of the hour" to train medical professionals in this important yet ignored aspect in clinical medicine. Of late, the medical system has witnessed an increase in the incidents of conflict between doctors and patients or their attendants. There has also been an increase in the number of lawsuits against doctors. Poor communication between doctors and patients is an important contributing factor. The practice of good communication skills in the medical profession is integral to the development of meaningful and trustworthy relationship between the doctors and patients and, thus, is beneficial to both of them.
- Effective communication has three basic components – verbal, non-verbal and para-verbal.
  - **Verbal component** deals with the content of the message including selection of the words. It covers information about the nature, course and prognosis of the disease; various treatment options available; nature, cost and yield of the investigations and risks/benefits of invasive procedures.
  - **Non-verbal component** includes body language like posture, gesture, facial expression and spatial distance. Although non-verbal component of the communication is frequently considered less important, evidence suggests that it significantly influences important outcomes like patient's satisfaction, adherence to advice and clinical outcome.
  - **Para-verbal component** includes tone, pitch, pacing and volume of the voice.
- There are several barriers to effective communication between patients and doctors. The most important one is lack of insight due to inadequate knowledge and training in communication skills. Many a time, doctors do not give enough heed to the importance of keeping patients adequately informed. Non-verbal components of the communications are frequently neglected. Language barrier is also important. It is not unusual for patients speaking in their local language and giving a tough time to doctors. Another important barrier is lack of adequate knowledge about the disease or treatment options. Finally, human failings like stress, tiredness or lack of time are major contributing factors in an overburdened setting.
- The importance of listening extends far beyond the academic and professional settings and is extremely important in creating a trustworthy doctor–patient relationship which is a prerequisite for therapeutic success. It is an active

process that involves imbibing all the information expressed verbally or non-verbally by the patient. It is a major part of communication process. It helps in better understanding of the patient's problem and finding better decisions. Studies exploring the reasons for filing litigations against doctors found that a significant proportion of the patients were dissatisfied because the doctor had not listened or understood their problem fully. Listening not only involves understanding the verbal component but also eliciting patient's attitudes, needs and motives behind the words. Some of the communication strategies that may help the doctor to improve listening skills are listed below:

1. Make the patient and the attendant comfortable. Never have discussions while walking in the corridors.
2. Show interest in what the patient is saying with your mannerism, body language and active involvement like leaning towards the patient.
3. Be careful not to interrupt him/her when he/she is expressing something.
4. While concluding, one must ask the patient, if he would like to add something more.
5. Respect the patient's confidentiality and maintain privacy. Patient should not be made to state the reason for their visit when other people are present.
6. Be the first one to greet the patient. Do not wait for the patient to speak because some patients will interpret your reticence as indifference. Shake hands and introduce yourself, wherever feasible and socially acceptable.
7. Be prepared and know the patient's name. Address a patient by his/her name whenever required. Do not fumble for name after the patient is in the room. If it is an old case, greet him and ask him how he is.
8. Establish eye contact and maintain it at reasonable intervals.
9. Put the patient at ease. Some patients may be nervous, so begin with a general non-medical inquiry in order to develop a comfortable scenario for the patient.
10. Pay attention to both the verbal and non-verbal clues from the patient and explore whenever there is any discrepancy between the two. Meanwhile, the physician too should be alert about his own non-verbal clues like body language, gestures, eye-contact.
11. Always provide information on what the patient wants to know and promptly respond to the patient's reaction.
12. Discuss nature, course and prognosis (both short term and long term) of the disease, treatment options available and necessity of the investigations.
13. Discuss in detail regarding necessity and feasibility of expensive investigations and drugs and their effect on main course and outcome of disease.
14. Involve the patient in the decision making. The treatment plan must conform to the patient's understanding, beliefs, cultural values and concerns.
15. Put additional efforts in motivating patients regarding adherence to lifestyle modifications.
16. Always convey details in simple language. The use of medical jargon and abbreviations can have a negative effect.

COMMUNICATING WITH A PATIENT'S ATTENDANTS

- This scenario usually arises when a doctor is treating an indoor patient. Attendants are apprehensive and at times full of doubts and queries. Communicating with the attendants assumes great importance especially when patient is critically ill or admitted in the ICU. The following tips can improve one's ability to communicate:
  1. Never be informal with them. Conduct conferences once and if possible twice daily.
  2. Talk about and appreciate the efforts made by them.
  3. Most of the attendants surf the Internet and gather lots of information. Try to satisfy their queries by giving better references.
  4. Always explain the dynamic nature of disease. This is especially important for critically ill patients.
  5. Second opinion should be sought proactively. This is important not only in patient management when one is in doubt but also helpful in building attendant's confidence. One will be more convinced and ready to accept bad outcome if the same fact is explained by more than one consultant.
  6. Never express shock. Try to convince that all efforts are being made to bring a situation under control or will be controlled.
  7. Consent taking is a very important part of counselling. Never neglect this and relegate it to paramedical staff or interns who may fail to explain convincingly.

COMMUNICATING WITH COLLEAGUES AND PEERS

- The following principles should be followed while interacting with colleagues, interns and students:
  1. Never talk disparagingly about your colleagues, or scold residents and students in front of patients or attendants. One should be extremely cautious while asking questions from Junior Residents on rounds. Patients may feel insecure in the absence of senior consultants who may not be present at all times. This may also create doubts in the minds of patients, if Junior Residents prescribe drugs for common complaints.
  2. Courtesy should be extended to all staff including nurses, paramedical staff and other supporting staff. Make them realise that they are a part of the team and their role and responsibility is also important. A system with effective teamwork can improve the quality of patient care and reduce workload among healthcare professionals.

3. Lead by setting examples. Supporting staff will never work with full sincerity unless and until they appreciate the hard work and ability of the doctor.
4. Try to teach them the principles of management of commonly encountered diseases in your ward. This will keep them motivated.
5. Audit and regular feedback improves in professional practice. Never delay to give appreciation, or positive criticism.

Breaking Bad News

- Bad news means any information that has a potential to have a devastating influence on one's life. However, its impact is highly dependent on the recipient's expectation and understanding.
- Disclosing bad news is a complex communication art that not only involves verbal component, but also includes empathetic response of the doctor to tackle the reaction. Studies have demonstrated that many doctors lack competence as well as confidence in their ability to divulge bad news, and there is a necessity to provide didactic training.
- Several protocols have been devised to guide doctors for acquiring this skill. It is useful to follow a strategic approach as described below while breaking bad news and provide information according to the patient's own knowledge or expectations, as well as to condense the emotional turmoil into an effective future management plan in the same setting.
    1. **Be primed up for the interview** – Breaking bad news is a daunting task and one should mentally rehearse the act of disclosure and the manner of reacting to the patient's emotions. Following key communication skills like maintaining privacy, sitting in a relaxed way with the patient, maintaining constant eye-to-eye contact, and avoiding any time pressure and interruptions, will allow an un-distracted and focussed discussion. If the patient wishes someone else to be with them, allow the patient to choose among relatives or friends.
    2. **Assess the patient's knowledge and attitude** – By asking open-ended questions, the doctor not only gains insight into the patient's perception of his medical problem, but also gets the opportunity to assess the patient's preparedness for the bad news.
    3. **Assess the patient's desire to get the level of detailed information** – Some patients may express the desire for full information about their diagnosis, prognosis and details of their illness, while others only want to have a broad idea.
    4. **Actual breaking of bad news** – It is better to plan an agenda with the patient, including diagnosis, treatment, prognosis and support or coping. An initial warning may decrease the shock that can follow the disclosure of bad news. Use of simple and non-technical words, giving information in small portions and periodic assessment of the impact are some of the communication tools that can be extremely useful.
    5. **Addressing the patient's emotions** – The patient's emotional reaction may vary from silence to disbelief, crying, denial or anger. It is the physician's duty to support the patient by making an empathic response. Moving closer to the patient, holding hands and using empathic statements help the physician to not only support the patient but also to acknowledge their own sadness and emotion. Validating responses help the patient to overcome and accept the reality. Sometimes, when the patient becomes silent or tearful, allow them time to recover. Exploratory questions may be helpful when the patient's reaction is ambiguous.
    6. **Summarising treatment plan** – It is important to formulate and discuss future plan of treatment with patients and/or attendants by involving them in the decision making. Those who are having a definite plan of action are less likely to get anxious or panic. Summarizing all the discussions at the end is extremely useful and helps in assessing, if the patient has understood the facts correctly or not.

FM 2.33 & FM 2.34: Core – Written/Viva Voce
- Demonstrate ability to use local resources whenever required like in mass disaster situations.

INTRODUCTION

- A **mass disaster** is defined as an event of serious magnitude causing severe damage to life and property.
- **Loss of life of 10 persons or more may be considered as a mass disaster**. Actually the number of victims involved is not important. A mass disaster is better defined as an incident in which so many people are injured that local emergency medical services are overwhelmed.
- A mass disaster could be of the following types*:
    - **Natural** – Floods, cyclones, earthquakes, drought, etc.
    - **Accidents** – Rail, air, road, sea, fire, etc.
    - **Industrial** – Gas leaks, explosions.
    - **Man-made** – Riot, war, terrorist attack, etc.
- There are two aspects to a mass disaster:
    - Preparation for disaster
    - Response to disaster
- The effectiveness of the response to a disaster is greatly enhanced by regular training exercises, continuous updating of plans and modifications of plans.
- The management of a mass disaster must be carried out by a well-coordinated team, consisting of any or all of the following:
    - Police
    - Ambulance service
    - Fire service
    - Military personnel

*Mnemonic: MANI.

- Forensic personnel
- Social workers
- Volunteers

FORENSIC ASPECTS

- Forensic team may consist of:
  - Forensic pathologists
  - Forensic odontologists
  - Fingerprint experts
  - DNA experts
  - Other experts, relevant to the nature of the disaster.
- A **temporary mortuary** should be constructed with facilities for refrigeration.
- There should be availability of tables or make-shift tables, instruments, gloves, cotton, packing and labeling materials, preservatives, disinfectants, antiseptics, whole-body size polythene bags or paper bags, sutures, needles and adequate water supply.
- Communication systems like telephones, computers, internet, etc., and adequate security arrangements should be there to avoid a **secondary disaster**.
- Examination of the scene of disaster (**Fig. 2.117**):
  - Examination of victims
  - Identification of the cause of death
  - Reconstruction of events

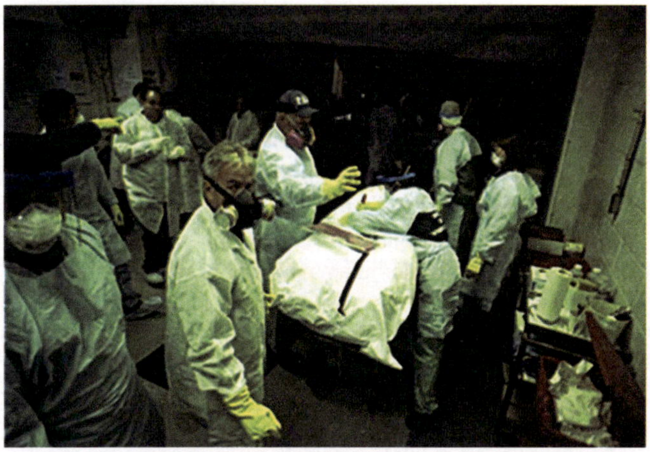

Fig. 2.117 Scene of a mass disaster

- Ensure the following measures:
  - Secure the disaster site.
  - Prepare a sketch plan of the site showing parts of the wreckage and position of the bodies.
  - Take photographs of the site.
  - Locate each body and label it with a "Mass casualty card", giving it serial number.
    - ***Note***: Mutilated bodies and fragmentary remains should also be labelled and numbered.
- Search for remains of explosive materials in case of explosions. The site may be required to be subjected to radiological examination which can help in the identification and detection of foreign bodies impacted in clothes or inside bodies.
- Clothes must be examined in detail, photographed and kept in safe custody for further identification by relatives.
- Personal properties such as identity card, documents that help in identification, jewellery such as rings, ear rings,etc., are very important to locate and preserve.
- Importance of identifying body remains:
  - Can help reconstruct the crime scene.
  - For the official death certificate to be issued, positive proof that the remains were found and identified is required.
  - Giving the victim's family members a sense of closure.
- Identifying criteria:
  - First option: Visual identification.
  - Second option: General and dental features.
  - Third option: Fingerprinting.
  - Fourth option: Radiological examination.
  - Final option: DNA fingerprinting.
- Diagnosis of the types of injuries: Nature, site, number, special characteristics, etc. Injuries will differ according to the type of disaster.
- Medical opinion can only be partial and contributory to other investigations. However, an opinion regarding the cause of disaster may be given in the case of airplane disasters, train mishaps and vehicular accidents, based on the following data:
  - Autopsy findings of pilot/driver:
    - Evidence of organic disease, like coronary occlusion, cerebrovascular accident or any other disease which could produce sudden collapse or blunting of mental faculties.
    - Evidence of poisoning due to alcohol or other psychotropic drugs affecting higher mental functions.
  - Autopsy findings of all victims:
    - Evidence of gun-shot injuries in case of air piracy.
    - Evidence of explosion injuries with retained explosive material, suggest an explosion.
- **Triaging**:
  - '**Triage**' is derived from Old French word "trier" which means "to sort". It is the process of sorting injured people into groups based on the need for, or likely benefit from immediate medical treatment. Triage is used in hospital emergency rooms, on battlefields, and at disaster sites when limited medical resources must be allocated.
  - **Sorting (Fig. 2.118)**: Green (Minimal Damage) – Yellow (Delayed Care) – Red (Immediate Attention) – Black (Deceased).
    - Green: Ambulatory patients (no impaired function, can self-treat or be cared for by non-professionals). Injuries are mostly in the form of abrasions, contusions, minor lacerations, etc.
    - Yellow: Can wait for expert care after simple first aid (dressing of wounds, application of splints).
    - Red: Critical victims (seriously injured, but have a reasonable chance of survival).

- Black: Victims showing obvious signs of death – unresponsive patients with no pulse, or with catastrophic head injuries and/or chest injuries.

FM 2.35: Core – Written/Viva Voce/OSPE (Objective Structured Practical Examination)

- Demonstrate professionalism while conducting autopsy in medicolegal situations, interpretation of findings and making inference/opinion, collection preservation and dispatch of biological or trace evidences.

Discussed under the following Competencies: FM 2.11–2.14.

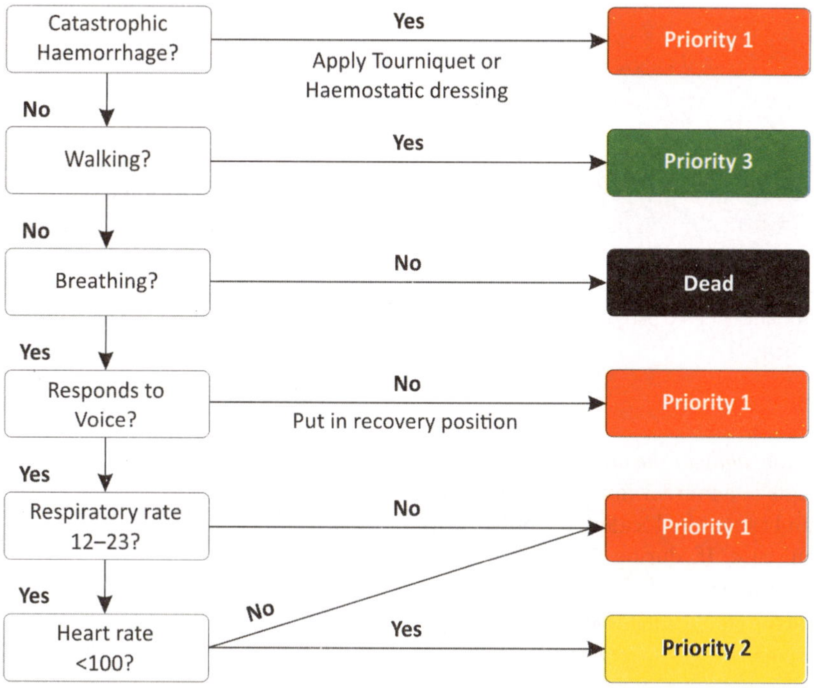

Fig. 2.118 Triaging in a mass casualty situation

Topic 3

CLINICAL FORENSIC MEDICINE

(Number of Competencies – 33: FM 3.1 to 3.33)

FM 3.1: Core – Written/Viva Voce/Skill Assessment
- **Identification**
  - Define and describe Corpus delicti
  - Establishment of identity of living persons including
    - Race
    - Sex
    - Religion
    - Complexion
    - Stature
    - Age Determination with regard to
      - Morphology
      - Teeth – eruption
      - Decaying remains
      - Bite marks
      - Bones – Ossification centres
      - Medicolegal aspects of age

CORPUS DELICTI

- **Corpus delicti** (Latin for '*body of the crime*') is one of the most important concepts in a murder investigation. When a person disappears and cannot be located, the police will file a 'missing person' case. If, during the course of the investigation, it is believed that he/she has been murdered, then a '**body of evidence**', including physical, demonstrative and testimonial evidence, must be obtained to establish that the missing individual has indeed been murdered before a suspect can be charged with homicide. This is referred to as **Corpus delicti**.
  - The best and easiest evidence establishment in these cases is the actual **dead body** of the deceased.
  - However, in the event that a dead body is not present or has not yet been discovered, it is possible to prove a crime took place, if sufficient **circumstantial evidence** is presented to prove the matter beyond a reasonable doubt. For example, the presence – at a missing person's home – of spilled human blood, identifiable as that person's, in large quantity, demonstrates – even in the absence of a corpse – the possibility that a fatal crime has occurred.
  - The British serial killer **John George Haigh** (Acid Bath Killer) destroyed the bodies of his victims with acid apparently because he thought that, in the absence of a corpse, murder could not be proven because there was no corpus delicti. Haigh had misinterpreted the Latin word *corpus* as a literal body, rather than a figurative one.
  - This had previously been the case, under **Matthew Hale's Rule** of "***no body, no crime***", but from the 20th century onwards, the law in many countries has been expanded to allow prosecution for murder even on circumstantial evidence. Sir Matthew Hale (1609–1676) was an influential but controversial British judge.

ESTABLISHMENT OF IDENTITY OF LIVING PERSONS

- **Identification** in the medicolegal sense refers to the determination of individuality of a person.
- It may be **complete** or **partial**.
  - In the case of living persons, as well as dead bodies recovered before the process of putrefaction has set in, identity can be fixed with respect to their name, age, sex, occupation, address, etc., with the help of their unique features. This is termed **complete identification**. Establishing complete identification is usually the responsibility of the police.
  - But, in cases of mutilated and highly putrefied bodies, as well as in skeletal remains, the police may require the help of a medical officer, or a forensic expert, who with his knowledge of anatomy can help provide certain information such as race, age, sex, stature, etc., by studying the morphology of the body parts. This is termed **partial identification**. Partial identification by a medical officer can provide some clues to the police for further investigation leading to complete identification.
- **The following factors can help in establishing the complete identity of a person, either living or dead**:
  - Race
  - Sex
  - Age
  - Hair
  - Anthropometry
  - Dactylography
  - Poroscopy
  - Footprints
  - Cheiloscopy
  - Rugoscopy
  - Tattoo marks
  - Scars
  - Occupational stigmata
  - Complexion & physical features

Race

Definition

- **Race** can be defined as "**a biological grouping within the human species distinguished or classified according to genetically transmitted differences**." Each race will have certain distinctive physical traits.

Classification

- The scientific classification of human racial types is based on certain combinations of fixed, inherited and measurable physical traits such as shape of the head, facial features, nose shape, eye shape and colour, skin colour, etc.
- Although difference of opinion exists regarding terminology and exact classification, the following divisions are generally accepted:
  - **Major groups** – ***Caucasoid, Negroid, Mongoloid, Australoid***
  - **Minor groups** – ***Indic, American Indian, Polynesian***

Some Characteristic Features of the Major Races

- **Caucasoid**:
  - These include European, Semitic (Arabs and Jews) and Indo-Aryan people.
  - Skin colour varies from very fair as in the case of North European people, to brown in the case of Indian and South West Asian people.
  - Hair is straight or wavy (sometimes frizzy), and may be blonde, brown or black.
  - Face is narrow to medium broad.
  - The nose is generally long and narrow.
- **Negroid**:
  - They chiefly inhabit Africa to the south of the Sahara, though some minor groups include the Negrito people of India and South East Asia, as well as the Melanesians of the South West Pacific.
  - Their skin colour varies from black to brown.
  - These people have broad, rather flat noses.
  - Their stature varies widely. The Pygmies of Central Africa are the shortest people in the world, while the Negroes of Sudan and Central Africa are among the tallest people in the world.
  - Face is narrow to medium-broad with prognathism.
  - Hair appears woolly, the colour is brown-black and texture is coarse.
- **Mongoloid**:
  - They are inhabitants of Northern, Eastern or South Eastern Asia. In fact, they were the original inhabitants of America.
  - The group includes Chinese, Japanese, Burmese, Thais, Vietnamese, and Malays, besides Eskimos, Red Indians, and American Indians of South America.
  - Their eyes have a characteristic fold of skin on the upper lid (epicanthic fold).
  - Hair is lank and straight.
  - Stature varies from short to medium.
- **Australoid**:
  - They are inhabitants of Southeast Asia, South Asia, Melanesia, Australia and other regions in East Asia.
  - Their skin colour is usually dark.
  - Hair is invariably curly.
  - Their stature is usually short.

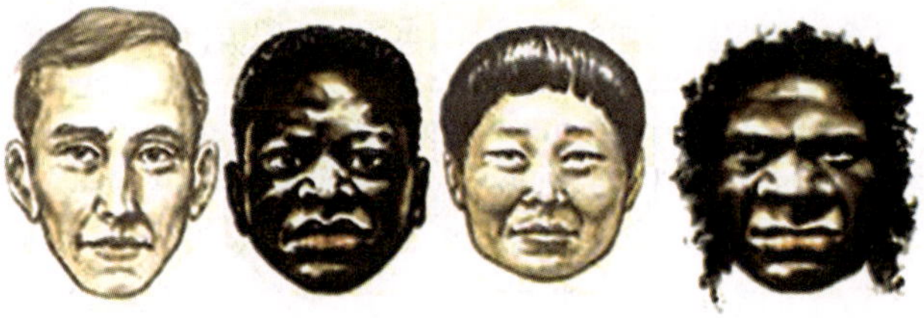

Fig. 3.1 Major human races of the world

Races of India:

- India has a diverse population and known to be one of the cradle lands of human civilisation. Ancient Indus Valley Civilisation was believed to have been of **Dravidian** origin in northern India.
- On the advent of **Indo-Aryan** race, and the conflicts between the two races, Dravidians were pushed to the south.

Identification of Race

- Race determination is mainly the domain of physical anthropologists. Due to global shrinkage and increasing incidence of mass disasters such as airplane crashes, etc., their help in identifying victims has become vital in many cases, which has led to the development of a specialised field, **Forensic Anthropology**.
- Race can be determined by studying
  - Variations in morphology.
  - **Osteometry**, i.e., measurement of various bones and studying the proportionalities to each other and
  - Multivariate discrimination function analysis.
- Krogman studied the morphological traits of the skull and outlined the essential descriptive morphology of the three main races. He further subdivided the **Caucasoids** into: **Nordic, Alpine** and **Mediterranean** groups on the basis of his findings.
- Attempts were also made by other investigators to differentiate the races on the basis of measurements of different **body parts**. Due to wide standard deviation, there is considerable overlap in the actual dimensions of various bones among the races, and hence the proportionality of different parameters was studied. This has led to the calculation of various indices such as **cephalic index, brachial index, crural index, inter-membral index, intra-membral index**, etc. (**Tables 3.1a & b**). The values of some of these indices for the three races – Asiatic Indians, Europeans & Negroes are mentioned in **Table 3.2**.
- **Scalp hair** also demonstrates characteristic features helpful in the determination of race (**Table 3.3**).

- Certain **dental characteristics** are also helpful in the determination of race.
  - The most distinctive feature is the '**shovel-shaped incisor**' seen among American Indians, Chinese and Palestinian Arab populations.
  - Other features like **cusp of Carabelli*** (**Fig. 3.2**), protostylid, cusp six & cusp seven, arrangement of groove patterns of molars, accessory ridges on canines, longitudinal tubercles in anterior teeth, etc., have also been studied for the discrimination of race.
  - The anterior curvature of the femur is said to be distinctive for the negroid race.

Sex

Situations where Sex Determination is Needed

- For the purpose of simple identification in the living, where the individual of one sex carries the features of the opposite sex.
- When a person appears to possess the primary sex organs of both the sexes.
- For the purpose of deciding whether an individual can exercise certain civil rights reserved to one sex only.
- For deciding questions relating to legitimacy, divorce, paternity, affiliation and also to some criminal offences.

Table 3.1a Various Indices

Race Indices	
Cephalic Index	$\frac{\text{Max Breadth of Skull}}{\text{Max. Antero-posterior Length of Skull}} \times 100$
Brachial Index	$\frac{\text{Length of Radius}}{\text{Length of Humerus}} \times 100$
Crural Index	$\frac{\text{Length of Tibia}}{\text{Length of Femur}} \times 100$
Inter-membral Index	$\frac{\text{(Length of Humerus + Length of Radius)}}{\text{(Length of Femur + Length of Tibia)}} \times 100$
Intra-membral Index	$\frac{\text{Length of Humerus}}{\text{Length of Femur}} \times 100$

Table 3.1b Cephalic Index

Type of Skull	Cephalic Index	Race
Dolico-cephalic (long-headed)	70–75	Pure Aryans, Aborigines & Negroes
Mesati-cephalic (medium-headed)	75–80	European and Chinese
Brachy-cephalic (short-headed)	80–85	Mongolian

Note*: *The* ***cusp of Carabelli**, or* ***Carabelli's tubercle****, or* ***tuberculum anomalum of Georg Carabelli*** *is a small additional cusp at the mesiopalatal line angle of maxillary first molars. Carabelli's cusp is most common among Europeans (75–85% of individuals).*

Table 3.2 Racial Differences from Osteometry

Index	Asiatic Indians	Europeans	Negroes
Brachial index	76.49	75.5	78.5
Crural index	86.49	83.3	86.2
Intermembral index	67.27	70.4	70.3
Intramembral index	71.11	69.0	72.4

Table 3.3 Racial Differences from Hair Analysis

Features	Negro	Caucasian	Mongolian
Diameter	60–90 mm	70–100 mm	90–120 mm
Cross-section	Kidney shaped	Oval	Round
Pigmentation	Dense & clumped towards the periphery	Evenly distributed towards the periphery	Dense auburn through the cross-section
Cuticle	–	Medium	Thick
Undulation	Prevalent	Uncommon	Rare

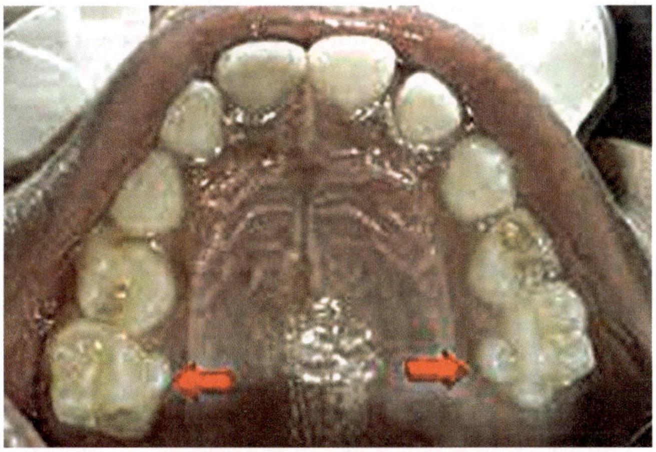

Fig. 3.2 Cusp of Carabelli (arrowed)

- Simple identification of dead individuals in an advanced state of decay, where primary sex organs are lost due to decomposition.

Determination of Sex in the Living

1. **Presumptive evidence of sex**: It is based on the outward appearance of the individual taking into account the clothing, general appearance of the face, the body contour, distribution of hairs including evidence of shaving, the habits, the voice, etc. It becomes unreliable when a person of one sex tries to conceal his own sex (***concealed sex***), and behaves like a person of the opposite sex.
2. **Probable evidence of sex**: It is based upon the possession of secondary sexual characteristics such as breast development, distribution of body hairs, muscular development and the presence of vagina in females and penis in males. Difficulty arises in the case of intersex states, when there is intermingling of sexes.
3. **Positive evidence of sex**: This is done by confirming the presence of ovaries in females, and testes in males, and by the presence of Barr bodies and Davidson bodies (**Fig. 3.3**).
   a. **Barr body** or **sex chromatin** is a distinctive basophilic, intranuclear structure usually located near the inner surface of nuclear membrane of the somatic cells of females, which is absent in males. It is presumed that this is due to the inactivation of an extra X chromosome, and the number of Barr bodies present is correlated with the number of X chromosomes as follows:

   $$B = X - 1$$

   (B = No of Barr bodies, X = No of X chromosomes)

   b. Davidson and Smith observed a sex difference in the morphology of polymorphonuclear leukocytes in females. Some polymorph nuclei demonstrate an additional lobe ("**drumstick**") which is rarely found in males. This has come to be called the "**Davidson body**".
   c. The Y chromosome present in some cells demonstrates fluorescence when stained with quinacrine.

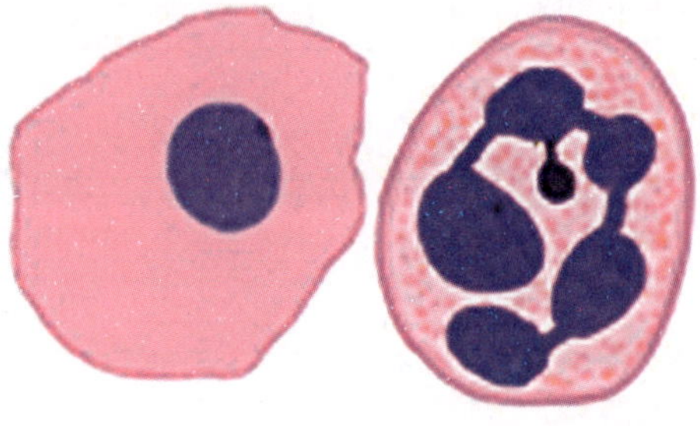

Fig. 3.3 Barr body (L) and Davidson body (R)

Intersex (Disorders of Sexual Differentiation)

- Sexual differentiation is a sequential and ordered process. Chromosomal sex, established at the moment of fertilization determines the gonadal sex, which in turn causes the development of phenotypic sex, in which male and female urogenital sex is formed.
- A disturbance in any process during embryogenesis may impair sexual differentiation. No matter how many X-chromosomes are present (47XXY, 49XXXY), a testis will develop as long as a normal Y chromosome is present. A normal testis is essential for the development of masculine characteristics. The absence of testes, as seen in females (and males in whom castration is done before puberty), will make a person feminine.
- **Classification of disorders of sexual development (DSD)***:
  - ***Disorders of chromosomal sex***:
    - Gonadal dysgenesis (Klinefelter syndrome)
    - Gonadal dysgenesis (Turner syndrome)
    - Mixed gonadal dysgenesis
    - True hermaphroditism
  - ***Disorders of gonadal sex***:
    - Pure gonadal dysgenesis
    - Dysgenetic testis
    - Absent testis syndrome
  - ***Disorders of phenotypic sex***:
    - *Female pseudohermaphroditism*:
      - Congenital adrenal hyperplasia
      - Non-adrenal female pseudohermaphroditism
      - Developmental disorders of mullerian duct
    - *Male pseudohermaphroditism*:
      - Abnormalities in androgen synthesis
      - Abnormalities in androgen action
      - Persistent mullerian duct syndrome
      - Developmental defect of male genitalia

Klinefelter Syndrome

- It is best defined as male hypogonadism that occurs when there are two or more X chromosomes and one or more Y chromosomes.
- This is the most common cause of hypogonadism in males. The incidence is 1 in 850 live male births.
- The classical pattern is associated with **47 XXY** karyotype.
- Characteristic features include:
  - Eunuchoid body with abnormally long legs.
  - Small atrophic testes often associated with a small penis.
  - Lack of such secondary sex characteristics as deep voice, beard and male distribution of pubic hair.
  - Gynaecomastia is a usual finding.
- It is the principal cause of male infertility.

Turner Syndrome

- This results from complete or partial monosomy of the X-chromosome, and is characterised primarily by hypogonadism in phenotypic females.
- It is the most common sex chromosome abnormality in females.
- Usual karyotype is **45 XO**.
- Characteristic features include:
  - Short stature
  - Low posterior hairline
  - Webbing of neck
  - Broad chest with widely spaced nipples
  - Cubitus valgus
  - Pigmented naevi
  - Peripheral lymphoedema at birth.
  - Coarctation of aorta is a common finding.
- It is the single most important cause of primary amenorrhoea.

Hermaphroditism

- The term "**true hermaphrodite**" implies the presence of both ovarian and testicular tissue.
- In contrast, a "**pseudo-hermaphrodite**" represents a disagreement between the phenotypic and gonadal sex.
  - Therefore, a **female pseudo-hermaphrodite** has ovaries but male external genitalia and
  - a **male pseudo-hermaphrodite** has testicular tissue but female type genitalia.
- **True hermaphroditism**:
  - It is an extremely rare condition.
  - In some cases, there is a testis on one side and an ovary on the other; whereas in other cases, there may be combined ovarian and testicular tissue known as ovotestes.
  - Karyotype: 46 XX in 50% of cases, and 46 XY in 25% of cases.
- **Female pseudohermaphroditism**:
  - Karyotype is 46 XX in all cases, and the development of gonads (ovaries) and internal genitalia are normal.
  - Only the external genitalia are ambiguous or virilized.
  - The basis of this disorder is excessive and inappropriate exposure to androgenic steroids during early foetal life.

**The new classification on Disorders of Sexual Development is given in Appendix IV. However, the older system is still popular in the forensic context.*

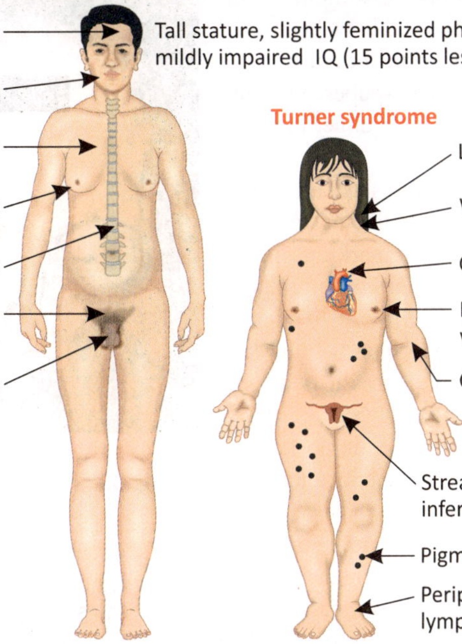

Fig. 3.4 Differences between Turner's and Klinefelter's syndromes

- **Male pseudohermaphroditism**
  - Karyotype is 46 XY.
  - Their gonads are exclusively testes, but the external genitalia are either ambiguous or completely feminine.
  - Commonest cause is defective virilization of male embryo, resulting from genetically determined defects in androgen synthesis or action, or both. **Table 3.4** provides a summary of Intersex.

Determination of Sex in the Dead

I. **In a Decomposed Body**:

a. Putrefaction starts early in the external genitalia altering their appearance.

b. Sometimes deliberate mutilation of external genitalia, as seen in sex crimes and destruction by carrion feeders (scavenging animals) soon after death, poses problems for identification.

c. In such circumstances, one must make a search for the ovaries.

d. A non-pregnant **uterus**, and uterus containing non-degenerative myomas are significantly resistant to putrefaction.

e. **Prostate** is also among the organs to putrefy last.

f. But when the primary sex organs are totally unidentifiable, one has to look for sexual characteristics in the skeleton.

II. **From Skeletal Remains**:

a. For a trained pathologist, it seldom poses a problem to determine sex from skeletal remains. The accuracy of estimating sex from skeletal remains depends upon the number of bones available.

i. According to Krogman, when the entire skeleton is available, sex can be determined with 100% certainty, from pelvis alone 95%, from skull alone 90%, from both skull & pelvis 98% and from long bones it can be done with 80% certainty.

Table 3.4 Sex Determination in Intersex

Intersex	Anatomical Sex	Nuclear Sex
Gonadal Agenesis	–	–
Gonadal Dysgenesis ▪ Turner's Syndrome ▪ Klinefelter's Syndrome ▪ True Hermaphroditism	 Female Male Bisexual	 – Female Female
Pseudo-Hermaphroditism ▪ Male ▪ Female	 Female Male	 Male Female

b. Sex differences in the morphology of skull and mandible are considered quite reliable, and have been used extensively for sex determination. While the female skull retains the gracile attributes seen in pre-pubescent skull, the male cranium becomes markedly rougher in adulthood at the site of muscle attachments.
   i. The important differentiating features include prominence of supraorbital ridges, glabella, mastoid process, digastric groove, muscular markings in the occipital area and frontal and parietal eminences (**Table 3.5**) (**Figs. 3.5 & 3.6**).

c. The pelvis is generally agreed to be the part of the skeleton best suited for sex determination as it is associated with female structural capability to bear children.
   i. The morphological features that are important for sex determination include greater sciatic notch, subpubic angle, pre-auricular sulcus, shape of pubis, etc. The shape of the greater sciatic notch is an important differentiating feature even in early foetal life. The other features become more pronounced after puberty due to the effect of hormones. The important differentiating features are given in **Table 3.6** (**Figs. 3.7 & 3.8**).

d. Because the differentiating features become more prominent after puberty, it is easier to sex an adult skeleton than to sex infant remains. Again towards old age, there occurs blurring of sexually dimorphic traits. So, the determination of sex from bones should ideally be limited to 15–55 years of age.

e. Although other bones (long bones, sternum and ribs) have also been investigated for their accuracy and reliability for sex determination, they are only used when the skull and the pelvis are not available for examination.

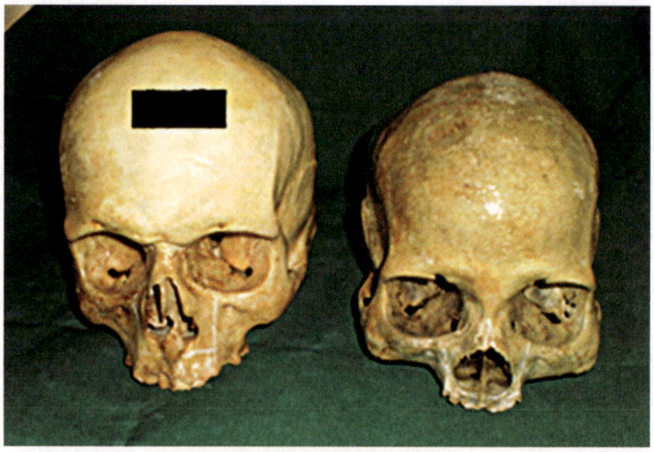

Fig. 3.6 Male and female skulls – Front view (*Courtesy*: *Dr Prateek Rastogi*)

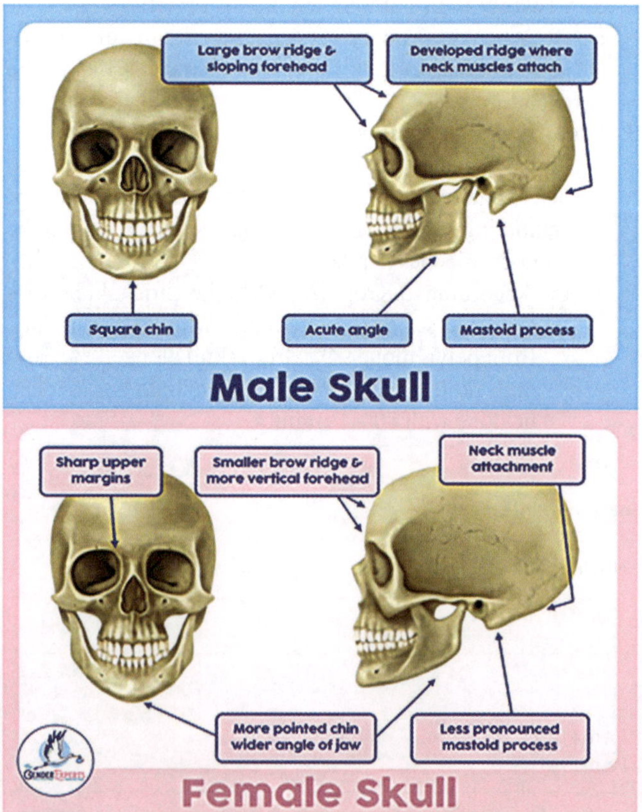

Fig. 3.5 Differences between male and female skulls

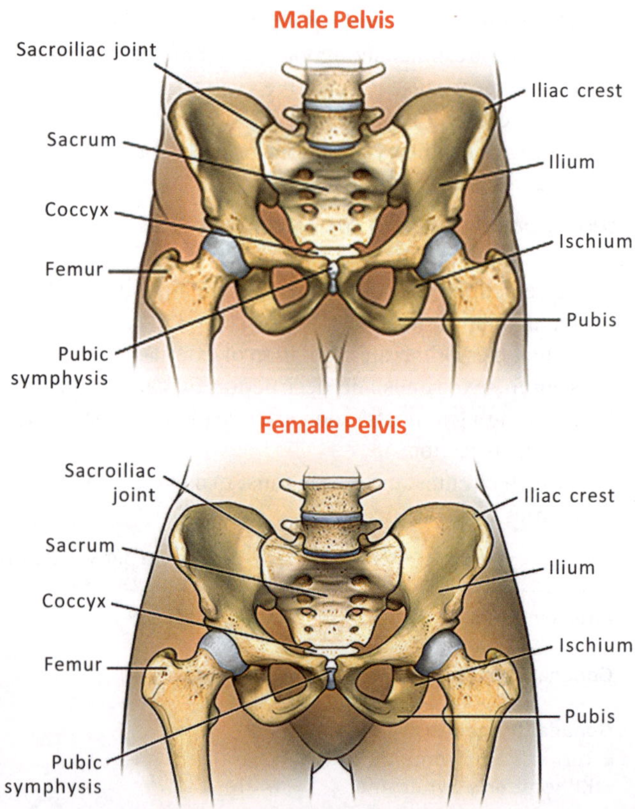

Fig. 3.7 Differences between male and female pelvis

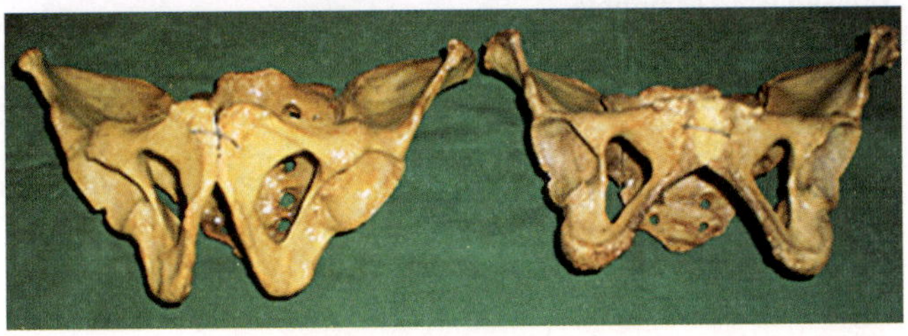

Fig. 3.8 Male and female pelvis – Front view (*Courtesy*: *Dr Prateek Rastogi*)

f. In addition to the qualitative assessment of sex from the skeleton, a quantitative approach can be used to "calculate" sex. Some important indices devised for this purpose are as follows:

i. **Sciatic notch index**:

$$\frac{\text{Width of notch (mm)}}{\text{Depth of notch (mm)}} \times 100$$

Male: 4–5; *Female*: 5–6

ii. **Washburn Ischiopubic index**:

$$\frac{\text{Pubic length (mm)}}{\text{Ischial length (mm)}} \times 100$$

Male: 73–94; *Female*: 91–115

iii. **Corporobasal sacral index**:

$$\frac{\text{Breadth of } 1^{st} \text{ sacral vertebra (mm)}}{\text{Breadth of base of sacrum (mm)}} \times 100$$

Male: 45; *Female*: 40.5

iv. **Sternal index**:

$$\frac{\text{Manubrial length (mm)}}{\text{Body length (mm)}} \times 100$$

Male: 46.2; *Female*: 54.3

Stature

- Estimation of stature or height of a person is subject to variations during life due to muscular relaxation and elasticity of intervertebral discs, but could still be valuable in identification.
- Stature estimation from **dismembered body parts** can be done on the basis of the ratio of the body part concerned, in relation to the entire body. Thus,

  Stature
  = 2 × (length of either arm) + 30 + 4 cm
  = 2 × (length from vertex to symphysis pubis)
  = 2 × (length from symphysis pubis to either heel)
  = 3.3 × (length from sternal notch to symphysis pubis)
  = 8 × (height of the skull)
  = 19/5 × (length of forearm)
- Generally, 2.5–4 cm is added to the stature calculated from skeletal remains in order to account for soft tissues.
- Stature can be estimated from skeletal remains quite accurately with the help of **regression formulae** using the length of long bones. The weight bearing long bones especially of the lower limbs are supposed to provide more reliable estimates of stature as compared to the other bones.
  - **Karl Pearson** (1899) developed regression formulae which became popular in the UK and other parts of the Western world. He utilized the data of another anthropologist (Rollet, 1888) and measured the stature and the lengths of the long bones of 50 male and 50 female French cadavers ranging in age from 24 to 99 years. Subsequently, he created tables for stature estimation (**Karl Pearson's formulae** for stature estimation).
  - **Dupertuis & Hadden** (1951) suggested using more than one long bone in the calculation of stature, and felt that the tibia and femur provided better estimates than radius and humerus. They derived regression equations for calculation of stature from a sample of 100 male Whites, 100 female Whites, 100 male Negroes and 100 female Negroes.
  - **Trotter & Gleser** (1952, 1958) studied the racial differences in stature calculation, and evolved regression formulae for the three major races, as well as the Mexican and Puerto Rican groups. Their studies are considered to be the most reliable for a Caucasian population, and are the most widely used method of estimating stature.* Later, **Trotter (1970) devised formulae which are today considered to be amongst the most accurate for stature estimation**.
  - **Steele** devised formulae to estimate **stature from fragmented bones**. He deduced the ratio of various segments of long bones in relation to their entire length, so that the length of a long bone could first be estimated from its fragments, which can then be applied to regression formulae to arrive at the stature.
- The bones must be measured in a dry state without cartilage, using a **Hepburn osteometric board** (**Fig. 3.9**).

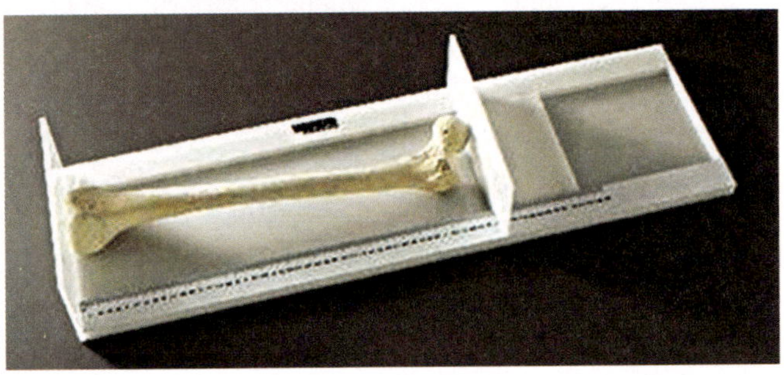

Fig. 3.9 Osteometric board

Pillay – Textbook of Forensic Medicine & Toxicology

Source: *Jantz RL. Modification of the Trotter and Gleser female stature estimation formulae. J Forensic Sci. 1992;37:1230–5.*

Table 3.5 Sex Differences in the Skull and Mandible

Trait	Sex	
	Male	Female
General size	Large	Small
Architecture	Rugged	Smooth
Supraorbital ridges	Medium to large	Small to medium
Mastoid processes	Medium to large	Small to medium
Frontal & parietal eminences	Small	Large
Orbits	Square, lower, smaller, with rounded margins	Rounded, higher, larger, with sharp margins
Forehead	Steeper, less rounded	More vertical and rounded
Cheek bones	Heavier, more laterally arched	Lighter, more compressed
Mandible	Larger, higher symphysis, broader ascending ramus	Small
Palate	Larger, broader, U shape	Small parabola
Occipital condyles	Large	Small
Teeth	Large, lower M1 often 5 cusped	Small molars, often 4 cusped

Table 3.6 Sex Differences in the Pelvis

Trait	Sex	
	Male	Female
Pelvis as a whole	Massive, rugged, marked muscle sites	Less massive, gracile, smoother
Symphysis	Higher	Lower
Subpublic angle	V-shaped	U-shaped, obtuse angle
Obturator foramen	Large, often ovoid	Small, triangular
Acetabulum	Large, directed laterally	Small, directed antero-laterally
Greater sciatic notch	Smaller, narrower, deeper	Larger, wider, shallower
Ischiopubic rami	Slightly everted	Strongly everted
Sacroiliac joint	Large	Wide
Pre & Post auricular sulcus	Not frequent	More frequent, better developed
Ischial tuberosity	Not everted	Everted
Sacrum	Longer, narrower, evenly distributed curvature, with 5 or more segments	Shorter, broader, marked curvature, with 5 segments
Pelvic brim	Heart shaped	Circular, elliptical
True pelvis, or cavity	Relatively smaller	Oblique, shallow, spacious

- The maximum length should be taken for all bones except femur and tibia, which are to be measured obliquely.
- Best results are obtained with lower limb bones, particularly, femur and tibia.

Age

Estimation of the age of an individual is usually done by studying the following:

1. Physical development.
2. Teeth.
3. Appearance and fusion of ossification centres.
4. Age-related changes.

Estimation of Age During Intra-uterine Life

- The age of a foetus can be assessed by studying the developing morphology, appearance of ossification centres in various bones, and also the germination of teeth (**Table 3.7**). The important ossification centres that need to be

Table 3.7 Age-related Changes in Foetus

Features	Months (IUL)						
	3	4	5	6	7	8	9
Length	9 cm	16 cm	25 cm	30 cm	35 cm	40 cm	45 cm
Weight	30–35 g	120–130 g	400 g	700 g	1 kg	1.5 kg	2–2.25 kg
Nails	Present in membranous form	–	Up to proximity of tips of fingers	–	Up to tips of fingers	–	Beyond the tips of fingers
Hair	–	Lanugo appears	Scalp hair appears	–	Scalp hair 1 cm long	Scalp hair 1.5 cm	Scalp hair 2 cm
Sex	–	Differentiable	–	Well differentiated	–	–	–
Eyelids	–	–	–	Adherent & eye lashes present	Non-adherent & eyelashes present	Well formed	
Brain	–	–	–	Sylvian fissure formed	–	–	–
Intestine	–	Meconium in upper part of small intestine	Meconium up to ascending colon	Meconium in transverse colon	Meconium in descen-ding pelvic colon		Meconium in rectum
Scrotum	–	–	–	Empty	–	Corru-gated	Occupied by testes
Testes	–	–	–	On psoas muscle	Near the internal ring	In canal (L before R)	In scrotum (L before R)
Centres of ossification	–	–	Centre for manubrium, 1st segment of sternum	–	Talus & 2nd & 3rd segments of sternum	–	Lower end of femur, and cuboid

studied for estimating foetal age include the talus, calcaneum, and tibial and femoral ends. These can be analyzed by dissection in the case of a dead foetus.

- **Haase's Rule***: Haase's rule enables us to calculate the age of a foetus in lunar months from the length of the foetus.
  - Until the foetus reaches the length of 25 cm, the square root of the crown–heel length is taken to arrive at the age.
  - When the length of the foetus is more than 25 cm, it is divided by 5.

Estimation of Age from Birth till 25 years

1. Physical Features

An approximate estimate of the age can be made from the height and weight of a person by referring to standard charts. A study of secondary sexual characteristics can be of added help.

2. Teeth

- The development of human dentition in three stages, viz deciduous dentition, mixed dentition and permanent dentition, follows a periodic sequence which can be utilised for a more or less accurate estimation of age. Data regarding the eruption and root calcification of deciduous and permanent teeth are mentioned in **Tables 3.8 & 3.9**.
- Differences between deciduous and permanent teeth are given in **Table 3.10**.
- An important point to remember in age estimation from dental eruption is with reference to the 3rd molar teeth, which have a predilection for either agenesis or impaction. In both cases, there will be **non-eruption of the 3rd molars**, but an X-ray of the jawbone will reveal impacted teeth, while agenesis will of course be associated with complete absence of the tooth concerned, even on X-ray. After the eruption of second molar, the ramus of mandible grows posteriorly for the third molar to erupt. This can be made out by placing the index finger behind the 2nd molar. Because the eruption of 3rd molar is very irregular, an X-ray of the jaw must always be undertaken to assess the calcification of 3rd molar, if spacing is present. If calcification is complete even without eruption of 3rd molar, age can be presumed to be more than 25 years.
- **Boyde's method**: Cross striations in the enamel of teeth represent daily incremental lines. The age of an individual can be calculated by counting the number of lines from the neonatal line onwards. This method is applicable mainly to infants. The age so calculated is accurate with an error of around 20 days.
- **Medicolegal importance of teeth**: Apart from estimation of age, dentition can be useful in a number of ways, and its study in relation to crime investigation has evolved into a new branch called **Forensic Odontology** (**Box 3.1** presents an overview).
  - Because teeth resist putrefaction and other destructive processes such as fire for a significantly longer period than most other structures in the body, they can be invaluable in the identification of decomposing or disintegrating remains. From the tooth pulp, tissues can be taken for determination of blood group, sex of the individual and also for DNA fingerprinting.

Table 3.8 Calcification and Eruption of Deciduous Teeth

Tooth	Calcification	Eruption	Calcification of Root Completed
Central incisor			
- Lower	5–6 months IUL	6–8 months	1.5–2 years
- Upper	5–6 months IUL	7–9 months	1.5–2 years
Lateral incisor			
- Upper	5–6 months IUL	7–9 months	1.5–2 years
- Lower	5–6 months IUL	10–12 months	1.5–2 years
First molar	5–6 months IUL	12–14 months	2–2.5 years
Canine	5–6 months IUL	17–18 months	2.5–3 years
Second molar	5–6 months IUL	20–30 months	3 years

****Note***: *Named after Carl Friedrich Haase (1788–1865), a German obstetrician.*

Table 3.9 Calcification and Eruption of Permanent Teeth

Tooth	Calcification	Eruption	Calcification of Root Completed
First molar	At birth	6–7 years	9–10 years
Central incisor	3–4 months	6–8 years	10 years
Lateral incisor	1 year	7–9 years	11 years
First premolar	1.5 years	9–11 years	12–13 years
2nd premolar	2 years	10–12 years	12–14 years
Canine	4–5 months	11–12 years	12–13 years
2nd molar	2.5–3 years	12–14 years	14–16 years
3rd molar	8–10 years	17–25 years	22–25 years

Table 3.10 Differences between Temporary Teeth and Permanent Teeth

Temporary Teeth	Permanent Teeth
Smaller in size, lighter and more delicate	Longer and larger, stronger and heavier
Anterior teeth vertically placed	Anterior teeth slightly inclined forward
China white in colour	Ivory white in colour
Neck is more constricted	Less constricted
X-ray reveals tooth germ below the tooth	

Box 3.1A—Forensic Odontology (Forensic Dentistry)

Definition: Application of dentistry in the investigation of crime and administration of justice.

Scope: Dental study can be extremely helpful in:

1. Identification of unknown dead body: This is done by comparing antemortem and postmortem records, or by DNA study of tooth pulp.
2. Identification of burnt, mutilated or decomposing remains (teeth are very resistant to decomposing or destructive processes).
3. Estimation of age, on the basis of eruption status, Gustafson's method, etc.
4. Identification of race, occupation, sex, etc., by study of characteristic features.
5. Identification of culprit through bite marks **(Box 3.1B)**.
6. Diagnosis of poisoning, e.g., lead poisoning leaves behind a bluish line on the gingival margins.

Charting of teeth

1. *Universal system*: Each tooth is given a number, 1 through 16 for upper jaw, beginning with right upper 3rd molar; and 17 through 32 for lower jaw, beginning with left lower 3rd molar, e.g., lower left canine is tooth no. 22 **(Fig. 3.1A-1)**.

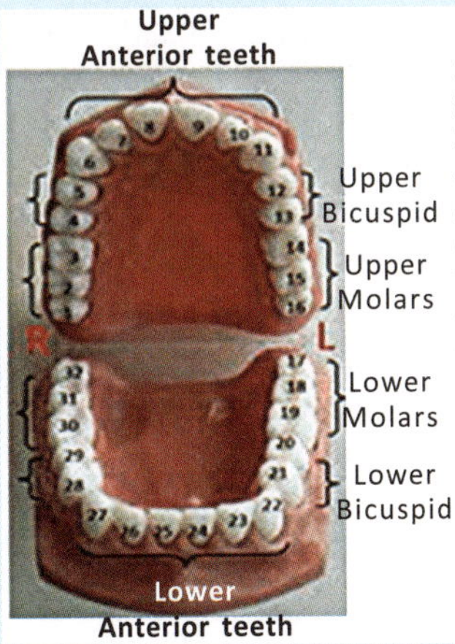

1, 17 – 3rd Molar (Wisdom teeth)
2, 18 – 2nd Molar (12-yr molar)
3, 19 – 1st Molar (6-yr molar)
4, 20 – 2nd Bicuspid (2nd premolar)
5, 21 – 1st Bicuspid (1st premolar)
6, 22 – Cuspid (canine/eye tooth)
7, 23 – Lateral incisor
8, 24 – Central incisor
9, 25 – Central incisor
10, 26 – Lateral incisor
11, 27 – Cuspid (canine/eye tooth)
12, 28 – 1st Bicuspid (1st premolar)
13, 29 – 2nd Bicuspid (2nd premolar)
14, 30 – 1st Molar (6-yr molar)
15, 31 – 2nd Molar (12-yr molar)
16, 32 – 3rd Molar (Wisdom teeth)

Fig. 3.1A-1. Universal system

2. *Palmer's notation*: The Palmer notation consists of a symbol (┘└ ┐┌) designating in which quadrant the tooth is found and a number indicating the position from the midline. Adult teeth are numbered 1–8, with deciduous (baby) teeth indicated by a letter A–E. Hence, the left and right maxillary central incisor would have the same number, "1", but the right one would have the symbol,

"┘", underneath it, while the left one would have, "└". Thus, lower left canine is designated ┌3.

3. *Haderup system*: Similar to Palmer's notation, except that it uses a + sign for upper teeth, and a – sign for lower teeth. The sign is placed before the number for left teeth, and after the number for right teeth. Thus, lower left canine is designated –3.
4. *Federation Dentaire Internationale (FDI) two-digit system*: Similar to Palmer's notation, but substitutes a number for quadrant sign: 1 for right upper, 2 for left upper, 3 for left lower and 4 for right lower quadrant. Thus, lower left canine is designated 33 **(Fig. 3.1A-2)**.
   For deciduous teeth: 5 for right upper, 6 for left upper, 7 for left lower and 8 for right lower quadrant. Thus, lower left permanent canine is designated 73.

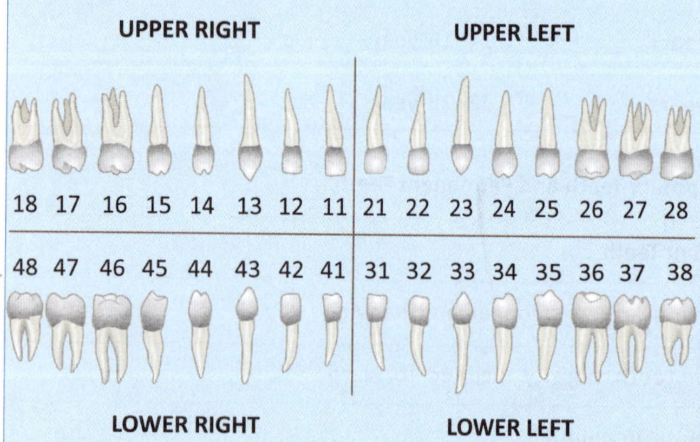

3.1A-2. FDI system

5. *Modified FDI system*: Same as above, except that right lower quadrant is 3, and left lower quadrant is 4 (zig-zag system). For deciduous teeth: 5 for right upper, 6 for left upper, 8 for left lower and 7 for right lower quadrant. Thus, lower left permanent canine is designated 43.

Box 3.1B—Forensic Odontology (Forensic Dentistry) Bite Mark Analysis

Bite Mark

- Bite mark is a special type of mechanical injury that results from biting with the teeth, and may be the result of attack by a human or animal.
- It is either a patterned abrasion or a contusion. If it is inflicted with great pressure or force, a laceration can result. It may occasionally involve loss of tissue, e.g., biting off fingers, nose, ears, etc.
- Medicolegally speaking, bite marks are inflicted during an assault offensively by the accused on the victim, and defensively by the victim on the accused. In sexual crimes, bite marks on the victim may be the offshoot of passion (love bite). Even in the case of consensual sex, love bites are common, and may in fact be inflicted by the female partner on the male as frequently as the other way around! **(Fig. 3.1B-1)**.
- Bite marks may also be encountered on inanimate objects such as fruits, cheese, chocolate, etc., left at the scene of a crime by the perpetrator **(Fig. 3.1B-2)**.

Bite Mark Analysis

- Careful examination of a bite mark can provide evidence to identify the accused. It can be photographed with a scale alongside, enlarged to actual size and then compared with the bite mark of the accused taken on a dental mould **(Fig. 3.1B-3)**. It is a highly specialized form of analysis, and must be undertaken only by a forensic odontologist.
- Although they are only a small portion of most forensic dentist's case load, bite marks represent the most challenging aspect of the discipline. In addition to the location of the bite mark, the type of severity of the injury may give investigators clues as to the mental state of the offender.
- Bite marks may be found on the flesh of victims of a violent attack, particularly on the face, breasts, trunk or buttocks. Alternatively, they may be found on the suspect, left by the victim during self-defense.
- Bite marks can be altered through stretching, movement or change in environment after the bite. There is also no set standard by which to analyse and compare bite marks.

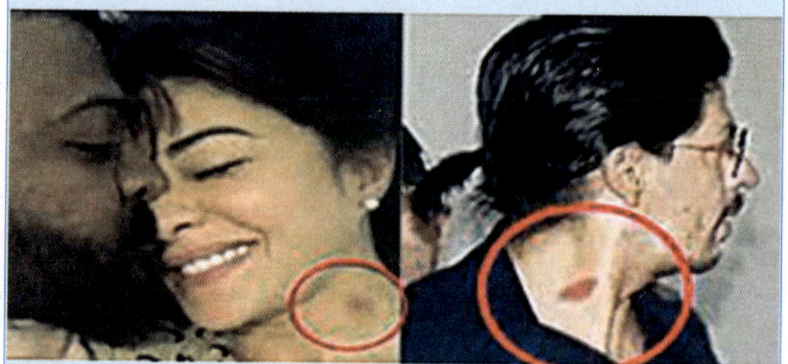

Fig. 3.1B-1. Love bite marks

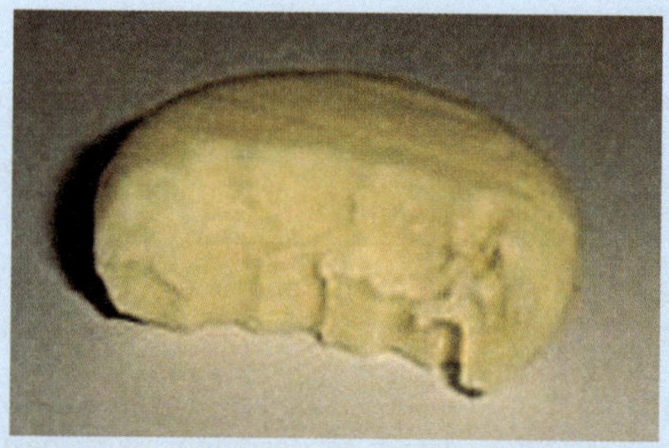

Fig. 3.1B-2. Bite mark on cheese left at scene of crime

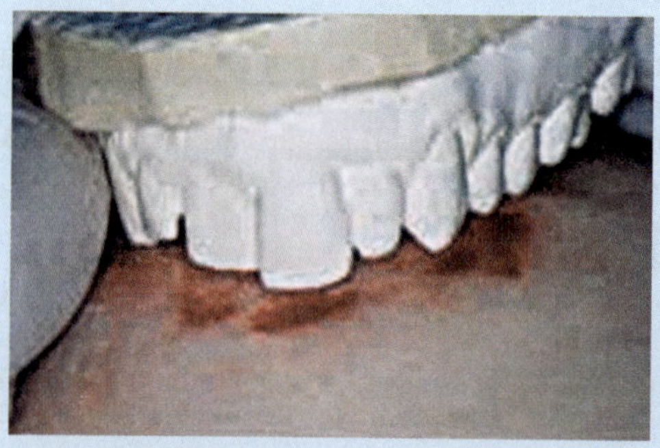

Fig. 3.1B-3. Bite mark analysis

- Factors that may affect the accuracy of bite mark identification:
  - Time-dependent changes of the bite mark on living bodies.
  - Effects of where the bite mark was found, damage on soft tissue and similarities in dentition among individuals.
  - Poor photography, impressions or measurement of dentition characteristics.
- Most bite mark analysis studies use porcine skin (pigskin), because it is comparable to the skin of a human, and it is considered unethical to bite a human for study purposes. Limitations to the bite mark studies include differences in properties of pigskin compared to human skin and the technique of using simulated pressures to create bite marks. Although similar histologically, pigskin and human skin behave in dynamically different ways due to differences in elasticity. Furthermore, postmortem bites on non-human skin display different patterns to those seen in antemortem bite injuries. Future research and technological developments may help reduce the occurrence of such limitations.
- In the past, the "direct method" compared a model of the suspect's teeth to a life-size photograph of the actual bite mark. Later, "indirect methods" were developed, which involve the use of transparent overlays to record a suspect's biting edges. Transparent overlays are made by free-hand tracing the occlusal surfaces of a dental model onto an acetate sheet. However, the use of transparent overlays is considered subjective and irreproducible because the tracing can be easily manipulated. Thus, photocopier-generated overlays were developed, where no tracing is used.
- While the photocopier-generated technique is sensitive, reliable, and inexpensive, new methods involving digital overlays have proven to be more accurate. Two recent technological developments include the 2D polyline method and the painting method. Both methods use Adobe Photoshop. Use of the 2D polyline method entails drawing straight lines between two fixed points in the arch and between incisal edges to indicate the tooth width. Use of the painting method entails coating the incisal edges of a dental model with red glossy paint and then photographing the model. Adobe Photoshop is then used to make measurements on the image. A total of 13 variables are used in analysis.

Criticism of Bite Mark Analysis

- Of late, the scientific foundation of forensic odontology, and especially bite mark comparison, has been called into question. In 2016, the President's Council of Advisors on Science and Technology (USA) declared that bite mark analysis had no scientific validity.
- Although bite mark analysis has been used in legal proceedings since 1870, it has become a controversial topic due to a variety of factors. Many investigators have shown that the accuracy of a bite mark on skin is limited at best. Skin is not a good medium for dental impressions; it is liable to have a number of irregularities present before the imprint, that could cause distortion. Also, bite marks can be altered through stretching, movement or a changing environment during and after the actual bite. Furthermore, the level of distortion tends to increase after the bite mark was made.
- Bite mark analysis is also controversial because dental profiles are subject to change. The loss of teeth or the alteration of arch configuration through a variety of procedures is common in human populations. The onset of oral diseases such as dental caries has been shown to alter the arch and tooth configuration and must be taken into account when comparing a dental profile to the bite mark.
- While the methods behind collecting bite mark evidence at the scene are leading toward greater standardization, the methodology behind analyzing bite marks is extremely variable because it depends upon the preference of the specific odontologist. As discussed earlier, there are several methods used to compare bite marks ranging from life-sized photographs to computer enhanced three-dimensional imaging. These methods vary in precision and accuracy, and there is no set standard by which to compare or analyze them. The lack of analytical standards leads to a wide array of interpretation with any bite mark evidence. Therefore, the interpretation of evidence lies largely on the expertise of the forensic odontologist handling the case.
- There have been several instances when forensic dentists have made claims, accusations and guarantees supported by bite mark evaluation that have been proven incorrect through other forensic sciences. DNA analysis has shed some light on the limitations of bite mark analysis because often the DNA from saliva surrounding the area of the bite mark proves to be a more reliable form of identification.

3. Appearance and Fusion of Centres of Ossification

- Development and growth of bones take place by various methods of ossification. The process of appearance and union of ossification centres follows a definite time sequence which can be utilised for age estimation. As a general rule, the ageing of bones is more precise with respect to the appearance of centres of ossification than it is with respect to the union of epiphyses.
- **Table 3.11** and **Fig 3.10** display the ages of appearance and fusion of ossification centres commonly utilised in age estimation.
- **Important Point**: Fusion of all epiphyses (ossification centres) is completed by
  - 16–17 years at elbow joint
  - 16–17 years at ankle joint
  - 17–18 years at hip joint
  - 18–19 years at knee joint
- One of the best methods of age estimation is undoubtedly the radiological survey of ossification status of various bones. In young children, radiological examination of hand (**Fig. 3.11**) and foot (**Fig. 3.12**) alone can be sufficient for accurate fixation of age (**Table 3.12**). Ossification status of pelvic skeleton is displayed in **Table 3.13**.

Table 3.11 Important Ossification Centres for Age Estimation

I. **Upper End of Humerus (Shoulder)**
   a. **Appearance**:
      i. Head – 1 year
      ii. Greater Tuberosity – 3 years
      iii. Lesser Tuberosity – 5 years
   b. **Fusion**:
      i. All 3 centres fuse together by 5–6 years
      ii. All centres fuse with shaft by 18–19 years

II. **Upper End of Femur (Hip)**
   a. Appearance:
      i. Head – 1 year
      ii. Greater Trochanter – 5 years
      iii. Lesser Trochanter – 12–14 years
   b. **Fusion**:
      i. All fuse with shaft at 17–18 years

III. **Elbow**
   a. **Appearance**:
      i. Capitulum: 1–2 years
      ii. Radial Head: 5 years
      iii. Internal (Medial) Epicondyle: 6–7 years
      iv. Trochlea: 9–11 years
      v. Olecranon (Upper End of Ulna): 9 years
      vi. External (Lateral) Epicondyle: 11 years
   b. **Fusion**:
      i. Capitulum, Trochlea and Lateral Epicondyle fuse together to form **Conjoint Epiphysis** at 14–15 years, and the conjoint epiphysis fuses with the shaft at 16 years.
      ii. Medial Epicondyle fuses separately with the shaft at 16–17 years.

IV. **Radius and Ulna**
   a. **Appearance**:
      i. Distal Radius: 1–2 years
      ii. Proximal Radius (Radial Head): 5 years
      iii. Distal Ulna: 5–6 years
      iv. Proximal Ulna (Olecranon): 9 years
   b. **Fusion**:
      i. Distal Radius: 18–19 years
      ii. Proximal Radius (Radial Head): 16–18 years
      iii. Distal Ulna: 17–18 years
      iv. Proximal Ulna (Olecranon): 16–18 years

V. **Knee**
   a. **Appearance**:
      i. Distal Femur: By birth
      ii. Proximal Tibia: At birth
      iii. Proximal Fibula: By 4 years
   b. **Fusion**:
      i. All fuse by 18–19 years
      Patella forms at 4 years (and attains adult contour at 14–16 years)

contd

VI. **Ankle**
   a. **Appearance**:
      i. Distal Tibia: 1 year
      ii. Distal Fibula: 1 year
      iii. **Tarsal Bones**
         1. Talus: 7th foetal month
         2. Calcaneum: 5th foetal month; Calcaneum (tuberosity): 6–8 years – unites by 14–16 years
         3. Cuboid: 9th foetal month
         4. Navicular: 3rd to 4th year
         5. Cuneiform:
            - Lateral: 1st year
            - Medial: 2nd to 3rd year
            - Intermediate: 3rd to 4th year
   b. **Fusion**:
      i. Distal Tibia and Distal Fibula fuse by 16–17 years

VII. **Wrist**
   a. **Appearance**:
      i. Distal Radius: 1–2 years
      ii. Distal Ulna: 5–6 years
      iii. Carpal Bones*
         1. **C**apitate: 1–3 months
         2. **H**amate: 2–4 months
         3. **T**riquetrum: 2–3 years
         4. **L**unate: 3–4 years
         5. **S**caphoid: 4–5 years
         6. **T**rapezium: 5–6 years
         7. **T**rapezoid: 6–7 years
         8. **P**isiform: 10–12 years
   b. **Fusion**:
      i. Distal Radius: 18–19 years
      ii. Distal Ulna: 17–18 years

Mnemonic to remember the order - **Clocks **H**ave **T**welve **L**etters, **S**ometimes **T**wo-**T**hree **P**endulums*

Table 3.12 Beginning of Ossification in Children

Age	Hand	Foot
5th to 6th month IUL	Whole hand cartilaginous	Calcaneum (body)
7th month IUL	Whole hand cartilaginous	Talus
9th month IUL	Whole hand cartilaginous	Cuboid
1st year	Capitate and hamate	Lateral cuneiform (1–2 years)
2nd year	First four metacarpal heads	Lateral cuneiform
3rd year	Triquetrum (2–3 years)	Medial cuneiform, tarsal, navicular
4th year	Lunate (4–5 years)	Intermediate cuneiform
5th year	Trapezium, carpal navicular	Scaphoid
6th year	Scaphoid (6–7 years)	–
8th year	Trapezoid	–
10th year	Pisiform (female 9–10 yrs, male 10–12 years)	Tuberosity of calcaneum

Table 3.13 Ossification in the Pelvis

Centre/Region	Appearance	Fusion/Union
Rami of pubis and ischium	–	6 years
Triradiate cartilage (acetabulum)	–	13–15 years
Iliac crest	14 years	20–21 years
Ischial tuberosity	16 years	18–20 years

Estimation of Age of an Individual over 25 years

1. Physical Features

Features like greying of hair, balding, decrease in stature, changes in the skin, arcus senilis (in the eyes), opacity of the corneal periphery, cataract, etc., give an idea of advancing age.

2. Changes in the Teeth

After the eruption and calcification of the 3rd molar (maximum 25 years of age), estimation of age in adults can be done based on the physiological changes of teeth. **Gustafson** (1950) used the following criteria (**APSRTC**) (**Fig. 3.13**):

a) *Attrition* – Wearing down of the incisal or occlusal surface of teeth.
b) *Paradentosis* – Loosening of teeth due to gum retraction.
c) *Secondary dentine* – Deposition of dentine in the pulp cavity.
d) *Root resorption.*
e) *Transparency of the root.*
f) *Cementum apposition* – Deposition of cementum in the root

Transparency of root has the highest correlation with age.*

Gustafson developed a ranking scale from 0 to 3 for each of the six criteria. By studying the cross-section (ground to 0.25-mm thickness) of a tooth microscopically, points are assigned to the various changes, and the total score obtained is applied to the following regression formula:

Total score = A + P + S + R + T + C
Age (years) = 11.43 + [4.56 × (total score)]
SE = 3.63

This has come to be known as the **Gustafson's method** of estimating age from teeth.

Mnemonic to remember the order of appearance of carpals: *Clocks Have Twelve Letters, Sometimes Two-Three Pendulums*:

1. Capitate
2. Hamate
3. Triquetral
4. Lunate
5. Scaphoid
6. Trapezium
7. Trapezoid
8. Pisiform

3. Changes in the Skeleton

i) ***Closure of skull sutures***: The closure of skull sutures seems to take place from the inner to the outer table, i.e., **endocranial to ectocranial surface**. Due to the phenomenon of **lapsed union**, i.e., incomplete union ectocranially, more reliance should be placed on endocranial closure. However, age evaluation by this method is generally not accurate, since it can only provide a range in decades. But, it can be considered partially corroborative in the presence of other features. The following points must be borne in mind:
   - The **metopic suture** which is present at birth between the right and left halves of the frontal bones, usually **closes by the age of 2–3 years**. However, in some cases it may persist throughout life (**metopism**) (**Fig. 3.14**).
   - **Basal suture of the skull** (basioccipital with basisphenoid) usually **closes by 18–21 years** (but can be delayed up to 40 years).
   - Closure of vault sutures rarely occurs before the age of 30 years.
   - Between 30 and 50 years, the sagittal and coronal sutures close endocranially. Ectocranial closure may or may not occur. The usual sequence is as follows (**Fig. 3.15**):
     - **Sagittal suture** closes in 3 phases – posterior third by **30–40 years**, anterior third by **40–50 years** and middle third by **50–60 years**.
     - **Coronal suture** closes by **40–50 years** (lower part) **and 50–60 years** (upper part).
     - **Temporal suture** closes by **60–65 years**.
   - In general, suture closure occurs a little **later in females** than in males.

ii) ***Age changes in the scapula***: **Stewart** summarised the age-related changes in the scapula as follows:
   - Lipping of the circumferential margin of the glenoid fossa and clavicular facet.
   - Appearance of facet on the underside of the acromial process.
   - Increasing demarcation of the triangular area at the base of the scapular spine.

**Source*: *Metzger Z, Buchner A, Gorsky M. Gustafson's method for age determination from teeth – a modification for the use of dentists in identification teams. J Forensic Sci. 1980;25:742–9.*

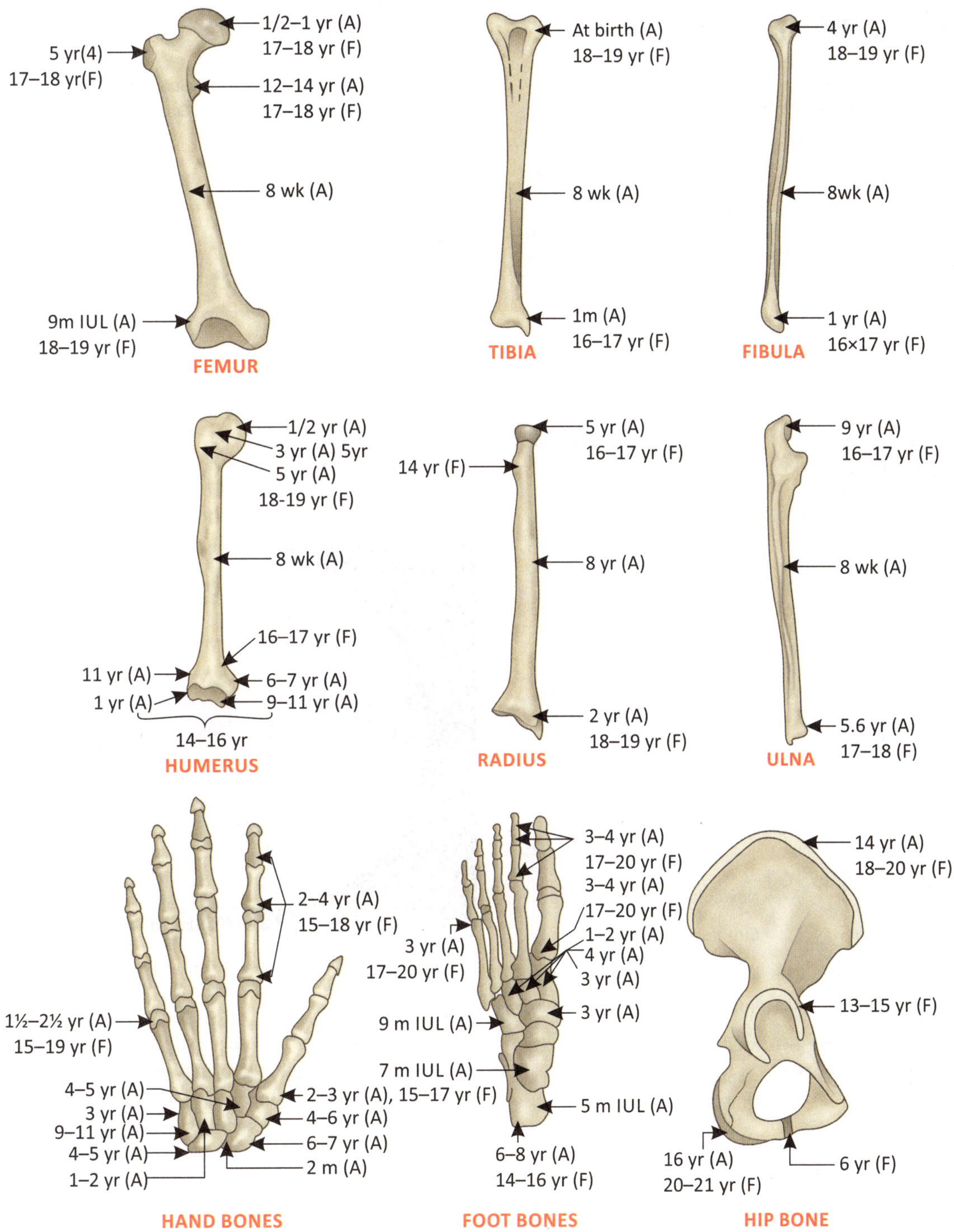

Fig. 3.10 Ages of appearance & fusion of ossification centres utilised in age estimation
(Illustration Courtesy: Dr Hareesh S Gouda & Dr Shashidhar C Mestri)

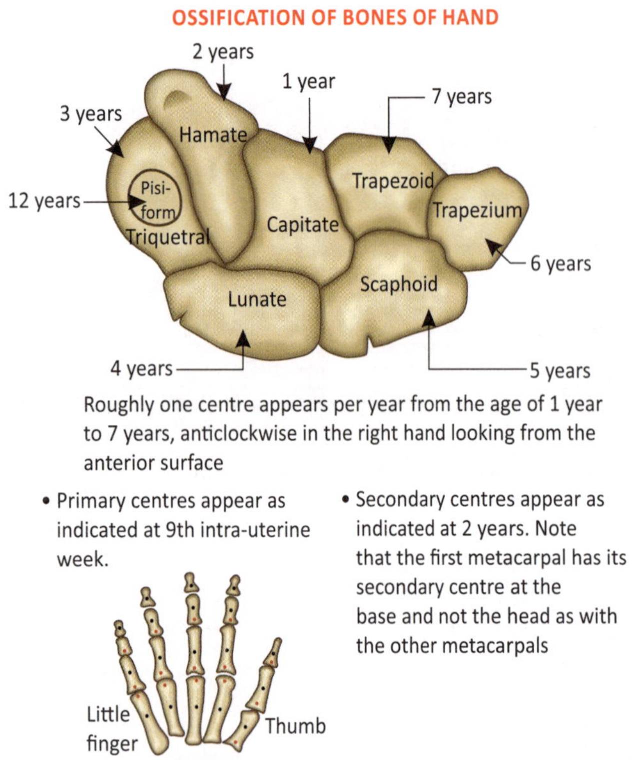

Fig. 3.11 Ossification of bones of hand

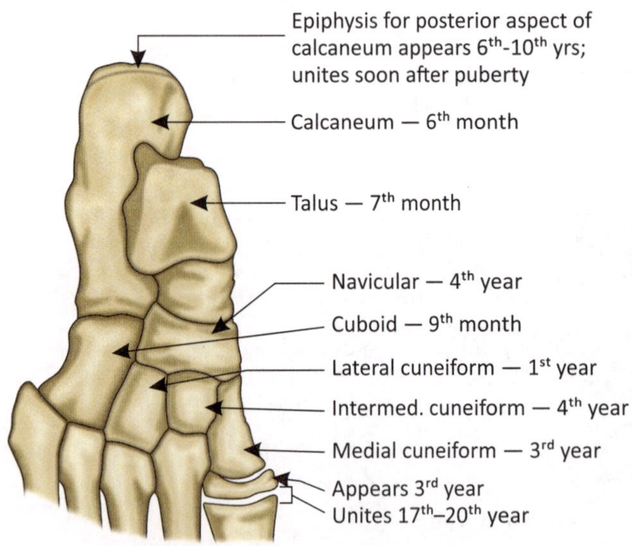

Fig. 3.12 Ossification of bones of foot

- Appearance of the cristae scapulae.
- Atrophy of the bone producing thinning, buckling and pleating of the infraspinous area.

These changes begin around **30 years** of age and become prominent at about **50 years** or more.

iii) ***Age changes in the sacrum***:
- The 5 sacral vertebrae are connected by cartilage until puberty, after which ossification starts from below upwards.
- **The sacrum becomes a single bone between 21 and 25 years** (though a gap may persist between S1 and S2 until 32 years due to lapsed union).

iv) ***Age changes in the symphysis pubis***: A study of the morphological changes of the articular surfaces of the innominate bone provides a reasonably good age indicator for adult remains. Variation in the face of the pubic symphysis, the anterior-most point of articulation between the two innominates in the pelvic girdle, is a common region analyzed for age determination. **Todd** (1920) outlined a 10-stage method for assessing this surface, based on a large sample of innominates.

Todd Method (main features are summarized in **Plate 3.1**):

Stage 1:

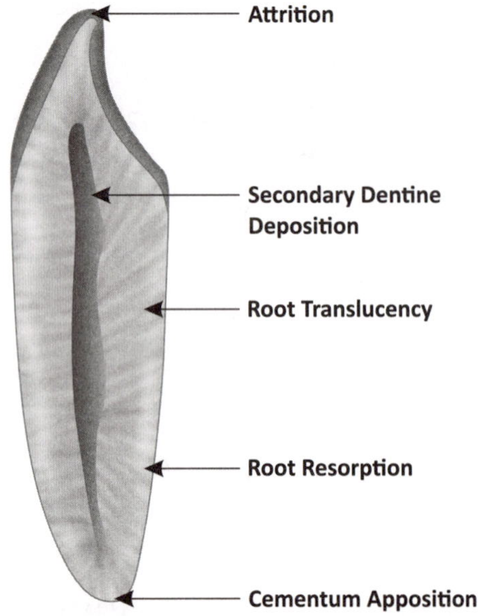

Fig. 3.13 Gustafson's criteria for age estimation (*Paradentosis is not represented here*)

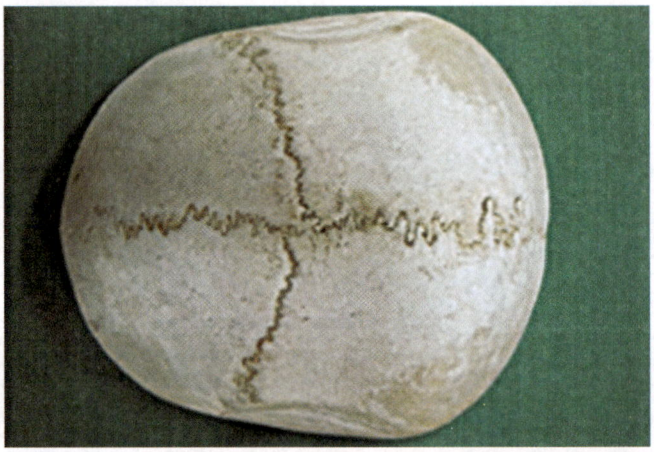

Fig. 3.14 Persistent metopic suture *(Courtesy: Dr Hareesh S Gouda & Dr Shashidhar C Mestri)*

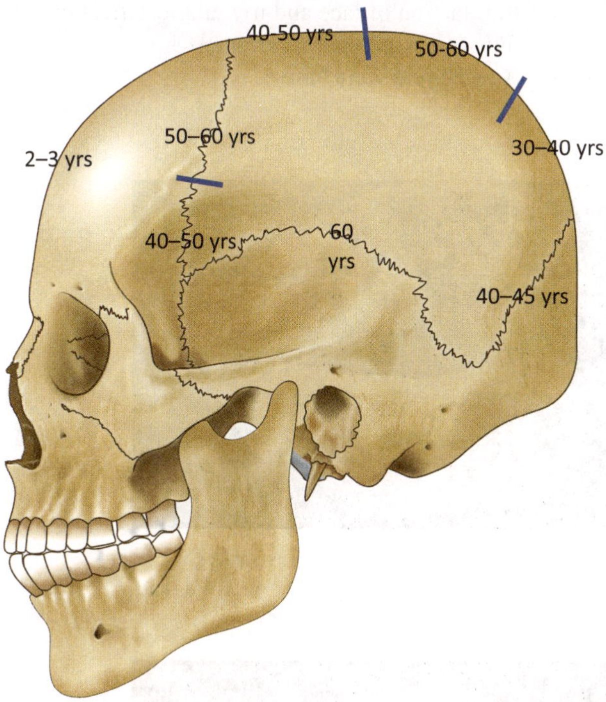

Fig. 3.15 Suture closure (*Illustration: Dr Hareesh S Gouda & Dr Shashidhar C Mestri*)

- Symphyseal face rugged, traversed by horizontal ridges separated by well-marked grooves.
- None of the following structures are present: nodules fusing with the surface, a delimiting margin or definition of extremities.
- Age: **18–19 years**.

Stage 2:

- Symphyseal surface still rugged. Horizontal grooves are becoming filled near their dorsal limit with new, finely textured bone.
- Bony nodules may be present, fusing with upper symphyseal face.
- Dorsal delimiting margin begins to develop.
- No delimitation of the extremities.
- Ventral bevel commences.
- Age: **20–21 years**.

Stage 3:

- Symphyseal face shows progressive obliteration of ridge and furrow system.
- Commencing formation of a dorsal platform.
- Bony nodules may be present.
- Definition of dorsal margin, with sharp lipping.
- Ventral bevel more pronounced.
- Extremities not delimited.
- Age: **22–24 years**.

Stage 4:

- Great increase of ventral bevelled area.
- Corresponding diminution of ridge and furrow formation.
- Complete definition of dorsal margin through the formation of the dorsal platform.
- Commencing delimitation of lower extremity.
- Age: **25–26 years**.

Stage 5:

- Little change in symphyseal face and dorsal platform.
- Margin more clearly defined and more sharply lipped.
- Lower extremity better defined.
- Upper extremity forming with or without the intervention of a bony nodule.
- Age: **27–30 years**.

Stage 6:

- Increasing definition of extremities.
- Development and practical completion of ventral rampart.
- Retention of some granular appearance of symphyseal face indicating that activity has not yet ceased. Failure of ventral aspect of pubis adjacent to ventral rampart to become transformed into a compact surface.
- Retention of the pectinate outline of the dorsal margin and slight ridge and furrow system.
- No lipping of ventral margin and no increased lipping of dorsal margin.
- Age: **30–35 years**.

Stage 7:

- Face and ventral aspect change from granular to fine-grained or dense bone.
- Slight changes in symphyseal face and marked changes in ventral aspect from diminishing activity.
- No formation of symphyseal rim.
- No ossification of tendinous and ligamentous attachments.
- Age: **35–39 years**.

Stage 8:

- Symphyseal face and ventral aspect of pubic bone generally smooth and inactive.
- Oval outline complete.
- Extremities clearly defined.
- No distinct "rim" to symphyseal face.
- No marked lipping of ventral or dorsal margin.
- Development of ossification in tendinous and ligamentous attachments, especially those of sacro-tuberous ligament and gracilis muscle.
- Age: **40–45 years**.

Stage 9:

- Symphyseal face presents a more or less marked rim.
- Dorsal margin uniformly lipped; ventral margin irregularly lipped.
- Age: **45–49 years**.

Stage 10:

- Ventral margin eroded at a greater or lesser extent of its length, continuing somewhat onto the symphyseal face.
- Rarefaction of face and irregular ossification. Disfigurement increases with age.
- Age: **50 years and above**.

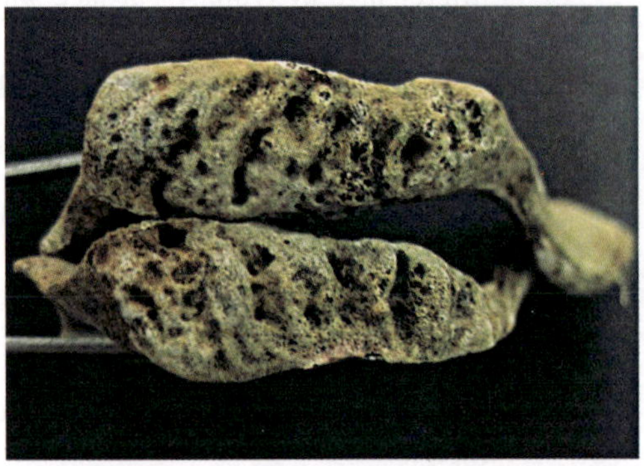

a) Transverse ridges across the symphyseal surface (2nd decade)

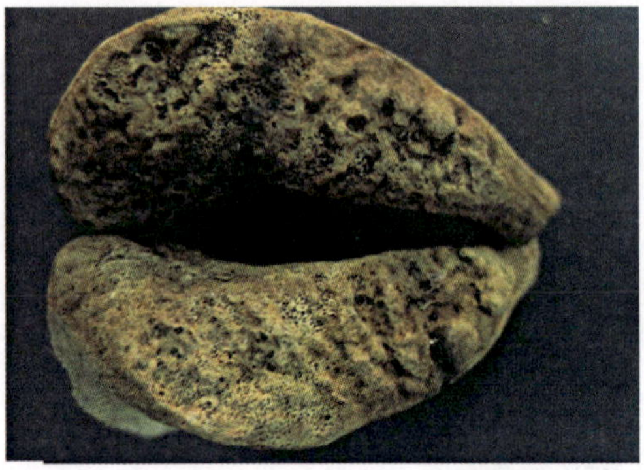

b) Gradual disappearance of symphyseal surface transverse ridges (2nd to 3rd decade)

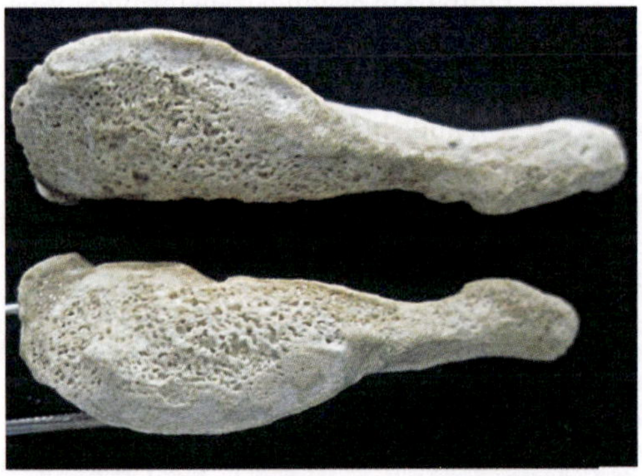

c) Granular sympyseal surface with well defined ventral & dorsal margin (4th decade)

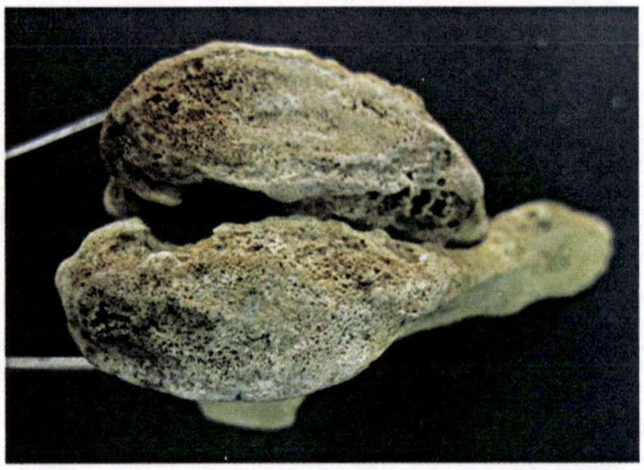

d) Beaded rim along the symphyseal margin (end of 5th decade)

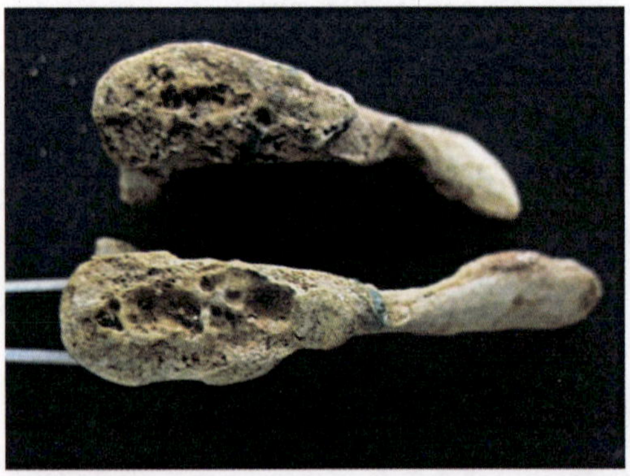

e) Erosion of symphyseal surface and breakdown of ventral margin (6th decade)

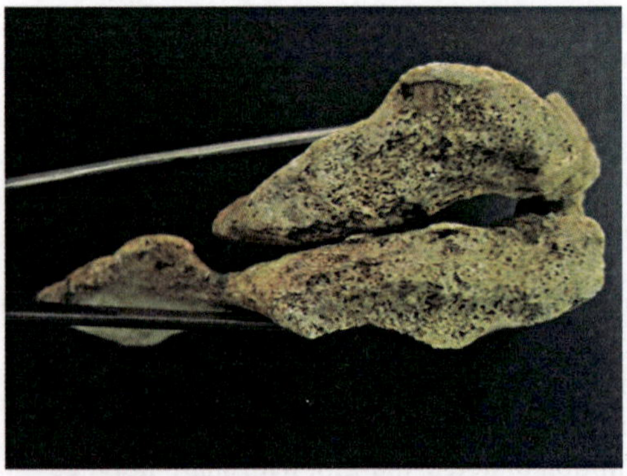

f) Irregular erosion of symphyseal surface (7th decade)

Plate 3.1: Pubic symphyseal changes
(*Courtesy*: *Dr Hareesh S Gouda & Dr Shashidhar C Mestri*)

v) ***Age changes in the sternum***:

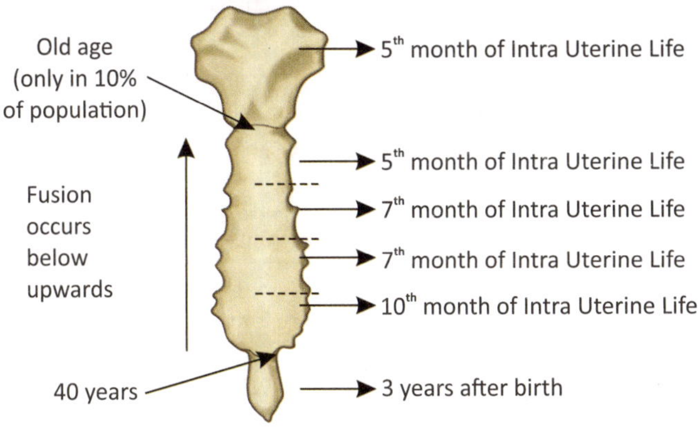

(*Illustration Courtesy*: *Dr Hareesh S Gouda & Dr Shashidhar C Mestri*)

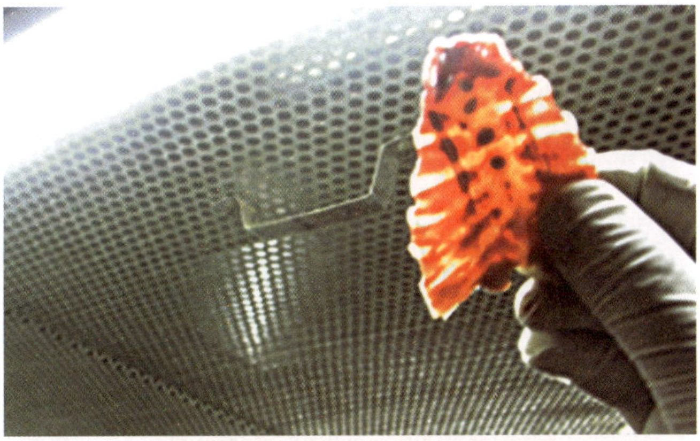

Fig. 3.16 Ossification centres – Sternum (*Courtesy*: *Dr Shashidhar C Mestri*)

Other factors that are helpful for the estimation of age:

- Thyroid and cricoid cartilages tend to ossify by 45–50 years.
- The fusion of cornua with the body of hyoid bone occurs after 40 years.
- Lipping of the body of lumbar vertebrae starts around 40–50 years of age.
- Atrophic changes in the intervertebral discs start around 50–60 years of age.
- Arcus senilis, i.e., an opaque zone around the periphery of cornea may be noticed around 60 years.
- Although greying of head or facial hair is not very reliable in the estimation of age, greying of pubic hair is more reliable, and usually starts after 60 years of age.

Medicolegal Importance of Various Ages

The medicolegal importance of various ages is outlined in **Table 3.13**.

> **FM 3.2: Core – Written/Viva Voce**
> - **Identification**
>   - Describe and discuss identification of criminals, unknown persons, dead bodies from the remains
>   - Hairs
>   - Fibres
>   - Teeth
>   - Anthropometry
>   - Dactylography
>   - Poroscopy
>   - Foot prints
>   - Scars
>   - Tattoos
>   - Superimposition

The importance of 'Teeth' in Identification has been discussed in great detail in the preceding Competency (FM 3.1). The remaining aspects listed under FM 3.2 will be discussed here.

HAIR & FIBRES

- The epidermal appendages referred to as hair, constitute a unique characteristic in human beings.
- Hair is known to resist putrefaction for a long time, and hence attempts were made to determine whether it could have the specificity of fingerprints in identification. Though this has now been proved wrong, a great deal of information can still be obtained from this trace evidence.
- Before trying to individualise a sample of hair, it is pertinent on the part of the forensic scientist to ascertain *whether it is really* ***hair****, or could it be some* ***fibre****?*
  - The distinct morphology of **hair** with the three layers, viz, cuticle, cortex and medulla, distinguishes it from **fibres** which are tubular and devoid of the three layers (**Fig. 3.17**).

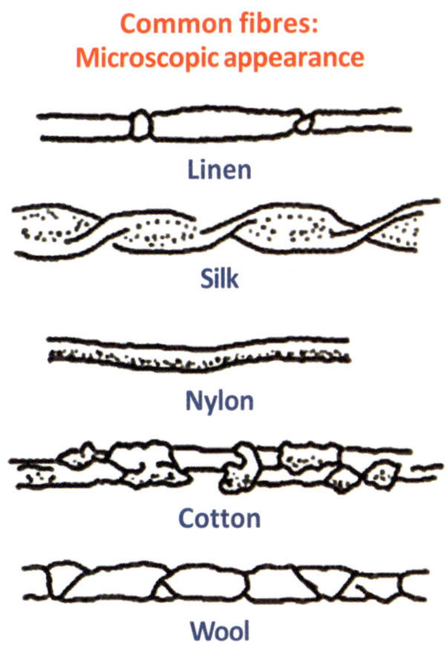

Fig. 3.17 Common fibres

Table 3.13 Medicolegal Importance (MLI) of Various Ages

Age	MLI	Section/Act	Remarks
>7 months IUL	Infanticide	Sec. 300 IPC	Viability is attained.
Child of any age	Endangering safety of railway passengers	Railways Act (1989)	Punishable for the offence.
<7 years	Criminal responsibility	Sec. 82 IPC	No criminal intent & not guilty of the crime.
7–12 years	Criminal responsibility	Sec. 83 IPC	Guilty of offence, if sufficient maturity and understanding is present.
<12 years	Consent	Sec. 89 IPC	Parent/Guardian must give consent for physical examination.
<14 years	Employment	Factories Act (1948)	Cannot be employed in factory jobs.
14–15 years	Employment	Factories Act (1948)	Non-hazardous jobs in the factory during daytime can be given.
>15 years	Employment	Factories Act (1948)	Can be employed, provided a fitness certificate is given.
<15 years (girls)	Rape	Sec. 375 IPC	Sexual intercourse with his own wife, with or without consent.
<18 years (girls)	Statutory rape	Sec. 375 IPC	Sexual intercourse with a girl, with or without consent.
<16 years (boys) <18 years (girls)	Kidnapping	Sec. 361 IPC	Taking away without the consent of the lawful guardian. 10 years imprisonment, with or without fine.
<18 years (girls)	Kidnapping	Sec. 366-A IPC	Procuring a girl for illicit intercourse. 10 years imprisonment, with/without fine.
>18 years	Consent	Sec. 87 IPC	Can consent to suffer any harm not intended or known to cause death/grievous hurt.
>18 years	Attainment of majority	Sec. 3 Indian Majority Act, 1875	Except those under the guardianship of court, can make a valid will, cast vote in election.
>18 years (girls)	Marriage	Prohibition of Child Marriage Act, 2006	–
>18 years	Employment	–	Minimum age to enter government service.
<18 years (both sexes)	Judicial punishment	Juvenile Justice (Care and Protection of Children) Act, 2015	Sent to a reformatory.
16–18 years (both sexes)	Judicial punishment	Juvenile Justice (Care and Protection of Children) Act, 2015 – Amendment	Will be tried as an adult for heinous crimes (rape or murder), but cannot be sentenced to death or life term
>21 years	Attainment of majority	Sec. 3, Indian Majority Act, 1875	For those under guardianship of court.
>21 years (boys)	Marriage	Prohibition of Child Marriage Act, 2006	–
<21 years (girls)	Kidnapping	Sec. 366-B IPC	Procuring girls from outside the country, or from Jammu & Kashmir for illicit intercourse. Punishment 10 years imprisonment with fine

- Cotton fibre: Flattened, twisted tubes
- Jute: Smooth without transverse lines
- Silk: Long clear threads without cells, smooth and finely striated
- Wool: Outer layer of flattened cells and overlapping margins

■ The next step involves **species identification**, i.e., determining whether it belongs to human or animal.

- **Human hair** (**Fig. 3.18**) is characterised by:
  - a thin medullary canal (sometimes discontinuous or fragmented or even absent altogether)
  - a broad cortex (usually 4 times as broad as medulla, or even more)
  - medullary index below 0.3
  - circular or oval cross section
  - evenly distributed pigmentation
  - cuticular scale type VII: short, thin and annular scales
  - precipitin test specific for humans

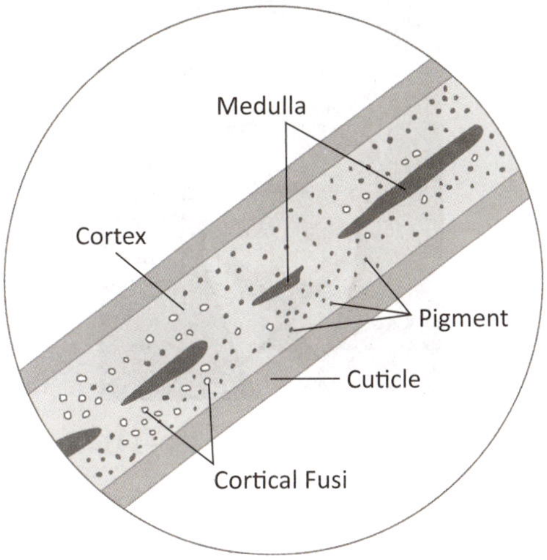

Fig. 3.18 Microscopic structure of human hair

- **Animal hair** (**Fig. 3.19**) is characterised by:
  - A wider medulla (sometimes filling the entire shaft).
  - Thin cortex (rarely twice as broad as medulla).
  - Medullary index above 0.5.
  - Pigmentation mainly around the medulla.
  - A variety of cuticular scale types: mainly large scales with wavy or step-like projections.
  - Colour changes along the hair shaft called "banding" is seen in certain animals.
  - Precipitin test is specific for the particular animal to which the hair belongs.
- Human scalp hair can be racially classified.
- Before attempting to compare the test hair from the exemplars, and individualise the hair sample, it is necessary to determine the **somatic** origin, i.e., the part of the body from which it originated.
- Differences between hair from various parts of the body:
  - ***Head hair*** – Long, taper gradually to the tip.
  - ***Beard & moustache*** – Thicker than any other body hair.
  - ***Eyebrows, eyelashes, nostrils*** – Stiff, thick and taper to a point.
  - ***Chest hair, armpit hair, pubic hair*** – Short, stout and curly (may show split ends).
  - ***Body hair from other parts*** – Fine, short, flexible and lack pigment cells in cortex.
- **Sex determination** of hair based on observations with reference to the length of hair, and the nature of cut ends, is not reliable.
  - Male hair is generally thicker, coarser and darker.
  - Refractive index appears to be one of the best criteria for sex determination, since a significant difference exists between male and female hair.
  - **Barr bodies** in root sheath cells (29 ± 5% in females; 6 ± 2% in males).

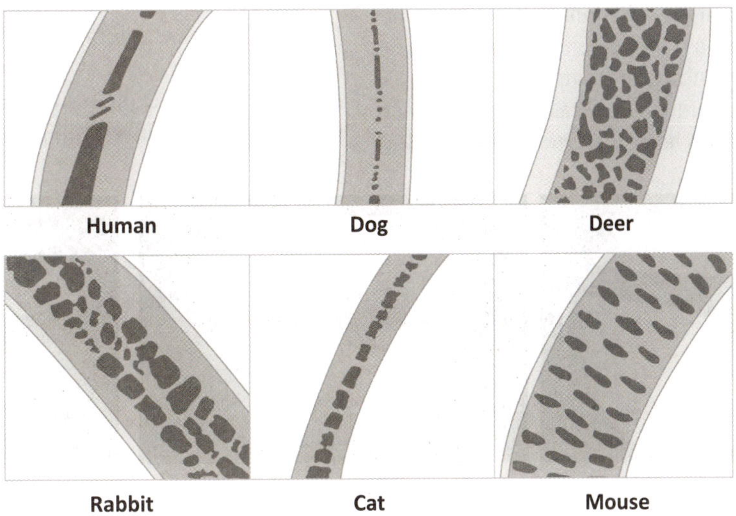

Fig. 3.19 Microscopic structure of various animal hairs

- **Estimation of age**:
    - Can be done only within wide limits, for instance, between hair of an infant or an adult.
    - Lanugo hair is seen in foetus and new born child: Fine, soft, non-pigmented and non-medullated.
    - Axillary and pubic hair are absent before puberty.
    - Hair turns grey usually after 40 years.
    - Roots of hair from a child dissolve fast in a solution of caustic potash, while that of an adult are resistant.
- Further steps in **individualisation** include:
    - ABO blood grouping.
    - Isozyme typing – PGM, RGD, EsD, AK, EAP, GLO, etc.
    - Identification of trace elements by neutron activation analysis.
    - Evidence of disease.
    - Evidence of application of dyes, henna, bleach, etc.

Medicolegal Importance of Hair (Fig. 3.20)

- Hair can be an important **aid in identification**: often identifiable on clothing, weapon, etc., in a case of assault.
- The **type of weapon** which caused injury in a particular case can sometimes be deduced by examining the tip of the hair. Neatly cut ends suggest the use of a sharp edged weapon, whereas crushed ends result from blunt force injury.
- Vehicle involved in a **hit-and-run incident** may be identified on the basis of hair from the pedestrian transferred to the vehicle.
- Singed hair is characteristic of **burns** and **contact firearm injuries**.
- In **rape**, there may be exchange of pubic hair between assailant and victim.
- In **bestiality**, there may be animal hair on the human, or human hair on the animal.
- **Nature of assault** may be determined by stains on the hair: seminal stain in rape, blood stain in assault, mud stain in struggle outdoors, etc.
- **Natural fall** or **pulled hair**: By examining the root of the hair, it is possible to opine as to whether it fell naturally or was pulled off forcefully during an assault.
- **Heavy metals** such as arsenic, as well as many **drugs of abuse** get deposited in the hair, thereby permitting the identification of poison or drug consumed. The deposition of arsenic at intermittent levels on the shaft can also give us useful information regarding the periods of ingestion of the poison.

ANTHROPOMETRY (BERTILLON SYSTEM)

- In the **Anthropometric system** devised by **Alphonse Bertillon (Fig. 3.21)** in **1882** and introduced in France in **1885**, criminal offenders were classified by certain measurements of specified parts of the body:
    - Total height
    - Span of arms
    - Height of trunk
    - Length and width of head
    - Length and width of right ear
    - Length of left foot
    - Length of left middle and ring fingers
    - Length of left forearm

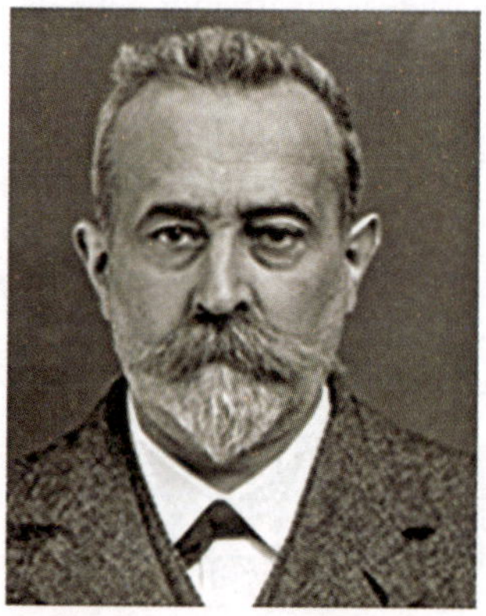

Fig. 3.21 Alphonse Bertillon (1853–1914) – French criminologist

- Along with these measurements, Bertillon used photography, now known as a **mugshot**, to complete this system of record.
- However, this method suffered from inherent defects, since cumbersome measurements were required to be made, sometimes leading to error. Also, the method was not applicable to children, and even to women. It was mostly designed for men who had reached full physical maturity and had short hair.

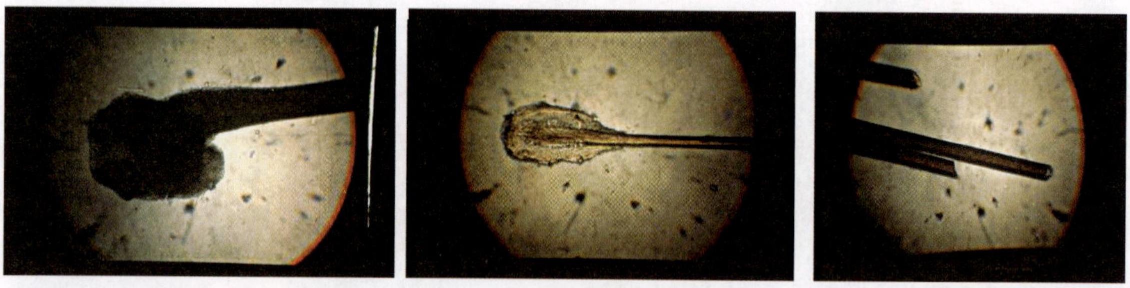

Burnt hair | Pulled hair | Cut hair

Fig. 3.20 Microscopic appearance of hair when it is burnt, pulled or cut (*Courtesy*: *Dr MB Rao*)

DACTYLOGRAPHY

History (Fig. 3.22)

- In 1880, **Henry Faulds**, a Scottish surgeon in a Tokyo hospital, published his first paper on the usefulness of fingerprints for identification and proposed a method to record them with printing ink. Returning to Great Britain in 1886, he offered the concept to the Metropolitan Police in London, but it was dismissed at that time. Up until the early 1890s police forces in the United States and on the European continent could not reliably identify criminals to track their criminal record.
- **Francis Galton** published a detailed statistical model of fingerprint analysis and identification in his 1892 book Finger Prints. He had calculated that the chance of a "false positive" (two different individuals having the same fingerprints) was about 1 in 64 billion.
- In 1892, **Juan Vucetich**, an Argentine chief police officer, created the first method of recording the fingerprints of individuals on file.
- In Kolkata, India, a Fingerprint Bureau was established in 1897, after the Council of the Governor General approved a committee report that fingerprints should be used for the classification of criminal records. The bureau employees **Azizul Haque** and **Hem Chandra Bose** have been credited with the primary development of a finger print classification system eventually named after their supervisor, **Sir Edward Henry**.

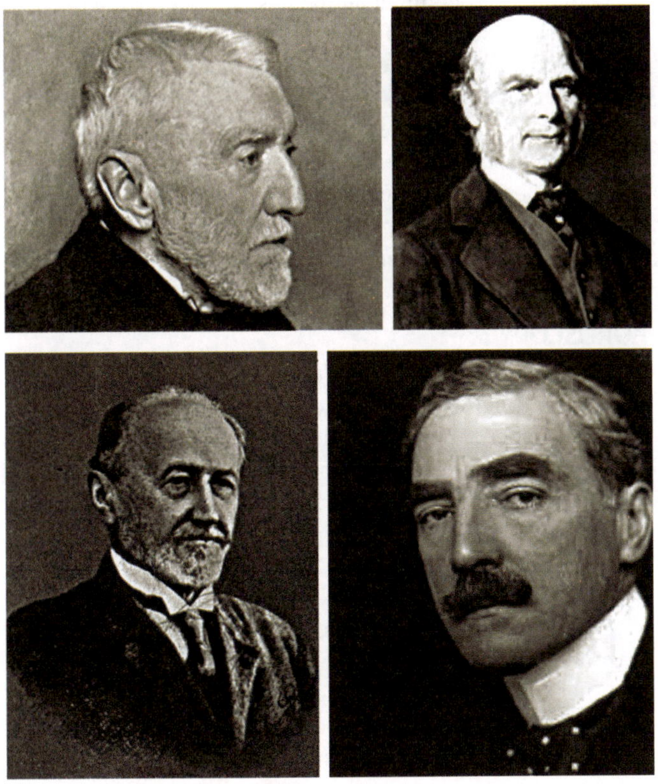

Fig. 3.22 Pioneers of dactylography (clockwise from top left): Henry Faulds; Francis Galton; Juan Vucetich; Edward Henry

Explanation

- **Dactylography** or the **fingerprint system** is based on the study of epidermal ridges and their configurations (***dermatoglyphics***) in the palms of the hands. The method can also be extended to the soles of the feet. This method of identification has superseded all the other methods for a variety of reasons:
  - Fingerprints are formed during intra-uterine life and remain constant throughout life.
  - They are highly individualistic even in monozygotic (identical) twins.
  - Fingerprint types can be coded in a form which can be easily filed and retrieved, and also can be teleprinted to various parts of the world.
  - They can be compared with latent prints which are developed with suitable reagents, left by the person at the scene of crime. (The credit goes to **Edmund Locard** for the recognition of 'chance' prints.)
- Today **fingerprints** (**Fig. 3.23**) are **classified** into **four major groups**:
  - ***Arches***
  - ***Loops***
  - ***Whorls***
  - ***Composites***
    - *Arches* are further classified as *plain* (*simple*) or *tented*
    - *Loops* as *radial* or *ulnar*
    - *Composites* can be either *central pocket loops*, *double loops* or *accidentals*.
- Loops are the commonest type (60–70%), followed by whorls (25–35%), arches (6–7%) and composites (1–2%).
- Individualisation is based not solely on the patterns but extends also to the counting of ridges between the core and the delta, and even the minutiae of ridges like ridge ending, bifurcation, spur formation, dots, lake formation, broken ridge, short ridge, etc.

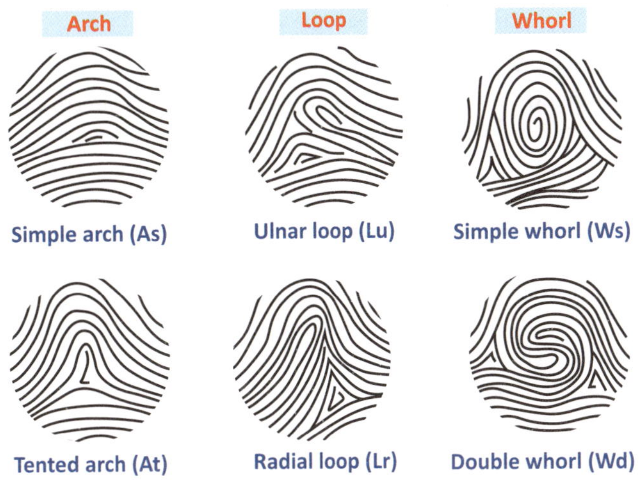

Fig. 3.23 Common types of fingerprint

- **16–20 points** of similarity in the minutiae are necessary to establish **positive identification**.
- Fingerprints encountered at a scene of crime can be classified in the following manner:
  - **Visible print**: Impression made by a finger contaminated with blood, paint, dust, dyes, etc., which can be recorded by photography with suitable use of lights and filters. It is also called a "**patent fingerprint**."
  - **Plastic print**: Impression made on a soft substrate like soap, wax, clay, etc., which can be recorded by photography or by means of a cast.
  - **Latent fingerprint**: Impression made due to deposition of sebaceous and sweat gland secretions, which has to be made visible by developing with reagents that vary according to the nature of the substrate, and recorded by photography and "lifting".
  - Some of the methods commonly used for developing latent prints include*:
    - ***Dusting***: Dusting with powders is the most basic and easiest form of lifting latent prints. Black powders are used on a large range of surfaces (**Fig. 3.24**). Fluorescent powder is used on dark surfaces.
    - ***Iodine fuming***: Typically used on paper surfaces. Iodine fumes stick to the outlines of the print to make it visible.
    - ***Superglue fuming***: Similar to iodine fuming. Items go into chamber and superglue is melted. Fumes make prints visible. Works best on plastics.
    - ***Ninhydrin method***: Works best on paper. Spray paper down with ninhydrin and place the piece of paper over steam. After some time, the fingerprints will become visible.
    - ***Silver nitrate method***: Similar to ninhydrin in that both are typically for paper. After spraying the paper down with silver nitrate, expose it to sunlight and the fingerprints will show up.
    - ***Crystal violet method***: Similar to ninhydrin and silver nitrate. Crystal violet is primarily for tape. Spray tape with crystal violet and wash excess off. Fingerprints will then become visible.

Applications of Fingerprinting

- Fingerprints collected at a crime scene, or on items of evidence from a crime, can be used to identify suspects, victims and other persons who touched a surface. No two fingerprints have ever been found identical in many billions of human and automated computer comparisons. Even in identical twins, fingerprints are dissimilar.
- Electronic fingerprint readers are increasingly being used for security applications such as identification of computer users (log-in authentication).
- Another recent use of fingerprints in a day-to-day setting has been the increasing reliance on biometrics where fingerprints and, to a lesser extent, iris scans are used to validate electronic registration, cashless catering, and library access, especially in schools and colleges in the West.

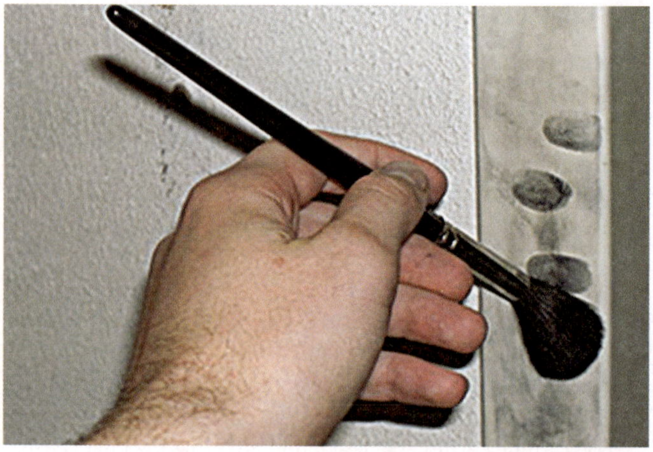

Fig. 3.24 Dusting for latent fingerprints with black powder

- The secretions, skin oils and dead cells in the fingerprint contain residues of various chemicals and their metabolites present in the body. These can be detected and used for forensic purposes. For example, the fingerprints of tobacco smokers contain traces of cotinine, a nicotine metabolite. By treating the fingerprint with gold nanoparticles with attached cotinine antibodies, and then subsequently with fluorescent agent attached to cotinine antibodies, a fingerprint of a smoker becomes fluorescent, while a nonsmoker's fingerprint stays dark. The same approach can be used for identifying heavy coffee drinkers, cannabis smokers and users of various other drugs. This application can perhaps be called "**dactylotoxicology**".
- In criminal cases, impressions of all 10 digits (fingers) are taken, but for civil purposes, only the left thumb impression is taken.

POROSCOPY

- The papillary ridges of epidermis are studded with minute pores through which sweat exudes out in life.
- The number of pores, as well as their size, shape and site in a given length of a ridge vary from person to person and are quite individualistic. In fact, they are as reliable as the minutiae of the ridges. This method of identification introduced by **Edmund Locard**, utilising the study of pores is called **poroscopy**.
- Poroscopy further enhances the reliability of latent fingerprints especially in cases of partial fingerprints where the usual comparison of minutiae cannot be resorted to.
- Since 9–18 pores (per mm) are present in a ridge, and each is unique in its characteristics, this method can lead to positive identification (**Fig. 3.25**).

Mnemonic to remember the different methods of lifting latent fingerprints: **DINCSS*
***D** = Dusting; **I** = Iodine fuming; **N** = Ninhydrin; **C** = Crystal violet; **S** = Superglue fuming; **S** = Silver nitrate.*

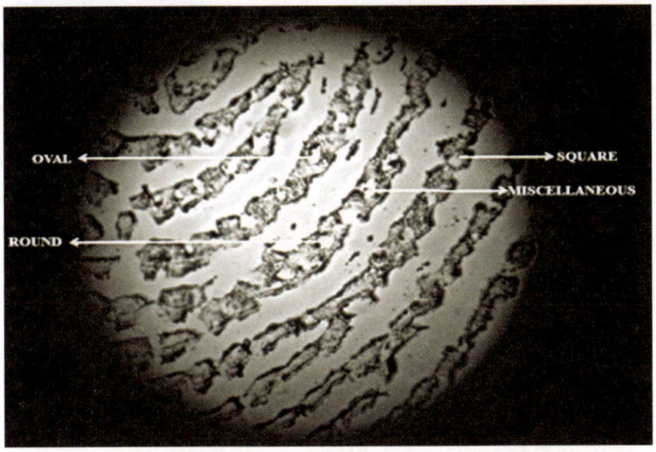

Fig. 3.25 Poroscopy: Various types of pores (*Courtesy*: *Dr Preethi DS, Dr Nithin MD, Dr Manjunatha B & Dr Balaraj BM*)

FOOTPRINTS

- Impressions of human feet on various substrates have been studied and have been found to be quite individualistic with reference to dermatoglyphics, various measurements and also the morphological analysis.
- Dermatoglyphics or the ridge pattern, if clearly visible on the substrate against a contrasting background, is highly individualistic. The comparison of the footprints of the suspect with the test print can be carried out in the same way as in the case of fingerprints. Latent prints are also developed in the same way.
- In the absence of ridge patterns, as happens often in substrates such as soil, sand, etc., the measurements like length and width of the foot, length and width of toes, toe pads, the angles of declination from each toe, and from the ball to its juncture with the arch, etc., aid in distinguishing the footprints of one individual from another.
- It may be possible to deduce the height of an individual from his footprint.* It has been suggested that stature of an individual constitutes **15% ratio of foot length**, i.e.,

$$\text{Stature} = \frac{\text{Maximum foot length}}{0.15}$$

- According to data from the University of Rhode Island (USA), the normal height-to-foot ratio is about **6.6:1**, which means 6.6 inches of height for 1 inch of foot length.
- The weight of a person can also be estimated by studying the foot outline ball width. It is around 60.5% ratio of the foot outline width in case of males above 14 years, and around 67% ratio in case of females above 14 years.
- In the case of a walking foot print, i.e., if a series of foot prints are available, it is possible to relate them with the gait pattern of the suspect. The weight distribution, length of the stride and presence of abnormalities can be studied.
  - The step length of an adult male is 63–70 cm, while that of an adult female is 45–55 cm.
- Footprints are recorded by photography or by making casts.

Applications of Footprinting

- When recovered at crime scenes or on items of evidence, sole and toe impressions are used in the same manner as finger and palm prints to effect identification.
- Footprints of infants, along with thumb or index fingerprints of mothers, are still commonly recorded in hospitals to assist in verifying the identity of infants.
- It is not uncommon for military records of flight personnel to include barefoot inked impressions. Friction ridge skin protected inside flight boots tends to survive the trauma of a plane crash (and accompanying fire) better than fingers.
- It is possible to deduce the height of a person from his footprint.

SCARS

- A scar is an acquired defect widely accepted as a marker of identification. The size, shape and location of a scar can aid in positive identification, especially if it is unusual or unsightly.
- A scar is the result of a repair mechanism to an injury involving the dermis of the skin. It is covered by epithelium and is devoid of pigmentation, sweat glands and hair follicles.
- Apart from aiding in identification, a scar can also give information regarding:
  - the nature of the injury, and
  - the causative agent
- The size and shape of a scar will be approximately the size and shape of the original wound. Hence, the nature of injury, as to whether it is an incised, lacerated, stab wound, etc., can be made out, which in turn can help predict the type of the weapon used to produce the injury (**Fig. 3.26**).
- The age of a scar usually correlates well with the time of infliction of the injury.

CHEILOSCOPY*

- Lip prints are similar to fingerprints and footprints in that individual characteristics are used for identification.
- The creases on the vermilion border of the lips, which appear as white areas in lip prints, and the raised reddish areas outlined by these creases, which appear as dark areas, are analogous to the furrows and ridges of friction ridge skin. The creases on the vermilion border are also referred to as grooves, furrows, wrinkles and valleys.

"Yes," he reported, after a short examination of the grass bed, "a number twelve shoe, I should say. If he was all on the same scale as his foot he must certainly have been a giant."

*- **Sherlock Holmes**, in The Adventure of Wisteria Lodge*

***From the Greek word 'cheiloswhich' which means lips.*

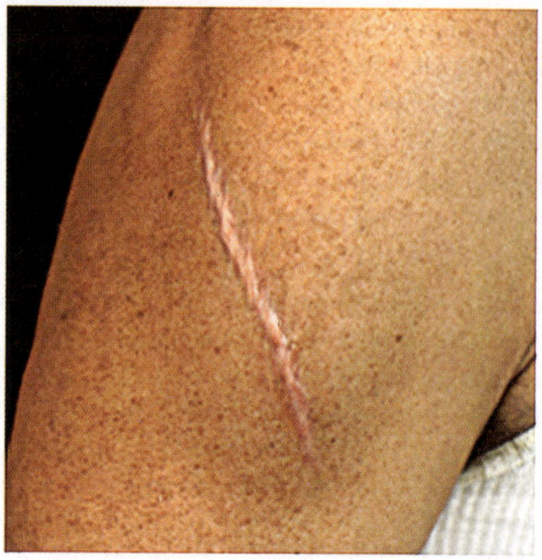

Fig. 3.26 Scar from a knife wound

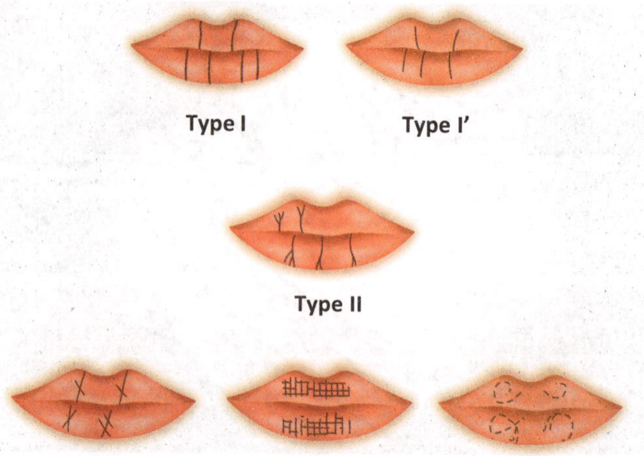

Fig. 3.27 Suzuki's classification of lip prints

- Lip prints are unique and do not change during the life of a person. It has been verified that they recover after undergoing alterations like trauma, inflammation and diseases like herpes, and that the disposition and form of the furrows does not vary with environmental factors.
- The lip prints of parents and children and those of siblings have shown some similarities, which can help in establishing relationships to a limited extent.
- It has also been suggested that variations in patterns among males and females could help in sex determination.
- Cheiloscopic patterns are classified as:
  - ***Linear***: Lines are predominant
  - ***Bifurcate***: Bifurcation of lines is dominant
  - ***Reticular***: Lines cross each other
- Apart from these class characteristics, 24 individual properties are distinguished in the same manner as the minutiae in the fingerprints.
- **Suzuki's classification** of lip prints (**Fig. 3.27**):
  - Suzuki divided lip prints into five main types:
    - Type I has an additional "sister group"; it is called Type Í (pronounced as "one-dash").
      - Type I represents a lip with clear-cut grooves running vertically over the lips.
      - Type Í has partial length grooves of Type I variety. They do not quite cover the entire breadth of the lips.
    - Type II comprises branched (or forked) grooves
    - Type III comprises intersected grooves, which look almost like crosses
    - Type IV comprises a reticular pattern much like a wire-mesh.
    - Type V includes all other patterns, which are mostly irregular patterns.
    - Different areas of lips may have different patterns. To simplify the study of lip prints in practice, the lips are divided into four quadrants. Each quadrant is then studied.
- Method of recording lip prints:
  - Lip prints can be collected from the suspect by
    - photographing the suspect's lips
    - applying red lipstick so that it can be obtained on paper or cellophane tape
    - or a non-porous surface such as mirror which can be photographed and enlarged, and subsequently overlay tracings can be made for comparison with crime scene sample.
- Three methods of cheiloscopic examination are generally employed for identification purposes:
  - Method of determining common features (similar to dactyloscopy): establishment of 7–9 fine characteristics leads to positive identification.
  - Method of photographic montage.
  - Contour method.

    The second and the third methods supplement each other, wherein the contour of the lips is compared.
- Apart from this, the substance forming the print, i.e., saliva, cosmetics, etc., can be identified which can act as corroborative evidence.

Applications of Cheiloscopy

- Lip prints have been studied in postmortem identification. Advances have been made in the techniques and dyes for developing lip prints. Software has been developed for the analysis of lip prints.
- However, limitations still exist in the use of lip prints. The permanent nature of lip prints requires more long term studies to be substantially documented. Advanced methods of developing lip prints at a scene of crime are still confined to research laboratories. Full utilization of lip depends to a high degree on the skill of members of law enforcement agencies.
- The problems involved in cheiloscopy are relatively little known and thus, so far lip prints have been used only occasionally despite their frequent occurrence at the scene of crime.

RUGOSCOPY (PALATOPRINTING)

- Palatal rugae are as unique to each individual as are lip prints.
- The use of human palatal rugae as a method of identification was suggested by **Harrison Allen** as early as **1889**.
- The advantages of palatal rugae as an ideal method of postmortem identification include:
  - They are protected from trauma by their internal location.
  - They are insulated from heat by the tongue and buccal fat pads.
  - No two palates are alike in their configuration. Study of the rugae pattern of twins showed that they are similar, but not identical.
  - Palatoprints do not change during growth.
- **Thomas & Kotze** have classified rugae into three types:
  - ***Primary Rugae***: 6–10 mm or more
  - ***Secondary Rugae***: 3–5 mm
  - ***Fragmented Rugae***: <3 mm
- The shape of the rugae could be either curved, wavy, straight or circular.

TATTOO MARKS

- A tattoo is a form of body modification made by inserting tattoo ink, dyes and/or pigments, either indelible or temporary, into the dermis layer of the skin to form a design. Tattoo artists create these designs using several processes of tattooing, including hand-tapped traditional tattoos and modern tattoo machine.
  - The most common method of tattooing in modern times is the electric **Tattoo machine**, which inserts ink into the skin via a single needle or a group of needles that are soldered onto a bar, which is attached to an oscillating unit. The unit rapidly and repeatedly drives the needles in and out of the skin, usually 80–150 times a second.
- Today, people choose to be tattooed for artistic, cosmetic, sentimental, memorial, religious and spiritual reasons, and to symbolize their belonging to, or identification with particular groups, including criminal gangs, or a particular ethnic group or law-abiding subculture. Tattoos may show how a person feels about a relative (commonly a parent or child) or about an unrelated person.
- Colouring pigments in common usage include carbon (black), cinnabar, vermilion (red), ochre (brown), chromic oxide (green), prussian blue (blue), etc.
- The permanence of the mark depends on the process followed, type of dye used and the depth of the skin involved. Stable pigments such as carbon, prussian blue, etc., impregnated into the deeper layers of the skin last longer.
- Even faint/disappeared marks of unstable pigments like cinnabar can be made out on histological study of the regional lymph glands.
- When tattoo marks are obscured by decomposition or mummification, they can be visualised by treating the area with 3% H_2O_2 which temporarily removes the products of decomposition.
- So-called permanent tattoo marks can be removed by surgical methods such as skin grafting, and also by laser beams, without leaving behind any mark. But crude methods of erasure like application of corrosives, burning, cautery, etc., will leave a permanent scar in that area.
- A tattoo mark can either be altered or superimposed over another design subsequently.
- A **temporary tattoo** is a non-permanent image on the skin resembling a permanent tattoo. As a form of body painting, temporary tattoos can be drawn, painted, airbrushed or needled in the same way as permanent tattoos, but with an ink which dissolves in the blood within 6 months.

Medicolegal Importance

- Apart from being a mark of identification by virtue of its size, shape, design, anatomical position, etc., tattoo marks can also provide additional information about an individual (**Fig. 3.28**):
  - Race, religion, nationality: The design may provide a clue to any of these.
  - Language.
  - The name tattooed could be that of a person associated/related to him.
  - The mental makeup and sexual preferences of the person can sometimes be made out, e.g., the blue bird design on the back of the hand at the base of the thumb and the forefinger, was once upon a time common among homosexuals.
  - The dates of personal events may be depicted in a tattoo mark.
  - Drug addicts often imprint tattoos over areas where multiple injection marks are present, in order to conceal them.
  - The social status to which the person belongs can be guessed by the nature of the dye used, the design and also the presence of complications arising out of employing unsterilised needles.

SKULL SUPERIMPOSITION

- Superimposition is a technique where a postmortem record is placed over a comparable antemortem record for comparison.

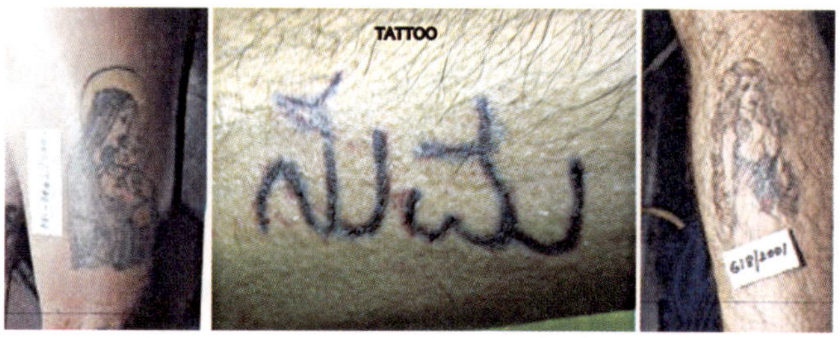

Fig. 3.28 Tattoo marks indicating religion, language, sexual orientation (*Courtesy: Dr EJ Rodrigues & Dr Shashidhar C Mestri*)

- **Skull superimposition (craniofacial superimposition) is the technique in which the skull to be identified is superimposed on a recent antemortem photograph of the suspected deceased.**
  - The antemortem photograph is enlarged to "life size", the enlargement factor being based upon the measurements of the fabric on the victim, or other measurable items seen in the photograph, or the focal length of the camera lens used, or the dimensions of the anterior teeth, etc.
  - The skull is adjusted in such a way that the inclination and orientation are the same as that of the head in the photograph. A life size picture is taken and superimposed on the transparency of the life size antemortem photograph, making allowances for soft tissue and hair thickness.
  - The anatomical landmarks compared for a positive match include the following: external auditory meatus, orbits, anterior nasal spine, chin point, angles of the mandible and zygomatic processes.
  - Arriving at a positive match does not always mean a positive identification, since a photograph of any other person with similar craniometry can produce a successful match with the same skull. Thus, this test can help in exclusion rather than conclusion.

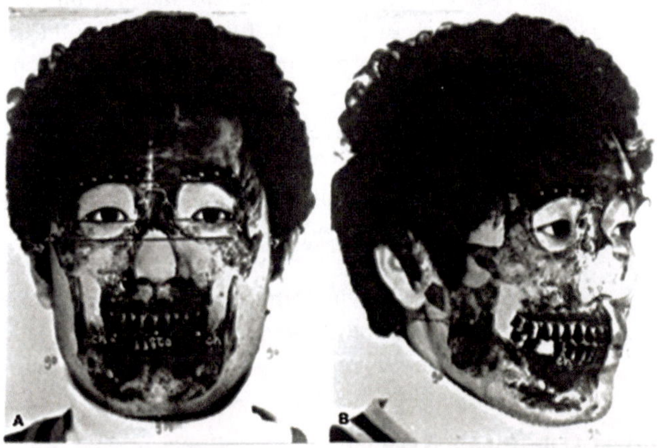

Fig. 3.29 **(A)** Frontal and **(B)** Oblique photographic superimposition images, showing a good match between skull and facial photographs

Disadvantages

- The major disadvantage in photographic superimposition is that a slight change in the enlargement of the antemortem photograph or a slight change in the angulation of the skull from that of the photograph can lead to major discrepancies resulting in a mismatch.
- Exact determination of the parameters however, results in loss of valuable time.
- These problems can be avoided by the use of video superimposition technique.

Video Superimposition

- The skull devoid of any extraneous soft tissue and foreign matter, is mounted on an adjustable support allowing movement in three planes. The antemortem photograph (preferably with the person smiling or displaying his teeth) is also mounted.
- A colour video camera, firmly mounted on a tripod, is aligned at right angles to the antemortem photograph. The centre of the lens should be at the same level as the horizontal centre of the photograph. The mounted skull is placed in a contrasting background, and a second camera similar to the first one, is aligned to the skull in the same way as the first camera to the photograph.
- The individual video signals from each camera are fed into a vision mixer so that a variety of functions like horizontal and vertical wiping, superimposition, and negative simulation can be performed.
- The skull is oriented on the adjustable mount as closely as possible to the angulation of the head in the photograph. The video pictures from both the cameras are relayed into the video mixer.
- By adjusting the mixer, the video picture of the antemortem photograph can be enlarged. If teeth are visible in both the skull and photograph, enlargement is carried out till the teeth in the antemortem photograph overlap the teeth in the superimposed picture. If teeth are not present or visible in either specimen, the enlargement factor is estimated by adjusting the vertical facial height of the photograph to the skull. The video mixer offers flexibility in making the adjustments and provides immediate results without having to process photographs or make tracings.
- After correct enlargements and orientation, superimposition is done, and features are compared with respect to the landmarks. The video mixer allows for the fading in and out of either the skull or the photograph, or for sweeping over each other in the vertical or the horizontal plane (**Fig. 3.30**). This procedure allows part of the skull or the photograph to be superimposed in either the vertical or horizontal plane on the video screen so that an accurate match is obtained.
- This technique can be video-taped for court purposes.

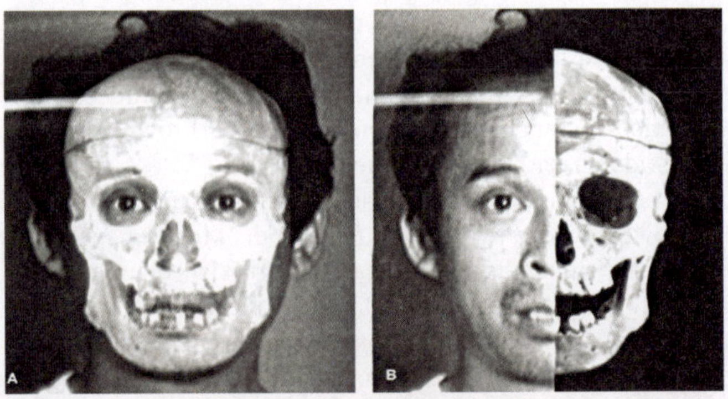

Fig. 3.30 Video superimposition showing **(A)** total mixing and **(B)** vertical wipe images of the skull and facial photograph

Computer-aided Superimposition

- Computer-aided craniofacial superimposition comprises **non-automatic** and **automatic** methods.
  - Non-automatic methods use some kind of digital infrastructure to support the craniofacial superimposition process, i.e., computers are used for storing and/or visualizing the data. However, they are characterized by the fact that their computational capacity to automate human tasks is not considered.
  - On the other hand, computer-aided automatic methods use computer programs to accomplish an identification sub-task itself.
- The most advanced method of computer-aided craniofacial superimposition is through the use of imaging tools provided by Adobe Photoshop® and Corel Draw® software packages.
- However, it is to be noted that this is not really an automatic method as images have to be manually resized, shifted and rotated by a process of trial and error. Thus, it is a time consuming and potentially error-affected process.

FM 3.3: Core – Written/Viva Voce/OSPE
(Objective Structured Practical Examination)
- **Mechanical Injuries and Wounds**
  - Define, describe and classify different types of mechanical injuries
    - Abrasion
    - Bruise (Contusion)
    - Laceration
    - Stab wound
    - Incised wound
    - Chop wound
  - Defense wound
  - Self-inflicted/fabricated wounds
- Mechanical Injuries and Wounds
  - Medicolegal aspects

MECHANICAL INJURIES AND WOUNDS

- **Trauma** is an insult to the state of well-being. This insult can be physical or mental. Usually, one is accompanied or followed by the other in negligible or substantial degree.
  - Physical trauma may manifest itself as a functional change, or structural (anatomical) change, or both.
  - The kind of physical trauma which causes structural (anatomical) change is called an **injury**. Injury may be associated with loss of tissue, or without recognisable loss (e.g., redness, oedema).
  - **Sec 44 IPC** defines an **injury** as "any harm whatever illegally caused to any person, in body, mind, reputation or property."
  - An injury which is associated with traumatic loss or discontinuity of tissue is called a **wound**.
  - In other words, *all wounds are injuries, but all injuries are not wounds*. However, injury and wound are often described as being synonymous. For the sake of convenience, the term 'injury' will be used interchangeably with 'wound' in this textbook even though it may not be accurate.
  - **Injuries** can occur due to natural causes (e.g., diabetic ulcer), or due to unnatural causes which may be **physical** (e.g., heat, cold, electricity, radiation, etc.), **chemical** (e.g., corrosives) or **mechanical** (e.g., weapons such as knife, stick, etc.).
    - A **mechanical injury** can be defined as "**Damage to any part of the body due to the application of mechanical force**." The damage referred to is loss or discontinuity of tissue.

CLASSIFICATION OF MECHANICAL INJURIES*

- Abrasion
- Contusion (Bruise)
- Laceration
- Incision
- Puncture (Stab)
- Fracture

Important!
- **Injuries** that result from **blunt force** comprise **abrasion, contusion, laceration** and **fracture**.
- **Injuries** that result from **sharp force** comprise **incision** and **stab**.
- **Bite marks** are a special category of injury that may be either an abrasion, contusion, or laceration, or a combination of all three.

Abrasion

- **An abrasion is the loss of superficial layers of skin or mucous membrane due to mechanical force.**
- Because of the corrugated nature of dermoid papillae, abrasions usually involve the corium of dermis. Since the blood vessels are confined to dermis, such involvement of corium seems to be the reason for the common occurrence of bleeding in abrasions. There is also oozing of lymph, which dries up after death making the abrasion firm, leathery or parchment-like.

Mechanism of Occurrence

- The mechanical force which causes an abrasion is either *friction* (sliding), or *pressure* (compression) applied on the body surface. Usually both these elements are present, with one predominating over the other.
- Friction-predominant abrasions are called **tangential abrasions**, while those which are compression-predominant, are referred to as **patterned abrasions**.

****Mnemonic***: *Ab Co La In Sta Fra (abcolainstafra).*

Tangential Abrasions

- **Scratch**: Linear abrasion produced by a narrow, sharp object such as a pin, needle, fingernail, etc., which is drawn across the skin superficially (**Fig. 3.31**).
- **Brush abrasion (graze or brush burn)**: This is produced when a rough object scrapes over the skin, or when the skin moves against a broad, rough surface (e.g., fall on a road) (**Fig. 3.32**). The terminal end of injury often shows a serrated border with piling of torn layers of skin, giving a fair indication of the direction of sliding movement.

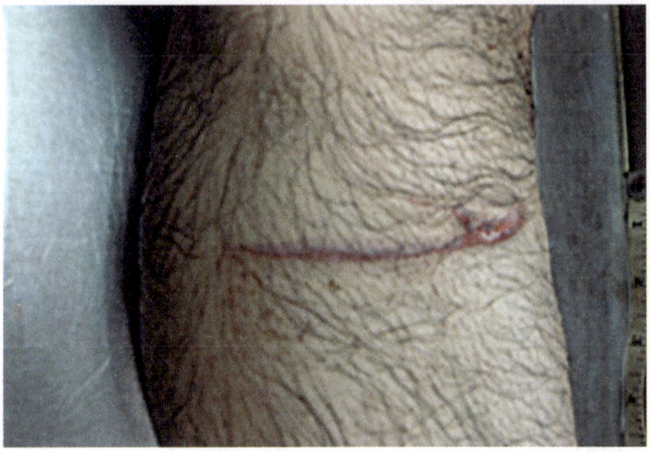

Fig. 3.31 Scratch abrasion (*Courtesy*: *Dr Prateek Rastogi*)

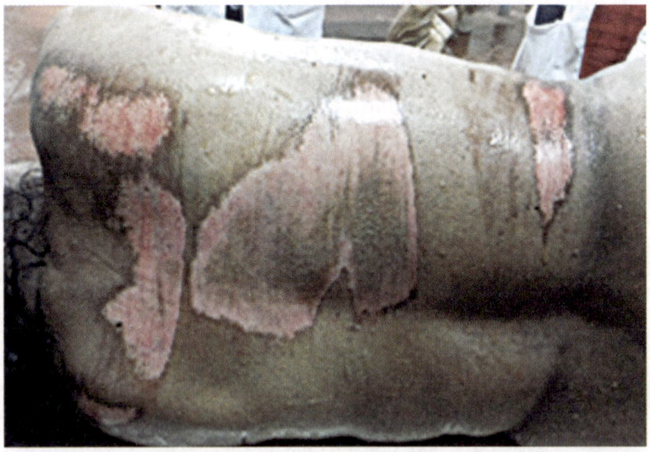

Fig. 3.32 Grazed abrasion (*Courtesy*: *Dr Jagadish Rao PP*)

Patterned Abrasions

- This is caused by pressure of an object on the skin resulting in a patterned injury.
- When the impact is vertical, the epidermis gets crushed, and an imprint of the impacting object is stamped upon the surface (e.g., radiator grill impression on the skin of a victim of vehicular impact). Such an injury produces a replica of the patterned surface of the causative object, and is called an **impact or imprint abrasion** (**Fig. 3.33**).
- In the absence of an impacting force, if there is merely sustained pressure, the resulting abrasion can still reflect the pattern of the object, and is referred to as a **pressure or contact abrasion** (e.g., ligature mark of hanging or strangulation) (**Fig. 3.34**).

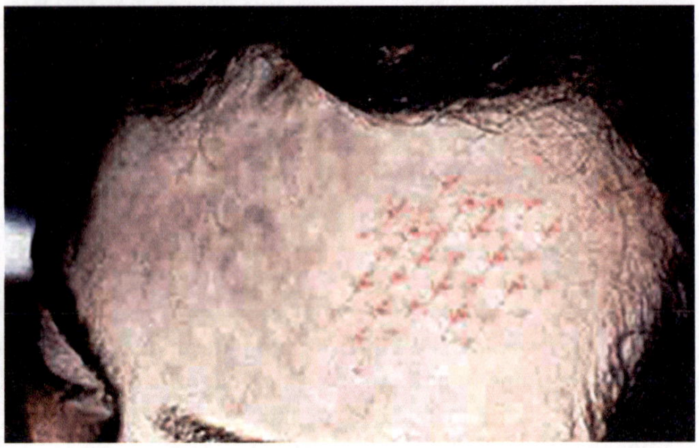

Fig. 3.33 Imprint abrasion

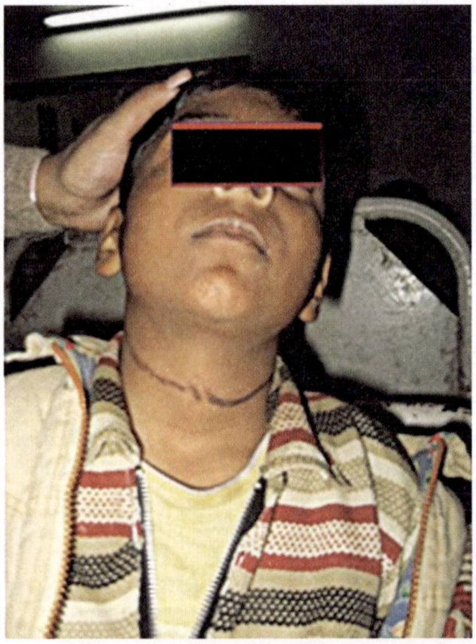

Fig. 3.34 Pressure abrasion – Ligature mark in survivor (accidental hanging while playing)

- In such **patterned abrasions**, the pressure of the object is mainly vertical, with the frictional (tangential) force being negligible.
- As the element of frictional force gradually increases, the abrasions begin to fail to exhibit the weapon pattern and are referred to as **non-patterned abrasions**.
- Depending on the presence and extent of crushing, a contused area can surround these abrasions to such an extent that in some cases, the contused area will be more marked than the abrasion, which is then called an ***abraded contusion***. Alternatively, if the abraded part is more prominent, it is more appropriately called a ***contused abrasion*** (**Fig. 3.35**).

A simple mnemonic to help remember the four important types of **abrasions** is **PIGS**:

P = Pressure; **I** = Impact; **G** = Graze; **S** = Scratch

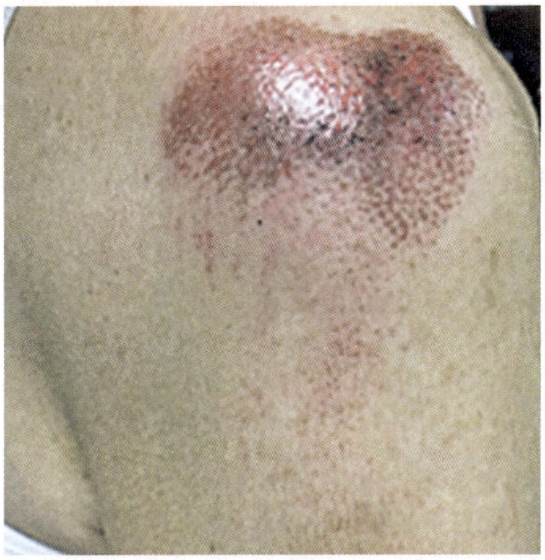

Fig. 3.35 Contused abrasion

Other Abrasions

- Abrasions can be induced after death. They are called **postmortem abrasions**.
  - They are quite common, and can occur due to mechanical force (e.g., dragging the body after death) or by animal action (e.g., ant bite) (**Fig. 3.36**).
  - Even the normal procedures of post-autopsy reconstruction and handling in the mortuary may cause dermal changes simulating abrasions, especially after washing with hot water.
  - While an abrasion caused during life is covered by scab due to coagulation of blood and lymph, and is associated with signs of inflammation, a postmortem abrasion does not demonstrate these features. In fact it usually appears pale and dry.
  - Ant bite marks are pale and irregular in shape, and are seen mainly in moist regions such as the areas around the eyes, nose, mouth, genitalia and axilla.
  - Abrasions produced immediately before or after death may be difficult to differentiate even by microscopic examination.
- An abrasion fabricated on the body by oneself, or with the help of another person, is called **fabricated abrasion**. In the former case, only accessible parts of the body are involved such as face, hands, etc. The motive for such fabrication can be serious or trivial.
- **Nappy abrasions** constitute a special variety of abrasion seen in infants due to excoriation of skin over areas usually covered by a nappy (groin and buttocks). They may be confused with antemortem violence when viewed at autopsy, unless the pathologist is vigilant. These abrasions generally appear yellowish or yellowish-brown, and lack apparent antemortem reaction.

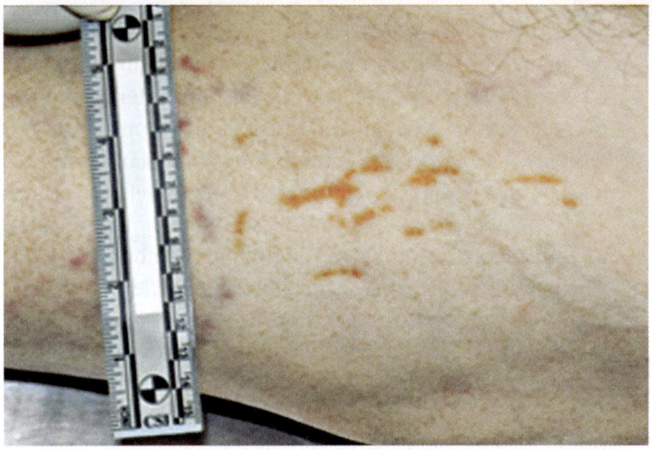

Fig. 3.36 Postmortem abrasions (ant bite marks)

Repair and Healing

- Healing involves two phenomena – contraction of the wound, and replacement of lost tissues.
- When fresh, an abrasion is bright red in colour.
- Scab forms by 12–24 hours. When fully formed, a scab is red in colour, and is moist, but it becomes reddish brown and dry by about 2–8 days (**Fig. 3.37**).
- Abrasions heal from the periphery by new growth of epithelial cells. Ordinarily, the scab falls off by about 7–8 days, leaving a pale area which may persist for a few days or weeks.
- A rough estimate of the age of an abrasion can thus be made from these features.
  - Earlier stages (before scab formation) can be assessed by histology. Infiltration by polymorphonuclear cells in a perivascular formation signifies that the wound is 4–6 hours old. At 12 hours, the wound shows three layers – a surface zone of fibrin and red cells, a deeper zone of polymorphonuclear cells, and a third layer of damaged, abnormally staining collagen.

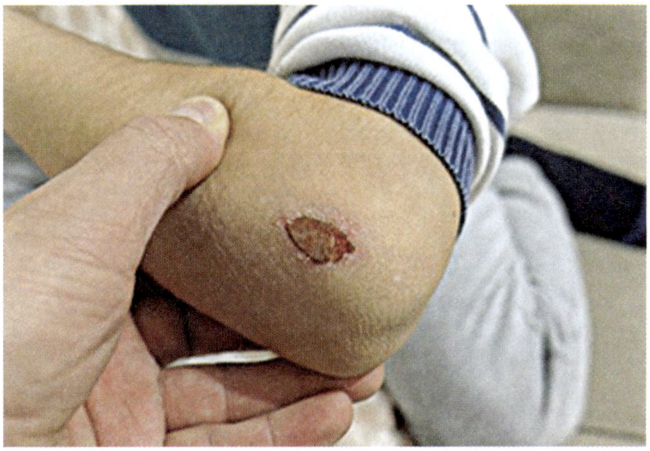

Fig. 3.37 Scab on abrasion

Medicolegal Significance

- An abrasion indicates the **site of contact** with an object. Occasionally, an abrasion may be the only external indication of a deep-seated injury. Abrasions are normally simple wounds. They are actually three dimensional, but for practical purposes they are considered to be two dimensional.
- The type of abrasion may reveal as to whether the **manner of contact** was a sliding one or compressing one.
- The pattern (if present), can help to some extent in deducing the **nature of the object**, e.g., the exact nature of vehicle involved in a "hit and run" case may be revealed by the radiator grill pattern.
- The stage of healing process could help in determining the **time of occurrence**. However, the determination of age of an abrasion is usually only approximate and is seldom accurate.
- The exact site of an abrasion can sometimes give valid information about the **nature of crime** (e.g., abrasions around the nose and mouth suggest smothering, while those around breasts and genitalia may suggest sexual assault). Abrasions on a suspected assailant may be the result of a struggle, and suggests evidence of resistance put forth by the victim. It is advisable to look for foreign material over abrasions (e.g., presence of mud particles indicates a fall in a muddy area).
- In the case of an assault, it is necessary to examine the fingernails of the victim and the accused, and to collect the debris from under each nail. Nail scratches may have been inflicted by both the victim and the accused on each other during the assault. There is a possibility of skin fragments being retained under the nails. Significant evidentiary material may be obtained from such retained tissue by microscopy and DNA typing to link the victim and the accused.

Contusion (Bruise)

- **A contusion is an extravascular collection of blood that has leaked from blood vessels damaged by mechanical impact of a blunt nature, without loss of continuity of tissues** (**Fig. 3.38**). The blood vessels involved are usually small arteries, veins or capillaries.

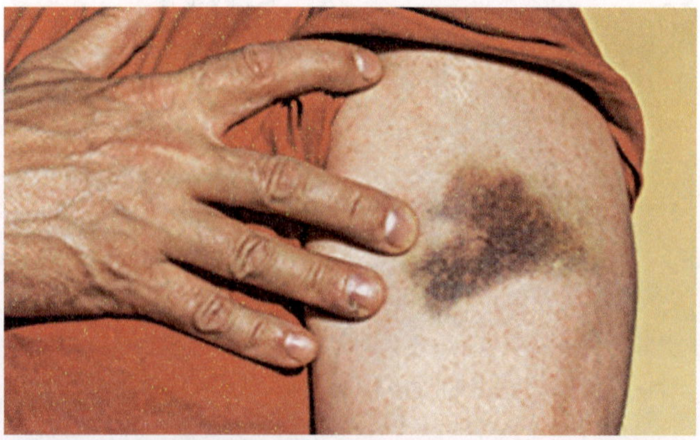

Fig. 3.38 Contusion (Bruise)

- A contusion is also referred to as a **bruise**.
- Contusions are usually situated in the subcutaneous tissue, but can also occur in various internal viscera.
- The term **ecchymosis** is used, if a contusion is smaller than a few millimeters in size, while pinpoint contusions are generally referred to as **punctate contusions** or **petechiae**. However, the latter term is usually restricted to haemorrhages resulting from bursting of congested capillaries, as in asphyxia, or bleeding points in the skin due to coagulation disorders, rather than those seen in trauma, since the nature of production is different.

Mechanism of Occurrence

- Extent of blood effusion resulting from damage to blood vessels depends on several factors:
  - ***Site*** of wound (effusion will be greater in lax tissues such as peri-orbital area),
  - ***Thickness*** of skin (effusion is lesser, if the dermis is thick, as in the palms and soles),
  - ***Resilience*** of the area (effusion is minimal in the yielding anterior abdominal wall),
  - ***Sex*** (females contuse more easily than males due to higher amount of adipose tissue) and
  - ***Age*** (children and aged individuals are more susceptible than young adults). Elderly people bruise easily due to increased fragility of blood vessels.
  - The degree of effusion is also directly proportional to the ***vascularity*** of the area, and the amount of ***force*** applied.
  - ***Diseases*** such as haemophilia, scurvy and leukaemia can aggravate effusion.
- A bruise will be less prominent, if it is situated in deeper tissues.
- Blood escaping from ruptured vessels usually percolates along the lines of least resistance. Hence, it is easily influenced by gravity. The site of a contusion, therefore does not necessarily indicate the site of application of force, e.g., black eye in head injury.
  - A "**black eye**" can be caused by a direct injury, or by gravitation of blood from a wounded scalp, or from a fractured orbit (**Fig. 3.39**).
  - A contusion appearing at a site remote from the site of application of force is called **percolated contusion** or **ectopic bruise**.
  - A deeply situated bruise may manifest externally only after several hours or days. Such a bruise is called a "**come-out bruise**." This may be due to haemolysis, wherein the freed haemoglobin stains the tissues more densely as time elapses.
- On certain occasions, the shape of a bruise may give information about the causative object.
  - Oval or rounded bruises caused by fingertips over the neck in throttling represent one such example.
  - Beating by a stick will produce linear contusions. Such bruises are called **patterned bruises**. They may also result from beating with a chain (**Fig. 3.40**).

- Sometimes, flat objects such as belts produce characteristic **tramline contusions** manifesting as two parallel linear contusions separated by a pale, undamaged section of skin (**Fig. 3.41**). Occasionally, rod-shaped objects may be responsible. They occur because at the site of impact, the blood is squeezed out from vessels without any leakage (due to lack of damage to the vessel walls), while at the edges, the vessel walls are torn because of stretching; as a result there is leakage of blood.

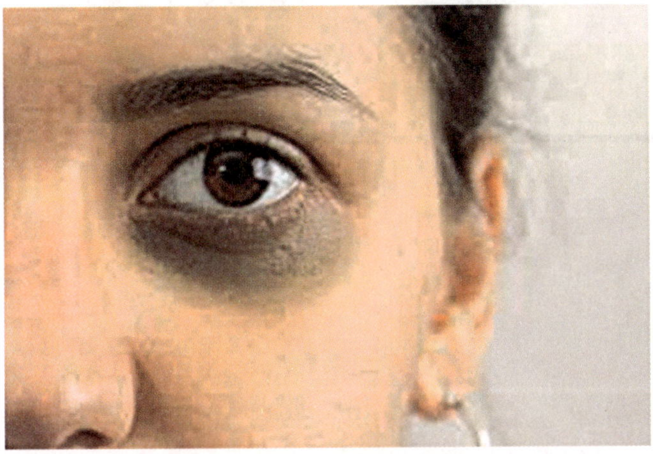

Fig. 3.39 Black eye

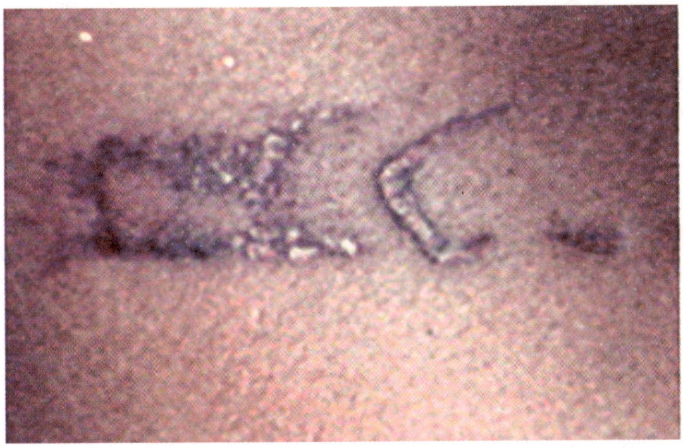

Fig. 3.40 Patterned contusion due to beating with a chain (*Courtesy*: *Dr Shashidhar C Mestri*)

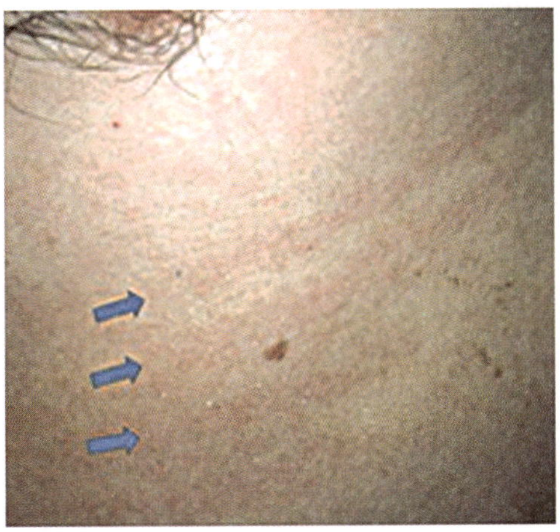

Fig. 3.41 Tramline contusions

- The size of a contusion may roughly correspond to the object causing it. This may give some clue regarding the weapon employed. Thus, a contusion caused by a stick is longer than it is broad. Its width usually corresponds to the diameter of the stick. With lapse of time however, the contusion may appear larger in size than it originally was, due to continued extravasation of blood and development of oedema.
- **Artificial bruise**: It is a lesion that is produced by applying the juice of an irritant plant, e.g., calotropis, marking nut, etc. Though, it has the superficial appearance of a bruise, and may be deliberately induced by a person on himself to substantiate a false allegation of assault against another person, it can be differentiated from a true bruise by the presence of blisters which are invariably present.

Repair and Healing

- After a lapse of some time, the red blood corpuscles in a bruise will begin to disintegrate by haemolysis, liberating haemoglobin, which in turn gets broken down into haemosiderin, haematoidin and bilirubin, by tissue enzymes and histiocytes. These pigments impart certain colour changes to a bruise which can be visualised, especially in the case of fair complexioned individuals (**Fig. 3.42**).
  - To begin with, the injury is **red** in colour.
  - It turns **bluish** in a day.
  - **Brownish** over the next 3 days (due to haemosiderin).
  - It turns **greenish** over the subsequent 3 days (haematoidin).
  - **Yellowish** in the final 2 days (bilirubin).
  - At the end of a fortnight, the original normal colour of the skin is restored, since these pigments get removed by phagocytosis.

  Colour changes (mnemonic): **RBBGY** – **R**ed, **B**lue, **B**rown, **G**reen, **Y**ellow
- In subconjunctival haemorrhage, due to diffusion of atmospheric oxygen, these colour changes may not be noticeable.
- Postmortem lividity (hypostasis) in the early stages can mimic a contusion, posing problems in interpretation. The important differentiating points are summarised in **Table 3.14**.
- Contusions can be produced after death, and are referred to as **postmortem contusions**. This is particularly likely when moderate force is applied over those areas where the skin is immediately subjacent to underlying bone (e.g., forehead). A severe blow to the body within a few hours of death can produce contusions in other parts of the body also, especially over an area of postmortem lividity. However, such contusions are devoid of swelling, and do not

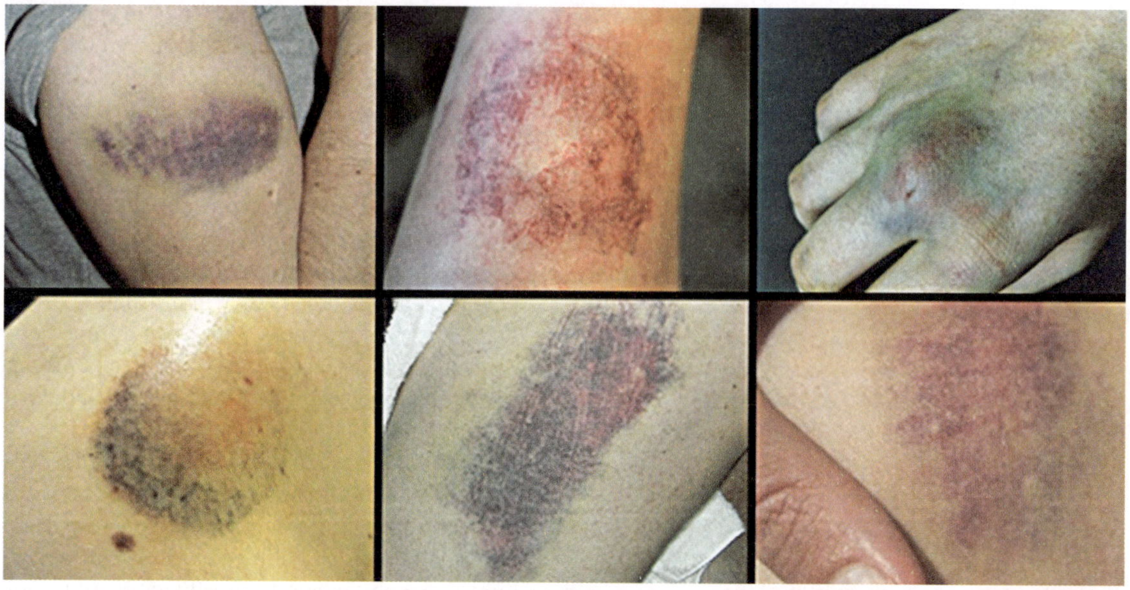

Fig. 3.42 Bruises at various stages of healing

Table 3.14 Differences between Contusion and Postmortem Lividity

	Contusion (Bruise)	Postmortem Lividity
Cause	Rupture of vessels and extravasation of blood	Engorgement of vessels due to pooling of blood
Site	Anywhere in the body	Only in dependent parts
Surface	Elevated	No elevation
Colour	Variable, depending on the age	Normally purple
On Incision	Shows extravasated blood in the cut tissues which cannot be washed off	Blood oozes out of cut vessels which can be easily washed off
Histology	Signs of inflammation present	No signs of inflammation

demonstrate inflammatory reaction. Their edges appear sharply demarcated.

Medicolegal Significance

- A contusion can give some clue about the **contact of a body with a blunt object**, and depending on the site of occurrence, to the **nature of crime** (e.g., contusions in and around the nose and lips suggest smothering).
  - However, a contusion need not necessarily indicate the exact site of contact with a blunt weapon, since it can appear at an area remote to the application of force.
- In several cases, the **nature of the object** used, and the degree of force applied can be reasonably presumed. However, the size of a contusion may be smaller or greater than the weapon producing it.
- Colour changes can help to deduce the **time of occurrence**. Contusions of markedly different colours on different parts of the body of the same individual suggest different times of occurrence, and are indicative of chronic abuse (e.g., *battered baby syndrome*). Since contusions sometimes become evident after a delay of variable period, a second examination is always advisable, whether the victim is alive or dead.
- If there is doubt as to whether a contusion is antemortem or postmortem in nature, it must be subjected to histopathological examination, which will reveal antemortem characteristics such as evidence of vital reaction, if the injury occurred before death.

Laceration

- **It is a type of mechanical injury where there is a rupture or tear of skin or deeper tissues, or both, due to application of blunt force.**
- Lacerated injuries are three dimensional with length, width and depth, and often have abraded margins, and irregular, contused edges.
- Since blood vessels are crushed, bleeding is usually not severe. However, substantial bleeding can occur, if blood vessels get torn partially.

- Foreign particles from the weapon or impacting surface are often present in the wound.
- The interior of the wound contains bridging strands of tissue which can be visualised clearly with a hand lens.
- The depth may not be uniform throughout the injury.

Classification

- Lacerated injuries can occur from splitting, stretching, grinding or compression force. Accordingly, they are classified as:
  - Split laceration (incised-looking laceration)
  - Stretch laceration
  - Cut laceration
  - Avulsion (grind laceration)
  - Tear

A simple mnemonic to help remember the 5 important types of **lacerations** is **CATSS**: **C** = Cut; **A** = Avulsion; **T** = Tear; **S** = Split; **S** = Stretch.*

Split Laceration

- In this type, the skin gets split due to compression between the weapon and underlying bone.
- The edges often appear clean cut on cursory inspection. Hence these injuries are also called **incised-looking lacerations**. However, a hand-lens examination will reveal contusion of edges and bridging of tissues.
- Common areas of involvement include scalp, lower jaw, shin, etc.
- A blunt blow over the parietal region may result in a split laceration with the so-called '**swallow tail**' appearance, especially if the impact is over the parietal **eminence** as the bone at that point has two diverging planes (**Fig. 3.43**).

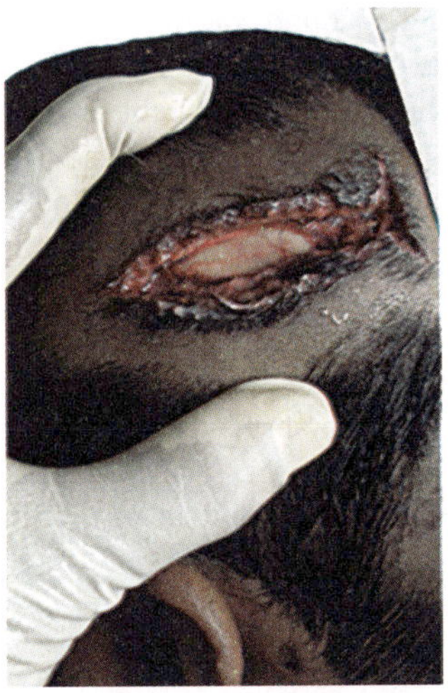

Fig. 3.43 Split laceration over parietal region with 'swallow tail' appearance (*Courtesy*: *Dr Girish Chandra YP*)

Stretch Laceration (Fig. 3.44)

- In this type, the skin gets stretched to a breaking point resulting in a laceration at that site. For example, pressure over the thigh which stretches the skin towards the knee can cause a laceration along the inguinal line.
- Ordinarily, unless great force is used, most lacerations require a firm base to act as an anvil for the skin and underlying tissues to be pinned against. But, this is not true for a stretch laceration.

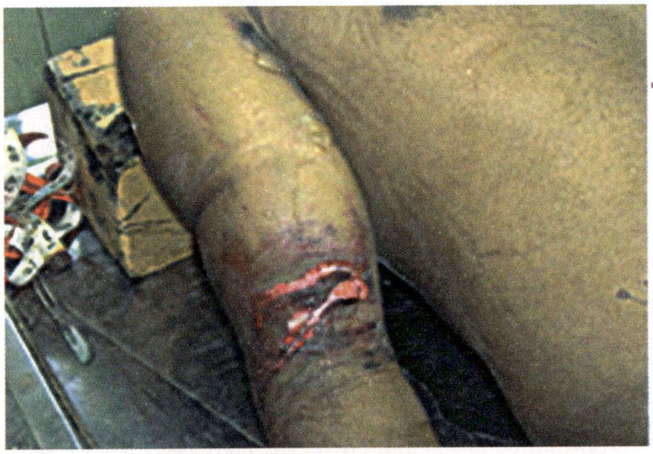

Fig. 3.44 Stretch laceration due to fractured humerus (*Courtesy*: *Dr Hareesh S Gouda*)

Avulsion (Grind Laceration) (Fig. 3.45)

- In this type, there is a separation of skin from underlying tissues due to the shearing or grinding action of a weight, e.g., the wheel of a heavy vehicle in a run-over injury.

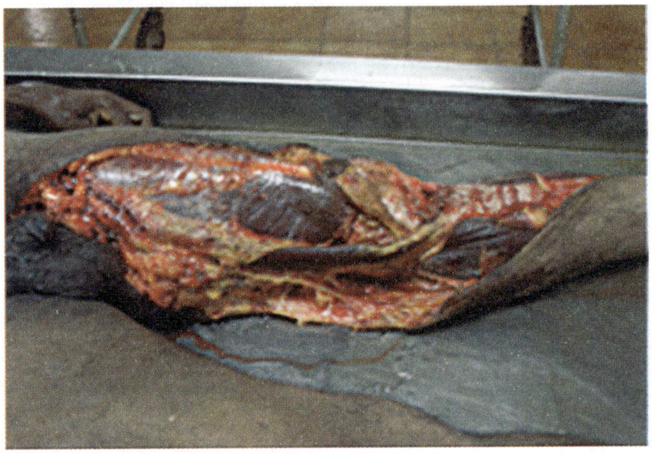

Fig. 3.45 Avulsed laceration due to run-over injury (*Courtesy*: *Dr Prateek Rastogi*)

**As stated under "Abrasion", the mnemonic to help remember the 4 important types of abrasions is PIGS; and as stated on this page, the mnemonic to help remember the 5 important types of lacerations is CATSS. So, be an animal lover! They help you remember important points!*

Cut Laceration

- This type of laceration results from the cutting action of a weapon which is not very sharp, e.g., a broken glass piece.
- It is a lacerated wound with profound and distinct contusion of edges.
- While incised wounds divide hairs cleanly, lacerations cause some hairs to be driven into the interior.

Tear*

- As the name suggests, this type of laceration results from tearing of tissues due to a relatively sharp force, which is not sharp enough to incise the tissues.

Other Types

- **Patterned laceration** – Lacerations usually do not reproduce the shape of the injuring object. However, rarely the shape is recognisable, as in the case of a hammer blow to the scalp. But, calculation of the exact size of striking surface in such cases can be misleading.
- **Postmortem laceration** – Lacerated injuries may be produced by terrestrial or aquatic animal action (rat, fish, crab, etc.) on corpses. Absence of vital reaction will assist in distinguishing them from antemortem lacerations. The edges may also show characteristic evidence of 'nibbling' or 'gnawing.' A running vehicle or train can cause extensive postmortem lacerations of a dead body lying in its path.

Repair and Healing

- Lacerated wounds often get infected, thus delaying the healing process.
- As they do not exhibit uniform healing pattern, age estimation is difficult and unreliable.
- Healing is by second intention.
  - It begins as phagocytosis to remove debris, followed by filling of the defect by granulation tissue.
  - Specialised tissues lost are repaired, and epithelium regenerated to cover the surface. A permanent scar is therefore inevitable.
  - The time frame will depend upon the extent and severity of the laceration.

Medicolegal Significance

- Areas of the body that are commonly the site of lacerations are those with **underlying bony support**, such as over the eyebrows, on the scalp and face, or over knees, shin, etc., whilst they are less common on areas of the body that are softer such as the buttocks.
- Lacerations are usually **accidental** or **homicidal**. Self-inflicted lacerations are uncommon.
- Foreign particles in these wounds may help to identify the **causative object**. Grease, mud, etc., may be seen in wounds of traffic accidents.
- The exact type of lacerated injury may provide a clue to the **nature of occurrence**.
- In the case of avulsions, the direction of force can often be ascertained.
- The site of the injury may provide some clue about the cause of death, e.g., lacerations of internal mucosa of lips may suggest smothering.
- Lacerated wounds of face constitute grievous hurt because of permanent disfiguration.

Incision (Incised Wound)

- **An incision (or incised wound) is a clean-cut separation of skin and deeper tissues, caused by a sharp cutting weapon, without loss of substance** (**Fig. 3.46**).

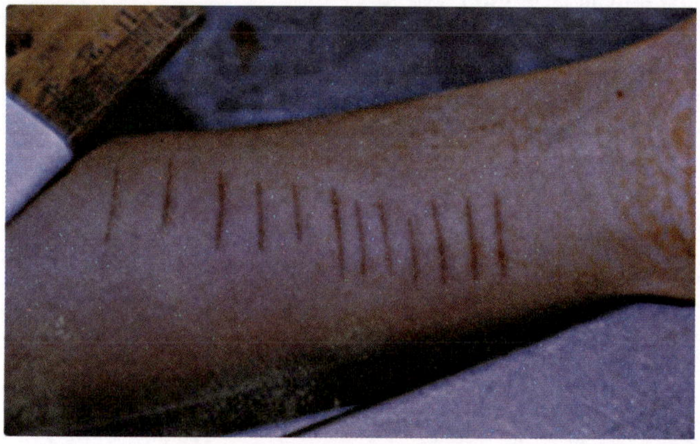

Fig. 3.46 Multiple superficial incised wounds (*Courtesy: Dr Pratik Patel*)

- The commencement of the wound is usually deep, gradually becoming shallower, and finally tailing off towards the end. This ***tailing*** of the wound indicates the site of withdrawal of the weapon from the body, suggesting the direction in which the wound was inflicted.
- The wound is generally straight and shows maximum retraction of the edges at the centre. In other words, the wound "***gapes***," because of which the width of the wound is greater than the width of the weapon causing it (**Fig. 3.47**). The gaping is more if the incision is made at right angles to the "**lines of cleavage**" (**cleavage lines of Langer**) (**Fig. 3.48**), and much less if it is parallel to these lines.
- The edges of the wound are clean cut and may be everted. Ordinarily, there is no bruising of the margins.
- An incised wound is necessarily longer than it is deep. In fact, the **length is the greatest of the three dimensions** (length, breadth/width, depth).
- It bleeds freely, as blood vessels are cleanly cut and not crushed.

Classification

- An incision produced by a light cutting weapon is smooth with minimal bruising of margins. Heavy cutting weapons such as an axe or cleaver produce distinct contusion of the

**Note: Pronounced as 'tare' and NOT 'teer' (like beer)! The latter 'tear' refers to lacrimal secretion which comes out of the eye when a student fails in such an easy subject as FMT!*

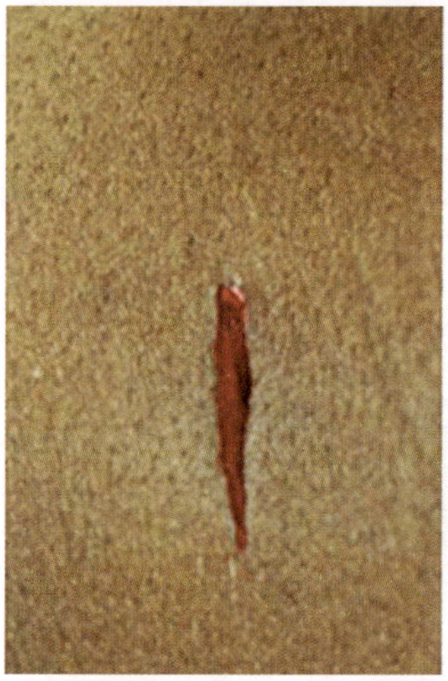

Fig. 3.47 Incised wound with gaping

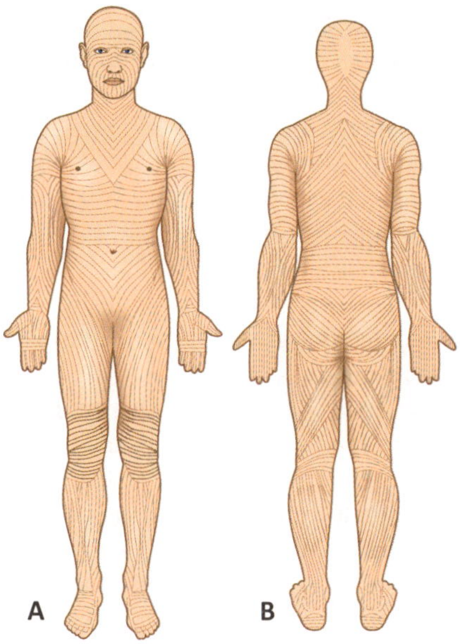

Fig. 3.48 Lines of Langer

edges, and the resulting injury is referred to as a **chop wound** (**Fig. 3.49**).

- Incised wounds produced over wrinkled skin may appear as lacerations, due to irregularity of edges, e.g., in the scrotum. A hand lens examination will help to differentiate them as incised wounds. Such wounds are sometimes called **lacerated-looking incised wounds**.

Repair and Healing

- In the case of an incised wound with very little damage to tissues on either side of the cut, healing occurs without delay, if the edges are apposed properly.
  - Small blood vessels which are cut get occluded by thrombosis. Fibrin precipitated locally will then link the two edges. Coagulated blood on the surface forms a scab and helps to keep the wound clean. This occurs within 12–24 hours.

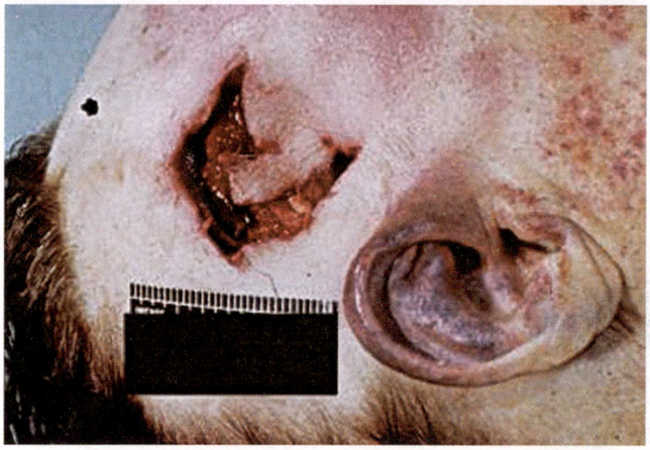

Fig. 3.49 Chop wound over head with claw hammer

  - Over the next few days, capillaries proliferate to bridge the gap, and fibroblasts secrete collagen.
  - In 3–5 days, vessels are thickened, and many of them get obliterated, which is followed by scar formation. This is usually complete by about the 6th day.
  - The scab over the wound then falls off, leaving behind a soft, tender, reddish scar, which in the course of weeks or months becomes whitish and firm.
  - Infection can however delay the healing process.

Medicolegal Significance

- Incised wounds invariably point to the use of a **cutting weapon** (light or heavy).
- The length, width or depth of an incised wound usually do not correspond to the length, thickness or width of the cutting object.
- **Tailing** gives an indication of the direction of movement of the cutting edge.
- The site may suggest the possible motive, intent or even the mental status of the assailant. For example, incised wounds concentrated over the genital area reveal a sex-related motive.
- Homicidal incised wounds sometimes suggest the disturbed mind of the assailant, which may vary from cold fury to irrational psychosis.

Stab (Puncture Wound)

- **Stab wounds are piercing wounds produced by sharp-pointed objects (e.g., knife, dagger, ice pick, fork, spear, sharpened bamboo stick, etc.).**
- The depth is necessarily greater than the surface length. In fact, **depth is the greatest of the three dimensions** (length, breadth/width, depth).
- Stab wounds are divided into:
  - **Penetrating wounds**, if they ***terminate*** in tissues, organ, or cavity (**Fig. 3.50**).
  - **Perforating wounds**, if they ***transfix*** them (through-and-through wounds). For example, stab wound piercing an upper arm completely, so that it goes in on one side, and comes out on the other side.

- In the former, there is only one surface wound, while in the latter, there will be two separate surface wounds, one caused by the *entry* and the other by the *exit* (**Fig. 3.51**).

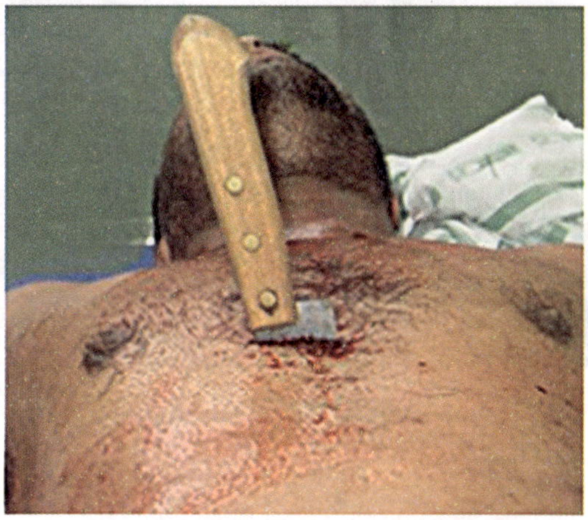

Fig. 3.50 Penetrating stab wound of chest

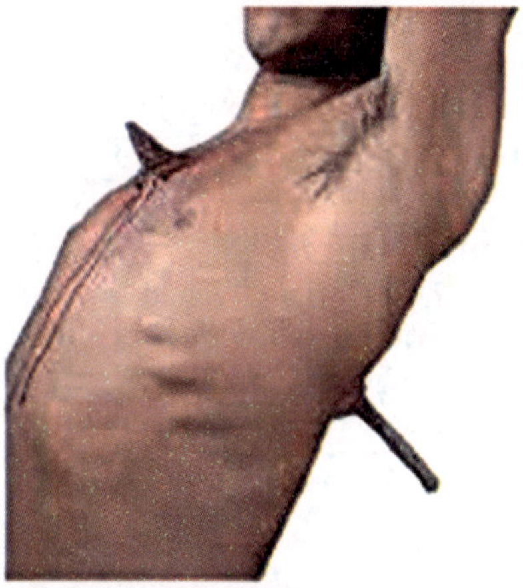

Fig. 3.51 Perforating stab wound of chest

- External bleeding may be slight, but internal bleeding can be very profuse.
- In perforating wounds, the wound of entry is usually larger than the wound of exit, because weapons used for stabbing usually taper towards the tip.
- The edges of the wound of entry are inverted, while they are everted in the wound of exit. Clothes may be pushed into the wound of entry.
- The direction in which the wound has been inflicted can be deduced by joining the wounds of entry and exit.
- **Incised-stab wound**: This starts as an incised wound and ends as a stab wound when there is a sudden thrust at the termination of the incised wound, or conversely it may begin as a stab wound, and then become an incised wound as the knife is pulled out with a little bit of dragging.

Medicolegal Significance

- The external appearance of a stab wound may sometimes give a clue regarding the kind of weapon used in inflicting it (**Fig. 3.52**).
  - Thus, a **knife** which has one sharp edge and a thicker, blunt edge, produces a wound which is usually **wedge shaped**.
  - On the other hand, a double-edged weapon such as a **dagger** will usually produce an **elliptical** wound.

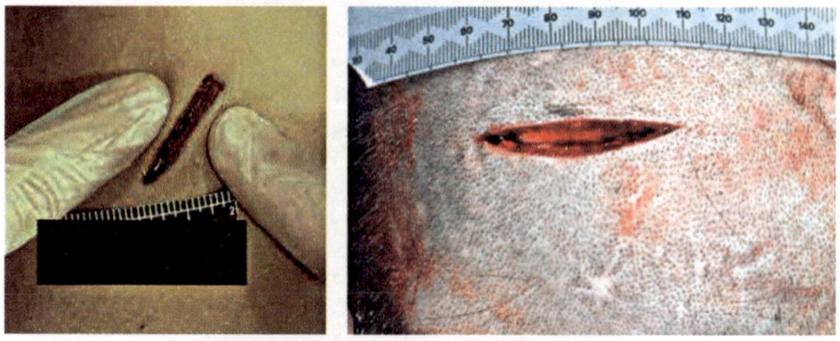

Fig. 3.52 Wedge shaped stab (left) and elliptical stab (right)

- The terminal ends of the injury may be sharp cut, square shaped, or rounded.
  - If both ends are sharp-cut, in all probability the weapon used was a double-edged one, even though a single-edged weapon can sometimes produce such an appearance due to splitting, or if the weapon possesses a curved beak. It can also occur if a single-edged weapon is tilted while being withdrawn.
  - Bruising around the stab wound may indicate that the weapon had been inserted up to the hilt.
- A round, pointed object such as a spear often produces a circular stab wound.
- A pointed weapon that is square-shaped in cross section, may produce a cross-shaped stab wound. Stabbing with a fork produces clusters of 2 or 3 small puncture wounds, depending upon the number of prongs on the fork.
- Small, slit-like stabs are produced by stabbing with a screwdriver. The exact shape will depend on the type of screwdriver (**Fig. 3.53**).

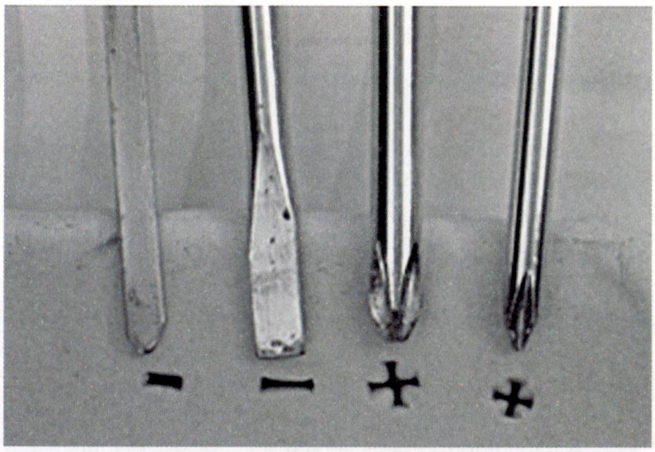

Fig. 3.53 Shape of stab wound with different screwdrivers

- A stab injury may not produce significant external bleeding, especially when the wound has entered a body cavity (**Fig. 3.54**). But, there may be extensive internal bleeding which can rapidly lead to death.

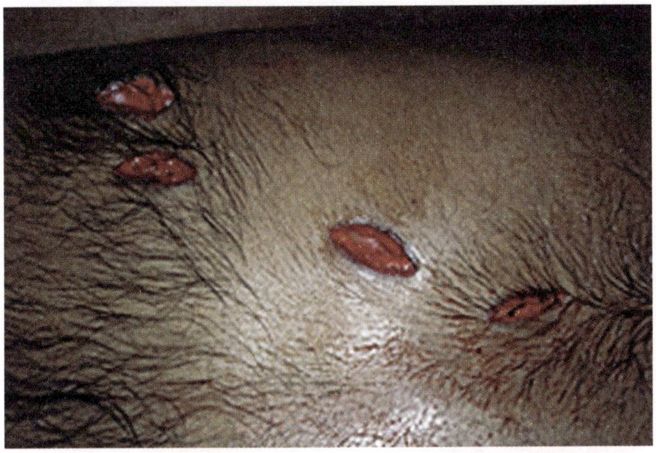

Fig. 3.54 Multiple abdominal stabs with minimal external bleeding (*Courtesy*: *Dr Prateek Rastogi*)

- If the weapon used to stab enters the skin obliquely, the edge of the wound on the side from which the weapon has entered becomes "***bevelled***," while the other edge overhangs the wound. From this, the direction in which the wound was inflicted may be ascertained.
- In the case of perforating stabs, direction is more easily ascertained, as the exit wound is invariably smaller than the entry, and appears everted.
- The depth of the wound may give an indication of the **minimum length of the weapon** used, provided the entry wound and the termination of the wound track are situated in non-yielding areas. If the punctured wound has made an entry through a yielding site (e.g., abdominal wall), or ends up in a cavity or a collapsible organ (e.g., lung), the deduction of depth becomes a matter of conjecture. The depth of the wound can be greater than the length of the weapon over yielding sites such as abdominal wall due to the compression of the wall downwards during the thrust, and its subsequent return to the normal position when the pressure is withdrawn. Similarly, collapse of lungs after sustaining stab injury over the chest (particularly on the front or lateral sides) may lend itself to wrong interpretation of the length of the weapon, since the distance between the chest wall and surface of lungs will be increased due to collapse.
- The length of a stab wound may be equal to the breadth of the stabbing weapon. However, it is usually lesser by 0.2 to 0.3 cm if the skin is elastic, while it may be greater if rocking of the object occurs during the course of stabbing.
- The width of a stab wound is usually greater than the thickness of the weapon, due to gaping.
- Stab wounds may be homicidal, accidental or suicidal. The presence of such wounds in inaccessible parts can help to exclude suicide. Also, suicidal stabs are usually single, and located characteristically on the left side of the chest.
- In some cases of stab homicides, the stabbing may have been done through a natural orifice (ear, nostril, vagina, rectum), or in unusual locations (axilla, nape of the neck) in order to conceal its presence. Such stabs are referred to as **concealed puncture wounds**.

Fracture

- **A fracture is a partial or complete break in a bone or tooth due to direct or indirect force.**
  - This is a type of injury that is always associated with a bone or tooth, and not with any other tissue or organ.
  - The term "fracture" is not used when a cartilage, ligament or tendon is affected, owing to lack of osseus tissue. The correct term would be a "tear" or "rupture."

Classification

Direct Fractures

1. ***Focal Fracture:***
   a. This is otherwise known as **tapping fracture**, and results from a small force applied to a small area.
   b. It is usually transverse.
   c. Injury to overlying soft tissues is minimal.
   d. Typically seen in regions such as the forearm or leg where two bones lie adjacent to each other, only one of the two bones being fractured, e g., while warding off blows during an attack.
2. ***Crush Fracture:***
   a. It results from application of a large force over a large area, and is typically **comminuted** in type, i.e., fragmented.
   b. Injury to surrounding soft tissues is usually extensive.
   c. If two bones lie adjacent to each other, both are involved, e.g., bumper fracture of the tibia and fibula in a pedestrian who has been hit by a car.
3. ***Penetrating Fracture:***
   a. It results from application of severe force over a small area.
   b. Bullet injury to a bone is a classical example of this type of fracture.

Indirect Fractures

1. ***Traction Fracture***: It results when a bone is pulled apart by traction, e.g., transverse patellar fracture due to violent contraction of quadriceps. It is also referred to as an **avulsion fracture**.
2. ***Angulation Fracture***: It occurs due to bending of a bone. The concave surface of the bend is compressed, while the convex surface is put under traction resulting in breakage.
3. ***Rotational or Spiral Fracture***: Here, the bone is twisted to produce a spiral fracture.
4. ***Vertical Compression Fracture***:
   a. In this type, there is an oblique fracture of a long bone such that the hard shaft of the bone is driven into the cancellous portion.
   b. It is sometimes encountered in the distal femur of a front seat passenger of a vehicle when there has been a collision, and his knee has impacted violently against the dashboard.

5. ***Angulation-Compression Fracture:*** Here, the fracture line is curved, with an *oblique* component due to compression, and a *transverse* component due to angulation.

Other Fractures

1. ***Greenstick Fracture***:
   a. It is an incomplete fracture involving only part of the thickness of a long bone.
   b. It is usually encountered in children whose bones are pliant rather than brittle.
   c. The usual cause is forcible angulation.
2. ***Simple and Compound Fractures***:
   a. A simple or closed fracture is one where the overlying skin is still intact.
   b. A compound or open fracture involves tearing of overlying tissues, including skin. The fractured ends often protrude through the defect. Such fractures are more prone for infection.
   c. In the case of the cranium, the term "compound" is used only when the dura is torn. It is not important whether the skin is intact or torn.

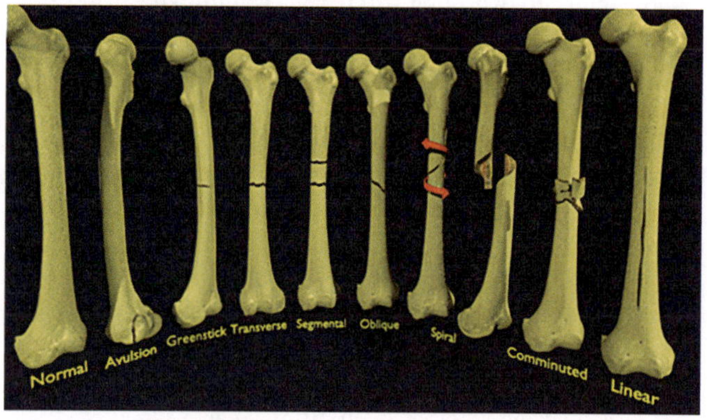

Fig. 3.55 Common types of fracture

Repair and Healing

- Healing of a fracture depends upon the age and nutritional status of the individual. In general, cancellous bone unites faster than cortical bone.
- There are five stages involved in the healing process:
  1. **Haemorrhagic phase**: There is haemorrhage at the site of fracture.
  2. **Proliferation phase**: A collar is formed around the fractured ends by proliferation of cells from periosteum and endosteum.
  3. **Callus phase**: Cellular elements give rise to osteoblasts and chondroblasts which produce a matrix of collagen and polysaccharide, impregnated with calcium. This is called "callus." In children, the callus is visible radiologically within 2 weeks of the fracture.
  4. **Consolidation phase**: The callus is transformed into mature bone which takes about 4–6 weeks in children, and approximately 3 months in adults.
  5. **Remodelling phase**: This is the final phase during which the mature bone is remodelled.

Medicolegal Significance

- Fracture of a bone, however trivial, constitutes **grievous hurt** according to law.
- From a study of the exact type of fracture, an idea about the causative force can be estimated, i.e., whether the force was direct or indirect, rotational or angular, etc.
- The site of fracture may help to indicate the cause of death, e.g., fracture of hyoid bone suggests throttling.
- The time of occurrence of a fracture can be estimated roughly from the stage of the healing process.

DEFENSE WOUND*

- A **defense wound** or **self-defense wound** is an injury received by the victim of an attack while trying to defend against the assailant.
- Such wounds are often found on the hands and forearms, where the victim has raised them to protect the head and face, or to fend off an assault (**Fig. 3.56**), but may also be present on the feet and legs where a victim attempts defense while lying down and kicking out at the assailant.
- The appearance and nature of the wound varies with the type of weapon used and the location of the injury, and may present as a laceration, abrasion, contusion or bone fracture. Where a victim has time to raise hands or arms before being shot by an assailant, the injury may also present as a gunshot wound.
- Severe laceration of the palmar surface of the hand or partial amputation of fingers may result from the victim grasping the blade of a weapon during an attack.
- The presence of defense wounds is highly indicative of homicide, and also proves that the victim was, at least initially, conscious and able to offer some resistance during the attack.
- Defense wounds may be classified as **active** or **passive**. A victim of a knife attack, for example, would receive active defense wounds from grasping at the knife's blade, and passive defense wounds on the back of the hand, if it was raised up to protect the face.

FABRICATED WOUND

- **Synonyms**: Fictitious wound/Forged wound/Invented wound
- **Definition**: **Fabricated wounds are produced by a person on his own body or by another with his consent.**
- **Types**:
  - ***Self-Inflicted***: Those inflicted by a person on his own body.
  - ***Self-Suffered***: Those inflicted by another person on the alleged victim.
- **Motive**:
  - To simulate a criminal offence in the form of a false charge of:

****Note***: *Also spelt as "Defence Wound".*

- Rape
- Assault or attempted murder
- Torture
- Conversion of simple injury into a grievous one

- To avert suspicion:
  - By the assailant to pretend self-defence.
  - Change the appearance of wounds, which might connect him with the crime.
  - By policemen and watchmen acting in collusion with robbers to show that they were defending the property.
  - In thefts by servants
  - By soldiers and prisoners to escape difficult tasks
  - Insurance frauds
  - Suicidal gestures, attempted suicide.

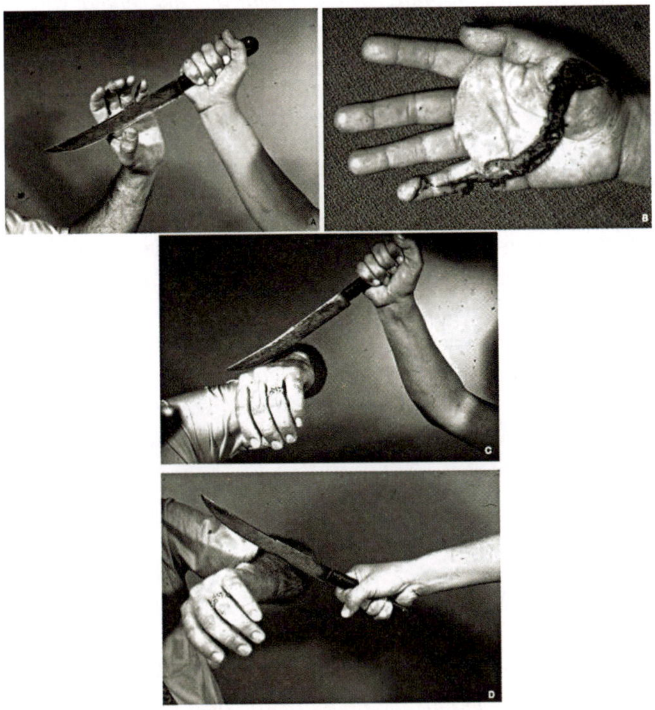

Fig. 3.56 Modes of sustaining defence wounds in a knife attack

- **Diagnosis**:
  - History of assault incompatible with injuries.
  - No damage, or inconsistent damage to clothes.
  - Most common nature of wound: Abrasions or superficial incised wounds. Less commonly, contusions, stab wounds and superficial burns. Lacerations and fractures are extremely uncommon.
  - Most commonly used weapons: Knife, razor, glass piece, scissors.
  - Most commonly involved body parts: Outer side of either arm, front and outer sides of either thigh, front of abdomen, chest, top of head, forehead, neck.

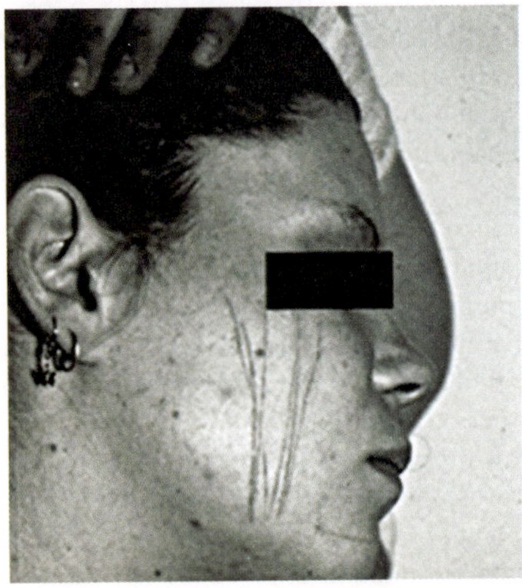

Fig. 3.57 Self-inflicted superficial incised wounds over face

FM 3.4: Core – Written/Viva Voce

- **Mechanical Injuries and Wounds**
  - Define
    - Injury
    - Assault
    - Hurt
  - Describe IPC sections pertaining to injuries

INJURY

- Defined in **Section 44** of Indian Penal Code (IPC): Denotes any harm, illegally caused to any person in body, mind, reputation or property.*

HURT

- Defined in **Section 319** of Indian Penal Code (IPC): Denotes any bodily pain, disease or infirmity caused to a person.**

GRIEVOUS HURT

- Defined in **Section 320** of Indian Penal Code (IPC).
- Denotes any of the following **8 clauses**:
  - Emasculation.
  - Permanent privation of the sight of either eye.
  - Permanent privation of the hearing of either ear.
  - Privation of any member or joint.
  - Destruction or permanent impairment of the powers of any member or joint.
  - Permanent disfiguration of the head or face (**Fig. 3.58**).
  - Fracture or dislocation of a bone or tooth.

*Any harm to BMRP – Body, mind, reputation or property.

**Any PDI – Pain, disease or infirmity.

- Any hurt which endangers life, or which causes the sufferer to be in severe bodily pain, or unable to follow his ordinary pursuits, during the space of 20 days.

- ***Important Points***:
  - Self-inflicted injuries are not covered by this definition.
  - Emasculation* means deprivation of masculine vigour (inflicting impotence by amputation of penis, or causing inability to take part in sexual intercourse by any means).
  - A crack fracture of bone which does not involve the medullary cavity will not be considered as fracture, for the purpose of this section.
  - A mere stay in hospital for 20 days or more will not constitute grievous hurt. It must be proved that during this period, he was in severe bodily pain or unable to follow his ordinary pursuits.
  - An injury may be construed as "simple" from the medical point of view, but legally it may fit one of the clauses (examples) under *Section 320 IPC*. The opinion of the doctor as to the nature of injury must always be as per legal definition.
  - The final opinion as to whether a particular injury is simple or grievous is left to the discretion of the court. The role of the doctor is only to guide and help the court in deciding the issue.

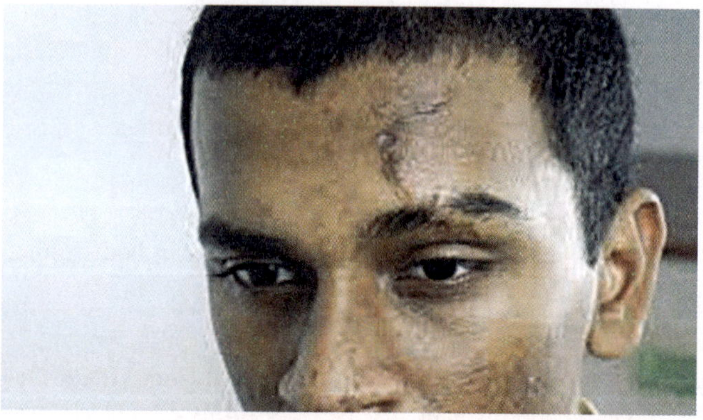

Fig. 3.58 Grievous hurt – Permanent disfiguration of face

VOLUNTARILY CAUSING HURT

- Defined in **Section 321** of Indian Penal Code (IPC): *Whoever does any act with the intention of causing hurt to any person, or with the knowledge that he is likely to cause hurt to any person, and does thereby cause hurt to any person, is said "voluntarily to cause hurt."*
- **Punishment for voluntarily causing hurt** (Section 323 IPC) – Imprisonment of either description for a term which may extend to one year, or with fine which may extend to one thousand rupees, or with both.

VOLUNTARILY CAUSING GRIEVOUS HURT

- Defined in **Section 322** of Indian Penal Code (IPC): *Whoever voluntarily causes hurt, if the hurt which he intends to cause or knows himself to be likely to cause is grievous hurt, and if the hurt which he actually causes amounts to grievous hurt, is said to "voluntarily cause grievous hurt."*
- **Punishment for voluntarily causing grievous hurt** (Section 325 IPC) – Imprisonment of either description for a term which may extend to seven years, and shall also be liable to fine.

VOLUNTARILY CAUSING HURT BY DANGEROUS WEAPONS OR MEANS

- Defined in **Section 324** of Indian Penal Code (IPC): *Whoever voluntarily causes hurt by means of any instrument for shooting, stabbing, or cutting, or any instrument which when used as a weapon of offence, is likely to cause death, shall be punished with imprisonment of either description for a term which may extend to three years, or with fine, or with both.*

VOLUNTARILY CAUSING GRIEVOUS HURT BY DANGEROUS WEAPONS OR MEANS

- Defined in **Section 326** of Indian Penal Code (IPC): *Whoever voluntarily causes grievous hurt by means of any instrument for shooting, stabbing or cutting, or any instrument which when used as a weapon of offence, is likely to cause death, shall be punished with imprisonment for life, or with imprisonment of either description for a term which may extend to ten years, and shall also be liable to fine.*

AMENDMENTS UNDER THE CRIMINAL LAW (AMENDMENT) ACT, 2013

Section 326A IPC

- **Voluntarily causing grievous hurt by use of acid**:
  - *Whoever causes permanent damage or deformity to, or burns or maims or disfigures or disables, any part of the body of a person, or causes grievous hurt by throwing acid on that person, or by using any other means, with the intention of causing such hurt, shall be punished with imprisonment (10 years to life), and with fine which may extend to 10 lakh rupees.*

Section 326B IPC

- **Attempt to cause grievous hurt by use of acid**:
  - *Whoever attempts to throw acid on any person, or use any other means, with the intention of causing permanent damage or deformity, or attempts to burn or maim or disfigure or disable a person, shall be punished with imprisonment (5–7 years), and shall also be liable to fine.*

**Note*: *Emasculation is different from castration, which refers to removal of testicles. Castration is covered by clause no. 4.*

- **Explanation 1**: For the purposes of Sections 326A and 326B, "acid" includes any substance which has acidic or corrosive character or burning nature, that is capable of causing bodily injury leading to scars or disfigurement or temporary or permanent disability.
- **Explanation 2**: "Permanent damage" includes deformity, or maiming, or burning, or disfiguring, or disabling any part of the body of a person.
- **Explanation 3**: Permanent damage or deformity shall not be required to be irreversible.

Important Points

So, after the amendments listed above, the following changes have come into effect:

- Earlier, only permanent disfiguration of face was considered as grievous hurt, but now any other part of the body by throwing acid is considered as grievous hurt.
- Even temporary disability due to throwing of an acid is covered under the amendments.
- Damage/deformity shall not be required to be irreversible.
- The punishments have been enhanced and may extend to life imprisonment, and a fine which may extend to 10 lakh rupees.
- Even an attempt to throw acid on any person is punishable.
- Offences under Sections 326A and 326B are **cognizable** and **non-bailable**.

ASSAULT

- Defined in Section 351 of Indian Penal Code (IPC): *Whoever makes any gesture, or any preparation, intending that it will cause any person present to apprehend that he is about to use criminal force to that person, is said to commit an* ***assault***.
  - **Explanation**: Mere words do not amount to an assault. But, the words which a person uses may give to his gestures or preparation such a meaning as may make those gestures or preparations amount to an assault.
  - **Examples**:
    - If A shakes his fist at Z, knowing it to be likely that he may thereby cause Z to believe that he is about to strike Z, A has committed an assault.
    - A begins to unloose the muzzle of a ferocious dog, knowing it to be likely that he may thereby cause Z to believe that he is about to cause the dog to attack Z. A has committed an assault upon Z.
    - A takes up a stick, saying to Z, "I will give you a beating". Here, though the words used by A could in no case amount to an assault, and though the mere gesture might not amount to an assault, the gesture explained by the words may amount to an assault.
      - When an assault is actually carried out, it is referred to as "physical assault".
    - If the physical assault is carried out with sexual intend, it is referred to as "sexual assault".

> FM 3.5: Core – Written/Viva Voce
> - **Mechanical Injuries and Wounds**
>   - Describe
>   - Accidental, suicidal and homicidal injuries
>   - Simple, grievous and dangerous injuries
>   - Antemortem and postmortem injuries

Injuries may be caused by human beings, animals or machines. Such infliction may be **accidental** or, if they have been caused by a human being, they could be **suicidal** or **homicidal**. These are covered by the term "**Manner of Death**".

HOMICIDE

- The term "**homicide**" means causing the death of a person by another person.
- The term "**dyadic death**" is used when homicide of a victim is followed by suicide of the perpetrator (formerly referred to as "**homicide-suicide**").

Classification

- **Lawful Homicide**
  - Justifiable
  - Excusable
- **Unlawful (Culpable) Homicide**
  - Amounting to Murder
  - Not Amounting to Murder

Lawful Homicide

- It refers to the causing of death of a person which is **permissible** or **excusable** by law.
  - The former is called **justifiable homicide**, e.g., judicial hanging.
  - **Excusable homicide** is that type of lawful homicide which is caused unintentionally by an act done in good faith, or in self-defence.

Culpable Homicide

- Defined in **Section 299** of IPC: *Whoever causes death by doing an act with the intention of causing death, or with intention of causing such bodily injury as is likely to cause death, or with the knowledge that he is likely by such act to cause death, commits the offence of* ***culpable homicide***.

Murder

- Defined in **Section 300** of IPC: *Except in the cases hereinafter mentioned,* **culpable homicide is murder**, *if*:
  - ***Firstly*** *– The act by which the death is caused is done with the* ***intention of causing death***, *or*
  - ***Secondly*** *– If it is done with the* ***intention of causing such bodily injury as is likely to cause the death*** *of the person to whom the harm is caused, or*
  - ***Thirdly*** *– If it is done with the* ***intention of causing bodily injury to any person which is sufficient in the ordinary course of nature to cause death***, *and*
  - ***Fourthly*** *– If the person committing the act* ***knows that it is so imminently dangerous that it must in all probability cause death*** *or such bodily injury as is likely to cause death.*

- **Exceptions**
  - **Culpable homicide is not murder**, if:
    - The offender, whilst deprived of the power of self-control by grave and sudden provocation, causes the death of the person who was responsible for the provocation, or causes the death of any other person by mistake or accident.
    - The offender, in the exercise (in good faith) of the right of private defence of person or property, exceeds the power given to him by law and causes death of the person without premeditation, and without any intention of doing more harm than is necessary for the purpose of such defence.
    - The offender, being a public servant acting for the advancement of public justice, exceeds the powers given to him by law, and causes death by doing an act which he, in good faith, believes to be lawful and necessary for the due discharge of his duty.
    - The offence is committed without premeditation in the heat of passion, in the course of a fight, without the offender's having taken undue advantage or acted in a cruel or unusual manner.
    - The person whose death is caused, being above the age of 18 years, suffers death or takes the risk of death with his own consent.
    - The death of a person other than the intended victim was caused inadvertently (**Section 301 IPC**).
- **Punishment for Murder**
  - Mentioned in **Section 302 IPC**.
    - Death (capital punishment), or imprisonment for life, and shall also be liable to fine.
- **Punishment for Murder by Life Convict**
  - Mentioned in **Section 303 IPC**.
    - Whoever, being under sentence of imprisonment for life, commits murder, shall be punished with death.
- **Punishment for Culpable Homicide Not Amounting to Murder**
  - Mentioned in **Section 304 IPC**.
    - Imprisonment for life, or imprisonment of either description for a term which may extend to 10 years, and shall also be liable to fine.

Dowry Death

- Defined in **Section 304B** of IPC: *Where the death of a woman is caused by any burn or bodily injury or occurs otherwise than under normal circumstances within 7 years of her marriage, and it is shown that soon before her death she was subjected to cruelty or harassment by her husband or any relative of her husband for, or in connection with any demand for dowry, such death shall be called "**dowry death**," and such husband or relative shall be deemed to have caused her death.*
- In cases of dowry death, the inquest should be conducted by a **magistrate** or police officer not below the rank of **deputy superintendent of police**.
- The postmortem examination should be carried out by a **panel of two doctors**, one of whom should preferably be a lady medical officer.

Harassment for Dowry

- Defined in **Section 498-A** IPC: *Whoever being the husband or the relative of the husband of a woman, subjects her to cruelty for the purpose of extracting dowry shall be punished with imprisonment for a term which may extend to 3 years, and shall also be liable for fine.*

ACCIDENT

- **Accidental death** is one where there was no intention to cause death of oneself, or by oneself of another.

Various kinds of accidents, including vehicular accidents such as road traffic accidents, are described under **Competency FM 3.12** *(page no. 205)*.

SUICIDE

- The deliberate act of taking one's own life is called "**suicide**."
- Common **reasons** for taking this extreme step include:
  - Endogenous depression
  - Depression arising out of sudden financial loss, bereavement, terminal illness, etc.
  - Escaping from huge debts which cannot be paid back, or from someone who is blackmailing the person for some illegal or immoral act.
  - Harassment of a married woman by husband for dowry ("dowry death").
  - Harassment of a person by someone for other reasons.
- Common **methods** of suicide in India include:
  - Hanging
  - Drowning
  - Poisoning
  - Immolation (burning)
  - Jumping from a tall structure (multi-storied building, bridge, mountain cliff, etc.)
  - Getting run-over by railway train
  - Cut throat injury, cutting wrists, etc. In such cases, tentative or hesitation cuts may be seen.
- **Legal Aspects**
  - ***Section 309 IPC*: Attempt to commit suicide** – *Whoever attempts to commit suicide and does any act towards the commission of such offence, shall be punished with simple imprisonment for a term which may extend to 1 year (or with fine, or with both).*
    - Although section 309 is still in effect, the **Mental Healthcare Act, 2017 (enacted July 2018)** has restricted its application. Thus, it has **decriminalized "attempted suicide"**.
    - The relevant provision of the new act states: Notwithstanding anything contained in Section 309 of the IPC, any person who attempts to commit suicide shall be presumed, unless proved otherwise, to have

severe stress and **shall not be tried and punished** under the said Code.

- The Mental Health Care Act does not repeal Section 309 of the Indian Penal Code, but merely provides the presumption of mental illness.

- ***Section 306 IPC*: Abetment of suicide** – *If any person commits suicide, whoever abets the commission of such suicide, shall be punished with imprisonment of either description for a term which may extend to 10 years, and shall also be liable to fine.*
- ***Section 305 IPC*: Abetment of suicide of child or insane person** – *If any person under 18 years of age, or any insane or mentally challenged person, or any person in a state of intoxication, commits suicide, whoever abets the commission of such suicide, shall be punished with death or imprisonment for life, or imprisonment for a term not exceeding 10 years, and shall also be liable to fine.*
- ***Section 304B IPC*: Dowry death** – *Where the death of a woman is caused by any burn or bodily injury or occurs otherwise than under normal circumstances within 7 years of her marriage, and it is shown that soon before her death she was subjected to cruelty or harassment by her husband or any relative of her husband for, or in connection with any demand for dowry, such death shall be called "**dowry death**," and such husband or relative shall be deemed to have caused her death.*
  - *Whoever commits dowry death shall be punished with imprisonment for a term which shall not be less than 7 years, but which may extend to imprisonment for life.*

SIMPLE INJURY

- There is no legal definition for Simple Injury or Hurt. Anything which is not grievous, or does not pose a threat to life, can be termed "Simple Injury or Hurt".
- However, there are legal definitions for **Hurt** (Section 319 IPC), and **Injury** (Section 44 IPC).

These terms have been discussed under **Competency FM 3.4**.

GRIEVOUS INJURY

Grievous Injury or more correctly, **Grievous Hurt** has been discussed under **Competency FM 3.4** *(page no. 163)*.

DANGEROUS INJURY

- There are three categories of **dangerous injuries***:
  - An injury, the result of which may possibly be death (**injury which endangers life**).
  - An injury as a result of which, death is not merely possible, but is likely (**injury which is likely to cause death**).
  - An injury as a result of which death is highly probable (**injury sufficient in the ordinary course of nature to cause death**).
- '**Endangering life**' is a much stronger expression than '**dangerous to life**'. An injury, however dangerous to life it may be, might not put life in a given case, in danger. The question is one of degree of gravity.
- An injury that definitely leads to death, e.g., decapitation, is referred to as "**necessarily fatal injury**."

ANTEMORTEM & POSTMORTEM INJURY

- **Antemortem injuries** occur before death, whereas **postmortem injuries** occur after death. The term "antemortem" refers to events occurring prior to death.
- In antemortem injuries, haemorrhage is associated with clotting in which clots are laminated, firm and variegated. Haemorrhage is characterized with copious amounts from arterial vessels.
- In postmortem injuries, slight haemorrhage occurs from the venous vessels in which clots are absent, or they are soft, non-laminated with friable chicken-fat (yellow) appearance.
- In addition, antemortem wound edges appear gaped, averted and swollen, whereas post-mortem wound edges are apposed without swelling.
- With regard to antemortem bruises, the appearance is usually indicative of the cause and time when the bruise occurred. In addition, the location of the bruise is considered quite useful in forensic examinations. Some body parts are more likely to sustain bruises than others. For instance, bruises are known to occur more readily where there is loose tissue such as eyebrows or subcutaneous fat than in areas where the tissue is strongly supported. Antemortem bruises can be differentiated from postmortem bruises with certainty by the use of the principal characteristics observed in histological aging. Ideally, histological ageing must always be used in dating antemortem bruises.
- Some of the most reliable methods applied in distinguishing antemortem from postmortem injuries include **enzyme histochemistry, microscopy** and **serology**.
- A related term is "**perimortem injury**" which refers to an injury sustained at or around the time of death (just before or after death). Such injuries may be very difficult to interpret.

Also refer **FM 2.14**: Postmortem artefacts *(page no. 62)*.

> **FM 3.6: Core – Written/Viva Voce**
> - **Mechanical Injuries and Wounds**
>   - Describe healing of injury and fracture of bones with its medicolegal importance

Discussed under respective type of mechanical injury (FM 3.3). *(page no. 151)*

**Source*: *Dasari Harish, Ajay Kumar, Akash Deep Aggarwal, Amandeep Singh. Dangerous injury or injury dangerous to life or grievous hurt endangering life: A dilemma. J Indian Acad Forensic Med. 2017;39:114–22.*

FM 3.7: Core – Written/Viva Voce
- Describe factors influencing infliction of injuries and healing, examination and certification of wounds
- Wound as a cause of death: Primary and Secondary

EXAMINATION AND CERTIFICATION OF WOUNDS

- Since the nature of infliction of mechanical injuries is either **accidental**, **suicidal** or **homicidal**, they are always associated with legal implications. Many such cases find their way to the criminal court. Therefore, a doctor who has examined and treated such cases will inevitably be called to give evidence as an **expert witness**. His opinion is often crucial to the final outcome. It is imperative that every doctor be familiar with the procedure of examination and recording of data. The following constitute some important points in this regard:
    - Every injury must be accurately documented as to the type, location, directions, dimensions, presence or absence of foreign bodies, time of infliction, etc. Measurements must be exact, and terms such as 'about,' 'approximately,' etc., must not be used.
    - As far as possible take photographs, or draw simple sketches of injuries.
    - While the primary duty of a doctor is to treat a patient, he must never neglect medicolegal requirements.
    - An **Accident cum Wound Certificate** is a medicolegal requirement to be recorded by the attending medical officer, especially by the first attending doctor, in full detail, in all cases irrespective of accident, suicide or homicide, when the doctor–patient relationship is established. It is to be prepared in duplicate, with the original furnished to the police as a confidential report when necessary, and the duplicate (carbon copy) to be retained in the institution under confidential safe custody. In India, the exact proforma differs from state to state, but is usually made available at both private and government hospitals. However, if a person is brought not as a patient but merely for certification of examination of wounds sustained, it is essential to insist on an official requisition from the police or court before commencing the examination to prepare the **wound certificate**. A sample of such a wound certificate is shown in **Box 3.2**. In such a case, a doctor–patient relationship is not necessarily established, and there is only doctor–subject relationship.
    - An informed written consent is a must only for wound examination in the scenario of doctor–subject relationship, and not in that of doctor–patient relationship. But if the person is under arrest, or if there is an order from court, the doctor can proceed with the examination even in the absence of consent. In fact, he is empowered "to use such force as is reasonably necessary for that purpose" (***Section 53 CrPC***). However, whenever a female is to be examined by such force, "the examination shall be made only by, or under supervision of, a female registered medical practitioner."
    - The doctor has to exercise maximum skill and care during management. Required investigations have to be undertaken. Dying declaration, if required, should be recorded in the usual manner.
    - It is desirable for a government doctor to intimate to the police, all wounded cases, irrespective of the manner and nature of occurrence. But, a private practitioner can abstain from such intimation in suicidal and accidental cases, if the patient does not give consent for such intimation.
    - As per ***Section 39 CrPC***, every citizen (including a doctor) has to give information about certain offences to the police. Such offences include **murder** (***Section 300 IPC***), **culpable homicide** (***Section 299 IPC***), **theft after preparation was made for causing death or hurt** (***Section 382 IPC***).
    - The duty of the doctor while examining a wounded subject is to record the wounds in detail and give necessary opinion. Recording and subsequent issue of the **wound certificate** is a must. The findings should be kept confidential. The wound certificate must be prepared in triplicate, under the seal and signature of the medical officer who prepared it. The original as well as one copy must be handed over to the police officer concerned in a sealed, addressed cover. The other copy is to be retained by the medical officer.

CONSEQUENCES OF INJURY (CAUSES OF DEATH FROM INJURY)

- A wound may heal, or may get complicated by processes other than healing.
    - Sometimes, there are undesirable sequelae, as in the case of healed ureteric rupture causing cicatrization which can result in hydronephrosis.
    - Keloid formation in scars can lead to permanent disfigurement.
    - The most serious consequence of an injury is of course the possibility of death.
    - Causes of death from wounds may be **primary** or **secondary**.

Primary (Immediate) Causes of Death

1. **Haemorrhage**
    - Bleeding from an injury (**primary haemorrhage**) may be external or internal. A sudden loss of 1000 cc of blood can result in shock and death. If the loss is spread over longer duration, the symptoms are less severe. However, advanced age and pre-existing morbid conditions can predispose to death. Also, effusion of even small amount of blood in certain situations can cause immediate death. An example is cardiac tamponade.
    - Bleeding occurring at a later stage due to infection, or due to dissolution of clot is called **secondary haemorrhage**.

Box 3.2—Wound Certificate

From **To**

Dr .... The Sub-Inspector of Police
....
....
....

Sir,

Sub: Issuance of wound certificate reg.
Ref: Requisition No. ...., dt. ....

Name of individual :
Sex :
Age :
Address :
Identification Marks : 1. ....
2. ....

Consent (*signature or thumb impression*)
Accompanying P.C. No., P.S. :
Brief History :

Date of Examination :
Time of Examination :
Beginning.............................
Conclusion ....

Place :

Injuries :

Nature	Size	Site	Simple/Grievous	Nature of Weapon	Dangerous Weapon or Not	Additional Remarks

Signature of Medical Officer
Date :
Name :
Designation :

2. **Injury to Vital Organs**
   - Severe injury to vital organs such as brain, heart or lungs can cause death irrespective of blood loss.
   - It is important to note that if the organ is diseased, even trivial trauma can result in fatal consequences.
3. **Neurogenic Shock**
   - The nervous control of cardiac and vascular functions is regulated by autonomic nervous system, and involves an optimum balance of two mutually antagonistic sympathetic and parasympathetic divisions. The former stimulates the cardiovascular system, while the latter exerts a tonic and inhibitory control over it, which is conservative-restorative in nature. The functioning of the cardiovascular system may be reflexly affected through the autonomic nervous system by factors such as emotion, variations in pressure in the carotid sinus, changes in the gaseous concentrations of blood, and excitation of peripheral afferent somatic or visceral nerves. These can cause either sympathetic stimulation or parasympathetic inhibition of cardiac function.

• **Emotion**: Psychic shock may lead to parasympathetic inhibitory effects, while fear and pain may lead to sympathetic stimulation.
• **Variations in pressure in the carotid sinus**: An increase in tension may lead to strong parasympathetic stimulation.
• **Gaseous concentrations in the blood**: Low oxygen and high carbon dioxide may cause sympathetic stimulation, acting directly on medullary centres

through chemoreceptors of the aortic and carotid bodies.

- **Excitation of peripheral nerves**: Stimulation of pressor and depressor afferent fibres can lead to either generalised vasoconstriction with raised blood pressure, or generalised vasodilatation with lowering of blood pressure. Weak stimuli cause depressor effects, while strong stimuli cause pressor effects. Severe pain as in squeezing the testicles, is an example of a strong stimulus.
- **Reflex autonomic stimulation**: Can lead to either sympathetic acceleration of pulse, myocardial contractility, generalised vasoconstriction and increased blood pressure, or parasympathetic reduction of pulse rate, myocardial contractility and central venous pressure, generalised vasodilatation, and decreased blood pressure.

4. **Air Embolism**
   - Injury to the veins in the neck or chest can lead to air embolism. Air is sucked in due to negative venous pressure. An air lock in the right chamber of the heart results in acute circulatory block.

Secondary (Delayed) Causes of Death

1. **Infection**
   - Various microorganisms can infect wounds. Prominent among them are bacteria such as *Staphylococci, Streptococci, Pseudomonas, Clostridium tetani* and *Clostridium welchii*. Cellulitis, abscess, gangrene, pyaemia, septicaemia and toxaemia are the sequelae.
   - Infection of the original injury with breakdown of sutures or blood clot can result in secondary haemorrhage.
2. **Thrombo-embolism**
   - Emboli and detached thrombi in injured veins can enter the right ventricle and (if large), can block the main pulmonary artery, or (if smaller), its branches. This can lead to cor pulmonale or pulmonary infarction. The time of occurrence is ordinarily 7–10 days after injury.
   - Leg vein thrombosis is a complication of injuries to lower limb leading to confinement in bed.
3. **Fat Embolism**
   - Fat can enter damaged veins at the site of injury from fractured long bones, or crushed fatty tissue. After passing through the heart, it can enter the systemic circulation.
   - Fat embolism may manifest as punctate haemorrhages in the brain or skin.
   - Oedematous fluid from cut surfaces of lungs may contain fat globules.
   - Urine may also contain fat globules.
   - Respiratory pathology is thought to result from the metabolism of neutral fat particles by lipase within the lungs, releasing free fatty acids and glycerol, which in turn cause severe inflammation of lung parenchyma, endothelial injury and increased capillary permeability.
   - Only when vital centres of brain are affected, death can be attributed to fat embolism.
   - **Fat embolism syndrome (FES)** is a serious manifestation of fat embolism, which appears as a combination of pulmonary, cerebral and cutaneous symptoms, including acute hypoxia, encephalopathy, thrombocytopenia and cutaneous petechial rashes.
4. **Crush Syndrome**
   - Crush syndrome occurs if a large bulk of muscle is crushed, as for example in vehicular run over injury, or injury due to falling masonry.
   - It is characterized by the development of profound shock.
   - The crushed limb becomes pulseless, and later red, swollen, and blistered. Nerve sensation and muscle power may be lost.
   - Crushing of muscles can liberate haem and myoglobin, which enter the circulation and get excreted through the kidneys. This can lead to acute tubular necrosis. Death may occur in a week's time. At autopsy, the kidneys appear large and bulky, and haem casts may be found in the distal convoluted tubules.
   - Amputation of the severely crushed limb above the site of compression is necessary to avoid development of crush syndrome. Cooling of the limb, and treatment for renal failure and shock are to be carried out in the event of the syndrome beginning to manifest.
5. **Other Causes**
   - Trauma can exacerbate an existing disease, e.g., tuberculosis.
   - Death can occur due to trauma to a diseased organ, e.g., malarial spleen.
   - Death can also occur from complications arising out of an injury, e.g., hypostatic pneumonia in bedridden victims of spinal cord injury.

Although not mentioned anywhere in the new curriculum (*very strangely indeed*), the concept of "Sudden Death" and its medicolegal importance needs to be understood by all doctors, and hence is being discussed here.

SUDDEN DEATH

Definition

- **Sudden death is defined as the sudden or unexpected termination of life of an apparently healthy individual, usually from some natural disease.**
  - It is usually taken to mean that death occurred unexpectedly, and within **24 hours after the onset of symptoms,** with or without known preexisting conditions. The emphasis is on the unexpected character, rather than the suddenness of the death. In fact, sometimes the individual may linger on for a few hours or days after the abrupt onset of illness.
- The expression '**sudden natural death**' means that the death was caused entirely by natural disease, and that it was not caused by trauma or poisoning.

Investigation

- The purpose of a medicolegal autopsy in sudden deaths is to determine whether violence or poisoning has been in any way responsible for the death. Absence of external evidence of injury does not preclude death from physical violence.
- The age of the deceased, authentic information as to past health status and the presence or absence of witnesses at the time of death are all helpful in deciding the necessity for an autopsy.
- Sudden deaths are more frequent in older individuals, and they usually take place under circumstances which arouse no suspicion. It is the sudden death of younger individuals that invariably arouses suspicion.
- Medical officers must never issue death certificate in a case of sudden death, and instead must suggest that an autopsy be done.
- When there is no apparent cause of death as revealed by the police inquest, and on external examination of the body, death due to natural causes should be suspected. In that case, a detailed examination of all the systems should be conducted. Each organ has to be weighed and the naked eye observations have to be recorded. Bits of tissues should be taken from all the organs. If there is difficulty in interpreting the morbid anatomical changes in any of the organs that organ as a whole can be preserved and despatched to the forensic pathologist for expert opinion.
  - The tissues for histopathological examination have to be collected in wide-mouthed glass bottles. The preservative used is 10% formalin. If bits of tissues are sent for examination, gross findings should be provided to the expert with the history of the case.
  - A peripheral blood smear should be taken for examination.
  - In all such cases, relevant viscera and body fluids must be preserved in saturated saline and despatched for chemical analysis.
  - Samples of blood must be collected for biochemical, haematological and microbiological examinations also. Sterile bottles have to be used for the collection of materials for microbiological examinations. If diseases like leukaemia are suspected, bone marrow should be taken.
- If injuries are present on the body, they should be examined and details recorded. Effort must be made to find out the cause of injuries found on the body by examination of the scene, interrogation of witnesses, etc.
- If, on the other hand, the natural cause of death was a result of the injury, the relation has to be established. Injuries can either precipitate or hasten death of a person who is already suffering from a disease. For example, trivial injuries may precipitate death by myocardial infarction in a person having coronary arteriosclerosis.

Causes

- Diseases of the cardiovascular system account for about 45% of sudden deaths, diseases of the respiratory system 25%, diseases of the nervous system about 20%, and the rest occur due to diseases of other organs.
- The most common causes appear to be:
  - Coronary artery disease with myocardial infarction.
  - Non-atherosclerotic coronary artery disease, cardiomyopathy, myocarditis.
  - Cerebrovascular accident (cerebral stroke).
  - Subarachnoid haemorrhage due to rupture of berry aneurysm.
  - Sudden rupture of a diseased blood vessel with fatal bleeding, such as the rupture of an aortic aneurysm.
  - Massive pulmonary embolism.
  - Acquired respiratory distress syndrome (ARDS) due to any cause.
  - Perforation of peptic ulcer.
  - Fulminating infectious disease without any recognizable symptoms until death, e.g., lobar pneumonia, bacterial endocarditis, etc.
  - A shift in the position of a viscus, causing sudden shock as in volvulus, strangulated hernia, twisted ovarian cyst, etc.
  - Anaphylactic shock due to any cause.
  - Sudden infant death syndrome.
- Since, a significant proportion of sudden deaths occurs due to myocardial infarction secondary to coronary artery disease, forensic pathologists must be able to clearly recognize evidence of the same at autopsy.
  - **Postmortem Demonstration of Myocardial Infarction**
    - The commonest lesion of the coronary artery is atherosclerosis. The anterior descending branch is most commonly involved, especially its proximal part. Atheromatous plaques developed in intima form the basis of thrombi which will produce occlusion (**Fig. 3.59**). The plaques can also rupture. If complete occlusion occurs, myocardial infarction results. Vegetations from bacterial endocarditis of the mitral or aortic valves may sometimes cause occlusion. The diagnosis of embolism can be made only if the source of embolus is established without doubt. When a thrombus is seen, histological examination should be done to confirm the diagnosis and also to find out whether it is a recent or old one.
    - Myocardial infarction refers to necrosis of the heart muscle. Usually, the apical portion of left ventricle, adjacent anterior wall, and interventricular septum are involved (**Fig. 3.60**). After the occlusion of the artery, the changes in the myocardium occur gradu ally. In sudden deaths, due to complete occlusion, there will not be any visible change in the heart muscle. Light microscopic changes will occur 6–8 hours after occlusion. Changes can be seen with the naked eye only after 24 hours.

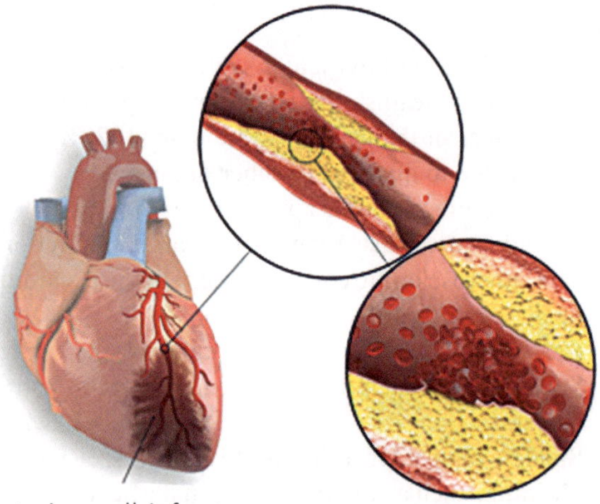

Fig. 3.59 Myocardial infarction

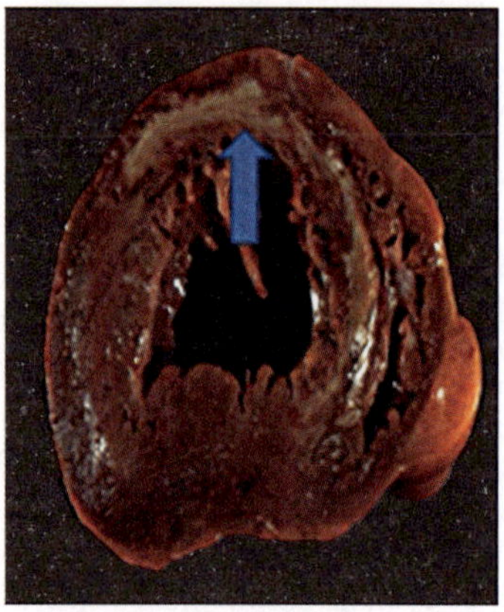

Fig. 3.60 Gross appearance of infarct

- Thus, in some cases of sudden death following coronary occlusion or stenosis, no evidence of myocardial infarction can be made out even by the most sensitive methods, especially if the interval between onset and death was too short. Death in such cases is attributable to ventricular fibrillation or damage to the conduction system. In many cases however, the infarct can be demonstrated by standard techniques.
- ***Enzyme histochemistry in myocardial ischaemia***: A number of enzymes have been studied in this context, but only a few are found useful in the study of autopsy material: maleic dehydrogenase (MDH), lactic dehydrogenase (LDH) and succinic dehydrogenase (SDH). Of the various methods, the triphenyl tetrazolium chloride (TTC) reaction is considered the most reliable.
- ***Best postmortem methods***: Of the various methods, the **triphenyl tetrazolium chloride (TTC) reaction (Fig. 3.61)**, and **acridine orange fluorescence study** are considered the most reliable postmortem methods of diagnosing myocardial infarction.

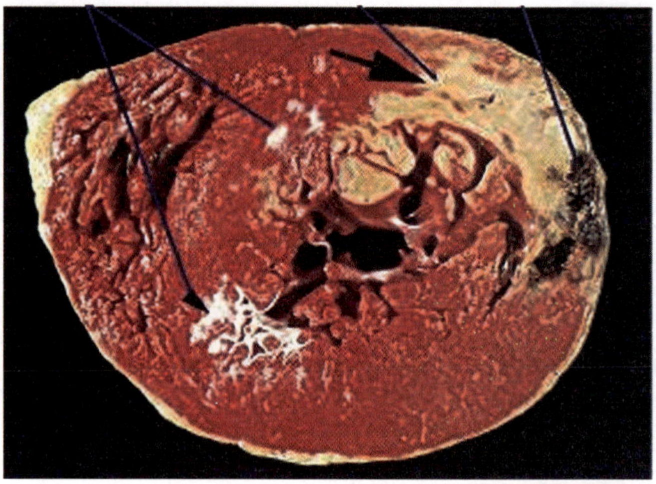

Fig. 3.61 Acute myocardial infarct – Lack of staining by triphenyl tetrazolium chloride in areas of necrosis

> **FM 3.8: Core – Written/Viva Voce**
> - **Mechanical Injuries and Wounds**
>   - Describe and discuss different types of weapons including dangerous weapons and their examination

INJURIES AND WEAPONS

The Indian Penal Code describes two types of weapons:

1. **Deadly weapon** (***Section 148 IPC***): Whoever is guilty of rioting, being armed with deadly weapon, which when used as a weapon of offence is likely to cause death, shall be punished with imprisonment for a term which may extend to 3 years, or with fine, or with both.
2. **Dangerous weapon** (***Sections 324 & 326 IPC***): **Described under Competency FM 3.4**. *(page no. 163)*
3. Weapons can also be classified as being **blunt**, **sharp** or **pointed**.
   a. They are further sub-divided into **light** and **heavy** weapons. The lightness or heaviness of a weapon is based on subjective opinion, since no optimum weight is prescribed by law for such classification.

> **FM 3.9: Core – Written/ Viva Voce**
> - **Firearm injuries**:
>   - Describe different types of firearms including structure and components
>   - Along with description of ammunition, propellant charge, and mechanism of firearms, different types of cartridges and bullets, and various terminologies in relation to firearm – calibre, range, choking

BALLISTICS

- **Ballistics is the science dealing with the study of firearms and ammunition**. It includes the study of the effects of discharging a firearm, projectile motion and factors affecting the efficacy of firing.

- **Sub-divisions**:
  - **Proximal (Internal) Ballistics**: The study of firearms and projectiles is called **proximal or internal ballistics**.
  - **Intermediate (External) Ballistics**: The study of the motion of a projectile after being ejected from the firearm till the time it hits the target is termed as **intermediate or external ballistics**.
  - **Terminal (Wound) Ballistics**: The study of injuries produced by firearms is referred to as **terminal or wound ballistics**, and is the exclusive realm of a forensic pathologist.

Proximal Ballistics

- In simple terms, a **firearm** is a mechanical device equipped to eject a **projectile** at high velocity in order to hit a target.

Ammunition

- The term **ammunition** of a firearm refers to the materials used for causing a detonation, along with the projectile.
  - One complete round of ammunition is called a ***cartridge***.
- The **projectile** is pushed out through a cylindrical tube which is called a ***barrel***.
  - If the barrel is grooved internally, it is a ***rifled firearm***.
  - If not, it is a ***smooth-bore firearm***.
- **Cartridge** (**Figs. 3.62 & 3.63**):
  - A **cartridge** consists of:
    - An outer ***case*** in which the explosive is stored, together with the chemicals required to ignite it, and the ***projectile***.
- The projectile is either a ***bullet*** or ***pellets (shot)***. The former is used in **rifled firearms**, and the latter in **smooth-bore firearms**.
  - The explosive is called ***propellant*** or ***gun powder***, while the igniting chemical is called ***detonator*** or ***primer***.
    - In short, **Cartridge = Case + Detonator + Propellant + Projectile**
  - **Cartridge Case**:
    - In **rifled firearms**, the cartridge case is made of an alloy of copper and zinc, while in **smooth-bore firearms** it is made of a special type of paper or cardboard.
    - In both types, the shape is **cylindrical**. One end of the case is closed with a plate of brass and is called the **base**, while the other end is open.
    - The cartridge case helps not only to keep the contents in place, but also provides a water-proof cover for them and protection against deterioration.
    - The **base** is **rimmed** in **revolver cartridge**, but **grooved (rimless)** in **pistol** and **automatic firearm cartridges** (**Fig. 3.64**).
  - **Detonator**:
    - It is also known as "**primer**."
    - Common **ingredients** comprise mercury fulminate (or lead azide), potassium chlorate and antimony sulphide. These chemicals are capable of rapid combustion.
    - They are stored in a small compartment attached to the base of the cartridge case called **percussion cap** which is made of copper. Hence, the detonator is also known as **cap composition**.
    - In most of the cartridges, the percussion cap is situated near the centre of the base, and are therefore referred to as **centre fire** cartridges, while in a few the whole of the base acts as a percussion cap and are known as **rim fire** cartridges.

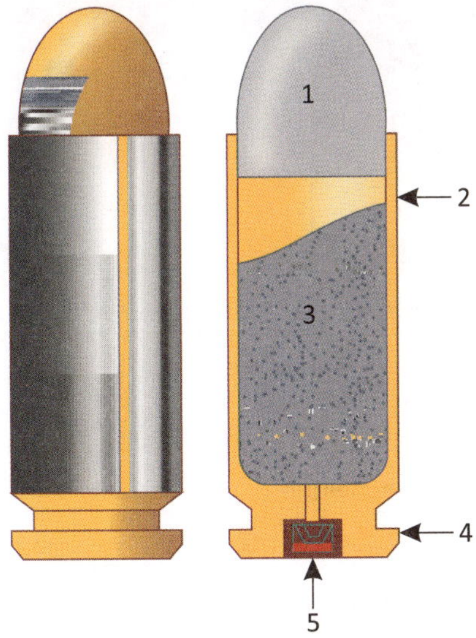

Fig. 3.62 Longitudinal section of rifled cartridge. 1. Bullet; 2. Cartridge case; 3. Propellant; 4. Rim; 5. Primer

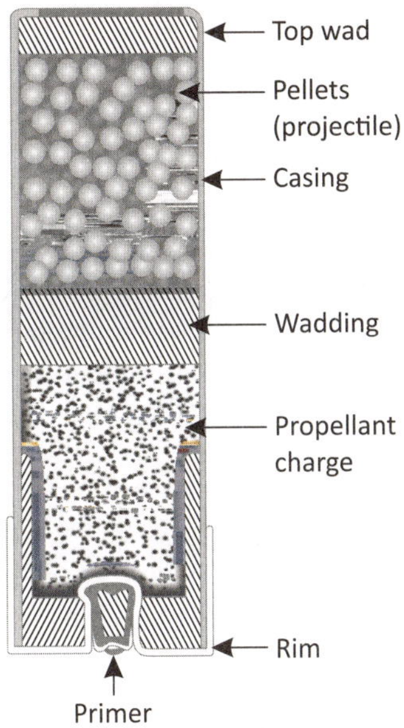

Fig. 3.63 Longitudinal section of shotgun cartridge

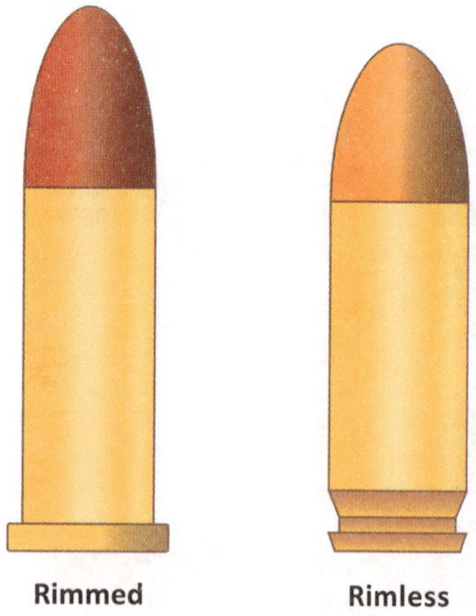

Fig. 3.64 Revolver cartridge (L); Pistol cartridge (R)

- **Propellant (Gun Powder)**:
  - This is situated in close proximity to the primer within the cartridge case.
  - There are three types of gun powder – **black powder**, **semi-smokeless powder** and **smokeless powder (Fig. 3.65)**.
  - **Black powder** is a mixture of 75% potassium nitrate, 15% charcoal and 10% sulphur.
  - **Smokeless powder** consists of nitrocellulose alone (*single base*), or nitrocellulose combined with nitroglycerine (*double base*).
  - **Semi-smokeless powder** consists of 20% smokeless powder and 80% black powder.
  - While all types of gun powder produce smoke, the smokeless variety does not produce as much smoke as black powder, and is the most effective type being capable of imparting higher velocity to the projectile.
  - The ignited primer causes combustion of gun powder by which hot gases under tremendous pressure are produced within the closed confines of the cartridge, propelling out the projectile with great velocity.
  - A single grain of black powder can produce 200–250 cc of gas composed of carbon monoxide, nitrogen, hydrogen, hydrogen sulphide and traces of methane and oxygen, while a grain of smokeless powder can generate 800–900 cc of gas.
- **Projectile**:
  - This is usually either a **bullet** or a bunch of **pellets (shot)**. The former is used in **rifled firearms**, while the latter is used in **smooth-bore weapons**.
  - Firearms meant to propel projectiles of less than one-inch diameter are called **small arms**. They may be hand operated, i.e., **hand arms** (e.g., pistol and revolver), or they may be placed against the shoulder and fired, i.e., **shoulder arms** (e.g., rifle, musket, shotgun, etc.). Hand arms are also referred to as **side arms**. In **country-made firearms**, unusual projectiles are often used, e.g., pieces of glass, cork, wood, nails, stones, etc.

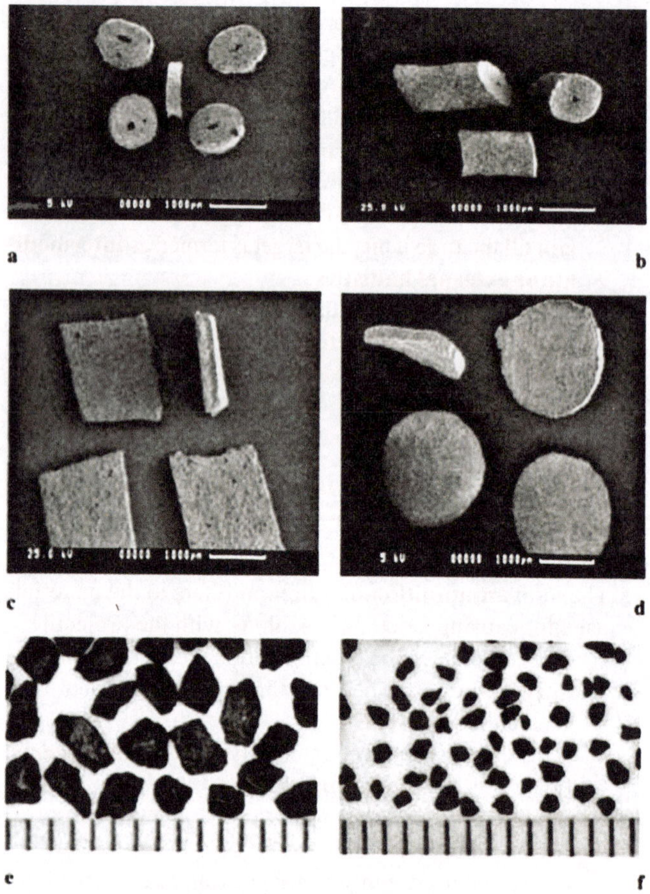

Fig. 3.65 Black and smokeless powders:
(a) "perforated disc" smokeless powder;
(b) "tube" smokeless powder;
(c) "cut square" smokeless powder;
(d) "disc" smokeless powder;
(e) Grade Fg black powder;
(f) Grade FFFG (3Fg) black powder

  - Normally, a bullet is held in the cartridge case by a groove called **cannelure**. As a result of the pressure generated by gases, the bullet gets released, and is pushed through the barrel and out of the muzzle with great velocity.
  - **Bullets** are usually made of lead with a coating of cupro-nickel alloy (**Fig. 3.66**). They are invariably conical in shape, in order to offer least resistance while travelling through air. The tip of a bullet is referred to as its **nose**.
  - Depending upon the size of the bullet, it can be short, medium or large, and as per the shape of the nose, it can be flat nosed, round nosed, hollow nosed or point nosed.
  - **Pellets** used in smooth-bore firearms are collectively referred to as **shot** (**Fig. 3.67**). Sometimes **slugs** may be used instead, which are much larger. A flat felt-disc or compressed paper or cardboard called **wad**

lies between the pellets and propellant. It is often called ***underwad***. There is another wad, termed the ***turnover wad*** or ***top wad***, situated over the lead shot, the purpose of which is to keep the shot in place. Wads not only hold the pellets and gun powder tightly in place, but also act as a piston sealing the bore effectively, thus preventing the expanding gases from escaping. This is known as **obturation** or **sealing** of the bore which is of vital importance. In order to lubricate the bore, wads are often impregnated with grease. In modern ammunition, plastic is being used increasingly commonly, and some of the older constituents are no longer present.

- Once a firearm has been discharged, the empty cartridge case is left behind in the chamber devoid of projectile, but with residues of primer and detonator still present. This is called **spent cartridge**. The spent cartridge has to be extracted from the chamber manually, or it may get ejected automatically (as in automatic firearms).

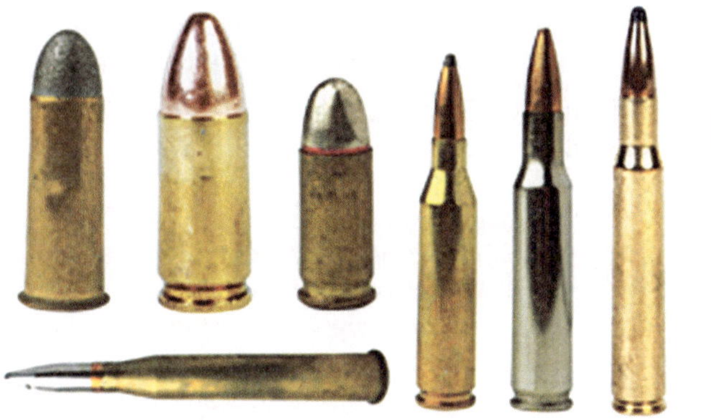

Fig. 3.66 Bullets

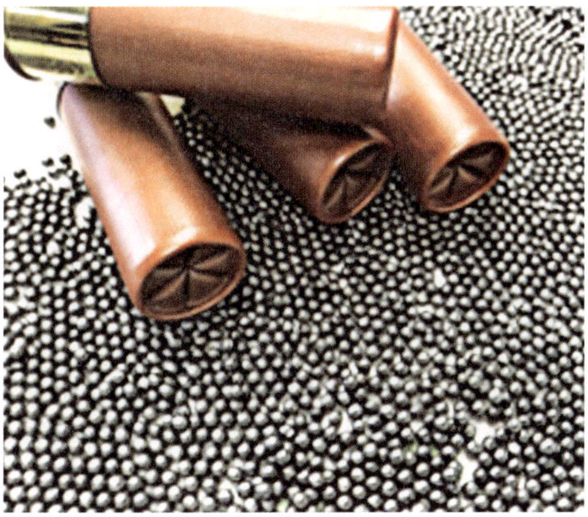

Fig. 3.67 Shotgun cartridges & pellets

Firearm **(Fig. 3.68)**

- Every **firearm** has a **chamber** in which the cartridge is normally lodged. The chamber leads into a hollow steel tube called the **barrel**. The projectile released from the cartridge in the chamber is forcefully pushed through the barrel by the expanding gases produced by the explosion of gun powder.
- The proximal end of the chamber has a minute hole, through which a pin moves forward to strike the base of the cartridge. This striking action produces heat which ignites the primer. This pin, known as **firing pin**, is activated by a spring connected to a trigger mechanism. The spring is released on pulling the **trigger**. The part which incorporates the firing pin, spring and trigger is called the **bolt**.

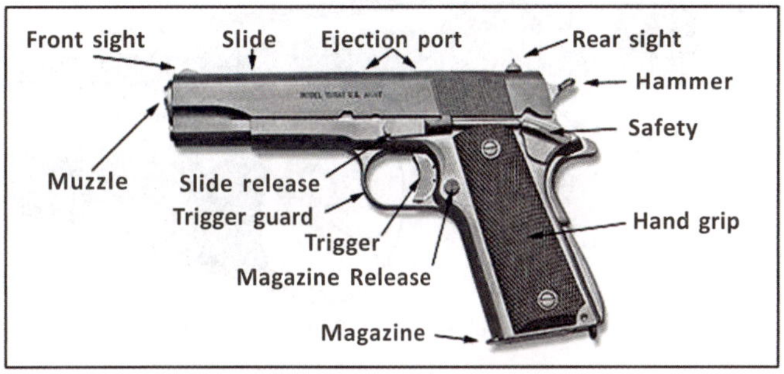

Fig. 3.68 Parts of a firearm

- **Barrel**:
  - It is a steel tube of varying length, and may be single or double.
  - The **chamber** constitutes the rear end of the barrel, and lodges the cartridge. This part is called the **breech**.
  - The front (distal) end of the barrel which is open to the exterior, is called the **muzzle**.
  - The term **bore** refers to that part of the barrel through which the projectile makes its exit.
  - The barrel may measure anything from 2.5 cm (1 inch) to 90 cm (3 ft). The tapering portion connecting the chamber with the bore is called the **leed** (**taper**).
  - In rifled firearms, the interior of the barrel is scored by a number of parallel, spirally twisted grooves called **rifling**, whereas in smooth-bore weapons the interior surface is smooth (**Fig. 3.69**).
- The rifling may be either clockwise or anti-clockwise.
- A cross-section of a rifled bore would reveal a series of elevations alternating with depressions (corresponding to the grooves). The former are called **lands**. The bullet is squeezed between the lands as it travels through the bore and since rifling is spiral, it imparts a spin or rotation to the projectile by which it acquires a gyroscopic steadiness, preventing it from wobbling.
  - In some smooth-bore firearms, the barrel becomes narrower towards the muzzle end. This is called **choking**.

Choking minimises dispersion of the pellets after they emerge from the barrel (**Fig. 3.70**).

- Depending upon the extent of narrowing, it may be either a ***full choke*** bore or a ***half (modified) choke*** bore.
- A barrel that is not choked is called ***cylinder bore***.
  - In some firearms (**paradox guns**), the bore is only partly smooth, while the remaining part is rifled.
  - If loading of a cartridge is done through the muzzle end of a firearm it is called a **muzzle loader**, and if it is done through the breech it is a **breech loader**.

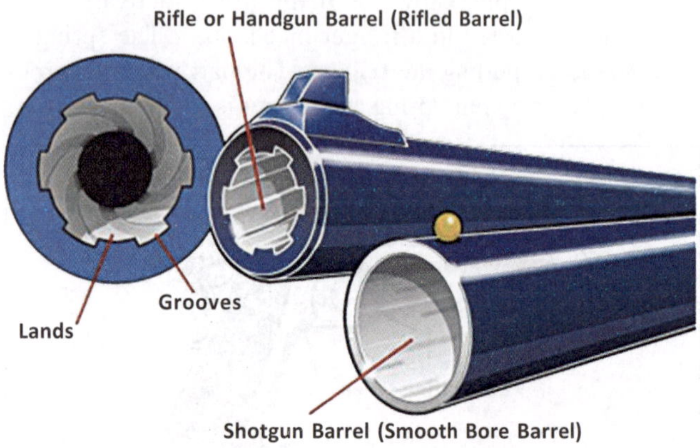

Fig. 3.69 Difference between the interior of barrel of a rifled and smoothbore firearm

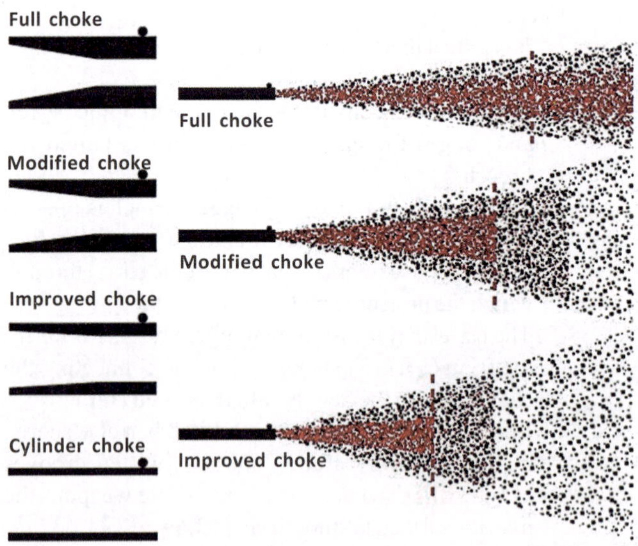

Fig. 3.70 Degrees of choking of a shotgun barrel

- **Bolt**:
  - This is also called **block** and is situated towards the breech end of the barrel. As described earlier, it consists essentially of a trigger, which when pulled releases the spring to activate the firing pin, which quickly moves forward to strike the base of the cartridge inside the chamber.
  - The trigger is usually surrounded by a trigger guard to prevent accidental firing.
  - In addition, there is a **safety catch** which prevents the gun from discharging even when the trigger is accidentally pulled.
  - The block also contains an **extractor** to remove the spent cartridge, and is fashioned into a grip or butt around the trigger mechanism, for holding the firearm.
  - The block can be opened to insert a fresh cartridge into the chamber manually or automatically.
  - In **automatic firearms**, the cartridges are arranged one below the other to form a **magazine**, which is attached to the block. If the trigger is pressed and the pressure is sustained, it will cause the continuous release of all the cartridges from the magazine until the latter becomes empty.
  - In **semi-automatic firearms**, only one cartridge at a time is released each time the trigger is pulled.
  - In **non-automatic firearms**, the spent cartridge has to be extracted manually each time after firing.

Classification of Firearms (Box 3.3)

1. **Rifled firearm**
   a. ***High velocity***:
      i. *Shoulder arms*, e.g., rifle
      ii. *Automatic weapons*, e.g., machine gun, sub-machine gun, sten gun, assault rifle, etc.
         - **Assault rifles** are selective-fire rifles* that use an intermediate cartridge (i.e., more power than a pistol but less than a standard rifle) and a detachable magazine. Assault rifles were first used during World War II. By the end of the 20th century, they had become the standard weapon in most of the world's armies, replacing semi-automatic rifles, battle rifles and sub-machine guns in most roles. Examples include the StG 44, AK-47 and the M16 rifle. The last mentioned was extensively used by the Americans in the Vietnam War.
   b. ***Low velocity***:
      i. *Hand arms*, e.g., revolver, pistol.
2. **Smooth-bore firearm (Shotgun)**
   a. ***Single barrelled*** or ***double barrelled***
   b. ***Breech loader*** or ***muzzle loader***
   c. ***Cylinder bore*** or ***choke bore***
3. **Air** or **gas operated firearm**: Generally referred to as ***air guns***, since most often compressed air is used to propel a projectile (usually ball bearings or pellets); these weapons

Note*: A ***selective-fire* firearm has at least two firearm modes, which are activated by means of a selector: ***burst fire mode***, which limits the maximum number of shots fired automatically, and ***fully automatic fire mode*** which enables continuous firing until either the feeding mechanism is emptied or the trigger is released.*

Box 3.3—Types of Firearms

1. **Pistol** is a miniature semi-automatic hand-arm with a small barrel.

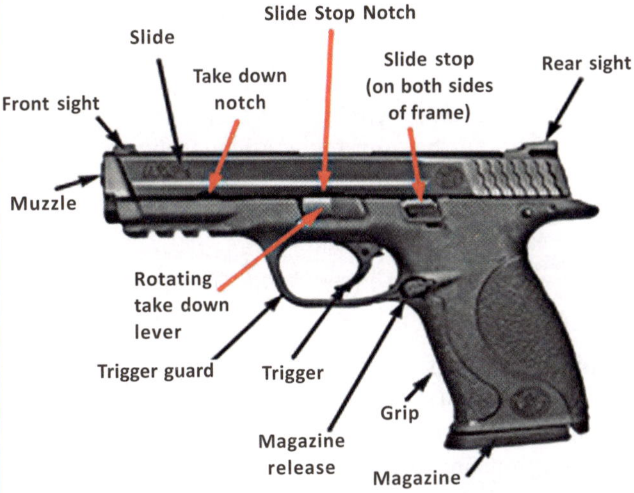

2. **Revolver** is a hand-arm with a revolving magazine cylinder filled with cartridges.

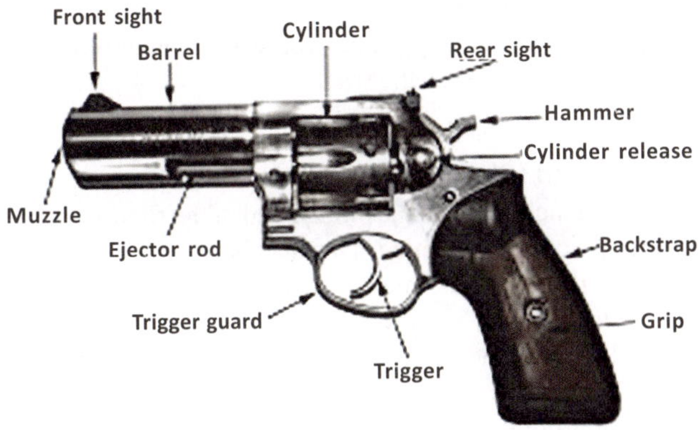

3. **Rifle** is a rifled shoulder-arm for long range firing. Effective range may extend to a mile.

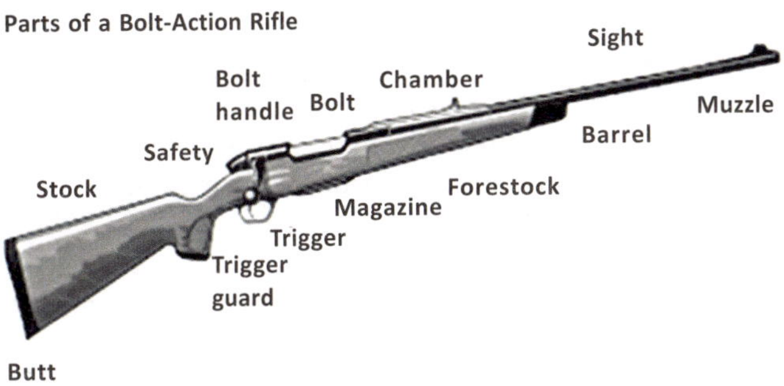

4. **Submachine gun** is an automatic rifled weapon, which can also be used as a self-loading firearm.

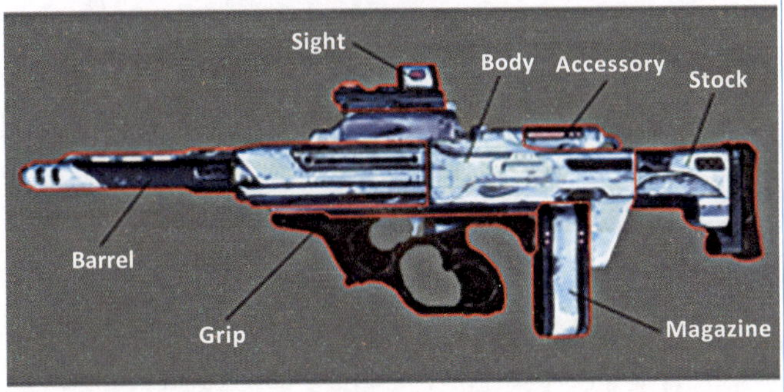

5. **Light machine gun (LMG)** is analogous to a rifle. It is of light weight and is capable of rapid uninterrupted fire with accuracy.

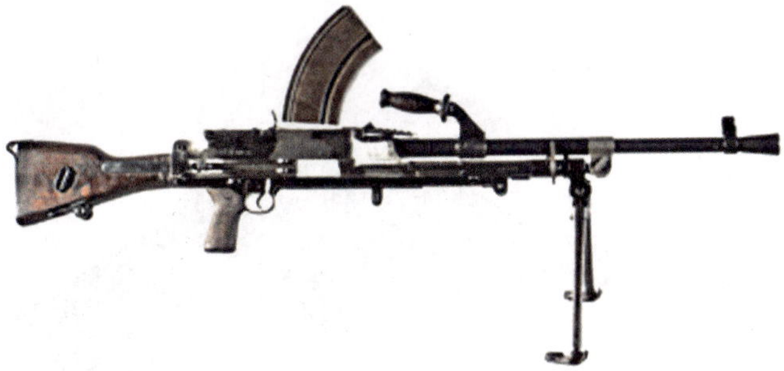

6. **Musket** is a smooth-bore shoulder-arm used for military purposes.

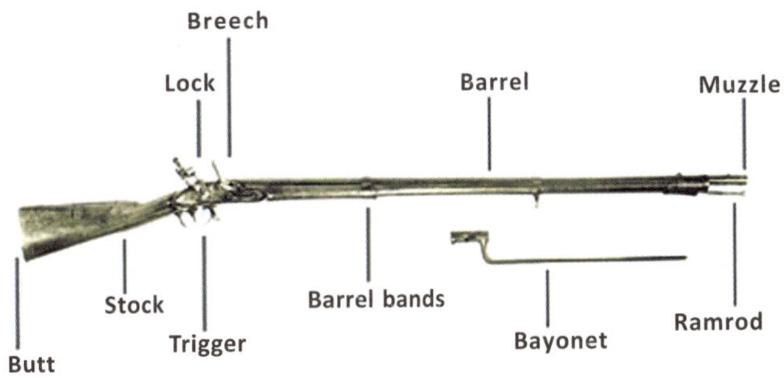

7. **Shotgun** is a smooth-bore shoulder-arm used for hunting.

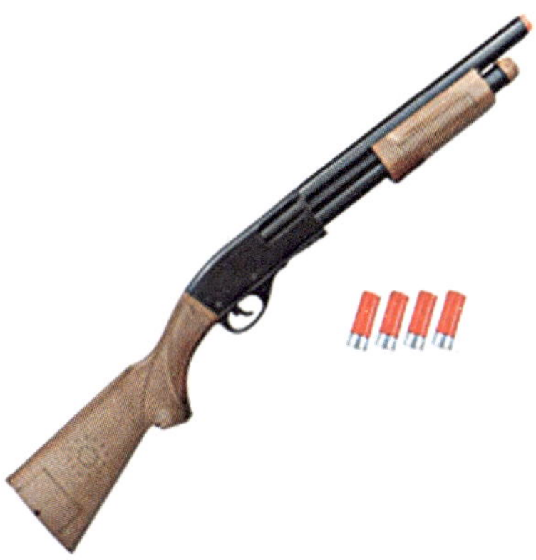

8. **Air gun** and **Air rifle** are suitable for small game hunting. Ball bearings or pellets are used, the propelling force being obtained through compressed air.

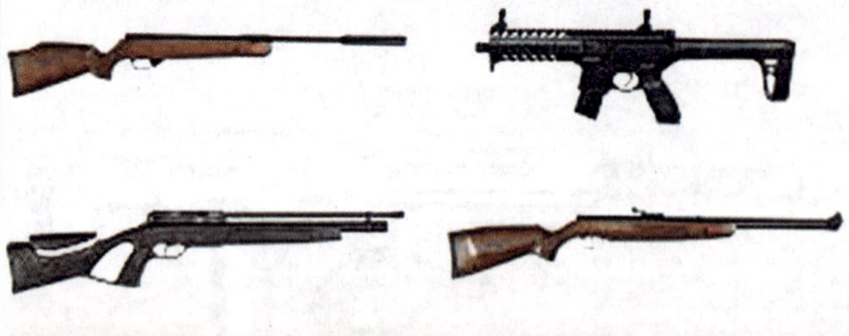

Types of Air Rifles

9. **Country-made firearms** are generally smooth-bore weapons that are crudely manufactured.

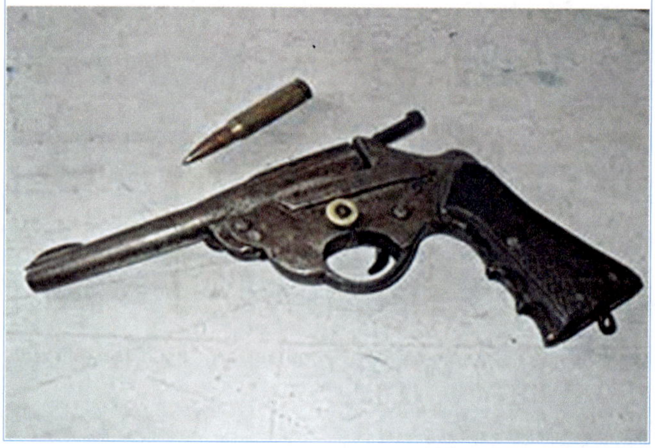

are by no means innocuous as generally believed. Fatalities have been reported.

4. **Country-made firearm**: Quite common in several rural parts of North India and some southern states. They are crude, smooth-bore weapons, but can be lethal. The ammunition is usually loaded through the muzzle end of the barrel.

Calibre of Firearm

- The **calibre** of a rifled firearm is usually expressed in terms of the inner diameter of the barrel, in fractions of an inch. Thus, we have the 0.303 and 0.22 rifle, meaning that the calibre is 0.303 of an inch and 0.22 of an inch, respectively. The measurement is made between two diametrically opposite lands and not between grooves.
- The **calibre** (or **gauge**) of a shotgun is expressed in terms of the number of balls of lead which can be made out of 1 pound (450 g) of the metal, so that each fits exactly into the bore of the weapon. If 12 balls of the same size can be accommodated, the calibre is referred to as **12 bore**. The other commonly available calibre of shotgun is **16 bore**. The actual calibre (in terms of inner diameter of the barrel) of a 12-bore gun is 1.850 cm (0.729 inch) while that of a 16-bore gun is 1.685 cm (0.663 inch).

Intermediate Ballistics

This is not very important for a forensic pathologist, and is the specialised field of a ballistics expert.

FM 3.10: Core – Written/Viva Voce/OSCE (Objective Structured Clinical Examination)

- **Firearm injuries**:
  - Describe and discuss wound ballistics:
    - Different types of firearm injuries, blast injuries and their interpretation
    - Preservation and despatch of trace evidence in cases of firearm and blast injuries
    - Various tests related to confirmation of use of firearms

Terminal Ballistics

- Forensic pathologists must have a thorough knowledge about **terminal ballistics**, which deals with the injuries resulting from firearms.
- The wound produced by a projectile (***bullet*** or ***shot***) as it enters the body is called the **entry wound**, and that by which the projectile leaves the body is the **exit wound**. Exit wound is generally absent in the case of shotgun injury, except in the region of the head.
  The path traversed by the projectile between the entry and exit wounds is called the **track**.

Rifled Firearm Injury

Entry Wound **(Figs. 3.71 & 3.72)**

- The distance between the muzzle end of the firearm and the target is called the **range**. This may be:
  - ***Contact range***, if muzzle end is in contact with body,
  - ***Close range***, if the range is within the distance travelled by flame,
  - ***Near range***, if it is within the distance travelled by unburnt or partially burnt gunpowder and
  - ***Distant range***, if it is beyond the range of flame, smoke, and gunpowder particles.
- During the bullet's attempt at perforating the skin while entering, due to the spin, the edge of the entrance wound may be abraded in the form of a collar, which is termed the **abrasion collar** or **areola**. In some cases, there is contusion instead of abrasion, in which case it is more appropriately called the **contusion collar**. The diameter of the entry hole together with the abrasion collar may give the approximate diameter of the bullet.
- The barrel of a firearm is generally lubricated between use. When such a weapon is fired, the bullet as it is propelled through the barrel, would naturally carry this lubricant (grease) on it, which subsequently gets deposited on the skin around the entrance wound. The spin of the bullet causes wiping of its surface on the skin while entering. This is called the **grease (or dirt) collar**.
- The abrasion and grease collars normally measure only about 0.3 cm and 0.7 cm, respectively.

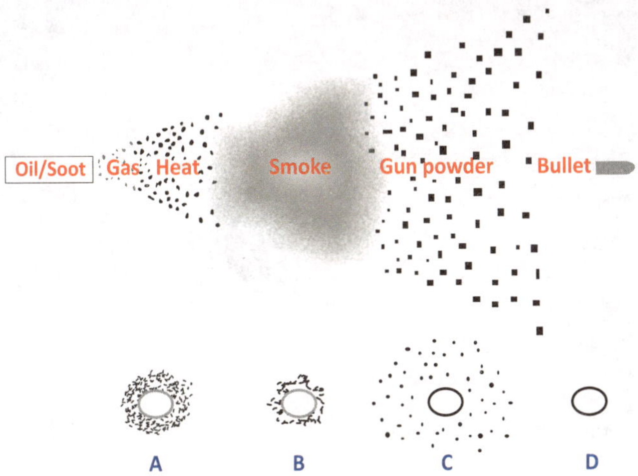

Fig. 3.71 Bullet entry wound characteristics at increasing range

- When both abrasion and grease collars are present, the grease collar is seen as the inner zone, while the abrasion collar constitutes the outer zone (**Fig. 3.73**).
- Burning (**scorching** or **singeing**) of skin and hair result from the flame that emerges from the muzzle, at the time of firing. Clothing around the entry wound may also show evidence of burning.
- **Tattooing (peppering** or **stippling)** results from grains of gunpowder being driven into the skin, each grain acting as a minute missile. Tattooing is seen on the skin as small, discrete, black specks which cannot be wiped off. The extent of tattooing will depend on the calibre of the weapon, the type of powder used, and the range. Tattooing may be absent if firing has taken place through clothing.
- **Blackening** or **smudging** results from a superficial deposit of smoke on the skin. In other words, it is only a carbonaceous deposit on the skin, and hence can be easily removed by wiping with a wet sponge. The intensity of

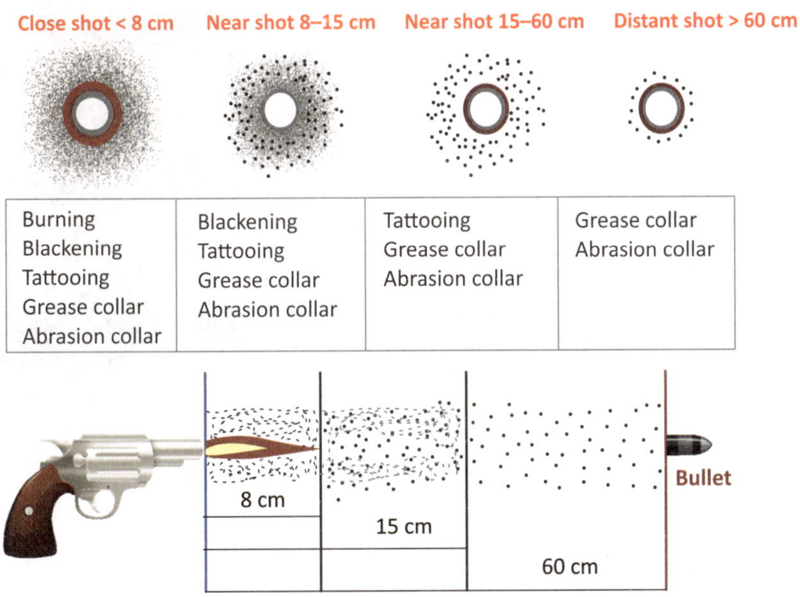

Fig. 3.72 Entry wound at various ranges for short-barrelled firearm (revolver, pistol)

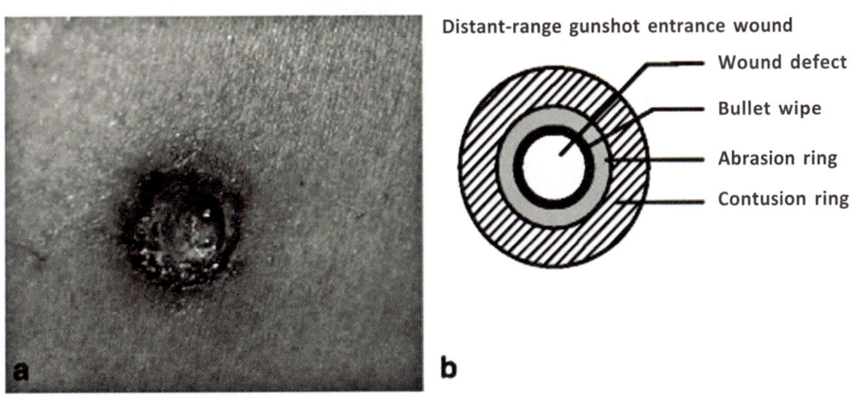

Fig. 3.73 Gunshot entry wound showing abrasion and grease collars

smudging will depend on the calibre of the weapon, the type of powder used, and the range. Thus, the greater the calibre of the weapon, the wider the area of blackening and vice versa. Similarly, if black powder is used, the blackening will be more clearly visible, than if smokeless powder had been employed. Smudging may be absent on skin if firing has taken place through clothing. The presence of blackening, especially when smokeless powder has been used, may not be clearly visible to the naked eye. In such cases, infrared or ultraviolet photography will help to visualise it.

- Since carbon monoxide is evolved on explosion of gun powder, the presence of this in the blood of the injured tissues at the entrance wound imparts a **cherry red colour** to the tissues.
- A **lead ring** or **metal ring** around the entry wound results from the deposition of very small quantities of lead or other metal in the form of a ring or collar, as the projectile enters the skin. The lead ring can be appreciated radiologically or by neutron activation analysis.
- Firearm wounds are generally easily recognised as such. But sometimes wounds caused by red hot pokers or a burning pointed stick may simulate bullet entry. However, in these wounds, there will be no evidence of tattooing or cherry red colour. Conversely, glancing injuries caused by rifled firearms may be confused with incised or lacerated wounds.
- **Contact shot**:
  - The firearm is placed in contact with the skin or clothing, and then fired. It is also known as a **point blank shot**.
  - A contact wound over a dense area such as the cranial vault is generally large and cruciate (cruciform, stellate, or star shaped), due to explosive effects of the gases liberated (**Fig. 3.74**).
  - Imprint of the muzzle of the weapon may be found stamped on the skin (**Fig. 3.75**).
  - Burning, blackening (smudging), and tattooing are slight or absent in the adjacent skin, since all the components of the explosion are driven into the wound.
  - The tissues are often saturated with carbon monoxide and therefore cherry red in colour.
  - Cranial contact wounds are generally seen on the forehead or temple.
  - Contact wounds over thin bone, chest or abdomen are usually circular in shape, and are surrounded by abrasion or contusion collar.
  - The overall diameter of the hole plus the collar represents the approximate diameter of the bullet.
  - Surrounding hair is singed.
- **Close shot**:
  - It means that the firearm was fired within the range of flame and powder blast, but was not in direct contact with the skin or clothing.
  - Flame travels approximately up to 8 cm in the case of revolver or pistol, and 15 cm in the case of rifle. The wound appears as a circular hole surrounded by scorching, singeing and smudging. These may be absent, if firing has occurred through clothing.
  - Abrasion collar, grease collar and tattooing are also present.
- **Near shot**:
  - It means that the firearm was fired outside the range of flame, but within the range of powder blast.
  - The entry wound is circular or oval in shape.
  - Unburnt powder grains and small metallic particles travel approximately up to 60 cm in the case of revolver and pistol, and 75 cm in the case of rifle. In practical situations, tattooing is seen up to a maximum distance of about 90 cm.
  - Singeing of hair and scorching are absent.
  - Smudging can occur up to a range of 30 cm. Beyond this it is not seen.
  - Grease collar and abrasion collar are present.

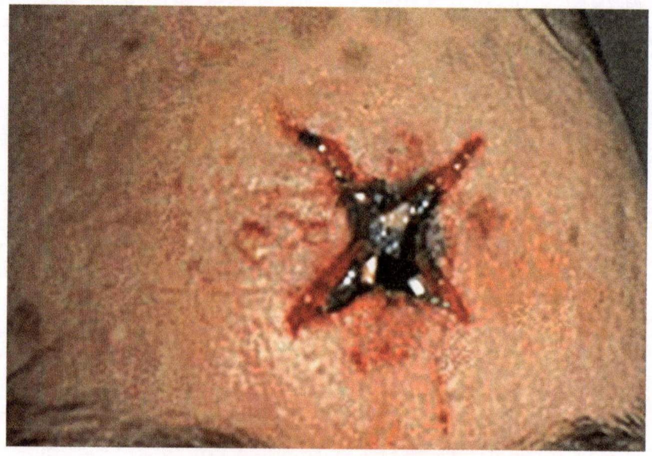

Fig. 3.74 Cruciate entry wound – forehead

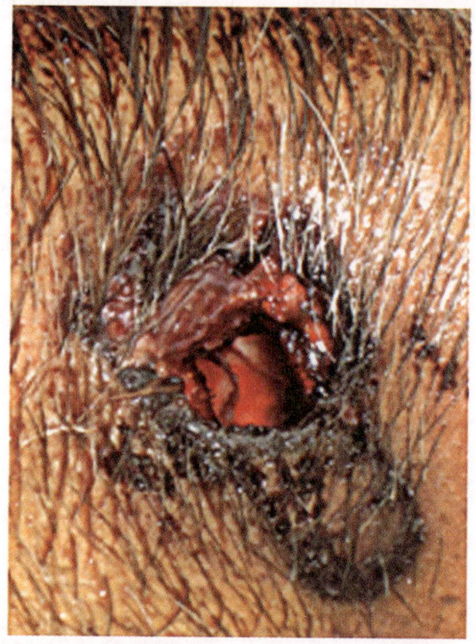

Fig. 3.75 Contact gunshot with muzzle and foresight imprint on skin (*Courtesy*: *Dr Girish Chandra YP*)

- **Distant shot**:
    - It means that the firearm was discharged outside the range of flame and powder blast (beyond 60 cm in the case of revolver and pistol; beyond 75 cm in the case of rifle).
    - The entry wound is circular with inverted margins (**Fig. 3.76**).
    - Scorching, tattooing and smudging are all absent.
    - Grease collar and abrasion collar are present.
    - Distant shot suggests a range beyond self-infliction. The range in any case of gunshot injury can be estimated accurately by test firing, using the same gun and similar cartridge at different ranges and comparing the effects with the wound present in the victim.

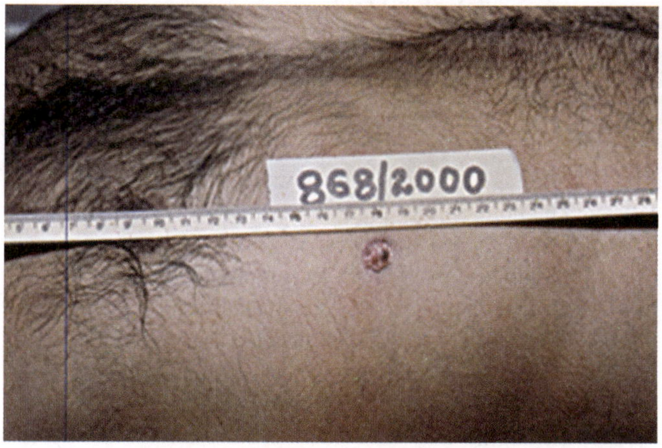

Fig. 3.76 Distant shot entry wound – rifled firearm (*Courtesy*: *Dr EJ Rodrigues*)

Exit Wound (**Fig. 3.77**)

- Exit wounds vary greatly in size, shape and configuration. They are usually larger than the corresponding wound of entry.
- Scorching, blackening and tattooing are absent, as also abrasion and grease collars.
- Edges are invariably everted. Bullet injury of the head usually causes inward bevelling of the skull at the entry, and outward bevelling at the exit wound.
- Salient differences between **entry** and **exit** wounds are mentioned in **Table 3.16**.

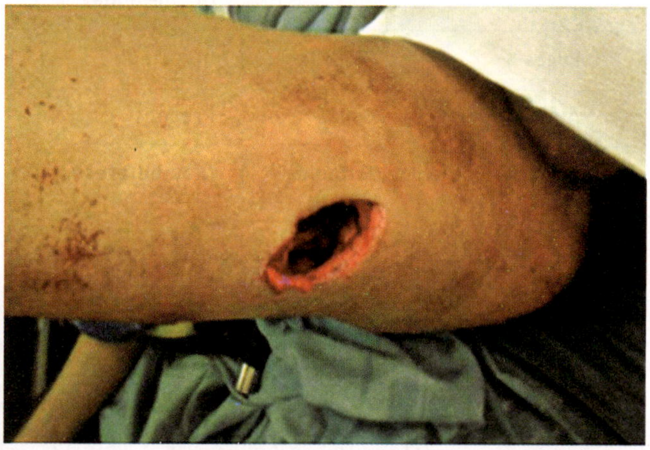

Fig. 3.77 Firearm exit wound

Track

- This is the **path** traversed by a projectile inside the body of a victim of gunshot injury, between the entry and exit wounds.
- In the case of low-velocity weapons, the track can be devious instead of straight.
- An X-ray prior to autopsy will assist significantly in locating bullets or pellets lodged in the body.
- When a projectile traverses through dense tissues such as muscle, liver, or spleen, shock waves are generated causing tissue damage even at a considerable distance away from the track (**temporary cavitation**).

Smooth-bore Firearm Injury

Entry Wound

- **Contact shot**:
    - The contact shot wound in the case of shotguns is

Table 3.15 Comparative Features of Discharge of Firearms

	Revolver/Pistol	Rifle	Shotgun
Muzzle velocity	Revolver: 150–180 m/sec Pistol: 300–360 m/sec	450–1500 m/sec	240–300 m/sec
Effective range	100 m	300 m (military rifle: 1000–3000 m)	30 m
Extension of flame	3 inches (8 cm)	12 inches (30 cm)	6 inches (15 cm)
Extension of smoke	6 inches (15 cm)	18 inches (45 cm)	12 inches (30 cm)
Extension of unburnt powder	24 inches (60 cm)	40 inches (100 cm)	35 inches (90 cm)

Table 3.16 Differences between Entry and Exit Rifled Firearm Injury

Characteristics	Entry Wound	Exit Wound
Size	Smaller than the diameter of the bullet	Larger
Edges	Inverted	Everted
Abrasion and Grease Collar	Present	Absent
Burning, Blackening, Tattooing	May be present	Absent
Bleeding	Less	More
Fat Extrusion	Absent	May be present
Cherry Red Colour	May be present	Absent
Lead Ring	May be present	Absent

usually a large, irregular hole, resulting from the explosive blast effect (**Fig. 3.78**).

- The edge of the defect is scorched by flame, and the skin surrounding it is blackened by smoke, and tattooed by unburnt powder.
- An imprint abrasion produced by the muzzle end may be seen.
- The shot (comprising a bunch of pellets) passes into the body as a solid mass.
- The injured tissue is usually cherry red in colour.
- Shotgun injury of the cranium is large and irregular, and fissured fractures often radiate outward from the margins. Sometimes a part of the head may be blown off.

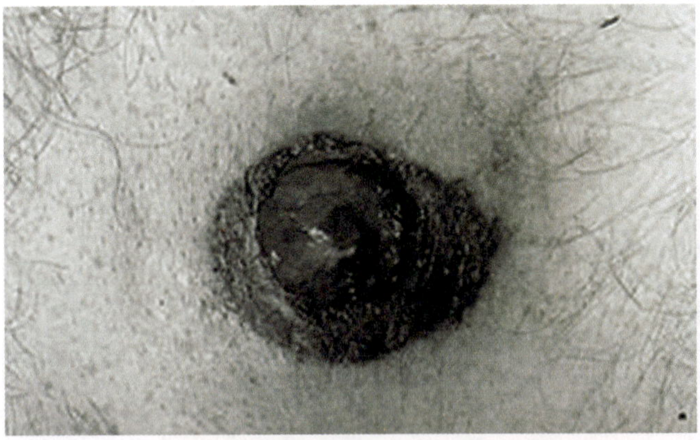

Fig. 3.78 Contact shotgun wound with scorching of edges

- **Close shot**:
  - This produces a circular defect with irregular inverted borders.
  - The edges are scorched due to flame, and smudged by smoke.
  - A fairly wide zone of tattooing may surround the edges of the wound.
  - Tissues often appear cherry red in colour.
  - The pellets enter the track en masse.
  - Sometimes, a shotgun may discharge parts of the cartridge case itself, such as fragmented cardboard, plastic or primer particles. At contact and close ranges, these may contribute to the wound.
- **Near shot**:
  - The wound is circular or oval in shape.
  - Smudging may be evident around the wound up to a maximum distance of 30 cm.
  - Sometimes the wad produces mild abrasions, if fired within a range of 30 cm.
  - Tattooing is present over a wide area.
  - The pellets travel in a compact mass up to a distance of about 45 cm, after which they begin to disperse (**Fig 3.79**). The entry wound is approximately 2.5 cm in diameter. If the shot enters at an angle < 90°, the shape of the wound may become triangular or semi-circular.

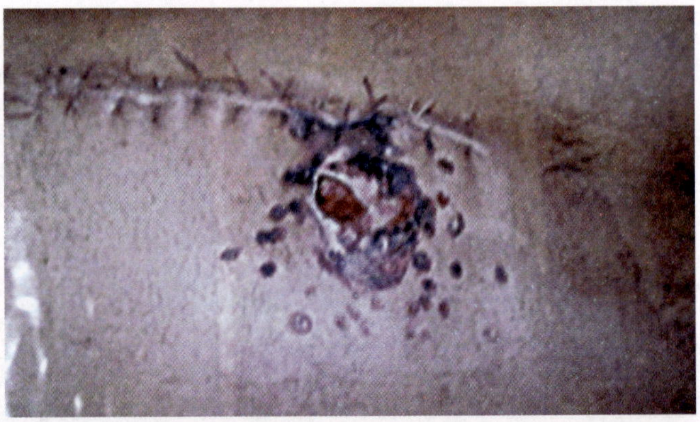

Fig. 3.79 Shotgun entry wound – Near shot with dispersion of pellets (*Courtesy*: *Dr Shashidhar C Mestri*)

- **Distant shot**:
  - Beyond a range of 2 metres, there will be no burning or blackening.
  - Tattooing is also rare.
  - But wad may be present in the wound (up to 5 metre range).
  - The dispersion of pellets becomes significant at ranges over 2 metres. Thereafter, the spread increases progressively, and the central defect diminishes in size proportionately. There is an old rule of thumb which states that *the diameter of the spread in inches is roughly equal to the range in yards multiplied by 1.5*.
  - At distant ranges (beyond 6–10 metres), the central hole may shrink to nothing. At such ranges the shot may not be lethal and the pellets, if they do penetrate the skin at all, may lie just in the subcutaneous tissue.

Medicolegal Aspects of Firearm Injury

- Legally, firearms are classified as dangerous weapons, and mere possession without license or authority becomes a cognisable offence.
- The following constitute some important medicolegal issues in firearm deaths:
  - The nature of firearm
  - The range of fire
  - The direction of fire
  - The place from where firing took place
  - The cause of death and
  - Whether the firing was an accident, homicide or suicide.
- **Nature of Firearm**:
  - It is important to know whether the firearm used was a rifled weapon or a smooth-bore weapon, and if it was a rifled weapon, whether it was a rifle, pistol or revolver.
  - An examination of the size of the **bullet** and its weight and calibre; the number, size and direction of the rifling marks on it; and the kind of metal it is made of, will all give clues regarding the weapon used. For example, a bullet of 0.7 cm diameter generally indicates that it has been fired from a weapon with a calibre of 0.7 cm. The diameter of a bullet is measured with a micrometer.
  - Bullets may be recovered at the scene of a shooting incident, or from a dead body during autopsy. Although a detailed examination of the bullet recovered at autopsy is within the province only of a ballistics expert, the medical officer conducting the autopsy should observe the following points (*details mentioned under* "Autopsy Procedure in Firearm Deaths", **Box 3.4**).
    - A bullet recovered from a dead body must not be washed or cleaned as this may remove the residue of any powder adhering to it. Instead, it should be dried without using heat and preserved for future examination by a ballistics expert.
    - He must handle the bullet carefully. Forceps or other metallic instruments must not be used in handling a bullet, for it will not only cause artefacts such as scratches on it, but also obliterate the existing rifling marks. Rubber-tipped forceps are best for handling projectiles.
    - The size of the bullet, its weight, calibre, the number, size and direction of rifling marks on it, the kind of metal of which it is made, any blunting of its nose, and other relevant details should be noted down. If the nose is blunted, it indicates that it had hit against a hard object. When a lead bullet strikes a person wearing clothes, the pattern of the weave of the clothing may sometimes be found stamped on the nose of the bullet.

Box 3.4—Autopsy Procedure in Firearm Death

Autopsy in a firearm death is of unique nature, where collection of evidentiary material is extremely important. It is the duty of the medical officer to meticulously collect and preserve every item that can help in the investigation. Some of the salient points to be remembered are as follows:

- Immediately after the dead body is received from the Police, an attempt must be made to detect primer residue in both the victim's hands (separately). Clean absorbent cotton buds or cotton gauze dipped in rectified spirit can be used to mop the hands. These are to be immediately transferred to cleaned glass bottles containing rectified sprit. Alternatively, the hands can be washed with rectified spirit, and the washing carefully collected in clean bottles.
- Punctures, stains, etc., on the clothing of the dead body are to be noted in detail, and subsequently photographed. The clothes must then be carefully removed, dried in shade and packed in paper bags.
- External injuries on the body should be recorded carefully and photographed. Entry wounds should be swabbed with absorbent cotton soaked in rectified spirit, which are then transferred to cleaned bottles containing rectified spirit.
- The dead body should be extensively X-rayed. Wet X-ray film must preferably be examined before commencing dissection. These films (after drying) should be marked with the following identifying characteristics: autopsy number, serial number, date, site, side and nature of view, and preserved as permanent records along with the autopsy report. X-rays are extremely helpful in revealing the exact path of the projectile within the body, or the extent of internal damage.
- The planned routine autopsy should immediately follow. All skin wounds as such should be dissected out carefully with surrounding tissue (minimum 2.5 cm thick). The dissected wound should be separately covered with absorbent cotton soaked in rectified spirit, and placed in suitable glass containers (containing rectified spirit). It is worthwhile to remember that some entry wounds may be hidden or inconspicuous, and a meticulous search of the entire body may be necessary to locate them.

contd.

- A thorough search should be made to retrieve all bullets (in rifled firearm death), or as many pellets as possible (in shotgun death) from the corpse. Foreign particles form wounds, if present, should be collected, placed in absorbent cotton, and secured in clean and empty cardboard boxes.
- A bullet recovered from a dead body must not be washed or cleaned, as this may remove the residue of any powder adhering to it. Instead, it should be dried without using heat and preserved. Bullets need to be handled carefully. Forceps or other metallic instruments must not be used, or they will cause not only artefacts such as scratches on it, which will interfere with rifling marks, but may in fact totally obliterate the existing rifling marks. Rubber-tipped forceps are best for handling projectiles. The size of the bullet, its weight, calibre, the number, size and direction of rifling marks on it, the kind of metal it is made up of, any blunting of its nose, etc., as well as other relevant details should be noted down. If the nose is blunted, it indicates that it had hit against a hard object. When a lead bullet strikes a person wearing clothes, the pattern of the weave of the clothing may sometimes be found stamped on the nose of the bullet.
- The bullet is marked by one's initials on its base with a sharp pointed instrument, to facilitate its subsequent identification in court, and not on its sides or nose, as this will obliterate other marks that may already be present. Bullets meant for future examination must be wrapped in absorbent cotton and preserved in empty cardboard boxes.
- Unfortunately, shotgun pellets cannot be traced to the offending weapon by means of ballistic marking, as in the case of bullets. However, a study of the wad used could help, since the prints on the top-wad and its diameter can connect it to the suspected weapon. The top-wad is almost always carried into the body along with the shot.
- At the end of the autopsy, all material objects collected should be packed, labelled, tied and sealed, and forwarded to the ballistics expert through proper channel, along with forwarding notes, and samples of labels and seal used. The following items must be submitted: the clothes of the victim, skin and tissues around the gunshot wounds, and recovered projectiles. Skin and tissues must be preserved in rectified spirit.
- The medical opinion should include information about not only the cause of death, but also (if possible) the kind of firearm involved, and the range and direction of fire. Opinion about the time of death, identity of the deceased, and the manner of death may also be added.

- The bullet is marked for future identification, by inscribing one's initials on its base with a sharp-pointed instrument, and not on its sides or nose, as this will obliterate other marks that may already be present.
- Bullets meant for future examination must be wrapped in absorbent cotton and preserved in empty cardboard boxes.

- The suspect weapon and the crime bullet are both examined by a ballistics expert. To find out whether the bullet recovered had been fired from the suspect weapon, **test firing** is done.
  - A test shot is fired from the weapon into a box called firing box, which is packed with cotton wool so that no distortion of the bullet occurs. The firing box is open at the side from which firing is done, and also at the opposite side.
  - The bullet so fired (test bullet) is recovered.
  - The test and crime bullets are then compared under a **comparison microscope** (**Fig. 3.80**). This is a kind of microscope under which two objects can be compared simultaneously. If the rifling marks are identical on the test and crime bullets, the inference is that the suspect weapon was the weapon used for the commission of the offence.
  - The number, width and depth of rifling marks on a bullet can be accurately examined under a Greenough type binocular microscope. The three-dimensional image afforded by such a procedure enables the operator to see the impressions more clearly.

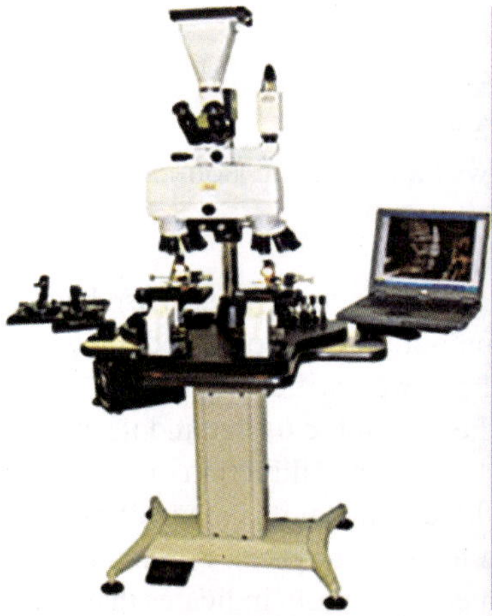

The comparison microscope is used to compare the individual characteristics of the "evidence bullet" to those of the "test bullet".

Fig. 3.80 Comparison microscope

- Examination of a **spent cartridge case** will also provide clues in identifying the crime weapon.
  - In the case of a shotgun cartridge, the name of the manufacturing firm and the calibre of the weapon for which it is intended, are generally imprinted on the casing.
  - Empty cases of revolvers have a rim at their base, while those of pistols do not.
  - The size of the spent case provides a clue regarding the calibre of the weapon.
  - In a revolver, the empty case usually remains within the weapon, so that it is rare to find it at the scene of crime.

- If an empty case is seen at the scene of crime, as in the case of a pistol or a rifle, it is generally found a few feet to the right of the spot where the weapon was discharged.
- The firing pin will make a dent on the base, which is peculiar to that weapon. The breech may also leave its marks on it.
- The state of chemicals inside can assist in knowing whether it was recently fired or not.
- All these points can help to identify a crime weapon. For future identification, a spent case is marked by scratching one's initials on its side.

- In a shotgun wound, the nature of the **shot**, e.g., lead pellets, glass beads or stones, may help in identifying the weapon. Factory-made shotgun cartridges use lead shot, while home-made ones employ glass beads or stones.
  - Lead pellets (and other kinds of shot) should be wrapped in absorbent cotton, placed in an empty cardboard box and preserved for examination.
  - Presence of **wad** at the scene of crime or in the dead body conclusively indicates that a shotgun had been employed. The diameter of the wad may give a clue regarding the calibre of the weapon. Wads are preserved in an empty cardboard box for future examination.
- Stains on the body of a victim can also provide help. Rifled weapons employ cartridges with smokeless powder which does not cause much blackening of the skin, because it burns up entirely, while the black powder of shotguns causes extensive smudging.

- **Range of Firing**:
  - The velocity of a rifle bullet is about 800 metres/second, and the range is 1000–3000 metres. The range of a revolver/pistol is up to 400–600 metres (effective or lethal range: 100 m).
  - Shotguns have an effective lethal range of only 30 to 40 metres, beyond which the pellets begin to disperse widely (**Fig. 3.81**). However, it is the most lethal weapon at close range.
  - The range of fire is deduced from the appearance of the entrance wound (*vide supra*). However, an accurate range of firing is usually better made out by **test firing**, than medical examination.
- **Direction of Fire**:
  - If there is no deflection of the projectile, a line joining the entrance wound with the exit wound in a dead body, or the area of lodgement of the bullet will give the direction of fire.
  - Cases of devious tracks, or deflection of projectile due to hitting an intervening object (**ricochet bullet**), can cause confusion in interpretation (**Fig. 3.82**).
  - An entry wound is circular if the projectile enters perpendicular to body surface and oval if entry is oblique. In the latter case, the edge on the side of the entry of the bullet appears bevelled, while the opposite edge becomes overhanging. In cases of oblique entry, the abrasion collar becomes eccentric, being wider at the side of entry.
- **Site of Firing**:
  - This will depend upon the calculation of range and direction of firing.
- **Cause of Death**:
  - Firearm injury can result in death due to haemorrhage, or damage to any of the vital organs such as the heart or the brain.
- **Manner of Death**
  - It must be deduced as to whether a particular case of firearm death was **accidental**, **suicidal** or **homicidal**. The

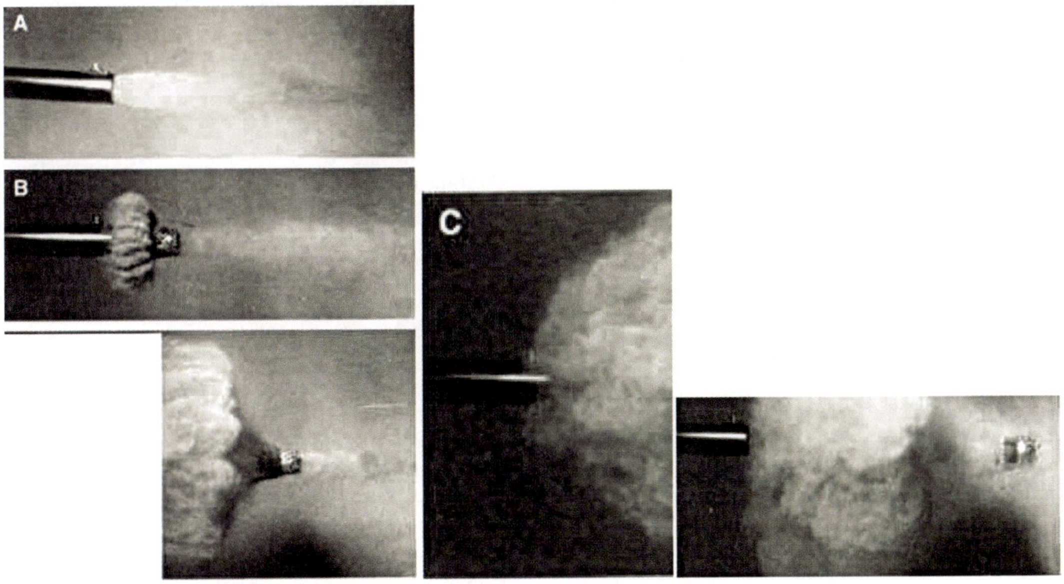

Fig. 3.81 Sequential images of a shotgun discharge

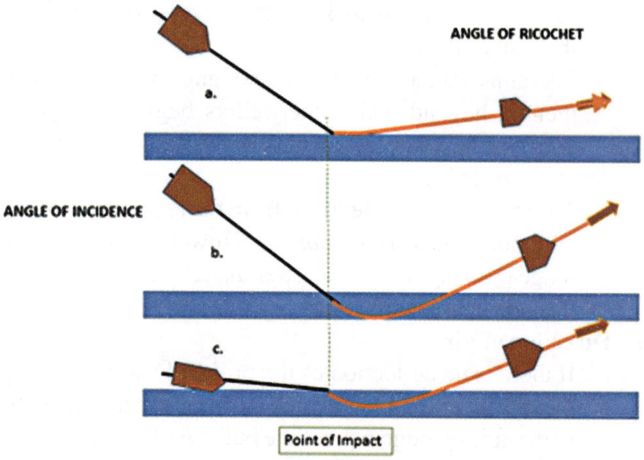

Fig. 3.82 Ricochet bullet – path depends on angle of impact on intervening object

important clues which can help to resolve this are mentioned in **Table 3.17**.

- The usual manner of death from firearms is either suicidal or homicidal, while accidental deaths are less common.
- Suicides often expose the site of election before shooting, as for example opening the shirt before placing the muzzle over the chest. They may also ensure that the muzzle is steady by holding the barrel by the non-firing hand, which may thus sustain burns from flame.
- Accidental deaths are often non-witnessed. However, firearm deaths almost always leave trace evidence from the weapon in or about the victim's body, which can be scientifically compared with the suspect weapon. In an accidental case, examination of the weapon may reveal clues about accidental discharge, such as defective safety catch, etc. Accidents usually occur from careless handling of the gun, or unfamiliarity with operation while cleaning, loading, or inspecting the firearm.

Tests Related to Confirmation of Use of Firearms

(Methods of finding out whether a person recently discharged a firearm)

- **Dermal Nitrate Test**:
  - When a person fires a gun, gunpowder residues will be invariably deposited in the hands because of leakage from the breech end of the weapon. The '**dermal nitrate test**' is often done on the hands of an accused to detect these residues (**Fig. 3.83**).
  - However, false-positive result can occur, if the hands are contaminated with tobacco, urine, etc.

Dermal Nitrate Test (Paraffin Test)

Method:
- Molten paraffin wax is brushed on the suspect's hand.
- After hardening, it is peeled off.
- The inner surface of the wax cast is then treated with diphenylamine or diphenylbenzidine reagent.
- 'Blue colour' develops wherever the powder residue is present.

Fig. 3.83 Dermal nitrate test

- **Other Tests**: The following tests are more sensitive and specific:
  - **Harrison and Gilroy's Test**:
    - The Harrison-Gilroy test checks for the presence of barium, antimony and lead on the hands. In this chemical test, the hands of the suspect are swabbed with gauze moistened with dilute hydrochloric acid.

Table 3.17 Differences between Accidental, Suicidal and Homicidal Firearms Wounds

Features	Accidental	Suicidal	Homicidal
Site of entry wound	Any part	Head or chest	Any part
Range	Close	Contact or close	Any range
Direction	Any direction	Upward or backward	Usually upward
Number of wounds	One	Usually one	One or multiple
Firearm residue on hand	Present	Present	Absent
Weapon at the scene	Present	Present	Usually absent
Location	Anywhere (usually home)	Usually home	Anywhere
Sex	Usually males	Usually males	Either sex
Motive	Absent	Depression, mental illness	Robbery, revenge, etc.

The gauze is allowed to dry and then treated with the chemical reagent triphenylmethylarsonium iodide. If antimony is present, the triphenylmethylarsonium iodide turns an orange colour.

- **Neutron activation analysis**
- **Automatic absorption spectroscopy**

Some other important ballistic information is mentioned in **Box 3.5**.

Box 3.5—Important Ballistic Trivia

Types of Bullet

- ***Dum-dum bullet*** – A type of bullet which is designed to explode on impact.
- ***Incendiary bullet*** – A hollow-point bullet which contains phosphorus.
- ***Frangible bullet*** – A bullet that is made of iron instead of lead, and fragments on impact.

Types of Lead Shot

- ***Dust shot*** – Consists of extremely fine particles.
- ***Bird shot*** – Consists of lead pellets of average diameter 3.5 mm. Used for small game hunting.
- ***Buck shot*** – Consists of large pellets of average diameter 6–8 mm. Used for big game hunting.
- ***Slug*** – Heavy projectile made of lead or copper designed for hunting large game.

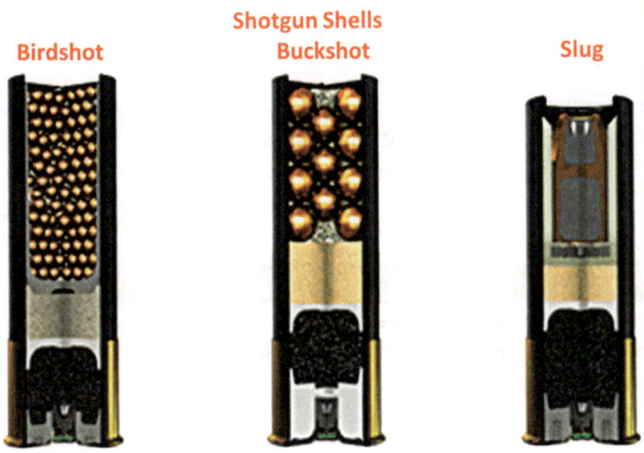

Unusual Ballistic Effects

1. ***Billiard ball effect*** – Extensive dispersion of lead shot because of the pellets striking against each other in flight. May give erroneous impression about the range of fire.

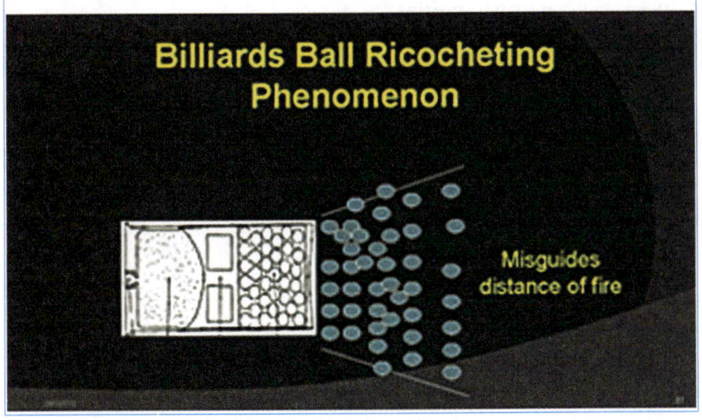

2. ***Balling of shot*** – The lead shot is bunched together for some distance during flight, resulting in much less dispersion than expected for that range.
3. ***Tandem bullet*** – Sometimes, when a firearm is discharged, the bullet does not emerge. On pulling the trigger again, two bullets may emerge, one behind the other. This happens in faulty or disused firearms.

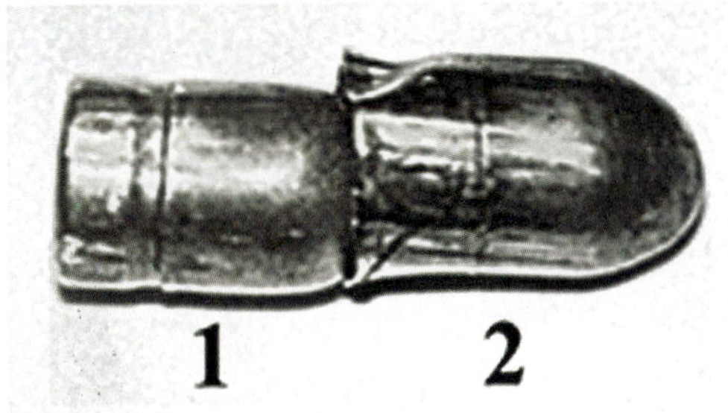

4. ***Tandem (Duplex) cartridge*** – A single cartridge contains two bullets, one behind the other, so that a single shot produces two separate entry wounds. Used in military rifles.

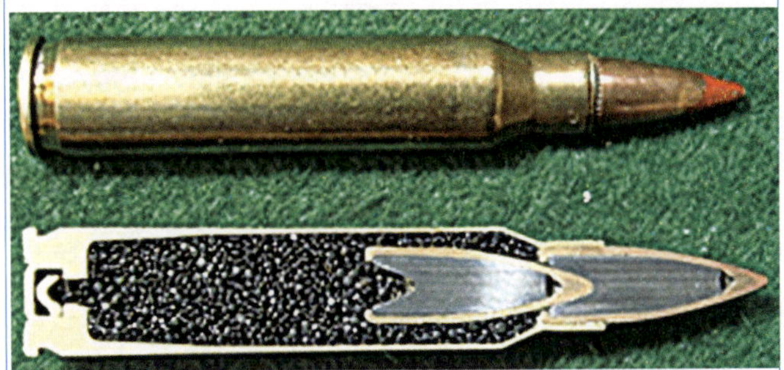

5. ***Shored exit wound*** – If the skin at the exit wound is supported against a wall, the wound may appear nearly circular with a surrounding margin of abrasion, simulating an entry wound.
6. ***Yawing bullet*** – A bullet that has an unsteady trajectory during flight.

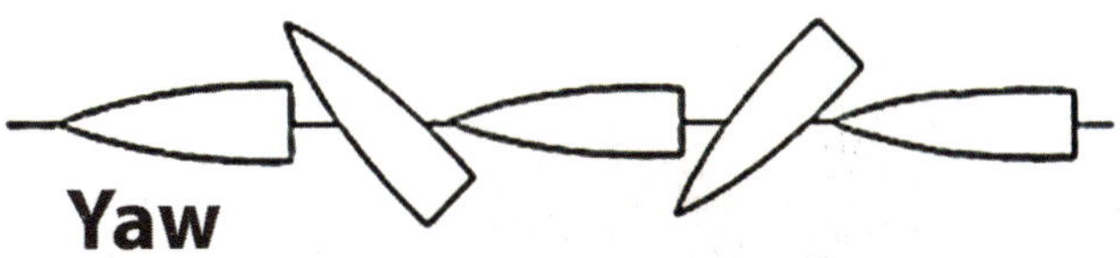

7. ***Tumbling bullet*** – A bullet that tumbles end-on-end (somersaults) during flight.

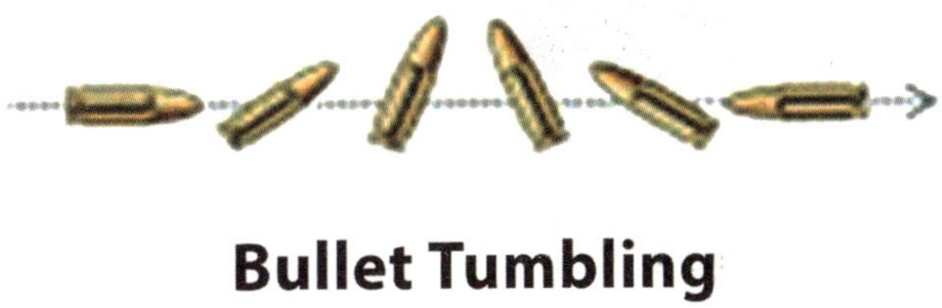

contd

8. ***Souvenir bullet*** – A bullet that remains in the body of a surviving victim of gunshot injury for a long time without producing any deleterious effects.

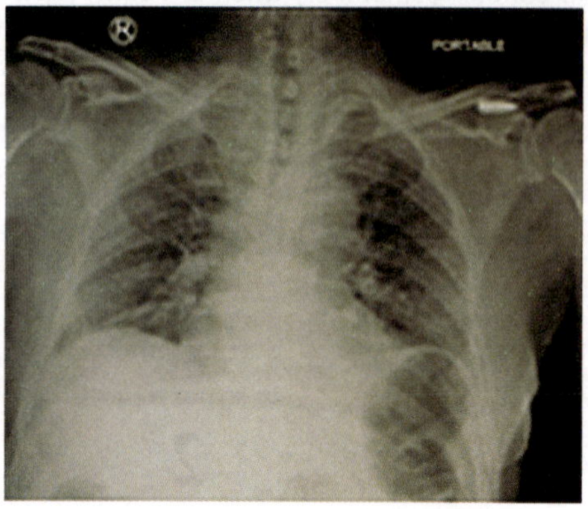

Souvenir bullet – near left shoulder

9. ***Kennedy phenomenon*** – Surgical intervention and alteration of a firearm wound, causing problems in medicolegal interpretation

EXPLOSIVE (BLAST) INJURIES

Common Explosives

- Nitroglycerine
- Trinitrotoluene (TNT)
- Pentaerythritol tetranitrate (PETN)
- Triacetone triperoxide (TATP)
- Cyclomethylene trinitramine (Cyclonite/RDX)

Classification of Blast Injuries (Fig. 3.84)

- **Primary blast injuries**: They are due to the direct effect of "blast overpressure." Injuries are caused by compressed air, which tends to affect air-filled organs such as the lungs, gastrointestinal tract, middle ear, etc.
- **Secondary blast injuries**: They are caused by flying objects generated by the blast.
- **Tertiary blast injuries**: These injuries occur when victims are thrown into the air and strike other objects.
- **Quaternary blast injuries**: These comprise injuries from fire, inhalation of toxic gases, etc.
- **Quinary blast injuries**: These comprise illnesses or diseases caused by chemical, biological or radiological substances ('dirty bombs').

Mechanisms of Death

- A minimum pressure of about 700 kilopascals (100 lb/sq inch) is needed for tissue damage in humans.
- In most explosions, pulmonary contusion, pneumothorax and abdominal injuries are the major reasons for mortality, while the middle ear is the organ that is most susceptible to the primary blast.
  - Pulmonary barotrauma is the most common *fatal* **primary blast injury**. This term encompasses pulmonary contusion, systemic air embolism, and free radical-associated injuries such as thrombosis, lipoxygenation and disseminated intravascular coagulation.
  - ARDS (acquired respiratory distress syndrome) may be the result of direct lung injury, or shock from other organ-system damage.
- Intestinal barotrauma is more common in underwater blasts. Colon is usually the most affected.
- Generally speaking, the intensity of an explosion declines as the cubed root of the distance from the explosion. In other words, a person 3 metres from an explosion experiences 9 times more overpressure than a person 6 metres

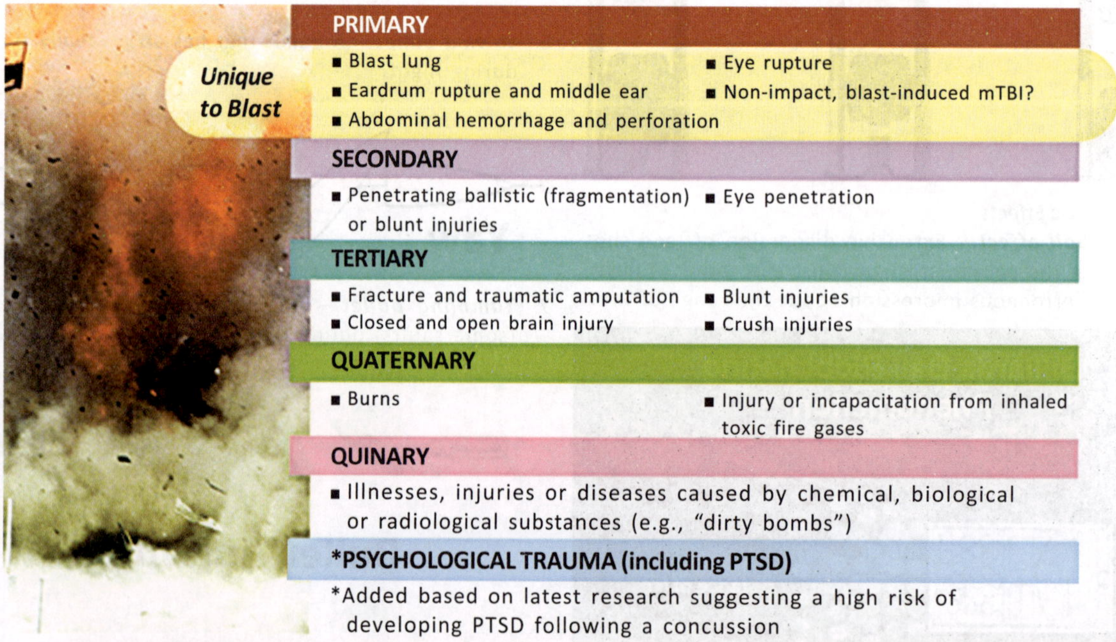

Fig. 3.84 Classification of blast injuries

away. Therefore, proximity of a person to the explosion is an important factor in primary blast injury.

- Solid surfaces reflect blast waves and increase the primary blast injury.
- Flying debris, shards of glass, metal objects, etc., impart **secondary blast injuries**, which can be lethal. They cause either blunt or penetrating injuries. Some terrorists deliberately add metal screws and nails to their explosives with the objective of enhancing lethality.
- A typical mixture of punctuate bruises, abrasions and puncture lacerations may be seen, referred to as the **Marshall's triad**.
- **Tertiary blast injuries** result from the victim flying through air and hitting against walls, trees, poles, etc.
- **Miscellaneous blast injuries** involving toxic inhalations, exposure to fire, toxins or radiations, traumatic asphyxia, crush injuries, etc., add to the overall catastrophic effect. Incomplete burning of plastic can release cyanides.

Medicolegal Significance

- Most explosive deaths are either homicidal (due to terrorist activity) or accidental. A few terrorist-related blasts may involve suicide bombers.
- In India, the incidence of blast injuries is varied and sporadic. States with terrorist problems report higher incidence, e.g., Jammu & Kashmir. Also, blasts related to fireworks cause a significant number of deaths in India, especially in Northern states during the festival of Diwali.
- Careful autopsy and practical use of laboratory rather than protocol tests are advisable in mass disasters (**Fig. 3.85**).
  - Identification of the dead assumes great importance, and is unfortunately extremely complex in large-scale explosions that cause mass casualties with dismemberment or fragmentation.
  - Blood tests for carboxyhaemoglobin, cyanides and phosphorus may be necessary, especially in closed-space explosions, or fire-related blasts.
  - Histopathology may help to detect ARDS, pulmonary contusion, or myoglobinuric renal failure resulting from crush syndrome.
  - Explosive residues will have to be collected for subsequent examination by experts in the field of explosives.
  - At the time of autopsy, the possibility of contamination of the body with chemical or radioactive material should be kept in mind.

FM 3.11: Core – Written/Viva Voce/
OSCE (Objective Structured Clinical Examination)/
OSPE (Objective Structured Practical Examination)

- **Regional injuries**:
  - Describe and discuss **regional injuries** to
    - Head (scalp wounds, fractures of skull, intracranial haemorrhages, coup and contre coup injuries)
    - Neck
    - Chest
    - Abdomen
    - Limbs
    - Genital organs
    - Spinal cord
    - Skeleton

REGIONAL INJURIES

Mechanical injuries can assume varying significance depending on the location, and the structure or organ that is involved. It would be pertinent therefore to discuss some common injuries in a **regionwise** manner.

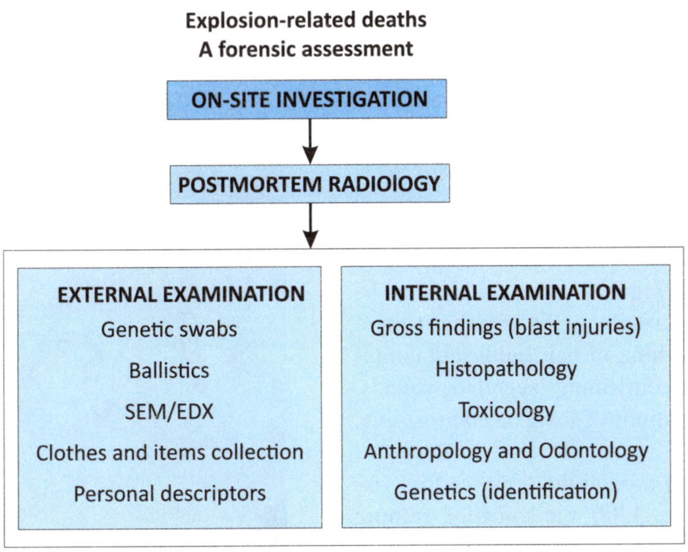

SEM—Scanning electron microscopy; EDX—Energy dispersive X-ray spectroscopy.

Fig. 3.85 Explosion-related deaths: A forensic assessment

Head

Mechanical force applied on the **head** can injure the:

- **Scalp**
- **Skull**
- **Meninges**
- **Brain** or related
- **Vessels** separately, or in combination.

Scalp

- Wounds of scalp can take the form of abrasions, incised wounds, lacerated wounds, contusions or puncture wounds. They are rendered more visible, if the scalp hair is shaven off (**Fig. 3.86**).

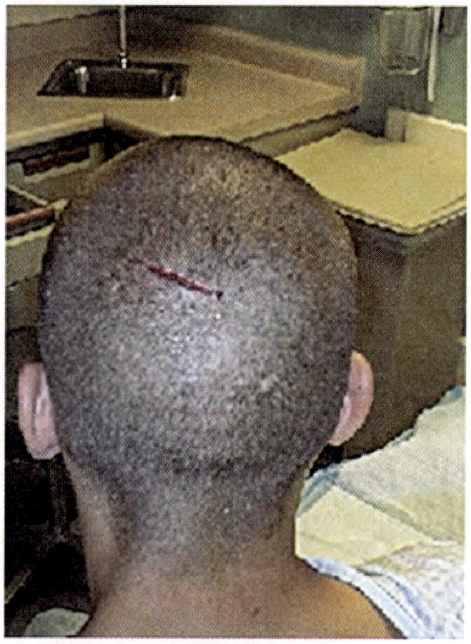

Fig. 3.86 Scalp wound rendered clear after removing hair

- Abrasions are relatively uncommon over the scalp because of the presence of hair.
- Incised wounds produced by light cutting weapons, and chop wounds produced by heavy cutting weapons can be differentiated by the presence or absence of contused edges. Incised wounds of head bleed profusely. However, wound healing is rapid when compared to other regions.
- Due to the close proximity to the skull bones, scalp lacerations are often **incised-looking lacerations**, which can be differentiated from true incised wounds only by using a hand lens (**Fig. 3.87**). Crushing of hair bulbs and contusion of the edges help in confirming lacerated wounds. Like incised wounds, lacerations of scalp bleed profusely.
- Contusion of scalp
    - Can percolate and settle around the orbit, and be visible as a **black eye** (**Fig. 3.88**), the so-called **ectopic contusion** or **ectopic bruise**. If it occurs around both eyes, it is called a "**spectacle haematoma**" (**Fig. 3.89**).
    - Superficial contusions appear as localised swellings on palpation, due to limitation by the fibro-fatty tissue.
    - Contusions deep to galea aponeurotica tend to become diffuse in nature due to the loose sub-aponeurotic tissue.
    - Puncture (stab) wounds of scalp may be incised- or lacerated-puncture wounds, of which the latter are more common. Such wounds invariably enter into the skull cavity to become penetrating wounds.

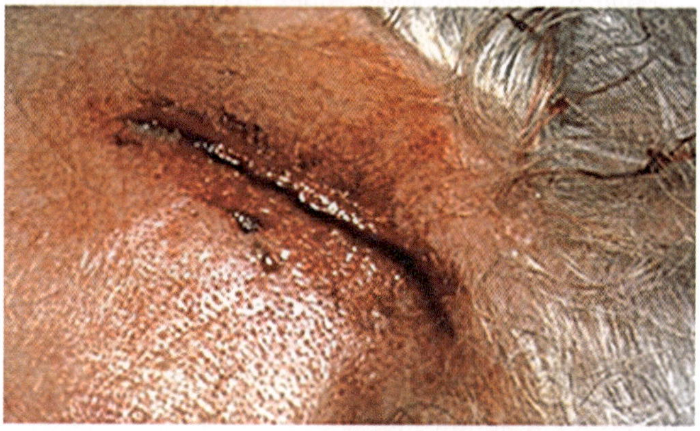

Fig. 3.87 Incised looking laceration

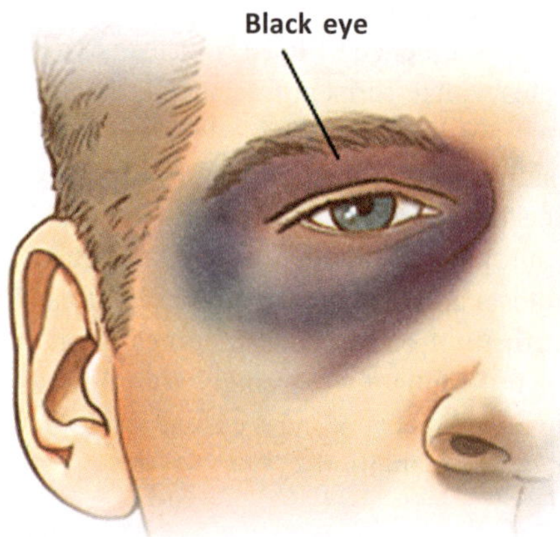

Fig. 3.88 Black eye

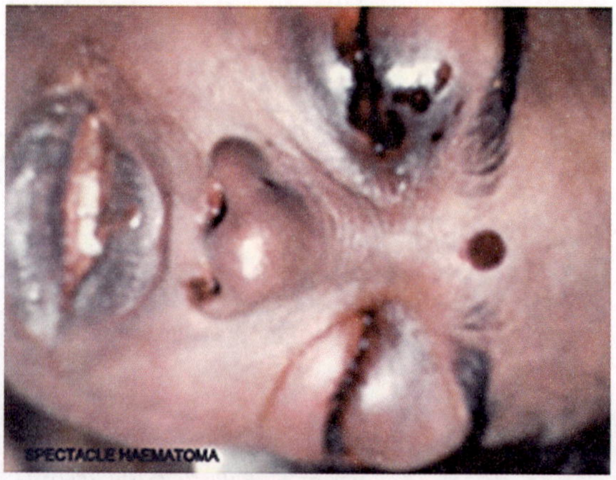

Fig. 3.89 Spectacle haematoma (*Courtesy*: *Dr Shashidhar C Mestri*)

Skull

- Fractures of skull could be due to direct impact (such as a blow), or due to indirect impact (such as a fall on the feet or buttocks).
- If the force of impact is less than the elasticity of the skull, in-bending of the bone at the site of impact alone is the result. The bone subsequently resumes its original position.
- A fracture results when the impact is greater than the elasticity of the bone. Experiments have proved that a force of 5 foot pounds can be sufficient to fracture the skull. However, the occurrence of fracture also depends upon the relative thickness and strength of the bone in different regions.

*Classification**

- **Fissured fracture**
  - Linear
  - Crack
  - Basilar
  - Ring (foraminal)
- **Comminuted fracture**
  - Depressed ('signature')
  - Non-depressed
  - Expressed
- **Gutter fracture**
- **Pond (indented) fracture**
- **Diastatic (sutural) fracture**
- **Perforating fracture**
- **Cut (chop) fracture**

Fig. 3.89b gives an overview of the current classification of skull fractures, which differs a little from the conventional classification.

Fissured Fracture

- It is a **linear fracture** involving both tables of skull, and is the commonest type of skull fracture.
- Such fractures can be straight, curved or irregular.
- They are produced ordinarily when the head hits against a hard surface, or when an object with a large striking surface hits the head with sufficient force.
- They can occur at the site of impact or some distance away, depending upon the temporary deformation of skull due to the applied force. They usually occur along the line of maximum stretching (**Fig. 3.90**).
- Fissured fractures can also occur as radiations from the sites of other types of skull fracture.
- **Basilar fractures** are fissured fractures that occur in the floor of the cranial vault (skull base), which require more force to cause than other areas of the neurocranium. Thus they are rare, occurring as the only fracture in only 4% of

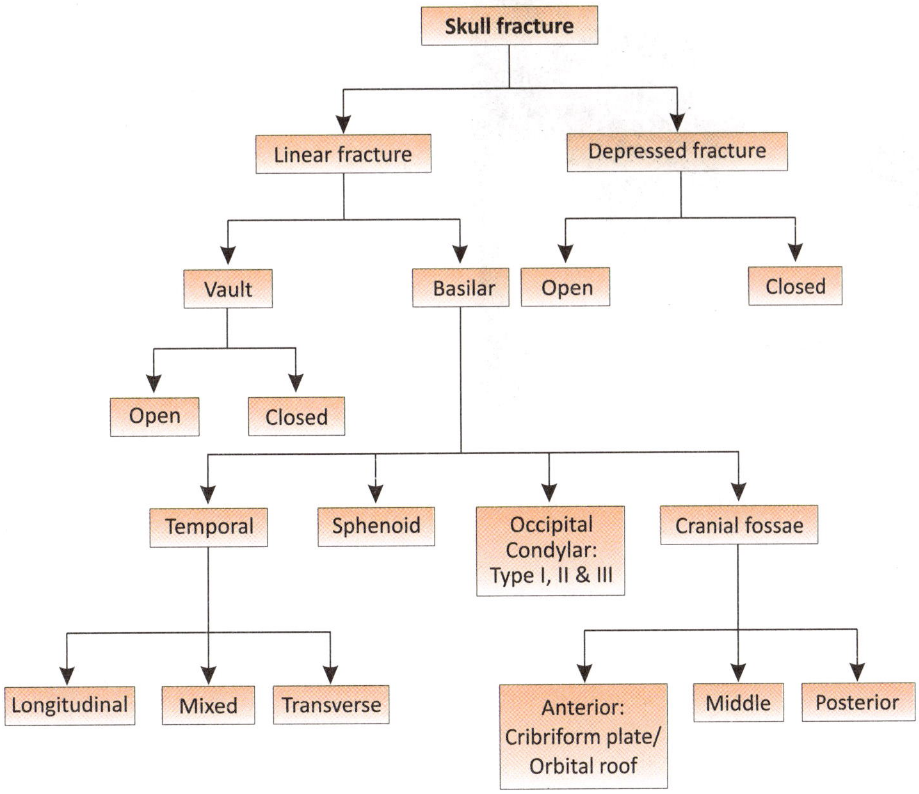

Fig. 3.89b Fractures of skull – current classification

***Mnemonic**: Fractures Can Get Painful; Delay Prevents Cure = Fissured Comminuted Gutter Pond Diastatic Perforating Cut.*

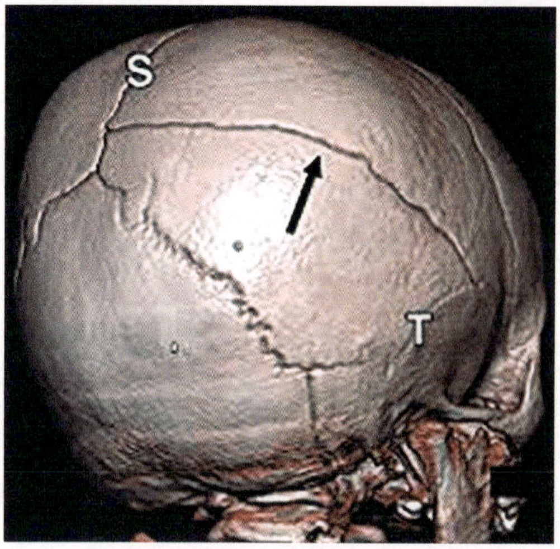

Fig. 3.90 Fissured fracture (*arrowed*)

head injury patients. Basilar fractures have characteristic signs:

- Blood in the sinuses, or cerebrospinal fluid leaking from the nose (**CSF rhinorrhoea**), or periorbital ecchymosis ('**raccoon eyes**') due to bruising around the eyes that result from blood collecting there as it leaks from the fracture site, in **anterior cranial fossa fracture** (**Fig. 3.91**).

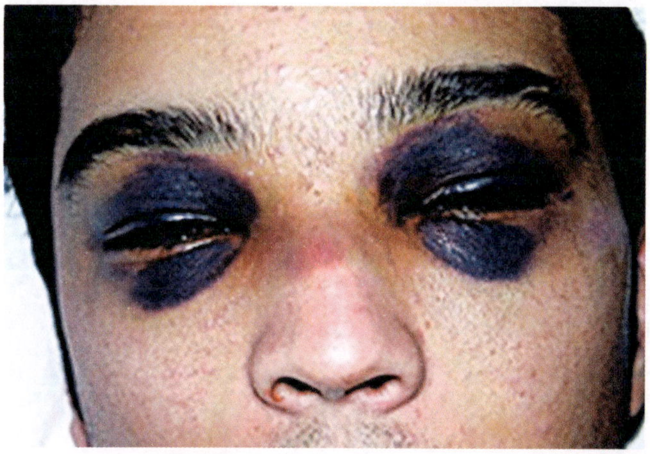

Fig. 3.91 Raccoon eyes

- CSF leaking from the ears (**CSF otorrhoea**) in **middle cranial fossa fracture**.
- Retroauricular ecchymosis ("**Battle's sign**") due to bruising over the mastoid process in **posterior cranial fossa fracture** (**Fig. 3.92**).

- A type of basilar fracture in the form of a circular fissured fracture occurring around the foramen magnum is sometimes referred to as a **ring fracture*** (**Fig 3.93**). Such a fracture results indirectly from the transmission of force through the vertebral column, as in the case of a fall on the feet or buttocks, or through the mandible as in the case of a blow to the chin.

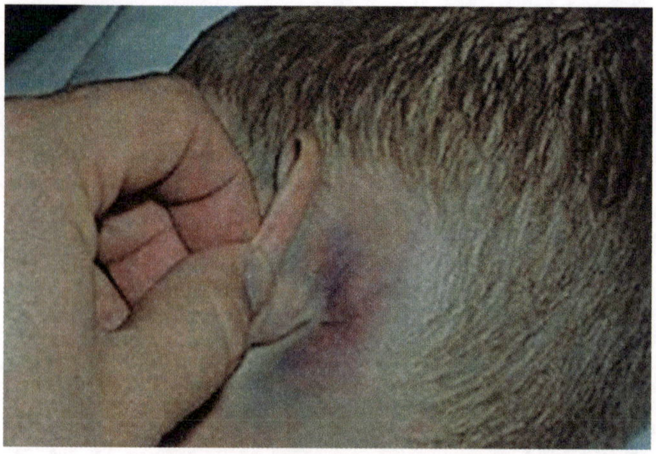

Fig. 3.92 Battle's sign

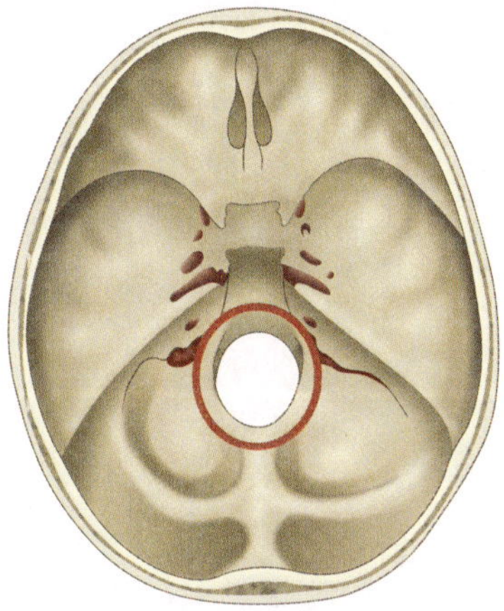

Fig. 3.93 Ring fracture – Base of skull

- A fissured fracture which involves only one table of the skull is referred to as a **crack fracture**. It is usually the inner table which fractures in such cases, since it is more brittle.

Comminuted Fracture

- The term "comminution" refers to fracture division of a bone into several fragments (three or more fragments).
- This results when a considerable force is applied over a relatively small area. Weapons with small striking surface like hammer are often the causative objects. Comminution can also be a complication of fissured fractures.
- Comminuted fractures can be with or without depression of the affected area. The former is called **depressed comminuted fracture**, while the latter is referred to as **non-depressed comminuted fracture**, or merely as a comminuted fracture.
  - ***Depressed comminuted fracture*** (*Fig. 3.94*): Local impact causes the outer table to be driven inwards. If the force is not absorbed in the dipole, the inner table also gets invaginated into the cranial cavity – both plates

**Note*: *Also called "Jeanneret fracture subtype II."*

therefore get comminuted, and thus a depressed comminuted fracture is produced.

- Such a fracture may provide a clue about the striking surface, i.e., the weapon used (**signature fracture**). For instance, a circular area of depressed comminuted fracture can indicate the application of a hammer.

- ***Non-depressed comminuted fracture***: In this type, there is no invagination of fractured segments. The fractured site appears in the form of several fissures arranged like a cobweb or "mosaic".
- ***Expressed fracture***: Those comminuted fractures where the free fragments come to lie outside the normal curvature of the cranium (as in pericranial tissue substance, cranial cavity, or outside the head) are called "expressed fractures."

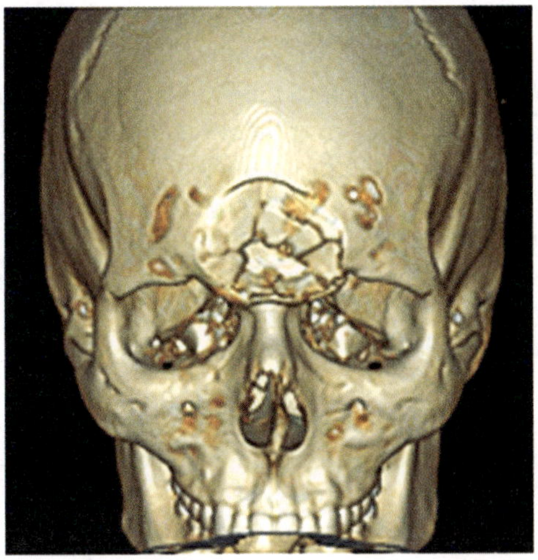

Fig. 3.94 Depressed comminuted fracture of frontal bone

Gutter Fracture

- If a weapon strikes the skull tangentially, the outer table alone may be fractured causing a deformity in the form of a gutter. The commonest example is a **glancing bullet injury**.

Pond or Ping-Pong or Indented Fracture

- Here, the applied mechanical force produces a mere indentation of the skull bones, without actual fracture (**Fig. 3.95**).
- This is due to the elasticity of skull, and is especially likely to occur in infants. Pond fractures can result from application of forceps during delivery.
- Fissured fractures may be present around the periphery of the dent.

Diastatic or Sutural Fracture

- This type of fracture constitutes a sutural separation occurring either alone (**Fig. 3.96**), or in the form of an extension of a fissured fracture.

Perforating Fracture

- It results from penetration of the skull by a sharp pointed object or a bullet. In the latter case, the entry causes more damage to the inner table than the outer table, while at the exit, the reverse effect is seen. Consequently, such wounds are funnel shaped with the broader end formed by the inner table in entry wounds, and by the outer table in exit wounds. This is called "bevelling" and can help in finding out the direction of firing.

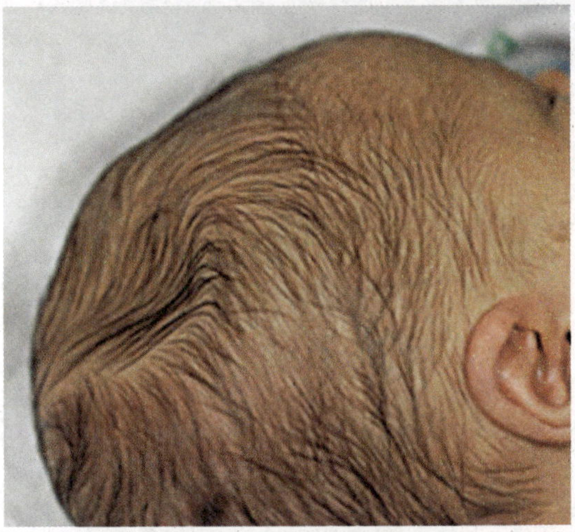

Fig. 3.95 Pond (ping pong) fracture

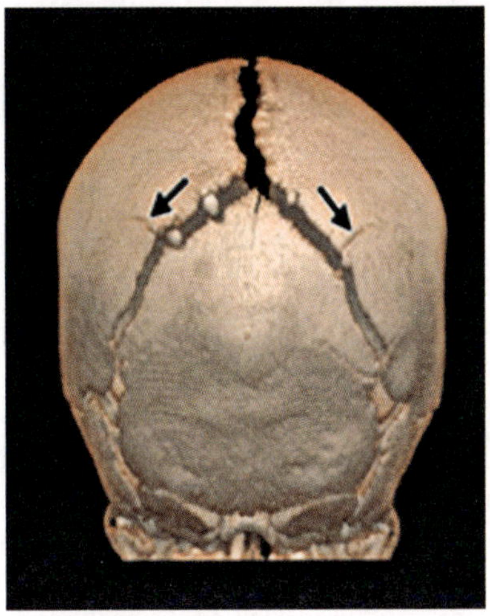

Fig. 3.96 Diastatic (sutural) fracture

- Pointed objects often produce clear cut openings, the size and shape usually corresponding to the dimensions of the causative weapon (**Fig. 3.97**).

Cut Fracture

- A heavy cutting weapon can cause straight chops of the skull, either involving the external plate alone, or sometimes affecting both the plates.
- In these fractures, except for the line of contact with the edge of the weapon, there may not be any lack of continuity of the bony substance anywhere.

Meninges

- Any of the three meninges can be torn by edges of fragmented pieces of skull or by penetrating objects.

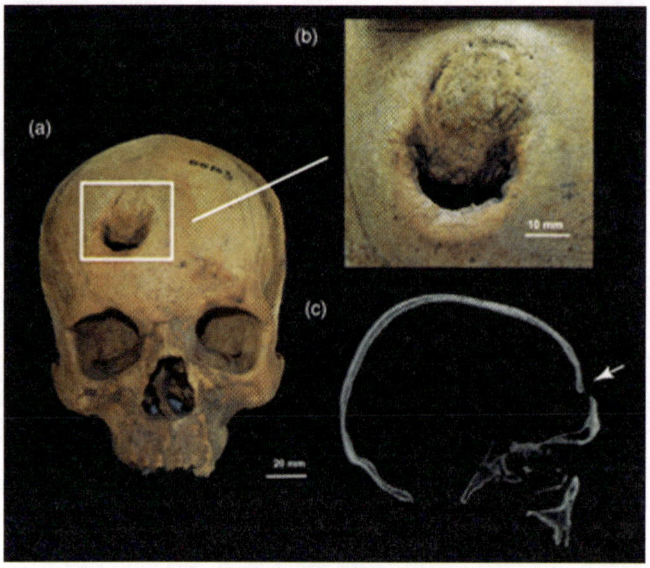

Fig. 3.97 Perforating skull fracture

- However, pia and arachnoid can also be ruptured due to accumulation of blood from beneath.

Brain

Traumatic Brain Injury (TBI)

- Traumatic brain injury (TBI), also known as **intracranial injury**, is an injury to the brain caused by an external force.
- TBI can be classified based on ***severity*** (ranging from mild traumatic brain injury [mTBI/concussion] to severe traumatic brain injury), ***mechanism*** (closed head injury or penetrating head injury) or ***other features*** (e.g., occurring in a specific location or over a widespread area).
- **Head injury** is a broader category that may involve damage to other structures such as the scalp and skull.
- TBI can result in physical, cognitive, social, emotional and behavioural symptoms, and outcomes can range from complete recovery to permanent disability or death.
- Causes include falling (accident), vehicle collisions and violence.
- Brain trauma occurs as a consequence of a sudden acceleration or deceleration within the cranium, or by a complex combination of both movement and sudden impact. In addition to the damage caused at the moment of injury, a variety of events following the injury may result in further injury. These processes include alterations in cerebral blood flow and intracranial pressure.
- Some of the imaging techniques used for diagnosis include computed tomography (CT) and magnetic resonance imaging (MRI).
- Preventive measures include use of seat belts and helmets, not drinking and driving, fall prevention efforts in older adults, and safety measures for children.
- Depending on the injury, treatment required may be minimal, or may include interventions such as medications, emergency surgery or surgery years later. Physical therapy, speech therapy, recreation therapy, occupational therapy and vision therapy may be employed for rehabilitation.
- TBI is a major cause of death and disability worldwide, especially in children and young adults. Males sustain traumatic brain injuries around twice as often as females. The 20th century saw developments in diagnosis and treatment that decreased mortality rate and improved outcomes.

Mechanism of Damage to Brain

- This is explained well by **Holbourn's hypothesis**:
  - In the case of a blow to the head, brain tissue gets injured when its constituent particles are pulled apart and do not join up subsequently. A shear strain type of deformation is thus produced in the brain tissue.
  - The forces transmitted from the skull to the brain act chiefly upon the surface of the brain. These forces are not evenly applied to the brain surface, but are maximally developed over those regions which are in close apposition to the projections of bony ridges or to the dural septa. Thus, these regions of the brain usually suffer more damage than other areas.
  - Actual physical disruption of cerebral tissue is caused by one of the following processes:
    - Compression of the constituent units while being forced together,
    - Tension in the units while being pulled apart and
    - Shifting or shear strain which causes adjacent units to move laterally.
- The brain can be damaged with or without skull fracture. Similarly, fracture of the skull can occur without damaging the brain.
  - In the case of a fractured skull, damage to the brain can sometimes result from fragments of bone.
  - Air can enter the ventricles from air sinuses leading to pneumocephalus.
  - Fracture of foramina can result in damage to cranial nerves.
  - Intracranial haemorrhages can occur from tearing of vessels following fractures, which further damages the brain by raising intracranial tension.
  - Bacterial entry can result in meningitis and brain abscesses.
- It is said that in general, injuries to the brain in the back of the head are more likely to be fatal than injuries to the brain in the front part of the skull.

Coup and Contrecoup Injury*

- A **coup injury** is one which occurs at the site of impact, while **contrecoup injury** occurs at a site opposite to the point of impact. For instance, a blow over the occiput may bruise the frontal poles of the brain.

**Note*: "Contrecoup" is spelt incorrectly in some books as "Counter Coup". There is no such term. The term "coup" and "contrecoup" are French for "blow" and "counter blow".*

- An impact on a stationary head causes the skull to move immediately in the direction of the force, but the brain lags behind for a brief period. The skull hits the brain at the site of impact leading to the development of a coup injury on the brain. This type of coup injury is referred to as an ***acceleration injury***. At the same time, vacuum is produced at the opposite site by the space created between the static brain and the forward displaced skull. This vacuum exerts a "suction effect" pulling the brain into that space to hit against the skull bone there, and thus producing injury to that part of brain leading to contrecoup injury formation.

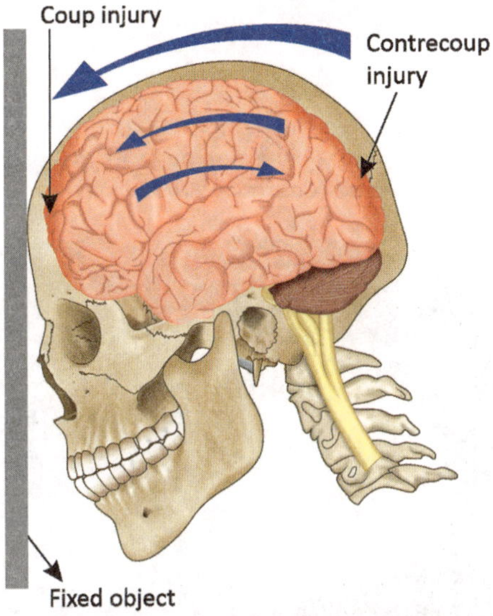

Fig. 3.98 Coup and contrecoup injury formation (*Courtesy*: *Patrick J Lynch*)

- Both coup and contrecoup injuries of brain can be in the form of contusions or lacerations.
- When a moving head strikes against a stationary object, the skull is suddenly brought to a stop by the impact, but the brain continues to move forward for a brief period, thereby hitting against the skull. This type of coup injury is termed a ***deceleration injury***.
- Forces leading to the rotation of skull cause the brain to slide or glide against fixed structures within the skull, resulting in shear strain injuries.
- Severe contrecoup injuries can result from a fall, even when coup injuries are absent or minimal.
- On the other hand, when the head is struck with an object, coup injuries are more common than contrecoup injuries. In a blow to a fixed head, contrecoup injuries may be totally absent.

Cerebral Concussion (Commotio Cerebri)

- This is a reversible or irreversible derangement of neuronal activity without demonstrable structural changes.
- Conventionally, cerebral concussion is clinically divided into three grades:
  - ***Grade I***: No loss of consciousness.
  - ***Grade II***: There is loss of consciousness, but for less than 5 minutes.
  - ***Grade III***: Unconsciousness for more than 5 minutes, associated with memory loss for more than 24 hours.
- In severe cases there can be total derangement of physiological activities leading to immediate death.
- In reversible cases, consciousness is regained.
- The cerebral irritation often due to cerebral oedema, manifests itself as constricted pupils, and altered blood pressure and respiration. Fluctuations in the level of consciousness can occur, as also post-traumatic and retrograde amnesia.
- During autopsy, the brain does not reveal any visible structural change. Occasionally, petechial haemorrhages may be seen.

Diffuse Neuronal Injury

- In this case, neurons and nerve fibres sustain injury in a diffuse manner when the force of impact is transmitted through the brain.
- This may be wholly or partly reversible.
- Rotational movements due to shear strains are the probable cause for this.

Diffuse Axonal Injury

- In this case, axons and vessels are disrupted as a result of impact. Deforming effect of shear strains is the main causative factor.
- **Diffuse axonal injury (DAI)** presents at the moment of impact.
  - **Mild grade** may present clinically as cerebral concussion.
  - **Severe grade** is associated with unconsciousness (without lucid interval). The coma usually lasts for more than six hours.
  - Additional clinical features that may be present include neurobehavioural manifestations, persistent vegetative state, and dementia.
  - At autopsy, petechial haemorrhages may be seen microscopically, due to damage to small blood vessels accompanying the axons. Occasionally, the petechiae may be seen even macroscopically. They are generally more frequent in the corpus callosum and over the dorsolateral aspects of pons, since these are the areas where axons are more susceptible to damage, due to greater length. Septum pellucidum and fornices may show tears leading to haemorrhages into lateral ventricles.
- Diffuse axonal and neuronal injuries are irreversible, and the damaged neurons are obliterated as time passes.

It is important to remember that the absence of histological changes in the brain differentiates cerebral concussion from diffuse neuronal and axonal injuries.

Cerebral Contusion

- Cerebral contusions are caused by blunt force injury to the head, and usually occur as circumscribed areas of brain

tissue destruction, resulting from extravasation of blood in traumatised tissues. They are often multiple and found mostly in the cortex, but may also occur in deeper tissues.
  - Cortical contusions are covered by a zone of intact cerebral tissue and are frequently wedge shaped. They are produced by distortion of skull, or by rotational movements of brain in relation to skull.
- Absorbed shock waves of trauma and penetrating injuries can also produce contusions.
- Subsequent infection can convert a contusion to a brain abscess.
- Older contusions appear yellow due to extravasated blood pigments. Occasionally, there may be cortical atrophy.

Cerebral Laceration

- Cerebral lacerations may occur with or without fractures of skull, and can be produced by the same mechanism as contusions.
- Lacerations are most commonly seen in regions of brain which are in close contact with projecting buttresses.
- Surface lacerations are accompanied by rupture of pia mater. Severed pial vessels can bleed and can increase the intracranial tension with fatal results.
- Healing occurs with gliosis, and cavities filled with yellow fluid may be formed in cases of extensive cell death.

Blood Vessels

Injury to intracranial blood vessels may manifest as any one of the following types of intracranial haemorrhages: **epidural (extradural)**, **subdural**, **subarachnoid**, **intracerebral** or **intraventricular haemorrhage**.

Epidural (Extradural) Haemorrhage (Figs. 3.99a & b)

- This type of haemorrhage occurs **between the skull and the dura mater** due to the rupture of diploic veins, venous sinuses or meningeal arteries. In the case of ruptured artery, the vessel most commonly involved is the **middle meningeal artery**, which usually gets cut at the sylvian point.
- A large haemorrhage (2 cm or more in thickness) in the extradural space leads to rapid compression of the brain, leading to fatal involvement of the vital centres in the medulla. The initial injury to the brain may cause unconsciousness due to cerebral concussion. Recovery may follow, but later the patient becomes unconscious due to compression of brain from accumulated blood. The intermediary period of consciousness between the two periods of unconsciousness is termed as **lucid interval**.* Because of this period of lucidity before death intervenes, it has been called "**Talk-and-die syndrome**".
- Extradural haemorrhage is almost always **traumatic**, and is more common in adults than in children.

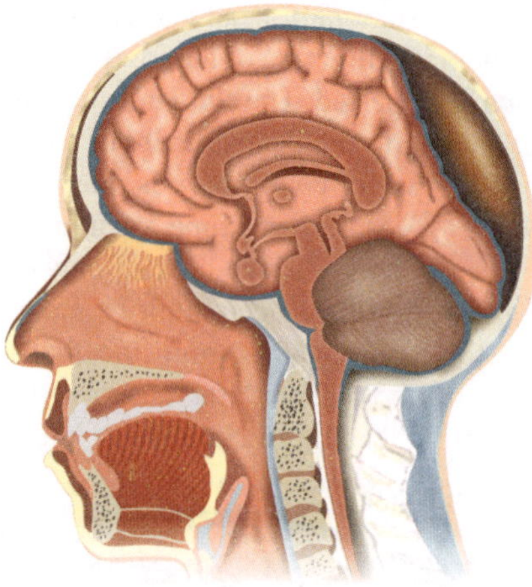

Fig. 3.99a Epidural haemorrhage in the occipital region (*Courtesy*: *Bruce Blaus*)

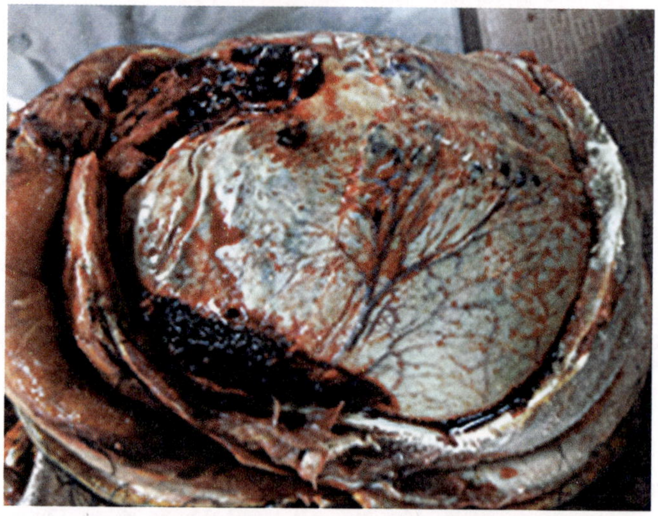

Fig. 3.99b Epidural haemorrhage in the frontal and temporal regions (*Courtesy*: *Dr Jagadish Rao PP*)

Subdural Haemorrhage (Fig. 3.100)

- This type of haemorrhage occurs **between the arachnoid and dura mater**. This could arise from tears in the dural venous sinuses or cortical veins, but the commonest cause is rupture of **bridging or communicating veins**.
- It can occur in either closed or open head injury.
  - Rapid accumulation of blood causing immediate brain compression is termed as **acute subdural haemorrhage**.
    - Unconsciousness, ipsilateral pupillary disturbance, hemianopia, speech defects, contralateral hemiparesis and urinary disturbance are the common features

**Note: This term is also used in forensic psychiatry, and refers to the period of sanity (lucidity) that is sometimes seen in a mentally ill person, during which period he appears to be quite normal. However, sooner or later he relapses into his original condition. Lucid interval in a mentally ill person is therefore totally unpredictable as to when it will occur, and how long it will last.*

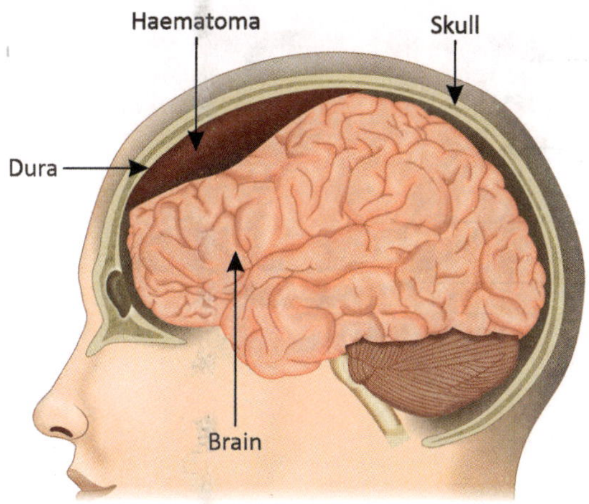

Fig. 3.100 Subdural haemorrhage in the fronto-parietal region

of acute subdural haemorrhage. Lucid interval is occasionally seen.

- In **subacute subdural haemorrhage**, the symptoms appear 2–14 days after injury.
- **Chronic subdural haemorrhage** takes several weeks for symptoms to commence, and the accumulation of blood is minimal to start with. Subsequent increase in the volume of the extravasation is characteristically slow.
    - Chronic subdural haemorrhage may either be symptomless, or manifest as recurrent headaches, convulsions (fits), altered mental status or focal neurological deficits such as aphasia, hemiparesis, etc.

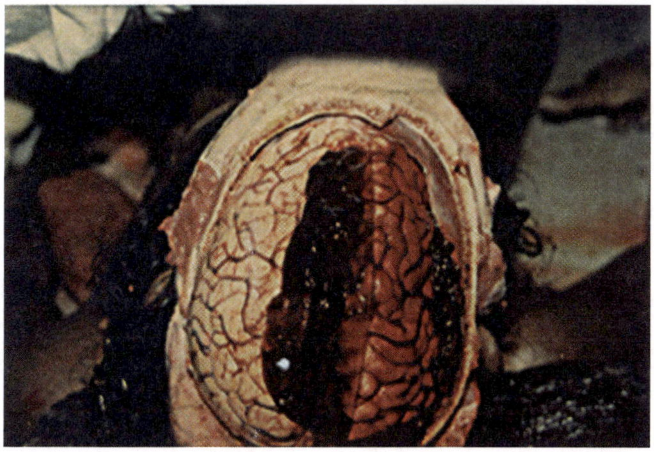

Fig. 3.101 Chronic subdural haematoma (*Courtesy*: *Dr Geetha O*)

- Subdural haemorrhage from natural causes is often bilateral, while the traumatic variety is usually unilateral.
- Subdural haematomas (**Fig. 3.101**) invariably become organised and encapsulated, into which bleeding can occur periodically from rupture of newly formed capillaries. Repeated bleeding and organisation causes progressive increase in size, and gives rise to a laminated appearance.

Subarachnoid Haemorrhage (Fig. 3.102)

- This type of haemorrhage occurs **between the arachnoid and the pia mater**, and usually arises from the rupture of **cerebral arteries** or **cerebral veins**. Blows to the neck can cause lacerations of vertebral artery with dissection of blood superiorly into subarachnoid space.
- The blood mixes with the CSF and gets distributed over the whole of the brain surface.
- Subarachnoid haematoma formation is extremely rare.
- Spontaneous subarachnoid haemorrhage can occur from natural causes as in rupture of congenital (berry) or infective (mycotic) aneurysms, in arteriovenous malformations, and also in bleeding disorders. **Berry aneurysms** are most common in the region of the **arterial circle of Willis** at the base of the brain. Even minor trauma can precipitate subarachnoid haemorrhage, if the arteries are weak, as in atherosclerosis. Minor trauma can also rupture basilar arteries in chronic alcoholics.
- Subarachnoid haemorrhage is said to be the most common intracranial lesion following head injury.
- It can be unilateral or bilateral, and may be localised or diffuse.
- Blood in the subarachnoid space is usually removed by phagocytosis, following the lysis of blood cells. About 1 month after injury, only yellowish brown areas of discolouration of the arachnoid may be left behind, which are referred to as **plaques jaunes**.

Intracerebral Haemorrhage

- This may be either a **parenchymatous haemorrhage**, or an **intraventricular haemorrhage**.
    - **Parenchymatous Haemorrhage (Fig. 3.103)**
        - This refers to haemorrhage in the brain tissue, and may arise directly from the trauma, in which case it usually occurs near the surface. It may be punctate, echymotic or larger (haematoma).
        - A single deep-seated parenchymatous haemorrhage is usually due to a disease process, and is often located in the internal capsule, basal ganglia or pons.
        - Multiple punctate haemorrhages may be seen in bleeding disorders, leukaemias, septicaemia, typhus, Caisson's disease, fat embolism and Wernicke's encephalopathy.
        - Traumatic intracerebral haemorrhages may or may not be associated with skull fracture.
        - Those haemorrhages occurring along the axis of transmission of mechanical force from coup site to the contrecoup site are termed **intermediate coup lesions**.
        - Occasionally, it takes several days for the haemorrhage to develop after a traumatic episode.
        - Sudden death is uncommon.
        - Minute haemorrhages occurring in the brain of a boxer due to repeated punches on the head can lead to mental changes and unsteady gait. This is called **punch drunkenness**.

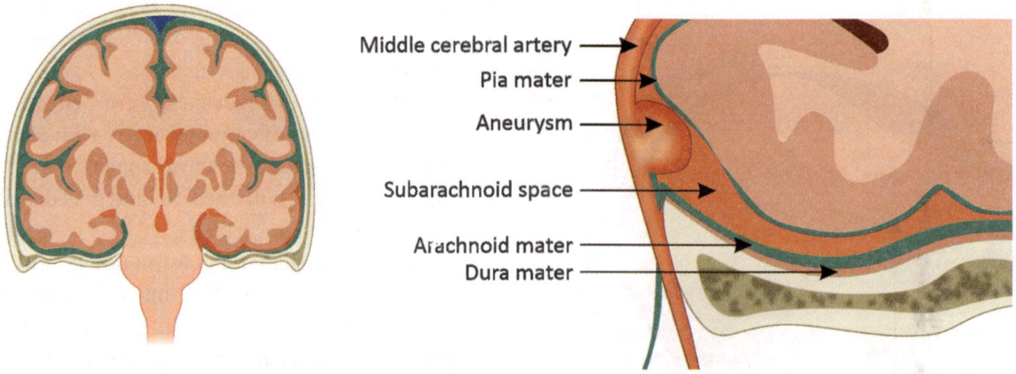

Fig. 3.102 Subarachnoid haemorrhage

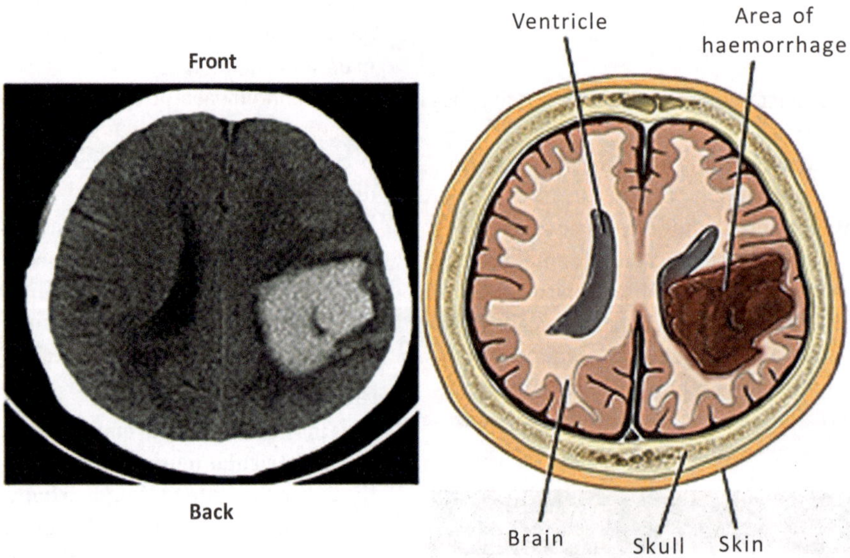

Fig. 3.103 Intracerebral (parenchymatous) haemorrhage – CT scan (L); Illustration (R)

- Today, this is referred to as **chronic traumatic encephalopathy**, or "**CTE**". It is an example of the cumulative damage that can occur as the result of multiple concussions or less severe blows to the head. The condition was previously referred to as "**dementia pugilistica**", or "**punch drunk**" syndrome, as it was first noted in boxers.
- The disease can lead to cognitive and physical handicaps such as Parkinsonism, speech and memory problems, slowed mental processing, tremor, depression and inappropriate behaviour. It shares features with Alzheimer's disease.
- **CTE** has been most commonly found in professional athletes participating in American football, rugby, ice hockey, boxing, professional wrestling, stunt performing, bull riding and other contact sports who have experienced repeated concussions or other brain trauma.
- Symptoms of **CTE** generally begin 8–10 years after experiencing repetitive mild traumatic brain injury.
  - **First stage** symptoms include deterioration in attention as well as disorientation, dizziness and headaches.
  - **Second stage** symptoms include memory loss, social instability, erratic behaviour and poor judgment.
  - **Third** and **fourth stages** include progressive dementia, slowing of muscular movements, impeded speech, tremors, vertigo, deafness and suicidality.
  - **Additional symptoms** include dysarthria, dysphagia and ocular abnormalities – such as ptosis.
  - This condition was first described by a Nigerian neuropathologist **Dr Bennet Omalu (Fig. 3.103A)** who worked on the case of American

football player Mike Webster, who had died following unusual and unexplained behaviour. The Hollywood film 'Concussion' (**Fig. 3.103B**) is a gripping drama film on Dr Omalu's groundbreaking discovery.

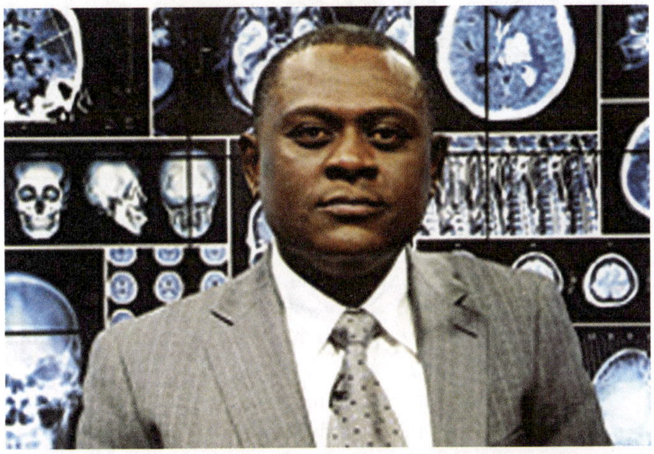

Fig. 3.103A Dr Bennet Omalu

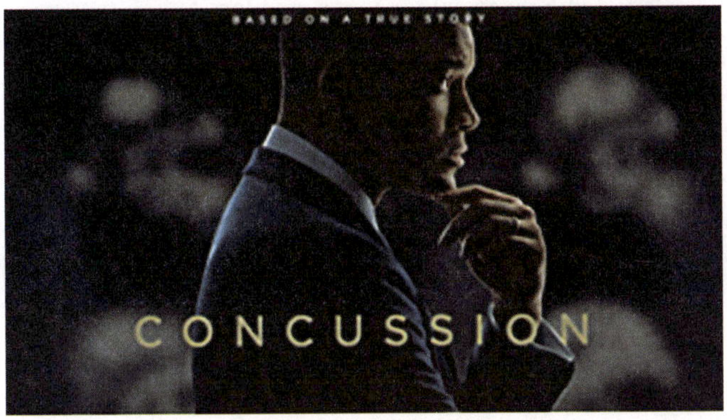

Fig. 3.103B Will Smith in the film 'Concussion'

- **Intraventricular Haemorrhage (Fig. 3.104)**
  - It is a collection of blood within the ventricular system, and may be associated with intracerebral or subarachnoid haemorrhage.

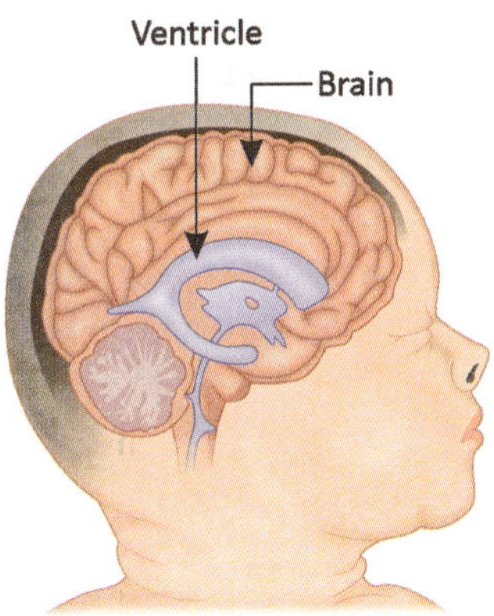

Fig. 3.104 Location of intraventricular haemorrhage

- However, it can occur as an isolated event, e.g., severe trauma, vascular malformations of choroid plexus, etc.
- When massive, intraventricular haemorrhage can be fatal due to impairment of circulation of cerebrospinal fluid and resultant hydrocephalus.

Face

- Injuries of face which cause permanent disfiguration represent **grievous hurt**. Such permanent disfiguration may be due to scar or keloid formation, or due to derangement or loss of tissues.
- **Le Fort fractures** are types of facial fractures involving the maxillary bone and surrounding structures in a usually bilateral and either horizontal, pyramidal or transverse way. Le Fort fractures are classic in facial trauma.
- Pulping of face can result from vehicular run-over injury, or blunt impact by a heavy stone.

Mouth and Nose

- Abrasions and contusions in or around the mouth and nose could suggest forceful opening of the mouth to administer something, or forcible closure of mouth and nose as in smothering. Superficial lacerations of inner aspects of lips can occur due to forceful apposition of lips against the teeth, especially against the free edges of the latter.
- Injuries to lips can also result from blunt impact such as fisting.
- Occasionally, the lips or nose may be cut off or bitten off as a revengeful act.
- Blunt trauma as in the case of a fall or blow, can cause injuries to nasal bones and teeth. Injuries which lead to fracture of jaw bones or nasal bones, or fracture/dislocation of teeth constitute grievous hurt, and are often accompanied by contusions or lacerations of lips and gums. If the cribriform plate of ethmoid bone is fractured, anosmia may result.
- Partial detachment of nasal mucous membrane leading to nasal bleeding occasionally occurs after blunt trauma to head, even without direct involvement of nose.

Eyes and Ears

- The term **black eye** refers to accumulation of blood around the eyeball and eyelids which manifests as a darkish discolouration around the eye. This can occur directly from blunt trauma over the eye, or indirectly as an **ectopic contusion** especially from the scalp.
- Trauma can also cause injuries to cornea, iris, lens and retina, or haemorrhage into anterior chamber. Retinal detachment and traumatic cataract are not uncommon sequelae of trauma.
- Penetrating injuries occasionally involve the eyes, sometimes leading to evisceration.
- Infections of eyeballs can spread to the brain and can lead to death by cavernous sinus thrombosis or meningitis. The uninvolved eye may suffer from sympathetic ophthalmia, leading to blindness of both eyes.

- Injury leading to permanent loss of vision of either eye or loss of hearing of either ear constitutes grievous hurt.
- Ears may be cut or chopped off, or bitten away as an act of revenge, or to forcibly remove ear rings.
- Abrasions, contusions and lacerations can occur to one or both ears, from accidents of different kinds.
- A hard blow to the ear can rupture the tympanic membrane and cause deafness.

Cheek

- Abrasions, contusions and lacerations of cheek can occur from blunt trauma.
- Bite marks can result from an assault, or may be the offshoot (ironically) of an act of love (*love bite*)!
- Cheek bones (malar bones) can fracture from direct or indirect violence. The fracture line in such cases is usually horizontal, and involves the posterior third of the malar skeleton.

Jaws

- Fractures of mandible are commonly vertical, and invariably result from direct trauma, e.g., fisting.
- A blow to the point of the chin can indirectly cause a **ring fracture** of the base of the skull.
- Comminuted fracture of the maxilla is not an uncommon occurrence in blunt force injuries to the face.
- Occasionally, there may be transmission of force to the cranial cavity leading to intracranial haemorrhages.
- Blood and dislocated teeth resulting from fracture of jaw bones may be ingested or even inhaled causing choking and death.

Neck

- Superficial wounds of the neck may or may not cause serious bleeding, but penetrating wounds (**Fig. 3.105**), incised wounds and deep lacerations produce copious bleeding due to severance of carotid and jugular vessels.
- Direct impact to hypopharynx can fracture the thyroid cartilage.
- Hyoid bone can fracture from blunt impacting force, or from blunt constricting force, as in hanging or strangulation. Scratch abrasions in the form of nail marks are good indicators of throttling (manual strangulation), while a pressure abrasion in the form of a ligature mark is pathognomonic for hanging or strangulation.
- A blow on the front of neck can precipitate vagal inhibition which can result in sudden unconsciousness or death.
- Choking due to blood can result from injuries to trachea and larynx.
- Laryngeal oedema is another serious complication of trauma to these areas.
- Incised wounds of the throat are not uncommon. Such **cut-throat wounds**, can be suicidal, homicidal or rarely accidental.
  - In a **suicidal** case, the person usually holds the weapon in his right hand and starts the incision from the left side of neck drawing it to the right. Tailing of the wound is therefore seen on the right side.

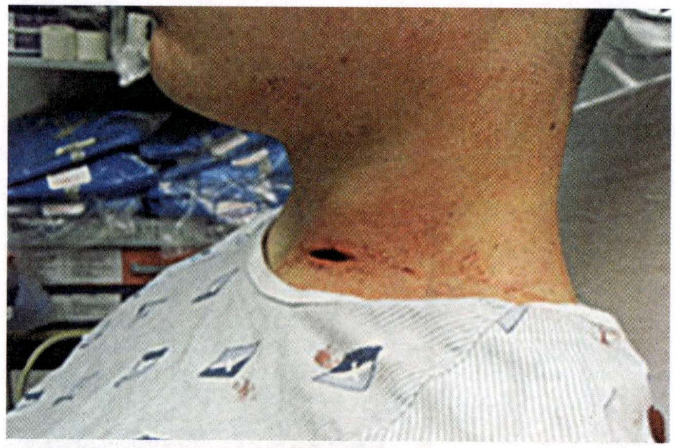

Fig. 3.105 Stab wound in the neck

  - Thyroid membrane and muscles are usually cut and the wound slopes towards the floor of the mouth.
  - Carotid arteries are not frequently injured as they slip backwards when the head is extended.
  - Bleeding is usually venous, and loss of consciousness is gradual.
  - However, death may take place quickly from air embolism, due to air being sucked in by negative pressure in the veins.
  - A person attempting suicide generally makes repeated horizontal, parallel, shallow, half-hearted cuts on the neck initially, before he picks up enough courage to make the final lethal cut sweeping across the neck. These preliminary shallow cuts which merge with the main wound represent hesitation or nervousness, and are therefore called **hesitation cuts**, **exploratory cuts**, **feeler strokes** or **tentative cuts**.
  - A **homicidal** cut throat wound is invariably very deep, and obviously lacks hesitation cuts. The direction is usually horizontal. The wound is often situated at the lower part of the neck (**Fig. 3.106**) and slopes away from the floor of the mouth. Carotid arteries are often severed.
  - Sometimes, air from wounded respiratory passages enters into the subcutaneous space resulting in ***subcutaneous emphysema***, which may dissect down into the mediastinum leading to ***mediastinal emphysema*** with respiratory obstruction.
  - The dome of the pleura, if penetrated through the neck can cause pneumothorax.
  - Aphonia and hoarseness of voice can occur, if recurrent laryngeal nerve is involved, resulting in the cadaveric position of vocal cords. Speech is impossible in cases of open wounds of larynx and trachea below the level of the vocal cords.
  - Injuries to postero-lateral aspect of neck can involve the brachial plexus leading to loss of function of the arm or hand.

- Infections from neck can spread to the mediastinum and cause a mediastinal abscess.

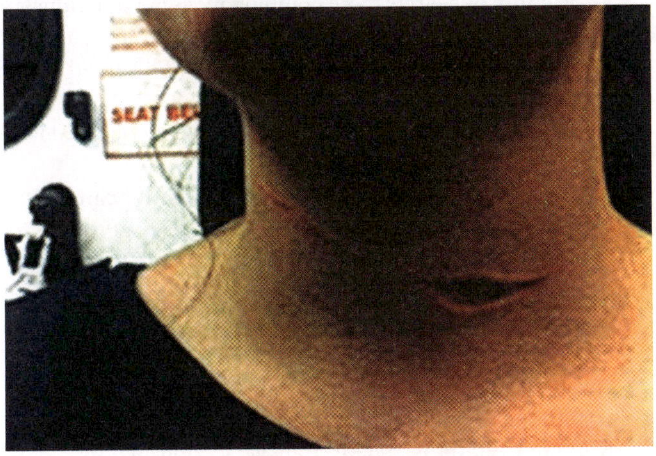

Fig. 3.106 Attempted homicidal cut throat injury

Table 3.18 summarises the salient differences between suicidal and homicidal cut-throat injury.

Chest

- Chest, although very elastic, becomes more fixed as age advances, and what would have been merely a temporary alteration in shape which would return to normal, will fracture under compression.
- External and internal injuries of chest often coexist, though this need not be the case always. Thus, serious internal injuries can occur without any external evidence of the same.
- Impact of a considerable nature can give rise to alternate compression and decompression. This leads to initial congestion followed by laceration and haemorrhage due to rupture of lung alveoli. Such sudden and swiftly acting trauma may not leave behind any external manifestation, but can still prove fatal after a lapse of time.
- Injuries of the chest may be penetrating ('open') or non-penetrating ('closed').

Chest Wall

- Breasts are common sites for wounds originating from a sexual act, e.g., nail marks and love bites.
- As far as fractures of ribs are concerned, they usually occur in regions of maximum stretch.
  - Thus, anteroposterior compression of chest which causes maximum stretch at mid-axillary level produces fractures in the mid-axillary line, while side-to-side compression causes maximum stretch at the necks and costochondral junctions resulting in fractures at these sites.
  - The 4th to 8th ribs are the commonest ribs to fracture. However, localised blunt trauma with reasonable force can involve any rib at any site.
  - Fractured ends of ribs sometimes project outwards or inwards causing injuries to the overlying or underlying membranes, tissues, muscles or organs.
  - Multiple rib fractures may give rise to **flail chest** or **stove-in chest** with consequent paradoxical respiration (**Fig. 3.107**).
  - Osteoporosis, osteomalacia and secondary malignancy are associated with fragility and easy fracture of ribs.
  - 3rd to 5th ribs of left side are often involved in external cardiac massage. Such fractures usually occur at costochondral junctions and are associated with negligible amount of blood infiltration.
  - Sternum is a bone which is not easily fractured. But, it can fracture from direct local force as in the case of an impact with the steering wheel of a vehicle in a collision accident. Such fractures usually occur at or near the

Table 3.18 Differences between Suicidal and Homicidal Cut-throat Wounds

Feature	Suicidal	Homicidal
Number	Usually multiple, of varying severity and depth	Single or multiple deep wounds
Hesitation cuts	Present	Absent
Tailing	Usually to the right	Either side
Slope	Towards the floor of the mouth	Away from the floor of the mouth
Position	Upper part of neck	Lower part of neck
Depth	Less	More
Direction	Usually oblique	Horizontal or oblique
Carotid arteries	Usually intact	Frequently cut
Bleeding	Usually venous	Mainly arterial

manubrio-sternal junction. Fractures of sternum are usually transverse in nature. Forces which result in hyperflexion or hyperextension of sternum are likely to result in fracture.

- Lacerated wounds involving chest wall and parietal pleura can lead to "open" pneumothorax.
- Severe blows on the chest wall may produce concussion of the chest, shock and death, even in the absence of structural damage to the viscera.

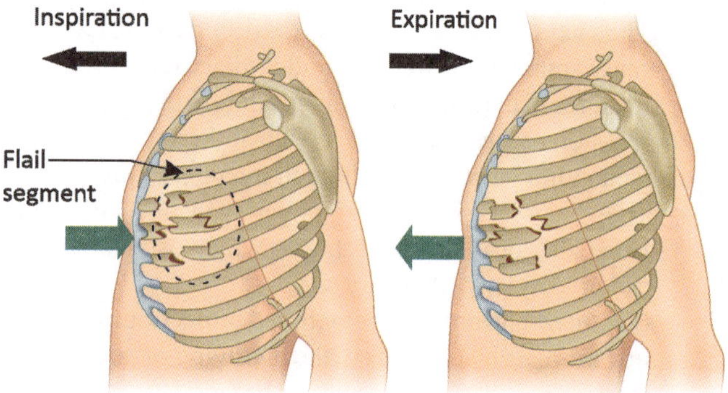

Fig. 3.107 Flail chest

Chest Cavity

- The lungs or the heart may get injured by blunt force applied on the chest, or from penetrating forces. They are especially susceptible to contusions (**Fig. 3.108**) or lacerations.
- Lung injury can be gross or microscopic, focal or diffuse, and located centrally or peripherally, or both. Trauma of substantial degree can produce multiple lacerations of lung (**Fig. 3.109**), or a single large irregular cavity, the latter being termed "traumatic cavitation." The pleura may or may not remain intact. Injury to lungs can result in pneumothorax, haemothorax, haemopneumothorax, interstitial and subcutaneous emphysema, mediastinal emphysema or obstruction of air passages. An injured lung may collapse.
- Injury to heart, especially stab injury, can result in serious consequences. As far as bleeding is concerned, injuries of atria are more dangerous than of ventricles, and those of right ventricle more dangerous than of left ventricle. The right ventricle is more prone for injuries, since it forms the major part of anterior surface of heart. If the injury to the heart is obliquely placed, there could be flap formation as a result of which bleeding is minimised, since the flap acts as a valve of occlusion during contraction of heart.
  - Penetrating injuries of heart inevitably penetrate the pericardium leading to accumulation of blood in the pericardial sac (**haemopericardium**) (**Fig. 3.110**), and subsequent escape from pericardial sac to pleural cavity (**haemothorax**).
  - In blunt injuries, the pericardium usually remains intact, while the heart itself may rupture leading to development of haemopericardium. Rapid accumulation of as little as 250–350 cc of blood can cause **cardiac tamponade**, i.e., progressive limitation of the pumping action of heart and eventual cardiac arrest.
  - Rupture of heart is more common in young individuals. Right atrium is most commonly involved in traumatic rupture, followed by right ventricle. A diseased heart may rupture even with trivial trauma.
  - In the old, blunt injuries can precipitate myocardial infarction.
  - Blunt injuries can also cause contusion of heart walls, septae, and papillary muscles. They can give rise to ventricular fibrillation or progressive circulatory failure.
  - In the case of a pericardial tear, the heart can herniate through it and get compressed – ***strangulation of heart***.
- Oesophagus, trachea, bronchi, bronchioles, aorta, vena cavae and pulmonary arteries can be injured by blunt or penetrating trauma.
- Rupture of aorta is usually transverse, and may be complete or partial (involving only the intima). It frequently occurs at the junction of the arch with the descending part.
- Ruptures of oesophagus usually occur in the form of longitudinal splits.
- The most common site of rupture of diaphragm due to blunt trauma is at or around the central tendon of the left side.

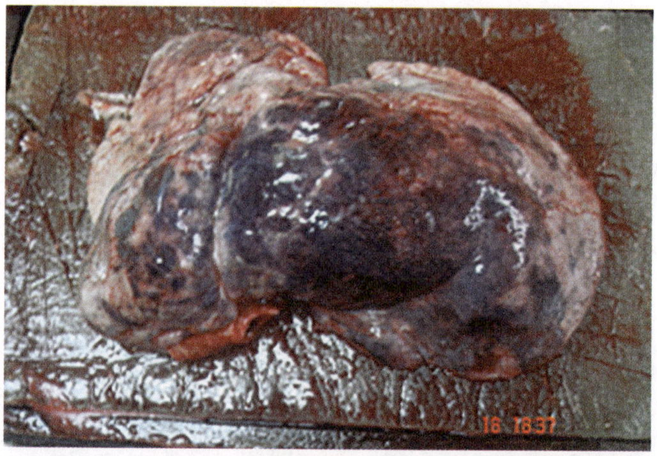

Fig. 3.108 Contused lung (*Courtesy*: *Dr Prateek Rastogi*)

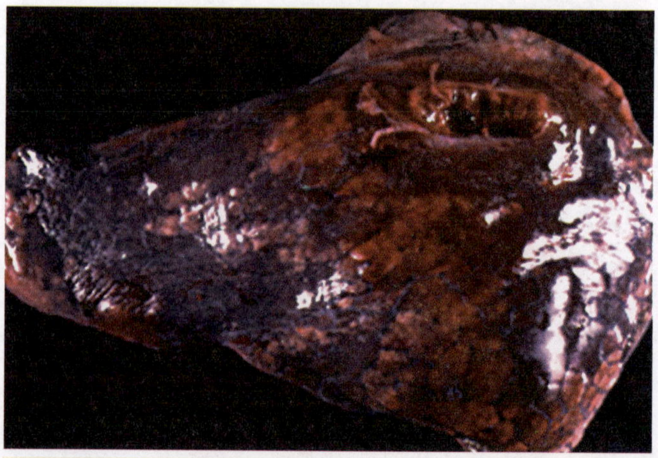

Fig. 3.109 Lacerated lung

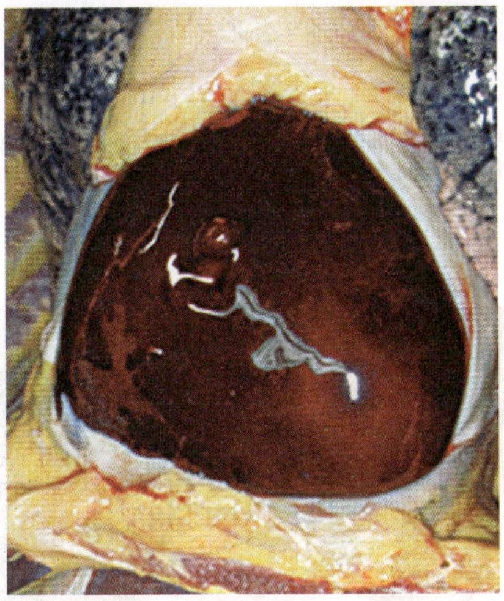

Fig. 3.110 Haemopericardium (*Courtesy: Dr Zachariah Thomas*)

Immediate or delayed herniation of abdominal viscera into the chest can occur in such a case.

- Injury to thoracic duct can lead to **chylothorax**.

Abdomen and Pelvis

Abdominal Wall

- The anterior abdominal wall easily yields to pressure, and hence usually escapes unscathed from blunt trauma. Contusion of anterior abdominal wall is therefore very rare, except in severe crushing injury as in the case of run-over injury by a vehicle. However, abrasions occur quite commonly.
- Following are some important points worth remembering:
    - Blunt trauma can result in extensive injuries of abdominal viscera even in the absence of any external injury.
    - The actual total depth of a penetrating wound of the abdomen can be exaggerated due to the yielding nature of anterior abdominal wall.
    - A blow to abdomen can cause death due to vagal inhibition.

Viscera

Oesophagus, Stomach and Intestines

- Rupture of stomach usually occurs in the pyloric region along the lesser curvature. This is due to deficient muscular layer in this region, as well as due to lesser elasticity. Since stomach wall can be contused from blunt trauma, delayed rupture can occur in such contused areas. Spontaneous rupture of stomach is extremely rare.
- Dissolution of distal end of oesophagus (oesophagomalacia), gastric fundus (gastric malacia) or both, may take place in some persons hours or days after sustaining cerebral trauma. This is believed to be brought about by neurogenic stimuli arising from the parasympatholytic centre of diencephalon.
- Intestines can rupture from blunt force either at the point of impact, or some distance away. The former shows clean edges, while the latter has a ragged appearance. Transverse ruptures of mesentery can lead to gangrene of a segment of intestine by transecting the supplying artery.

Liver and Spleen

- **Liver** is an organ which is very vulnerable to injury.
    - Laceration (**Fig. 3.111**) or rupture mainly occurs over anterior and inferior surfaces of the right lobe. The direction of rupture depends upon the direction of pressure. For example, if the force compresses the lower part of the liver, a transverse rupture results. If the right lobe alone is compressed, a vertical rupture occurs between right and left lobes.
    - Hepatic ruptures can be transcapsular, subcapsular, or central (**Fig. 3.112**).
    - Ribs can also cause injury to liver.
    - Diseased liver (e.g., due to fatty change, malaria, etc.), ruptures easily by trauma.
    - Ruptured liver usually causes substantial haemoperitoneum.

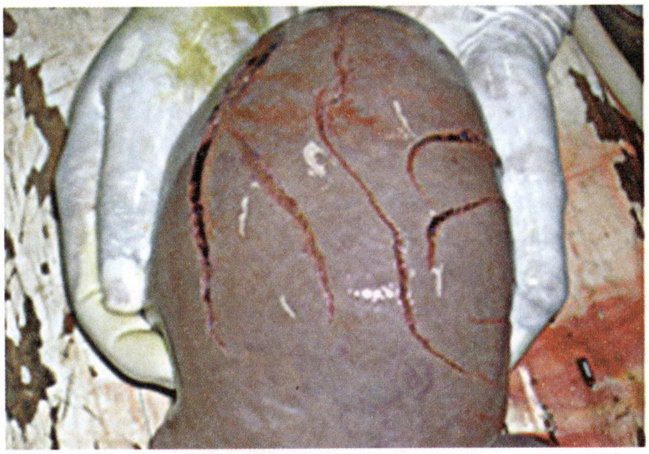

Fig. 3.111 Lacerated liver (*Courtesy*: *Dr Hareesh S Gouda*)

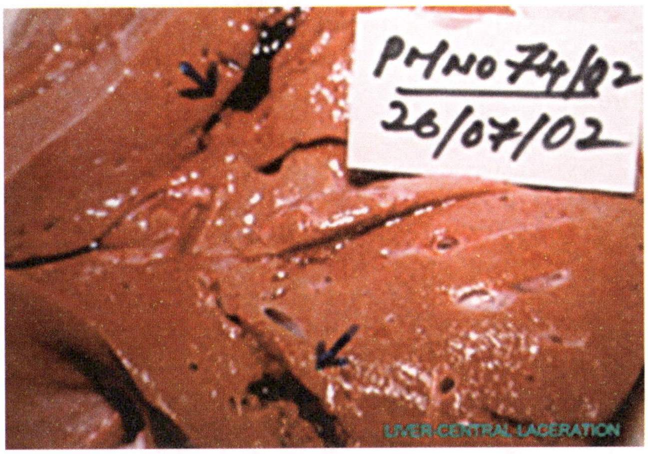

Fig. 3.112 Cut-section of liver – central laceration (*Courtesy*: *Dr Shashidhar C Mestri*)

- **Spleen** is easily injured from trauma due to either blunt force or penetrating injury.
  - The degree of damage varies from laceration of capsule to pulverisation. Bleeding is characteristically profuse.
  - Malarial or leukaemic spleen is extremely susceptible to traumatic rupture. Such a diseased spleen can sometimes rupture in situations of strong muscular contractions as in coughing or defaecation.
  - The concave surface is more prone for rupture.
  - Splenic ruptures result in haemoperitoneum.
  - Ribs can cause laceration of spleen.

Urinary Tract

- Rupture of urinary bladder often accompanies pelvic fractures, especially if the bladder happened to be full at the time of the incident. Even violent muscular contractions can lead to rupture of a full bladder.
- Ruptured bladder is usually accompanied by extraperitoneal extravasation of urine or blood.
- Shock, bleeding, peritonitis and urinary tract infection are common complications.
- Urethra usually ruptures in the region of the membraneous part, and may accompany pelvic fracture, or result from the application of blunt force in the perineum. Female urethra may be ruptured during a violent act of rape. Falling astride a projecting object is a frequent reason for rupture of male urethra.
- Lacerations of the kidneys can be transcapsular, subcapsular or transrenal.

Genitalia

- External genitalia can suffer different types of injuries, especially related to violent sexual act or sexual jealousy.
- Squeezing the testicles can be fatal due to reflex cardiac inhibition.
- Criminal amputation of male genitalia can cause death from bleeding.
- Self-inflicted injuries to genitalia are sometimes encountered in mentally ill persons.
- Attempted criminal abortion or self-introduction of foreign objects can lead to injuries of female genitalia.

Limbs

- Any type of wound can occur to the limbs, from blunt injuries to sharp incisions. Direct and indirect trauma can produce different types of injuries to muscles. Tetanus, gas gangrene and renal failure may follow.
- Muscles may sustain severe crush injuries even though the skin may be intact (due to elasticity of the latter). Thighs with intact skin can accommodate even up to one litre of blood resulting from rupture of vessels due to a crushing force. This can be fatal. Even multiple superficial soft tissue injuries due to blows or kicks can cause death, though the bones may be intact. Ligaments can undergo avulsion.
- Blunt injury to the limbs is extremely common, especially in traffic accidents. Fracture of femur or the bones of the lower leg resulting from the impact of a vehicle against a pedestrian is often referred to as a **bumper fracture**.
- Wounds sustained by a victim while trying to defend himself from an attack by raising his hands (**Fig. 3.113**), or attempting to wrest the weapon away from the assailant (**Fig. 3.114**), are called **defence wounds**. They are usually seen on the palms, and inner aspects of forearms.

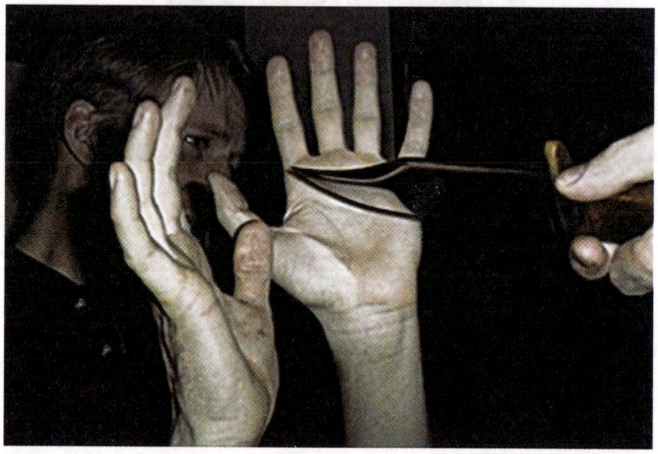

Fig. 3.113 Mode of sustaining defence wound in a knife attack

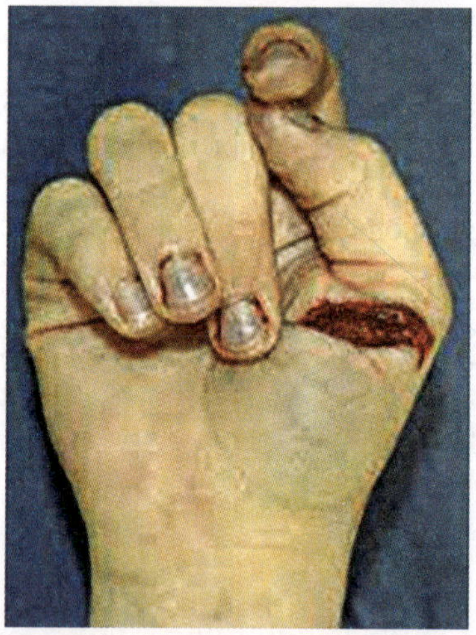

Fig. 3.114 Defence wound sustained when trying to grasp weapon in a knife attack

Vertebral Column

- A useful categorization of vertebral column injuries is to divide them into fractures, dislocations and fracture-dislocations. Such injuries can occur to the vertebral column due to direct or indirect mechanical force, which may or may not involve the spinal cord.
- Commonest site of traumatic damage to the vertebral column is the lumbar region.
- Spinal cord is rarely injured without associated fractures of vertebral column.

- A sudden drop from a height of more than 5–7 feet in a case of hanging can cause dislocation between 2nd and 3rd, or 3rd and 4th cervical vertebrae, resulting in sudden death. Dislocation of atlas, with or without fracture of odontoid process, is a potentially lethal injury.
- Fractures of vertebrae can be one of the following three types:
  - ***Wedge compression fracture*** (vertebral bodies are compressed from above and below)
  - ***Comminuted fracture***
  - ***Fracture-dislocation*** (sliding of one vertebra over another).
- A direct impact usually causes comminuted fracture, while an indirect impact, as in a fall on the feet or buttocks causes wedge compression fracture.
- Hyperflexion or hyperextension of neck can result in cervical vertebral column injury and is called **whiplash injury** (**Fig. 3.115**):
  - It is due to sudden strain affecting nerves, bones, muscles, discs, and tendons of the neck due to a sudden and violent jerk of the neck forwards and backwards. As a result, the muscles and nerves may be torn or stretched, and bones slightly displaced, thus irritating nerves, interfering with blood flow and nerve impulse transmissions.
  - Whiplash injury can be extremely uncomfortable and may last for some time. The symptoms may appear immediately or after several weeks.
  - Common symptoms include dizziness, headaches; stiffness of neck, jaw, shoulder or arm; pain in the neck, shoulder, upper limb or lower back; numbness including pins and needles in upper arm, diminished ability to bend, nausea, vomiting, blurred vision, ringing in ears, lack of concentration, memory loss, tiredness, sleeplessness and irritability.
  - Fatal contusion or laceration of the spinal cord can occur in whiplash injuries in the absence of any fracture of the vertebral column. Involvement of the cord above the level of the 5th cervical vertebra can be fatal due to damage to phrenic nerve. Lower level involvement can cause quadriplegia.

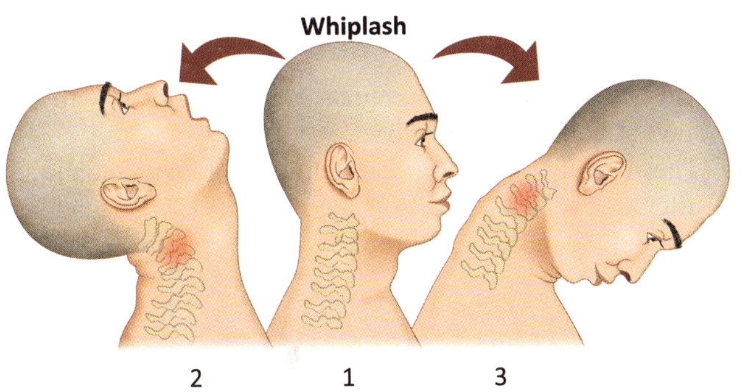

Fig. 3.115 Mechanism of whiplash

- Paraplegia, quadriplegia, and respiratory and urinary infections invariably follow vertebral column and spinal cord injuries.
- Sacral segment involvement can lead to impotence in a male victim.
- Blunt force over vertebral column can lead to concussion of spinal cord without visible injury to vertebrae. This is called **railway (railroad) spine** due to its frequent occurrence in railway accidents. Commonest region affected is the lumbo-sacral spine resulting in paraplegia, bladder disturbances and impotence. Since concussion is spontaneously reversible, these abnormalities are usually only temporary.

FM 3.12: Core – Written/ Viva Voce/
OSCE (Objective Structured Clinical Examination)/
OSPE (Objective Structured Practical Examination)
- **Regional injuries:**
  - Describe and discuss
    - Injuries related to fall from height
    - Vehicular injuries
      - Primary and secondary impact injuries
      - Secondary injuries
      - Crush syndrome
      - Railway spine

REGIONAL INJURIES

Fall from Height*

- **Situations/Causes:**
  - Fall from tall trees.
  - Fall from high-rise buildings/bridges: The victims are usually construction workers. Suicides constitute only a minority of these cases.
- Two types of injury result from falls from heights: injury resulting from **direct impact** and **deceleration** injury. The injuries resulting from direct impact are mostly fractures. The body position at the time of impact is very crucial. The deceleration forces immediately post-impact, result primarily in visceral and internal injury, including cerebral injury.
- Height of descent, body landing position, impact surface and clothing worn by the victim, all have varying effect on the extent and distribution of skeletal injuries, soft tissue injuries and visceral damage.
- Most of the severe injuries are sustained at the site of primary impact.
- In the majority of cases, the site of primary impact is the head, followed by trunk impact and buttock impact. Incidence of leg impact is usually less.

****Source***: Adapted partly from Jagannatha SR, Pradeep Kumar MV, Naveen Kumar T, Ananda K, Venkatesha VT. Injuries due to fall from height – a retrospective study. J Forensic Med Toxicol. 2010;27:47–50.*

- Head injury takes the form of fractures, intracranial bleeds and brain injury.
- Fractures of spine are quite common:
  - Cervical and upper thoracic spine is usually affected in primary head impact, while lower thoracic and lumbar vertebrae are involved in primary trunk impact.
  - Fracture of sacrum is a salient feature in buttock impacts.
  - In leg impacts, cervical vertebrae are commonly involved. This is due to transmission of force from the feet upwards through the vertebral column.
- Fracture of ribs is often seen in primary trunk impacts, usually at three sites: front, back and the posterior axillary line. The side of trunk impact can be found out from the sites of rib fracture. Fracture of clavicle and sternum are frequently seen associated with rib fractures. Sternal fractures are invariably associated with injuries to lungs and heart.
- Fractures of humerus, ulna and radius are also seen in many cases. As also, pelvic fractures, which are especially common in primary buttock impact. Fracture of femur is more common in primary leg impacts. Fracture of lower leg bones is less common. Fracture of calcaneum is an indication of feet impact (**Fig. 3.116**).
- Visceral injuries are common, involving internal organs like lungs, heart, liver, spleen, intestines and urinary bladder. Rupture of heart and aorta can occur. Liver injuries are most often encountered in primary trunk and buttock impacts. Injury to kidneys is rare.
- **Medicolegal Importance**:
  - Falls from heights are most commonly due to accidents in children.
  - Suicide among adolescents and adults – usually by jumping from a high rise building or a bridge.
  - Accidental falls among construction workers, tree climbers (toddy tappers, fruit pickers).
  - Homicide (rare) – pushing or throwing somebody off a high rise building.

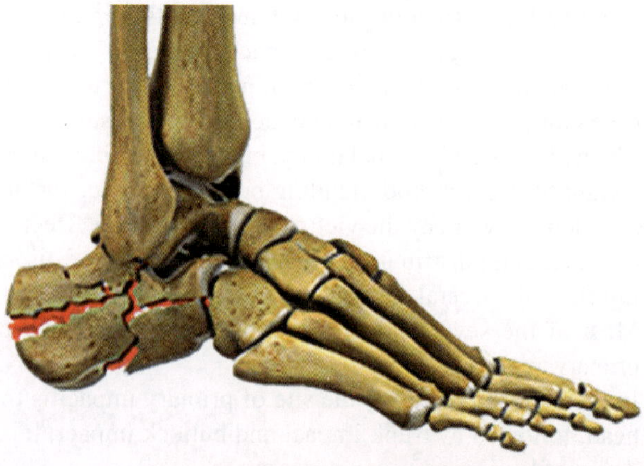

Fig. 3.116 Fracture of calcaneum – fall from height

Vehicular Injuries

Road Traffic Accidents

- Numerically, **road traffic accidents** account for the great majority of accidental deaths world-wide.
- The purpose of forensic examination in traffic accidents is to determine the nature and manner of causation of injuries on a pedestrian, or the occupant or rider of a vehicle. At times, it may be necessary to reconstruct the details of an accident on the basis of the pattern of injuries, especially if there are no eyewitnesses.
- In traffic accidents, apart from examination of injuries sustained, a doctor has to observe whether the driver or pedestrian was suffering from any disease or disability, or if there is evidence of intoxication, and if so, whether the accident could have been a result of that.
- Identification of the vehicle involved in a **hit and run** case may be assisted by looking for trace evidence that is likely to have been exchanged between the victim and vehicle at the time of impact (**Locard's principle of exchange**).

Pedestrian Injuries

Classification

- Primary impact injuries
- Secondary impact injuries
- Tertiary impact injuries (*formerly called "Secondary injuries"*)
- Run over injuries

Primary Impact Injuries

- These are produced by the initial contact with the vehicle, and may be in the form of abrasions, lacerations or contusions. Occasionally, patterned injuries are seen.
- Often, legs may get fractured in the region of impact with the bumper of the vehicle, usually tibia-fibula (**bumper fracture**).
- Direct impact on the thorax not only results in fracture, but also may rupture the aorta.
  Direct impact on the hips may cause fracture of the vertebral column and pelvis.

Secondary Impact Injuries

- They are caused by subsequent contact of body with vehicle after the primary impact.
- They usually result from the victim being flung into the air after the primary impact and subsequently landing against the hood, windscreen or roof of the vehicle.
- Head injuries are common.

Tertiary Impact Injuries

- These injuries are caused by striking against objects or surfaces other than the vehicle, such as the kerb, road surface or street poles.
- Grazed abrasions, flaying injuries, etc., due to being dragged on the road are common (**Fig. 3.119**).

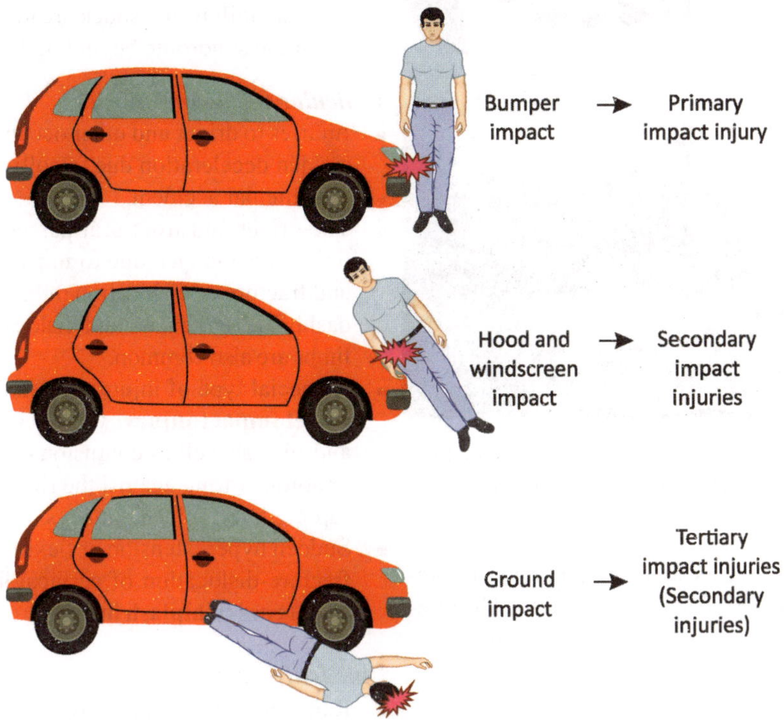

Fig. 3.117 Mode of sustaining primary and secondary impact injuries

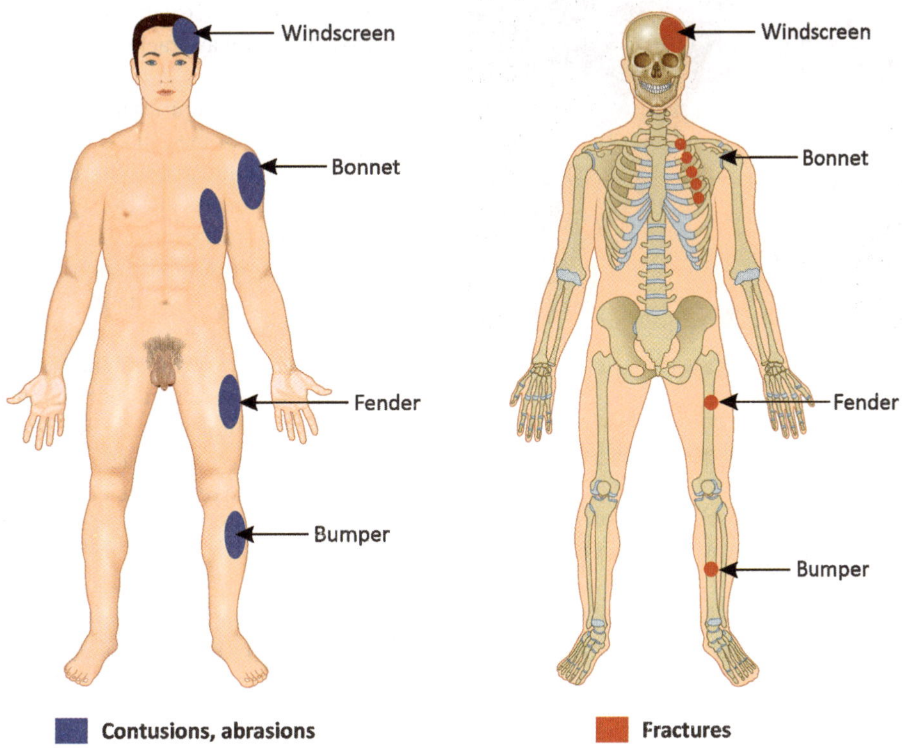

Fig. 3.118 Regions of body involved in vehicular impact

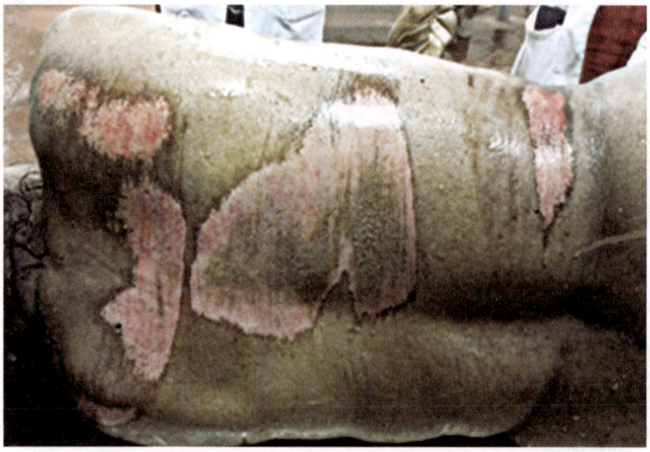

Fig. 3.119 Grazed abrasions over back due to dragging on road surface (*Courtesy: Dr Jagadish Rao PP*)

Run Over Injuries

- Abrasions in the form of grazes, and impact or imprint abrasions of the tire marks may be seen (**Fig. 3.120**). The rotator effect against a fixed limb often causes avulsion laceration. If head is involved, complete avulsion of the ear may occur. If abdomen is involved, intestines may get extruded.

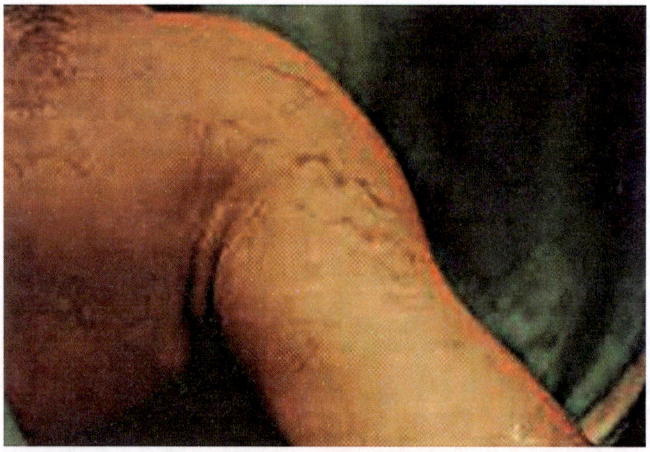

Fig. 3.120 Tyre impression – run over injury

- **Crush syndrome** occurs if a large bulk of muscle is crushed.
  - It is characterized by the development of profound shock.
  - The crushed limb becomes pulseless, and later red, swollen and blistered. Nerve sensation and muscle power may be lost.
  - Crushing of muscles can liberate haem and myoglobin, which enter the circulation and get excreted through the kidneys. This can lead to acute tubular necrosis. Death may occur in a week's time. At autopsy, the kidneys appear large and bulky, and haem casts may be found in the distal convoluted tubules.
  - Amputation of the severely crushed limb above the site of compression is necessary to avoid development of crush syndrome. Cooling of the limb, and treatment for renal failure and shock are to be carried out in the event of the syndrome beginning to manifest.

Vehicular Occupant Injuries

- Injuries to driver and other occupants are mostly related to sudden deceleration due to collision, the commonest type of vehicular accident.
- The driver and front seat passenger often sustain lacerations over the face due to impact against the windscreen, and fracture or dislocation of hip due to hitting against the dashboard. Fractures and dislocations of upper and lower limbs are also common.
- A special type of injury seen in the driver is the **steering wheel impact injury**, which causes fractures of sternum and ribs, as well as contusion or even rupture of the heart or aorta. Hitting against the rim of the steering wheel may rupture liver, spleen, kidneys or duodenum.
- Sudden hyperextension or flexion of the neck may result in fracture-dislocation of cervical spine and injuries of the spinal cord (**whiplash injury**).

Rail Traffic Accidents

- Railway accidents may involve a person who is not an occupant of the train (e.g., someone who is attempting to cross railway tracks), as well as one who is an occupant (passenger, driver, etc.).
- **Accident involving a non-occupant**:
  - Such a victim is usually someone who is attempting to cross the railway tracks. He is invariably either hit or run over.
  - Primary impact injuries may be sustained over the front, back, or one or the other side of the body.
  - After being hit, if he is thrown clear, he can sustain secondary injuries due to impact against the rail tracks, the ground, rocks or boulders, posts or trees. If he is run over by the train, the injuries are usually in the form of decapitation, amputations, etc., at various levels, transection of trunk, etc., which can be either instantly fatal, or extensively mutilating.
  - Decapitation alone without the presence of other injuries usually indicates suicide (**Fig. 3.121**), wherein the victim has lain on the tracks with the neck on one of the tracks, and the rest of the body lying outside the tracks. In such a case, there is usually generalized pallor of organs.
- **Accident involving an occupant**:
  - Passengers of a railway train can sustain injuries when the train collides with another, or if it derails at high speed.
  - Generally, they take the form of blunt injuries due to falling out of berths, or being knocked about violently, or heavy luggage falling on them, etc.
  - Blunt force over vertebral column can lead to concussion of spinal cord without visible injury to vertebrae.

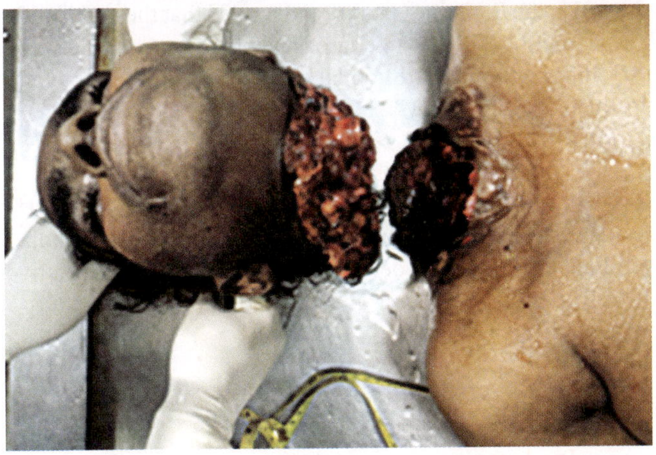

Fig. 3.121 Decapitation – Railway suicide (*Courtesy*: *Dr Jagadish Rao PP*)

This is called **railway (railroad) spine** due to its frequent occurrence in railway accidents. Commonest region affected is the lumbo-sacral spine resulting in paraplegia, bladder disturbances and impotence. Since concussion is spontaneously reversible, these abnormalities are usually only temporary.

- Occasionally, a passenger who is hanging out of a compartment door, or peeping out injudiciously may hit against posts or trees.
- Electrocution, or death by burns, or drowning in a lake or river (if the train falls off a bridge), etc., can also occur in train accidents.

Air Traffic Accidents

- Aviation injuries characteristically involve large numbers of occupants, and are almost always highly mutilating, with a high degree of possibility for dismemberment or even fragmentation.
- The actual nature of injuries will depend on the circumstances.
    - If decompression of a large aircraft cabin occurs at high altitude, victims may be sucked out and fall to their death; others may suffer from barotrauma or physical trauma from being thrown about within the cabin.
    - When an aircraft hits the ground, the effects will depend upon the speed and angle of impact. Injuries result mainly from extreme deceleration, and are usually of severe nature.
    - An aircraft which crashes or sustains a mid-air collision almost inevitably will burst into flames, and the occupants could get extensively burnt, or even reduced to ashes.
- Identification of each and every passenger and crewmember is the main aim of the autopsy in aircraft accidents, and is often a daunting task.
- Other important objectives include the evaluation of flight crew for evidence of disease, disability or drug abuse that could have contributed to the mishap, and the overall reconstruction of events leading to the accident.
- A significant number of aircraft accidents occur at the time of take-off or landing. The various causes of aircraft accidents include:
    - Mechanical defects of aircraft
    - Signalling defects of airport
    - Errors on the part of pilot or other flight crew
    - Collision
    - Climatic disturbances such as storm, or lightning
    - Of late, terrorist activity has become a common cause of aircraft mishaps.
        - A new and bizarre twist to aircraft crashes is the possibility of deliberate crashing of the aircraft by the pilot or co-pilot killing all crew and passengers on board. This may be an act of terrorism, or an act of suicide-mass homicide.

Waterway Accidents

- In waterway accidents, fatalities occur most commonly due to drowning rather than due to injuries.
- However, the violent rocking of vessels in storm or collision may cause blunt injuries to the occupants by being thrown about, or due to luggage falling on them, etc.

IMPORTANT: The National Medical Commission (NMC), after consulting an expert committee, has recommended **modifications in the CBME curriculum** to address issues related to the LGBTQ community on **18th Aug 2022**.

This book incorporates all the modifications and requests medical teachers to impart only these currently accepted perspectives, and refrain from conveying obsolete information. They must **NOT** set questions which are based on the original (unmodified) curriculum in examinations.

Modified FM 3.13: Core – Written/Viva Voce/ OSCE (Objective Structured Clinical Examination)/ OSPE (Objective Structured Practical Examination)

- Describe:
  - Various sections of IPC & CrPC related to the definition of rape and sexual assault.
  - Medical examination of rape victim and accused of rape.
  - Police information by the doctors.
  - Medical care with recent amendments notified till date.
- Describe the relevant provisions of POCSO Act related to:
  - Medical examination
  - Emergency medical care
  - Police information

- The law in India **till recently** permitted only heterosexual natural sexual intercourse (i.e., penile-vaginal sexual intercourse) between man and wife. **A sexual offence was therefore defined as any form of sexual intercourse which departs from this norm, and is consequently contrary to law.** However, a landmark decision of the Supreme Court of India permitting also consensual homosexual acts in private between adults (over the age of 18 years) challenges this archaic definition, which must now be re-phrased as follows:
  - **A sexual offence is today defined as any form of sexual intercourse which is contrary to heterosexual natural sexual intercourse (i.e., penile-vaginal sexual intercourse) between man and wife, and consensual homosexual acts in private between adults (over the age of 18 years).**
  - The relevant portion of the section of **Indian Penal Code (377)** that criminalised homosexuality has now effectively been **de-criminalised.**
- **Sexual offences** are today classified as:
  - Rape
  - Indecent assault
  - Incest
  - Bestiality
- **Homosexuality and oral sex (buccal coitus) are no more to be designated as "unnatural sexual offences".** On 6th Sept 2018, the Supreme Court of India ruled that the application of Section 377 IPC to consensual homosexuality between adults was unconstitutional, "irrational, indefensible and manifestly arbitrary".
- But, Section 377 remains in force relating to sex with minors, non-consensual sexual acts and bestiality.
- **Adultery is no more a criminal offence.** On 27th Sept 2018, the Supreme Court struck down Section 497 of the Indian Penal Code (which deals with adultery) as being violative of Articles 14, 15 & 21 of the Constitution.
- **Sexual paraphilias***
  - Fetishism/Transvestism
  - Sadism/Masochism
  - Voyeurism/Exhibitionism
  - Paedophilia
  - Miscellaneous disorders: necrophilia, necrophagia, etc.

SEXUAL OFFENCES

Rape

Definition

- As per **Sec 375 IPC**, rape is defined as unlawful sexual intercourse by a man with a woman
  - Against her will
  - Without her consent
  - With her consent, when her consent is obtained by
    - Force
    - Fear
    - Fraud
  - With or without her consent
    - When she is of unsound mind or intoxicated
    - When she is under 18 years of age. **The Criminal Law (Amendment) Act, 2018** has increased the previous recommended age of consent from 16 to 18 years, which means any sexual activity irrespective of the presence of consent with a woman below the age of 18 will constitute **statutory rape.**
- **Sec 375 IPC** also explains that **mere penetration** is sufficient to constitute the offence of rape, and provides an **exception** to the age of valid consent to sexual intercourse by a female, i.e., *sexual intercourse by a man with his own wife, the wife being not less than 18 years of age, is **not** rape.* **In 2017, the Supreme Court increased the consent age of wife from 16 to 18 years.**
  - In other words, **marital rape is not a crime under 375 IPC**, unless the wife is less than 18 years of age.
  - Such cases must be dealt with under the **Protection of Women from Domestic Violence Act 2005.**
  - However, Section 376A criminalizes the rape of a judicially separated wife.
  - The **Criminal Law Amendment Act 2013** (further amended in **2018**) has expanded Section 375 **to include**

***Note**: *Today, terms such as **perversion** and **deviation** must not be used in the medical context. The correct term for these acts is "**paraphilia**".*

acts in addition to vaginal penetration. The definition is now broadly worded with acts like

- Penetration of penis, or any object, or any part of body to any extent, into the vagina, mouth, urethra or anus of another person or making another person do so; penetration means "penetration to any extent", and lack of physical resistance is immaterial for constituting an offence.
- Applying mouth or touching private parts constitutes the offence of **sexual assault**.

- It must be emphasized here that **rape is not a medical term, but a legal concept**.
- Before proceeding any further, it would be pertinent to critically analyse from a medical viewpoint the provisions of **Sec 375, IPC**:
  - **Firstly**, to constitute rape, sexual intercourse must be **unlawful**, i.e., between two persons who are not lawfully married. It must be noted that coitus between a man and a woman who are not lawfully married (either to each other or to anybody else), is not "unlawful" as long as such coitus takes place by mutual consent. Such sexual intercourse is, however, considered by orthodox societies as **illicit**, i.e., not permitted, and is called "**fornication**".
    - However, coitus between man and wife also amounts to **rape**, if the wife is less than 18 years of age, because Indian law considers that, in view of her tender age and consequent immaturity of mind, the act may affect her body and mind adversely; hence, the husband has no absolute right to coitus with her.
  - **Secondly**, a **man** is defined in the Indian Penal Code as *a male human being of any age.* Therefore, there is, as per Indian law, no age below which a "man" cannot be charged with the offence of rape, unless Secs 82 and 83 IPC can be applied, the latter stating that "*Nothing is an offence which is done by a child above 7 years of age and under 12, who has not attained sufficient maturity of understanding to judge the nature and consequences of his conduct.*"
    - The question of *minimum age* of the woman does not arise, because victims of rape have ranged from infants to the old and infirm.
  - **Thirdly**, there is bound to be some confusion between "will" and "consent" because in the minds of most people, the two words are synonymous. The two, however, differ considerably in that "will," in this context, is most simply explained as *desire, wish or choice*, whereas "consent" is defined as *compliance or approval of what is done or proposed by another*. Therefore, a person may be willing to do something, but may not agree to do it. On the other hand, one may not be willing to do something, yet may comply, for whatever reason, with what is demanded.
    - It is important to note that ***legally valid*** consent by a woman to sexual intercourse, whether implied or expressed, **must be given before the act – that obtained subsequent to the act is not acceptable to a court of law**.
    - Till recently, Indian law also required that unwillingness or lack of consent by the woman must be proven by signs of resistance on her person, such as damage to her clothing or injuries on her body. However, this is possible only if the victim was in a position to put up a fight; it would be futile to search for such evidence if the victim had changed her clothing after the incident, or was unable to resist because of fear, fraud, impersonation, unsoundness of mind, etc. Today, most courts go by the oral evidence of the victim together with scientific evidence of sexual intercourse.
  - **Fourthly**, Sec 375 explains that **mere penetration** (even up to the vulva) is sufficient to constitute the offence of rape – neither injury to the external genitalia, nor rupture of the hymen, nor penetration into the vagina, nor seminal emission is essential. Similarly, the inability to achieve or sustain erection does not preclude the inability to commit rape, and the presence of abrasions, and absence of a uniform layer of smegma over the glans penis indicate only complete sexual intercourse, not rape.
    - **The Criminal Law Amendment Act 2013 (further amended in 2018)** has **extended** the term **'rape'** to include acts in addition to vaginal penetration, including **penetration of penis, or any object or any part of body to any extent, into the vagina, mouth, urethra or anus of another person or making another person do so**.
- The **punishment** for **rape** is prescribed in **Sec 376 IPC** (*see below*).

Box 3.6—Summary of Amended 375 IPC

A man is said to commit "rape", if he:

1. Penetrates his penis, to any extent, into the vagina, mouth, urethra or anus of a woman or makes her to do so with him or any other person; or
2. Inserts, to any extent, any object or a part of the body, not being the penis, into the vagina, the urethra or anus of a woman, or makes her to do so with him or any other person; or
3. Manipulates any part of the body of a woman so as to cause penetration into the vagina, urethra, anus or any part of body of such woman, or makes her to do so with him or any other person; or
4. Applies his mouth to the vagina, anus, urethra of a woman, or makes her to do so with him or any other person,

Under the circumstances falling under any of the following seven descriptions:

1. Against her will.
2. Without her consent.

contd.

3. With her consent, when her consent has been obtained by putting her or any person in whom she is interested, in fear of death or of hurt.
4. With her consent, when the man knows that he is not her husband and that her consent is given because she believes that he is another man to whom she is, or believes herself to be lawfully married.
5. With her consent when, at the time of giving such consent, by reason of unsoundness of mind or intoxication or the administration by him personally or through another of any stupefying or unwholesome substance, she is unable to understand the nature and consequences of that to which she gives consent.
6. With or without her consent, when she is under eighteen years of age.
7. When she is unable to communicate consent.

Explanations

1. For the purposes of this section, "vagina" shall also include labia majora.
2. Consent means an unequivocal voluntary agreement when the woman by words, gestures or any form of verbal or non-verbal communication, communicates willingness to participate in the specific sexual act.
   a. Provided that a woman who does not physically resist to the act of penetration shall not by the reason only of that fact, be regarded as consenting to the sexual activity.

Exceptions

1. A medical procedure or intervention shall not constitute rape.
2. Sexual intercourse or sexual acts by a man with his own wife, the wife not being under 18 years of age, is not rape.

Recent Amendments to Laws Relating to Sexual Offences

Recent sensational rape cases such as the **Nirbhaya case (2012)**, **Unnao case (2017) and Kathua case (2018)** triggered widespread public outrage, and led the government of India to bring in radical changes in the form of **Criminal Law Amendment Act 2013** and **2018**.

Criminal Law Amendment Act, 2013

The Criminal Law Amendment Act, 2013 was the outcome of the **Nirbhaya Case of 2012**:

- On 16th Dec 2012, a 23-year-old woman, a physiotherapy student, was gang raped by six men on a bus in the outskirts of Delhi. She had boarded with a male friend on the way home.
- The six men included a driver and a juvenile. Firstly, the men started abusing them, passing obscene remarks, and then they assaulted her male friend and dragged her to the back of the bus to commit rape. She was brutally beaten and raped, and the perpetrators inserted a rod into her body and then, both of them were thrown naked in the middle of the highway.
- On 29th Dec 2012, the woman, **Jyoti Singh** (named **Nirbhaya** by the media) (**Fig. 3.122**), succumbed to her injuries in a hospital in Singapore due to internal bleeding, multiple organ failure and cardiac arrest.

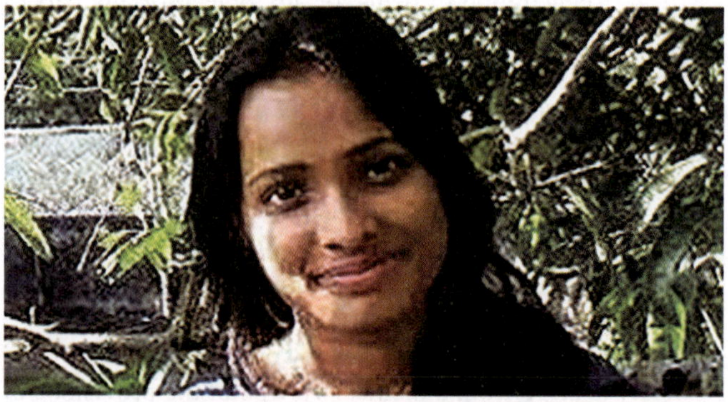

Fig. 3.122 Jyoti Singh (Nirbhaya)

- All the accused were arrested and charged with sexual assault and murder. One of the accused, Ram Singh, died in police custody from possible suicide on 11th March 2013. The rest of the accused went on trial in a fast-track court; the prosecution finished presenting its evidence on 8th July 2013. On 10th Sept 2013, the four adult defendants – Pawan Gupta, Vinay Sharma, Akshay Thakur and Mukesh Singh (Ram Singh's brother) (**Fig. 3.123**) – were found guilty of rape and murder, and were sentenced to death. On 18th Dec 2019, the Supreme Court of India rejected the final appeals of the condemned perpetrators of the attack, and the four adult convicts were executed by hanging on 20th March 2020, while the juvenile convict was given the maximum sentence of 3 years imprisonment in a reform facility, as per the Juvenile Justice Act.
- As a result of widespread rage and protests, a judicial committee was set up to study and take public suggestions for the best ways to amend laws to provide quicker investigation and prosecution of sex offenders. After considering about 80,000 suggestions, the committee submitted a report which indicated that failures on the part of the government and police were the root cause behind crimes against women.
- In 2013, the **Criminal Law (Amendment) Act, 2013** was passed, and several fast-track courts were created to hear rape cases.
- Provisions added or amended in the **Indian Penal Code (IPC)** after the Act was passed include the following:

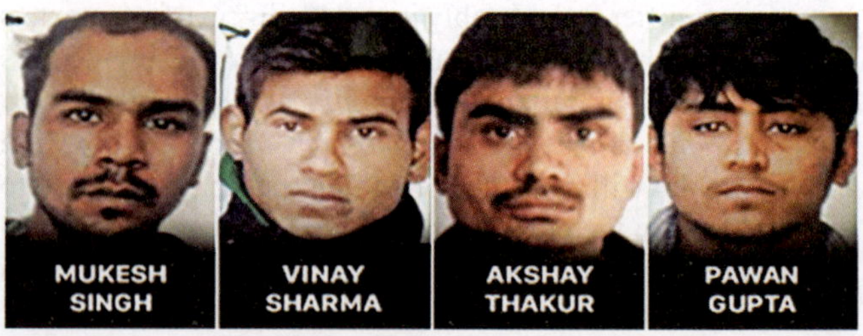

Fig. 3.123 The adult convicts

- ***Acid attack***:
  - These provisions were added to the Code as a consequence of the case of *Laxmi v. Union of India* (2015), in which a 16-year-old girl was attacked with acid. After this incident, the need for stringent provisions to counter the said offence was realised.
  - Under **Section 100**, a ground was added in the general exception of the "right to private defence", that is, an act of throwing acid or an attempt to throw acid. It means a person can now use the right to private defence in the case of an acid attack.
  - New provisions, namely, Section 326A and Section 326B, were inserted.
    - **Section 326A** makes the offence of "acid attack" punishable by a minimum of 10 years imprisonment extending to life imprisonment and a fine.
    - **Section 326B** makes the attempt to throw acid an offence punishable by a minimum of 5 years extending to 7 years imprisonment and a fine.
- ***Sexual offences***: This Amendment inserted four other sexual offences in view of the rising statistics of sexual harassment cases in the country. These are:
  - **Sexual harassment (Section 354A)**: This Section includes acts like making physical contact, demanding sexual favours and showing pornography to a woman by a man. For these offences, a man can be punished with rigorous imprisonment, which may extend to 3 years. It also covers the offence of making sexually-coloured remarks to a woman, for which there is imprisonment which may extend to 1 year.
  - **Assault or criminal force with intent to disrobe a woman (Section 354B)**: This Section makes an act of assaulting or threatening a woman using criminal force to disrobe her or forcing her to be naked punishable by a minimum imprisonment of 3 years, which may extend to 7 years, and a fine.
  - **Voyeurism (Section 354C)**: The word "voyeurism" literally means "an act of gaining pleasure from watching others naked or engaged in sexual activity." This Section makes any such acts committed by a man, punishable by a minimum of 1-year imprisonment, which may extend to 3 years, and a fine. It can also include the act of watching or taking photos of a woman when they are engaged in private activity. If a man is convicted of the same offence more than once, he shall be punishable with a minimum of 3 years of imprisonment, which may extend to 7 years.
  - **Stalking (Section 354D)**: This Section includes the act of following or attempting to make contact with a woman who has already shown disinterest in a man, or monitoring her use of the internet, email or other electronic communication means. This conduct by any man will be punishable by imprisonment which may extend to 3 years, and for repeated offenders, the punishment will be imprisonment which may extend to 5 years and a fine. There are some exceptions to this offence; that is, these acts will not amount to "stalking", if the man proves his act for the following reasons:
    - If the man was entrusted with preventing or detecting a crime by the State,
    - If the man has done such acts under any law, or while complying with any condition under any law,
    - If it was reasonable and justified.
  - The Criminal Law Amendment Act, 2013 widens the ambit of the offence of "**rape**" so as to provide harsher punishments for the more grievous acts. It also enlarged the provision to cover certain non-penetrative acts like oral sex and inserting any object or any other part of the body into a woman's body as an offence under the definition of "rape" under **Section 375**. Although under Section 376, the punishment for the offence of "rape" was not enhanced (after the Criminal Law Amendment Act 2018, it was increased to a minimum of 10 years imprisonment – life imprisonment), this Amendment of 2013 added provisions and enhanced punishment for more grievous forms of rape, as laid out in **Table 3.19**.
- ***Provisions for the authorities***:
  - **Section 166A** and **Section 166B** were inserted after the amendment to make the authorities, like public servants or hospital authorities, liable if they failed to discharge their duties against the victims of the crime.
    - **Section 166A** holds any public servant liable, if they failed to obey the directions of law or to conduct an investigation wherever it necessitates, or especially if failed to register an FIR in cases of sexual offences under Section 154 of the Code of Criminal Procedure. Any such public servant would be liable for the punishment of imprisonment for a minimum of 6 months which may extend to 2 years and a fine.
    - **Section 166B** similarly, holds the hospital management or staff liable, if they failed to provide proper treatment free of cost, including first aid, to the victim of the cases of sexual offences, as provided under Section 357C of the Code of Criminal Procedure. It is irrelevant whether the hospital is a private or public hospital. Any such contravention would be punished with imprisonment, which may extend to 1 year or a fine or both.
- ***Provisions added or amended*** in the **Code of Criminal Procedure (CrPC)** after the Act was passed include the following:
  - The Criminal Law Amendment Act 2013 has made changes to the Code of Criminal Procedure, 1973 so as to provide a congenial atmosphere for women

Table 3.19 New Provisions and Enhanced Punishments for Grievous Forms of Rape

Section	Offence	Punishment
Section 376A	Causing death or resulting in a persistent vegetative state of the woman	Rigorous imprisonment for a minimum of 20 years which may extend to life imprisonment, or death sentence.
Section 376B	Sexual intercourse by the husband during separation	Imprisonment for a minimum of 2 years which may extend to 7 years and a fine.
Section 376C	Sexual intercourse by a person in authority (fiduciary relationship, public servant, jail authorities, institutions for women and children or hospital authorities)	Rigorous imprisonment for a minimum of 5 years which may extend to 10 years and a fine.
Section 376D	Gang rape	Rigorous imprisonment for a minimum of 20 years, which may extend to life imprisonment.
Section 376E	Repeat offenders	Life imprisonment or death sentence.

while conducting investigations, trials and examinations. Some key changes made in the Code are as follows:

- Section 154 and Section 161 were amended to include the provision which requires the recording of the statements of the victim to be done by only a female police officer. In addition, Section 154 also provides that if the victim is mentally or physically disabled, then for the comfort of the victim, the recording of statements should be done at their residence or any other convenient place in the presence of an interpreter or special educator, and that the recording should be videotaped.
- Section 164 also added the provision for the assistance of an interpreter or special educator and videography of the statements. Moreover, it also held the statements under Section 164 to be considered as statements in lieu of examination-in-chief that can be cross-examined at the time of trial.
- Section 273: It was amended to include the provision which requires the court to take appropriate measures so that women under the age of 16 years and victims of rape or sexual offences should not be confronted by the accused while assuring the right of cross-examination to the accused.
- Section 357C: It added the provision which requires hospitals, whether public or private, to provide treatment, free of cost, to the victims of sexual offences and to inform about the case to the police authorities immediately.
- Section 197: This Section requires sanction from the government to prosecute judges, magistrates or public servants who are accused of any offences which they have committed in the discharge of their official duty. This Amendment adds 'explanation' in this Section stating that in cases of sexual offences, no previous sanction is required to be taken from the respective governments for the prosecution of public servants, magistrates and judges.
- Section 309: Clause (1) was amended for this Section to include the provision which requires that all the proceedings related to inquiry or trial should be completed within a period of 2 months from the date of the charge sheet, in the cases of sexual offences.

- ***Provisions added or amended*** in the **Indian Evidence Act (IEA)** after the Act was passed include the following:
  - Exclusion of previous sexual experiences in evidence:
    - Section 53A was added in the Act which declares that during prosecution for sexual offences, the character of the person or the previous sexual experiences of the victim is irrelevant as the evidence for the consent or quality of the consent of the victim.
    - Presumption of the absence of consent – **Section 114A** was added in the Act, which states that it was sufficient for the victim of the sexual offences to state before the court in her evidence that she had not consented to the sexual intercourse so as to presume the absence of consent in the case.
    - Nature of the questions asked in cross-examination – **Section 146** of the Act was amended to include the provision which states that no questions can be asked from the victims of sexual offences during cross-examination which are im-

moral in nature or which are related to previous sexual experiences of the victim so as to prove the consent or test the quality of the consent by the victim.

- Provision for dumb witnesses – Under **Section 119**, the witnesses who are unable to communicate verbally can give their statements in other ways, by writing, by signs, etc., which shall be deemed as oral evidence, and such witnesses should provide the assistance of an interpreter or special educator, and such statements shall be videotaped.

- ***Provisions added or amended*** in the **Protection of Children from Sexual Offences Act (POCSO), 2012** after the Act was passed include the following:
  - **Section 42** of this Act was amended in order to declare that if the offence was committed under the POCSO Act and the same offence is also punishable under provisions related to sexual offences in the Indian Penal Code, the offender shall be given the punishment under this Act or the Indian Penal Code, whichever provides graver punishment for such an offence.

Criminal Law Amendment Act, 2018

The Criminal Law Amendment Act, 2018 was the outcome of the **Unnao Case of 2017** and **Kathua Case of 2018**:

- *Unnao Case of 2017*:
  - The **Unnao rape case** refers to the gang rape of a 17-year-old girl on 4th June 2017 in Unnao, Uttar Pradesh. On 16th Dec 2019, former BJP MLA **Kuldeep Singh Sengar** (**Fig. 3.124**) was convicted for the rape and sentenced to life imprisonment. Further, Sengar was found guilty in the death of the girl's father in judicial custody.
  - Two charge sheets had been filed in the case. The first charge, filed by the Central Bureau of Investigation on 11th July 2018, accused Sengar of the rape. The second was filed 2 days later accusing Sengar, his brother, three policemen and five other individuals of framing the rape survivor's father as the perpetrator.
  - The rape survivor attempted to immolate herself at the residence of Yogi Adityanath, the Chief Minister of Uttar Pradesh, on 8th April 2018. Her father died in judicial custody shortly thereafter. These incidents brought public attention to the case, and the incident was widely reported on in the national media in April 2018.
  - Following a truck collision on 28th July 2019, resulting in the serious injury of the victim and death of two relatives, it was revealed that the family had been threatened and had written to the Chief Justice of India for help. On 31st July 2019, the Supreme Court and Chief Justice acknowledged the case.

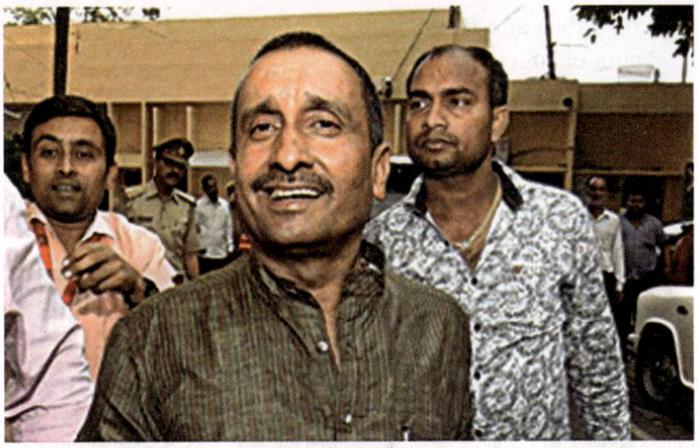

Fig. 3.124 Kuldeep Singh Sengar

- *Kathua Case of 2018*:
  - The **Kathua rape case** involved the abduction, gang rape and murder of an 8-year-old girl (**Fig. 3.125**) by six men and a juvenile, in Jan 2018 in Rasana village near Kathua in Jammu and Kashmir. A charge sheet for the case was filed, the accused were arrested and the trial began in Kathua on 16th April 2018. The victim belonged to the nomadic Bakarwal community. She had disappeared for a week before her body was discovered by the villagers a kilometer away from the village. The incident made national news when charges were filed against seven men in April 2018. The arrests of the accused led to protests by people, who sought justice for the victim. The gang rape and murder, as well as the support the accused received by some politicians, sparked widespread outrage in India and world-wide. On 10th June 2019, six of the seven defendants were convicted (**Fig. 3.126**) and one acquitted. Three of those convicted were sentenced to life imprisonment and the remaining 3–5 years.

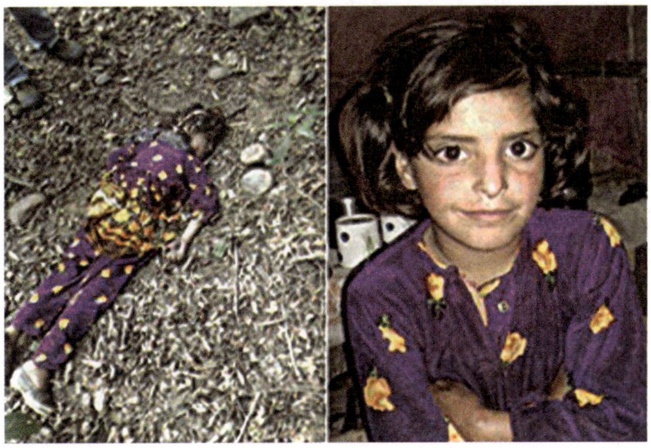

Fig. 3.125 Kathua case – the victim

- The Ministry of Law and Justice introduced the Criminal Law Amendment Bill, 2018 in Lok Sabha on 23rd July , 2018, and the same was passed on 30th July and 6th August by

Lok Sabha and Rajya Sabha, respectively. This Act made major changes to:
- Indian Penal Code (IPC)
- Criminal Procedure Code (CrPC)
- Indian Evidence Act (IEA)
- Protection of Children from Sexual Offences (POCSO) Act

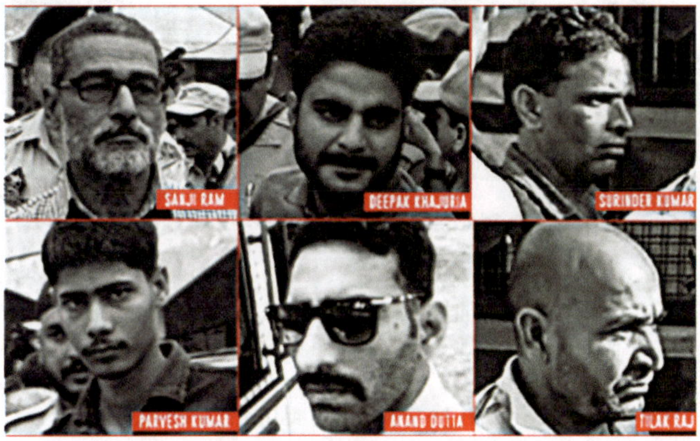

Fig. 3.126 Kathua case – the convicts

- ***Salient Features of Criminal Law Amendment Act, 2018*:**
  - Anyone who commits the offence of rape shall be punished for a minimum period of 10 years (earlier it was 7 years).
  - If any person rapes a girl under 16 years of age, minimum punishment will be imprisonment for 20 years.
  - If any person rapes a girl under 12 years of age, minimum punishment will be rigorous imprisonment for 20 years, or imprisonment for life, or may be liable for the death penalty.
  - For offence of rape with a girl below 16 years, **anticipatory bail** will not be granted to the accused.
  - Convicted person is bound to compensate the victim, and such compensation will be used for the victim's medical expenses and for rehabilitation.
  - If the offence of rape is committed by a Police Officer (irrespective of the place), he shall be punished by rigorous imprisonment for a minimum period of 10 years.
  - All rape investigations must be completed within **2 months** after the FIR is lodged.
  - For an offence of rape, the time to dispose of appeal starts after 6 months.
  - Gang rape of girl below 16 years of age will be punished with rigorous imprisonment for life, and will also be liable for fine.
  - Gang rape of girl below 12 years of age will be punished with rigorous imprisonment for life, with fine or may be liable for the death penalty.
- ***Amendments in the Indian Penal Code*:**
  - **Three new sections** have been added:
    - **376AB**: Whoever, commits rape on a woman under 12 years of age shall be punished with rigorous imprisonment for a term which shall not be less than 20 years, but which may extend to imprisonment for life, and with fine, or with death.
    - **376DA**: Where a woman under 16 years of age is raped by one or more persons constituting a group or acting in furtherance of a common intention, each of those persons shall be deemed to have committed the offence of rape and shall be punished with imprisonment for life, and with fine.
    - **376DB**: Where a woman under 12 years of age is raped by one or more persons constituting a group or acting in furtherance of a common intention, each of those persons shall be deemed to have committed the offence of rape and shall be punished with imprisonment for life, and with fine, or with death.
  - **Three sections** have been **amended**:
    - **166A**: Whoever, being a public servant—
      1. knowingly disobeys any direction of the law which prohibits him from requiring the attendance at any place of any person for the purpose of investigation into an offence or any other, or
      2. knowingly disobeys, to the prejudice of any person, any other direction of the law regulating the manner in which he shall conduct such investigation, or
      3. fails to record any information given to him under sub-section (1) of section 154 of the Code of Criminal Procedure, 1973, in relation to cognizable offence punishable under section 326A, 326B, 354, 354B, 370, 370A, 376, 376A, 376AB, 376B, 376C, 376D, 376DA, 376DB, 376E or 509, shall be punished with rigorous imprisonment for a term which shall not be less than 6 months, but which may extend to 2 years, and shall also be liable to fine.
    - **228A**:
      1. Whoever prints or publishes the name or any matter which may make known the identity of any person against whom an offence under section 376, 376A, 376AB, 376B, 376C, 376D, 376DA, 376DB, 376E is alleged or found to have been committed (hereafter, in this section referred to as the victim) shall be punished with imprisonment of either description for a term which may extend to 2 years and shall also be liable to fine.
      2. Nothing in sub-section (1) extends to any printing or publication of the name or any matter which may make known the identity of the victim if such printing or publication is
         - by or under the order in writing of the officer-in-charge of the police station or the police officer making the investigation into such offence acting in good faith for the purposes of such investigation; or
         - by, or with the authorisation in writing of, the victim; or

- where the victim is dead or minor or of unsound mind, by, or with the authorisation in writing of, the next-of-kin of the victim: Provided that no such authorisation shall be given by the next-of-kin to anybody other than the chairman or the secretary, by whatever name called, of any recognised welfare institution or organisation.

- 376 (punishment for rape):
  1. Whoever, except in the cases provided for in sub-section (2), commits rape, shall be punished with rigorous imprisonment of either description for a term which shall not be less than 10 years, but which may extend to imprisonment for life, and shall also be liable to fine.
  2. Whoever—
     - being a police officer, commits rape,
       - within the limits of the police station to which such police officer is appointed; or
       - in the premises of any station house; or
       - on a woman in such police officer's custody, or in the custody of a police officer subordinate to such police officer; or
     - being a public servant, commits rape on a woman in such public servant's custody or in the custody of a public servant subordinate to such public servant; or
     - being a member of the armed forces deployed in an area by the Central or a State Government commits rape in such area; or
     - being on the management or on the staff of a jail, remand home or other place of custody established by or under any law for the time being in force or of a women's or children's institution, commits rape on any inmate of such jail, remand home, place or institution; or
     - being on the management or on the staff of a hospital, commits rape on a woman in that hospital; or
     - being a relative, guardian or teacher of, or a person in a position of trust or authority towards the woman, commits rape on such woman; or
     - commits rape during communal or sectarian violence; or
     - commits rape on a woman knowing her to be pregnant; or
     - commits rape, on a woman incapable of giving consent; or
     - being in a position of control or dominance over a woman, commits rape on such woman; or
     - commits rape on a woman suffering from mental or physical disability; or
     - while committing rape causes grievous bodily harm or maims or disfigures or endangers the life of a woman; or
     - commits rape repeatedly on the same woman,

     shall be punished with rigorous imprisonment for a term which shall not be less than 10 years, but which may extend to imprisonment for life, and shall also be liable to fine.
  3. Whoever, commits rape on a woman under 16 years of age shall be punished with rigorous imprisonment for a term which shall not be less than 20 years, but which may extend to imprisonment for life, and shall also be liable to fine. Provided further that any fine imposed under this sub-section shall be paid to the victim.

- *Amendments in the Indian Evidence Act*:
  - **Two new sections** have been added:
    - 53A: In a prosecution for an offence under section 354, 354A, 354B, 354C, 354D, 376, 376A, 376AB, 376B, 376C, 376D, 376DA, 376DB or 376E of the IPC, or for attempt to commit any such offence, where the question of consent is in issue, evidence of the character of the victim or of such person's previous sexual experience with any person shall not be relevant on the issue of such consent or the quality of consent.
    - 146: When a witness is cross-examined, he may, in addition to the questions herein-before referred to, be asked any questions which tend—
      1. to test his veracity,
      2. to discover who he is and what is his position in life, or
      3. to shake his credit, by injuring his character, although the answer to such questions might tend directly or indirectly to incriminate him or might expose or tend directly or indirectly to expose him to a penalty or forfeiture.

      Provided that in a prosecution for an offence under section 376, 376A, 376AB, 376B, 376C, 376D, 376DA, 376DB or 376E of the Indian Penal Code, or for attempt to commit any such offence, where the question of consent is an issue, it shall not be permissible to adduce evidence or to put questions in the cross-examination of the victim as to the general immoral character, or previous sexual experience, of such victim with any person for proving such consent or the quality of consent.

- *Amendments in the Code of Criminal Procedure*:
  - **Following sections** have been **amended**:
    - Section 173: Investigation of an offence under section 376AB, 376B, 376C, 376D, 376DA and 376DB or section 376E of the IPC shall be completed within 2 months.
    - Sections 374 & 377: Appeal shall be disposed of within 6 months from the date of filing of such appeal.

- **Section 438**: Provides that nothing in this section shall apply to any case involving the arrest of a person on accusation of having committed an offence under sub-section (3) of Section 376, 376AB, 376DA, 376DB of the IPC.
- **Section 439**: The High Court and the Sessions Court shall, before granting bail to a person who is accused of an offence triable under sub-section (3) of Sections 376, 376AB, 376DA, 376DB, give notice of the applicant for bail to the public prosecutor within a period of 15 days from the date of receipt of such notice.

- ***Amendments in the Protection of Children from Sexual Offences (POCSO) Act, 2012***:
  - There is a change in **Section 42** of POCSO Act, 2012. This section deals with **Alternative Punishment** and Sections 376A, 376C, 376D were substituted with 376A, 376AB, 376B, 376C, 376D, 376DA and 376DB of Indian Penal Code.

> **FM 3.14: Core – Written/Viva Voce/ OSCE (Objective Structured Clinical Examination)**
> - **Sexual Offences**
>   - Describe and discuss the following:
>   - Examination of a victim of alleged rape.
>   - Preparation of report, framing the opinion.
>   - Preservation and despatch of trace evidence in such cases.

MEDICOLEGAL EXAMINATION OF AN ALLEGED VICTIM OF RAPE (Fig. 3.127)

- In the past, rape survivor examination was recommended to be done only after receiving police requisition. **Today, police requisition is not mandatory for a rape survivor to seek medical examination and care**. The doctor should examine such cases, if the survivor reports to the hospital first without FIR. He can then inform the police accordingly as per the request of the patient.
- A survivor may come to the hospital only for treatment of the effects of assault. Under section 39 CrPC the doctor is not bound to inform such cases to the police. Informed refusal for not informing the police should however be documented. **Neither the court nor the police can force a rape survivor to undergo medical examination.** It has to be with her/parental/guardian's informed consent (depending on age).
- A physician's responsibilities in the medicolegal examination of the victim of an alleged sexual assault are both **therapeutic**, in ameliorating the physical and emotional consequences of the incident, as well as **evidentiary**, in order to facilitate the scientific investigation of the crime.
- **Written informed consent** of the victim to examination and treatment, as well as for the collection of material evidence, duly **witnessed**, must be obtained if she is over the age of **12 years**. If the victim is less than 12 years of age, or is mentally unsound, the consent of the parent or guardian must be obtained. In case an invasive procedure needs to be performed, age of consent is **18 years**. Invasive procedures include per-vaginal, per-speculum, per-rectal examinations. Noninvasive procedures include physical examination and evidence collection from exposed parts of the body.
- A **support person** (e.g., family member or rape counsellor) and/or a **female nurse** must be present throughout, not only to assist the examining physician (who must preferably be a female), but also to prevent allegations of sexual assault against the physician (if this happens to be a male), and to provide emotional support to the victim.
- The medicolegal examination should include complete **history, physical examination** and **collection of material evidence** for laboratory examination, to establish the following crucial points:
  - Did sexual intercourse occur?
  - If yes, was this sexual intercourse forced on the alleged victim?
  - Was the alleged victim a virgin prior to the commission of the alleged offence?*
  - If the validity of consent is the question
    - how old is the victim?
    - was she of sound or unsound mind (whether due to mental disease or intoxication) at the time of commission of the alleged offence?
  - How many assailants were there?
  - Is it possible to identify the assailant from material evidence gathered?
  - Are there any sequelae of the alleged offence (e.g., sexually transmitted disease, pregnancy or psychological trauma)?
  - How much time has elapsed between commission of the alleged offence and medicolegal examination?

History

The purpose of the history (which includes a general medical history, a sexual history, and a history of the incident) is to gather information that will help the medical and legal management of the case.

General Medical History

- Past medical history of injury or illness (particularly disorders which may have an adverse effect on the alleged victim, e.g., bleeding disorders).
- Is the victim on any medication?

Sexual History

- Has the victim attained menarche?
  - If yes, what is the frequency and regularity of menstruation?
- Has the victim been sterilized, or does she use any contraceptives?

**Note*: *Controversial; deemed irrelevant and inappropriate by most investigators today.*

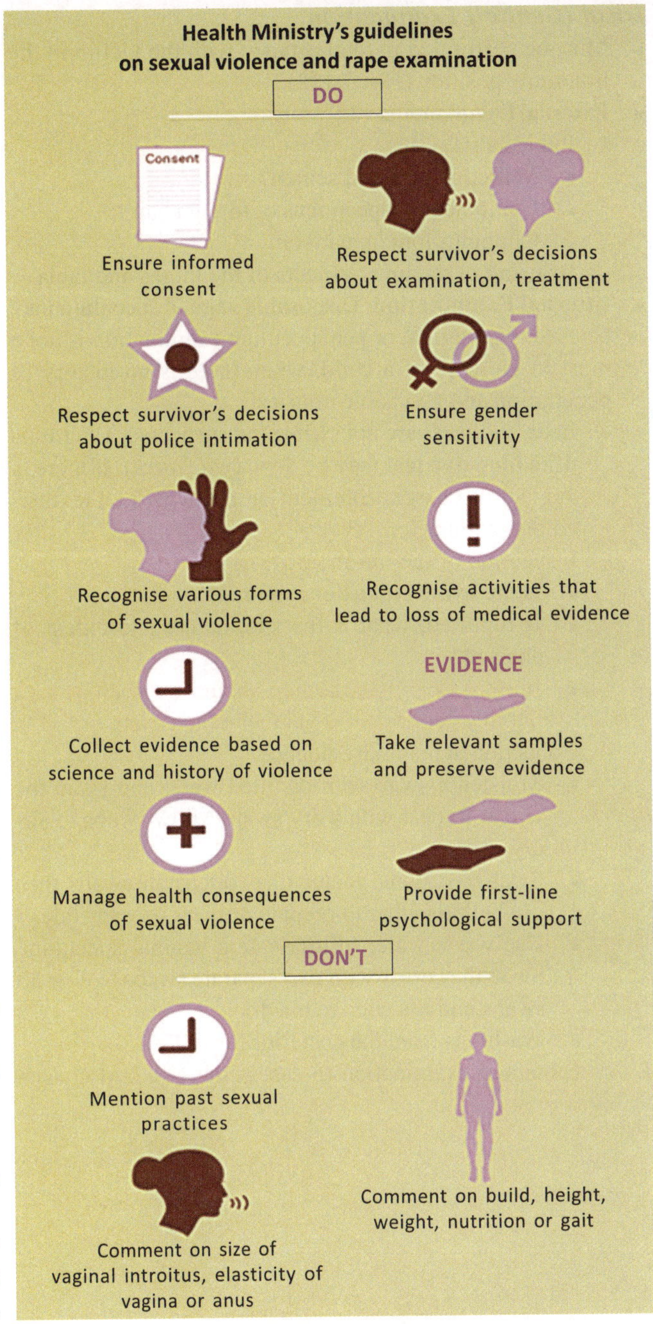

Fig. 3.127 Health Ministry's Guidelines on sexual violence and rape examination

- Marital and obstetric history (where applicable):
  - Number of pregnancies, and the result of each.
  - Most recent consensual sexual intercourse.
  - Existence and onset of any symptoms or signs of pregnancy.
  - Patient's attitude to pregnancy and its prevention or termination by therapeutic measures.
- Past history of venereal disease:
  - If there is past history, whether treated or not, and if yes, where and when, and whether the patient was cured completely.

History of the Incident

- Time and location of the alleged assault.
- Specific nature of the alleged assault.
- Whether penetration was vaginal, oral or anal.
- Whether penetration was accomplished/attempted with penis, finger, any other object.
- Whether she experienced pain at the time of the incident or subsequently.
- Whether or not body fluids were left in/on the victim.
- Whether or not instruments and/or restraints were used.
- Number of assailants, and their physical description, if she is able to recall such information.
- Whether she resisted – in which manner?
- Was there use of condom and/or foam or jelly or lubricant?
- Whether or not there were any activities which could possibly interfere with the collection of material evidence (change of clothing, bathing, douching, urinating, defaecating, etc.).

Physical Examination

It must be conducted gently, but firmly, in the presence of a female nurse, explained step by step after ensuring total privacy, and thorough enough to note any abnormalities resulting from the sexual assault.

General Examination

- Take the victim's (or that of the parent/guardian) written informed consent.
- Assess and record the victim's general appearance (disarrangement or damage to, or any stains on clothing; demeanour of the victim, signs of emotional distress, gait, etc.).
- Record vital parameters (blood pressure, pulse, temperature and respiration).
- Record at least two marks of identification.
- Request the victim to stand on a large clean white sheet of paper, and to undress herself, and collect any material that falls onto the paper in the process.
- Examine the fingernails for any damage, and for any material which may have accumulated under them, which must be scraped off into cellophane packets (to be sealed, labelled and forwarded to the Forensic Science Laboratory for examination).
- Record the presence of fresh/dried stains of blood, semen, dirt, mud, grass, etc., on the surface of the body; these too, must be swabbed/scraped off into appropriate containers, sealed, labelled and despatched to the Forensic Science Laboratory.
- Carefully examine and meticulously record external injuries (signs of restraint, bite marks, scratches, contusions, etc.).
- Follow-up examination for injuries: If there are deep bruises or contusions, signs of injury will usually show only after 48 hours. Therefore, it is mandatory to repeat the examination of the survivor for recording the appearance of bruises. Bite marks may not be obvious immediately following an assault, but may become more apparent with time.

Local (Genital) Examination

- Must be performed in total privacy with the victim in the lithotomy position (**Fig. 3.128**).
- **External Examination**:
  - Pubic hair:
    - Matted with blood/semen?
    - Combings for specimens of foreign hair
    - Clippings for comparison.
  - Bruising of the inner aspects of the thighs and labia.
- **Internal Examination**: Disposable vaginal speculum may be used. Per vaginal or per speculum examination is not a must in the case of a child, when there is no history of penetration and no visible injuries.
  - In case injuries are not visible but suspected, **1% toluidine blue dye test** may be done (*vide infra*). If there is vaginal discharge, comment on the type, i.e., texture, colour, odour, etc.
  - Inspection of the introitus:
    - Is the hymen intact or ruptured?
    - If ruptured, what is the site, nature and extent of damage?
    - Presence of intact hymen should be documented, but does not rule out vaginal penetration.
  - Collection of material evidence:
    - Moisten a swab with distilled water and swab the vulva. Repeat with a dry swab. Allow swabs to air-dry.
    - Swab the vaginal vault with two separate swabs, then use both together to prepare a smear on one slide.
    - Use warm water to lubricate a vaginal speculum. Swab the cervix with two separate swabs. Allow all swabs and the slide to air-dry.
    - Washings from the posterior fornix.
  - Bimanual examination to assess the size and consistency of the uterus, signs of pre-existing pregnancy, and tenderness resulting from trauma sustained during the assault.
  - **Anoscopic examination** need only be used in cases of anal bleeding, or severe anal pain, or if the presence of a foreign body in the rectum is suspected.
  - **Colposcopic examination** (only when facility available) (**Fig. 3.129**) is required to be done when injuries are not appreciated by naked eye examination and when collection of photographic evidence is required.
  - **Toluidine blue dye test**: Toluidine blue dye is used to assist in the identification of recent genital and perianal injuries. After the initial examination of the posterior fourchette and fossa navicularis and the collection of swabs, apply 1% aqueous solution of toluidine blue dye to the posterior fourchette and fossa navicularis. After allowing a minute for the dye uptake, remove the excess with lubricant, such as K-Y jelly or 10% acetic acid. Dye uptake is considered positive and affirms injury when there is residual blue colouring of the laceration or its border after the excess dye has been removed. Abrasions from forced cunnilingus can result in a diffuse pattern of dye uptake.
  - **The previously recommended 'two-finger test' should not be performed in cases of sexual assault as information about past sexual conduct has been considered irrelevant to the case in several judgments (Section 146 of the Indian Evidence Act & deletion of Sub-section (4) of Section 155). The National Medical Commission has also denounced it.* The test itself has no scientific validity and is subjective. On the basis of such a test, no doctor can conclude that a victim is habituated to sexual intercourse**.

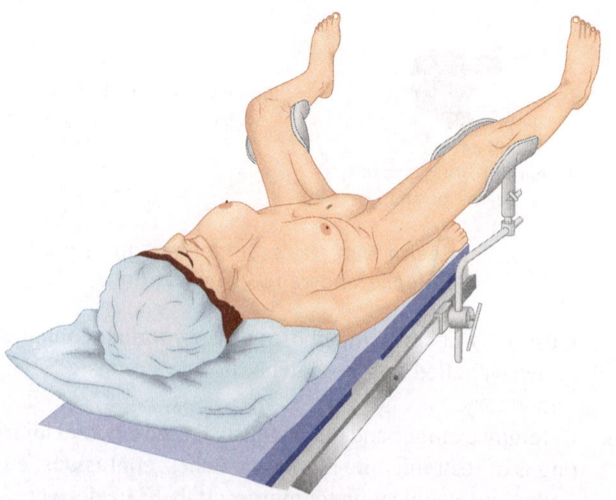

Fig. 3.128 Lithotomy position

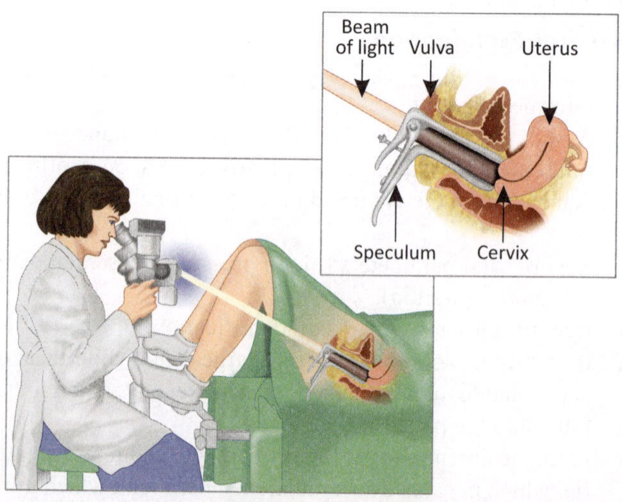

Fig. 3.129 Colposcopy

**Source*: Advisory No. U. 11029/49/2022/UGMEB dated 18.08.2022 from National Medical Commission (Undergraduate Medical Education Board), New Delhi.

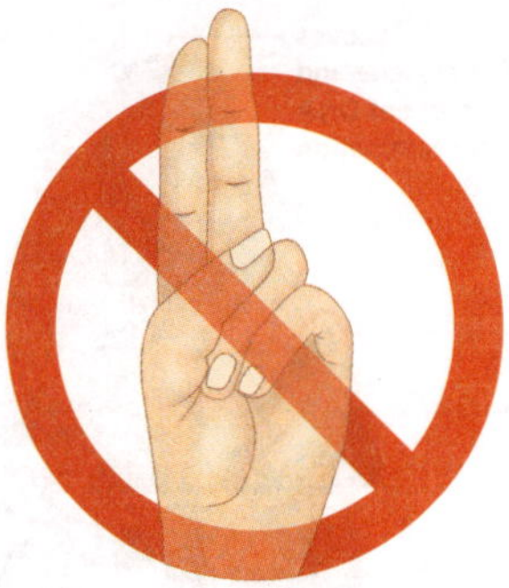

Two Finger Test

Laboratory Investigations

- All material evidence collected during the general and local examinations must enter a **chain of evidence** by proper sealing and labelling, with the name, case number, date and time of collection, and the name and designation of the examining physician, and despatched to the nearest Forensic Science Laboratory through the police constable concerned.
- **A checklist** of the said material evidence, for ready reference, is as follows:
  - **Clothing** that is torn, blood stained or soiled.
  - **Foreign debris**: Hair, fibres and fresh/dried secretions on the surface of the body.
  - **Fingernail scrapings**.
  - **Combings** from pubic hair, and **clippings** of the victim's pubic hair for comparison.
  - **Washings** from the posterior fornix and vagina, for histochemical and histological examination for the detection of the constituents of seminal fluid.
  - **Vaginal swabs**
    - For the detection of *Mycobacterium smegmatis*, and for the presence of sexually transmitted disease (by Gram's staining and culture of secretions).
    - Inspection of a **wet mount** slide of vaginal swabs under light microscope (for sperms):
    - The presence of motile sperm in the vaginal pool is the best indication of recent ejaculation. The absence of motile sperm, however, does not negate the possibility of recent ejaculation as sperm may become non-motile within hours of entering the vaginal environment.
    - Place a drop of normal saline or buffered nutrient medium on the slide to preserve the motility of the sperm. A glucose fortified solution of balanced salts, such as Ringer's, Tyrode's or Dulbecco's at normal osmolality, pH 7.2–7.4 is recommended. Prepared solutions of media designed to enhance sperm survival during microscopic examinations are commercially available.
    - Select one of the swabs collected from the vaginal pool and roll the swab back and forth in the drop to transfer cellular debris to the medium. Place a cover slip on the slide.
    - Examine the wet mount slide within 5–10 minutes using a biological microscope at 400 power, or by using a phase contrast or other "optically staining" microscope to determine whether or not motile or non-motile sperms are present.
  - **Blood** for grouping, baseline serology for sexually transmitted disease, and presence and levels of ethanol and/or other intoxicating agents.
  - **Urine** for the presence and levels of ethanol and/or other intoxicating agents, and pregnancy tests.
    - In addition to clinical implications, presence of ethanol and/or drugs in the patient's blood or urine or vomitus may have legal significance. The assailant may have used drugs to subdue the victim (**drug-facilitated sexual assault**). The victim may have lost the ability to make rational decisions, or to offer resistance, or she may have lost consciousness, or may have no recollection of events. There may not be any physical or genital injuries in such cases. Drugs such as marijuana (cannabis), cocaine, methamphetamine, benzodiazepines and gamma hydroxy butyrate (GHB) can be detected through testing blood and urine samples.
- In 2019, the Ministry of Home Affairs, Govt of India distributed special kits to states and union territories to help forensic investigation of sexual assault cases. These '**Sexual Assault Evidence Collection Kits (SAECK)**' or '**rape investigation kits**' are designed to carry out immediate medico-legal investigation and aid in furnishing evidence in sexual assault and rape cases. The contents include swabs, speculum, gloves, forceps, gauze, specimen containers, slides, etc. (**Fig. 3.130**). However, there are doubts as to whether they are being utilized.

Opinion*

Following opinions may be drawn as per the available findings:

1. If there are recent genital and/or physical injuries (fresh injuries) with wet vaginal/anal smear detecting spermatozoa, the opinion could be stated as '**There is evidence suggestive of recent forceful vaginal/anal intercourse**."
2. If there are genital/physical injuries but no evidence of spermatozoa in the wet smear, it does not rule out forced penetrative sex. So, the opinion should be stated as "**There are signs of use of force/forceful penetration of vagina/anus, however the opinion regarding penetrative intercourse is reserved pending availability of FSL reports**."
3. If there are only physical injuries and no genital injuries, and no evidence of spermatozoa in the wet smear, it does not rule out forced penetrative sex. So, the opinion should be stated as "**There are signs of use of force, however the opinion regarding penetrative intercourse is reserved pending availability of FSL reports**."

***Note**: *Do not use the term "rape" anywhere in a medical/medico-legal report. It is purely a legal term.*

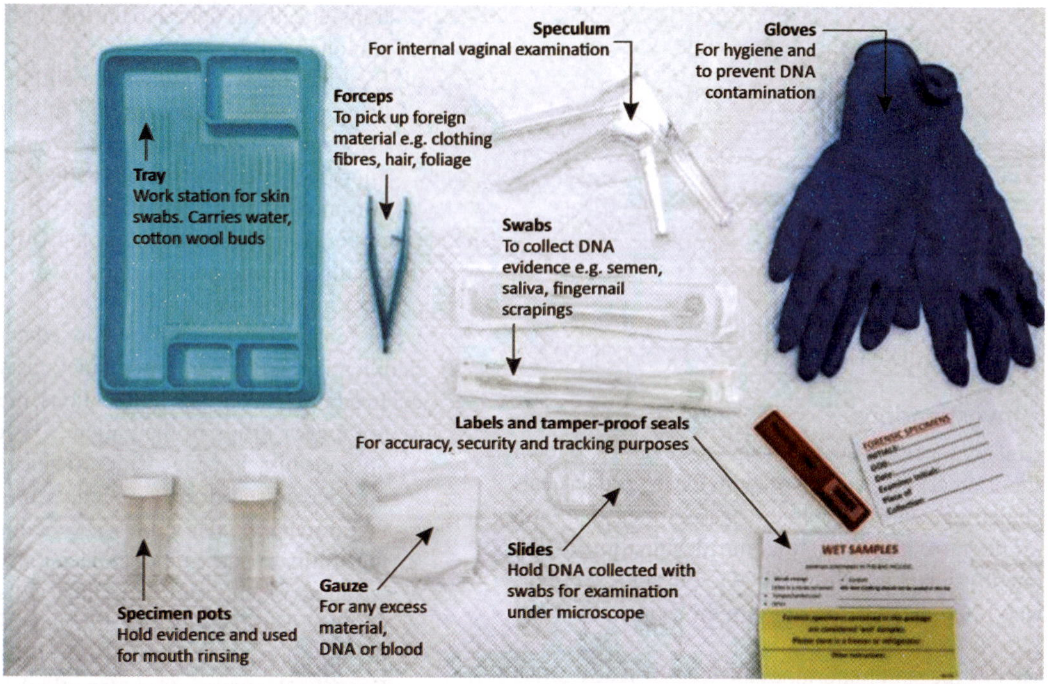

Fig. 3.130 Contents of the 'Rape Kit'

4. If there are only genital injuries but no physical injuries, and no evidence of spermatozoa in the wet smear, it does not rule out forced penetrative sex. So, the opinion should be stated as "**There are signs of use of force/forceful penetration of vagina and/or anus; however, the opinion regarding penetrative intercourse is reserved pending availability of FSL reports**".
5. If there is evidence of spermatozoa in the wet smear of vagina, but no physical and genital injuries then the opinion could be stated as, "**There are signs of recent sexual intercourse. However, opinion regarding forceful sexual intercourse will be given after the follow-up examination**".
   If there are normal exam findings, i.e., there are no physical and genital injuries, no evidence of spermatozoa in the wet smear, the opinion could be stated as "**On examination, the findings are within normal limits which neither refute nor confirm forceful sexual intercourse. However, final opinion regarding penetrating intercourse is reserved pending till availability of FSL reports and opinion regarding application of force will be given after follow up examination**".

MEDICOLEGAL EXAMINATION OF ACCUSED IN A CASE OF ALLEGED RAPE

- If the accused in a particular case of rape is produced for medicolegal examination (conducted under **Secs 53** and **54** of the **Code of Criminal Procedure**), it is preferable that the same physician who examined the victim also examines the accused, for better correlation. However, it is not mandatory.
- The objectives of the medicolegal examination do not differ significantly from that of the examination of the victim, except that such sequelae of the incident as signs of pregnancy cannot obviously be looked for!
- Answers to the following questions must be sought:
  - **Did the accused take part in sexual intercourse?** This can be determined by:
    - Examination of the clothing and undergarments for recent seminal stains.
    - Absence of smegma under the prepuce: smegma is a thick, cheesy secretion with a disagreeable odour, consisting of desquamated epithelial cells and smegma bacilli (*Mycobacterium smegmatis*), which is generally wiped off during sexual intercourse. However, its absence is not conclusive evidence of sexual intercourse, since during the customary daily bath, the prepuce is expected to be retracted and any accumulated smegma washed away. On the other hand, the actual presence of smegma can be taken as evidence that the person did not participate in sexual intercourse.
    - Examination of the surface of the shaft of the penis for the presence of vaginal epithelial cells: Since these have a high glycogen content, whether or not they have been transferred to the penile shaft (as per Locard's principle of exchange), can be assessed by wiping the shaft with a clean moist filter paper, which is then exposed to vapours of Lugol's iodine. A brown colour indicates a positive test (**Lugol's iodine test**).
    - Fresh/Dried bloodstains, which may be from the victim, or of the accused himself from injuries sustained, such as tearing of the frenulum.
    - It must be noted that the defence often raises the

plea that the accused was impotent, and, therefore, could not have committed the offence. However, since potency is the usual and normal state in man, it will always be presumed to be so, unless the contrary is proved by the accused. Also, as per the current legal definition of rape, penile erection and penetration are not essential to be proved. **Therefore, conducting a "potency test" is redundant and meaningless.**

- **If yes, was this sexual intercourse forcible?**
  - If the victim offered resistance to the assault, or if there was considerable disproportion between the size of the genitalia of the assailant and victim, the assailant may have sustained injuries such as
    - Scratches on the face
    - Bite marks on his upper limbs or elsewhere
    - Frenular tears or grazed abrasions on the shaft of the penis, etc.
- **What was the mental status of the accused at the time of commission of the alleged offence?**
  - The answer to this question is relevant to the criminal responsibility of the accused, as determined by **Secs 84 & 85, IPC**, which do not hold a person responsible for an act if, at the time of committing it he was, by reason of unsoundness of mind or forced intoxication, unable to understand the nature or consequences of what he was doing, or that he was doing what was either wrong or contrary to law.
- **Was the accused suffering from any sexually transmitted disease which he may have communicated to the victim?**
  - This can be determined by:
    - Serological examination of the blood
    - Bacteriological examination of a urethral swab
- **How much time has elapsed between commission of the alleged offence and medicolegal examination?**
  - This is probably the most difficult question to answer, unless the age of injuries proven to be sustained by him during the alleged offence can be estimated with any degree of accuracy.

In conclusion, it can be stated that courts of law consider rape as *"the easiest charge to make and the most difficult to refute."*

> **FM 3.15: Core – Written/Viva Voce/ OSCE (Objective Structured Clinical Examination)**
> - Sexual Offences
>   - Describe and discuss examination of accused and victim of sodomy.
>   - Preparation of report, framing of opinion.
>   - Preservation and despatch of trace evidence in such cases.
>
> **and**

> **Modified FM 3.16: Core – Written/Viva Voce**
> - Describe and discuss informed consent in sexual intercourse.
> - Describe and discuss histories of gender and sexuality-based (sexual orientation) identities and rights in India.
> - Describe history of decriminalisation of 'adultery' and consensual adult homosexual sexual behaviour.
> - Describe sexual offences with its medicolegal significance:
>   - Forced/Non-consensual penetrative anal sex.
>   - Forced/Non-consensual oral sexual acts with animals/bestiality/zoophilia.
>   - Forced/Non-consensual insertion of fingers or objects.
>   - Forced/Non-consensual touching or groping or disrobing ('indecent assault').

ADULTERY

- **Adultery was a criminal offence under Section 497 of IPC, until it was quashed by the Supreme Court of India on 27th Sept 2018 as unconstitutional.**
  - **Sec 497 IPC** states that, *"Whoever has sexual intercourse with a person whom he knows or has reason to believe to be the wife of another man, without the consent or connivance of that man, such sexual intercourse not amounting to rape, is guilty of the offence of adultery."*
    - **This section has been struck down by the Supreme Court.**
  - **Sec 498** describes the offence of enticing, or taking away, or detaining with criminal intent, a married woman.
- The Supreme Court called the law unconstitutional because it "treats a husband as the sole master." **However, adultery is still sufficient grounds for divorce as ruled by the Supreme Court.**
- **Fornication** (sometimes confused with adultery) refers to consensual sexual intercourse between two people not married to each other. It is not an offence as per the Indian Penal Code, but is considered "immoral" by conservative societies.

INCEST

- **Incest** is defined as **sexual relationship between two close relatives who are usually within the prohibited degrees of relationship to get married**.
- The meaning of the expression "closely related" does, of course, differ from country to country, so that incest is punishable by legislation and constitutes a valid ground for divorce, and is prohibited by religious laws (by annulment of marriage) in many developed countries.
- However, in India and in many other Asian countries, incest per se is **not** a criminal offence (unless it also amounts to rape or child sexual abuse) because of the social acceptability of intracaste marriage.
- When it is without consent or is forced, it is considered **incestuous rape**. This term is also applied if consent, even

though it was obtained, is invalid, e.g., if the victim was under 18 years of age.

- The Indian Penal Code does not directly mention incest, but any such offence shall attract **Section 376(2)(f)**, which reads as follows:"...*being a relative, guardian or teacher of, or a person in a position of trust or authority towards the woman, commits rape on such woman, shall be punished with rigorous imprisonment for a term of not less than 10 years, and may extend to life imprisonment with a fine.*"
- Incest in any form is not socially accepted in India and is viewed as a taboo. But, different communities interpret such restrictions differently. For example, cross-cousin marriages are prohibited in North India, but the same is allowed in some communities in South India.
- Incest most frequently occurs between members of a nuclear family, and the victims are most often children. Notable examples include:
  - Between father and daughter (e.g., the ***Electra complex***, derived from the Greek myth of Electra, who wanted her brother to avenge the death of their father by killing their mother).
  - Between mother and son (e.g., the ***Oedipus complex***, named after the Greek mythical character Oedipus, who unknowingly kills his father, and marries his mother).
  - Between brother and sister (e.g., "***Pharaonic incest***," derived from the practice in ancient Egypt in which royal brothers and sisters married each other).
  - **Table 3.20** lists the main differences between Oedipus Complex and Electra Complex. It is to be noted however, that most psychiatrists today consider these conditions as fanciful theories rather than scientific facts.
- **In circumstances where the child is a victim of forced incest, it is called "juvenile incest."** The POCSO (Protection of Children from Sexual Offences) Act, 2012, just like the Indian Penal Code, does not per se mention incest, but Section 5(n) and Section 9(n) of the Act deals with such crimes.
  - Section 5(n) reads as follows: "....*whoever being a relative of the child through blood or adoption or marriage or guardianship or in foster care or having a domestic relationship with a parent of the child or who is living in the same or shared household with the child, commits* ***penetrative sexual assault*** *on such child shall be punished with rigorous imprisonment for a term which shall not be less than 20 years, but which may extend to imprisonment for life, and shall also be liable to fine, or with death.*"
  - Section 9(n) reads as follows: "....*whoever, being a relative of the child through blood or adoption or marriage or guardianship or in foster care, or having a domestic relationship with a parent of the child, or who is living in the same or shared household with the child, commits* ***sexual assault*** *on such child shall be punished with imprisonment of either description for a term which shall not be less than 5 years, but*

Table 3.20 Oedipus complex versus Electra complex

OEDIPUS COMPLEX	ELECTRA COMPLEX
Oedipus complex is a Freudian concept that describes a child's sexual desire for the parent of the opposite sex and sense of rivalry with the parent of the same sex	Electra complex is a non-Freudian concept that describes a girl's adoration and attraction to her father and resentment, hostility and rivalry towards her mother
Introduced by Sigmund Freud in 1899	Introduced by Carl Jung as a female counterpart of Oedipus complex
Traditionally used to describe a boy's attraction towards the mother and sense of rivalry with father	Describes a girl's attraction towards the father and sense of rivalry with mother
Boys experience castration anxiety	Girls experience penis envy

which may extend to 7 years, and shall also be liable to fine."

- Factors promoting the perpetration of incest:
  - Marital discord leading to frequent quarrels between husband and wife, and lack of a healthy sexual relationship.
  - Overcrowding by close relatives within the same house.
  - Lack of parental supervision over children.
  - Low morality and delinquency in a family.

MALE HOMOSEXUALITY

- **Sexual relationship between two males is referred to as male homosexuality.**
- On 6th Sept 2018, the Supreme Court of India ruled that the application of Section 377 IPC to consensual homosexual sex between adults was unconstitutional, thereby **decriminalising homosexuality**.
  - However, Section 377 remains in force relating to sex with minors, non-consensual sexual acts and bestiality.
- Penile-anal intercourse is one manifestation of male homosexuality and is called **sodomy**. It derives its name from a historical city (Sodom) mentioned in the Bible, where it was supposed to have been prevalent.
  - Heterosexual penile-anal intercourse is called **buggery**.
- The person who performs the act is called the ***active agent***, while the other partner (who may or may not have consented to the act) is termed the ***passive agent***.
  - If the passive agent is a child, the practice is known as **paederasty** (and is one form of paedophilia).
  - Habitual passive agents are called ***catamites*** (also *fairies*, *gays* or *queens*, in the West); in our country, ***hijras*** (castrated males), and ***zenanas*** (male transvestites) sometimes prostitute themselves as passive agents.

History of Decriminalisation of Consensual Adult Homosexuality (Box 3.7)

- Section 377 of the IPC introduced in 1861 during the British rule of India (modelled on the Buggery Act 1533) makes sexual activities "against the order of nature" illegal.
- Portions of the section were first struck down as unconstitutional with respect to gay sex by the Delhi High Court in July 2009. That judgement was overturned by the Supreme Court on 11th Dec 2013. The Court held that amending or repealing section 377 should be a matter left to Parliament, not the judiciary.
- On 6th Feb 2016, a 3-member bench of the Court reviewed petitions submitted by the Naz Foundation, and decided that they would be reviewed by a 5-member constitutional bench.
- On 24th Aug 2017, the Supreme Court upheld the right to privacy as a fundamental right under the Constitution in the landmark Puttaswamy judgement. The Court also called for equality, and condemned discrimination, stating that the protection of sexual orientation lies at the core of the fundamental rights, and that the rights of the LGBT population are real and founded on constitutional doctrine.
- In Jan 2018, the Supreme court agreed to hear a petition to revisit the 2013 Naz Foundation judgment.
- On 6th Sept 2018, the Court ruled unanimously in Navtej Singh Johar v. Union of India that Section 377 was unconstitutional "in so far as it criminalises consensual sexual conduct between adults of the same sex". The judgment was given by a five judges bench, including the then Chief Justice of India Dipak Misra.

Circumstances of Commission of Homosexual Acts

- Penile-anal sexual intercourse is viewed today by psychologists as a **variation of normal sexual behaviour** (and *not* as a perversion) that is widely prevalent because it is closest to heterosexuality in offering sexual gratification with a usually willing human subject.
- Most people are said to have subconscious or unconscious homosexual desires.
- Isolation of males from females (or vice versa), as in boarding schools, prisons, defence establishments, ships on long voyages, etc., frequently leads to temporary homosexuality.
- Even though '**homophobia**' is today still prevalent in India, and public discussion of homosexuality in India is inhibited by the fact that sexuality in any form is rarely discussed openly, attitudes towards homosexuality have shifted dramatically. In particular, there have been more depictions and discussions of homosexuality in the Indian news media, in films, and on streaming platforms (e.g., Netflix).
- Lesbian, gay, bisexual and transgender (**LGBT**) rights in India have historically and culturally been accepted under the 'Hijra' concept. India is one of the few countries in the world to legally recognize a **third gender**. Tamil Nadu was the first state to introduce a transgender (hijra/aravani) welfare policy. According to the transgender welfare policy, transgender people can access free Sex Reassignment Surgery (SRS) in the Government Hospital; free housing programme; various citizenship documents; admission in government colleges with full scholarship for higher studies; alternative sources of livelihood through formation of self-help groups (for savings), and initiating income-generation programmes.
  - Hijras have been legally granted voting rights as a 'third sex' since 1994.
  - On 15th April 2014, the Supreme Court of India declared transgender people as a socially and economically backward class entitled to reservations in education and jobs, and also directed union and state governments to frame welfare schemes for them.

Box 3.7—Twists and turns against 150-year-old ban on homosexuality

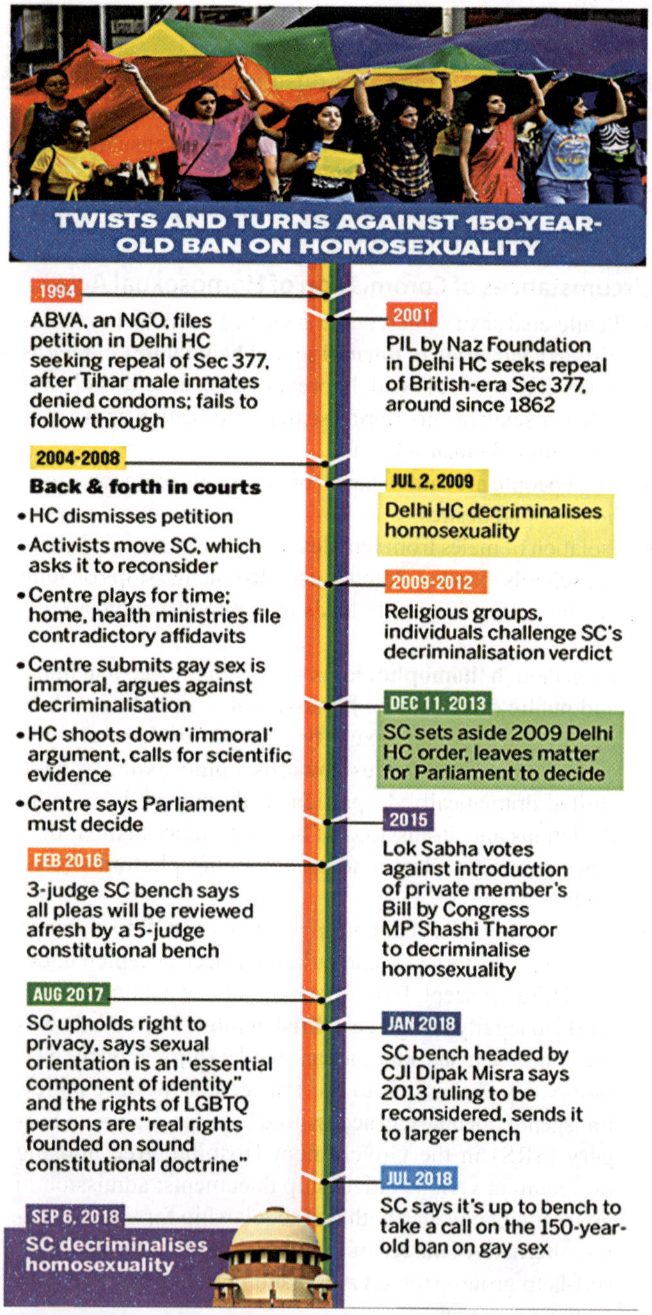

Medicolegal Examination of an Alleged Victim of Forced/Non-consensual Penetrative Anal Sex (Sodomy)*

- **Written requisition** for the examination from the police or magistrate.
- **General information** (name, age, sex, occupation, address of normal residence, marital status).
- Express written informed **consent**, duly witnessed.
- **History** as per that taken from a victim of alleged rape, modified according to the sex and age of the victim.
- **Gait**: Normal, or broadbased and painful.
- **Examination of clothing** for:
  - Damage
  - Loose pubic hairs
  - Stains of blood/semen/lubricant/faeces
- **General physical examination**, including:
  - At least two marks of identification, and
  - Any injuries indicating resistance.
- **Local examination** (in knee-elbow position)
  - ***Victim Not Used To Sodomy***
    - Pain/Tenderness during examination.
    - Smears of lubricant and loose foreign pubic hairs around/in the anus.
    - Perianal abrasions (whose severity is dependent on the relative proportion between the size of the penis of the assailant and the anal sphincter of the victim, and are therefore most marked in children).
    - Perianal bruising, and extension of injuries into the anal canal.
    - Anal lacerations – Usually triangular and based at the external sphincter, with the sides extending horizontally inward, but rarely more than 2–3 cm, because penile penetration would have been limited by a strong contraction of the sphincter ani. These lacerations will result in bleeding onto the thighs and clothing.
    - Digital examination per rectum: Usually very painful.
    - Fresh/Dried semen around/in the anus, if present, should be swabbed/scraped off, appropriately packed, sealed, labelled and sent through the accompanying police officer, to the Forensic Science Laboratory for serological and microscopic examination.
  - ***Habitual Passive Agent***
    - Bloodstains are usually not observed.
    - Loose foreign pubic hairs and smears of lubricant may or may not be present.
    - Perianal hair is usually shaved.
    - The person does not experience any pain or tenderness during examination, and the external sphincter relaxes reflexly when bimanual traction is applied to the buttocks (***lateral traction test***).
    - Funnel-shaped depression of the buttocks towards the anus.
    - Perianal skin may be thickened and keratinised from constant friction.
    - Anus:
      - Dilated and patulous
      - Loss of rugosity of mucous membrane
      - Fresh or old fissures/sinuses (tunnelling)
    - Rectum: Prolapse of mucosa, which is usually thickened, with disappearance of radial folds.

****Note***: *Referred to as "Buggery", if it is a case of heterosexual penile-anal intercourse.*

- Evidence of sexually transmitted disease (e.g., condylomata acuminata, chancre/chancroid, gonorrhoeal discharge, etc.) may or may not be present.
- Digital examination per rectum: Relatively painless.

Medicolegal Examination of Alleged Assailant of Forced/Non-consensual Penetrative Anal Sex (Sodomy)

Examination of the alleged assailant/active agent proceeds exactly in the same manner as that of the medicolegal examination of the accused in a case of alleged rape, except that the shaft of the penis may reveal traces of faecal matter and/or lubricant instead of vaginal epithelial cells.

Medicolegal Aspects

- Penile-anal intercourse between consenting adults is now legally permissible in India, provided it is practiced in private.
- The marriage contract gives implied consent only for sexual intercourse per vaginum, not per anum.
  - If the husband forces his wife (who is unwilling) to submit to anal intercourse (especially repeatedly or persistently), it can constitute valid grounds for divorce.
- Homosexual jealousy often leads to intense emotional upheaval, and can result in suicide or homicide.

FEMALE HOMOSEXUALITY

- Also referred to as **lesbianism**, **sapphism**, **tribadism**.
- Typically, it involves kissing, cuddling, mutual masturbation and occasionally an active–passive relationship, by biclitoral/digital/lingual-vaginal stimulation, or the use of vibrators or artificial phalluses (*dildos*).
- A preferentially active lesbian, who is often a transvestite or transsexual, is known as a ***butch*** or ***dyke***, while the usually passive agent is called a ***femme***. These are however degrading expressions that must not be used in scientific discussions on female homosexuality.

Medicolegal Aspects

- In the same way as male homosexuality, female homosexuality has also been **de-criminalised** by the Supreme Court of India on 06th Sept 2018, provided both partners are mutually consenting adults.
- Forced lesbian acts are extremely difficult, if not impossible to prove, unless
  - Traces of fresh/dried saliva or buccal mucosal cells can be detected on/around the external genitalia, or
  - Injuries result from the use, or forcible introduction into the vagina, of an artificial phallus.
- Because habitually active lesbians are strongly averse to heterosexual relationships (passive agents are usually less so and, in fact, frequently **bisexual**), continued lesbianism can be valid grounds for divorce or annulment of marriage.
- Morbid jealousies, as frequent in lesbianism as in male homosexuality, may lead to homicide, suicide or suicide pacts.

Conversion Therapy

- In Feb 2014, the Indian Psychiatric Society (IPS) issued a statement in which it stated that there is no evidence to prove that homosexuality is unnatural: "Based on existing scientific evidence and good practice guidelines from the field of psychiatry, the Indian Psychiatric Society would like to state that there is no evidence to substantiate the belief that homosexuality is a mental illness or a disease."
- In June 2018, IPS reiterated its stance saying: "Certain people are not cut out to be heterosexual and we don't need to castigate them, or punish them, or ostracize them".
- Despite this statement from the IPS, conversion therapies are still performed in India. These practices usually involve electroconvulsive therapy (which may lead to memory loss), hypnosis, the administration of nausea-inducing drugs or more commonly talk therapy, where the individual is told that homosexuality is caused by "insufficient male affirmation in childhood" or "an uncaring father and an overbearing mother".
- Conversion therapy can lead to depression, anxiety, seizures, drug use and suicidal tendencies for the individuals involved.
- **In 2022, the National Medical Commission banned the practice of 'conversion therapy'**, following the Madras High Court ruling in *S Sushma v. Commissioner of Police*.

BUCCAL COITUS* (ORAL SEX)

- Also quite quaintly (and inappropriately) called the "Sin of Gomorrah" because of the alleged prevalence of the practice in Gomorrah, the Biblical twin city of Sodom.
- The outdated term "**buccal sex**" denotes penile/vaginal buccal sexual intercourse, and can therefore be performed by both males and females.
  - Buccal-penile intercourse is called **fellatio**. The partner who performs the act is known as the "fellator"; the one on whom it is performed is the "fellatee."
  - Buccal-vaginal stimulation is referred to as **cunnilingus**.
- Although formerly considered as a sexual deviation/perversion, psychiatrists and psychologists today view buccal coitus, or more properly, "**oral sex**" as a part of normal sexual foreplay.

Medicolegal Aspects

- Provided the act (oral sex) is performed by mutual consent of two adults, buccal coitus is permissible in India and is no more considered "unnatural".
- Forced or non-consensual oral sex is punishable, as well as oral sex with minors.
- Under the Hindu Marriage Act, insistence on buccal coitus, if it is non-consensual and repetitive, would constitute a valid ground for divorce.

**What a terribly outdated expression! As doctors we should strive to avoid using archaic terms out of a sense of false modesty. The term "oral sex" is always to be preferred.*

- The only material evidence of commission of the offence would be
  - Spermatozoa of the fellatee in the mouth of the fellator
  - Fresh/Dried saliva or buccal mucosal cells on the penis of the fellatee, or on the external genitalia or the vulva of the subject of cunnilingus.
  - As any of these would be unobtainable under ordinary circumstances (unless the participants were caught in the act), it is generally practically impossible to prove a charge of buccal coitus in a criminal court of law.

Gender and Sexuality Based (Sexual Orientation) Identities and Rights in India

- **Lesbian**, **Gay**, **Bisexual**, **Transgender (LGBT)** rights in India have been evolving rapidly in recent years. However, Indian LGBT citizens still face social and legal difficulties not experienced by non-LGBT persons.
- India has repealed its colonial-era laws that directly discriminated against homosexual and transgender identities and also explicitly interpreted Article 15 of the Constitution to prohibit discrimination on the basis of sexual orientation and gender identity. But, many legal protections have not been provided for, including same-sex marriage.
  - On 12th June 2020, the Uttarakhand High Court acknowledged that while same-sex marriage may not be legal, cohabitation and "live-in relationships" are protected by the law.
  - Amidst strong political movements in favour of LGBT rights, people are more accepting of same-sex relationships. LGBT people in India are increasingly gaining tolerance and acceptance, especially in large cities.
- In **2018**, in the landmark decision of **Navtej Singh Johar v. Union of India**, the Supreme Court of India decriminalised consensual homosexual intercourse by reading down Section 377 of the Indian Penal Code and excluding consensual homosexual sex between adults from its ambit.
- On 4th February 2021, the Allahabad High Court ruled that firing and discriminating against a person in employment on the basis of sexual orientation is a violation of Navtej Singh Johar v. Union of India ruling of the Supreme Court, hence extending the anti-discriminatory provisions to employment everywhere.
- Transgender people in India are allowed to change their legal gender post-sex reassignment surgery under **Transgender Persons (Protection of Rights) Act, 2019**, and have a constitutional right to register themselves under a third gender. Additionally, some states protect **hijras**, a traditional third gender population in South Asia through housing programmes, and offer welfare benefits, pension schemes, free operations in government hospitals as well as other programmes designed to assist them.
  - The **Transgender Persons (Protection of Rights) Act, 2019** defines transgender persons as those "whose gender does not match the gender assigned to that person at birth, and includes trans-men or trans-women, persons with intersex variations, gender-queers, and persons having socio-cultural identities such as kinnar, hijras, aravani and jogta".
  - A person would have the right to choose to be identified as **male**, **female** or "**transgender**". However, transgender people are required to go to a district magistrate to have their gender identity certified, and require proof of sex reassignment surgery.
  - The Act bans discrimination against transgender people in
    - educational establishment and services
    - employment
    - healthcare services
    - access to the "use of any goods, accommodation, service, facility, benefit, privilege or opportunity dedicated to the use of the general public or customarily available to the public"
    - the right to movement
    - the right to "reside, purchase, rent or otherwise occupy any property"
    - the opportunity to stand for or hold public or private office, and in government or private establishments.
- Thomas Trace Beatie, born as Tracy Lagondino in 1974, grew up in Honolulu, Hawaii. Assigned female sex at birth, Beatie underwent sex reassignment surgery involving a double mastectomy, also known as "top surgery, and officially changed his sex marker from "female" to "male" on his state and federal identity documents in 2002. However, he retained his female reproductive organs, which later allowed him to become pregnant. Beatie married Nancy Gillespie in 2003. The couple moved to Oregon, in 2005. When the two decided to start a family, Beatie chose to carry the child, since Nancy was unable due to a prior hysterectomy. Beatie suspended testosterone hormone treatment in order to conceive, and became successfully pregnant afterwards, twice with donor sperm, delivering both children without complications. Guinness World Records named Beatie the "**World's First Married Man to Give Birth**" in 2010.
- In India, the first transgender couple to get married were Zahad, a 23-year-old trans man and Ziya Paval, a 21-year-old trans woman, both from Kerala. Zahad subsequently became pregnant and gave birth at the Kozhikode Government Medical College Hospital on 08th Feb 2023.

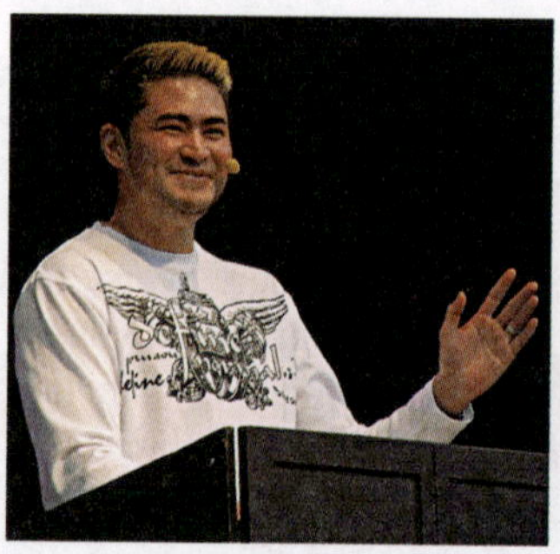

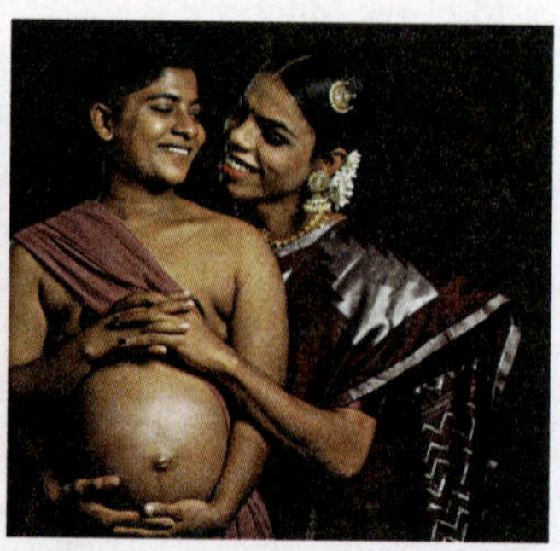

Thomas Beatie (L) and Zahad & Ziya (R)

BESTIALITY

(Sexual Acts with Animals; Zoophilia)

- **Zoophilia** is a paraphilia involving a sexual fixation on non-human animals.
- **Bestiality** is cross-species sexual activity between humans and non-human animals.
  - The terms are often used interchangeably, but some researchers make a distinction between the attraction (zoophilia) and the act (bestiality). Bestialists rape or abuse animals, while zoophiles form an emotional and sexual attachment to animals.
- **Faunoiphilia** refers to sexual arousal from watching animals mate with each other.
- There are a few references in Hindu scriptures to religious figures engaging in symbolic sexual activity with animals such as explicit depictions of people having sex with animals included amongst the thousands of sculptures of "Life events" on the exterior of the temple complex at Khajuraho. The depictions are largely symbolic depictions of the sexualization of some animals and are not meant to be taken literally. In fact, as per some Hindu scriptures, having sex with animals, especially a cow, leads one to hell.
- The animals usually selected for bestiality (sexual acts with animals):
  - **By males** – cows, mares, bitches, female sheep/goats/donkeys and large birds.
  - **By females** (far less common) – bulls, horses, dogs and male sheep/goats/donkeys.
- Just as any animal may be used by a male, so also sexual intercourse may be effected through any of its natural orifices, i.e., the vagina or anus.

Psychological Aspects and Circumstances of Commission

- Of all the sexual offences, bestiality is the least common.
- It is characteristically the act of an isolated, simpleminded, aberrant farmworker, who is the object of ridicule and/or ill treatment by his fellow men, or by women (in which case he feels frightened and incapable of approaching the opposite sex). He then overcomes his rejection and humiliation by sexual intercourse with an available and usually compliant animal companion. An element of revenge, if present, is usually manifested as sadism (*vide infra*).
- Bestiality may also be the product of a superstition among some ignorant males that sexual intercourse with a female donkey cures gonorrhoea!

Medicolegal Aspects

- Bestiality is a criminal offence worldwide. In India, it is punishable under Sec 377 of the IPC.
- Bestiality is a valid ground for annulment of marriage.
- The offence is difficult to prove (unless the accused is caught in the act), not the least because one of the parties is incapable of expression.
- The following general findings may be observed on medicolegal examination of the accused:
  - Young adult male, often (but not always) mentally challenged or mentally abnormal.
  - Injuries inflicted by the animal, if it resisted the act by kicking and/or biting.
  - Hair/feathers and/or bloodstains of the animal on the clothing or person of the accused.
- Human seminal stains may be present in or around the genitalia of the animal.

INDECENT ASSAULT

(Forced/Non-consensual Groping, Touching, Disrobing)

- It is necessary to differentiate **sexual assault** from **indecent assault** as both do not mean the same.
  1. Sexual assault is a broad term which mainly covers the offence of rape, but can also include indecent assault.
- The offence of "**indecent assault**" is defined in **Section 354 of the IPC** as follows: "*Whoever assaults or uses criminal force to any woman, intending to outrage her modesty, shall be punished with imprisonment of not less than 1 year, but which may extend to 5 years, and shall also be liable to fine*".
- It is a cognizable and non-bailable offence.
- What exactly amounts to "outraging the modesty of a woman" has not been clearly stated in Sec 354 IPC. But, it can include verbal obscenity, obscene gestures, inappropriate touching or groping, lewd remarks, displaying vulgar images, etc.
- **Sec 354A** deals with **sexual harassment**:
  1. A man committing any of the following acts—
     i. physical contact and advances involving unwelcome and explicit sexual overtures; or
     ii. a demand or request for sexual favours; or
     iii. showing pornography against the will of a woman; or
     iv. making sexually coloured remarks, shall be guilty of the offence of sexual harassment.
  2. *Punishment*—
     i. Sexual harassment of the nature of unwelcome physical contact and advances or a demand or request for sexual favours or showing pronography: up to 3 years or fine or both.
     ii. Sexual harassment of the nature of making sexually coloured remark: up to 1 year or fine or both.
  3. **Sec 354B** deals with **assault with intent to disrobe a woman**: Any man who assaults or uses criminal force to any woman, or abets such act with the intention of disrobing or compelling her to be naked, shall be punished with imprisonment of either description for a term which shall not be less than 3 years but which may extend to seven years, and shall also be liable to fine.
  4. **Sec 354C** deals with **voyeurism** (*see page no. 213*).
  5. **Sec 354D** deals with **stalking** (*see page no. 213*).

Modified FM 3.17: Core – Written/Viva Voce

- Describe the difference between Paraphilia and Paraphilic disorder.
- Describe paraphilic disorder as per the latest guidelines of DSM & ICD and describe medico-legal implications of paraphilic disorder by referring scientific literature and legal justification (if any).
- Describe and discuss the various paraphilias in the context of informed consent during any sexual interaction.

PARAPHILIA & PARAPHILIC DISORDER

Definitions

As per *Diagnostic and Statistical Manual of Mental Disorders*, 5th edition (*DSM-5*) 2013:

- **Paraphilia**: A paraphilia is any intense and persistent sexual interest other than sexual interest in genital stimulation or preparatory fondling with phenotypically normal, physically mature, consenting human partners.
- Paraphilias are no more termed "perversions" or "deviations". Such terms must NOT be used in the scientific context.
- Paraphilia is not ipso facto a psychiatric disorder, while **paraphilic disorder** is a condition associated with unusual sexual desires that cause distress or impairment to the individual, or harm to others.
- **DSM-5 specified paraphilic disorders**:
    1. Voyeuristic disorder (spying on others engaged in private activities)
    2. Exhibitionistic disorder (exposing the genitals)
    3. Frotteuristic disorder (touching or rubbing against a non-consenting individual)
    4. Sexual masochism disorder (undergoing humiliation, bondage or suffering)
    5. Sexual sadism disorder (inflicting humiliation, bondage or suffering)
    6. Paedophilic disorder (sexual focus on children)
    7. Fetishistic disorder (using non-living objects or having a highly specific focus on non-genital body parts)
    8. Transvestic disorder (engaging in sexually arousing cross-dressing)
    9. Other specified paraphilic disorders:
        i. Zoophilia (animals)
        ii. Scatalogia (obscene phone calls)
        iii. Necrophilia (corpses)
        iv. Coprophilia (faeces)
        v. Klismaphilia (enemas)
        vi. Urophilia (urine)

Voyeuristic Disorder (Voyeurism)

- **Voyeurism** (which is almost exclusively seen in males) refers to the repetitive seeking out of situations in which unsuspecting women might be observed when they are grooming themselves, undressing, bathing or copulating.
- A male voyeur is sometimes referred to as a **Peeping Tom**, named after a person who, in the legend of Lady Godiva, watched her during her naked ride on horseback, and was struck blind.
    - **Lady Godiva** (died between 1066 and 1086) was a late Anglo-Saxon noblewoman who was the wife of Leofric, Earl of Mercia. Today, she is mainly remembered for a legend dating back to at least the 13th century, in which she rode naked – covered only in her long hair – through the streets of Coventry to gain a remission of the oppressive taxation that her husband, Leofric, imposed on his tenants (**Fig. 3.131**). The name "Peeping Tom" for a voyeur originates from later versions of this legend, in which a man named Thomas watched her ride and was struck blind or dead.

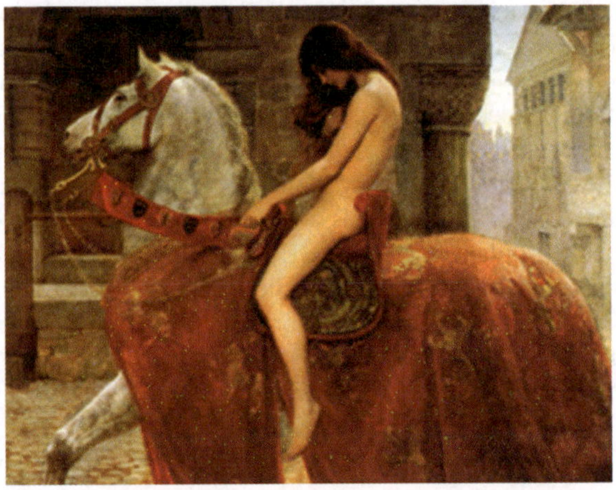

Fig. 3.131 Lady Godiva (*painting by John Collier*)

- Voyeurism can take several forms, but its principal characteristic is that the voyeur does not normally relate directly with the subject of his or her interest, who is often unaware of being observed. The voyeur may observe the subject from a distance, or use stealth to observe the subject with the use of two-way mirrors, camera, videos, etc. Today, mobile phones (which are invariably fitted with cameras) are commonly misused for this purpose. The diagnosis of "voyeurism" does not apply to people who experience sexual arousal simply by seeing nudity or sexual activity. The aspect of **spying** is central to paraphilic voyeurism.
- Voyeurism has high prevalence rates in most studied populations. Research shows that up to 65% of men engage in peeping, which suggests that this behaviour is widely spread throughout the population.
- Voyeurs usually do not come in conflict with the law, unless they are caught in the act of spying. They are more often considered to be a public nuisance than a social menace. However, some voyeurs gradually become bolder and may venture into **exhibitionism**.
- As per **Section 354C**, a man committing the offence of voyeurism would be liable for imprisonment not less than 1 year, and which may extend up to 3 years for the first offence, and shall also be liable to fine, and for any subsequent conviction would be liable for imprisonment for not

less than 3 years, and which may extend up to 7 years and with fine.

Exhibitionistic Disorder (Exhibitionism)

- **Exhibitionism** refers to sexual gratification obtained by repeated acts of exposing one's genitals to a stranger or unsuspecting person (usually of the opposite sex).
  - **Flashing** is the display of bare breasts by a woman with an up-and-down lifting of the shirt, blouse, or bra, or a man exposing his genitals (**Fig. 3.132**).
  - **Mooning** is the display of one's bare buttocks by pulling down trousers and underwear.
  - In either case, there may not be any sexual connotation, but may be merely an attention-getting gambit. Mooning is sometimes resorted to as an offensive gesture.
  - **Streaking** is the act of taking off one's clothes and running naked through a public place. It is purely an attention-seeking gambit, and almost never has sexual connotations.

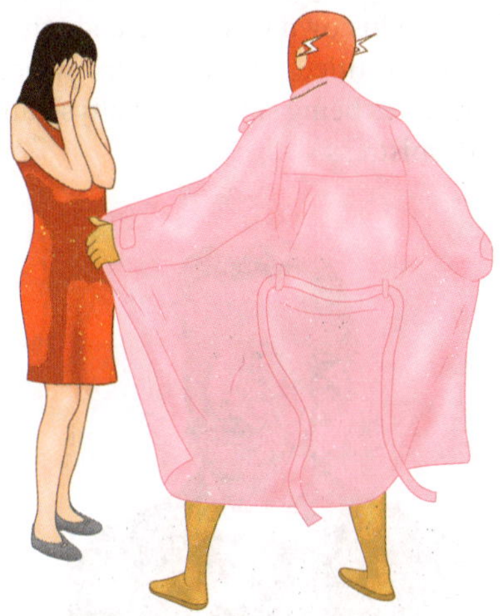

Fig. 3.132 Exhibitionism (*'Flashing'*)

- Exhibitionism is only considered a paraphilic disorder when the practice begins to interfere with the quality of life, or normal functioning capacity of the individual.
- Because of the tendency for repeated exposure, true exhibitionists (who do it for sexual gratification) sooner or later get arrested and charged with the offence of "**indecent exposure**" under **Sec 294 IPC**:
  - Whoever, to the annoyance of others:
    - does any obscene act in any public place (indecent exposure), or
    - sings, recites or utters any obscene song, ballad or words, in or near any public place,
  - shall be punished with imprisonment of either description for a term which may extend to 3 months, or with fine, or with both.
- Like voyeurism, exhibitionism can lead to paedophilia, as in many cases, the victim is a child.

Frotteuristic Disorder (Frotteurism)

- **Frotteurism** is a paraphilic disorder in which rubbing, usually one's pelvic area or erect penis, against a non-consenting person leads to sexual gratification. It may involve touching any part of the body, including the genital area. A person who practices frotteuristic acts is known as a **frotteur**.
- The DSM called this sexual disorder by the name **frottage** until the third edition (DSM III-R), but changed to **frotteurism** in the fourth edition (DSM-IV) and now uses the term **frotteuristic disorder** in the fifth edition (DSM-5). Nevertheless, the term frottage still remains in some law codes, where it is synonymous with the term frotteurism.
- Today, the term **frotteurism (Fig. 3.133)** is usually applied specifically to the act of rubbing any part of the body, including the buttocks, breasts, abdomen, thighs, feet, hands, legs or sexual organs against the sexual organ of another person; this is done whether naked or clothed, and is more commonly known as **dry humping** or **dry sex**. When frottage includes genital-genital rubbing, it is sometimes called **genito-genital** or **GG rubbing**.

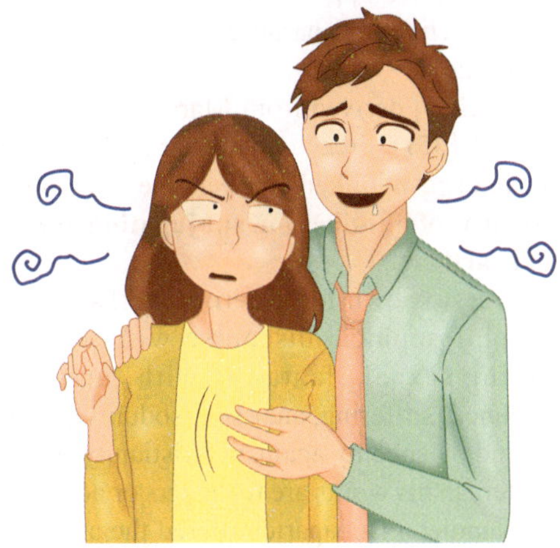

Fig. 3.133 Frotteurism

- **Toucherism** ("**Groping**") (**Fig. 3.134**) is a related disorder in which sexual arousal is based on grabbing or rubbing one's hands against an unexpecting (and non-consenting) person. It usually involves touching breasts, buttocks or genital areas, often while quickly walking across the victim's path. Some psychologists consider toucherism a manifestation of frotteurism, while others distinguish the two.
- The majority of frotteurs are male and the majority of victims are female.
- This activity is often done in circumstances where the victim cannot easily respond, in a public place such as a crowded train or bus or mass gathering.
- Frotteurism is one form of sexual crime, and is usually booked under "**indecent assault**".
- Treatment of frotteuristic disorder involves cognitive

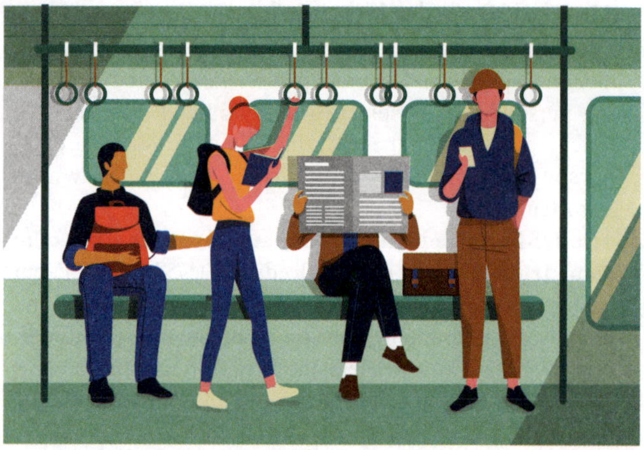

Fig. 3.134 Toucherism ('Groping')

behavioural therapy coupled with the administration of medications such as selective serotonin reuptake inhibitors (SSRIs).

Sexual Sadistic Disorder (Sadism) and Sexual Masochistic Disorder (Masochism)

- These represent two opposite and separate aspects of the self, i.e., the active and passive poles of a subjugation-humiliation axis.
- The term **sadism**, derived from Marquis de Sade (1740–1814) **(Fig. 3.135)** a French novelist, is applied to **sexual arousal and orgasm linked to the active infliction, in fantasy or reality, of humiliation, subjugation or torture of the sexual partner**.
  - Sade is best known for his erotic works, which combined philosophical discourse with pornography, depicting sexual fantasies with an emphasis on violence, suffering, anal sex (sodomy), child rape, crime and blasphemy against Christianity. Many of the characters in his works are teenagers or adolescents. In 1801, Napoleon Bonaparte ordered the arrest of Sade, expressing outrage after he had been sent a copy of one of his novels. Despite having no legal charge brought against him, Sade was incarcerated in various prisons and an insane asylum for about 32 years of his life, until his death in 1814.

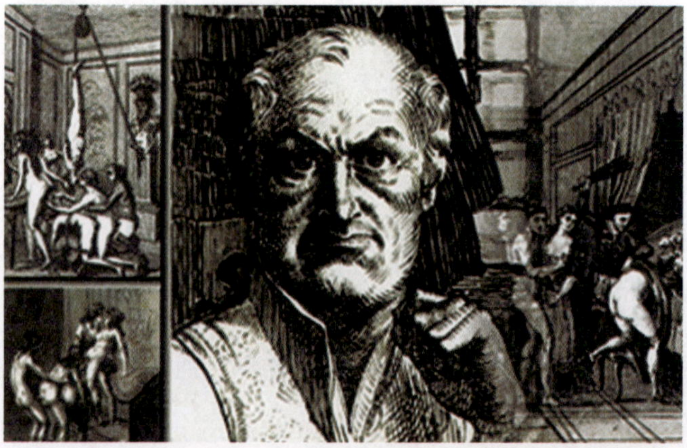

Fig. 3.135 Marquis de Sade (*with illustrations from some of his books*)

- The term **masochism** is named after Leopold von Sacher-Masoch (1836–1895) **(Fig. 3.136)**, an Austrian writer and journalist, who enjoyed being humiliated and subjugated by women. It is the direct reciprocal of sadism, and is defined as **sexual excitement linked with the passive experience of physical or emotional humiliation, subjugation, torture or danger**.
  - Leopold von Sacher-Masoch was born in Lemberg, Galicia (now Poland), on Jan 27th 1836, in a respectable family of Slavic and Bohemian ancestry. During his lifetime, Sacher-Masoch was well known as a man of letters, in particular a utopian thinker who espoused socialist and humanist ideals in his fiction and non-fic tion. Sacher-Masoch's fantasies and fetishes (especially for dominant women wearing fur) were expressed in many of his writings. He did his best to live out his fantasies with his own mistresses and wives. His most famous novel is titled "Venus in Furs' which deals with a man who likes being subjugated physically and sexually by his mistress.

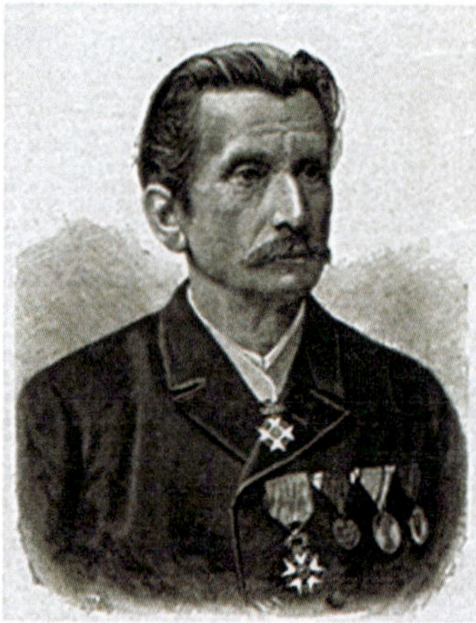

Fig. 3.136 Leopold von Sacher-Masoch

- Both are included under a broader entity often referred to as **BDSM**, which is a compound acronym derived from the terms **bondage** and **discipline**; **dominance** and **submission**; **sadism** and **masochism**.
  - BDSM is not a form of sexual abuse – although some BDSM activities may appear to be violent or coercive, such activities are conducted with the consent of all partners involved.
- Neither sadism nor masochism is exclusively male or exclusively female, but sadistic practices are more common among men, and masochistic practices are more frequently observed in women.
- **Medicolegal Aspects**
  - Prevalence figures of both sadism and masochism are

underestimated, because the acts are usually by mutual consent, and therefore are not reported.

- Masochism comes to medical and legal attention when the degree of tolerable suffering is unknowingly exceeded, with tragic results.
- A sadist may be sought by law enforcement personnel only in cases of brutality, marital cruelty, rape or **lust murder** (i.e., homicide committed in the pursuit of sexual arousal and orgasm).
- Some serial killers are sexual sadists by nature.

Paedophilic Disorder (Child Sexual Abuse; Paedophilia)

- **Paedophilia** (or **pedophilia**) is generally defined as a psychological disorder in which an adult experiences a sexual preference for prepubescent children.
- In law enforcement, the term "paedophile" is generally used to describe those accused or convicted of the sexual abuse of a minor (including both prepubescent children and adolescent minors younger than the local age of consent). Most paedophiles are men, though there are also women who have paedophilic tendencies.
- Paedophilic crimes may be perpetrated within a family (amounting to **incest**), or among acquaintance groups, or by strangers. In all cases, the offence is punishable, under **Sec 376, IPC**, if the victim is a female, or **Sec 377, IPC**, if male.
- **Child sexual abuse** includes a variety of sexual offences, including:
  - **Sexual assault** – A term defining offences in which an adult touches a minor for the purpose of sexual gratification; for example, rape (including sodomy), and sexual penetration with an object.
  - **Sexual molestation** – A term defining offences in which an adult engages in non-penetrative activity with a minor for the purpose of sexual gratification; for example, exposing a minor to pornography or to the sexual acts of others.
  - **Sexual exploitation** – A term defining offences in which an adult victimizes a minor for sexual gratification or profit; for example, prostituting a child, and creating or trafficking in child pornography.
  - **Sexual grooming** – Defines the social conduct of a potential child sex offender who seeks to make a minor more accepting of their advances, for example in an online chat room.
- Aggression and sadism are inherent components of paedophilia. These may be subconscious, under control or open. Only a few paedophilic encounters result in injuries and/or death, but a victim may be badly beaten, or killed, if the assailant is a cold-blooded killer or a lust murderer, or panics after the act.
- The effects of child sexual abuse include depression, post-traumatic stress disorder, anxiety and physical injury to the child, among other problems such as transmission of venereal disease.
- The Parliament of India passed the '**Protection of Children Against Sexual Offences Act, 2012' (POCSO Act)** relating to child sexual abuse which came into effect on **14th Nov, 2012**. The new Act provides for a variety of offences under which an accused can be punished.
  - It recognizes forms of penetration other than peno-vaginal penetration.
  - It criminalizes acts of immodesty against children.
  - With respect to **pornography**, the Act criminalizes even watching or collection of pornographic content involving children.
    - Section 13 of the POCSO Act states that anyone who uses a child for pornographic purposes by either representing the sexual organs of the child or using a child in real or simulated sexual acts or representing a child indecently or obscenely in programmes or advertisements on television or on the internet, commits the offence under this section and is liable in accordance with Sections 14 and 15 of the POCSO Act.
  - Section 3 of the POCSO Act defines **penetrative sexual assault**, and Section 4 lays down the punishment, which was made more stringent by the 2019 amendment.
  - Section 5 lays down the criteria for **aggravated penetrative sexual assault**. For example, penetrative sexual assaults on a child by a police officer within the vicinity of a police station, by armed forces within the limits of their area, by a public servant, by the staff of jails, hospitals or educational institutions are all considered aggravated penetrative sexual assault and are punishable under Section 6 of the Act.
  - Section 7 defines **sexual assault** as "*Whoever, with sexual intent, touches the vagina, penis, anus or breast of the child or makes the child touch the vagina, penis, anus or breast of such person or any other person, or does any other act with sexual intent which involves physical contact without penetration.*"
  - Sections 9 and 10 lay down criteria for **aggravated sexual assault** on a child.
  - Section 11 defines **sexual harassment**. There are six clauses which constitute sexual harassment of a child:
    - Uttering any word or making any sound or exhibiting any object with sexual intent to a child.
    - Making a child to exhibit his/her body, so that it is seen by the offender or any other person.
    - Showing a child any form or media for pornographic purposes.
    - Constantly watching or stalking a child directly or online.
    - Threatening to use a real or fabricated depiction of any part of the body of the child, or the involvement of the child in a sexual act through electronic, film or digital media.
    - Enticing a child for pornographic purposes.
  - The Act does not create any distinction between the victim or the perpetrator on the basis of their gender.

This overcomes one of the biggest shortcomings of the Indian Penal Code's provisions. The court can even convict women for engaging in child sexual abuse incidents.
- Makes abetment of child sexual abuse an offence.
- Sexual abuse cases often happen behind closed doors and the elders attempt to hide these incidents due to the stigma that is attached to these crimes. Consequently, for the effective implementation of the POCSO Act, reporting of these incidents by the third parties who have the knowledge or apprehension of such offences, has been made mandatory under Sections 19 to 22 of the Act.
- Provides for various procedural reforms, making the tiring process of trial in India considerably easier for children.
    - The statement of the child is to be recorded at his/her place of residence and as far as possible by a woman police officer.
    - The officer who is to record the statement of the child should not be wearing a uniform.
    - The officer should ensure that the child does not come in contact with the accused during the examination.
    - A child is not to be detained in the police station at night.
    - The officer should ensure that the identity of the child is not revealed.
    - The statement of the child is to be recorded in the presence of a person in whom the child has trust, for example, a parent.
    - The statement of the child is to be recorded via audio–video electronic means.
    - The assistance of translators or interpreters should be taken wherever necessary.
    - Frequent breaks must be allowed during the trial.
    - The special court has to ensure that the child is not called to repeatedly testify in the trial court.
    - Aggressive questioning of the child is not permitted during the trial.
- Section 23 of the Act outlines the procedure to be followed by the media, and imposes the duty to refrain from revealing the victim's identity unless the Special Court has allowed the disclosure.
- The main criticism is that the Act has criminalized consensual sexual intercourse between two people below the age of 18, while previously (under the Indian Penal Code) it was 16 years.
    - Section 2(1) (d) of the POCSO Act defines a child as *any person below the age of eighteen years*. This implies that offences perpetrated against anyone of the age less than 18 years are punishable under the POCSO Act.

Fetishistic Disorder (Fetishism; Fetichism)

- The essential feature of this condition is the **sexual focus on parts of the body not normally associated with sexual arousal** (e.g., hair, foot, toes, etc.), **or on inanimate objects intimately associated with the human body** (handbag, glove, underwear, shoe/slipper, etc.).
- Sexual activity may be directed toward the fetish itself, or may be part of sexual intercourse, and the preferred fetish or class of fetishes is usually constant over a period of time.
- One of the most commonly encountered is 'foot fetish', characterized by a pronounced sexual interest in feet (**Fig. 3.137**).
- Fetishism does not ordinarily contravene law, unless
    - The constant search for a particular fetish leads to theft or mischief.
    - Repeated insistence on the use of fetishes by a non-consenting spouse is cited by him/her as grounds for divorce.

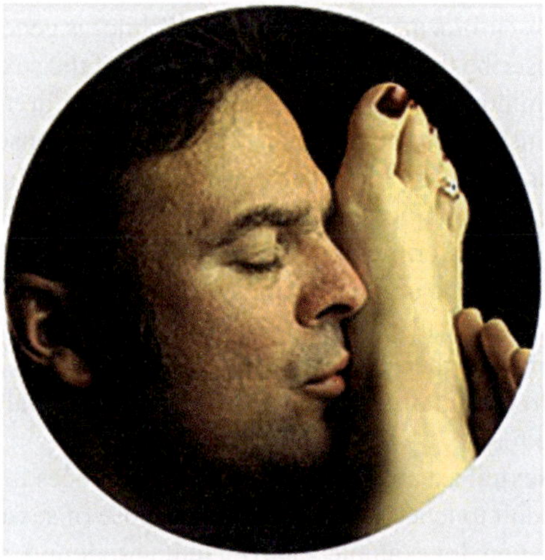

Fig. 3.137 Foot fetish

Transvestic Disorder (Transvestism)

- Also called "**cross-dressing**" or **Eonism**, after the Chevalier d'Eon de Beaumont (1728–1810, a noted practitioner who was a French diplomat; he lived the latter part of his life dressed constantly as a female) (**Fig. 3.138**).

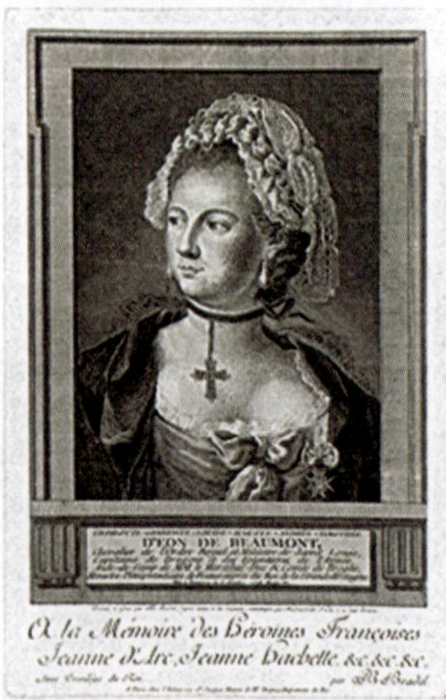
D'EON DE BEAUMONT
A la Mémoire des Héroïnes Françoises
Jeanne d'Arc, Jeanne Hachette, &c. &c. &c.

Fig. 3.138 Portrait of Chevalier d'Eon de Beaumont

- It is defined as **fantasised or actual dressing in the clothing of the opposite sex, for the purposes of sexual arousal,** and as an adjunct to masturbation or sexual intercourse.
- The following points must be noted:
  - Male preponderance.
  - Commencement of the transvestic syndrome at around puberty (but frank dressing in women's clothing does not begin until mobility and relative independence from parents is well established).
  - Transvestism is also seen in girls, but it seems to start later than in boys, is nowadays easily disguised because of unisex clothing, and has an uncertain outcome.
  - At first glance, **transvestism** and **trans-sexualism** appear to be quite similar. However, there are distinct differences between the two conditions. Until recently, trans-sexualism has been included as a part of transvestism but the difference lies mainly in the different degrees of desire held by the individual.
    - **Trans-sexualism** involves a more permanent desire to be the other sex, whereas
    - **Transvestism** involves only the desire to dress in clothes typically worn by the other sex.
    - **Transgender** is the state of one's gender identity or gender expression not matching one's assigned sex. Transgender is independent of sexual orientation; transgender people may identify as heterosexual, homosexual, bisexual, etc.
      - **Gender dysphoria** or **gender identity disorder (GID)** is the dysphoria (distress) a person experiences as a result of the sex and gender they were assigned at birth. In these cases, the assigned sex and gender do not match the person's gender identity, and the person is **transgender**. There is evidence suggesting that those who identify with a gender different from the one they were assigned at birth may do so not just due to psychological or behavioural causes, but also biological ones related to their genetics or exposure to hormones before birth.
- '**Drag**' is a term that is used to refer to the clothing associated with one gender when worn by a person of another gender. '**Drag queen**' refers to a gay man who dresses in drag, either as part of a performance or for personal fulfillment (**Fig. 3.139**). Though a good portion who wear women's clothing are straight men, the term 'drag queen' distinguishes them from transvestites, transsexuals or transgender people. Doing drag here often includes wearing dramatically heavy makeup, wigs and prosthetic devices as part of the costume. While some male music celebrities wear exaggerated feminine clothing as part of their show, they are not necessarily drag queens. Females who dress in drag are called '**drag kings**'.
- **Medicolegal Aspects**:
  - Transvestite behaviour (both by males and females) was until the 1960s seen as an expression of homosexuality or suppressed homosexual impulses. However, it is known today that most homosexuals are not transvestites. Transvestites are generally heterosexual males who wear traditionally feminine clothing as a form of sexual arousal. They distance themselves strictly from both homosexuals and transsexuals, and usually also deny any fetishistic intentions.
  - Transvestism does not cause any problems, if it is practiced privately. A male transvestite who flaunts himself in public may be considered to disturb the peace by so doing. In our country, long accustomed to male transvestism under such circumstances as religious festivals and Ramlila performances, and used to the presence of **hijras** and **zenanas**, it is unlikely to deserve a second glance.
  - However, if a male spouse persistently indulges in transvestism, even in private and refuses to participate in normal sexual intercourse, it would obviously constitute a ground for divorce, or even annulment of marriage.

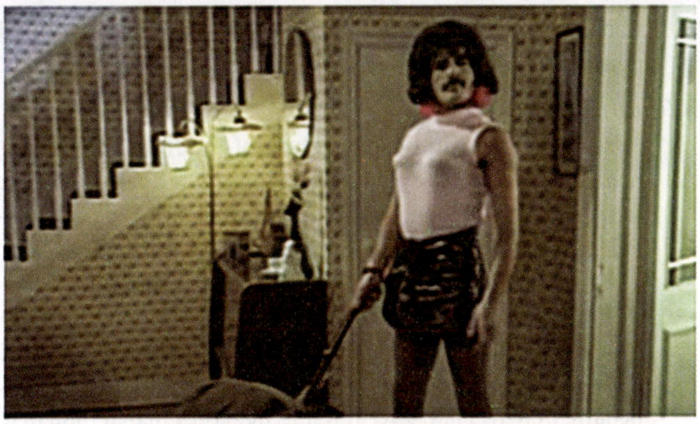

Fig. 3.139 Freddie Mercury (of the rock band Queen) in drag, for the song *"I want to break free"*

Hijra

- In the Indian subcontinent, **hijras** are eunuchs, intersex people or transgender people who live in communities that follow a kinship system known as guru-chela system. Also known as **aravani**, **aruvani** and **jogappa**, the hijra community in India prefer to call themselves "**kinnar**", referring to the mythological beings that excel at song and dance.
- Hijras are officially recognised as a **third gender** in the Indian subcontinent, being considered neither completely male nor female.
- Many hijras today live in well-defined and organised all-hijra communities, led by a "guru". These communities have consisted over generations of those who are in abject poverty, or who have been rejected by or fled their family of origin. Some work as sex workers.
- In general, hijras have been assigned male at birth, with only a few having been born with intersex variations. Some hijras undergo an initiation rite into the hijra community called "nirvaan", which involves the removal of the penis, scrotum and testicles.
- In April 2014, the Supreme Court recognised hijras,

transgender people, eunuchs and intersex people as a "**third gender**" in law.

Zenana

- A **zenana** or **kothi** in the culture of the Indian subcontinent, is a man or boy who takes on an "effeminate" role in same sex relationships, often with a desire to be the penetrated member in sexual intercourse.
- The original meaning was intended as a slur, similar to "fag" or "sissy".
- Zenanas or Kothis differ from Hijras in the sense that they do not live in the kind of intentional communities that hijras usually live in. They are similar to the Hijra in that they may take a same-sex lover for a period of time, and they may perform sexual favours for men through prostitution.

Scatalogia

- **Scatalogia** or more precisely, **Telephone Scatalogia** refers to **obscene phone calls** or unsolicited phone calls, where a person uses foul or sexual language to interact with someone who may be known to them, or who may be a complete stranger. The motive is sexual arousal or sexual pleasure, and is considered by some to be a form of **exhibitionism**.
- From the viewpoint of the recipient of the calls, obscene calls may be considered to be a form of sexual harassment, stalking or both.
- Generally, unwilling recipients of obscene phone calls are advised to simply hang up on obscene callers and then report the incident to the telephone company or the police. Even when Caller ID is not shown, calls are logged by the telephone company, so the perpetrator's phone number can be discovered. However, many people who regularly engage in obscene phone calls use payphones or prepaid cell phones, and in these cases, a more extensive investigation is necessary. The prevalence of internet telephony, and sophisticated international operations have also stymied the investigation of nuisance phone calls.
- Most of the perpetrators are male, and they are often emotionally or behaviourally maladjusted. Some of them may have been victims of sexual abuse.
- Many of these culprits feel inadequate, have feelings of isolation, have trouble forming relationships and consider making obscene phone calls to be the only way that they can sexually express themselves.
- Obscene phone calls must be differentiated from "prank calls".
  - A **prank call** (also known as a **crank call**) is a telephone call intended by the caller as a practical joke played on the person answering. It is often a type of nuisance call.

Phone Sex

- **Phone sex** is a conversation between two or more people by means of the telephone, which is sexually explicit and is intended to provoke sexual arousal in one or more participants. All parties participate voluntarily; it is typically accompanied by masturbation.
- As a practice between individuals temporarily separated, it is as old as dial telephones, on which no operator could eavesdrop (1930s–1950s). In the later 20th century, businesses emerged offering, for a fee, sexual conversations with a **phone sex worker**.
- Phone sex takes imagination on both individuals' part, as each party imagines "virtual sex". The sexually explicit conversation takes place between two or more persons via telephone, especially when at least one of the participants masturbates or engages in sexual fantasy.

Necrophilia

- **Necrophilia (necrolagnia, thanatophilia)** is a paraphilic disorder that is characterized by sexual attraction towards a corpse, or a sexual act involving a corpse.
- It is almost exclusively encountered in males, and is usually associated with psychiatric issues.
- **Necrophagia** is an extreme degree of necrophilia wherein the individual who is often a sadist, derives sexual gratification by mutilating the genitals or other body parts of a corpse, and eating them.
- Both acts are punishable under **Sec 297 IPC** (apart from other sections as applicable), which states that *"Whoever with the intention of...(offering) any indignity to any human corpse...shall be punished with imprisonment of either description for a term which may extend to one year, or with fine, or with both*".
- **Lee Mellor's typology of homicidal necrophiliacs** consists of 8 categories (A–H) and is based on the combination of two behavioural axes:
  - ***Destructive*** (offender mutilates the corpse for sexual reasons) – ***preservative*** (offender does not), and
  - ***Cold*** (offender uses the corpse sexually 2 hours or more after death) – ***warm*** (offender uses the corpse sexually less than 2 hours after death).
  - This renders four categories (A–D) to which Mellor adds an additional four (E–H):
    - Category A (cold/destructive)
    - Category B (cold/preservative)
    - Category C (warm/destructive)
    - Category D (warm/preservative)
    - Category E (dabblers): Transitory opportunistic sexual relations with corpses, but do not prefer them.
    - Category F (catathymic): Commit postmortem sex acts only while in a sudden impulsive state.
    - Category G (exclusive necromutilophiles): Derive pleasure purely from mutilating the corpse.
    - Category H (sexual cannibals & vampires): Sexually aroused by eating human body parts.
- **Jeffrey Dahmer** (1960–1994), also known as the **Milwaukee Cannibal** or the **Milwaukee Monster**, was an American serial killer and sex offender who killed and dismembered 17 men and boys between 1978 and 1991. Many of his later murders involved necrophilia and cannibalism, and the preservation of body parts—typically all or part of the skeleton.

- He was played by Peter Evans in the Netflix adaptation titled "*Monster – The Jeffrey Dahmer Story*" (**Fig. 3.140**).

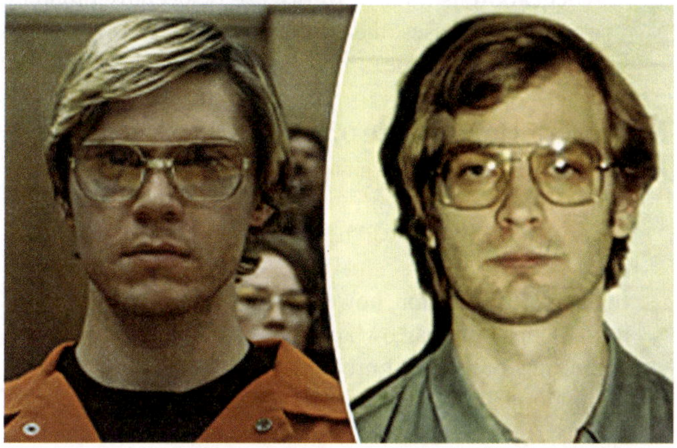

Fig. 3.140 Peter Evans (L) as Jeffrey Dahmer (R)

Coprophilia

- **Coprophilia** (**scatophilia** or **scat**) is a paraphilia involving sexual arousal and pleasure from faeces (feces).
- The diagnosis is made if the behaviour, sexual urges or fantasies cause clinically significant distress or impairment in social, occupational or other important areas of functioning.

Klismaphilia

- **Klismaphilia** is a paraphilia involving enjoyment of, and sexual arousal from enemas.
- Klismaphiles gain sexual satisfaction relating to enemas through fantasies, or by actually receiving or giving one.
- Sadomasochistic activities may incorporate enemas for erotic humiliation, or for physical discomfort.

Urophilia

- **Urophilia** (**urolagnia**) associates sexual excitement with the sight or thought of urine or urination, and may also refer to such behaviours or acts.
- During the activity, urine may be consumed or the person may bathe in it. Other variations include arousal from wetting or seeing someone else urinate in their pants or underclothes, or wetting the bed.
- "Golden shower" is slang for the practice of urinating on another person for sexual pleasure.
- Other forms of urolagnia may involve a tendency to be sexually aroused by smelling urine-soaked clothing or body parts. In many cases, a strong correlation or conditioning arises between urine smell or sight, and the sexual act.

Modified FM 3.18: Core – Written/Viva Voce
- Describe and discuss how 'signs' of virginity (so-called 'virginity test', including finger tests on female genitalia) are unscientific, inhuman and discriminatory.
- Describe and discuss how to appraise the courts about the unscientific basis of these tests, if the court orders it.
- Describe legitimacy and its medicolegal importance.

VIRGINITY

- **Virginity**, also referred to as **chastity**, is defined as "the state of being ***virgo intacta***, i.e., one who has never had sexual intercourse."
- In contrast, **defloration** refers to the "deprivation of virginity; the rupture of the hymen, either in coitus or in vaginal examination."
- From the medicolegal point of view, the term "**virginity**" has been applied to females in the context of penile-vaginal intercourse.
- **The National Medical Commission has stated in the modified Competency No. FM 3.18: 'Signs' of virginity (so-called 'virginity test', including finger tests on female genitalia) are unscientific, inhuman and discriminatory.**
  - **Therefore, 'signs of virginity' will not be discussed here at all, and teachers of FMT are advised not to teach these obsolete concepts to medical students. Asking questions pertaining to these concepts is also prohibited by the NMC.**

Medicolegal Aspects of Virginity

- In **civil cases**, whether a woman is a virgin or not may have to be decided in instances of:
  - **Nullity of marriage**, where virginity is proof of *non-consummation*,
  - **Divorce**, when deliberate withholding of a non-virgin state before marriage may be cited as grounds and
  - **Defamation of character**, when a woman brings an action for tort for illegal damage to reputation, against a person who has alleged that she is not a virgin.
- In **criminal cases**, loss of virginity may be offered as an *index* of sexual intercourse to substantiate a charge of **rape**.

HYMEN

- The **hymen** is a thin (but firm) fold of connective tissue, covered by mucous membrane, about 1 mm in overall thickness, situated at the vaginal orifice.
- Commonly, it is deficient anteriorly, and usually has a **central aperture**, but may be any of the following types (**Fig. 3.141**):
  - **Annular** – the hymen forms a ring around the vaginal opening.
  - **Semilunar or Crescentic** – forms a crescent shape, like a half moon, above or below the vaginal opening.
  - **Cribriform** – characterized by many small holes.
  - **Septate** – a piece of hymen makes a septum, or bridge, across the vaginal opening.
  - **Subseptate** – same as septate hymen, but does not make a bridge all the way across (similar view on examination as one gets when viewing the throat, with the uvula hanging down).
  - **Fimbriate** – makes an irregular pattern around the vaginal opening.
  - **Denticular** – so-called because it looks like a set of teeth surrounding the vaginal opening.
  - **Infundibuliform** – funnel-shaped.

- **Labial hymen** – the opening is in the form of a vertical slit in the centre, giving the hymen an appearance of a third set of vulvar lips.
- **Imperforate** – does not have any opening, and needs surgical correction before menarche for menstrual flow to occur.
- Occasionally, the hymen may be **congenitally absent**, which need not be a matter of concern at all.

Causes of Hymenal Rupture

- As a result of sexual intercourse, the hymen is usually torn posteriorly, with unilateral or bilateral tears extending to the point of its attachment to the vaginal wall. These ruptures bleed freely when fresh, and heal by scar formation.
- After the delivery of a child per vaginum, the hymen is almost completely torn, leaving only small remnants called "**caruncula e myrtiformes**"or "**carunculae hymenalis**."
- In a **true virgin**, the hymen may be ruptured because of:
  - **Trauma**, due to
    - An accidental fall on a protruding substance/object (this is not usually possible by strenuous physical exercise or by merely forcible separation of the thighs).
    - Instrumental masturbation with large foreign bodies (provided the instrument or object enters deep enough. Digital masturbation, unless practiced with two or more fingers, does not usually rupture the hymen).
    - Careless insertion of sanitary tampons.
    - Surgical operation for imperforate hymen.
    - Per vaginal examinations on a virgin.
    - The introduction of foreign bodies for reasons other than those described above, e.g., the insertion of sola pith into the vagina of very young girls to render them suitable for sexual intercourse.
  - **Ulceration** as a result of disease (especially diphtheria). In such cases, the entire hymen is destroyed leaving only scar tissue.

Medicolegal Importance of Hymen

- Besides being of limited anatomical value, the hymen, from a medicolegal viewpoint, is a **grossly overrated piece of tissue** – even experts can never be certain of virginity because of false virginity and hymenoplasty (surgical repair). In this latter condition, however, the hymen is usually taut, has an unusually narrow aperture, and exhibits fine scars at the sites of repair of previous tears.
- It is important to remember that the annular type hymen may appear intact even when sexual intercourse has taken place (especially when there is only a thin rim of hymen), while the fimbriated type may appear torn even in the intact state.
- It is also important to remember that the intact state of hymen must never be given any importance while examining an alleged victim of rape: rape can be accomplished by acts which do not damage the hymen at all, and this is explicitly stated in the Criminal Law Amendment Act (2013 and 2018).
- **Doctors must refrain from deducing any kind of evidentiary value to the status of hymen in a victim of rape.**

The "Two-finger Test"

- The two-finger test is an unscientific and regressive procedure that involves the insertion of two fingers into a person's vagina to gauge the laxity of vaginal muscles, thereby determining her 'virginity'. It is based on the patriarchal assumption that a woman who is sexually active is less likely to have been sexually assaulted; several judg-

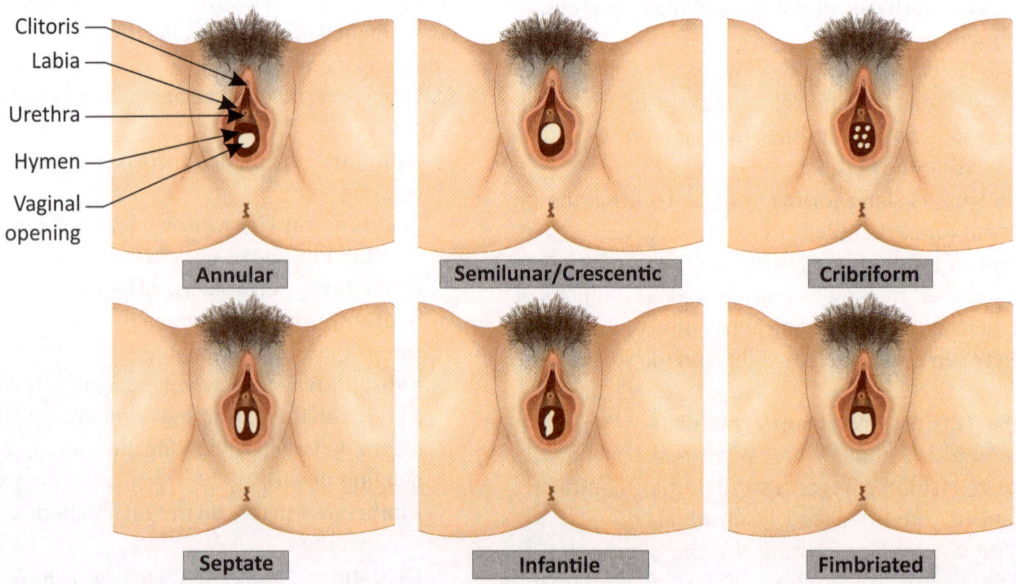

Fig. 3.141 Common types of hymen

ments and research have shown that a person's sexual history have no bearing on sexual assault.

- This test, also called 'virginity test', and in medical terms, 'per-vaginum examination'—is aimed at checking the presence/absence of hymen and whether the vaginal muscles are loose or not, to gauge sexual assault. However, the test is unscientific because the hymen can rupture due to several reasons other than sexual intercourse, including playing sports, riding a bicycle, using tampons or during medical examinations.
- The Supreme Court had deemed the practice of performing the atrocious "Two-finger test" unconstitutional way back in 2013, and yet many doctors continued stubbornly to subject rape victims and even other women to this degrading, humiliating and unscientific method of ascertaining as to whether she was a 'virgin' or not, until finally the **National Medical Commission came out with a notice banning this practice,*** which is now considered as professional misconduct.
- On **31st Oct 2022, the Supreme Court of India explicitly banned the "Two-finger test"** and directed the Union Govt, as well as State Govts to ensure that the guidelines formulated by the Department of Health and Family Welfare (prohibiting the practice) are circulated to all Govt and private hospitals across the country.

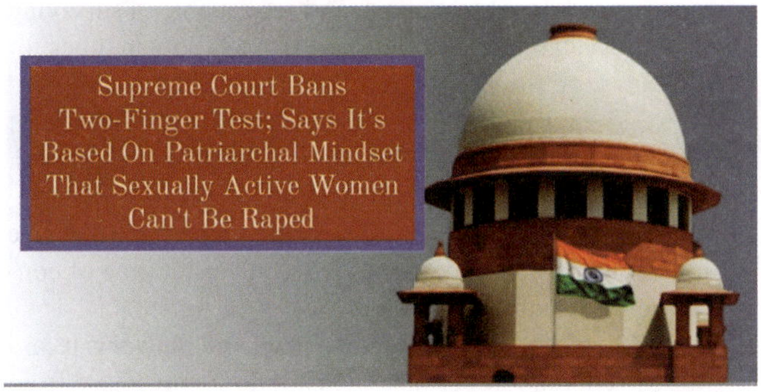
Supreme Court Bans
Two-Finger Test; Says It's
Based On Patriarchal Mindset
That Sexually Active Women
Can't Be Raped

LEGITIMACY

Definition

- **Legitimacy** is the status of a child born during the continuance of a valid marriage between the mother and any man, or within 280 days after its dissolution if the mother remains unmarried, unless it is shown that the parties to the marriage had no access to each other at any time when the child could have been conceived. Such a child is deemed to be "**legitimate**".
- Conversely, **illegitimacy** is the status of a child born outside marriage, such a child being known as an **illegitimate child (bastard,** love child)**.

Medicolegal Aspects

The question of determination of legitimacy may arise in the following cases:

1. Inheritance of property
2. Affiliation case
3. Supposititious child
4. Nullity of marriage
5. Divorce
6. Posthumous child

Inheritance of Property

- As per law, only a legitimate child (born within wedlock) can inherit the property of its father. However, the Supreme Court in 2008 held that if a man and woman live together and cohabit for a long period as husband and wife, there is a presumption of a valid marriage between them and that a child born out of such relationship would be legitimate and have inheritance and succession rights (see **Box 3.7** for succession laws in India).
- Under Section 12 of the Hindu Adoptions and Maintenance Act 1956, an adopted son or daughter is also entitled to succeed to the estate of his adoptive parents. Adoption can only be recognized if it is permitted by statute or accepted by custom. In India, the only religion that maintains a statutorily recognized right to adopt is the Hindu religion under the Hindu Minority and Guardianship Act, 1956. Barring Muslims, adoption in India in respect of all religious communities is governed by the Guardians and Wards Act, 1890. The Act contains no reference to domicile, nationality, residence, etc., as a condition precedent to their applicability.
- Personal laws of Muslims, Christians, Parsis and Jews do not recognize complete adoption.

Affiliation/Adoption Cases

- These are the suits instituted for fixing the paternity of an illegitimate child upon a certain individual as he is bound, under Section 125 of the Code of Criminal Procedure 1973, to support his illegitimate child which is unable to maintain itself, irrespective of age.
- A first class Magistrate may make a monthly allowance for the maintenance of such a child. In determining the amount of maintenance under the Hindu Adoptions and Maintenance Act, 1956, the court has to consider the position and status of the parties and reasonable wants of the claimant, the value of the claimant's property, and any income derived from it, and the number of persons entitled for maintenance. In determining the amount of maintenance, only the necessities of life, namely, food, clothing and lodging are taken into consideration and not luxuries.
- Adoption under the Hindu Minority and Guardianship Act 1956, and the Guardian and Wards Act 1890 is a private action, and as such does not require the intercession of a court except when the minor is offered for adoption by a

*****Source**: Advisory No. U. 11029/49/2022/UGMEB dated 18.08.2022 from National Medical Commission (Undergraduate Medical Education Board), New Delhi.*

******Note**: A term that is considered taboo by many, and therefore must not be used in academic or scientific context.*

guardian appointed by a will or other instrument, or appointed or declared by the court.

Box 3.7—Succession Laws in India

- **Minor children**: According to the Indian Succession Act, 1956, and the Indian Succession (Amendment) Act, 2005, children (boys or girls) have a right to the father's ancestral property by birth. The parents' self-acquired property can be given to anyone they want through a written will. However, if they die intestate, i.e., without a will, the children being Class I heirs have a first right to their property. If, on the other hand, the children are minors, they do own the property but cannot legally manage it. In this case, a legal guardian, or one appointed by the court, has to file a petition in court to manage the property on behalf of the minor child till such time that the child becomes an adult.
- **Children of divorcees**: If the parents are divorced, the children still have a legal right to their property. The normal succession laws as per one's religion apply in such cases. So the child has a right over the ancestral property, and in case of a self-acquired property, if the father dies intestate, he has the first right over it since he is a Class I heir. Of course, if the property is self-acquired, the father can give it to anyone he wants during his lifetime via a written ill.
- **Adopted children**: Adopted children have the same inheritance rights as the biological children and are entitled to a share in their adoptive parents' property. So if the adoptive parent passes away intestate, the adopted child can stake the same claim to property as the biological child. However, according to the Hindu Adoptions and Maintenance Act, 1956, after adoption, the child loses the right to stake a claim in the property of his/her own biological parents. But, if the biological parents want to voluntarily leave such property or a share in it to the child, they can do so.
- **Children of live-in couples**: Live-in relationships have not been granted any legal status or acceptance under the Hindu Succession Act, Islamic Law or the Christian Personal Law. However, according to the Supreme Court ruling of 2008, a child born to a couple in a live-in relationship would have the same right of inheritance as a legal heir. A subsequent Supreme Court ruling of 2015 declared that an unmarried couple that has been living together for a long time can be considered married. Hence, offspring of such a couple will have the right to his/her father's self-acquired property.

Suppositious/Fictitious Child

- A woman may feign a pregnancy, followed by a fake delivery and later produce a child claiming it to be her own in order to extort money by blackmail, or divert succession of property. Such a child is called a **suppositious** or **fictitious child**.

Nullity of Marriage

- If a mother delivers a child the intrauterine age of which is greater than the period intervening between the marriage and delivery, the marriage in such a case may be nullified on the grounds of immorality.

Divorce

- If the intrauterine age of a child is proved to be greater than the period of access between the parents, dissolution of marriage is allowed by the court on the grounds of adultery.

Posthumous Child

- A **posthumous child** is one who was conceived when the father was alive, but was born after the death of his father.

Investigation of Legitimacy

- The following medicolegal issues have to be considered in these cases:
  - The average duration of pregnancy
  - The maximum period of pregnancy
  - The minimum period of pregnancy of viability of foetus
  - Paternity
  - Unusual forms of pregnancy
- **Average duration of pregnancy**: It is the period that ordinarily elapses between conception and delivery. This period is estimated from the date of conception from single coitus and arrest of menstruation. However, neither of them is reliable. Single coitus does not fix the date of conception, but merely the date of insemination. Modern observers agree that spermatozoa retain their activity in the vagina for 2–3 days at the most, and are capable of surviving in the cervical canal, uterine cavity and fallopian tubes for 4–5 days, or slightly longer. But, conception usually occurs 2–3 days after coitus, as spermatozoa are capable of retaining their power of fertilization for about that period. They lose their power of fertilization long before their motility disappears. However, non-motile spermatozoa may be found even up to 15 days or so. So, the exact time of conception is usually not known.
- **Period between last menstrual period and delivery**: It cannot be relied upon because menstruation may cease from other causes and may continue even after pregnancy has commenced, and impregnation may occur at any period during the menstrual period. So exact period is not known, but can be calculated from experience, i.e., 280 days or 40 weeks.
- **Maximum period of pregnancy**: No fixed limit is laid in India, England or USA. English Courts have accepted up to 349 days as maximum period, the child being legitimate. Some studies indicate that even a period of 354 days is not impossible.
- **Minimum period of pregnancy for a foetus to be viable**: Legitimacy may be disputed when a child is born within a short time of the husband and wife living together, after a long separation. So the important question is, whether it is possible for a fully developed child to be born before the usual period of gestation is completed. Age of viability is generally taken to be 210 days, but even at 180 days it can be viable, and capable of living a separate existence.
- **Paternity**:

- The word 'paternity' literally means 'fatherhood', but the term is used here in a broader sense to mean 'parenthood'. The supposed parent may or may not be the real father.
- The question of **disputed paternity** may arise in cases of
  - Illegitimacy
  - Posthumous birth
  - Suppositious child
  - Nullity of marriage
  - Divorce
  - Inheritance of property
  - Guardianship
  - Maintenance
- Paternity can be determined by the following methods:
  - Paternal likeness of features or developmental defects.
  - Blood grouping
  - Human Leucocyte Antigen (HLA) typing
  - DNA Typing (DNA Profiling)
- **Parental likeness of features or developmental defects**: The child may resemble his parents in features, figure, complexion, gestures, voice, manners, gait, colour of skin, hair, iris and other personal peculiarities, including developmental defects. But it is not essential, as in **atavism**, the child may not resemble his immediate parents but resembles his grandparents due to inheritance of certain characters from the remote rather than immediate ancestors. This is due to chance combination of genes or presence of genes which are expressed in the child when the environmental conditions become favourable.
- **Blood grouping**: Blood typing based on the ABO blood group system, is not an accurate method for determining paternity. Power of exclusion of paternity by ABO grouping is only about 30%. It cannot be used to prove paternity.
- **Serological testing**: Serum testing uses the Rhesus (Rh) factor, and the MNS, Kell and Duffy blood group systems, but it eliminates only about 40% of the entire male population from being the possible father. Serological testing cannot be used to prove paternity.
- **HLA typing**: HLA testing can eliminate up to 80% of the male population from being the possible father, and in some cases it is possible to produce a probability of paternity of up to 90%. But, it is almost never conclusive.
- **DNA typing**: This is the most conclusive method of determining paternity or maternity of a child.
  - The question of **disputed maternity** arises in following circumstances:
    - When two women claim the same child.
    - Interchange of newborn children in a maternity home or hospital, either intentionally or accidentally.
    - In the case of a supposititious child.

FM 3.19: Core – Written/Viva Voce
- **Discuss the medicolegal aspects of:**
  - Pregnancy and delivery
  - Signs of pregnancy
  - Precipitate labour
  - Superfoetation and superfecundation
  - Signs of recent and remote delivery in living and dead

PREGNANCY

(GESTATION, FOETATION, GRAVIDITY)

- **Pregnancy** is the physiological condition of having a developing embryo or foetus in the body, from the time of fertilisation of an ovum by a spermatozoon until the birth of a child.
- Since, it is not possible to determine the precise moment at which the spermatozoon fertilises the ovum, the exact moment of commencement of pregnancy is usually uncertain. About 7 days after fertilisation, the ovum reaches the uterine cavity and implants itself in the uterine wall.
- In obstetric practice, it is customary to estimate the **expected date of delivery** by employing the **Naegele's rule**. This rule estimates the expected date of delivery (EDD) from the first day of the woman's last menstrual period (LMP) by adding a year, subtracting three months and adding seven days to that date. This approximates to the average normal human pregnancy which lasts 40 weeks (280 days) from the LMP, or 38 weeks (266 days) from the date of fertilization. Another method is by adding 9 months and 7 days to the first day of the last menstrual period.
- It is also customary to divide the duration of pregnancy into "trimesters," to facilitate both ease of diagnosis and awareness of the problems particular to each stage of pregnancy.

Diagnosis of Pregnancy

In medicolegal cases involving the issue of pregnancy, the woman in question may be sent to a registered medical practitioner for examination and certification as to whether she is really pregnant or not (the expressed written consent of the woman, duly witnessed, is mandatory). To perform this duty, one must be familiar with the symptoms and signs of pregnancy, as well as the laboratory and other examinations that are useful in the diagnosis of pregnancy. These may be classified under three heads: **presumptive**, **probable** and **positive**.

Presumptive Evidence of Pregnancy

This is based largely on the **signs** and **symptoms** experienced by the woman.

Presumptive Signs of Pregnancy

1. **Secondary amenorrhoea**: Though strongly suggestive of pregnancy, this is not reliable until 10 or more days have passed after the expected date of the first day of menstruation. It must be noted that:
   a. There are rare instances of pregnancy in women who have never menstruated or who are supposedly menopausal.

b. Menstruation may continue even after conception.
c. There are several causes for amenorrhoea other than pregnancy, e.g., environmental, nutritional, organic diseases such as severe anaemia and tuberculosis, and psychic causes.

2. **Mammary changes**: They are more marked in primigravidae (women who are pregnant for the first time):
   a. Progressive enlargement and tenderness.
   b. Easily visible superficial veins.
   c. In the 2nd month, hyperpigmentation of the areolae and nipples, with the appearance of **Montgomery's tubercles** (raised spots due to enlargement of the sebaceous glands).
   d. From the 4th month onwards, **colostrum**, which consists of free fat globules and large phagocytic cells filled with droplets of fat, can be squeezed from the breasts.
3. **Changes in the vagina**:
   a. **Jacquemir's/Chadwick's sign**, i.e., bluish discolouration of the vaginal mucosa (this is not a reliable sign, since it can be caused by anything that obstructs proper venous return).
   b. **Barnes' sign**, i.e., flattening of the anterior vaginal wall because of upward tilting of the cervix.

Presumptive Symptoms of Pregnancy

1. **Morning sickness**: It refers to the nausea, often followed by vomiting, soon after waking, and which usually disappears on its own later on during the pregnancy. Like many other presumptive symptoms, this is not to be relied on because it is seen mostly in primigravidae, may not occur in all cases, and may also be a symptom of several gastrointestinal disorders. It may occasionally persist as **hyperemesis gravidarum**.
2. **Disturbances in micturition**: Such as increased frequency during the first trimester, a return to normal as the uterus grows into the abdomen, and reappearance of the increased frequency at or near the end of term because of the descent of the foetal head into the pelvis.
3. **Easy fatiguability, hypersalivation, unusual appetite** and **increased irritability**.

Probable Evidence of Pregnancy

Probable Signs of Pregnancy

1. **Abdominal changes**:
   a. Progressive enlargement after the 12th week, so that the umbilicus becomes flush with the skin.
   b. Increased pigmentation (**Fig. 3.142**):
      i. **Linea nigra** (dark vertical line from above umbilicus to the pubis)
      ii. **Striae gravidarum** ("stretch marks")
      iii. **Linea albicans** (old, silvery white striae)
2. **Changes in the uterus**:
   a. Mucus becomes a thick and viscid plug, blocking the cervical canal.

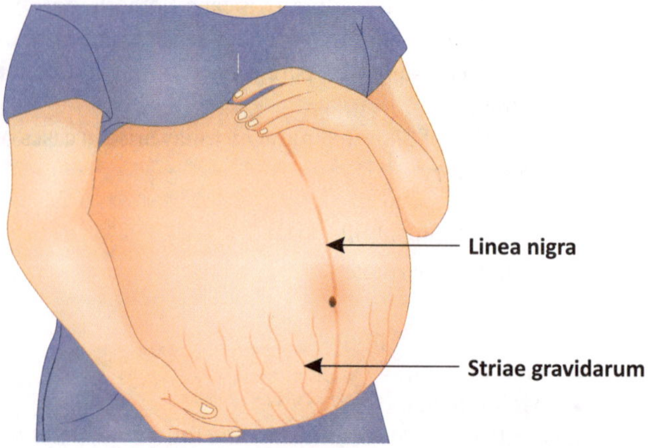

Fig. 3.142 Skin changes in pregnancy

   b. **Goodell's sign** (softening of cervix because of increased vascularity) can first be appreciated at 6–8 weeks. The cervix becomes more and more patulous as pregnancy advances, but this change may also occur in acute cervicitis, haematometra and in women who are long-term regular users of combined contraceptives.
   c. Towards term, there is apparent shortening of the cervix, the cervical canal becomes circular and the external os admits the tip of a finger with ease and to a greater depth.
   d. **Uterine souffle*** (a soft, blowing murmur, synchronous with the maternal pulse, which can be heard with a stethoscope applied just above the midline of the inguinal ligament) is usually audible from the 16th week onwards.
   e. **Hegar's sign** (softening and easy compressibility of the lower uterine segment) first appears at 6–8 weeks. This sign is elicited by introducing two fingers of one hand into the posterior fornix while the other hand rests on the pelvis just above the pubic symphysis. On pressing upwards with the first hand, it appears as if there is no intervening uterus between the two hands.
   f. **Braxton Hicks' sign**: The appreciation of intermittent painless contractions of the uterus from the 16th week onwards by palpation of the abdomen, occurring at intervals of 5–20 minutes, each lasting for about 1–5 minutes.
   g. **Ballottement** (tossing of a ball), i.e., the method of eliciting the presence of the foetus floating in the liquor amnii. This can be determined either **externally** or **internally**.
      i. ***External ballottement*** is elicited by placing the palms of both hands over the abdomen on either side of the midline, and pushing firmly with one hand towards the other, where upon the impetus thus given to the foetal head can be felt against the other.
      ii. ***Internal ballottement*** is done by inserting two fingers of one hand into the posterior fornix and pushing sharply upwards. The foetal head will first move

*****Note***: *Pronounced "soofl" not "soufflay" which is a French dish!*

upwards in the liquor, then settle down onto the fingers.

Probable Symptoms of Pregnancy

1. The only **symptom** that could be taken as probable evidence of pregnancy is **quickening**, i.e., the first perception of foetal movements by the mother. This is possible from the 16th to 20th week onwards, and increases in intensity as pregnancy advances.

Laboratory Investigations

1. Laboratory investigations for pregnancy all depend upon increased levels of **human chorionic gonadotropin (HCG)** in the urine, using either **biological** or **immunological methods**. The morning midstream urine of the woman suspected to be pregnant is used for these tests.
   a. The **biological (animal) tests**, which are easy to perform but time-consuming, include:
      i. **Ascheim-Zondek** (female mouse) **test**
      ii. **Friedman** (female rabbit) **test**
      iii. **Hogben** (female toad or frog) **test**
      iv. **Galli-Mainini** (male toad) **test**

   All these tests are, however, obsolete and only of historical interest, having given way to the immunological tests.

   b. The **immunological tests** are much faster, more specific, less cumbersome, more sensitive, and do not require laboratory animals, equipment or special skills. All these tests take advantage of the antigenic properties of HCG. They include:
      i. **Haemagglutination** (Prognosticon) **test**
      ii. **Latex-agglutination** (Gravindex) **test**, which can deliver a result in 2 hours, and its improvement, the **Pregcolor test**, which can be read in **2 minutes**.
      iii. **Radioreceptor assay**, which is highly sensitive and 98% accurate. However, all these HCG-based tests will also be positive in those conditions in which abnormal or pathological products of conception are formed, viz., hydatidiform mole and chorionepithelioma. Further, false positives could also occur because of the biological and immunological similarities between HCG and luteinising hormone (LH).

Positive Evidence of Pregnancy

Absolute/Certain/Conclusive/Sure signs can be grossly appreciated only from the 4th to 5th month (16th to 20th week) of gestation onwards. They include:

1. **Foetal parts and foetal movements**, discernible by bimanual palpation. This may be difficult when the abdominal wall is fatty, or in hydramnios.
2. **Foetal heart sounds**, with a normal rate of 120–160 per minute, which sound like the muffled ticking of a watch. These can be heard on auscultation of the abdominal wall with a foetoscope. Foetal heart sounds can be detected much earlier, if more advanced techniques are used, e.g., at 10–12 weeks by Doppler principle with ultrasound, at about 8 weeks by pulse-echo and real-time sonography and even as early as 7 weeks by echocardiography.
3. **Radiological demonstration of the foetal skeleton**, which, although possible in some cases at the 20th week of pregnancy, is contraindicated during the first trimester. By ultrasonography, a small white gestational ring can be seen as early as the 6th week of gestation, and distinct echoes from the embryo within this gestational ring can be discerned by careful scanning 2 weeks later.

Medicolegal Aspects of Pregnancy

Civil Cases

- Malicious persons may allege either verbally (*slander*) or in writing (*libel*), that an unmarried woman or widow is pregnant, in which case she would definitely want to vindicate herself.
- A concealed pregnancy before marriage, or after marriage by a person other than the lawfully wedded spouse, would constitute valid grounds for divorce.
- The duration of pregnancy assumes importance when the legitimacy of a **posthumous child** (one born after the death of its father) is questioned.

Criminal Cases

- Pregnancy is positive proof of sexual intercourse in a trial for rape.
- Pregnancy may be a motive for the suicide of a married or unmarried woman, or for the murder of a married woman by her husband, when it is the result of an illicit sexual relationship.
- Such a situation has also driven women to criminal abortion and to foeticide or infanticide.

Civil and Criminal Cases

- A woman may feign pregnancy (a condition termed **pseudocyesis**, or false/imaginary pregnancy) in order to:
  - Avoid capital punishment (because the unborn child is innocent of any crime its mother may have committed, and must not be punished for it, the death sentence is either commuted to imprisonment for life, or is postponed till after the delivery of the child).
  - Compel a person to marriage.
  - Secure more maintenance in a case of divorce.
  - Pseudocyesis is also encountered in sterile or infertile women who long for children.
- Also to be considered here are the conditions of **superfoetation** (where two or more pregnancies result from the fertilisation of two or more ova of ***different*** ovulatory periods), and **superfecundation** (in which two or more ova of the ***same*** ovulatory period are fertilised by ***separate*** acts of sexual intercourse with the same person, or two different persons) (**Fig. 3.143**).
  - Although superfoetation is theoretically possible, it has not been demonstrated beyond doubt in human females (though it is known to occur in certain lower animals, e.g., mares).
  - On the other hand, superfecundation is not only a more likely possibility, but has also been described in literature.

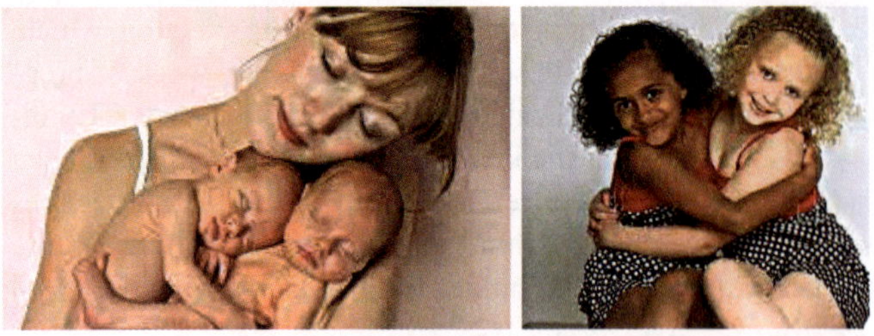

Fig. 3.143 Superfecundation – (a) same father; (b) two separate fathers

DELIVERY

- **Delivery** is defined as complete evacuation of a foetus (that has attained viability) and other products of conception from within the uterus and genital passages into the external environment.
- This process may be spontaneous or assisted.
- When delivery occurs after the full period of gestation, i.e., 280 days, it is called a "**full-term delivery**." If it occurs earlier or later than this, it is said to be "**pre-term/premature**" and "**post-term/postmature**", respectively.

Symptoms and Signs of Recent Delivery in the Living (At Full Term)

Symptoms of Recent Delivery in the Living

1. **Fatigue**, which is most pronounced immediately after delivery, and more so when labour has been prolonged.
2. **Loss of weight** mainly because of expulsion of the contents of the uterus.
3. **Diuresis** during the 2nd to 5th day, because of physiological reversal of the increased intracellular fluid during pregnancy.
4. **Afterpains** experienced by primiparae as tonic contractions, and by multiparae as vigorous contractions, at intervals. They are occasionally painful and/or severe, become mild after 3 days, and usually disappear after 7 days, but may last longer in some patients.
5. A sharp **rise in temperature** for the first 24 hours postpartum (*milk fever*) – any fever which lasts longer is most likely due to infection.
6. **Transient depression**, a common feature which is usually self-limiting and responsive to treatment or reassurance, but may progress to **puerperal (postpartum) psychosis**, as a result of which the mother may neglect, ill-treat or even kill her child.

Signs of Recent Delivery in the Living

1. In the **breasts**, similar to those of pregnancy, but more marked (**colostrum** can be squeezed out for the first 2 days, after which it is replaced by mature milk).
2. In the **abdomen**, which remains soft and flabby for several weeks (although tone and contour can often be regained by exercise), displays silvery-white **linea albicantes**, and, when Caesarean section has been performed, the operative incision in the lower segment.
3. In the **vagina and its outlet**, which may display the following features:
   a. **Smooth-walled, relaxed and wide** (the width progressively decreases, but nulliparous dimensions are never regained).
   b. **Ironed-out rugae** (reappear by the 3rd week in primiparae, but never in multiparae).
   c. **Lacerated walls** which heal rapidly.
   d. **Carunculae myrtiformes** of the hymen.
   e. The **labia** in primiparae, appear swollen, tender, gaping, bruised and/or lacerated.
   f. The **perineum**, which shows ruptures of the fourchette and posterior commissure with or without a sutured/healing incision of episiotomy.
   g. **Lochia**, i.e., an alkaline discharge with a peculiar, sour, disagreeable odour, consisting of red blood cells, leukocytes, shreds of decidua, epithelial cells and bacteria. The appearance of this discharge changes as the puerperium progresses, so that
      i. for the first few days, it is red (*lochia rubra*),
      ii. from the 5th to 10th days, it is watery and pale (*lochia serosa*),
      iii. from the 10th day onwards, it becomes thicker, scantier, and white or yellowish-white (*lochia alba*) and
      iv. it disappears in 2–3 weeks.
4. In the **cervix** (which is thin, collapsed and flabby soon after delivery):
   a. **External os**:
      i. shows lacerations of its outer margins(these heal rapidly to leave permanent bilateral depressions) and
      ii. contracts slowly, so that for the first 2 days, it admits 2 fingers easily, and at the end of 1 week, 1 finger with difficulty.
   b. The **walls** simultaneously thicken to re-establish the cervical canal.
5. In the **uterus**: because of ***involution***, the fundus of the uterus keeps dipping progressively after delivery (**Fig 3.144**):
   a. Immediately after delivery – midway between the umbilicus and symphysis pubis.
   b. 12 hours after delivery – above the umbilicus.

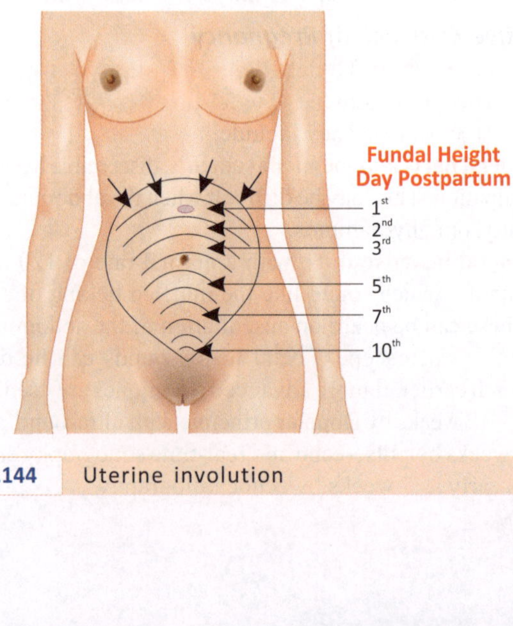

Fig. 3.144 Uterine involution

c. After that – the fundus descends about one fingerbreadth every 24 hours.
d. After the 10th day of postpartum – the uterus should not be palpable abdominally.
e. In 5–6 weeks postpartum, it attains its normal non-pregnant size (**Table 3.21**).

Laboratory Investigations

- The **biological tests** for pregnancy are positive for about 7 to 10 days after delivery.

Signs of Recent Delivery in the Dead

1. Besides observing the gross changes in the breasts, abdomen, the vagina and its outlet, and the cervix, and palpating the uterus per abdomen, the **uterus**, **ovaries** and **peritoneum** are also examined.
2. The weights and dimensions of the involuting uterus are listed in **Table 3.21**.
3. Morphology of the involuting uterus:
   a. If lower segment caesarean section has been performed, its fresh or healing incision will be seen.
   b. *Cut section* soon after delivery shows:
      i. anterior & posterior walls each 4–5 cm thick
      ii. a body made up mostly of myometrium, lined by basal deciduas
      iii. a placental site about the size of a palm, which rapidly decreases in size and
      iv. an ischaemic appearance because the vessels are compressed by the contracting myometrium.
   c. *Cut section* 2–3 days after delivery shows that the remaining decidua has differentiated into two layers:
      i. a superficial layer which is necrotic (shed in lochia) and
      ii. a basal layer, which is the foundation of a new endometrium.
   d. *Cut section* 2 weeks after delivery shows:
      i. that the rapidly growing endometrium has covered the entire surface except for the placental site, and
      ii. a placental site 3–4 cm in size.
   e. At 6 weeks after delivery, even the placental site gets covered by new endometrium.
4. The ovaries and fallopian tubes are congested. On microscopic examination, an intact or degenerating corpus luteum can be seen.
5. The peritoneum covering most of the uterus is folded and wrinkled.
6. The broad and round ligaments are lax; they take a long time to recover their pre-pregnancy consistency.

Signs of Remote Delivery in both the Living & the Dead

1. These include the permanent morphological alterations that have been previously described, with linea albicantes of the breasts and slight concavity inwards of the inner surface of the uterus.
2. If there is any doubt from naked-eye appearances as to whether delivery has taken place or not, the endometrium must be examined under the microscope for the presence of trophoblastic endothelium and chorionic villi.

Medicolegal Aspects of Delivery

Civil Cases

In civil cases, whether a woman has delivered or not needs to be determined in instances of:

1. **Feigned delivery**, when a woman pretends to have been pregnant for some time and later produces a child, alleging that it is hers to claim property of a deceased husband. Such a child is called a **suppositious child**.
2. **Affiliation cases** (*affiliation = adoption*), in which a woman claims that her child has been fathered by a person who is not her wedded spouse, or by a husband who has subsequently divorced her, and who must therefore adopt the child as his own and pay for its upkeep.
3. **Contested legitimacy of a child**, when, as part of the evidence that a child was born of a particular woman and her husband, it must be proven that the woman did indeed deliver a child at the time claimed by her.

Table 3.21 Weight and Dimensions of Involuting Uterus

Duration after Delivery	Weight	Dimensions
Freshly delivered	1000–2000 g	Variable
Immediately after delivery	Variable, but less than above	22 cm × 15 cm
2–3 days postpartum	Variable, but still less	Less than above
End of the 1st week	500 g	13–15 cm × 8 cm
End of the 2nd week	300 g	10 cm × 5 cm
Soon thereafter	100 g or less	Variable, but less than above
5–6 weeks	Normal non-pregnant weight	Normal non-pregnant size

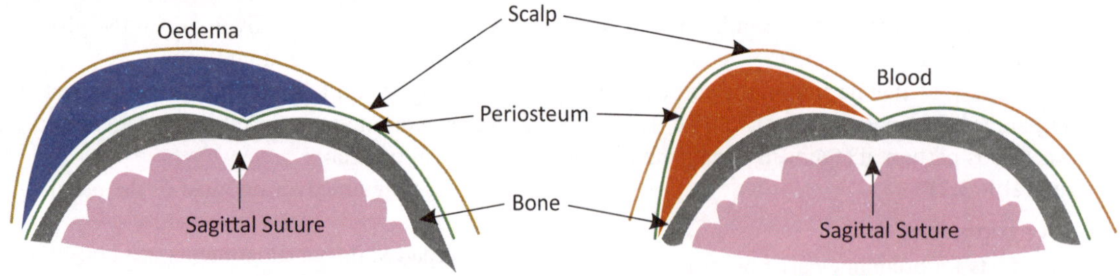

Fig. 3.145 Caput succadeneum versus Cephalohaematoma

Criminal Cases

In criminal cases, the question of delivery assumes importance in trials for:

1. **Abortion** and **infanticide**.
2. **Concealment of a child** begotten out of an illicit sexual relationship.
3. When an **affiliation case** proceeds to the degree of **blackmail**.

PRECIPITATE LABOUR

- **Precipitate labour** is said to occur when all the stages of labour merge with each other, and the birth takes place in an abnormally short time.
- The mother may experience mild pain which she may attribute to a distended rectum, and therefore she may attempt to defaecate, as a result of which the child may be born into the lavatory pan. The child may sustain skull fractures or bleed from the torn end of the umbilicus. It may inhale faecal matter which may be demonstrable in the lungs.
- Precipitate labour occurs when the pelvis is roomy and the foetus is very small. In such cases, ***caput succedaneum*** or ***cephalohaematoma*** which are pointers to obstructed labour, are absent.
  - **Caput succedaneum**: Swelling (oedema) on the top of the scalp that is usually noticeable at birth. This swelling causes the scalp to feel spongy, does cross suture lines, and starts to go down soon after birth. Caput resolves in 1–7 days.
  - **Cephalohaematoma**: Accumulation of blood deep to the scalp, and is limited to suture lines. It takes 1–3 months to resolve and shows colour changes similar to a bruise.

> FM 3.20: Core – Written/Viva Voce
> - Discuss disputed paternity and maternity

DISPUTED PATERNITY/MATERNITY

- When a child is born he/she carries the DNA of both parents. The man who has contributed his sperms is considered to be the **biological father**.
- A **paternity dispute** occurs when the father claims that he is not the biological father of that child and refuses to take the responsibility of maintaining or bringing up the child, even though the mother claims that he is the biological father of her child.
- A **maternity dispute** occurs when there is a baby mix-up in a hospital, which may be accidental or deliberate.
- The question of **disputed paternity** may arise in the following cases:
  - Illegitimacy
  - Posthumous birth
  - Suppositious child
  - Nullity of marriage
  - Divorce
  - Inheritance of property
  - Guardianship
  - Maintenance
- It is well known that only a **legitimate child** can inherit the parental property. However, the Supreme Court ruled in 2015 that if a man and woman who are unmarried stay together for a long time and behave like a married couple, then there is presumption of a valid marriage and the child born will be considered legitimate, and will have the right to inheritance and succession. Under Section 3(57) of the General Clauses Act, 1897, the definition of son includes an adopted son and under Section 12 of the Hindu Adoption and Maintenance Act, 1956, an adopted son or daughter is entitled to succeed to the estate of his adoptive parents.

Methods of Resolving Disputed Paternity/Maternity

1. **Evaluating morphological similarities between the child and parent**: Every trait is transferred from parents to children. Each parent contributes equally in the formation of the zygote. So, it is normal that the child represents the characteristics of its biological parents. The dominant characteristics are expressed phenotypically. The child resembles his/her parents with regard to features like figure, skin colour, nose form, eyes, stature, hair, etc. Deformities or developmental details are also sometimes seen in the child. Some diseases also are transferred from parents to children.
2. **Serological approach**: Involves study of blood groups.
3. **Immunological approach**: Involves Human Leukocyte Antigen (HLA) typing.
4. **DNA typing (DNA profiling)**: It is the most conclusive method.

FM 3.21: Core – Written/Viva Voce
- Discuss:
  - Pre-conception and Pre-natal Diagnostic Techniques (PC&PNDT) Act, 1994
  - Prohibition of Sex Selection Act, 2003
  - Protection of Women from Domestic Violence Act, 2005

PRE-CONCEPTION & PRE-NATAL DIAGNOSTIC TECHNIQUES (PCPNDT) ACT, 1994 & PROHIBITION OF SEX SELECTION ACT, 2003

- The **Pre-conception & Pre-natal Diagnostic Techniques (PCPNDT) Act, 1994** is an Act of the Parliament of India enacted to stop female foeticides and arrest the declining sex ratio in India.
  - The Act **bans prenatal sex determination**. Every genetic counselling centre/genetic laboratory/genetic clinic engaged in counselling or conducting pre-natal diagnostic techniques, like in vitro fertilisation (IVF) with the potential of sex selection (pre-implantation genetic diagnosis) before and after conception, comes under purview of the PCPNDT Act, and are banned.
- The main purpose of enacting the Act is to ban the use of sex selection techniques after conception, and prevent the misuse of prenatal diagnostic techniques for sex selective abortions.
- "**Sex selection**" refers to any act of identifying the sex of the foetus and elimination of the foetus, if it is of the unwanted sex.
- Offences under this act include:
  - Conducting prenatal diagnostic techniques in unregistered units.
  - Conducting PND test for any purpose other than the one mentioned in the Act.
  - Sale, distribution, supply, renting, etc., of an ultrasound machine or any other equipment capable of detecting sex of the foetus.
- The Act regulates the use of pre-natal diagnostic techniques like ultrasound and amniocentesis, by allowing their use only to detect:
  - genetic abnormalities
  - metabolic disorders
  - chromosomal abnormalities
  - congenital malformations
  - haemoglobinopathies
  - sex linked disorders.
- No person, including the one who is conducting the procedure as per the law, will communicate the sex of the foetus to the pregnant woman or her relatives by words, signs or any other method.
- Any person who advertises pre-natal and pre-conception sex determination facilities in the form of a notice, circular, etc., or advertises through any media in electronic or print form, can be imprisoned for up to 3 years and fined Rs. 10,000.
- The Act mandates compulsory registration of all diagnostic laboratories, genetic counselling centres, genetic laboratories, genetic clinics and ultrasound clinics.
- The Act was amended in 2003 as: **Prohibition of Sex Selection Act 2003**, in order to improve the regulations:
  - Amendment of the Act mainly covers bringing the technique of pre-conception sex selection within the ambit of the Act.
  - Bringing ultrasound within its ambit.
  - Empowering the central supervisory board, and constitution of state level supervisory boards.
  - Provision for more stringent punishments.
    - Persons seeking to know the sex of the foetus: 3 years imprisonment and/or fine of Rs. 50,000 for the first offence. For subsequent offences, 5 years imprisonment and/or fine of Rs. 1,00,000. The pregnant woman herself is considered innocent under the Act, unless and until proved otherwise. It is presumed that she has been compelled to undergo sex determination tests by her husband and relatives.
    - Persons connected with advertising of sex selection/sex determination services: 3 years imprison ment and/or a fine of Rs. 10,000, with additional fine for continuing contravention at the rate of Rs. 500 per day.
- The Act was further amended in 2004 as the **Pre-Conception and Pre-natal Diagnostic Techniques (Regulation and Prevention of Misuse) (PCPNDT) Act, 2004** to deter and punish prenatal sex screening and sex selective abortion.

PROTECTION OF WOMEN FROM DOMESTIC VIOLENCE ACT, 2005

- The **Protection of Women from Domestic Violence Act, 2005** is an Act of the Parliament of India enacted to protect women from domestic violence. It came into force on 26th Oct 2006.
- The Act provides a definition of "**domestic violence**" for the first time in Indian law, with this definition being broad and including not only physical violence, but also other forms of violence such as emotional/verbal, sexual and economic abuse.
- The aggrieved person is defined as "any woman who is, or has been, in a domestic relationship with the respondent, and who alleges to have been subjected to domestic violence by the respondent."
- This law protects not only women from violence within their husband–wife relationships, but also women living in the same home with people with whom they are in a domestic relationship with.
  - This protects women from violence within their relationships by marriage (e.g., husband–wife, daughter-in-law with father-in-law/mother-in-law, etc.), relationships by blood (father–daughter, sister–brother), relationships by adoption (adopted daughter–father) and even relationships in the nature of marriage (live-in relationships).

- **Domestic violence** is defined by Section 3 of the Act as "any act, omission or commission or conduct of the respondent shall constitute domestic violence in case it:
  - harms or injures or endangers the health, safety, life, limb or well-being, whether mental or physical, of the aggrieved person, and includes causing physical abuse, sexual abuse, verbal abuse, emotional abuse and economic abuse; or
  - harasses, harms, injures or endangers the aggrieved person to coerce her or any other person related to her, to meet any unlawful demand for any dowry or other property or valuable security."
- Pursuant to Chapter III of the Act, the aggrieved person has the right to:
  - Apply for a protection order, an order for monetary relief, a custody order, a residence order and/or a compensation order;
  - Free legal services under the Legal Services Authorities Act, 1987;
  - File a complaint under section 498A of the Indian Penal Code.

> **FM 3.22: Core – Written/Viva Voce**
> - **Define and discuss:**
>   - Impotence
>   - Sterility
>   - Frigidity
>   - Sexual dysfunction
>   - Premature ejaculation
> - **Discuss:**
>   - Causes of impotence and sterility in male and female

IMPOTENCE*

- Impotence, in its simplest meaning, is the inability to perform the act of coitus. Since in this act, the male is usually the active partner and the female is relatively passive, the term **impotence** is generally applied to **the inability of the male to achieve and/or maintain penile erection and thus engage in copulation**.
- Today the term "**erectile dysfunction**" is preferred, which is defined as **male sexual dysfunction involving inadequacy of erection, or problems with emission, ejaculation or orgasm**.
- Impotence may be either temporary or permanent.

Causes of Impotence

Physiological Causes

- ***Extremes of age*** – Very young infant, very old male. This is however not the rule, and infants as well as old individuals may be quite potent.

Organic Causes

- Due to structural abnormalities in the reproductive system.
  - ***Congenital:***
    - Klinefelter's syndrome
    - Primary testicular failure
    - Cryptorchidism
    - Congenital deformities (e.g., phimosis, epispadias, etc.)
  - ***Acquired:***
    - Partial/Total amputation of the penis
    - Pre-pubertal castration
    - Local diseases (e.g., large hydrocoele, filariasis, infections such as gonorrhoea and carcinomata).

Atonic Causes

- Due to paralysis of the motor nerves supplying the genitalia without evidence of any lesion of the central nervous system.
  - ***Traumatic:***
    - Blow to the external genitalia
    - Injury to the cauda equina
  - ***Pharmacogenic:***
    - Excessive doses or prolonged use/abuse of sedatives, parasympatholytic agents, ethanol, opiates, cocaine, etc.
  - ***Diseases:***
    - Autonomic neuropathies of varying aetiology, or tumours of the cauda equina.

Paretic Causes

- Due to lesions in the central nervous system or spinal cord.
  - Hemiparesis or paraplegia, as a result of either trauma or a cerebrovascular accident.
  - General paralysis of the insane (tertiary syphilis).

Functional Causes

- They are dependent upon the mental complex, and are usually due to:
  - Fear, timidity and anxiety, all of which are responsible for what is commonly described as ***first-night*** or ***bridegroom impotence***.
  - Aversion to a particular female (***impotentia quoad persona*** or ***quoad hanc*** or ***quoad hunc***) or to females in general (***sexual aversion disorder***, defined as a "persistent or recurrent aversion to, and avoidance of all genital sexual contact with a sexual partner").
  - Excessive passion (leading to premature ejaculation).
  - Sexual overindulgence.

The commonest reason for impotence in males is generally due to one of the above *functional* causes.

Medicolegal Importance of Impotence

Civil Cases

- Legally, a marriage is a contract between man and wife, in which sexual union between the two is presumed to take place periodically (**consummation**).
  - If there is any cause, in either partner, which prevents such sexual intercourse (such as impotence existing either before or at the time of the marriage), the marriage

*__Note__: *It is __not__ "Impotency" as mentioned in some textbooks. "Potency" is correct, but "Impotency" is wrong.*

cannot be consummated and can therefore be declared to be **null and void**.

- However, when impotence develops after the marriage has been consummated, it can only be cited as grounds for **divorce**, whether or not the consummation has resulted in conception and the production of offspring.
- A marriage that has been declared "**null and void**," i.e., a "**void marriage**," is one that is totally **invalid** as per law. In other words, even though it may have been solemnized by religious rites or by formal registration, the two individuals cannot be considered as husband and wife.
- On the other hand, the term "**divorce**" refers to the dissolution of a previously **valid** marriage between two individuals who were husband and wife.
- **Table 3.22** mentions the important grounds under which a spouse can file for **nullity** (void marriage) or divorce.

- In a case of **disputed paternity**, the putative father may claim that he is impotent, and therefore could not have fathered the child.
- A man may claim **compensation** for an injury that has allegedly rendered him impotent.

Criminal Cases

- In criminal cases of alleged **natural or unnatural sexual offences**, the accused may plead that he is impotent, and so cannot be charged with the crime.

Important Points

1. The role of a registered medical practitioner in the cases listed above is obvious. However, in no instance can he positively conclude that a person is potent. If on examination, he finds that a male is physically normal in all respects, including development of secondary sexual characteristics and external genitalia, and if all the causes of impotence enumerated above are excluded, he is justified in opining that he "***finds nothing to suggest that the person is incapable of participating in normal sexual intercourse***." In other words, a **medical certificate of potency** should be couched in **double negative language**.
2. But, if there is gross anomaly such as amputation of penis or emasculation, he can opine conclusively that the said individual ***is incapable of participating in normal sexual intercourse***.
3. It is however the opinion of some experts that there is nothing wrong in exceptional cases, in giving an opinion that a particular individual ***is capable of participating in sexual intercourse*** if there is convincing evidence that the individual is potent (**Box 3.8** recounts an interesting true anecdote).

Box 3.8—A Clearly Potent Man

Prof Keith Simpson (1907–1985) was one of the most renowned British forensic pathologists of his time (*see figure*).

In one case relating to an alleged rape committed by a man, he was called to examine the accused for evidence of potency. It was essential in those days to prove that a man was capable of sexual intercourse to get a conviction, if he was accused of rape. Generally, a doctor would be called to examine him, and if there was no evidence to suggest impotence, would certify that there was "nothing to suggest that the person is incapable of participating in normal sexual intercourse". This would mean indirectly that the accused was potent. However, almost never would a doctor directly certify a male as potent.

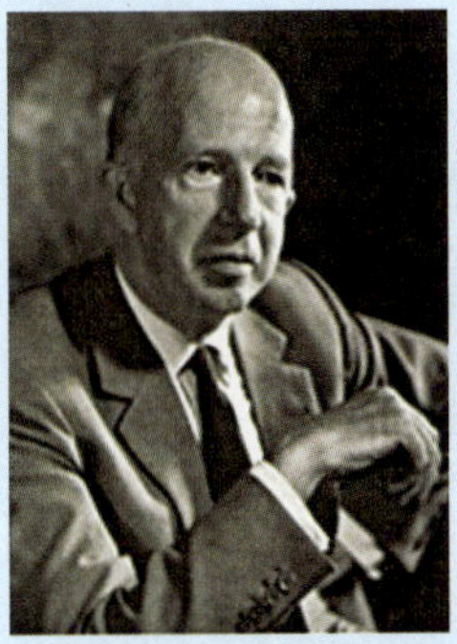

Prof Keth Simpson

But surprisingly, Prof Simpson mentioned in his opinion in this case that the accused male was indeed capable of participating in sexual intercourse, and that he was definitely potent. When the case came up for trial, the defence lawyer asked Prof Simpson while he was on the witness stand, to clarify as to how he could be so certain that the accused was potent.

Prof Simpson replied, "In the course of the medical examination, I performed a per rectal examination to assess the status of his prostate. During this procedure, I noted that he had got an erection, which indicated clearly that he was potent."

The lawyer looked at the professor for a moment and then turned around and proclaimed sarcastically to those present in the courtroom, "According to the learned professor, each time this man has to have an erection, the good doctor has to come and put his finger in his rectum!" The court dissolved in loud laughter, but Prof Simpson remained unperturbed.

When the laughter subsided, he said calmly, "That is not entirely correct Sir. Your finger will do equally well!"

This of course brought the house down.

Potency Test

- Indian legal system makes it mandatory to medically examine any accused of rape as well as other forms of sexual assault. The accused is brought under police custody for conducting the medical examination, which includes general physical examination, **potency test** and evidence collection. The medical examination report of the accused is labelled as the "***Potency Test Report***".
- But, as per the changed definition of rape after Criminal Law (Amendment) Act, 2013, **potency test stands irrelevant in rape cases because the changed law does not require peno-vaginal intercourse to call it as rape**.

- However, even after the change in definition of rape and laws related to it, potency test is still being carried out as part of the medical examination of an accused.
- It is important to understand that potency depends on various anatomical, physiological, pathological and psychological factors. To correctly diagnose/rule out organic impotence (erectile dysfunction), other than general physical examination, the following tests/investigations need to be performed:
  - Blood tests:
    - Serum testosterone and sex hormone binding globulin – to exclude endocrine causes.
    - Fasting glucose and glycated haemoglobin (HbA1c) – to exclude latent diabetes mellitus.
    - Lipid profile – for deranged lipid profile.
    - Thyroid hormones – for hypogonadal patients.
    - Follicle stimulating hormone – for patients with special clinical conditions.
  - Nocturnal penile tumescence
  - Duplex ultrasonography
  - Intracavernosal testing with vasoactive substance
  - Cavernosometry – used to test for venous leaks.
  - Cavernosography – radiographic visualization of the cavernous penile tissues using contrast material in order to exclude structural abnormalities within the cavernous tissues.
  - Penile arteriography
  - Spongiosography
- Even after undertaking this battery of tests, and getting normal results for the extensive list of investigations mentioned above, which can only exclude organic causes of sexual dysfunction, an accused man can still be impotent due to functional reasons.
- The possession of virility and power neither requires to be, nor can be, proved to exist by any physician, but is supposed to exist just like any other normal function. If the genitals are normal, an opinion of impotence cannot be given. The amended Section 375 of IPC implies that a man will be held guilty of committing rape even if he inserts his fingers, or any object inside the vagina, anus or mouth of the victim. Therefore, peno-vaginal intercourse is not essential to call it 'rape'. A person, who is unable to get a penile erection can also perform and be accused of rape. One can sexually assault a female even without the involvement of the penis.
- The cost of investigations and manpower involved must always be taken into consideration, whenever the police insist on performing "potency testing" of the accused. Many of the tests need to be done by a radiologist or urologist who will not only do the examination but will also attend the court summons in future. In a developing country like India, where the health sector is already struggling due to lack of funds and manpower, there is no justification of diverting so many resources to one issue which ultimately does not have any impact over the fate of the case in the court of law.
- The potency examination of a rape accused can be compared to another redundant and now condemned medical examination test called "***the two finger test***" that was used to be done on a victim of rape. In the same way that this test is today considered demeaning and humiliating to the female, a rape accused also has all the fundamental rights

Table 3.22 Legal Grounds for Nullity of Marriage (Void Marriage) and Divorce

Nullity (Void Marriage)	Divorce
1. Either party has a spouse living at the time of the marriage	1. Adultery
2. The parties are within prohibited degree of relationship (consanguinity) to each other	2. Cruelty
3. Impotence on the part of either spouse from the time of marriage leading to non-consummation	3. Desertion
4. Either party was mentally unsound from the time of marriage	4. Conversion to another religion
5. Consent of either party was obtained by force or fraud	5. Mental unsoundness developing after marriage
6. Either party was below the legal age for marriage	6. Venereal disease in a communicable form
	7. Renunciation (turning "sanyasi")
	8. Either spouse not being heard of for 7 years or more
	9. Husband found guilty of rape, sodomy or bestiality
	10. Mutual consent

granted by the constitution of India, including the right to dignity. Therefore, there is no justification in subjecting a rape accused to the so-called ***potency testing***, which must be undertaken only in rare cases where there are sufficient grounds to indicate that it may be of help.

FRIGIDITY

- **Frigidity** is the correct term for impotence in the female. In other words, it refers to a **difficulty or inability to take part in sexual intercourse by a female.**
- Like male impotence, frigidity could be either temporary or permanent.

Causes of Frigidity

- **Permanent frigidity** is invariably psychogenic in nature, resulting most often from either sexual abuse during childhood, or a traumatic sexual assault during adulthood, manifesting as either a
  - **Sexual aversion disorder**: Persistent or recurrent aversion to, and avoidance of all genital sexual contact with a sexual partner.
  - **Female sexual arousal disorder**: Persistent or recurrent lack of a subjective sense of sexual excitement and pleasure in a female during sexual activity.
- **Temporary frigidity** manifests only as **female sexual arousal disorder**. It may be due to either:
  - **Dyspareunia**, a term loosely used to describe both difficult and painful coitus, or
  - **Vaginismus**, which is hyperaesthesia leading to painful spasms of the sphincter vaginae and levator ani, with simultaneous spasmodic contractions of the adductor muscles of the thighs and the erector spinae, making penetration impossible.
    - **Vaginismus** may be:
      - ***Primary*** (where there is no organic lesion)
      - ***Secondary*** (due to a painful local inflammation or lesion, or during menstruation)
      - ***Psychogenic*** (due to fear, timidity, or anxiety).

Medicolegal Importance of Frigidity

- If a woman is so frigid as to prevent sexual intercourse after being married, preventing it from being consummated, such a marriage can be declared by a court of law to be **null and void**.
- But, if the frigidity develops after the marriage has been consummated, it can only be cited as grounds for **divorce**, whether or not the consummation has resulted in conception and the production of offspring.

STERILITY (ABSOLUTE INFERTILITY)

- **Sterility** is defined as **the incapability of fertilisation or reproduction**. However, the term "sterility" has fallen out of favour, and has been replaced by the phrase "**absolute infertility**."
  - **Absolute infertility** in the **male** is the *inability to fertilise the ovum.*
    - Impotence and absolute infertility may co-exist, but not invariably – a person may be potent but sterile; conversely, he may be impotent, but not necessarily sterile.
  - **Absolute infertility** in the **female** is her *inability to conceive, due to inadequacy in genital structure or function.*
- **Absolute infertility** is complete and usually irremediable. On the other hand, **relative infertility**, which is the diminished capacity to produce offspring, can often be corrected. A forensic expert's opinion is usually sought only in cases of absolute infertility (either male or female). Opinions regarding relative infertility are better given by a practising-genitourinary surgeon or obstetrician.

Causes of Absolute Infertility in the Male

1. **Azoospermatogenic** (total failure to produce living spermatozoa)
   a. ***Seminiferous tubular necrosis***, e.g., Klinefelter's syndrome.
   b. ***Germinal aplasia***, either idiopathic, or due to the XYY syndrome, or exposure to radiation/drugs.
   c. ***Arrest of maturation***, as in varicocele.
   d. ***Endocrinopathies***.
2. **Oligospermatogenic** (failure to produce living spermatozoa in sufficient numbers)
   a. ***Congenital conditions***, e.g., Frohlich's and Klinefelter's syndromes, primary testicular failure and cryptorchidism.
   b. ***Acquired conditions***, e.g., general debilitating diseases, local diseases such as adolescent mumps orchitis/tuberculous epididymo-orchitis/varicocele/carcinomata, and drug-induced (nicotine, alcohol, cannabis, cocaine).
3. **Asthenospermatogenic** (defects in sperm movement)
   a. Idiopathic
   b. Spermatozoal structural defects
   c. Antisperm antibodies
   d. Genital tract infections
   e. Prolonged abstinence
4. **Normospermatogenic**
   a. Structural/Functional abnormalities in the male
   b. Abnormal coital habits (including poor timing)
   c. Acrosomal defects in the spermatozoa
   d. Immunological causes
   e. Unexplained causes
5. **Absent ejaculation** due to
   a. Surgery (e.g., vasectomy)
   b. Vascular occlusion
   c. Diabetes mellitus
   d. Psychological disturbances
   e. Drug-induced

Causes of Absolute Infertility in the Female

1. **Organic Causes**:
   a. ***Congenital defects***:
      i. of the **vagina**, which may not have developed at all,

may not be canalised, may be septate, or may manifest an imperforate hymen.

ii. of the **cervix**, which may be elongated or conical, or may have a pinhole os (hostile cervical mucosa may also obstruct/impede penetration of the ovum by the sperm).

iii. of the **uterus**, which may be either absent or retroflexed.

iv. of the **fallopian tubes**, which may be stenosed (an extremely rare condition).

b. ***Acquired causes***:

i. Diseases of genital tract, e.g., gonorrhoea leading to salpingitis.

ii. Diseases of ovaries, uterus or fallopian tubes.

iii. Exposure to radiation.

iv. Exposure to drugs.

2. **Hormonal dysfunction** leading to menstrual irregularities may occur from pituitary dysfunction, adrenogenital syndrome or prolonged use of contraceptives.
3. **Chromosomal abnormalities**, e.g., Turner's syndrome.

Medicolegal Aspects of Sterility (Absolute Infertility)

Civil Cases

- The putative father, in a suit of disputed paternity, may plead that he is sterile, and so could not have fathered the child.
- A patient may claim damages for loss/diminution of reproductive capability as a result of professional negligence during a surgical operation.
- Absolute infertility in the male is the prime indication for artificial insemination (donor) or adoption of a child.

Criminal Cases

- Battery or criminal negligence may be cited as the cause for the incapability of a male for fertilisation, or of a female for conception.

Investigation of a Case of Sterility (Absolute Infertility)

- In both **males** and **females**, a detailed physical and marital history, general examination and scrutiny of secondary sexual characteristics are mandatory. A psychological assessment may also be carried out when indicated.
- In the **male**, the specific investigations to be conducted include:
  - ***Initial basic laboratory evaluation***
    - of seminal fluid for its physical characteristics, morphology and motility of spermatozoa, and presence and level of fructose; and
    - of hormonal levels with particular reference to follicle stimulating hormone (FSH), gonadotropin and gonadotropin-releasing hormone (GnRH), testosterone and prolactin and luteinising hormone (LH).
  - ***Transrectal ultrasonography (TRUS)*** to detect the absence of or anatomical abnormalities of the seminal vesicles or ejaculatory ducts.
  - ***Second-level testing*** (not all patients need these):
    - to rule out antisperm antibodies
    - leucocyte staining of semen
    - testicular biopsy
    - vasography
    - functional evaluation of spermatozoa
- In the **female**, the specific investigations to be conducted include:
  - ***Evaluation of ovulation*** by several methods, including basal body temperature charting, and testing of urinary LH, mid-luteal progesterone levels, endometrial biopsy, and ultrasonic monitoring of the development and disappearance of the ovarian follicles.
  - ***Evaluation of the fallopian tubes*** by hysterosalpingogram using either oil or water-based dyes, to determine the patency of the fallopian tubes as well as the shape of the uterus. It is generally performed in the early follicular phase of the cycle, once menstrual bleeding ceases.
  - ***Laparoscopy*** may be indicated when clinical examination or prior investigations have raised a suspicion of pelvic pathology, or when all other investigations have proved normal.
  - ***Additional investigation*** of the functional relation between spermatozoa and ova may be performed when considered absolutely necessary.

SEXUAL DYSFUNCTION

Explanation

- **Sexual dysfunction** is difficulty experienced by an individual or partners during any stage of normal sexual activity, including physical pleasure, desire, preference, arousal or orgasm.
- The World Health Organization defines sexual dysfunction as a "person's inability to participate in a sexual relationship as they would wish". This definition is broad and is subject to many interpretations.
- A diagnosis of sexual dysfunction under DSM-5 requires a person to feel extreme distress and interpersonal strain for a minimum of 6 months (except for substance- or medication-induced sexual dysfunction).
- The term sexual disorder may not only refer to physical sexual dysfunction, but to paraphilias as well; this is sometimes termed **disorder of sexual preference**.

Types

Sexual Desire Disorders

- **Sexual desire disorders** or **decreased libido** are characterized by a lack of sexual desire or libido for sexual activity, or of sexual fantasies. The condition ranges from a general lack of sexual desire, to a lack of sexual desire for the current partner. The condition may have started after a period of normal sexual functioning, or the person may always have had an absence or a lesser intensity of sexual desire.
- **Causes** vary considerably, but include a decrease in the production of normal oestrogen in women or testosterone in both men and women. Other causes may be ageing, fa

tigue, pregnancy, medications or psychiatric conditions, such as depression and anxiety.

Sexual Arousal Disorders

- **Sexual arousal disorders** were previously known as **frigidity** in women and **impotence** in men, though these have now been replaced with less judgmental terms.
  - Impotence is now known as **erectile dysfunction**, and
  - Frigidity has been replaced with a number of terms describing specific problems that can be broken down into four categories as described by the DSM-5: **lack of desire, lack of arousal, pain during intercourse** and **lack of orgasm**.
- For both men and women, these conditions can manifest themselves as an aversion to and avoidance of sexual contact with a partner. In men, there may be partial or complete failure to attain or maintain an erection, or a lack of sexual excitement and pleasure in sexual activity.
- There may be physiological origins to these disorders, such as decreased blood flow or lack of vaginal lubrication. Chronic disease can also contribute, as well as the nature of the relationship between the partners.
- Additionally, the condition **post-orgasm illness syndrome (POIS)** may cause symptoms when aroused, including adrenergic-type presentation: rapid breathing, paraesthesia, palpitations, headaches, aphasia, nausea, itchy eyes, fever, muscle pain and fatigue.
  - From the onset of arousal, symptoms can persist for up to a week in patients.
  - The aetiology of this condition is unknown; however, it is believed to be a pathology of either the immune system or autonomic nervous systems. It is not thought to be psychiatric in nature, but it may present as anxiety relating to coital activities and thus may be incorrectly diagnosed as such. There is no known cure or treatment.
- **Erectile dysfunction**
  - Erectile dysfunction (ED), or **impotence**, is a sexual dysfunction characterized by the inability to develop or maintain an erection of the penis. There are various underlying causes of erectile ED including: damage to anatomical structures, psychological causes, medical disease, as well as use of certain drugs. Many of these causes are medically treatable.
  - Psychological erectile dysfunction can often be helped by almost anything that the patient believes in; there is a very strong placebo effect. Physical damage can be more difficult to treat.
  - The introduction of perhaps the first pharmacologically effective remedy for impotence, **sildenafil** (trade name **Viagra**), in the 1990s caused a wave of public attention, propelled in part by the newsworthiness of stories about it and heavy advertising.

Orgasm Disorders

- **Anorgasmia**:
  - Anorgasmia is classified as persistent delays or absence of orgasm following a normal sexual excitement phase in at least 75% of sexual encounters.
  - The disorder can have physical, psychological or pharmacological origins. SSRI antidepressants are a common pharmaceutical culprit, as they can delay orgasm or eliminate it entirely. A common physiological culprit of anorgasmia is menopause; one in three women report problems obtaining an orgasm during sexual stimulation following menopause.
- **Premature ejaculation**:
  - Premature ejaculation is when ejaculation occurs before the partner achieves orgasm, or a mutually satisfactory length of time has passed during intercourse. There is no correct length of time for intercourse to last, but generally, premature ejaculation is thought to occur when ejaculation occurs in under 2 minutes from the time of the insertion of the penis. For a diagnosis, the patient must have a chronic history of premature ejaculation, poor ejaculatory control and the problem must cause feelings of dissatisfaction as well as distress for the patient, the partner or both.
- **Post-orgasmic disorders**:
  - Post-orgasmic disorders cause symptoms shortly after orgasm or ejaculation. **Post-coital tristesse (PCT)** is a feeling of melancholy and anxiety after sexual intercourse that lasts for up to 2 hours. Sexual headaches occur in the skull and neck during sexual activity, including masturbation, arousal or orgasm.
  - In men, **postorgasmic illness syndrome (POIS)** causes severe muscle pain throughout the body and other symptoms immediately following ejaculation. These symptoms last for up to a week.
  - **Dhat syndrome** is another condition which occurs in men. It is a culture-bound syndrome which causes anxious and dysphoric mood after sex. It is distinct from the low-mood and concentration problems (acute aphasia) seen in POIS.

Sexual Pain Disorders

- Sexual pain disorders in women include **dyspareunia** (painful intercourse) and **vaginismus** (involuntary painful spasms of vaginal walls that interfere with intercourse).
  - Dyspareunia may be caused by insufficient lubrication (vaginal dryness) in women. Poor lubrication may result from insufficient excitement/stimulation, or from hormonal changes caused by menopause, pregnancy or breastfeeding. Irritation from contraceptive creams can also cause dryness, as can fear and anxiety about sex.
  - It is unclear exactly what causes vaginismus, but it is thought that past sexual trauma (such as rape or abuse) may play a role.
- In men, structural abnormalities of the penis like **Peyronie's disease** can make sexual intercourse difficult and/or painful. The disease is characterized by thick fibrous bands in the penis that lead to excessive curvature during erection.

Risk factors include genetics, minor trauma, chronic systemic vascular diseases, smoking and alcohol consumption.

- **Priapism** is a painful erection that occurs for several hours and occurs in the absence of sexual stimulation. This condition develops when blood gets trapped in the penis and is unable to drain. If the condition is not promptly treated, it can lead to severe scarring and permanent loss of erectile function. Individuals with sickle-cell disease and those who use certain medications can often develop this disorder.

> **FM 3.23: Core – Written/Viva Voce**
> - **Discuss:**
>   - Sterilization of male and female
>   - Artificial insemination
>   - Test tube baby
>   - Surrogate mother
>   - Hormonal replacement therapy

STERILIZATION

Definition

- **Sterilization** (*also spelled 'sterilisation'*) is a medical method of birth control that leaves a person unable to reproduce.
  - Sterilization methods include both surgical and non-surgical, and exist for both males and females.
  - Sterilization procedures are intended to be permanent; reversal is generally difficult or impossible.

Methods

- Commonest methods include **tubal ligation** for women and **vasectomy** for men.
- **Tubal ligation**:
  - The fallopian tubes, which allow the sperm to fertilize the ovum and would carry the fertilized ovum to the uterus, are closed (ligated).
  - This generally involves a general anaesthetic and a laparotomy or laparoscopic approach to cut, clip or cauterize the fallopian tubes.
- **Vasectomy**:
  - The vasa deferentia, the tubes that connect the testicles to the prostate, are cut and closed. This prevents sperm produced in the testicles from entering the ejaculated semen (which is mostly produced in the seminal vesicles and prostate).
    - Although the term vasectomy is established in the general community, the correct medical terminology is **vasoligation**.
- **Other Methods**:
  - **Hysterectomy** in females: The uterus is surgically removed, permanently preventing pregnancy and some diseases such as uterine cancer.
  - **Castration** in males: The testicles are surgically removed. This is frequently used for the sterilization of animals, but rarely for humans.
  - **Transluminal Methods**:
    - Transluminal procedures are performed by entry through the female reproductive tract. These generally use a catheter to place a substance into the fallopian tubes that eventually causes blockage of the tract in this segment. Such procedures are generally called non-surgical as they use natural orifices and thereby do not necessitate any surgical incision.
    - The **Essure procedure** is one such transluminal sterilization technique. In this procedure, polyethylene terephthalate fibre inserts are placed into the fallopian tubes, eventually inducing scarring and occlusion of the tubes. However, in April 2018, the FDA restricted the sale and use of Essure. On July 20, 2018, Bayer announced the halt of sales in the US by the end of 2018.
    - Quinacrine has also been used for transluminal sterilization, but despite a multitude of clinical studies on the use of quinacrine and female sterilization, no randomized, controlled trials have been reported to date and there is some controversy over its use.
  - **Pharmacological Method**: There is no working "sterilization pill" that causes permanent inability to reproduce. Most of the drugs that are claimed to cause sterilization either do not work, or are associated with serious adverse effects.

Types

- ***Voluntary sterilization***:
  - **Personal choice**: Because of the emphasis placed on childbearing as the most important role of women, not having children was traditionally seen as a deficiency or due to fertility problems. However, better access to contraception, new economic and educational opportunities, and changing ideas about motherhood have led to new reproductive experiences for women, particularly for women who choose to be childless.
  - **Financial**: Some women state the lack of financial resources as a reason why they choose to remain childfree.
  - **Physiological**: Physiological reasons, such as genetic disorders or disabilities, can influence whether couples seek sterilization. Couples may choose sterilization in order to concentrate on caring for a child with a disability and to avoid withholding any necessary resources from additional children. Technological advancements have enabled the use of carrier screening and prenatal testing for the detection of genetic disorders in prospective parents or in their unborn offspring.
- ***Promoted sterilization***:
  - **Compulsory sterilization**: Compulsory sterilization -refers to governmental policies put in place as part of human population planning, or as a form of eugenics (improving hereditary qualities of a race or breed by controlling mating) to prevent certain groups of people from reproducing.

- **Incentive-based sterilization**: Some governments in the world have offered and continue to offer economic incentives to using birth control, including sterilization. For countries with high population growth and not enough resources to sustain a large population, these incentives become more enticing. While these policies are controversial, the ultimate goal is to promote greater social well being for the whole community.

Effects

- *Physical*:
  - Among women who had interval tubal sterilization, studies have shown a null or positive effect on female sexual interest and pleasure. Similar results were discovered for men who had vasectomies. Vasectomies did not negatively influence the satisfaction of men and there was no significant change in communication and marital satisfaction among couples as a result. Tubal sterilization is an effective procedure, but pregnancy can still occur in about 1 out of 200 women.
  - Some potential risks of tubal sterilization include:
    - Bleeding from a skin incision or inside the abdomen.
    - Infection.
    - Damage to other organs inside the abdomen.
    - Side effects from anaesthesia.
    - Ectopic pregnancy.
    - Incomplete closing of a fallopian tube that results in pregnancy.
  - Some potential risks of vasectomies include:
    - Pain continuing long after surgery.
    - Bleeding and bruising.
    - Inflammatory reaction to sperm that spill during surgery called "sperm granuloma".
    - Infection.
    - Additionally, the vas deferens may grow back together, which could result in unintended pregnancy.
- *Psychological*:
  - **Depression**: If an individual goes into the procedure after being coerced, or with a lack of understanding of the procedure and its consequences, he or she is more likely to suffer negative psychological consequences afterwards.
  - Because sterilization is a largely irreversible procedure, **post-sterilization regret** is a major psychological effect. The most common reason for post-sterilization regret is the desire to have more children.
- *Familial*:
  - Some people believe that sterilization gives women, in particular, more control over their sexuality and their reproduction. This can lead to **empowering women**, to giving them more of a sense of ownership over their body, as well as to an improved relationship in the household. Many women report feeling more sexually liberated after being sterilized, as there is no concern of a pregnancy risk. By eliminating the risk of having more children, a woman can commit to a long-term job without a disruption of a maternity leave in the future. Sterilization eliminates the need for potential abortions, which can be a very stressful decision overall.
  - **Relationship with spouse**: In countries that are more entrenched in the traditional patriarchal system, female sterilizations can inspire abusive behaviour from husbands for various reasons. Sterilization can lead to distrust in a marriage if the husband then suspects his wife of infidelity. Furthermore, the husband may become angry and aggressive, if the decision to be sterilized was made by the wife without consulting him. If a woman marries again after sterilization, her new husband might be displeased with her inability to bear him children, causing tumult in the marriage. Sexual activity remains fairly constant and marital relationships do not suffer, as long as the sterilization decision was made collaboratively between the two partners.
  - **Children**:
    - Especially in countries that give parents incentives for family planning and for having fewer children, it is advantageous to existing children to be in smaller families.
    - In more rural areas where families depend on the labour of their children to survive, sterilization could have more of a negative effect. If a child dies, a family loses a worker.

ASSISTED REPRODUCTION

Artificial Insemination

- The oldest and simplest method to conceive a child by artificial means is **artificial insemination**, defined as **the introduction of semen into the vagina other than by coitus** **(Fig. 3.146)**.
- The procedure employs a sterile syringe to introduce 1 mL of semen into the uterus at about the time of ovulation. The semen should be collected by masturbation into a wide-mouthed sterile glass container, after 3 days' abstinence. The specimen should be used within 2 hours of collection, during which it should be subjected to examination to ensure its normalcy with respect to its physical characteristics and the quality of spermatozoa (number, morphology and motility).
  - If the semen used for this purpose is derived from the woman's husband himself, the procedure is called **homologous artificial insemination (AIH)**.
  - If it is obtained from a person other than the husband, the method is termed **heterologous artificial insemination**, or, for differentiation from the first type, **artificial insemination (donor) (AID)** (**Fig. 3.147**). The use of frozen semen stored in sperm banks for heterologous artificial insemination is becoming increasingly popular, as is pooling of the husband's semen with that of a donor (which is psychologically advantageous to both the husband and his wife).
- The **indications** for artificial insemination include

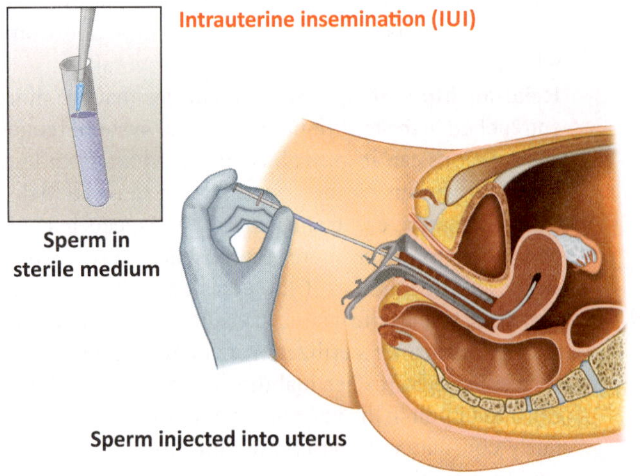

Fig. 3.146 Artificial insemination

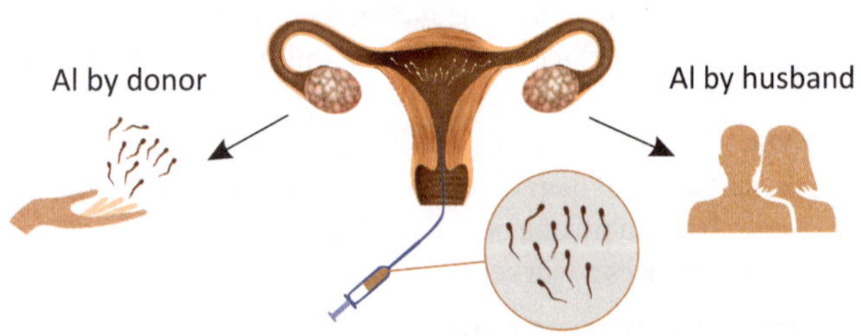

Fig. 3.147 Types of artificial insemination

- For AIH: An impotent but fertile husband.
- For AID:
  - A sterile husband
  - Genetic defects in the husband, carrying a high risk of mortality, which would definitely be transmitted to the child (e.g., blood dyscrasias)
  - Rh incompatibility between husband and wife, which would result in erythroblastosis foetalis in the child.

Ethical Aspects of Artificial Insemination

- Homologous artificial insemination is not associated with significant legal or ethical problems, so no special precautions are called for.
- On the other hand, when AID is contemplated, the registered medical practitioner who undertakes the procedure must observe with greatest care, the following precautions in the selection of the donor, lest he be accused of ethical malpraxis:
  - The expressed written informed consent of both the recipient and her husband, and of the donor and his wife.
  - Absolute confidentiality must be maintained:
    - Neither should the identity of the donor be revealed to the recipient, her husband or their children;
    - Nor should the identities of the recipient, her husband or the child be made known to the donor, his wife, or children.
  - The donor
    - Should be less than 40 years of age,
    - Should not be related by blood to either the recipient or her husband (however, it is preferable that he resemble the husband physically, socially and intellectually as closely as is possible),
    - Should be in sound physical and mental health, and should be free of hereditary, familial and sexually transmitted diseases and
    - Should be potent and fertile (if married, he should have at least two healthy children of his own).

Medicolegal Aspects of Artificial Insemination

- The medicolegal aspects of artificial insemination vary from country to country. Although practised widely in the West, it has not gained much popularity in India (except in veterinary practice).
- Strangely, even abroad, it has no definitive legal sanction in statutory or case law. Thus, multiple legal questions arise about the procedure:
  - **Does artificial insemination (donor)**
    - Amount to **rape** or **adultery**?: *Not in India, where sexual intercourse is necessary to constitute the offence.*
    - Constitute a valid ground for **divorce** by reason of adultery?: *Again, this is not a valid reason (because of the definition of the offence), unless the procedure was performed without the expressed written informed consent of the husband.*
    - Lead to **annulment of marriage** by reason of non-consummation?: *This question would definitely arise if the husband was both impotent and sterile prior to the marriage. However, no such instance seems to have been reported to date, for obvious reasons.*
  - Is a child born of artificial insemination **legitimate**?: *Peculiarly, the law says "No," regardless of whether the child was born of AIH or AID! This view raises further queries, such as:*
    - If the husband is not the father of the child, then who is? Or is the child to be considered fatherless? This is an anomaly, because no child can be begotten without a father (at least, until the advent of cloning!).
    - Would naming the father of the child born of AID, as the father in legal documents (birth certificate, applications for various purposes, etc.), amount to a false declaration?
    - How could the child lawfully inherit the property of the "father"?
    - The general consensus of opinion as to the above question of **legitimacy** and its corollaries is that while in India there is no legislation regarding artificial insemination, a child born as a result of artificial insemination is considered as legitimate, provided the child was born during lawful wedlock, or the child was legally adopted by its parents, so that

- the husband is legally considered as the father of the child, even though he may not have contributed to its conception, and
- the child can lawfully inherit the property of its parents, or be entitled to maintenance should its parents divorce.

- Does sexual intercourse between a child born of AID and the children of the donor born in wedlock amount to incest?: *Theoretically it would, but practically, the probability of such an event is extremely remote.*

- Finally, it must always be kept in mind that the physician who conducts an artificial insemination can be held liable for civil negligence, indecent assault or breach of trust, unless he:
  - exercises the utmost skill and care in the selection of a donor, and in the performance of the procedure,
  - ensures that a registered nurse is present throughout the procedure,
  - himself conducts the delivery of the child conceived by the procedure which he has performed and
  - maintains all records pertaining to the procedure meticulously and in the strictest confidence.

Other Methods of Assisted Reproduction

- In vitro fertilisation and embryo transfer (IVF-ET)
- Gamete intra-fallopian transfer (GIFT)
- Pronuclear stage tubal transfer (PROST)
- Micromanipulation techniques: zona drilling, partial zona dissection, perivitelline sperm transfer (PST) and intra-cytoplasmic sperm injection (ICSI).

Test Tube Baby

- **In vitro fertilisation (IVF)** is a process of fertilisation where an egg is combined with sperm in vitro ("in glass"). The process involves monitoring and stimulating a woman's ovulatory process, removing an ovum or ova (egg or eggs) from her ovaries and letting sperm fertilise them in a culture medium in a laboratory. After the fertilised egg (zygote) undergoes embryo culture for 2–6 days, it is transferred by catheter into the uterus, with the intention of establishing a successful pregnancy.
- IVF is a type of assisted reproductive technology used for infertility treatment and gestational surrogacy. A fertilised egg from a donor may implant into a surrogate's uterus, and the resulting child is genetically unrelated to the surrogate. Some countries have banned or otherwise regulate the availability of IVF treatment, giving rise to **fertility tourism**. Restrictions on the availability of IVF include costs and age, in order for a woman to carry a healthy pregnancy to term.
- Children born through IVF are commonly called **test tube babies**.
- The term "**test-tube baby**," prior to the development of in vitro fertilization technologies in the 20th century, was used to refer to babies born as a result of artificial insemination.
  - **William Pancoast**, an American physician, performed the first artificial insemination that led to a successful birth in **1884**, marking the birth of the first test-tube baby.
- By the middle of the 20th century, in vitro fertilization had been thoroughly researched and reported on, though no successful human reproduction had occurred from its practice. However, the successful fertilization and reproduction of various species of animal besides humans through in vitro fertilization was common practice by 1960.
- It was not until **25th July 1978** with the work of two British medical researchers, **Patrick Steptoe** and **Robert Edwards**, that the revised definition of test-tube baby became a reality. With their work, the first child born from a zygote fertilized outside of a human body was created.
- The first test-tube baby born via in vitro fertilization was **Louise Brown (25 July, 1978)** (**Fig. 3.148**). Shortly after her birth, discussion of both legal and ethical implications regarding the existence of test-tube babies began in the international media as well as in scientific journals. These debates continue to this day as the ongoing research of embryos and reproduction leads to the development of new medical practices.

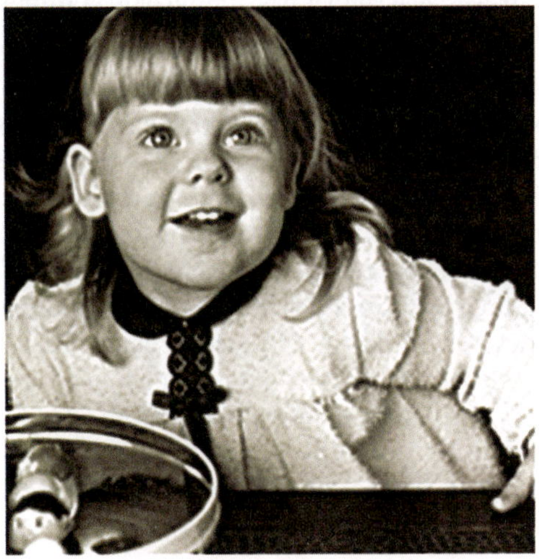

Fig. 3.148 Louise Brown

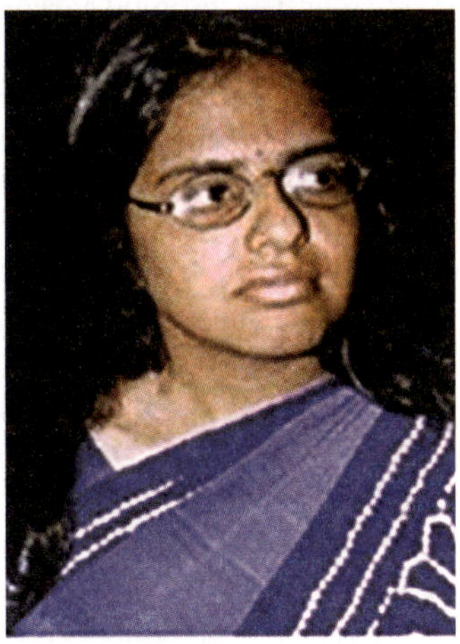

Fig. 3.149 Kanupriya Agarwal (Durga)

- In India, **Dr Subhash Mukherjee** became the first physician to successfully produce a test-tube baby: **Kanupriya Agarwal** who was born on **October 3, 1978**.

SURROGACY

Definition

- **Surrogacy** is an arrangement whereby a woman (**surrogate mother**) agrees to bear a child for another person or persons, who will become the child's parent(s) after birth. Surrogacy is considered one of many assisted reproductive technologies.
- People may seek a surrogacy arrangement when:
  - pregnancy is medically impossible
  - pregnancy risks are too dangerous for the intended mother
  - a single man or a male couple wish to have a child.
- In surrogacy arrangements, monetary compensation may or may not be involved. Receiving money for the arrangement is known as **commercial surrogacy**.

Methods

- Surrogacy may be either **traditional** or **gestational**, which are differentiated by the genetic origin of the egg.

Traditional

- A **traditional surrogacy** (also known as **partial, natural** or **straight surrogacy**) is one where the surrogate's egg is fertilised by the intended father's or a donor's sperm.
- Insemination of the surrogate can be either through sex (**natural insemination**) or **artificial insemination**.
- Using the sperm of a donor results in a child who is not genetically related to the intended parent(s). If the intended father's sperm is used in the insemination, the resulting child is genetically related to both the intended father and the surrogate.

Gestational

- **Gestational surrogacy** (also known as **host** or **full surrogacy**) takes place when an embryo created by in vitro fertilization (IVF) technology is implanted in a surrogate, sometimes called a **gestational carrier**.
- Gestational surrogacy has several forms, and in each form, the resulting child is genetically unrelated to the surrogate:
  - The embryo is created using the intended father's sperm and the intended mother's eggs;
  - The embryo is created using the intended father's sperm and a donor egg;
  - The embryo is created using the intended mother's egg and donor sperm;
  - A donor embryo is transferred to a surrogate. Such an embryo may be available when others undergoing IVF have embryos left over, which they donate to others. The resulting child is genetically unrelated to the intended parent(s).
- A gestational carrier should preferably be between the ages of 21 and 45, has had one full-term, uncomplicated pregnancy where she successfully had at least one child, and has had no more than five deliveries or three Caesarean sections.
- The International Federation of Gynaecology and Obstetrics recommends that the surrogate's autonomy should be respected throughout the pregnancy even if her wishes conflict with what the intended parents want.
- The most commonly reported motivation given by gestational surrogates is an altruistic desire to help a childless couple. Other less commonly given reasons include enjoying the experience of pregnancy, and financial compensation.

Risks

- The embryo implanted in gestational surrogacy faces the same risks as anyone using IVF would. Pre-implantation risks of the embryo include unintentional epigenetic effects, influence of media which the embryo is cultured on and undesirable consequences of invasive manipulation of the embryo.
- Children born through singleton IVF surrogacy have been shown to have no physical or mental abnormalities compared to those children born through natural conception. However, children born through multiple gestation in surrogate mothers often result in preterm labour and delivery, resulting in prematurity and physical and/or mental anomalies.

Indications

- Opting for surrogacy is often a choice made when women are unable to carry children on their own. This can be for a number of reasons, including
  - Abnormal uterus
  - Complete absence of uterus either
    - Congenitally (also known as Mayer-Roakitansky-Kuster-Hauser syndrome) or
    - Post-hysterectomy: Women may have a hysterectomy due to complications in childbirth such as heavy bleeding or a ruptured uterus. Medical diseases such as cervical cancer or endometrial cancer can also lead to surgical removal of the uterus.
- Past implantation failures, history of multiple miscarriages, or concurrent severe heart or renal conditions that can make pregnancy harmful may also prompt women to consider surrogacy.
- The biological impossibility of single men and same-sex couples having a baby also may indicate surrogacy as an option.

Psychological Issues

- Anthropological studies of surrogates have shown that surrogates engage in various distancing techniques throughout the surrogate pregnancy so as to ensure that they do not become emotionally attached to the baby.
- Some surrogates describe feeling empowered by the experience.

- Although gestational surrogates generally report being satisfied with their experience as surrogates, there are cases in which they are not. Unmet expectations are associated with dissatisfaction. Some women do not feel a certain level of closeness with the couple and others do not feel respected by the couple. Some gestational surrogates report emotional distress during the process of surrogacy.
- Gestational surrogates may struggle with postpartum depression and issues with relinquishing the child to their intended parents.

Legal Issues

- The legality of surrogacy varies around the world. Many countries do not have laws which specifically deal with surrogacy. Some countries ban surrogacy outright, while others ban **commercial surrogacy** but allow **altruistic surrogacy** (in which the surrogate is not financially compensated).
- In 2005, the Govt of India approved the 2002 draft of the National Guidelines for the Accreditation, Supervision and Regulation of ART Clinics in India.
- In 2013, surrogacy by foreign homosexual couples and single parents was banned.
- In 2015, the government banned commercial surrogacy in India and permitted entry of embryos only for research purposes. Shortly thereafter in **2016**, a **Surrogacy (Regulation) Bill** was introduced in parliament, and was passed by Lok Sabha in 2019, proposing to permit only heterosexual Indian couples married for at least 5 years with infertility problems to access altruistic or unpaid surrogacy and thereby further banning commercial surrogacy. The bill would require to be passed by the Rajya Sabha, before it becomes an act and thereby a law.
- The citizenship and legal status of the children resulting from surrogacy arrangements can be problematic. In some countries, the child will not be a citizen of the country in which he/she is born because the surrogate mother is not legally the parent of said child. This could result in a child being born without citizenship.

Ethical Issues

- Those who view surrogacy as a social justice issue argue that it leads to the exploitation of women in developing countries whose wombs are commodified to meet the reproductive needs of the more affluent. While opponents of this stance argue that surrogacy provides a much-needed source of revenue for women facing poverty in developing countries, others purport that the lack of legislation in such countries often leads to much of the profit accruing to middlemen and commercial agencies rather than the surrogate mothers themselves.
- Human rights activists express concern over the conditions under which surrogate mothers are kept by surrogacy clinics which exercise much power and control over the process of surrogate pregnancy. Isolated from friends and family and required to live in separate surrogacy hostels on the pretext of ensuring consistent prenatal care, it is argued that surrogate mothers may face psychological chal lenges that cannot be offset by the (limited) economic benefits of surrogacy.
- The relevance of a woman's consent in judging the ethical acceptability of surrogacy is another point of controversy within human rights circles. While some hold that any consensual process is not a human rights violation, other human rights activists argue that human rights are not just about survival but about human dignity and respect. Thus, decisions cannot be defined as involving agency if they are driven by coercion, violence or extreme poverty, which is often the case with women in developing countries who pursue surrogacy due to economic need or aggressive persuasion from their husbands.
- Some feminists also argue that surrogacy is an assault to a woman's dignity and right to autonomy over her body. By degrading impoverished women to the mere status of "baby producers", commercial surrogacy has been accused by feminists of commodifying women's bodies in a manner akin to prostitution. Some feminists also express concerns over links between surrogacy and patriarchal expressions of domination as numerous reports have been cited of women in developing countries coerced into commercial surrogacy by their husbands wanting to "earn money off their wives' bodies".

Religious Issues

Different religions take different approaches to surrogacy, often related to their stances on assisted reproductive technology in general.

1. **Catholicism**: The Catholic Church is generally opposed to surrogacy which it views as immoral and incompatible with Biblical texts surrounding topics of birth, marriage and life. Additionally, the practice of in vitro fertilisation involved in gestational surrogacy is generally viewed as morally impermissible due to its removal of human conception from the sacred process of sexual intercourse.
2. **Hinduism**: Surrogacy and other scientific methods of assisted reproduction are generally supported within the Hindu community. Nonetheless, Hindu women do not commonly use surrogacy as an option to treat infertility, despite often serving as surrogates for Western commissioning couples. When surrogacy is practiced by Hindus, it is more likely to be used within the family circle as opposed to involving anonymous donors.
3. **Islam**: The Islamic community has largely outlawed the practice of surrogacy. Many Muslim groups claim that surrogate motherhood is not permitted under Islamic law because it is akin to zina (adultery) which is strictly prohibited in the Muslim religion. This is based on the fact that in gestational surrogacy, the surrogate carries the fertilized egg of someone who is not her legal husband, thus transgressing the bounds of the Quran.

HORMONE REPLACEMENT THERAPY

- **Hormone replacement therapy (HRT)**, also known as **menopausal hormone therapy** or **postmenopausal hormone therapy**, is a form of hormone therapy used to treat symptoms associated with female menopause. These symptoms can include hot flashes, vaginal atrophy, accelerated skin aging, vaginal dryness, decreased muscle mass, sexual dysfunction and bone loss. They are in large part related to the diminished levels of sex hormones that occur during menopause.
- The main hormonal medications used in HRT for menopausal symptoms are oestrogens and progestogens, among which progesterone is the major naturally-occurring female sex hormone and also a manufactured medication used in menopausal hormone therapy. Though both can have symptomatic benefits, progestogen is specifically added to oestrogen regimens when the uterus is still present. Unopposed oestrogen therapy promotes endometrial thickening and can increase the risk of cancer, while progestogen reduces this risk. Androgens like testosterone are sometimes used as well.
  - **Oestrogens** – Bioidentical oestrogens like oestradiol and oestriol, animal-derived oestrogens like conjugated oestrogens (CEEs) and synthetic oestrogens like ethinylestradiol.
  - **Progestogens** – Bioidentical progesterone, and progestins (synthetic progestogens) like medroxyprogesterone acetate (MPA), norethisterone and dydrogesterone.
  - **Androgens** – Bioidentical testosterone and dehydroepiandrosterone (DHEA), and synthetic anabolic steroids like methyltestosterone and nandrolone decanoate.
- Studies suggest that, when initiated within 10 years of menopause, HRT reduces all-cause mortality and risks of coronary disease, osteoporosis and dementia; after 10 years the beneficial effects on mortality and coronary heart disease are no longer apparent, though there are decreased risks of hip and vertebral fractures and an increased risk of venous thromboembolism when taken orally.
- **Contraindications**:
  - *Absolute contraindications*:
    - Undiagnosed vaginal bleeding
    - Severe liver disease
    - Pregnancy
    - Severe coronary artery disease
    - Aggressive breast, uterine or ovarian cancer
  - *Relative contraindications*:
    - Migraine headaches
    - History of fibroids or breast/ovarian cancer
    - Venous thrombosis
    - Active gallbladder disease
    - Early endometrial cancer

> FM 3.24: **Non-Core – Written**
> - Discuss the relative importance of surgical methods of contraception (vasectomy and tubectomy) as methods of contraception in the National Family Planning Programme.

- Surgical methods of contraception (sterilization) comprise terminal methods such as **vasectomy** and **tubectomy**.

The **National Family Planning Programme** carries the following below-mentioned guidelines.

GUIDELINES FOR CASE SELECTION FIT FOR STERILIZATION

- The partners should be married.
- Male partner should be at least 22 years old and ideally be below the age of 60 years.
- Female partner should be below the age of 49 years and above the age of 22 years.
- The couple should have at least one child whose age is above 1 year, unless the sterilization is medically indicated.
- Both partners must not have undergone sterilization in the past (*not applicable in the cases of failure of previous sterilization*).
- The couple must be in a sound state of mind so as to understand the full implications of sterilization.
- Mentally ill persons must be certified by a psychiatrist, and a statement should be given by the legal guardian/spouse regarding the soundness of the individual's state of mind.
- A relevant medical history, physical examination and laboratory investigations need to be completed to ascertain eligibility for surgery.

ADVANTAGES OF TERMINAL METHODS OF STERILIZATION

- Does not require sustained motivation.
- It is the most effective method of contraception.
- Low rate of complications, if the surgery is correctly performed.
- Does not require any action at the time of intercourse.
- Compensation is paid under Government of India Family Planning Insurance Scheme and the amount is revised from time to time.

DISADVANTAGES OF TERMINAL METHODS OF STERILIZATION

- Need for a trained doctor for performing the surgery.
- Need for facilities for the surgery.
- Reversibility is difficult.
- Does not protect against STD/HIV.

Vasectomy (Male Sterilization)

- Vasectomy is preferable to tubectomy (female sterilization) as it is easier, safer and cheaper.
- **Method**:
  - The vas is clamped at two points.
  - A piece of approximately 1 cm is resected from the segment between the two clamps.

- The cut ends are ligated.
- The ends are folded onto themselves and sutured in that position.
- The removed section is gently squeezed onto a glass slide, stained with Wright's stain, and examined under the microscope to confirm that the removed part is the vas only and not any other structure.
- The individual must be warned that he is not immediately rendered sterile after vasectomy.
- He should use another method of contraception till azoospermia is established. This takes approximately 30 ejaculations.
- He must report back for stitch removal on the 5th post-operative day.
- The individual should be warned that there is a small possibility of re-canalization of the vas, which may result in failure of contraception. His written consent should include the acknowledgement of having received this information.
- He should report for semen analysis after 3 months.

- **No-scalpel Vasectomy (NSV)**
  - No-scalpel vasectomy is a refined approach for isolating and delivering the vas, and uses only vasal-block anaesthesia.
  - NSV neither requires any scalpel cut on the skin nor any skin stitch after completion of the procedure. Therefore it is much less painful and faster than conventional vasectomy.
  - In the no-scalpel vasectomy technique, the provider grasps the vas deferens with specially designed forceps and makes a tiny puncture in the skin at the midline of the scrotum with a special surgical instrument.
  - In March 1992, NSV was officially included in the National Family Planning Programme of India.

Tubal Ligation (Female Sterilization)

- The female herself can give the consent for sterilization. Consent of the spouse is not essential.
- There are two surgical procedures which are used for female sterilization:
  - **Laparoscopy** – This involves inserting a laparoscope into the abdomen, through a small incision. The laparoscope enables the doctor to view and occlude the fallopian tubes with Fallope ring.
  - **Mini laparotomy (Minilap)** – This involves making a small incision in the abdomen. In this, a portion of the fallopian tube is ligated and incised.
- Sterilization surgery can be performed:
  - As an interval procedure: This is known as "**interval sterilization**." This should be performed within 7 days of the menstrual period (because this is the follicular phase and the ovulation is yet to occur).
  - **Postpartum sterilization**: This is done after 24 hours and within 7 days of the delivery.
  - **At the time of an MTP**: Can be done concurrently with the MTP.
  - **Following a spontaneous abortion**: Provided that the client is medically fit.
  - **Concurrent with other surgery**: LSCS (lower section caesarean section), salpingectomy or ovarian cystectomy.
- Eligibility for performing these surgeries:
  - **Minilap**: An MBBS doctor after training and certification in minilap laparoscopic sterilization.
  - **Laparoscopy**:
    - DGO
    - MD (Obs & Gyn)
    - MS (Surgery) with training in laparoscopic sterilization.
    - MBBS with experience in minilap followed by training in laparoscopic sterilization.
  - In addition, these doctors should be on the district panel and this panel is to be updated 6 monthly.
- Recommended venue:
  - If no pre-existing medical conditions require special arrangements:
    - Minilap Tubectomy can be provided in basic health facilities such as PHC/CHC/district hospitals where surgery can be done. These include both permanent and temporary facilities that can refer the woman to a higher level of care in case of emergency.
    - Laparoscopy requires a better equipped centre, where the procedure is performed regularly.

FM 3.25: Non-Core – Written
- Discuss the major results of the National Family Health Survey.

NATIONAL FAMILY HEALTH SURVEY-5

- The 2019–20 National Family Health Survey (NFHS-5), the fifth in the NFHS series, provides information on population, health, and nutrition for India and each state and union territory.
  - Like NFHS-4, NFHS-5 also provides district-level estimates for many important indicators.
- All five NFHS surveys have been conducted under the stewardship of the Ministry of Health and Family Welfare (MoHFW), Govt of India. MoHFW designated the International Institute for Population Sciences (IIPS), Mumbai, as the nodal agency for the surveys.
- The findings were released in Dec 2020.
- The NFHS provides estimates on key indicators related to population, family planning, child and maternal health, nutrition, adult health, and domestic violence, among others. The following are some salient findings for the various states on indicators related to: (i) population, (ii) health and nutrition, (iii) access to infrastructure and (iv) gender.

- **Population**:
  - Use of family planning methods increased; most states reduced their total fertility rate (TFR),* below the target of 2.1. Bihar's TFR declined from 3.4 (in NFHS-4) to 3. All other medium and large states in the survey (i.e., population above 1 crore) have a TFR below the replacement level rate of 2.1.
  - All states (except Mizoram) have seen an increase in the use of family planning methods. Goa (42%-point) and Bihar (32%-point) have seen the highest increase in the use of family planning methods.
- **Sex ratio at birth**: This has declined in a few states.
  - Sex ratio at birth is the number of female children born per 1000 male children born. This is below 950 for seven states (of the 17 states for which data have been released). In three states, the ratio is below 900 (Goa: 838, Himachal Pradesh: 875 and Telangana: 894).
  - The most notable decline was in Goa (from 966 to 838) and Kerala (from 1047 to 951). Only Tripura has a sex ratio at birth above 1000 (i.e., more females born than males).
- **Health and Nutrition**:
  - The infant mortality rate (IMR), i.e., number of infants who die before reaching the age of 1 year per 1000 live births, declined across states; however, malnourishment among children is increasing. Assam was one of the states with the largest drop in IMR, from 48 deaths (per 1000 live births) to 32 deaths. IMR remains high in Bihar (47 deaths per 1000 live births).
  - Nutritional status of children below 5 years of age is however worsening. Stunting or chronic malnutrition (i.e., low height with respect to age) has increased in 11 of the 17 states. The proportion of children who are underweight (low weight with respect to age) has increased in 11 of the 17 states. In Bihar and Gujarat, 40% or more of the children under the age of 5 years are underweight.
  - Obesity is rising for both men and women across all states. The proportion of women and men, between the age of 15–49 years, who are overweight or obese have increased across nearly all states (except Gujarat and Maharashtra). Overweight or obesity is measured through the Body Mass Index of persons.

▪ In Andhra Pradesh, Goa, Karnataka, Telangana, Kerala and Himachal Pradesh, nearly one-third of men and women (between 15 and 49 years of age) are overweight or obese.
  - **Access to Infrastructure**: In this item, certain indicators related to access to infrastructure for households are assessed. These include access to electricity, improved source of drinking water, improved sanitation facility (includes flush system, ventilated pit or composting toilet), and clean fuel for cooking (LPG/natural gas or biogas).
    - Access to electricity, improved source of drinking water and sanitation facility has increased. The proportion of households with electricity and improved drinking water source has increased across all states. Households with an improved sanitation facility has also increased across all states. About 99% households in Kerala have an improved sanitation facility, while only 49% households have it in Bihar.
    - Similarly, the proportion of households using clean fuel for cooking has also increased across nearly all states. Telangana has seen a nearly 25%-point increase in access to improved sanitation facility and clean cooking fuel as compared to NFHS-4.
    - The proportion of women who have a savings or bank account has increased across all the 17 states. Bihar (51%-point) and Manipur (39%-point) have seen the highest increase in this regard. Across all 17 states, close to 80% women now have a savings or bank account, except in Gujarat (70%) and Nagaland (64%).
    - However, the proportion of women who own a house or land (including joint ownership) has declined in 9 of the 17 states. Tripura, Maharashtra and Assam have seen a large decline in women owning house/land.
  - **Gender Related Indicators**: In this item, the following indicators are assessed: (i) use of hygienic methods of protection during menstrual period among women between 15 and 24 years of age, and (ii) spousal violence among married women.
    - Use of hygienic methods of protection during menstrual period has increased across states. The largest increase was seen in Bihar and West Bengal (28%-point). However, it still remains low in Bihar (59%), Assam and Gujarat (66%).
    - Gender-based violence still remains high, and has increased in some states. The proportion of married women (between 18 and 49 years of age) who have ever faced spousal violence has increased in 5 states. In Karnataka, it has doubled, from 21% to 44%. More than a third of the married women face spousal violence in Karnataka (44%), Bihar (40%), Manipur (40%) and Telangana (37%).

FM 3.26: Core – Written

▪ Discuss:
  - National Guidelines for accreditation, supervision & regulation of ART Clinics in India.

****Note***: *TFR is the average number of children born to a woman in her life time. Governments set targets for TFR for the purpose of population control. TFR of 2.1 is considered as the replacement level fertility rate at which population stability is achieved (i.e., population replaces itself).*

NATIONAL GUIDELINES FOR ACCREDITATION, SUPERVISION & REGULATION OF ART CLINICS IN INDIA, 2005

- Drafted by the Indian Council of Medical Research (ICMR) and National Academy of Medical Sciences (NAMS).
- The term "Assisted Reproductive Technology (ART)" is taken to encompass all techniques that attempt to obtain a pregnancy by manipulating the sperm and/or oocyte outside the body, and transferring the gamete or embryo into the uterus.

Levels of ART Clinics

- ***Primary (Level 1a) Infertility Care Units***:
  - Clinics where preliminary investigations are carried out, and type and cause of infertility diagnosed.
    - This could be a doctor's consulting room, such as a gynaecologist's or a physician's consulting room, or even a general hospital.
  - The gynaecologist or the physician in charge of a Level 1A infertility care unit should have an appropriate postgraduate degree.
- ***Primary (Level 1b) Infertility Care Units***:
  - These units would be required to have, in addition to what has been stated for Level 1A, more advanced facilities and shall need accreditation.
  - Such clinics must be under the supervision of a gynaecologist with a postgraduate degree.
- ***Secondary (Level 2) Infertility Care Units***:
  - These units must have infrastructure for further in-depth investigation and extended treatment of infertility, except where oocytes are handled outside the body.
- ***Tertiary (Level 3) Infertility Care Units***:
  - Such units must have diagnostic and therapeutic facilities at the highest level of specialization. The clinic should have access to accredited semen bank, or laboratory.

Minimal Physical Requirements for an ART Clinic

- ART clinic of Level 2 or Level 3 should have a non-sterile and a strictly sterile area. Some of the spaces could be combined, as long as such a step does not compromise the quality of service. However, the space provision for the sterile area cannot be combined with those for the non-sterile area, and vice-versa.
- For level 1B infertility care units, a strictly sterile area will not be required. The space requirement, however, will include a reception area, a waiting room for the patients, and a consulting room for the gynaecologist.

Non-Sterile Area

The non-sterile area must include:

- A reception and waiting room for patients.
- A room with privacy: for interviewing and examining male and female partners independently.
  - Evaluation of infertility necessitates history taking of the most intimate sexual practices between the couples. This is followed by close examination of the reproductive tract and sexual organs. Adequate measures must be taken to ensure that history taking and examination are carried out in strict privacy, maintaining the dignity of the patients.
  - In case a male doctor examines a female patient, there must always be a female attendant present.
  - The room must be equipped with an examination table and gynecological instruments for examining the female per vaginum, an appropriate ultrasonographic machine with a probe for transvaginal examination of the female, and examination of the testes and male reproductive tract. A colour Doppler would be useful but not essential.
- General-purpose clinical laboratory.
- Store room:
  - A well-stocked store for keeping essential stock of especially those items that have to be imported, precluding the need to be caught short in the middle of treatment.
  - Facilities must be available for storing sterile (media, needles, catheters, petri dishes) and non-sterile material under refrigerated and non-refrigerated conditions as appropriate.
- Record room:
  - Record keeping must be computerized as far as possible so that data is accessible retrospectively for analysis or when called upon by the supervisory agency. Besides containing essential details of the patient's records, such files must contain history of the cause of infertility as diagnosed earlier, results of new diagnosis if relevant, the treatment option best suited for the particular patient, the treatment carried out and the outcome of treatment, and follow-up if any.
- Autoclave room: A separate facility must be available for sterilizing and autoclaving all surgical items, as well as those to be used in the in vitro culture laboratory.
- Steps for vermin proofing: Adequate steps should be taken to make the whole clinic vermin proof, with suitable traps for preventing insects and other forms of unwanted creatures entering the clinic.
- Semen collection room: This must be a room with privacy, and should be located in a secluded area close to the laboratory. Such a facility must be available in-house rather than having the patient collect the sample and bring it to the laboratory for analysis as, in the latter case, semen quality and identity is likely to be compromised. Procedures for collection of semen as described in the WHO Semen Analysis Manual must be followed with special reference to the type of container used; these containers must be sterile, maintained at body temperature and nontoxic. This room must have a washbasin with availability of soap and clean towels. The room must also have a toilet and must not be used for any other purpose.
- Semen processing laboratory: There must be a separate room with a laminar air flow for semen processing, preferably close to the semen collection room. This laboratory must also have facilities for microscopic examination of post-coital test smears. Care must be taken for the safe

disposal of biological waste and other materials (syringes, glass slides, etc.). Laboratory workers should be immunized against hepatitis B and tetanus.
- Clean room for IUI: There must be a separate area/room with an appropriate table for Intra-Uterine Insemination (IUI).

Sterile Area

The sterile area shall house the operation theatre, a room for intrauterine transfer of sperm or embryos and an adjoining embryology laboratory. Entry to the sterile area must be strictly controlled by an anteroom for changing footwear, area for changing into sterile garments and a scrub-station. The sterile area must be air-conditioned where fresh air filtered through an approved and appropriate filter system is circulated at an ambient temperature.

- Operation theatre: Must be well equipped with facilities for carrying out surgical endoscopy and transvaginal ovum pick-up.
- Room for intrauterine transfer of embryo: Must be a sterile area having an examination table on which the patient can be placed for carrying out the procedure, and rest undisturbed for a period of time.
- Embryology laboratory complex:
  - Must have facilities for the control of temperature and humidity, and must have filtered air with an appropriate number of air exchanges per hour.
  - Walls and floors must be composed of materials that can be easily washed and disinfected; use of carpeting must be strictly avoided.
  - The embryology laboratory must have the following:
    - Laminar flow bench with a thermostatically controlled heating plate
    - Stereo microscope
    - High-powered binocular light microscope
    - 'High resolution' inverted microscope with phase contrast or Hoffman optics, preferably with facilities for video recording
    - Micromanipulator (if ICSI is done)
    - CO_2 incubator, preferably with a back up
    - Hot air oven
    - Laboratory centrifuge
    - Equipment for freezing embryos in a programmed manner
    - Liquid nitrogen cans
    - Refrigerator
  - Appropriate steps need to be taken for the correct identification of gametes and embryos to avoid mix-ups. All material from the operation room, culture dishes and Falcon tubes for sperm collection (including lids), must bear the name of the patient. In the incubator, identified oocytes and sperm should be kept together on the same tray and double-checked. Pipettes used should be disposed off immediately after use.
  - The embryology laboratory must have a daily logbook in which all the day's activities are recorded, including the performance of the equipment.

Ancillary Laboratory Facilities

- Hormone and other assays: The infertility clinic must have ready access to laboratories that are able to carry out immunoassays of hormones (FSH, LH, Prolactin, hCG, TSH, Insulin, Estradiol, Progesterone, Testosterone and DHEA) and tests such as for HIV and Hepatitis B.
- Microbiology and histopathology: Another important facility in an ART clinic (or easily accessible to it) would be that of a microbiology laboratory that can carry out rapid tests for any infection, and a clinical chemistry laboratory. Facilities for carrying out histopathological studies on specimens obtained from the operation theatre would also be desirable.
- Maintenance of the laboratories: Each laboratory should maintain in writing, standard-operating manuals for the different procedures carried out in the laboratory. It should be ensured that there is no "mix up" of gametes or embryos. The patient's name should be clearly labelled on all the tubes, dishes and pipettes containing the gametes and embryos. All pipettes should be immediately discarded after use. Laminar flowhoods, laboratory tables, incubators and other areas where sterility is required must be periodically checked for microbial contamination using standard techniques, and a record of such checks must be kept. A logbook should be maintained which records the temperature, carbon dioxide content and humidity of the incubators and the manometer readings of the laminar air flow. All instruments must be calibrated periodically (at least once every year) and a record of such calibration maintained.
- Quality of consumables used in the laboratory: All disposable plasticware must be procured from reliable sources after ensuring that they are not toxic to the embryo. Culture media used for processing gametes or growing embryos in vitro should be preferably procured from reliable manufacturers. Each batch of culture medium needs to be tested for sterility, endotoxins, osmolality and pH.

Essential Qualifications of the ART Team

- **Gynaecologist**:
  - Minimal qualification (for Level 1B, 2 or 3 clinic) is a diploma or degree in gynaecology.
  - Additional experience should include knowledge about:
    - Male and female infertility.
    - Diagnostic methods for determining the cause of infertility.
    - Reproductive endocrinology.
    - Gynaecological ultrasonography.
  - Responsibilities:
    - Interviewing the infertile couple.
    - Physical examination of the female.
    - Deciding on the tests to be carried out, interpreting them and treating medical disorders (infections, endocrine anomalies).
    - Carrying out laparoscopy or sonohystero-salpingography for determining the status of the uterus and the fallopian tube.

- Carrying out AIH, AID, IUI, IVF or ICSI as the case may warrant.
- Maintaining all records of diagnosis, treatment given and consent forms.

- **Andrologist**:
  - In India, it is a urologist who often takes on the task of treating male infertility. Such individuals must receive additional training in diagnosis of various types of male infertility covering psychogenic impotence, anatomical anomalies of the penis which disable normal intercourse, endocrine factors that cause poor semen characteristics and/or impotence, infections and causes of erectile dysfunction.
  - He/She must have knowledge of ultrasonographic or vasographic studies of the reproductive system, and the principles of semen analysis. He/She should be familiar with relevant surgical procedures.
  - An individual may act as an andrologist for more than one clinic but each clinic where the andrologist works must own responsibility for the andrologist and ensure that the andrologist is able to take care of the entire work load of the clinic without compromising on the quality of service.
- **Clinical Embryologist**:
  - Must be knowledgeable in mammalian embryology, reproductive endocrinology, genetics, molecular biology, biochemistry, microbiology and in vitro culture techniques.
  - Must also be familiar with ART. He/She must be either a medical graduate or have a degree or a doctorate in an appropriate area of life sciences.
  - An embryologist must not be associated with more than two centres at any given time.
- **Counsellor**:
  - Counselling for ART is not taught as a separate subject anywhere. A person who has at least a degree in Social Sciences, Psychology, Life Sciences or Medicine, and a good knowledge of the various causes of infertility and its social and gender implications, and the possibilities offered by the various treatment modalities, should be considered as qualified to occupy this position.
  - The person should have a working knowledge of the psychological stress that would be experienced by potential patients, and should be able to counsel them to assuage their fears and anxiety and not to have unreasonable expectations from ART.
- **Programme Co-ordinator/Director**
  - The programme co-ordinator/Director should have a post-graduate degree in an appropriate medical or biological science. In addition, he/she must have a reasonable experience of ART.
  - He/She should be able to co-ordinate the activities of the rest of the team and take care of staff administrative matters, stock keeping, finance, maintenance of patient records, statutory requirements and public relations.

> **FM 3.27: Core – Written/Viva Voce**
> - Define, classify and discuss:
>   - Abortion
>   - Methods of procuring abortion
>   - MTP Act
>   - Criminal abortion

ABORTION

Definition

- **Abortion* is defined as the premature expulsion of products of conception from the uterus, at any time before the complete period of gestation.**
- By convention however, **abortion** is the term used to denote termination of pregnancy during the first trimester, while that occurring in the second trimester is called **miscarriage** and that occurring in the last trimester of pregnancy is called **premature birth**.

Classification

- **Abortion** is classified into two types: **natural** and **artificial**.
  - **Natural (spontaneous) abortion** occurs invariably in the first trimester of pregnancy.
  - **Causes**:
    - Maternal Infections: Rubella, cytomegalovirus, malaria, toxoplasmosis.
    - Maternal Hypoxia & Shock: Respiratory diseases, heart failure, severe anaemia.
    - Trauma: Direct trauma to the abdominal wall may result in abortion.
    - Immunological: Anti-phospholipid antibody increases the risk of abortion.
    - Toxic Agents: Environmental toxins such as lead, arsenic, tobacco, alcohol and caffeine increase the risk of abortion.
  - **Artificial abortion** is that which is **deliberately induced**.
    - It is further subdivided into justifiable (therapeutic) and criminal:
      - **Therapeutic Abortion**: Carried out for medical reasons (usually a threat to the mother's life).
      - **Criminal Abortion**: Before medical termination of pregnancy became a legal option, women were not allowed to abort, unless there was a proven threat to life. Those women who were denied legal abortion (unmarried females, widows and rape victims), therefore had to resort to alternative means of abortion, i.e., criminal abortion.
      - Nowadays, criminal abortion has come to mean the termination of pregnancy by the woman herself, or by another party not qualified to perform

*Note: *The word 'abortion' is derived from the Latin word 'aboriri', which means "to get detached from the proper site".*

the termination, or when it does not conform to the MTP Act of 1971.

Methods of Procuring Abortion

First Trimester Medical Abortion

- **Abortion Pill (Mifepristone; Misoprostol)**
  [*Approximately up to 4–7 weeks after the start of the LMP (Last Menstrual Period)*]
  - These drugs are only approved for women up to the 49th day after the start of their last menstrual period.
  - The procedure usually requires 3 clinic visits:
    - On the first visit, the woman is given the pill.
    - 2 days later, if the abortion has not occurred, she is given a drug which induces uterine contractions, causing it to expel the embryo.
    - The last visit is to determine, if the procedure has been completed.
  - The abortion pill will not work in the case of an ectopic pregnancy.

First Trimester Surgical Abortion

- **Dilatation and Curettage**
  [*Approximately up to 7–12 weeks after LMP*]
  - This surgical abortion is done early in the pregnancy, up until 12 weeks after the woman's last menstrual period.
  - The cervix is dilated, the curettage tool is inserted, and the developing foetus is "scraped" out from the uterus (**Fig. 3.150**).
- **Suction Curettage (Vacuum Aspiration)**
  [*Approximately up to 6–14 weeks after LMP*]
  - This is the most common surgical abortion procedure.
  - Because the foetus is larger, the doctor must first stretch open the cervix using metal rods, under local or general anaesthesia.
  - The doctor then inserts a hard plastic tube into the uterus, and connect it to a suction device (**Fig. 3.151**). The suction pulls the foetus' body apart and out of the uterus.

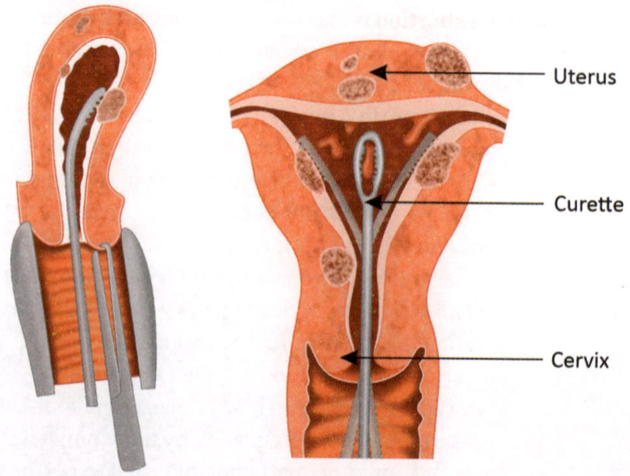

Fig. 3.150 Dilatation and Curettage

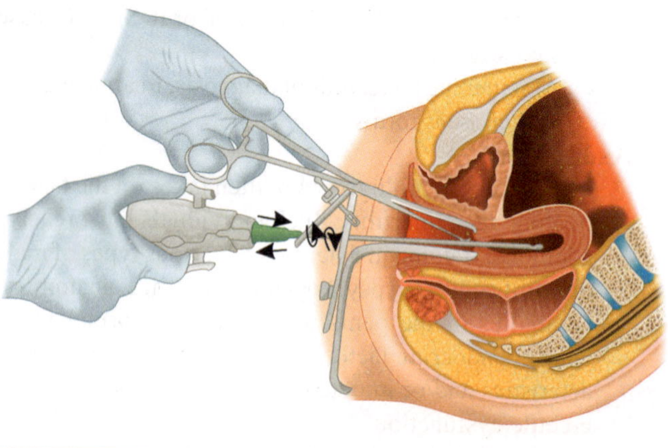

Fig. 3.151 Suction Curettage (Vacuum Aspiration)

  - Alternatively, a curette may be used to scrape the products of conception out of the uterus.

Second Trimester Surgical Abortion

- **Dilatation and Evacuation (D&E)**
  [*Approximately up to 13–24 weeks after LMP*]
  - This surgical abortion is done during the second trimester of pregnancy. At this point in the pregnancy, the foetus is too large to be broken up by suction alone and will not pass through the suction tubing.
  - In this procedure, the cervix must be opened wider than in a first trimester abortion. This is done by inserting a ***laminaria tent***, a day or two before the abortion.

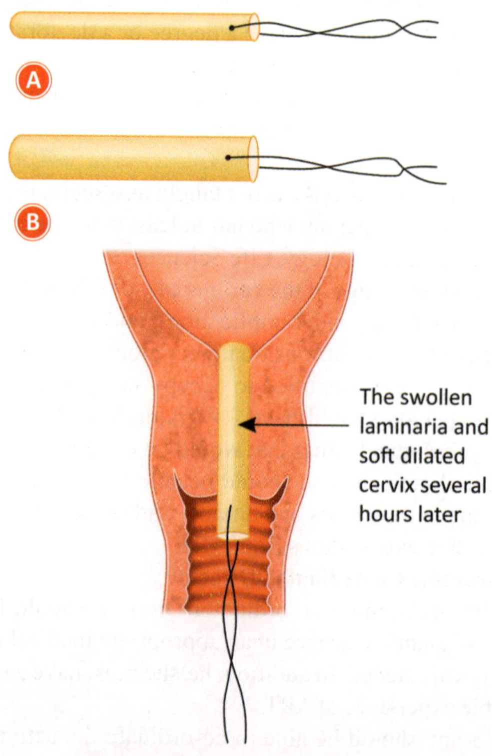

Fig. 3.152 Dilatation and Evacuation (D&E) with Laminaria

- A laminaria tent is a small rod of dehydrated seaweed that when inserted in the cervix, rehydrates, absorbing the water from the surrounding tissue in the woman's body (**Fig. 3.152**). Laminaria expands up to 10 times its original size, slowly opening the cervix, and when removed, creates easier access to the uterus.
- Once the cervix is stretched open, the foetal parts are pulled out with forceps.
- A curette is also used to scrape out the contents of the uterus, removing any remaining tissue.

Third Trimester Surgical Abortion

- **Late Term Abortions**
  [*Approximately 20 weeks after LMP to full-term*]
  - These procedures typically take place over 3 days, use local anaesthesia, and are associated with increased risk to the life and health of the mother.
  - On the first day, under ultrasound guidance, the foetal heart is injected with a medication that stops the heart and causes the foetus to die.
  - Also over the first 2 days, the cervix is gradually stretched open using laminaria.
  - On the third day, the amniotic sac is burst and drained.
  - The remainder of the procedure is similar to the D&E procedure.
  - An alternative procedure involves inducing labour (using oxytocin).

Complications of Therapeutic Abortion

Immediate Complications

- Haemorrhagic shock
- Perforation of uterus, peritoneum or intestine
- Laceration of cervix or vagina
- Incomplete abortion
- Embolism
- Thrombophlebitis

Delayed Complications

- Pelvic inflammatory disease
- Menstrual irregularities
- Sterility
- Endometritis
- Cervicitis
- Vaginitis

Medical Termination of Pregnancy Act (1971, Amended 1975, 2002, 2021)

- The **MTP Act** of **1971** was passed to **liberalise** abortions in India, on the basis of clearly specified guidelines. It is not an Act that outright legalizes abortion. This liberalisation was decided upon with the idea of saving the lives of millions of women, who would otherwise resort to criminal abortion out of desperation, thereby succumbing to its complications. As per this Act, pregnancy can be terminated on the following **grounds**:
  - **Therapeutic**: If the pregnancy, when allowed to continue, is likely to endanger the life of the woman, or cause serious injury to her physical or mental health.
  - **Eugenic**: If there is evidence to suggest that the child to be born would suffer from severe physical or mental abnormalities, e.g., the mother has contracted any of the TORCH group of infections (toxoplasmosis, rubella, cytomegalovirus or herpes) in the first trimester.
  - **Humanitarian**: When pregnancy results from rape.
  - **Social**: If pregnancy has resulted due to contraceptive failure in a married woman, or if there are severe economic constraints in bringing up a child which can cause substantial burden on the family.
- **Qualifications Required**: As per the Act, a medical officer is qualified to perform MTP if:
  - He/She, as a registered medical practitioner, has assisted in at least 25 cases of MTP in a recognised hospital.
  - He/She is a specialist with MD (obstetrics) or DGO qualification, or has 6 months of experience as a house surgeon in obstetrics, in a recognised hospital.
- **Place**: MTP can be carried out in any government hospital, or non-government institution, provided that a license has been procured from the Chief Medical Officer of district.
- **Consent**: Any woman over the age of 18 years can give written consent for an abortion. In the case of a minor or a mentally ill woman, the consent of the guardian/parent is required.
- **Duration of gestation**: For a pregnancy of below 12 weeks duration, one medical officer alone can take the decision of performing an abortion, while if it is between 12 and 20 weeks, two medical officers are required to terminate the pregnancy. However, if it is an emergency situation, a pregnancy exceeding 20 weeks can be terminated even if only one doctor is available. **(All these have been changed in the 2021 amendment of the Act – *see below*).**
- **2002 amendments**:
  - No termination of pregnancy shall be made in accordance with this Act at any place other than:
    - a hospital established or maintained by the Government, or
    - a place for the time-being approved for the purpose of this Act by the Government or a District Level Committee constituted by that Government with the Chief Medical Officer or District Health Officer as the Chairperson of the said Committee.
    - Notwithstanding anything contained in the Indian Penal Code, the termination of pregnancy by a person who is not a registered medical practitioner shall be an offence punishable with rigorous imprisonment for a term which shall not be less than 2 years but which may extend to 7 years under that Code, and that Code shall, to this extent, stand modified.
    - Whoever terminates any pregnancy in a place other than that mentioned in this Act, shall be punishable

with rigorous imprisonment for a term which shall not be less than 2 years but which may extend to 7 years.
- Any person being the owner of a place which is not approved as per this Act, shall be punishable with rigorous imprisonment for a term which shall not be less than 2 years but which may extend to 7 years.

- **2021 amendments**:
  - **Termination due to failure of contraceptive method or device**:
    - Under the Act, a pregnancy may be terminated up to 20 weeks by a married woman in the case of failure of contraceptive method or device. It allows unmarried women to also terminate a pregnancy for this reason.
  - **Opinion needed for termination of pregnancy**:
    - Opinion of one Registered Medical Practitioner (RMP) for termination of pregnancy up to 20 weeks of gestation.
    - Opinion of two RMPs for termination of pregnancy of 20–24 weeks of gestation.
    - Opinion of the State-level medical board is essential for a pregnancy to be terminated after 24 weeks in case of substantial foetal abnormalities.
  - **Upper gestation limit for special categories**:
    - Upper gestation limit is increased from 20 to 24 weeks for special categories of women, including survivors of rape, victims of incest and other vulnerable women (differently-abled women, minors, among others).
  - **Confidentiality**: The name and other particulars of a woman whose pregnancy has been terminated shall not be revealed, except to a person authorised in any law that is currently in force.
- **Medical Termination of Pregnancy Regulations 2003**: Issued under the Act to enable women to access safe and legal abortion services.

Criminal Abortion

Definition

- **Any abortion conducted outside the purview of the Medical Termination of Pregnancy Act is called criminal abortion.**

Common Methods

- When the pregnancy is in its initial stages, heavy physical exercise, hot baths, ingestion of purgatives, etc., are some of the (useless!) methods advocated by criminal abortionists.
- When the pregnancy is in a more advanced stage, **abortifacient drugs** or **mechanical trauma** are favoured.
  - **Abortifacient drugs** are quaintly classified as **ecbolics** and **emmenagogues**:
    - **Ecbolics** stimulate uterine contractions and bring about abortion. Ergot preparations are usually used for this purpose. Lead oleate is also used, which is toxic to the foetus leading to its death. It may cause lead poisoning in the mother. Pituitary extract administered parenterally behaves in the same way as oxytocin.
    - **Emmenagogues** are drugs which promote uterine congestion and bleeding, resulting in the expulsion of products of conception. Examples include borax, oil of savin, rue, laburnum and sanguinarine.
    - Other abortifacient drugs (which act indirectly) include:
      - **Genito-urinary tract irritants** such as cantharides, turpentine oil, etc., which act by producing inflammation of the genito-urinary tract, thereby reflexly irritating the uterus and stimulating its contractions.
      - **Gastro-intestinal tract irritants** such as tartar emetic, which can also cause reflex contractions of uterine muscle fibres. Plant irritants such as seeds or unripe fruit of papaya and methi seeds (fenugreek). Calotropis is also commonly used.
      - **Systemic poisons** such as the salts of arsenic, lead, copper, antimony and mercury.
  - **Mechanical trauma**: When drugs fail to bring about abortion, mechanical trauma is resorted to.
    - This may take the form of primitive, and often barbaric, methods of rupturing the membranes with the help of knitting needle, stick, metal wire, coat hanger, screwdriver, etc. Once the membranes are ruptured, the products of conception get expelled.
    - Sometimes hot water, Savlon or Dettol is injected under pressure, using a Higginson's syringe. Lysol, cresol, formalin or potassium permanganate may also be used. This process of injecting a fluid under pressure is called **syringing**. At times, instillation of hot water has resulted in death due to vagal inhibition, or due to embolism. A visit to the scene of the crime may reveal the presence of a syringe or remnants of the fluid used.
    - Some abortionists insert foreign bodies such as a stick, in order to dilate the cervix. More commonly, a laminaria tent is inserted into the cervix. **Laminaria** or **Sea-tangle tent** is a type of seaweed. Each "tent" is a cylinder about 5–10 cm long made from the dried stalk of the marine plant *Laminaria digitata*. It is inserted into the cervical canal when it is dry, and slowly expands as it absorbs water, dilating the cervix. This results in expulsion of the foetus. Other substances that have been used include sola pith, compressed sponge, bark of the slippery elm, etc.
      - **Abortion stick**: This is a method favoured by untrained midwives (dais) in the rural areas. A thin stick about 12 inches long is wrapped in gauze or cotton wool. It is then dipped in an irritant solution like the juice of marking nut, or calotropis, or the paste of some metallic salt. The stick is then inserted into the cervix or vagina. It causes ulceration, bleeding from the os and expulsion of

the foetus. At times, death of the woman takes place due to systemic absorption of the irritant or due to septicaemia. The application of potassium permanganate crystals can be extremely dangerous, causing ulceration, haemorrhage and toxic effects due to systemic absorption.

- **Cupping**: A lighted wick is placed over the hypogastrium and a cup is inverted over it. This creates a negative pressure, and when the cup is pulled suddenly, partial separation of placenta can result.
- Other methods resorted to by criminal abortionists include introduction of pastes, curetting, application of electrical current locally, or insufflation of air.

Complications of Criminal Abortion

- **Immediate Complications**:
  - Haemorrhage due to perforation of vessels.
  - Shock due to vagal inhibition resulting from instrumentation, or insertion of objects into the genital tract.
  - Fat embolism may occur while syringing with soapy liquid.
  - Air embolism due to insufflating air inadvertently into the uterine cavity during amateur procedures.
- **Delayed Complications**:
  - Septicaemia
  - Tetanus
  - Endotoxic shock
  - Renal failure
  - Meningitis, hepatitis, etc.

FM 3.28: Core – Written/Viva Voce
- Describe investigation of death due to criminal abortion with special reference to gathering evidence in the:
  - Living
  - Dead
- Describe duties of doctor in a case of abortion.

INVESTIGATION OF DEATH DUE TO CRIMINAL ABORTION

- Criminal abortion is punishable under various sections of the **Indian Penal Code (IPC)**:
  - **312** (Causing miscarriage) – Whoever voluntarily causes criminal abortion is liable for imprisonment up to 3 years and/or fine. The imprisonment may extend up to 7 years, if the woman is 'quick with child'. It is necessary that the woman should be pregnant and abortion carried out with her consent.
    - Here, the term 'with child' means pregnant, and 'quick' means the woman should have felt the child move within her.
  - **313** (Causing miscarriage without consent) – If miscarriage is carried out without the consent of the woman, the imprisonment may be extended up to 10 years.
  - **314** (Death caused by act done with intent to cause miscarriage) – If death of the woman takes place as a result of miscarriage, the minimum punishment would be 10 years.
  - **315** (Act done with intent to prevent the child being born alive, or to cause it to die after birth) – A person doing an act to prevent a child from being born alive, or causing it to die soon after its birth is liable for punishment up to 10 years imprisonment.
  - **316** (Causing death of a quick, unborn child) – Causing death of a quick, unborn child amounts to culpable homicide, and the punishment may extend up to 10 years imprisonment.

Medical Evidence of Abortion

In a Living Victim

- The breasts show pigmentation.
- Secretion of milk or colostrum from the nipple.
- Linea nigra and/or albicans may be present.
- In advanced pregnancy, the uterus may be palpable even after abortion.
- Congestion of the labia majora and minora is often present.
- Tags of membrane may be found in the uterus.
- Ulceration or erosion of the vagina or cervix may be noted.
- A swab taken from the cervical canal may help in detecting the chemical used for syringing.
- Blood or urine should be tested for HCG. Urine examination will reveal high levels of HCG up to 7 days.
- An ultrasound scan should be taken to study the uterus and appendages.
- Aborted material, if available, should be subjected to visual and histological examination.

In a Dead Victim (Autopsy Findings)

In addition to the above findings, the following may be observed:

- The face may appear pale or bluish.
- Undergarments may show blood clots and fragments of products of conception.
- Examination of the genitalia often reveals congestion of the labia, and injury to the posterior commissure.
- The abdominal cavity may contain clotted blood.
- Perforation of pelvic organs may have occurred. There may be evidence of peritonitis.
- Uterus may show the presence of paste, or marks of instrumentation.
- In the case of intrauterine infection, the uterus will be swollen, spongy and discoloured. Serosal surface may be brownish, especially in clostridial infections. The endometrium may exhibit foul-smelling purulent discharge.
- Vaginal fluid should be collected for chemical analysis. Swabs should be taken for microbiological examination. If air embolism is suspected, X-rays or CT scans must be taken.
- Uterus and ovaries may also be sent for chemical analysis to detect the presence of abortifacients.
- Spontaneous (natural) abortion should be differentiated from criminal abortion.
  - Histological examination of the expelled products of conception may be helpful. Blighted embryo, degenerative

changes in the chrorionic villi, hydatidiform mole, attenuated trophoblastic layer and myxomatous avascular stroma indicate spontaneous abortion.
- Macerated foetus and macerated placenta are also indicative of natural abortion.
- Foetal abnormalities are often associated with natural abortion.

DUTIES OF A MEDICAL PRACTITIONER IN CRIMINAL ABORTION

- When a lady comes to a doctor with history of incomplete abortion attempted by an abortionist or by herself, the medical practitioner must make a detailed note of the circumstances and the method employed to procure abortion.
- If death is imminent, he must record a dying declaration.
- If the patient dies, he must not issue a death certificate, but report to the police and arrange for an autopsy to be done.

> **FM 3.29: Core – Written/Viva Voce**
> - Describe and discuss:
>   - Child abuse
>   - Battered baby syndrome

CHILD ABUSE (NON-ACCIDENTAL INJURIES IN CHILDREN)

- Child abuse can take the following forms:
  - Physical abuse
  - Neglect
  - Sexual abuse
  - Emotional abuse

Physical Abuse & Neglect

Battered Baby Syndrome

Synonyms

- Non-accidental Injury of Childhood, Caffey's Syndrome, Child Abuse Syndrome, Maltreatment Syndrome.

Definition

- A **battered baby or child** is one that suffers repetitive physical injuries inflicted by a parent or guardian, which are non-accidental in nature.
- Such children usually belong to broken families, low socioeconomic strata and may be illegitimate or unwanted.
- The physical findings will not corroborate the history (of accident) given by the parents.
- One of the first to recognise child abuse at the hands of its parents was paediatric radiologist **John Caffey** who in 1946 described six cases of multiple fractures in the long bones of infants who had chronic subdural haematomas – classic signs of physical abuse. In 1956, Caffey made a statement about child abuse in a speech before the Congress of the British Institute of Radiology by urging early diagnosis to save abused children from further injury. Hence, the name "**Caffey's syndrome**".*

Manifestations

The signs to look for in a suspected victim of battering:

- The body language of the child may reflect fear and despair.
- Bruises around the wrist, forearm, thighs and ankles, which form 'handles' for adults to grip and swing the child.
- The buttocks may show burns or whip marks.
- The face and lips may be bruised. There may be bruising or laceration inside the oral cavity (**Fig. 3.153**).
- Circular bruises of 1–2 cm size, called 'six-penny bruises,' which occur due to the poking of adult fingers on chest, abdomen and thighs.
- Bruises of different periodicity on the same child with a history inconsistent with the findings.
- Crack fractures of the skull bones associated with intracranial haemorrhages.
- Multiple rib fractures may be seen, which may be fresh or show healing process (**Fig. 3.154**).

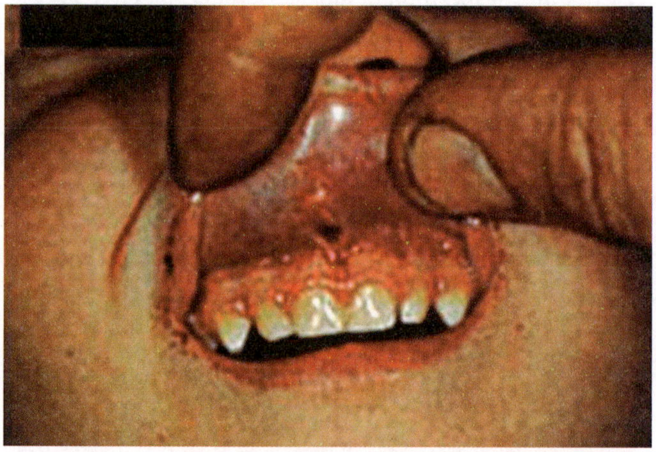

Fig. 3.153 A case of battered baby: Frenulum tear

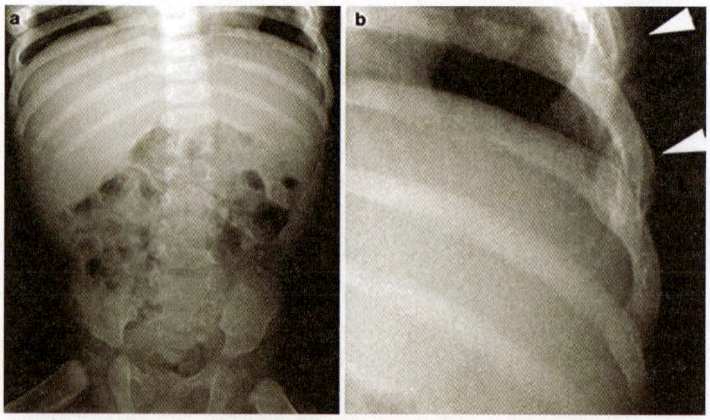

Fig. 3.154 (a) KUB in a child showing evidence of healing rib fractures bilaterally, just at the top edges of the image. (b) Magnified view of the left ribs demonstrates healing rib fractures (arrowheads)

**Note: Not to be confused with Caffey's disease, also known as Infantile Cortical Hyperostosis, which is a rare, benign, inflammatory gene-related disorder of infants that causes bone changes, soft tissue swelling and irritability.*

- Limb fractures are mostly in the region of the metaphysis and epiphysis of growing bones. Periosteal elevations may be seen.

Cinderella Syndrome

- Sometimes in a family, a single child is chosen to receive the battering.
- The child (commonly the youngest or eldest) is repeatedly thrashed, while the other children of the same family are spared.
- Occasionally, it may take the form of deliberate neglect, wherein the child is ignored, while all attention is showered on the siblings.

Shaken Baby Syndrome (Fig. 3.155)

Definition

- **Shaken baby syndrome** is a serious and clearly definable form of child abuse. It results from extreme rotational cranial acceleration induced by violent shaking or shaking/impact.
- It most often involves children younger than 2 years, but may be seen in children up to 5 years old.
- It occurs commonly, yet may be misdiagnosed in its most subtle form, and under-diagnosed in its most serious form.

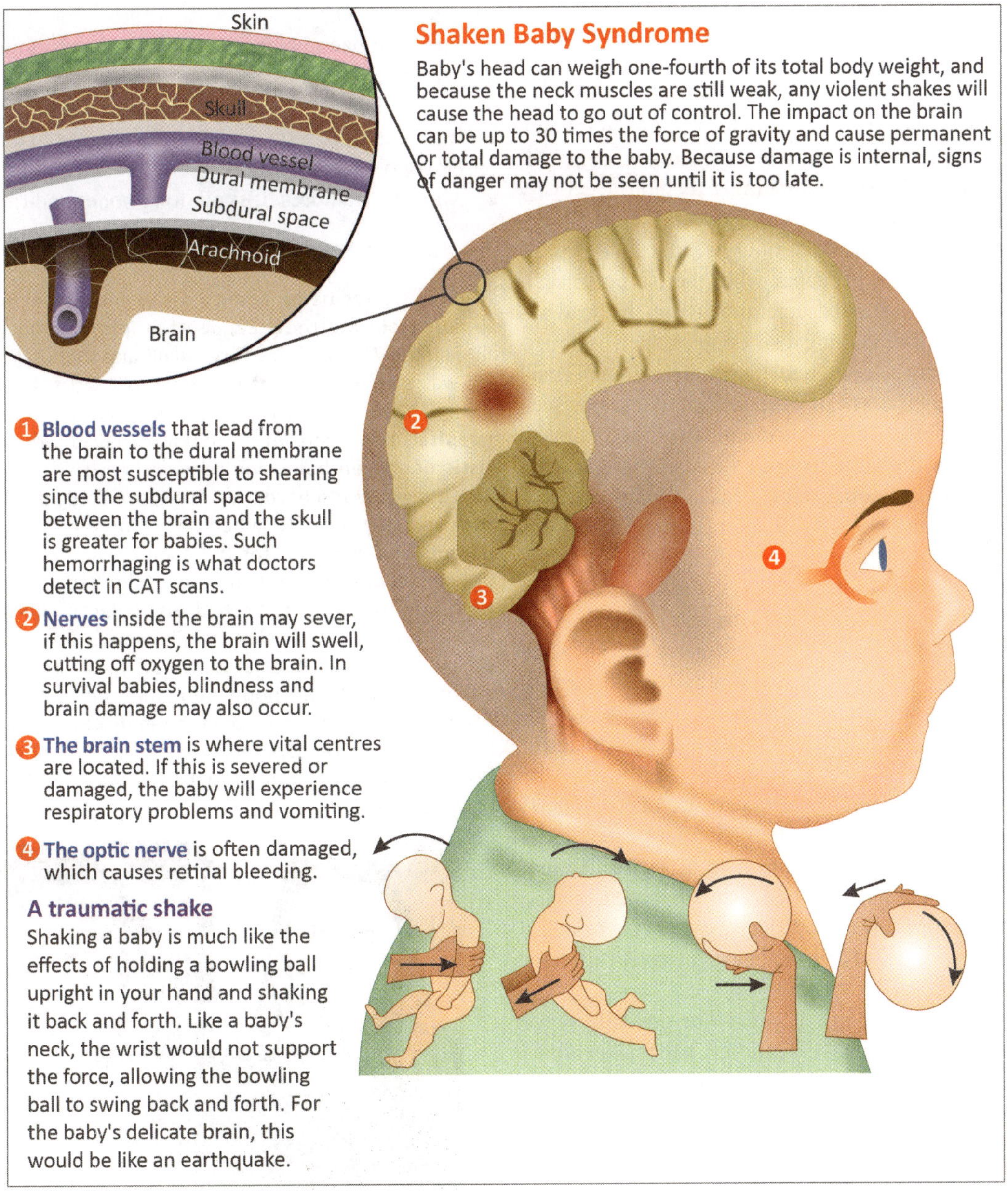

Fig. 3.155 Mechanics of Shaken Baby Syndrome

Clinical Features

- In 1973, paediatric radiologist **John Caffey** popularized the term "**whiplash shaken baby syndrome**" to describe a constellation of clinical findings in infants, which included retinal haemorrhages, subdural and/or subarachnoid haemorrhages, and little or no evidence of external cranial trauma.
- Shaken baby injuries usually occur in children younger than 2 years old, but may be seen in children up to the age of 5.
- A victim of sub-lethal shaking may have a history of poor feeding, vomiting, lethargy and/or irritability occurring for days or weeks.
- The constellation of these injuries does not occur with short falls, seizures or as a consequence of vaccination (as often alleged by the guilty parent/guardian).
- Shaking by itself may cause serious or fatal injuries. In many instances, there may be other forms of head trauma, including impact injuries. Thus, the term **shaken/slam syndrome** (or **shaken-impact syndrome**) may more accurately reflect the age range of the victims (who are not always babies) and the mechanisms of injury seen.
- Injuries are most likely to happen when there is both acceleration (from shaking) and deceleration (from the head hitting something). Even hitting a soft object, such as a mattress or pillow, may be enough to injure newborns and small infants. The result is a type of whiplash, similar to that seen in some automobile accidents. A number of factors make infants highly vulnerable to such forces. For example, children's brains are softer, their neck muscles and ligaments are weak and not fully developed, and their heads are large and heavy in proportion to their bodies.
- When an infant or toddler is shaken, the brain bounces back and forth against the skull. This can cause cerebral contusion, oedema and intracerebral haemorrhage. The large veins along the outside of the brain may tear, leading to further bleeding, swelling and increased pressure (subdural haematoma). This can cause permanent brain damage or death.
- Shaking an infant or small child may cause other injuries, such as damage to the neck, spine and eyes. Eye damage is very common and may result in loss of vision (retinal haemorrhage). Such shaking often results from tension and frustration generated by a baby's incessant crying or irritability, though crying is of course not a legal justification for such violence.
- Caretakers at risk for abusive behaviour generally have unrealistic expectations of their children, and may exhibit a role reversal whereby caretakers expect their needs to be met by the child.

Investigations

- CT scan is generally the method of choice for demonstrating subarachnoid haemorrhage, or other kinds of intracranial bleeding. The scan should be repeated after a time interval, or if the neurologic picture changes rapidly.
- MRI is of great value as an adjunct to CT in the evaluation of brain injuries in infants.
- At times, the clinical signs suggest meningitis, and a spinal tap yields bloody cerebrospinal fluid. Centrifuged spinal fluid that is xanthochromic should raise the suspicion of cerebral trauma that is at least several hours old, and not the result of a traumatic spinal tap.
- Because of confusing respiratory symptoms, chest X-rays should be obtained, which may appear normal, or show unexplained rib fractures. A skeletal survey of the hands, feet, long bones, skull, spine and ribs should be obtained as soon as the infant's medical condition permits. Skull films complement CT bone windows in detection of skull fractures.

Autopsy Features

- Subdural haemorrhage (most prominent in the interhemispheric fissure).
- Cerebral oedema with subarachnoid haemorrhage.
- Intracranial or retinal haemorrhages, which may be unilateral or bilateral.
- Multiple fractures of skull, long bones and ribs.

Box 3.8—Matthew Eappen Case

Five days after being admitted to a hospital in Boston, USA, 8-month-old Matthew Eappen fell into a coma and died on 9th Feb 1997, from a fractured skull and subdural haematoma. He was also found to have a fractured wrist, an unexplained injury from a month earlier. An ophthalmologist at the hospital, observed retinal haemorrhages judged characteristic of shaken-baby syndrome.

Louise Woodward, an 18-year old girl had been babysitting the child when this happened as the latter's parents had gone out for the evening. In a statement to the police, Woodward said that she "plopped the baby on the bed", indicating that she had just "placed the baby on the bed". However, in addition to "plopping" him on the bed, the police maintained that she also said that she dropped him on the floor at one point and that she had been "a little rough" with him. The police officer who interviewed her immediately after the incident stated that she never used the word plopped, but in fact said that she "dropped" the baby on the bed.

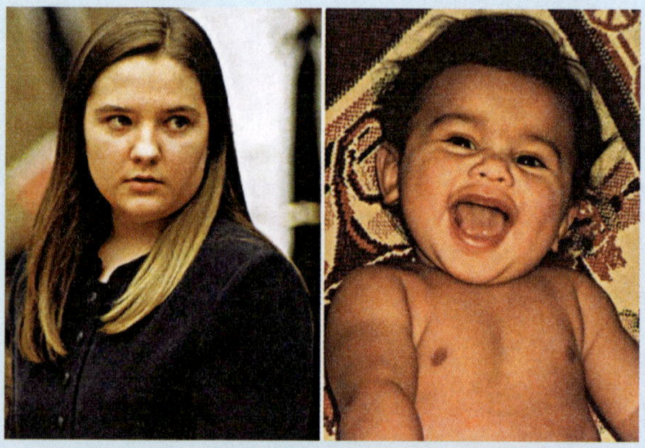

Louise Woodward (L) and Matthew Eappen (R)

contd.

Woodward was arrested on 5th Feb and held for assault and battery initially, then murder when Matthew died. A grand jury decided on a first-degree murder charge in March. She was denied bail and held until trial in a maximum-security unit in jail.

On 30th Oct 1997, the jury found her guilty of second-degree murder, and sentenced her to life in prison with a minimum of 15 years to be served.

On 10th Nov, at a post-conviction relief hearing, Woodward's conviction was reduced to involuntary manslaughter, the Judge stating that "there was no evidence of malice". Woodward's sentence was reduced to time served (279 days) and she was freed.

FM 3.30: Core – Written/Viva Voce

- Describe and discuss issues relating to:
  - Torture
  - Identification of injuries caused by torture and its sequelae
  - Management of torture survivors

DEFINITION OF TORTURE

- As per the **Tokyo Declaration** of the **World Medical Association** in **1975**, **torture** is defined as **the deliberate and wanton infliction of physical or mental suffering by one or more persons acting alone, or on the orders of any authority, to force another person to yield information or confession, or for any other reason**.

AIMS OF TORTURE

- **To obtain information**:
  - By criminal gangs, terrorist organizations, etc., to ferret out some specific information.
  - If a person is suspected to be involved in anti-national or terrorist activity, government organizations may themselves indulge in infliction of torture.
- **To force a confession**:
  - A person may be tortured in order to force him/her to confess to a crime.
- **To obtain testimony incriminating others**: In some cases, a victim is forced into signing documents incriminating other people, whether they are involved or not, in order to build a case against them.
- **To take revenge**: Sometimes, a victim is tortured merely to take revenge, which may be not only against the individual concerned, but also the family members of the victim, or even an entire community. For example, raping an enemy's wife or daughter, kidnapping family members, etc.
- **To spread terror in the community**:
  - Common in dictatorial regimes – Anybody who dares to raise his/her voice against the regime, may be tortured mercilessly.
  - If the victim dies, his body may be displayed to the community openly, with evidence of torture.
  - This creates terror in the minds of the people, and nobody would then dare to rise up against the regime.
- **To destroy the personality**:
  - People with leadership skills gathering support against a dictatorial regime may sometimes be arrested, kidnapped and tortured, so that they are transformed into weak and submissive individuals.

METHODS OF TORTURE

Physical Torture

1. ***Physical Torture that causes Severe Pain***:
   a. **Beating** – By using sticks, cables, whips, etc.
   b. **"Falanga" Torture** – Also called "falaka", "foot whipping" or "bastinado." It involves beating on the soles of the feet (**Fig. 3.156**). The person may become disabled for a long time.
   c. **Finger Torture** – Pencils or similar objects are placed in between two fingers and squeezed hard. Sometimes, the fingers are twisted to cause severe pain.
   d. **Cold Torture** – Victim is made to lie on an ice slab without clothing, or on a cold and damp floor.
   e. **Heat Torture** – Victim is suspended upside down very near to fire, or cigarette burns are inflicted.

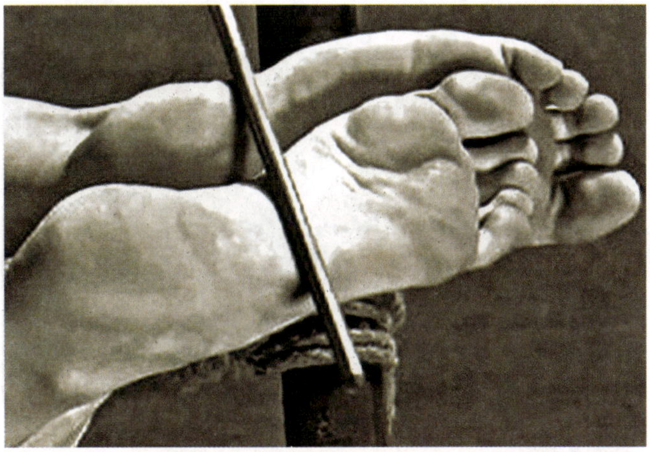

Fig. 3.156 Falanga or Falaka

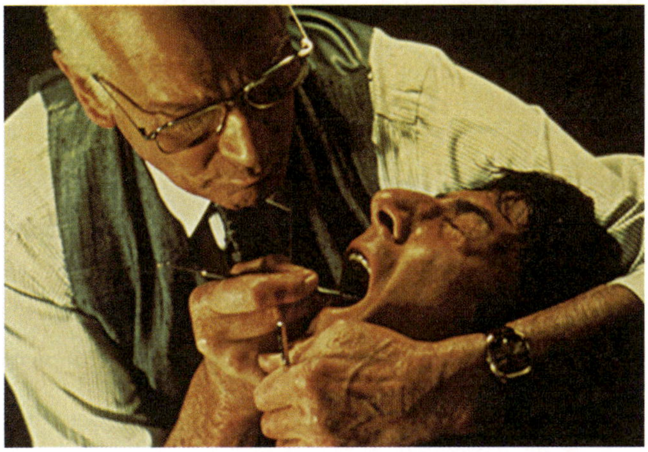

Fig. 3.157 Dental torture – from the film "Marathon Man" [*in the pic*: *Laurence Olivier* (L) and *Dustin Hoffman* (R)]

f. **Dental Torture** – Pulling out teeth by clips or forceps, or drilling into a tooth without anaesthetic (**Fig. 3.157**). Sometimes, the victim is asked to chew hard on small stones, metal pieces, etc.

2. ***Physical Torture that causes Fear of Imminent Death***:
   a. **Electrical Torture**:
      i. Electric shock is applied to sensitive parts of the body such as nipples, genitals, etc.
      ii. Sometimes, the victim is tied to a metallic bed and electricity is passed, causing shock all over the body.

   b. **Sham Execution** – Victim is sometimes blind folded and asked to stand before a wall, and then threatened that a vehicle is going to hit him. The victim hears the sound of a vehicle very near to him, and coming towards him, causing fear and shock.

   c. **Waterboarding** – This is a form of torture that consists of immobilizing the victim on his back with the head inclined downwards, and then pouring water over the face and into the breathing passages (**Fig. 3.158**). By forced suffocation and inhalation of water, the subject experiences drowning, and believes that he is about to die.

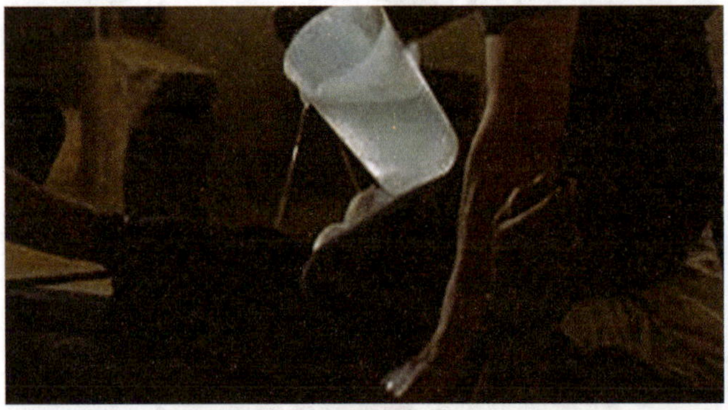

Fig. 3.158 Waterboarding torture – from the film "Zero Dark Thirty"

3. ***Physical Torture that causes Severe Exhaustion***:
   a. **Physical Exhaustion** – The victim may be asked to stand in the hot sun on one leg for a long time, or he may be asked to stretch out both his hands holding heavy bricks or stones.

   b. **Forced Labour** – The victim is made to work very hard without food or water.

   c. **Dunking** – The victim is immersed into a vat of water, or a pond, and taken out after some time, and given the ability to confess. If he does not confess, he is submerged again.

4. ***Physical Torture that causes Mutilation or Permanent Disability***:
   a. "**Telefono**" – In this method, simultaneous beating of both ears with the palms of the hands is done, causing rupture of tympanic membranes.

   b. **Mutilation** – Chopping off ears, nose, fingers, etc. (**Fig. 3.159**).

   c. **Disfiguration** – Throwing acids or corrosives over face and other parts of the body, causing severe burns leading to disfiguration.

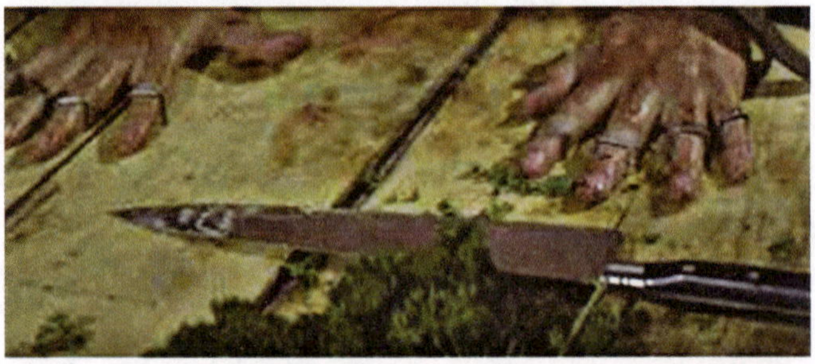

Fig. 3.159 Finger chopping scene from the film "The Passage"

Mental Torture

1. ***Deprivation Techniques***:
   a. **Sensory deprivation** – Victim may be blindfolded for a long time.

   b. **Perceptual deprivation** – Inducing confusion and disorientation in the victim, for example, by frequent transfer of the victim from one place to another, after blindfolding him.

   c. **Social deprivation** – Solitary confinement in a dark environment (**Fig. 3.160**).

   d. **Deprivation of basic needs** – Withholding food, water, toilet facilities, etc.

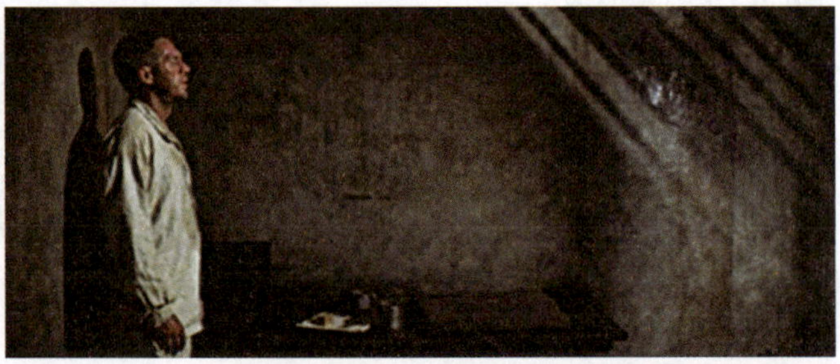

Fig. 3.160 Solitary confinement from the film "Papillon" [*in the pic*: *Steve McQueen*]

2. ***Coercion Techniques***:
   These methods involve the compelling of a victim to perform or witness certain acts, which can cause mental anguish, e.g.,
   a. Coercion to commit blasphemous acts.
   b. Coercion to witness torture of other victims.
   c. Coercion to torture other victims.

3. ***Communication Techniques***: The victim is mentally tortured by exposure to a variety of confusing or false communications, such as:
   a. **Misinformation** – Giving false information to victim regarding tragedy involving close relatives such as wife or children, which causes mental anguish.

Sexual Torture

Sexual Torture using Instruments

- Infliction of injuries to private parts of male or female victim, forcible introduction of rods, bottles, or batons in the rectum or vagina, mutilation of breasts or genital organs, etc.

Sexual Torture without the Use of Instruments

- The victim may be forced to:
  - undress in front of others
  - raped in front of others
  - photographed in humiliating positions or situations
  - sexually tortured by trained animals.

Pharmacological Torture

- This method may employ psychotropic or other drugs, to induce pain and cause compliance with the torturer's goals.
- Victim may be forcibly injected with addictive drugs to get him dependent, and then denied the drug and forced to go through withdrawal unless he provides what the torturer wants.

CONSEQUENCES OF TORTURE

Physical Consequences

- **Early consequences**: Injuries in the form of abrasions, bruises, lacerations, incised wounds, dislocations, fractures, etc.
- **Late consequences**: Infections, scars, mal-united bones, disfiguration of the face, impairment of hearing or vision, etc.

Psychological Consequences

- Anxiety, depression, sleep disturbances, alcohol/drug abuse, seizures, low self esteem, stress disorders, etc.

Social Consequences

- Social stigma, employment problems, negativity in social activities, etc.

TREATMENT OF TORTURE VICTIMS

Principles of Treatment

- Developing a good rapport with the victim.
- Empathising with the victim and his/her family.
- Avoiding situations or objects that remind the victim of the torture event.
- Punctuality in keeping appointments with the victim, and his/her family, should be strictly maintained.
- Doctors, psychologists, social workers, physiotherapists, nurses and legal experts must work together in close collaboration, for maximum efficacy.

> FM 3.31: Non-Core – Written/Viva Voce
> - Torture and Human Rights
>   - Describe and discuss guidelines and protocols of National Human Rights Commission regarding torture.

- The Manual on Effective Investigation and Documentation of Torture and Other Cruel, Inhuman or Degrading Treatment or Punishment, commonly known as the **Istanbul Protocol**, is the first set of international guidelines for documentation of torture and its consequences. It became an official United Nations document in 1999.
  - The Istanbul Protocol is intended to serve as a set of international guidelines for the assessment of persons who allege torture and ill treatment, for investigating cases of alleged torture, and for reporting such findings to the judiciary and any other investigative body.
- Torture is prohibited for the signatories of the **United Nations Convention Against Torture (UNCAT)**, which has 163 state parties. India is one of only five countries that are yet to ratify this 1987 UN convention.
- Torture is not criminalised in Indian law as a separate or special offense, but there are provisions in the Indian Penal Code (Sections 330 & 331) for penalising acts that can be considered as torture, with 7 and 10 years of imprisonment, respectively, if proven guilty.
  - **Sec 330 IPC**: Voluntarily causing hurt to extort confession, or to compel restoration of property.
  - **Sec 331 IPC**: Voluntarily causing grievous hurt to extort confession, or to compel restoration of property.
- **National Human Rights Commission Guidelines**
  - The National Human Rights Commission (NHRC) of India is a Statutory public body constituted on 12th Oct 1993.
  - Guidelines on Custodial Deaths/Rapes:
    - Cases of death due to police action are to be reported to the commission by the SSP/SP of the district within 48 hours of the incident.
    - Cases of custodial deaths/rapes are to be reported to the commission by the DM and SPs within 24 hours of their occurrence.
    - Chief Ministers and Administrators are required to send a 6 monthly statement of all cases of deaths in police action in the States/UTs to the Commission.
    - Women Police officers should be associated where the arrested person is a woman. The arrest of women between sunset and sunrise should be avoided.
    - Where children or juveniles are arrested, no force or beating should be administered.
    - The arrested person can demand that a friend/relative/person known to him be informed of the fact of his arrest and the place of his detention.
    - Whenever some person is arrested by police, there must be proper entry in Daily Diary Report (DDR).
    - It is mandatory to the police to send the arrestee remanded to the police custody for medical examination by a doctor on the panel or approved doctors and is to be repeated every 48 hours.
    - The person under arrest must be produced before the appropriate court within 24 hours of the arrest (Secs 56 and 57 CrPC).

- The arrested person should be permitted to meet his lawyer at any time during the interrogations.
- The interrogation should be conducted in a clearly identifiable place, which is accessible, and the relatives/friend for the person must be informed of the place of interrogation.
- 'Lie detector test' should not be administered without the consent of the accused. Consent should be recorded before a Judicial Magistrate and the accused should be duly represented by a lawyer.

For the NHRC protocol on the conduct of medicolegal autopsy in a case of death in police custody or following violation of human rights, refer FM 2.15 *(page no. 64)*.

FM 3.32: Core – OSPE/Viva Voce

- Demonstrate professionalism while:
  - Preparing reports in medicolegal situations.
  - Interpretation of findings and making inference/opinion.
  - Collection preservation and dispatch of biological or trace evidence.

This Competency is related to AETCOM, and is a practical/viva question that must not feature in written examinations (as per the new curriculum).

FM 3.33: Core – Written/Viva Voce

- Should be able to demonstrate professionalism while dealing with victims of torture and human right violations, sexual assaults, psychological consultation, rehabilitation.

Even though this Competency is related to AETCOM, and is essentially a practical/viva question, it can feature in written examinations also (as per the new curriculum).

For the explanation of these aspects, the reader is directed to refer the relevant Competencies that deal with the following topics: Torture (FM 3.30 and 3.31) and Sexual Offences (FM 3.13 to FM 3.16).

Topic 4

MEDICAL JURISPRUDENCE (MEDICAL LAW & ETHICS)

(Number of Competencies – 30: FM 4.1 to 4.30)

> FM 4.1: Core – Written/Viva Voce
> - Describe:
>   - Medical Ethics
>   - Explain its historical emergence

MEDICAL ETHICS

Medical Jurisprudence

('*Juris*' = law, and '*Prudence*' = knowledge)

- **Medical jurisprudence is the study of law in relation to medicine**.
  - In other words, ***it deals with the legal aspects of medicine such as the legal rights, privileges, duties and obligations of a medical practitioner***.
- **Medical ethics is an applied branch of ethics which deals with the practice of clinical medicine and related scientific research**.
  - Historically, the first code of medical ethics, **Formula Comitis Archiatrorum**, was published in the 5th century, during the reign of the king Theodoric.
  - In the medieval and early modern period, the field was enriched by Islamic scholars such as:
    - **Ishāq bin Ali al-Rohawi** – 9th century, who wrote **Adab al-Tabib** (Practical Ethics of the Physician), the first Arabic book dedicated to medical ethics),
    - **Avicenna** or more correctly, **Ibn Sina** – 980-1037 CE (who wrote *The Book of Healing and The Canon of Medicine*) (**Fig. 4.1**) and
    - **Abū Bakr al-RāzĪ** (known as **Rhazes** in the West) – 865-925 CE, a Persian physician, as also
    - Jewish thinkers such as **Maimonides** or more correctly, **Moses ben Maimon** – 1138-1204 and

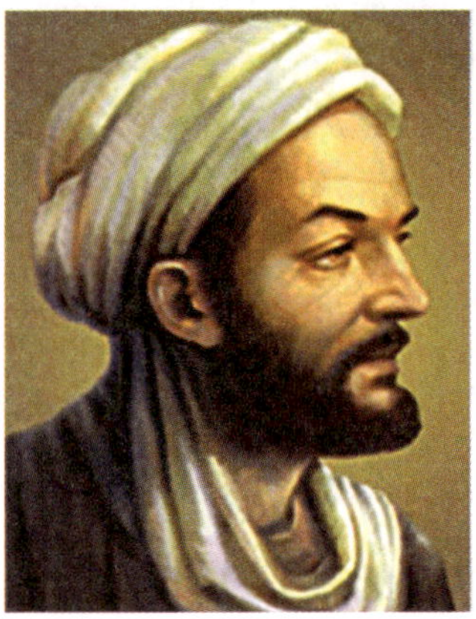

Fig. 4.1 Avicenna (Ibn Sina)

    - Roman (Italian) Catholic thinkers such as **Thomas Aquinas** – 1225-1274.
  - In England, **Thomas Percival** (**Fig. 4.2**), a physician and author, crafted the first modern code of medical ethics. He drew up a pamphlet with the code in 1794 and wrote an expanded version in 1803, in which he coined the expressions "medical ethics" and "medical jurisprudence".
  - In 1815, the **Apothecaries Act** was passed by the Parliament of the United Kingdom. It introduced compulsory apprenticeship and formal qualifications for the apothecaries of the day under the license of the Society of Apothecaries. This was the beginning of regulation of the medical profession in the UK.
  - In 1847, the **American Medical Association** adopted its first code of ethics, with this being based in large part upon Percival's work.
  - In the 20th century, a distinctively Protestant approach was articulated by thinkers such as **Joseph Fletcher**.
  - In the 1960s and 1970s, building upon liberal theory and procedural justice, much of the discourse of medical ethics went through a dramatic shift and largely reconfigured itself into **Bioethics**.

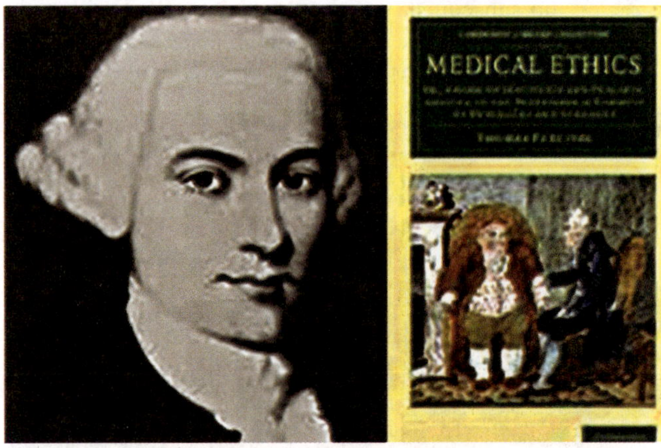

Fig. 4.2 Thomas Percival

  - Since the 1970s, the growing influence of ethics in contemporary medicine can be seen in the increasing use of **Institutional Review Boards** to evaluate experiments on human subjects, the establishment of hospital ethics committees, the expansion of the role of clinician ethicists and the integration of ethics into many medical school curricula.
  - **Medical ethics** is based on a **set of values** that professionals can refer to in the case of any confusion or conflict. These values include the **respect for autonomy**,

non-maleficence, beneficence and **justice**. It is important to note that these four values are not ranked in order of importance or relevance and that they all encompass values pertaining to medical ethics.

- The general principles mentioned in the **Hippocratic Oath** were brought up-to-date by the World Medical Association several years ago.
  - The modernised versions of the **Hippocratic Oath** comprise the **Declaration of Geneva** (as adopted by the third General Assembly of the World Medical Association at Geneva, Switzerland, in **September 1948**), and the
  - **International Code of Medical Ethics** (as adopted by the fourth General Assembly of the World Medical Association held in London, in **October 1949**).
- Each country has its own code of ethics, usually modelled on the lines of the International Code. In fact, India can boast of an oath proposed by **Maharshi Charak**, thousands of years ago!
  - **Maharshi Charak** (somewhere between 100 and 200 CE) (**Fig. 4.3**) was one of the principal contributors to Ayurveda. He is known as an editor of the medical treatise entitled ***Charaka Samhita***, one of the foundational texts of classical Indian medicine and Ayurveda.
  - The National Medical Commission (NMC) recommended the code of ethics propounded by Maharshi Charak (***Charak Shapath***) as a replacement for Hippocratic Oath for medical students in India earlier on, but because of the ensuing controversy, came up subsequently with "**Physicians Pledge**" which is based on the Declaration of Geneva as amended by the World Medical Association in 2017.

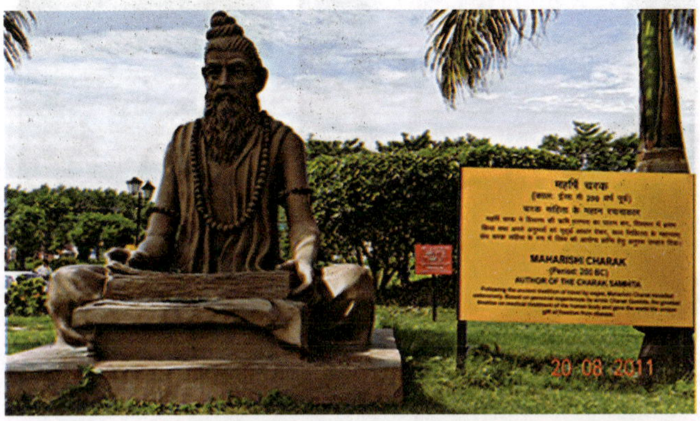

Fig. 4.3 Charaka sculpture – Patanjali Yogpeeth campus, Haridwar, Uttarakhand

FM 4.2: Core – Written/Viva Voce
- Describe:
  - Code of Medical Ethics 2002
  - Conduct, etiquette and ethics in medical practice
  - Unethical practices
  - Dichotomy

CODE OF MEDICAL ETHICS 2002

- **FULL TITLE**: **Indian Medical Council (Professional Conduct, Etiquette and Ethics) Regulations, 2002**
- Published in Part III, Section 4 of the Gazette of India, dated **6th April, 2002**.

Salient (Important) Points

General Principles

1. ***Character of the physician***:
   - The prime object of the medical profession is to render service to humanity; reward of financial gain is a subordinate consideration.
   - Whoever chooses this profession assumes the obligation to conduct himself in accordance with its ideals. He must keep himself pure in character and be diligent in caring for the sick.
2. ***The physician's responsibility***:
   - Physicians should merit the confidence of patients entrusted to their care, rendering to each a full measure of service and devotion.
   - They should continuously try to improve medical knowledge, and should make available to their patients and colleagues the benefits of their professional attainments.
3. ***Advertising***:
   - Solicitation of patients (either directly or indirectly by a physician, group of physicians or institutions) is unethical.
   - A physician shall not make use of lay channels so as to invite attention to himself or to his professional position, skill, qualifications or achievements that could result in his self-promotion.
   - A medical practitioner is however permitted a formal announcement in press regarding the following:
     - When starting practice
     - Change of type of practice
     - Change of address
     - Temporary absence from duty
     - Resumption of practice
4. ***Payment for professional service***:
   - Remuneration received for his service should be in the form and amount specifically announced to the patient at the time the service is rendered.
   - It is unethical to enter into a contract of "no cure, no payment."
5. ***Patents and copyrights***:
   - A physician may patent surgical instruments, appliances and medicines, or copyright applications, methods and procedures. The use of such patents or copyright, or the receipt of remuneration from them which retards or inhibits research, or restricts the benefits derivable therefrom are unethical.

The Code of Medical Ethics 2002 is now called "National Medical Commission Registered Medical Practitioner (Professional Conduct) Regulations 2023." Detailed draft available online in the NMC website.

6. ***Running an open shop (dispensing drugs and appliances) by physicians***:
   - A physician should not run an open shop for sale of medicines prescribed by physicians other than himself, or for sale of medical and surgical appliances.
7. ***Rebates and commissions***:
   - A physician shall not give, solicit or receive, nor shall he offer to give, solicit or receive any gift, commission or bonus with respect to referring, recommending or procuring of any patient for medical, surgical or other treatment.
   - Nothing in this section however, shall prohibit payment of salaries by a qualified physician to other duly qualified person rendering medical care under his supervision.
8. ***Secret remedies***:
   - The prescribing or dispensing by a physician of secret medicines or other secret remedial agents of which the composition is not revealed, or the manufacture or promotion of such products is unethical.
9. ***Evasion of legal restrictions***:
   - The physician will observe the laws of the country in regulating the practice of medicine, and will not assist others to evade such laws.
   - He should be cooperative in the observance and enforcement of sanitary laws and regulations in the interests of public health. A physician should observe the provisions of State Acts such as Drugs Act, Rules and Regulations made by the General Govt/State Govt, or local administrative bodies for the protection and promotion of public health.
10. ***Obligations to the sick***:
    - Though a physician is not bound to treat each and everyone asking for his service except during emergencies, for the sake of humanity and the noble traditions of the profession, he should not only be ever ready to respond to the call of the sick and the injured, but should also be mindful of the high character of his mission, and the responsibility he incurs in the discharge of his professional duties.
11. ***Patience, delicacy and secrecy***:
    - Patience and delicacy should characterize the physician.
    - Confidence concerning individual or domestic life, entrusted by patients to the physician, and defects in the disposition or character of patients observed during medical attendance should never be revealed, unless their revelation is required by laws of the state.
12. ***Prognosis***:
    - The physician should neither exaggerate nor minimize the gravity of a patient's condition. He should assure himself that the patient, his relatives or his responsible friends have such knowledge of the patient's condition as will serve the best interests of the patient and his family.
13. ***Treatment rules***:
    - Once having undertaken a case, the physician should not neglect the patient, nor withdraw from the case without giving notice to the patient or his relatives sufficiently long in advance of his withdrawal, to allow them to secure another medical attendant.
14. ***Upholding the profession***:
    - All physicians are expected to uphold the dignity and honour of the profession.
15. ***Membership in societies***:
    - For the advancement of his profession, a physician should affiliate with medical societies and contribute his time, energy and means, so that these societies may represent the ideals of the profession.
16. ***Safeguarding the profession***:
    - Every physician should aid in safeguarding the profession against admission to it of those who are deficient in moral character or education.
    - A physician should not employ in connection with his professional practice, any attendant who is neither registered nor enlisted under the Medical Act in force, and should not permit such persons to attend, treat or perform operations upon patients in respect of matters regarding professional discretion or skill, as it is dangerous to public health.
17. ***Exposure of unethical conduct***:
    - A physician should expose without fear or favour, incompetent or corrupt, dishonest or unethical conduct on the part of members of the profession.
18. ***Dependence of physicians on each other***:
    - Though there is no rule that a physician should not charge another physician for his services, he should cheerfully and without recompense give his professional services to other physicians or his dependents, if they are in his vicinity.
19. ***Compensation of expenses***:
    - A physician should consider it a pleasure and privilege to render free service to all other physicians and their immediate family dependents.
    - When a physician is called from a distance to attend or advise another physician or his dependents, reimbursement should however be made of travelling and other incidental expenses.
20. ***Consultations***: In case of serious illness, especially in doubtful or difficult conditions, the physician should request consultation.
    - Rules relating to consultation:
      - In every consultation, the benefit to the patient must be of first importance.
      - Utmost punctuality must be observed in meetings for consultation.
      - With reference to consultations, no insincerity, rivalry or envy should be indulged in. Due respect should be observed towards the physician in charge of the case, and no statement or remark be made which would impair the confidence reposed in him.

- Difference in opinion should not be divulged unnecessarily, but should be expressed frankly and impartially.
- When a physician has been called as a consultant, none but the rarest and most exceptional circumstances would justify that consultant taking charge of the case. He must not do so merely on the solicitation of the patient or his friends.
- When a patient is referred to a specialist by the attending physician, a statement of the case should be given to the specialist who should communicate his opinion in writing in a closed cover directly to the attending physician.

21. ***Appointment of substitute***:
    - Whenever a physician requests another physician to attend to his patients during his temporary absence from his practice, professional courtesy requires the acceptance of such appointment consistent with his other duties.
    - The physician acting under such an appointment should give the utmost consideration to the interests and reputation of the absent physician.
    - All such patients should be restored to the care of the latter upon his return.
22. ***Visiting another physician's case***: A physician called to visit a patient who has recently been under the care of another physician for the same illness should not take charge of, nor prescribe for such patient, except
    - in case of emergency, when he should communicate to the former explaining the circumstances under which the patient was seen and treatment given,
    - or when the physician has relinquished his case,
    - or when the patient has notified such physician to discontinue his services.
23. ***Obstetric cases***: If a physician agrees to attend to a woman during her pregnancy, he must make himself available whenever necessary. Inability to do so on an excuse of any other engagement is not tenable, except when he is already engaged on a similar, or other serious case.
24. ***Physicians as citizens***:
    - Physicians as good citizens possessed of special training should advise concerning the health of the community wherein they dwell.
    - They should operate especially with the proper authorities in the administration of sanitary laws and regulations.
25. ***Public health***:
    - Physicians, especially those engaged in public health work, should enlighten the public concerning quarantine regulations, and measures for the prevention of epidemic and communicable diseases.
    - At all times, the physician should notify the public health authorities of every case of communicable disease in his care, in accordance with the laws, rules and regulations of the health authorities.
    - When an epidemic occurs, a physician must continue his work without regard to the risk to his own health.
26. ***Relationship with pharmacists***: Physicians should recognize and promote the practice of pharmacy as a profession, and should recognize the cooperation of the pharmacist in education of the public concerning the practice of ethical and scientific medicine.

CONDUCT, ETIQUETTE & ETHICS IN MEDICAL PRACTICE

Principles of Medical Ethics

Beneficence, non-maleficence, autonomy and justice constitute the four principles of ethics.

1. ***Beneficence***:
   a. The principle of **beneficence** is the **obligation of a physician to act for the benefit of the patient** and ensure the following: prevent harm, remove conditions that will cause harm, help persons with disabilities, and help persons in danger. It is worth emphasizing that, in distinction to non-maleficence, the language here is one of positive requirements.
   b. The principle calls for not only just avoiding harm, but also to benefit patients and to promote their welfare.
2. ***Non-maleficence***:
   a. The principle of **non-maleficence** is the **obligation of a physician not to harm the patient**. This includes the following directives – do not kill, do not cause pain or suffering, do not incapacitate, do not cause offense and do not deprive others of the quality of life.
   b. The practical application of non-maleficence is for the physician to weigh the pros and cons of all interventions and treatments, to avoid those that are inappropriate, and to choose the best course of action for the patient.
3. ***Autonomy***:
   a. The philosophical underpinning for **autonomy**, and accepted as an ethical principle, is that all persons have intrinsic and unconditional worth, and therefore, should have the power to make rational decisions and moral choices, and each should be allowed to exercise his or her capacity for self-determination. This ethical principle was affirmed in a court decision by Justice Cardozo in 1914 with the dictum, "**Every human being of adult years and sound mind has a right to determine what shall be done with his own body**".
   b. Autonomy, as is true for all four principles, needs to be weighed against competing moral principles, and in some instances may be overridden; an obvious example would be if the autonomous action of a patient causes harm to another person(s).
   c. The principle of autonomy does not extend to persons who lack the capacity (competence) to act autonomously; examples include infants and children and incompetence due to developmental, mental or physical disorder.
   d. In countries with ancient civilizations like India, rooted

beliefs and traditions, the practice of **paternalism** by physicians emanates mostly from beneficence. However, culture is not static and autonomous, and changes with other trends over passing years. It is presumptuous to assume that the patterns and roles in physician-patient relationships that have been in place for a half a century and more still hold true. Therefore, a critical examination of paternalistic medical practice is needed for reasons that include technological and economic progress, improved educational and socioeconomic status of the populace, globalization and societal movement towards emphasis on the patient as an individual, than as a member of a group.

e. Respecting the principle of autonomy obliges the physician to disclose medical information and treatment options that are necessary for the patient to exercise self-determination and supports informed consent, truth-telling, and confidentiality.

f. **Informed Consent**: The requirements of an informed consent for a medical or surgical procedure, or for research, are that the patient or subject (i) must be competent to understand and decide, (ii) receives a full disclosure, (iii) comprehends the disclosure, (iv) acts voluntarily and (v) consents to the proposed action.

g. **Truth-telling**: A vital component in a physician-patient relationship is "truth-telling"; without this component, the physician loses the trust of the patient. An autonomous patient has not only the right to know (disclosure) of his/her diagnosis and prognosis, but also has the option to forgo this disclosure. However, the physician must know which of these two options the patient prefers. In Western countries, full disclosure to the patient, however grave the disease is, the norm now. Providing full information, with tact and sensitivity, to patients who want to know is mandatory.

   i. In contrast to Western countries, full disclosure to the patient is highly variable in other countries such as India. A continuing pattern in these countries is for the physician to disclose the information to the family and not to the patient. The likely reasons for resistance of physicians to convey bad news are concern that it may cause anxiety and loss of hope, some uncertainty on the outcome, or belief that the patient would not be able to understand the information or may not want to know. However, this does not have to be a binary choice, as careful understanding of the principle of autonomy reveals that autonomous choice is a right of a patient, and the patient, in exercising this right, may authorize a family member or members to make decisions for him/her.

h. **Confidentiality**: Physicians are obligated not to disclose confidential information given by a patient to another party without the patient's authorization. An obvious exception (with implied patient authorization) is the sharing of necessary medical information for the care of the patient from the primary physician to consultants and other health-care teams. In the present-day, modern hospitals with multiple points of tests and consultants, and the use of electronic medical records, there has been an erosion of confidentiality. However, individual physicians must exercise discipline in not discussing patient specifics with their family members or in social gatherings, and social media.

   i. There are some noteworthy **exceptions to patient confidentiality**. These include, among others, legally required reporting of gunshot wounds and sexually transmitted diseases and exceptional situations that may cause major harm to another (e.g., epidemics of infectious diseases, partner notification in HIV disease, relative notification of certain genetic risks, etc.).

4. ***Justice***:

   a. **Justice** is generally interpreted as fair, equitable and appropriate treatment of persons. Of the several categories of justice, the one that is most pertinent to clinical ethics is ***distributive justice***. Distributive justice refers to the fair, equitable and appropriate distribution of health-care resources determined by justified norms that structure the terms of social cooperation. Although this important health-care policy discussion exceeds the scope of this book, a few examples on issues of distributive justice encountered in hospital and office practice need to be mentioned. These include:

      i. allotment of scarce resources (equipment, tests, medications, organ transplants)
      ii. care of uninsured patients and
      iii. allotment of time for outpatient visits (equal time for every patient? based on need or complexity? based on social and or economic status?).

   b. Difficult as it may be, and despite the many constraining forces, physicians must accept the requirement of fairness contained in this principle. Fairness to the patient assumes a role of primary importance when there are conflicts of interests. A flagrant example of violation of this principle would be when a particular option of treatment is chosen over others, or an expensive drug is chosen over an equally effective but less expensive one because it benefits the physician, financially or otherwise.

Medical Etiquette

Medical etiquette refers to the conventional laws of courtesy observed between members of the medical profession.

- Every medical practitioner should treat his colleagues in the same way as he would have them treat him, i.e., with courtesy and grace.
- In 1803, Thomas Percival wrote a classic essay on medical ethics that endorsed complimentary professional care to "all members of the profession, including physicians and surgeons, together with their wives and children, who should be attended gratuitously."
- In 1847, the American Medical Association's Code of Ethics similarly endorsed waiving charges for services to other

physicians and their families. This is likely the first modern-day documentation of the philosophy.

- Among physicians, it has been historically traditional to provide medical care at nil or reduced cost to physician colleagues and their immediate family members. The custom dates back to Hippocrates. However, there is no law against doctors treating other doctors or their family members for a charge, as it avoids questions of objectivity, and the danger of emotional attachment colouring assessment and treatment.
- In 1994, the American Medical Association issued a Code of Medical Ethics Opinion advising that free-of-charge and reduced rate services were not an ethical requirement, and that physicians can use their own judgment when deciding to extend such professional courtesy.

UNETHICAL PRACTICES & DICHOTOMY

Discussed under FM 4.5 (*vide infra*).

> **FM 4.3: Core – Written/Viva Voce**
> - Describe the functions and role of:
>   - Medical Council of India
>   - State Medical Councils

The Indian Medical Council (IMC) or Medical Council of India (MCI) was a body that was intimately concerned with the medical profession, and was governed by the Indian Medical Council Act (1956) (modified in 1964, 1993 and 2001). **However, the MCI was disbanded in 2010, and functioned under a Board of Governors until 2012, when a new council was formed.** This was in turn abolished and the **National Medical Commission (NMC)** was established under the **National Medical Commission Act of 2019**. The NMC came into existence on **25th Sept 2020**, and is today the country's apex regulator of medical education and profession.

The Medical Council of India (MCI) does not exist anymore.

NATIONAL MEDICAL COMMISSION

The **National Medical Commission (NMC)** is a statutory body established under the **National Medical Commission Act of 2019**, and came into force on **25th Sept 2020**.

It is the country's apex regulator of medical education and profession.

Composition

- 33 members: 1 Chairman, 10 ex-officio members, 22 part time members (19 nominated by States and Union Territories).
- Chairperson, Secretary and some part time members are appointed by the Central Govt on the recommendations of a Search Committee.

Powers/Functions

- Observance and promotion of professional ethics in the medical profession, and provision of care by medical practitioners.
- Assess requirements in healthcare, including human resources.
- Develop a road map for meeting the above requirements.
- Frame guidelines for determination of fees and other charges in respect of 50% of seats in private medical institutes and universities which are governed by the provisions of the NMC Act.
- Grant limited license to practice medicine at mid-level as a Community Health Provider (CHP) who is qualified as per prescribed criteria, and can prescribe specified medicines independently in primary and preventive healthcare.
- Conduct National Eligibility-cum-Entrance Test (NEET) and regulate the manner of conducting counselling by the designated authority for admission to UG and PG courses, as well as super speciality seats in all medical institutes.
- Conduct National Exit Test (NExT), a common final year UG medical examination for granting license to practise medicine as medical practitioners, and for enrolment in State or National Medical Register.

Differences between the NMC and the erstwhile MCI are laid out in **Table 4.1**.

Autonomous NMC Boards

Each Autonomous Board comprises of a President, 2 whole-time members and 2 part-time members.

Undergraduate Medical Education Board

- Grants recognition to undergraduate medical qualifications.
- Develops and maintains competency based dynamic curriculum for addressing the needs of primary health services, community medicine and family medicine.
- Frames guidelines, minimum requirements and standards for setting up medical institutes, conducting courses and examinations, and norms for infrastructure, faculty and quality of education.
- Facilitates faculty training and development, research, and international student and faculty exchange programmes.

Postgraduate Medical Education Board

- Grants recognition to postgraduate and super-speciality medical qualifications.
- Develops and maintains competency based dynamic curriculum to impart appropriate skills, knowledge, attitude, values and ethics.
- Frames guidelines, minimum requirements and standards for setting up medical institutes, conducting courses and examinations, and norms for infrastructure, faculty and quality of education at postgraduate level.
- Facilitates faculty training and development, research and international student and faculty exchange programmes.
- Facilitates and promotes postgraduate courses in family medicine.

Medical Assessment and Rating Board

- Grants permission for establishment of new medical institutes, or to start any postgraduate course, or to increase the number of seats.
- Carries out inspections of medical institutes for assessing and rating.

Table 4.1 Differences between NMC Act and MCI Act

S. No.	NMC Act	MCI Act
1	Governing body under the NMC Act is the NMC	Governing body under the IMC Act was the MCI
2	All members of NMC will be appointed or nominated by the Central Govt	MCI was mostly comprised of members who were elected from amongst members of the medical faculty of Universities and State Medical Registers/Councils
3	Section 5 of NMC Act provides for the composition of a seven-member Search Committee, which shall include the Chairperson, part-time members and the Secretary, who shall be appointed by the Central Govt on the recommendations of the Search Committee	No such provision existed under the IMC Act
4	Provides for constitution of Autonomous Boards	No such provision
5	Introduction of Exit Exam for all candidates	Only for graduates with foreign medical qualifications

Ethics and Medical Registration Board

- Maintains a National Register of all licensed medical practitioners.
- Regulates professional conduct, promotes medical ethics and exercises appellate jurisdiction with respect to actions taken by any State Medical Council.

Medical Advisory Council

Composition

- Chairperson and all members of the NMC (as ex-officio members).
- Chairman of University Grants Commission.
- Director of National Assessment and Accreditation Council.
- Other members to be nominated by State Governments, Ministry of Home Affairs, State Medical Councils and Central Government.

Functions

- Acts as the primary platform through which the States and Union Territories may put forth their views and concerns before the NMC, and helps in shaping the overall agenda, policy and action relating to medical education and training.
- Advises the NMC on measures to determine and maintain minimum standards in all matters relating to medical education, training and research, and on measures to enhance equitable access to medical education.

STATE MEDICAL COUNCIL

- Every state in India has a State Medical Council (SMC), located usually in the capital of that state.
- It is composed of members of the medical profession elected from among themselves, as well as those nominated by the State Government.
- A President and a Vice President are elected by the members from amongst themselves.

Functions of the State Medical Council

1. ***Medical Register***
   a. The SMC maintains a register containing the names, addresses, and qualifications of those medical practitioners who have registered with the council.
   b. It also contains the date on which a particular degree was obtained, and the name of the university which conferred it.
   c. This register is maintained by a Registrar who is appointed by the council. On receiving further qualifications, the medical practitioner concerned must inform the Registrar of the same.
   d. The Registrar is expected to inform the IMC without delay, all the additions and amendments made from time to time in the State Medical Register.
2. ***Disciplinary Control***
   a. The council exercises disciplinary control over registered medical practitioners, and has the power to delete the names of those found guilty of professional misconduct. Such deletion may be temporary or permanent.
   b. If an appeal is made by an aggrieved medical practitioner against the punishment awarded, and if the IMC makes a recommendation in favour of the appellant, his name will be restored in the State Medical Register.
3. ***Warning Notice***
   a. The council makes clear disclosure of those practices it considers as constituting **infamous conduct** (**Box 4.1**). It issues a warning to the registered medical practitioners found indulging in unethical practice, and advises them to conduct themselves according to the ethical norms prescribed by the council.
   b. It is important to note that a **warning notice** is different from a **warning**.
      i. The **warning notice** is a list of offences which are considered as infamous conduct (**Box 4.1**). This list

is given to doctors at the time of registration with the State Medical Council, and later periodically.

ii. On the other hand, a **warning** is a cautionary notice given by the SMC after judicial enquiry, on finding a doctor guilty of infamous conduct.

Box 4.1—List of acts mentioned in Warning Notice, contravention of which will attract disciplinary action (Infamous Conduct, Professional Misconduct)

- ***Adultery or improper conduct or association with a patient***
- ***Conviction by a court of law for offences involving moral turpitude:*** Such offences include theft, perjury, bigamy, rape, etc.
- Issuance of fraudulent professional certificates, reports, and other documents: Such documents include certificates and reports relating to
  - Births, deaths or disposal of the dead
  - Mental Health Act
  - Factory Acts
  - Public Health Act
  - Workmen's Compensation Act
  - Notifiable diseases
  - Employees' State Insurance Act
  - Sickness or fitness certificates

  Issuance of fraudulent certificates relating to any of the above will attract disciplinary action. A registered medical practitioner must maintain a Register of Medical Certificates in which all details must be entered of certificates issued.

  Whenever a medical certificate is issued, the identification marks of the patient must be mentioned, and his signature or thumb impression taken on the certificate or report.
- ***Contravention of provisions of the Drugs Act***
- ***Selling scheduled poisons or drugs*** to the public under the cover of his qualifications, except to his patients.
- **Association** with unqualified person to perform abortion, or any illegal operation, or operations for which there is no medical or surgical indication.
- ***Advertisement***
  - A physician should not contribute to the lay press articles, and give interviews regarding diseases and treatment which may have the effect of advertising himself or soliciting practice for himself. But, there is no restriction in writing to the lay press under his own name on matters of public health and hygienic living, or to deliver public lectures, give talks on radio or public broadcast system for the same purpose and send announcements of the same to the lay press.
  - An institution run by a physician for a particular purpose such as a maternity home, private hospital, etc., may be advertised in the lay press, but such advertisements should not contain anything more than the name of the institution, type of patients admitted, facilities offered and residential fees. Name of either the superintendent or the doctors attending to the patients should not appear in the advertisement.
  - It is improper for physicians to use an unusually large signboard, or write on a signboard anything other than his name, qualifications obtained from a recognized university or statutory body, titles and name of his specialty. It is improper to affix a signboard on a chemist's shop, or in places where he does not reside or work.
  - It is improper for a physician to exhibit publicly the scale of his fees. But, there is no objection to the same being put up in the physician's waiting room or consultation chamber.
- ***Contravention of professional secrecy***
  - A physician must not disclose the secrets of a patient that have been learnt in the exercise of his profession. Such matters can be disclosed only in a court of law under orders of the presiding judge.
  - A physician must not publish photographs or case reports of his patients in any medical or other journal in a manner by which their identity could be made out without their permission. If the identity is not disclosed, consent is not necessary.
- ***Refusal on religious grounds*** to give assistance in matters relating to birth control, sterility, therapeutic abortion, etc., when there is medical indication.
- ***Failure to obtain consent*** from husband, wife, parent, guardian or patient himself, as the case may be, before performing a surgical operation. Consent of both husband and wife is mandatory for any operation that can result in sterility of either party.
- ***Employing touts or agents*** to procure patients.
- ***False claims of specialist status***, unless the physician has undergone the requisite training programme in a recognized institute.

FM 4.4: Core – Written/Viva Voce
- Describe the Indian Medical Council Register

INDIAN MEDICAL REGISTER

- The National Medical Commission (NMC) maintains a register containing the names, addresses and qualifications of all medical practitioners who have registered themselves with any state medical council.
- When a medical graduate with a recognised medical qualification registers himself with any State Medical Council (SMC) after paying the prescribed fee, notification is sent to the NMC and his name gets registered in the Indian Medical Register also.
- Similarly, if the name of a medical practitioner is erased from the State Medical Register for any reason, it is automatically deleted from the Indian Medical Register also.

FM 4.5: Core – Written/Viva Voce
- Rights/Privileges of a medical practitioner
- Infamous conduct
- Disciplinary Committee, disciplinary procedures, warning notice and penal erasure

RIGHTS AND PRIVILEGES OF A REGISTERED MEDICAL PRACTITIONER

There are certain rights and privileges that accrue to a medical practitioner as a result of registration in a medical council, and they are as follows:

- Right to **practice the profession** anywhere in India.
- Right to **add professional titles** to his name.
- Right to **choose patients**.
- Right to **prescribe or dispense medicines**.
- Right to **perform a surgical operation**.
- Right to **seek government employment** as a doctor.
- Right to **issue birth, sickness, insanity and other certificates** which will be held valid in a court of law.
- Right to **give evidence as an expert witness** in a court of law.
- Right to **possess, dispense or prescribe drugs** listed in the **Dangerous Drugs Act**.
- Right to **claim payment of fees** for professional services rendered.

What About Using the Red Cross Emblem?

- The objectives of the Red Cross Society are closely allied with those of the medical profession. This has led to the mistaken belief on the part of some doctors that they are entitled to use the Red Cross emblem. This belief is erroneous, and in fact the law prohibits its misuse by medical practitioners.
- The Red Crescent emblem is used in 33 Islamic countries in place of the Red Cross because of perceived religious connotations relating to the latter, while neutral countries use the Red Crystal emblem (**Fig. 4.4**).

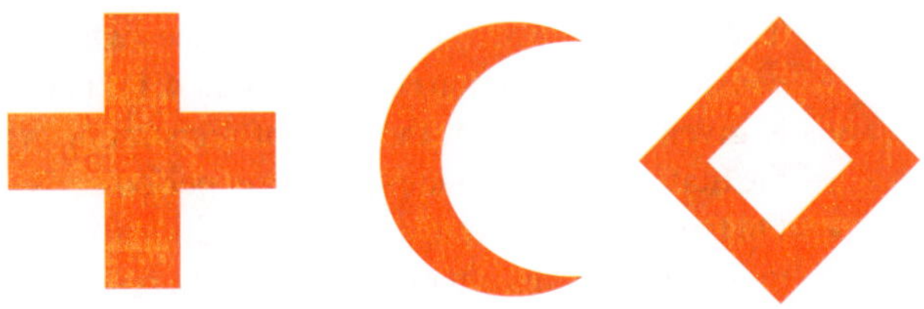

Fig. 4.4 (L to R): Red Cross, Red Crescent, Red Crystal

The right to display the Red Cross emblem (a red cross on a white background) can be exercised only by the members of the medical division of the armed forces of a country and the Red Cross Society (**Fig. 4.5**). The International Committee of the Red Cross (ICRC) is a private humanitarian institution founded in 1863 in Geneva, Switzerland, by Henry Dunant and Gustave Moynier. Its 25-member committee has a unique authority under International Humanitarian Law to protect the life and dignity of the victims of international and internal armed conflicts.

As per the **Geneva Convention Act 1960** (to which India is a signatory), *Sec 12* prohibits the use of the Red Cross emblem and all other allied emblems for any purpose whatsoever, without approval of the Government of India, while *Sec 13* lays down the penalty for unauthorised use. The punishment may take the form of a fine (up to Rs. 500), as well as forfeiture of the goods upon or in connection with which the emblem, designation or wording was used by that person.

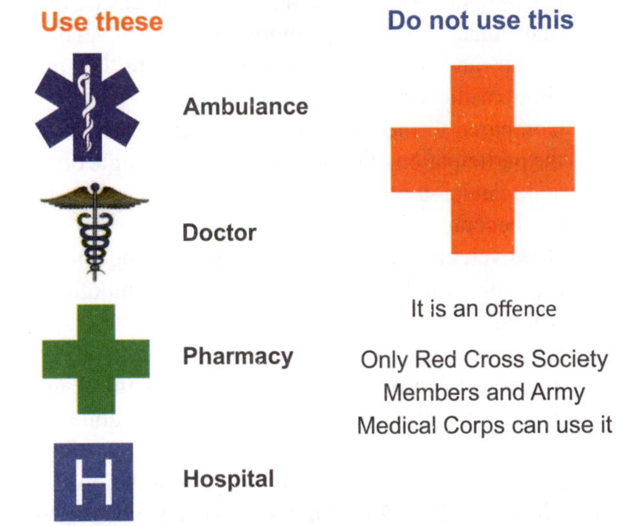

Fig. 4.5 Usage of various symbols in healthcare

INFAMOUS CONDUCT (PROFESSIONAL MISCONDUCT)

Any act or behaviour of a doctor which is considered disgraceful or dishonourable by his professional colleagues of good repute, amounts to professional misconduct or infamous conduct.

Such cases, when brought to the notice of a State Medical Council, will be examined to determine if the doctor is guilty, and if so, to decide on the punishment. The procedure of enquiry is mentioned on *page no. 286*.

It is not possible to enumerate all the situations in which a doctor may be charged with professional misconduct, but the general categories of serious professional misconduct include the following (*many of which have already been described in the foregoing sections*):

1. **Abortion**
   Illegal termination of pregnancy is considered as an act of professional misconduct, i.e., contravention of the rules laid out in the ***Medical Termination of Pregnancy Act 1971*** (*page no. 267*).
2. **Adultery**
   A medical practitioner must maintain the highest standards of moral integrity. He should not misuse his position to commit adultery with his patients, or their relatives or attendants.
3. **Alcohol**
   Attending to patients under the influence of alcohol is strictly prohibited.
4. **Addiction**
   By virtue of his profession, a medical practitioner has easy access to various kinds of drugs. He can be punished for professional misconduct, if he resorts to drug abuse.
5. **Advertising**

- The rigid attitude of the past towards advertisement of one's professional skills and ability is gradually being replaced by more liberal views. This change in attitude has become inevitable because of the increasing impact of the media on the community, increasing level of education, and heightened awareness of the lay public about medical matters.
- Compared to the past when anonymity was absolute, the participation of medically qualified people on radio and television programmes, and in newspaper articles has become an everyday occurrence.
- However, **canvassing for patients** is wrong and unacceptable, whether it is done by word of mouth, or in writing.
- It is also not correct on the part of a doctor to **advertise a change of consulting hours through a public notice or in a newspaper**. This should only be done by an individual notice to the existing patients, or by displaying a note at the doctor's office or consultation room.
- The **scale of professional fees** must never be disclosed in public.
- **Name boards** must be modest in size, colour and lettering.
- **Personal achievements** in surgery or medical treatment must never be advertised.

6. **Association**
   - Association with unqualified persons to promote one's practice is perhaps still in vogue, but it undoubtedly amounts to professional misconduct.
   - Similarly, engaging unqualified persons in technical positions is undesirable and unethical.
   - ***Dichotomy*** or ***fee splitting*** is also considered highly unethical. Dichotomy refers to receiving or giving commission to colleagues, pharmacists, manufacturers of drugs, etc., for professional favours.
     - A doctor is expected to provide the best medical treatment available for his patients. If he is not competent or qualified to handle a particular case, then he should refer it to the specialist concerned.
     - It is objectionable to ask for a share in fees from the doctor to whom the case was referred. By fee-splitting, the doctor is receiving fees for work that he has not done, and hence it is unethical.

The examples cited above are sometimes referred to as the **6 A's** of **professional misconduct**.

Some other practices amounting to professional misconduct include:

- Ownership of a shop selling pharmaceutical drugs, or medical or surgical appliances.
- Assisting unqualified persons (i.e., without recognised qualifications) in the treatment of patients. This is referred to as ***Covering***.
- Associating with bodies or societies comprising unqualified persons who are engaged in "training" health professionals.
- Violation of the provisions of the Drugs Acts in vogue.
- Performing surgical operations when they are not required or indicated.
- Issuing false or fraudulent medical certificates.
- Withholding information about notifiable diseases from public health authorities.
- Disclosure of professional secrets (*vide infra*).
- Refusal to render professional service on grounds of religion, nationality, language or community.
- Violation of the provisions of ***The Pre-Conception and Pre-Natal Diagnostic Techniques (Prohibition of Sex Selection) Act, 1994*** (refer **Annexure I**).

Disciplinary Measures

- Every State Medical Council exercises disciplinary control over registered medical practitioners, and has the power to delete the names of those found guilty of professional misconduct. Such deletion may be temporary or permanent.
- If an appeal is made by an aggrieved medical practitioner against the punishment awarded, and if the IMC makes a recommendation in favour of the appellant, his name will be restored in the State Medical Register.
- **Warning Notice**
  - The council makes clear disclosure of those practices it considers as constituting **professional misconduct** or **infamous conduct** (**Box 4.1**). It issues a warning to the registered medical practitioners found indulging in any of these practices, and advises them to conduct themselves according to the ethical norms prescribed by the council.
  - It is important to note that a **warning notice** is different from a **warning**.
    - The **warning notice** is a list of offences which are considered as infamous conduct (**Box 4.1**). This list is given to doctors at the time of registration with the State Medical Council, and later periodically.
    - On the other hand, a **warning** is a cautionary notice given by the SMC after judicial enquiry, on finding a doctor guilty of infamous conduct.
- **Procedure of Disciplinary Action**
  - The State Medical Council initiates disciplinary action in any of the following situations:
    - When a complaint is made by a person or persons against a registered medical practitioner.
    - When a court of law convicts any registered medical practitioner for an offence involving moral turpitude.
  - The complaint is received by the Registrar. He submits the complaint to the President who refers it to a subcommittee or an executive committee.
  - The committee examines the complaint and decides whether it is necessary to take action against the medical practitioner concerned. If there is *prima facie* evidence of misdemeanor, a notice is issued to the medical practitioner to be present on a specified day to face the charges.

- The defendant medical practitioner and his legal advisor should be present on the appointed day. First, the charges are read out with relevant details. The counsel for the complainant outlines the nature and substance of allegations with relevant evidentiary material. Then the defendant (registered practitioner) or his legal advisor rebuts the charges.
- After hearing both sides, the members of the council are asked to express their opinion. The judgement is based on the majority view.
- If the council finds *prima facie* evidence, and a majority of the members feel that the offence is proved, the guilty registered medical practitioner is punished in one of the following ways:
  - **Warning**: A warning is issued to the medical practitioner to conduct himself according to the expectations of ethical standards prescribed by the council.
  - **Temporary erasure**: The name of the medical practitioner is erased from the register for a specified period after which it is restored.
  - **Penal erasure**: The name is permanently removed from the register. This is also known as ***professional death sentence***.

> FM 4.6: Core – Written/Viva Voce
> - Duties of a medical practitioner towards patients
> - Duties of a medical practitioner towards society

DUTIES AND RESPONSIBILITIES OF A MEDICAL PRACTITIONER/PHYSICIAN

Character of Physician

- A physician shall **uphold the dignity and honour of his profession**.
- The physician shall **keep himself pure in character** and be **diligent in caring for the sick**.
- Physicians should try **continuously to improve medical knowledge and skills**. The physician should **practice methods of healing founded on scientific basis** and should not associate professionally with anyone who violates this principle.
- For the advancement of his profession, a physician should **affiliate with associations and societies of allopathic medical professions** and involve actively in the functioning of such bodies.
- A physician should **participate in professional meetings** as part of Continuing Medical Education programmes, for at least 30 hours every 5 years, organized by reputed professional academic bodies or any other authorized organisations. The compliance of this requirement shall be informed regularly to the National Medical Commission or the State Medical Councils as the case may be.
- **Maintenance of medical records**:
  - Every physician shall **maintain the medical records** pertaining to his/her indoor patients for a period of 3 years from the date of commencement of the treatment **in a standard proforma.**
  - If any request is made for medical records either by the patients/authorised attendant or legal authorities involved, the same may be duly acknowledged and **documents shall be issued within a period of 72 hours**.
  - A Registered Medical Practitioner shall **maintain a Register of Medical Certificates** giving full details of certificates issued. When issuing a medical certificate he/she shall always **enter the identification marks of the patient** and keep a copy of the certificate.
  - Efforts shall be made to **computerize medical records** for quick retrieval.
- **Display of registration numbers**:
  - Every physician shall **display the registration number** accorded to him by the State Medical Council/Medical Council of India in his clinic and in all his prescriptions, certificates, money receipts given to his patients.
- Physicians shall **display as suffix to their names only recognized medical degrees** or such certificates/diplomas and memberships/honours which confer professional knowledge or recognizes any exemplary qualification/achievements.*
- Every physician should **prescribe drugs with generic names** and he/she shall ensure that there is a **rational prescription** and use of drugs.
- Every physician should maintain the **highest quality assurance in patient care**.
- **Exposure of unethical conduct**: A physician should expose, without fear or favour, incompetent or corrupt, dishonest or unethical conduct on the part of members of the profession.
- **Payment for professional services**: A physician should **announce his fees before rendering service** and not after the operation or treatment is under way. It is unethical to enter into a contract of "no cure, no payment".
- The physician shall **observe the laws of the country** in regulating the practice of medicine and shall also not assist others to evade such laws.

Duties of Physicians to their Patients

Obligations to the Sick

- Though a physician is not bound to treat each and every person asking his services, he should not only **be ever ready to respond to the calls of the sick and the injured**, but should be mindful of the high character of his mission

Note*: *This **does not include mere membership of a professional society, e.g., MAFMT (Member of Association of Forensic Medicine & Toxicology). Such suffixes are **unethical**. Memberships that are conferred only upon clearing an examination, and offer the status of an additional qualification, however can be used, e.g., MRCP (Member of the Royal College of Physicians). Such suffixes are **ethical**.*

and the responsibility he discharges in the course of his professional duties.

- A physician advising a patient to seek service of another physician is acceptable; however, in case of emergency a physician must treat the patient. **No physician shall arbitrarily refuse treatment to a patient**. However for good reason, when a patient is suffering from an ailment which is not within the range of experience of the treating physician, the physician may refuse treatment and refer the patient to another physician.
- A medical practitioner having any **incapacity detrimental to the patient** or which can affect his performance vis-à-vis the patient is **not permitted to practice his profession**.
- **Patience, delicacy and secrecy**:
    - Confidences concerning individual or domestic life entrusted by patients to a physician and defects in the disposition or character of patients observed during medical attendance should never be revealed unless their revelation is required by the laws of the State.
    - Sometimes, however, a physician must determine whether his duty to society requires him to employ knowledge, obtained through confidence as a physician, to protect a healthy person against a communicable disease to which he is about to be exposed.
- Prognosis: The physician **should neither exaggerate nor minimize the gravity of a patient's condition**.
- The **patient must not be neglected**: Once having undertaken a case, the physician should not neglect the patient, nor should he withdraw from the case without giving adequate notice to the patient and his family.
- **Engagement for an obstetric case**: When a physician who has been engaged to attend an obstetric case is absent and another is sent for and delivery accomplished, the acting physician is entitled to his professional fees, but should secure the patient's consent to resign on the arrival of the physician engaged.

Duties of Physician in Consultation

- **Unnecessary consultations should be avoided**:
    - However, in case of serious illness and in doubtful or difficult conditions, the physician should request consultation, but under any circumstances such consultation should be justifiable and in the interest of the patient only and not for any other consideration.
    - Consulting pathologists/radiologists or asking for any other diagnostic Lab investigation should be done judiciously and not in a routine manner.
    - Consultation for patient's benefit: In every consultation, the benefit to the patient is of foremost importance. All physicians engaged in the case should be frank with the patient and his attendants.
- **Utmost punctuality** should be observed by a physician in making themselves available for consultations.
- **Statement to patient after consultation**:
    - All statements to the patient or his representatives should take place in the presence of the consulting physicians, except as otherwise agreed. The disclosure of the opinion to the patient or his relatives or friends shall rest with the medical attendant.
    - Differences of opinion should not be divulged unnecessarily but when there is irreconcilable difference of opinion the circumstances should be frankly and impartially explained to the patient or his relatives or friends. It would be open to them to seek further advice as they so desire.
- **Treatment after consultation**: No decision should restrain the attending physician from making such subsequent variations in the treatment if any unexpected change occurs, but at the next consultation, reasons for the variations should be discussed/explained. The same privilege, with its obligations, belongs to the consultant when sent for in an emergency during the absence of attending physician. The attending physician may prescribe medicine at any time for the patient, whereas the consultant may prescribe only in case of emergency or as an expert when called for.
- **Patients referred to specialists**: When a patient is referred to a specialist by the attending physician, a case summary of the patient should be given to the specialist, who should communicate his opinion in writing to the attending physician.
- **Fees and other charges**:
    - A physician shall **clearly display his fees** and other charges on the board of his chamber and/or the hospitals he is visiting.
    - A physician shall write his name and designation in full along with registration particulars in his prescription letter head.

Responsibilities of Physicians to Each Other

- A physician should consider it as a **pleasure and privilege to render gratuitous (free) service to all physicians and their immediate family dependants**.
- **In consultations, no insincerity, rivalry or envy should be indulged in.**
- When a physician has been called for consultation, the Consultant should normally not take charge of the case, especially on the solicitation of the patient or friends. The Consultant **shall not criticize the referring physician**. He/She shall discuss the diagnosis treatment plan with the referring physician.
- **Appointment of substitute**: Whenever a physician requests another physician to attend his patients during his temporary absence from his practice, professional courtesy requires the acceptance of such appointment only when he has the capacity to discharge the additional responsibility along with his/her other duties. The physician acting under such an appointment should give the utmost consideration to the interests and reputation of the absent physician and all such patients should be restored to the care of the latter upon his/her return.
- **Visiting another physician's case**: When it becomes the duty of a physician occupying an official position to see

and report upon an illness or injury, he should communicate to the physician in attendance so as to give him an option of being present. The medical officer/physician occupying an official position should avoid remarks upon the diagnosis or the treatment that has been adopted.

Duties of Physician to the Public & to the Paramedical Profession

- Physicians, as good citizens, possessed of special training **should disseminate advice on public health issues**.
- Physicians, especially those engaged in public health work, **should enlighten the public concerning quarantine regulations and measures for the prevention of epidemic and communicable diseases**.
- **When an epidemic occurs a physician should not abandon his duty for fear of contracting the disease himself**.
- **Physicians should recognize and promote the practice of** different paramedical services such as, **pharmacy and nursing** as professions and should seek their cooperation wherever required.

> **FM 4.7: Core – Written/Viva Voce**
> - Describe and discuss ethics related to HIV patients

HUMAN IMMUNODEFICIENCY VIRUS & ACQUIRED IMMUNE DEFICIENCY SYNDROME (PREVENTION & CONTROL) ACT – 2017 (HIV/AIDS PREVENTION ACT – 2017)

- **Human Immunodeficiency Virus & Acquired Immune Deficiency Syndrome (Prevention & Control) Act – 2017 (HIV/AIDS Prevention Act – 2017)** is an act of the Parliament of India that provides for controlling and preventing of HIV/AIDS, and securing the rights of individuals diagnosed with HIV/AIDS.
- It received Presidential assent on 20th April 2017, and became effective from 10th Sept 2018.
- The Act prohibits discrimination against persons living with HIV/AIDS for the purposes of employment, provides for access to educational establishments of such persons, along with access to healthcare and insurance services, renting property or running for public or private office.
- The law also prohibits any form of expression that is deemed as inciting hatred against people infected with HIV/AIDS.
- Testing for HIV requires specific and informed consent of the person being tested, and for any research and information sharing. Conducting an HIV test, medical treatment or research on a person without their informed consent is unlawful.
- The Act prohibits a person from being forced to disclose their HIV/AIDS status, unless mandated by a court order.
- The Act also protects the rights of HIV/AIDS affected minors to shared household.
- No informed consent is required by licensed blood banks, or for medical research and epidemiological purposes where an HIV test is conducted anonymously and not specifically for the purpose of identifying an HIV positive individual.
- The Act penalises propagation of hate against HIV/AIDS affected persons with fine and imprisonment for a term of 3 months up to 2 years.
- The Act makes anti-retroviral treatment (ART) a right for all HIV/AIDS affected persons.
  - Article 14 of the Constitution of India guarantees the right of equality to every person, which includes treatment for HIV/AIDS patients. Articles 15 and 16 protect patients against any forms of discrimination.
- The Act also mandates for the central and state governments to provide HIV prevention, testing, treatment and counselling services to affected individuals.

> **FM 4.8: Core – Written/Viva Voce**
> - Describe the Consumer Protection Act – 1986 (Medical Indemnity Insurance, Civil Litigations and Compensations)
> - Workman's Compensation Act
> - Employees State Insurance Act

CONSUMER PROTECTION ACT – 1986 (COPRA)

- The **Consumer Protection Act – 1986 (COPRA)** is an Act by the Parliament of India to protect the interests of consumers in India.
- It has been repealed by the **Consumer Protection Act, 2019**.
- It was enacted for the establishment of consumer councils and other authorities for the settlement of consumer's grievances and matters connected with it.
- **District Consumer Disputes Redressal Forum (DCDRF)**: Also known as the "**District Forum**" established by the State Government in each district of the State. The State Governments may establish more than one District Forum in a district. It is a district-level court that deals with cases valuing up to Rs. 1 crore.
- **State Consumer Disputes Redressal Commission (SCDRC)**: Also known as the "**State Commission**" established by the State Government in the State. It is a state-level court that takes up cases valuing from Rs 1 to 10 crores.
- **National Consumer Disputes Redressal Commission (NCDRC)**: Also known as the "**National Commission**" established by the Central Government. It deals with matters of more than Rs. 10 crore.

Objectives

The objectives of the Central Council is to promote and to protect the rights of the consumers such as:

- The right to be protected against the marketing of goods and services which are hazardous to life and property.
- The right to be informed about the quality, quantity, potency, purity, standard and price of goods or services, as the case may be to protect the consumer against unfair trade practices.
- The right to be assured, wherever possible, access to a variety of goods and services at competitive prices.

- The right to be heard and to be assured that consumer's interest will receive due consideration at appropriate forums.
- The right to seek redressal against unfair trade practices or restrictive trade practices or unscrupulous exploitation of consumers.
- The right to consumer education.

Jurisdiction/3-Tier System of Council Courts

Jurisdiction of District Forum

- Subject to the other provisions of this Act, the **District Forum** shall have jurisdiction to entertain complaints where the value of the goods or services and the compensation, if any, claimed **does not exceed rupees one crore**.
- A complaint shall be instituted in a District Forum within the local limits of whose jurisdiction the opposite party actually resides, or carries on business, or has a branch office.
- Consumer courts do not have jurisdiction over matters where services or goods were bought for a commercial purpose.

Jurisdiction of State Commission

- Subject to the other provisions of this Act, the **State Commission** shall have jurisdiction to entertain:
  - complaints where the value of the goods or services and compensation, if any, claimed **exceeds rupees one crore but does not exceed rupees ten crores** and
  - appeals against the orders of any District Forum within the State.

Jurisdiction of National Commission

- Subject to the other provisions of this Act, the **National Commission** shall have jurisdiction to entertain:
  - complaints where the value of the goods or services and compensation, if any, claimed **exceeds rupees 10 crores** and
  - appeals against the orders of any State Commission.

Consumer Protection Act & Medical Profession

Definitions

- **Consumer in Medical Profession**
  - A patient who pays to get services of doctor/hospital.
  - Any person who pays for the patient, legal heirs/representatives of such patients.
  - In case of death of patient who was a consumer, legal heirs (representatives) of the deceased will be considered as "consumer".
  - If the payment has been made by any person who is not a legal heir of the deceased, he too will be considered as "consumer".
- **Complaint**
  - Any allegation in writing, made by a complainant that the services hired or agreed to be hired or availed of by him suffer from deficiency in any respect.
- **Complainant**
  - A consumer.
  - The Central Government or any State Government.
  - Any registered voluntary consumer association.
  - One or more consumers, having the same interests.
- **Service**
  - Service means any description which is made available to potential users, and includes the provision of facilities in connection with banking, financing, insurance, transport, medical, etc., but does not include the rendering of any service free of charge, or under a contract of personal services.
- **Medical negligence**
  - Medical negligence or malpractice – lack of reasonable care and skill or wilful negligence on the part of a doctor in the treatment of a patient whereby the health or life of the patient is endangered.

Features

- **Personnel liable**
  - All medical/dental practitioners doing independent medical/dental practice, unless rendering only free service.
  - All Private hospitals charging patients.
  - All hospitals having free as well as paying patients, and all the paying and free category patients receiving treatment in such hospitals.
  - Medical/Dental practitioners and hospitals paid by an insurance firm for the treatment of a client, or an employment for that of an employee.
- **Procedure**
  - Complainant files a written complaint before the Forum/ Commission, which admits the complaint and sends a written notice to the opposite party asking for a written response to be submitted within 30 days.
  - Proceedings will be conducted thereafter based on evidence in the form of interrogatories, expert evidence, medical literature, and judicial decisions.
  - If the Forum/ Commission is satisfied that any of the allegations contained in the complaint about the services are proved, it will issue an order to the opposite party directing him/her to pay compensation to the consumer.
  - Where the defendant fails to comply, it is punishable with imprisonment for a term which will not be less than 1 month but which may extend to 3 years, or with fine which is not less than Rs 2,000, but which may extend up to Rs 10,000, or with both.
  - Every complaint must be decided within 90 days from the date of receipt of notice by opposite party, where there is no requirement for testing of sample, etc. In the event of such a requirement, the prescribed time is 5 months.
  - There is a provision for filing appeal against the verdict within 30 days:
    - Appeal against the decision of the District Forum can be filed before the State Commission.
    - Appeal against the decision of the State Commission to the National Commission.

    - Appeal against the decision of the National Commission to the Supreme Court.
    - Appeals must be disposed of within a period of 90 days.
  - A complaint must be filed within 2 years from the date on which the cause of action has arisen.
  - Dismissal of frivolous or vexatious complaints: the complaint is dismissed and an order is made that the complainant pays a cost, not exceeding 10,000 rupees, to the opposite party.

Medical Indemnity Insurance

- In the context of medical malpractice actions, hospitals can be held directly liable for their own negligence, as well as be held "vicariously" liable for the negligent actions of an employee. So, a hospital is legally liable for any malpractice committed by a physician, nurse, or other health care providers who are employed by the hospital.
- Doctors are probably the only professionals who face the risk of a financial liability in the course of practising their profession.The amount they can be sued for can be very high. Doctors therefore, require special insurance so that they can protect themselves both financially and legally when they are sued for negligence.
  - **Professional or Medical Indemnity** is an insurance plan to financially safeguard medical practitioners against legal costs and claims for compensation by patients in case of a legal row. Indemnity is a special contractual obligation of one party to compensate the loss incurred by the aggrieved party.
  - The scope of Medical Indemnity Insurance is to provide cover for the extent of financial damage for the loss caused to the victim against unintentional errors and omissions by the doctor, insured qualified and nonqualified employees, and staff. It also covers the cost of defending oneself in the court of law (Cost of Decree).
  - The plan covers liabilities for a year from the point of subscription. However, the policy does not cover criminal actions.
  - The policy will pay the sum insured that has been set as a limit. The expense over and above the sum insured has to be borne by the doctor. The sum insured is referred to as the **Limit of Indemnity**. This limit is fixed per accident and per policy period.
  - Indemnity insurance policies should be taken for doctors and hospital with staff separately and should be renewed every year to meet the claims arising out of the Consumer Protection Act (CPA).
  - Various organizations in India render indemnity insurance policies for medical practitioners:
    - Indian Medicolegal Consulting Services or Professional protection groups
    - IMA National Professional Protection Scheme
    - Professional Indemnity Policies by National General Insurance companies.

WORKMEN'S COMPENSATION ACT – 1923

- The early version of the Workmen Compensation Act was framed after noticing factory labourers' exposure to danger due to advanced machinery in the late 1880s.
- But according to the Compensation Act of 1884, employers were responsible for compensation only when a fatal accident took place.
- The government then formed a committee of experts from various fields, and enacted the **Workmen's Compensation Act – 1923**.
- In **2010**, the act came to be known as the **Employee's Compensation Act**.

Scope

- This act is applicable to any workers who work in an industry mentioned in the act.
- The act protects only those injuries caused by accidents during employment, and such accidents are subject to certain exceptions.
- It is mainly meant for the employees working in factories, mines, docks and other establishments mentioned under Schedule II of the Act, which also includes drivers, mechanics, helpers or persons connected with motor vehicles, captains or other crew members on aircraft. It also applies to persons hired to work abroad.
- The Act does not apply to members of the armed forces, and workmen who get covered under the Employees State Insurance Act.

Objectives

- To provide compensation at the time of an accident.
- Ensure that workmen have a sustainable life after an injury caused during their employment.

Liability of the Employer for Compensation

- Section 3 of the Employee's Compensation Act deals with 'Employer's Liability for Compensation'.
  - ***Conditions***:
    - The personal injury caused to an employee due to an accident should have occurred during employment.
    - In the case of an occupational disease, the disease should have been caused due to exposure during employment.
    - The claim application must be submitted within 2 years from the accident date. In the case of occupational disease: 2 years from the first date when illness occurred.
  - ***Calculation of compensation***:
    - Section 4 of the Employee's Compensation Act outlines the amount of compensation to be paid by the employer.
      - *In case of death of an employee*: An amount equal to 50% of the employee's monthly wage that gets multiplied with relevant factors (minimum amount payable is 1,20,000 rupees).
      - *In case of permanent or total disablement*: An

amount that is equal to 60% of monthly wages paid to the employee who is injured, the amount to be multiplied with relevant factors (minimum amount payable is 1,40,000 rupees).
  - *In case of permanent partial disablement*: Compensation percentage payable gets specified as the percentage of the loss of earning capacity caused by the injury.
  - *In case of temporary disablement*: An amount equal to the half-monthly payment equal to 25% of the employee's monthly wages.
  - *The Central Government changed the rules* for the calculation of compensation of employees under the Workmen's Compensation Act – 1923 in the year 2020. Minimum wages, which was Rs. 8000/- earlier, were increased to Rs. 15,000/-.
- ***Conditions when employer is not liable to pay compensation***:
  - If the injury does not result in partial or total disablement of the employee for more than 3 days.
  - Any injury that does not result in partial, total disablement of employee.
  - Injury or death was caused due to:
    - The employee being under the influence of alcohol or drugs during the time of the accident.
    - The employee was not following rules or orders that the employer had expressly framed for the employee's safety.
    - The employee had removed the safety guard willingly, provided for their safety.

EMPLOYEES STATE INSURANCE ACT – 1948

- Employees' State Insurance Corporation (ESIC) established by the ESI Act is a statutory body under the Ministry of Labour and Employment, Govt of India. As it is a legal entity, the corporation can raise loans and take measures for discharging such loans with the prior sanction of the central government, and it can acquire both movable and immovable property, and all incomes from the property shall vest with the corporation.
- The corporation can set up hospitals either independently or in collaboration with state government or other private entities.

Benefits

- As per Section 46 of the ESI Act, 1948, six benefits are envisaged to its subscribers:
  - Medical benefit
  - Sickness benefit
  - Maternity benefit
  - Disablement benefit
  - Dependants benefit
  - Other benefits
- For all employees earning Rs. 21,000 or less per month as wages, the employer contributes 3.25% and the employee contributes 0.75% (total share 4%). This fund is managed by the ESI Corporation (ESIC) according to rules and regulations stipulated in the ESI Act 1948, which oversees the provision of medical and cash benefits to the employees and their family. ESI scheme is a type of social security scheme for employees in the organised sector.
- The employees registered under the scheme are entitled to medical treatment for themselves and their dependents, unemployment cash benefit in certain contingencies, and maternity benefit in case of women employees.
- In case of employment-related disablement or death, there is provision for a disablement benefit and a family pension, respectively.
- Outpatient medical facilities are available in ESI dispensaries and through specified registered medical practitioners. Inpatient care is available in ESI hospitals and hospital annexes. In addition, several state government hospitals also have beds for the exclusive use of ESI beneficiaries. Cash benefits can be availed in any of 830 ESI centres throughout India.
- Recent years have seen an increasing role of information technology in ESI, with the introduction of "Pehchan smart cards" as a part of Project Panchdeep. In addition to insured workers, poor families eligible under the Rashtriya Swasthya Bima Yojana can also avail facilities in ESI hospitals and dispensaries.
- ESI Corporation also runs medical, nursing and paramedical colleges in some ESI hospitals across India. Presently, there are 11 medical colleges and 2 dental colleges established by the ESI Corporation. These colleges admit students on the basis of marks obtained in the competitive examinations conducted at the central level, the National Eligibility cum Entrance Test (NEET-UG).

> **FM 4.9: Non-Core – Written/Viva Voce**
> - Describe the medicolegal issues in relation to family violence, violation of human rights, NHRC and doctors.

FAMILY VIOLENCE (DOMESTIC VIOLENCE; INTIMATE PARTNER VIOLENCE)

- **Domestic violence includes any form of violence suffered by a person from a biological relative, but typically is the violence suffered by a woman by male members of her family or relatives.**
- Although men also suffer domestic violence, the law under IPC 498A specifically protects only women. Specifically, only a woman can file a case of domestic violence.
- There are several domestic violence laws in India. The earliest law was the **Dowry Prohibition Act 1961** which made the act of giving and receiving dowry a crime. In an effort to bolster the 1961 law, two new sections, **Section 498A** and **Section 304B** were introduced into the **Indian Penal Code** in **1983** and **1986**. The most recent legislation is the **Protection of Women from Domestic Violence Act (PWDVA) 2005**.

Definition

- Domestic violence is currently defined in India by the Protection of Women from Domestic Violence Act of 2005. According to Section 3 of the Act, "any act, omission or commission or conduct of the respondent shall constitute domestic violence in case it:
  a) harms or injures or endangers the health, safety, life, limb or well-being, whether mental or physical, of the aggrieved person, and includes causing physical abuse, sexual abuse, verbal and emotional abuse and economic abuse; or
  b) harasses, harms, injures or endangers the aggrieved person with a view to coerce her or any other person related to her to meet any unlawful demand for any dowry or other property or valuable security; or
  c) has the effect of threatening the aggrieved person or any person related to her by any conduct mentioned in clause (a) or clause (b); or
  d) otherwise injures or causes harm, whether physical or mental, to the aggrieved person."
- Jammu and Kashmir, which has its own laws, enacted the Jammu and Kashmir Protection of Women from Domestic Violence Act, 2010.

Forms

Physical Violence

- Physical injury is the most visible form of domestic violence. The scope of physical domestic/intimate partner violence includes slapping, pushing, kicking, biting, hitting, throwing objects, strangling, beating, threatening with any form of weapon, or using a weapon.
- Physical injuries as a result of domestic violence against women are more obvious than psychological ones, and can be more easily discerned by health professionals as well as courts of law in the context of legal prosecution.

Emotional Abuse

- Emotional abuse has been gaining more and more recognition in recent years as a common form of domestic violence (and therefore a human rights abuse) within the private home throughout developing nations such as India. Psychological abuse can erode a woman's sense of self-worth and can be very harmful to overall mental and physical wellbeing.
- Emotional/psychological abuse can include harassment; threats; verbal abuse such as name-calling, degradation and blaming; stalking; isolation.

Sexual Assault

- Domestic sexual assault is a form of domestic violence involving sexual/reproductive coercion and **marital rape**.
- Under Indian law, marital rape is not a crime, except during the period of marital separation of the partners. Section 375 of the Indian Penal Code (IPC) considers forced sex in marriages as a crime only when the wife is below 15. Thus, marital rape is not a criminal offense under IPC. Marital rape victims have to take recourse to the Protection of Women from Domestic Violence Act 2005 (PWDVA). However, it offers only a civil remedy for the offence.

Honour Killing

- **An "honour killing" is the practice wherein an individual is killed by one or more family member(s), because he or she is believed to have brought shame on the family.**
- The shame may range from refusing to enter an arranged marriage, having sex outside marriage, being in a relationship that is disapproved by the family, starting a divorce proceeding, or engaging in homosexual relations.
- Such cases are reported with terrible regularity from various parts of India. A fairly recent case is recounted in **Box 4.2**.

Dowry-related Abuse and Deaths

- In almost all Indian families, the ritual of taking dowry has caused serious problems. A newly married bride suffers domestic violence in the form of harassment, physical abuse or death when she is thought to have not brought enough dowry with marriage.
- Some cases end up in suicides by hanging, self-poisoning or by fire. In dowry deaths, the groom's family is the perpetrator of murder or suicide.
- Dowry deaths in India are not limited to any specific religion, and it is found among Hindus, Muslims, Sikhs and others.
- The **Dowry Prohibition Act 1961**, prohibits the request, payment or acceptance of a dowry, "as consideration for the marriage", where "**dowry**" is defined as a gift demanded or given as a precondition for a marriage.
  - Gifts given without a precondition are not considered dowry and are legal.
  - Asking or giving of dowry can be punished by imprisonment of up to 6 months or a fine.
  - Murder and suicide under compulsion are addressed by India's criminal penal code.
- The law was made more stringent with **Section 498A of Indian Penal Code**.
- Under the **Protection of Women from Domestic Violence Act 2005 (PWDVA)**, a woman can seek help against dowry harassment by approaching a domestic violence protection officer.

Effects

- Physical health outcomes include injury (from lacerations to fractures and internal organ injuries), unwanted pregnancy, gynaecological problems, STDs including HIV, miscarriage, pelvic inflammatory disease, chronic pelvic pain, headaches, permanent disabilities, asthma, irritable bowel syndrome, self-injurious behaviours (smoking, unprotected sex).
- Mental health effects can include depression, fear, anxiety, low self-esteem, sexual dysfunction, eating disorders, obsessive-compulsive disorder or post traumatic stress disorder. Fatal effects can include suicide, homicide, maternal mortality or HIV/AIDS.

Box 4.2—The Goygaon Horror

In a macabre case of 'honour killing', the Maharashtra Police on 6th Dec 2021 arrested an 18-year-old youth and his mother for allegedly beheading his elder sister with a sickle. The incident happened on 5th Dec afternoon in the small agricultural village of Goygaon in Vaijapur tehsil of Aurangabad.

Hours after committing the gruesome murder, the accused Sanket Mote, 18, along with his mother Shobha Mote, 40, surrendered to the police and confessed to their crime.

The Goygaon Police said, preliminary investigations indicated a case of 'honour killing' as the accused and his mother were enraged after the victim Kirti, 19, and her boyfriend Ajay Thore, 23, both living in the same village, eloped on June 21.

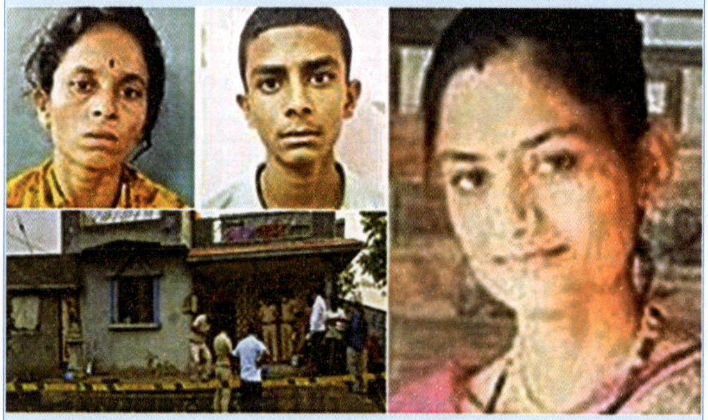

Clockwise from above left: Shobha Mote, Sanket Mote, Kirti and the scene of the murder

A few days before the gruesome murder, the couple arrived back at the village after getting married at Alandi, Pune, 6 months ago, against the wishes of her family as the boy's reputation was allegedly shady. Upon learning of their return, the mother–son duo went to meet the girl (Kirti) at her husband's home and hinted at a rapprochement, following which she went to the kitchen to prepare tea and snacks for them.

The mother–son followed her to the kitchen, where Shobha Mote grabbed her legs, while Sanket whipped out a sickle and beheaded his sister.

Later, the mother–son threw Kirti's head outside the house and went to the police station to give themselves up and admitted to the crime.

In Goygaon, sometime later, horrified neighbours saw the woman's head outside the home and the headless body lying inside in a pool of blood and alerted the police.

NATIONAL HUMAN RIGHTS COMMISSION (NHRC)

- The **National Human Rights Commission (NHRC) of India** is a statutory public body constituted on **12th Oct 1993** under the Protection of Human Rights Act of 1993 (amended in 2006 and 2019).
- The NHRC is responsible for the protection and promotion of human rights, defined as "Rights relating to life, liberty, equality and dignity of the individual guaranteed by the constitution of India".

Functions of NHRC

- Proactively or reactively inquire into violations of human rights by government of India or negligence of such violation by a public servant.
- Recommend measures for effective implementation of human rights.
- Review the factors including acts of terrorism that inhibit the enjoyment of human rights and recommend appropriate remedial measures
- Undertake and promote research in the field of human rights.
- Visit jails and study the condition of inmates.
- Engage in human rights education among various sections of society and promote awareness of the safeguards available for the protection of these rights through publications, the media, seminars and other available means.
- Encourage the efforts of NGOs and institutions that work in the field of human rights voluntarily.

Composition

- A Chairperson, who has been a Chief Justice of India or a Judge of the Supreme Court.
- One member who is, or has been, a Judge of the Supreme Court of India and one member who is, or has been, the Chief Justice of a High Court.
- Three Members, out of which at least one shall be a woman to be appointed from amongst persons having knowledge of, or practical experience in, matters relating to human rights.
- In addition, the Chairpersons of National Commissions, viz., National Commission for Scheduled Castes, National Commission for Scheduled Tribes, National Commission for Women, National Commission for Minorities, National Commission for Backward Classes, National Commission for Protection of Child Rights; the Chief Commissioner for Persons with Disabilities serve as ex-officio members.

Upholding the Dignity and Protecting the Rights of the Dead

- There is no specific law in India for protecting the rights of the dead. However, the courts have time and again reiterated to uphold the dignity and protect the rights of the dead. The Supreme Court of India in the landmark case of Parmanand Katara v. Union of India in 1989 recognized that the right to life, fair treatment and dignity, extends not only to a living person but also to a dead body. These rights have been derived from Article 21 of the Constitution of India.

Basic Principles for Upholding the Dignity & Protecting the Rights of the Dead

A. **General**:
1. No discrimination in treatment of the body in any form – Ensure that the dead body is properly preserved and handled irrespective of religion, region, caste, gender, etc.
2. No physical exploitation – Any form of physical exploitation of the body of the dead violates the basic right of the deceased person.

3. Decent and timely burial/cremation.
4. Justice in case of death due to crime – The dead have the right to receive justice in cases where death occurs due to crime.
5. Implementation of legal will – The will, if any, left by the dead must be respected and honoured.
6. No defamation after death – The deceased person should not be defamed by any kind of statement or visible representation, made or published intending to harm his/her reputation.
7. No breach of privacy – The deceased person has the right to privacy, i.e., the right to control the dissemination of information about one's privacy.

B. **Hospital Administration**:

1. Clothing of the dead body: Clothing of the deceased should be collected, examined as well as preserved and sealed by the doctor conducting the autopsy, and should be sent for further examination at the concerned forensic science laboratory. Further, it should be covered in special Body Bags for proper transportation.
2. Storage of unclaimed bodies: Unclaimed bodies must be stored under safe conditions in a deep freezer to prevent any decay or damage.
3. Segregation and arrangement of the dead bodies: It must be ensured that the bodies are segregated based on gender and are kept in a dignified manner by avoiding piling up.
4. Release of dead bodies: The hospital administration should be explicitly prohibited from deliberately retaining any dead body on the count of pending bill payment. Hospitals must hand over the body to the family of the deceased or to the civic body (if it is an unclaimed body) in a dignified way.
5. Licensure for use of unclaimed bodies: Hospitals that utilise unclaimed bodies for academic, research and training of medical students must have valid license for the same.

C. **Medical Practitioners**

1. Implementation of the ethical guidelines of ICMR: All medical practitioners must follow the guidelines of the ICMR while dealing with the claimed as well as unclaimed dead bodies.
2. Announcement of death: After death, it must be officially pronounced/declared by a doctor without any delay.
3. Forensic Medicine Department and Practitioners:
   a. Trained and qualified professionals: Only trained and qualified professional in forensic medicine should perform the autopsy procedure and the use of inappropriate tools such as a hammer, etc., should be avoided.
   b. Video-filming and photography of postmortem examination: In case of custodial death where there is a requirement of postmortem examination, NHRC guidelines for video-filming and photography should be complied with accordingly.
   c. Handing over the body to the family: It must be ensured that the external appearance of the deceased and the incisions on the body must be hidden by clothes while handing over the body to the family/relatives.
   d. Timely autopsy: It must be ensured that the postmortem examination is done without any delay, so that funeral arrangements are not delayed.
   e. Protection of personal and genetic information: Genetic data obtained through DNA profiling must be handled carefully and confidentially as the same may be required to trace the identity of unclaimed dead bodies. For this, data banks should be properly maintained to store the genetic data and biological samples of unclaimed bodies, as per the existing laws.

D. **Mortuary Services**

1. Mortuary hygiene: Regular mopping and cleaning of mortuary should be undertaken so that dead body remains are preserved in a proper, clean environment, thereby maintaining its dignity.
2. Secured information: The facility should maintain confidentiality of clinical records and must have a mechanism for guarding information related to the deceased, especially for cases that are stigmatized and socially criticised, such as that of HIV and suicidal cases.
3. Maintaining privacy of premises: Postmortem room should not come under the direct line of sight of the general public/visitors. To ensure the same, provision of curtain, screen or buffer area may be made in a postmortem room.
4. Removing physical/infrastructural barriers: The facility must have infrastructure for delivery of assured services, to meet the prescribed norms. All basic requirements must be available and maintained as per the Indian Public Health Standard Guidelines for District Hospitals for management of dead bodies.
5. Sensitization of the staff: The mortuary administration may sensitize the staff from time to time to train them in handling of dead bodies, and deal with the attendants of the deceased with sensitivity.

E. **Police**

1. No delay in postmortem: The police administration should ensure that there is no undue delay in calling a forensic team to the crime scene and in transferring the body of the deceased for postmortem examination. Transfer of the dead body to the hospital administration and submission of the complete inquest form should be done within the stipulated period of time.
2. Handling of the dead body: In cases where death has occurred due to fire accidents, self-immolation, murders, death due to sexual offences, custodial deaths, suicides, road and other accidents, the body of the deceased must be covered, handled with respect and sent to mortuary immediately for performing the autopsy procedures.

3. Identification of the dead bodies: For identification of the dead bodies, labelling of a unique body code, technical photographs, other data from the dead bodies may be collected and stored under the police record for identification and further transfer of the dead body to the family.
4. Availability of body bags & basic forensic kits: 'Body bags' and basic forensic kits to be made available at police stations to maintain the sanctity of the body and collection of evidence from the incident site, if it is a case of homicide/accident/unnatural death.
5. Keeping the dead bodies in the mortuary: It may be ensured that the dead bodies do not remain in the mortuary for more than 72 hours. In case of an unidentified body, the police should make serious efforts for its identification and disposal accordingly in a dignified manner.
6. Photography: Video-filming and photography of the postmortem examination should be done by a person trained in forensic photography and videography.

FM 4.10: Core – Written/Viva Voce
- Describe communication between doctors, public and media.

This issue has been dealt with under FM 4.6: Duties of a medical practitioner towards patients and society *(page no. 287)*.

It involves attitudinal, ethical and communication (AETCOM) domains. It can be learnt/taught in the form of role play based on various kinds of scenarios.

FM 4.11: Core – Written/Viva Voce
- Describe and discuss euthanasia.

EUTHANASIA

(MERCY KILLING, ASSISTED SUICIDE, PHYSICIAN-ASSISTED SUICIDE, AID-IN-DYING, SELF DELIVERANCE)

Origin

- The word **euthanasia** is derived from the Greek, and means a "**good death**", though it has undergone considerable distortion over a period of time to assume its present day meaning of "mercy killing".

Definition

- Euthanasia refers to the infliction of a **painless death on an individual suffering from severe, intractable pain or discomfort, arising out of a terminal illness or condition**.

Classification*

- ***Voluntary***: The dying individual consents to the act.
- ***Non-voluntary***: The dying individual is incapable of giving or refusing consent, e.g., an irreversibly comatose patient.
- ***Involuntary (Compulsory)***: Decision by society to terminate the life of an individual.
- ***Active***: Inflicting painless death by an act of commission, e.g., injection of a lethal dose of barbiturates.
- ***Passive***: Inflicting painless death by an act of omission, e.g., withdrawal of life support to a comatose patient.
- ***Paediatric***: Euthanasia administered to seriously sick or deformed infants.
- ***Geriatric***: Euthanasia administered to seriously sick, aged individuals.
- ***Battlefield***: Euthanasia administered to severely wounded or handicapped individual.

Arguments in Favour of Euthanasia

- The medical ethos of the "**sanctity of life**" implying the unqualified duty to preserve life at all costs, has come under increasing challenge. There is a perceptibly growing movement away from a rigid obligation on the part of a doctor to preserve life "at all costs", towards a more flexible duty to provide good palliative terminal care. Terminal illness is considered best treated by providing optimum conditions for death rather than by the use of increasingly invasive techniques to prolong some sort of existence. A conscious, dying patient can make his own decision, since patient's autonomy is today considered to be the cornerstone of ethical medical practice. To continue to treat in the face of contrary instructions can attract legal liabilities, though the exact position is still not clear-cut in India.
- In many Western countries, it is generally accepted that there is no moral obligation on the part of a doctor to preserve life at the expense of suffering, and if in the course of good terminal care, the use of drugs inadvertently hastens death, this is ethically acceptable within the doctrine of "**double effect**," i.e., an ill effect is morally acceptable as long as there is a greater, intended good effect from an action.
  - This concept was first given legal sanction in relation to euthanasia by **Justice Devlin** in the ***Bodkin Adams case* (1957)**, when he remarked, "The doctor is entitled to relieve pain and suffering even if the measures he takes may incidentally shorten life."
    - **John Bodkin Adams** (1899–1983) (**Fig. 4.6**) was a British general practitioner, convicted fraudster and suspected serial killer. Between 1946 and 1956, 163 of his patients died while in coma, which was deemed to be worthy of investigation. In addition, 132 out of 310 patients had left Adams money or items in their will.
    - Adams was tried and acquitted for the murder of one patient in 1957, while another count of murder was withdrawn by the Prosecution in what was later described as "an abuse of process" by the presiding judge Patrick Devlin, causing questions to be asked in Parliament of the United Kingdom about the prosecution's handling of events. Adams was found guilty in a subsequent trial of 13 offences of prescription drug fraud, lying on cremation forms,

**Mnemonic* (to help remember the 8 categories): VIP BAN PG.

obstruction of justice during a police search and failing to keep a dangerous drugs register. He was struck off by the General Medical Council in 1957, but was reinstated in 1961.

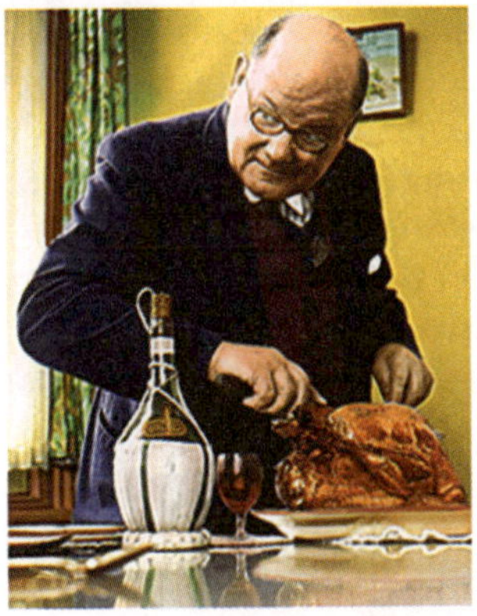

Fig. 4.6 John Bodkin Adams: Celebrating his acquittal in 1957

- The trial also had several important legal ramifications. It established the "**doctrine of double effect**", whereby a doctor giving treatment with the aim of relieving pain may lawfully, as an unintentional result, shorten life. Secondly, because of the publicity surrounding Adams's committal hearing, the law was changed to allow defendants to ask for such hearings to be held in private.

- The possibility of maintaining "physiological life," i.e., the continuation of the body functions by artificial means, while the patient remains unconscious over a period of months or years, has introduced a new dimension into the debate – "**quality of life**". Clearly, the sustaining of physiological functions with no prospect of recovery of consciousness or contact with the patient's environment has led to considerable debate as to whether or not such support systems should be continued, and who should be responsible for the decision to turn off such systems.
- Views vary widely, but there is a substantial proportion of population in countries such as the USA which favours the view that support systems can be switched off by attending doctors with consent from the victim's relatives, in certain cases.
- The case of ***Karen Ann Quinlan*** is representative of this. Karen (**Fig. 4.7**), a 21-year-old girl fell into a coma after imbibing an overdose of alcohol and drugs on 15th April, 1975. She passed into "persistent vegetative state" from which recovery was extremely remote. Her parents, both devout Roman Catholics, were initially hopeful of a miracle, but as the months passed by, they realised that this was only wishful thinking, and that their daughter was never going to come back to meaningful existence. They requested that life support systems prolonging the futile ordeal be switched off. The doctors attending on the case refused, and the issue was taken to court. In 1976, the New Jersey Supreme Court delivered a verdict in favour of Karen's parents. However, while the support systems were subsequently switched off, artificial feeding was not stopped, and Karen continued to "live" for nearly 10 years before her heart finally stopped in 1985. The case however served to focus medical attention on a topic that had for decades been considered taboo.

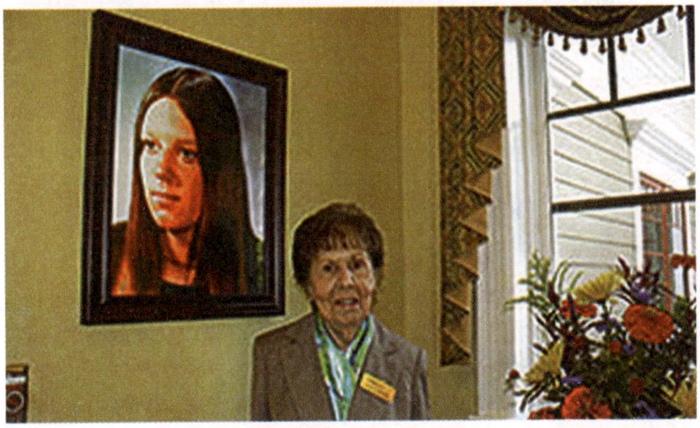

Fig. 4.7 Karen Ann Quinlan's mother in front of the framed picture of her daughter

- Today, not only in the case of terminally unconscious patients, but also in conscious patients (who are suffering from an intractable, painful, terminal illness), euthanasia is being increasingly considered as applicable, provided the patient concerned makes the request, and he is judged to be of sound and rational mind. Withdrawing treatment and allowing a patient to die (passive euthanasia) is therefore not perceived as repugnant anymore in certain situations. In fact in several Western countries, adult individuals over a specified age can execute a "**living will**" or "**advance directive**" which entitles him to refuse treatment any time in future in the event of a catastrophic accident or natural disease.
- While passive euthanasia has been accorded some semblance of acceptance in certain situations by most people, active euthanasia is in the centre of a heated (and often bitter) debate, with vociferous sections of the population in India and elsewhere either strongly advocating or condemning its practice.
  - Despite its unresolved status, active euthanasia is being employed without serious legal difficulties in some countries, e.g., USA, Sweden, etc.
  - Some countries have virtually legalised active euthanasia, if performed by a physician under strict guidelines (**physician-assisted suicide**), e.g., Holland, Belgium and Luxembourg.
  - Some parts of the world have enacted legal statutes, e.g., **The Death with Dignity Act (1994)** of the State of Oregon, USA, and The Northern Territory of Australia, which was however overturned by the Australian Senate in 1997.
  - Holland practices physician-assisted suicide openly ever since the Royal Dutch Medical Association officially endorsed it in 1984, and the parliament approved the practice, provided it was done within a framework of specified guidelines.
- Countries that have **legalized voluntary, active euthanasia**

(in some cases, physician-assisted suicide) as of 2022: Netherlands, Belgium, Canada, Colombia, Luxembourg, Australia (some states), New Zealand, Spain.*

- In 2021, a Peruvian court allowed euthanasia for a single person, Ana Estrada.

- Switzerland and **death tourism**: Hundreds of Europeans travel to Zurich to end their lives because of '***Dignitas***', an organization set up in 1998 to help people with terminal illnesses. They are provided with a lethal dose of barbiturates which they have to take themselves. In fact, in several other European countries, assisted suicide is not illegal and can have the involvement of non-physicians.

Arguments Against Euthanasia

- The opponents of euthanasia (particularly *active euthanasia*) state that there are moral, religious and ethical objections which cannot be ignored. They argue that no one has the right to take away the life of an individual, not even the individual himself. The concept of "**sanctity of life**" is inviolable and doctors having taken an oath (the Hippocratic Oath) "to preserve life at all costs", cannot justify allowing a patient to die either through active or passive means.
- It is also true that doctors are not omniscient; there have been several cases where a patient certified as terminally ill, has survived and led a reasonably fulfilling existence for several years with good palliative care. The classical example is that of renowned physicist **Stephen Hawking** who was diagnosed with motor neurone disease, when he was in his twenties and given 2 years to live. He went on to live for decades and contributed significantly to our understanding of cosmic physics.
  - However, "**Right to Die**" activists argue that he must not be held up as an example to encourage doctors to prolong life at all costs, as his is an exceptional case. Besides, they go on to state that just as Hawking has been given the right to live in spite of a debilitating illness that has no known cure, another individual in the same situation should be given the choice of whether he would like to live (right to life) or die (right to die). There should not be compulsion either way. Even if a patient does have only a few months to live, adequate medical care can in most cases serve to make him reasonably comfortable for the remaining period till natural death supervenes. The emphasis therefore should be on improving palliative care, rather than improving methods of terminating life.
- A disturbing feature that has come to light in those countries where physician-assisted euthanasia has been accorded legal sanction, is the impatience (and sometimes greed) of the relatives of a dying patient who happens to be affluent, in pressing ahead with "euthanasia" for their own selfish ends. In such cases the patient's "**right to die**" is subtly converted to a "**duty to die**", pressure being brought on the hapless victim to accede to the infliction of "painless death".

Current Legal Status in India

- On 9th **March 2018**, the Supreme Court of India **legalised passive euthanasia** by means of the withdrawal of life support to patients in a permanent vegetative state. The decision was made as part of the verdict in a case involving **Aruna Shanbaug**, who had been in a "persistent vegetative state (PVS)" until her death in 2015 (**Box 4.3**).
- The Supreme Court specified two irreversible conditions to permit Passive Euthanasia Law in its earlier 2011 Law:
  - The brain-dead for whom the ventilator can be switched off.
  - Those in a "persistent vegetative state (PVS)" for whom the feed can be tapered out and pain-managing palliatives be added, according to laid-down international specifications.
  - The same judgement-law also asked for the scrapping of IPC 309, the code which penalises those who survive suicide-attempts. In December 2014, government of India declared its intention to do so.
- **Active euthanasia**, including the administration of lethal compounds for the purpose of ending life, is still **illegal** in India, and in most countries.
- In 2018, the Supreme Court of India declared that if strict guidelines are followed, the government would honour "**living wills**" allowing consenting patients to be passively euthanized, if the patient suffers from a terminal illness or is in a vegetative state.
  - However, there were a number of cumbersome conditions, and a Constitution Bench of the Supreme Court modified the directions relating to advance medical directives or living wills issued in the 2018 judgement, on a request by the Indian Council for Critical Care Medicine, making the entire process much easier. The order was issued on **24th Jan 2023**.

Box 4.3—Aruna Shanbaug Case

Aruna Shanbaug was a nurse working at the King Edward Memorial Hospital, Parel, Mumbai. On 27th November, 1973 she was strangled and sodomized by Sohanlal Walmiki, a sweeper. During the attack, she was strangled with a chain, and the deprivation of oxygen left her in a vegetative state. She was treated at KEM ever since the incident and was kept alive by feeding tubes.

On behalf of Aruna, her friend Pinki Virani, a social activist, filed a petition in the Supreme Court arguing that the "continued existence of Aruna is in violation of her right to live in dignity".

The Supreme Court made its decision on 7th March 2011. The court rejected the plea to discontinue Aruna's life support but issued a set of broad guidelines legalising

contd.

Mnemonic to remember the names of the countries: NBC CLANS passive euthanasia in India. The Supreme Court's decision to reject the discontinuation of Aruna's life support was based on the fact that the hospital staff who were treating and taking care of her did not support euthanizing her.

Aruna died from pneumonia on 18th May 2015, after being in a coma for a period of 42 years.

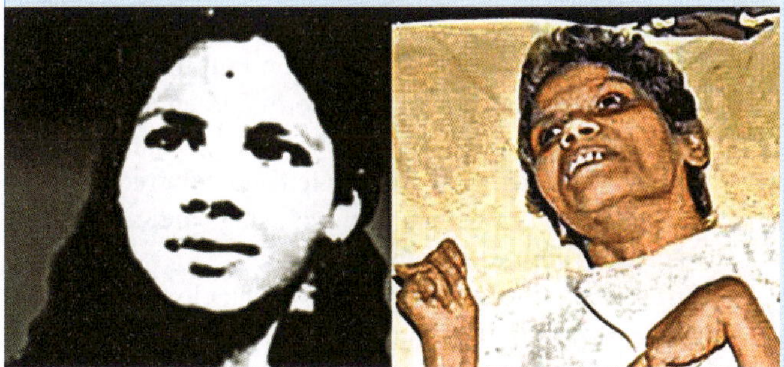

Aruna Shanbaug as a young woman (L); in vegetative state (R)

Chronology of Euthanasia (Summary of important events from early 20th century)

Year	Developments
1906	First euthanasia bill drafted in the USA (Ohio), but it does not succeed.
1935	World's first euthanasia society is founded in London.
1938	The Euthanasia Society of America is founded in New York
1967	The first "living will" is written by American attorney Louis Kutner.
1974	The Euthanasia Society in New York is renamed the Society for the Right to Die.
1976	First international meeting of Right to Die groups.
1978	A Broadway play *"Whose Life is it Anyway"*? about a quadriplegic wanting to die is staged for the first time. It goes on to become a massive hit and is followed by its movie version in 1982.
1980	Hemlock Society (advocating euthanasia) is founded in California by journalist Derek Humphry.
1980	World Federation of Right to Die Societies is formed in Oxford, England.
1984	The Netherlands Supreme Court approves voluntary euthanasia under certain conditions.
1990	Dr Jack Kevorkian (Michigan, USA) assists for the first time, in the death of a patient. Over the next 9 years, he assists in a total of 130 deaths. He will be tried 4 times before finally being convicted in his 5th trial, in April 1999 for 2nd degree murder and sentenced to 10–25 years in prison.
1991	Derek Humphry publishes *"Final Exit"*, a how-to book on self deliverance. It quickly tops the US best-seller list, and is subsequently translated into 12 languages.
1999	Dr Kevorkian sentenced to 10–25 years in prison for 2nd degree murder of Thomas Youk suffering from motor neurone disease. The videotape of Youk's death had been telecast on national television, provoking public outrage.
2000	The Netherlands becomes the first country in the world to legalize physician-assisted suicide.

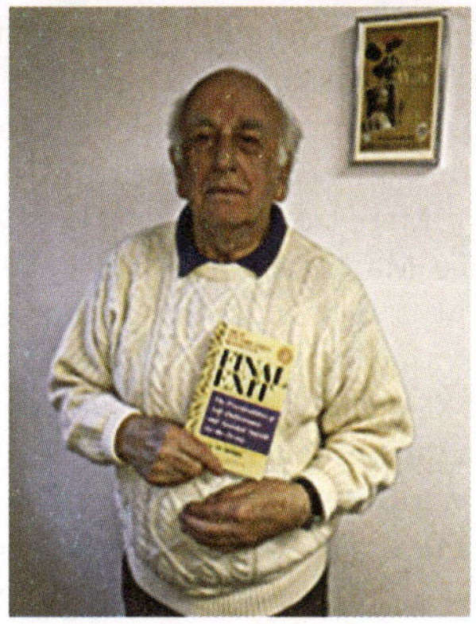

Derek Humphry in 2017, holding a copy of his bestselling 1991 book, *Final Exit*

2000	The Switzerland-based Dignitas, a legal euthanasia centre begins its operations under the lax euthanasia laws of the country, and as of 2008 has assisted nearly 900 deaths. However, a clear-cut law legalizing physician-assisted suicide has so far not been passed in Switzerland.
2005	Terri Schiavo collapses in her Florida home in full cardiac arrest on 25th Feb, 1990. She suffers massive brain damage due to lack of oxygen and, after 2½ months in a coma, her diagnosis is changed to vegetative state. For the next 2 years doctors attempt therapy, hoping to return her to a state of awareness. In 1998 Schiavo's husband, Michael, petitions the Court of Florida to remove her feeding tube. He is opposed by Terri's parents, who argue that she is conscious. The court determines that she would not wish to continue life-prolonging measures, and on April 24, 2001, her feeding tube is removed for the first time, only to be reinserted several days later. On Feb 25, 2005, a County judge orders the removal of Terri Schiavo's feeding tube. Several appeals follow. After all these fail, staff at the hospice facility where Terri was being cared for disconnect the feeding tube on March 18, 2005. Terri dies on March 31, 2005.
2007	Dr Jack Kevorkian is released from prison after serving 8 years.

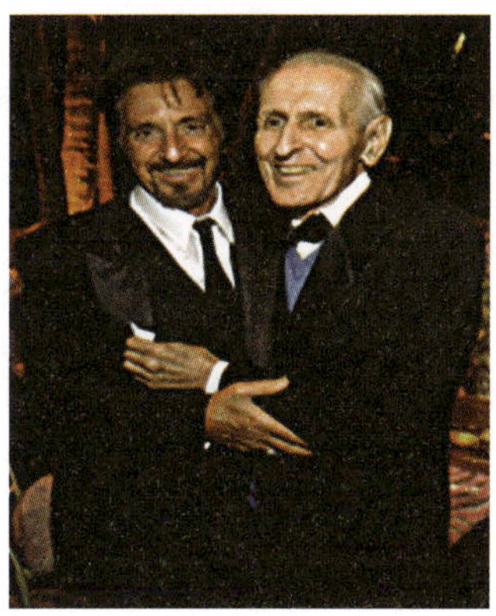

Jack Kevorkian (R) with Al Pacino at the premiere of his biographical film

2008 'Exit International' founded by Dr Philip Nitschke, an Australian physician, devises "Exit Bag" for euthanasia, which utilises nitrogen for causing rapid death. Earlier devices include Thanatron (Jack Kevorkian), Mercitron (Jack Kevorkian) and Deliverance Machine (Philip Nitschke).

2009 Pinki Virani, a journalist and euthanasia activist in India, files a petition in the Supreme Court to stop doctors of KEM hospital (Mumbai) from force feeding Aruna Shanbaug, and allow her to finally die a dignified natural death.

2010 Al Pacino plays Jack Kevorkian in the HBO Film *"You Don't Know Jack"*. He wins the Emmy for Outstanding Lead Actor, along with the Golden Globe award in 2011 for his role as Kevorkian.

2011 Jack Kevorkian dies at the age of 83 (from natural causes).

2011 The Supreme Court of India turns down the plea of Pinki Virani to stop doctors of KEM hospital (Mumbai) from force feeding Aruna Shanbaug. Strangely, while the Supreme Court disallows withdrawal of life support for Aruna, it lays down guidelines for passive euthanasia.

2015 Aruna Shanbaug passes away in hospital without ever regaining full control of her mental faculties.

2017 Philip Nitschke invents the Sarco pod (Pegasos; Suicide pod) a euthanasia device consisting of a 3D-printed detachable capsule mounted on a stand that contains a canister of liquid nitrogen which causes painless death by inert gas asphyxiation. The decrease in oxygen levels occurs rapidly which prevents panic, sense of suffocation and struggling before unconsciousness, known as the "hypercapnic alarm response" caused by the presence of high carbon dioxide concentrations in the blood.

2018 The Supreme Court of India legalises passive euthanasia, and approves the concept of 'Medical Directive' or 'Living Will'.

2023 A Constitution Bench of the Supreme Court simplifies the procedure for implementing living wills on a request by the Indian Council for Critical Care Medicine.

FM 4.12: Core – Written/Viva Voce

- Discuss legal and ethical issues in relation to stem cell research

STEM CELL RESEARCH

- In multicellular organisms, **stem cells** are undifferentiated or partially differentiated cells that can differentiate into various types of cells and proliferate indefinitely to produce more of the same stem cell (**Fig. 4.8**). They are the earliest type of cell in a cell lineage.
- They are found in both embryonic and adult organisms, but they have slightly different properties in each.
  - They are usually distinguished from **progenitor cells**, which cannot divide indefinitely.
  - And **precursor** or **blast cells**, which are usually committed to differentiating into one cell type.
- In mammals, roughly 50–150 cells make up the inner cell mass during the blastocyst stage of embryonic development, around days 5–14. These have stem-cell capability.
  - In vivo, they eventually differentiate into all of the body's cell types (making them **pluripotent**). This process starts with the differentiation into the three germ layers – the ectoderm, mesoderm and endoderm – at the gastrulation stage.
  - However, when they are isolated and cultured in vitro, they can be kept in the stem-cell stage and are known as **embryonic stem cells (ESCs)**.
- **Adult stem cells** are found in a few select locations in the body, known as **niches**, such as those in the bone marrow or gonads. They exist to replenish rapidly lost cell types and are **multipotent** or **unipotent**, meaning they only differentiate into a few cell types or one type of cell.
  - In mammals, they include, among others, ***hematopoietic stem cells***, which replenish blood and immune cells, ***basal cells***, which maintain the skin epithelium, and ***mesenchymal stem cells***, which maintain bone, cartilage, muscle and fat cells.
  - Adult stem cells are a small minority of cells; they are vastly outnumbered by the progenitor cells and terminally differentiated cells that they differentiate into.

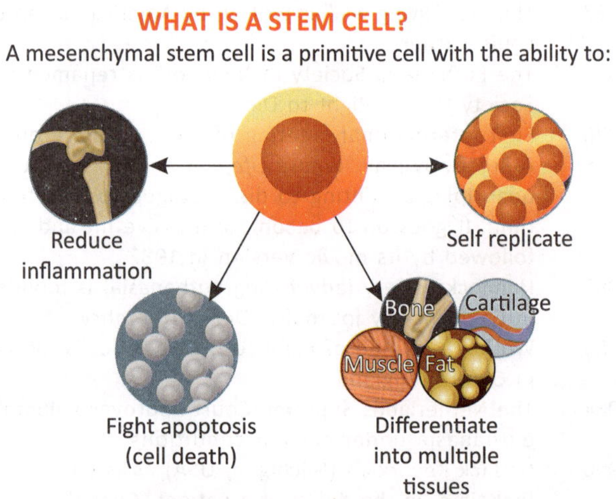

Fig. 4.8 Stem cell functions

- Research into stem cells grew out of findings by Canadian biologists Ernest McCulloch, James Till and Andrew Becker at the University of Toronto and the Ontario Cancer Institute in the 1960s.
- As of today, the only established medical therapy using stem cells is **hematopoietic stem cell transplantation**, first performed in 1958 by French oncologist Georges Mathé.
- Since 1998, however, it has been possible to culture and differentiate human embryonic stem cells (in stem-cell lines). The process of isolating these cells has been controversial, because it typically results in the destruction of the embryo.
  - Sources for isolating ESCs have been restricted in some

European countries and Canada, but others such as the UK and China have promoted the research.

- **Somatic cell nuclear transfer** is a cloning method that can be used to create a cloned embryo for the use of its embryonic stem cells in stem cell therapy.
- In 2006, a Japanese team led by Shinya Yamanaka discovered a method to convert mature body cells back into stem cells. These were termed **induced pluripotent stem cells (iPSCs)**.
- Since pluripotent stem cells have the ability to differentiate into any type of cell, they are used in the development of medical treatments for a wide range of conditions.
  - Treatments that have been proposed include treatment for physical trauma, degenerative conditions and genetic diseases (in combination with gene therapy). Yet further treatments using stem cells could potentially be developed due to their ability to repair extensive tissue damage.
- Great levels of success and potential have been realized from research using adult stem cells. In early 2009, the FDA approved the first human clinical trials using embryonic stem cells.
- Only cells from an embryo at the morula stage or earlier are truly totipotent, meaning that they are able to form all cell types including placental cells. Adult stem cells are generally limited to differentiating into different cell types of their tissue of origin. However, some evidence suggests that adult stem cell plasticity may exist, increasing the number of cell types a given adult stem cell can become.

Controversy (Ethical & Legal Issues)

- The **stem cell controversy** is the consideration of the ethics of research involving the development and use of human embryos. Most commonly, this controversy focuses on **embryonic stem cells**.
  - Not all stem cell research involves human embryos. For example, adult stem cells, amniotic stem cells and induced pluripotent stem cells do not involve creating, using or destroying human embryos, and thus are minimally, if at all, controversial.
  - Many less controversial sources of acquiring stem cells include using cells from the umbilical cord, breast milk, and bone marrow, which are not pluripotent.
- Destruction of a human embryo is required in order to research new embryonic cell lines. Much of the debate surrounding human embryonic stem cells, therefore, concern ethical and legal quandaries around the destruction of an embryo. Ethical and legal questions central to the controversy include the following:
  - What point does one consider life to begin?
  - Is it justified to destroy a human embryo though it has the potential to cure a number of patients and further our understanding of disease?
- Political leaders debate how to regulate and fund research studies that involve the techniques used to remove the embryo cells. No clear consensus has so far emerged.
  - Much of the criticism has been a result of religious beliefs and, in the most high-profile case, US President George W Bush signed an executive order banning the use of federal funding for any stem cell lines other than those already in existence.
  - This ban was in part revoked by his successor Barack Obama, who stated: "As a person of faith, I believe we are called to care for each other and work to ease human suffering. I believe we have been given the capacity and will to pursue this research and the humanity and conscience to do so responsibly."
- Stem cell debates have motivated and reinvigorated the **anti-abortion movement**, whose members are concerned with the rights and status of the human embryo as an early-aged human life. They believe that embryonic stem cell research profits from and violates the sanctity of life and is tantamount to murder.
  - The fundamental assertion of those who oppose embryonic stem cell research is the belief that human life is inviolable, combined with the belief that human life begins when a sperm cell fertilizes an egg cell to form a single cell.
  - The view of those in favour is that these embryos would otherwise be discarded, and if used as stem cells, they can survive as a part of a living human person.
- **Arguments in favour of stem cell research**:
  - Medical researchers widely report that stem cell research has the potential to dramatically alter approaches to understanding and treating diseases, and to alleviate suffering (**Fig. 4.9**). In the future, most medical researchers anticipate being able to use technologies derived from stem cell research to treat a variety of diseases and impairments. Spinal cord injuries and Parkinson's disease are two important examples.
  - Embryos are not equivalent to human life, as they are still incapable of surviving outside the womb (i.e., they only have the potential for life).
  - More than a third of zygotes do not implant after conception. Thus, far more embryos are lost due to chance than are proposed to be used for embryonic stem cell research or treatments.
  - Blastocysts are a cluster of human cells that have not differentiated into distinct organ tissue, making cells of the inner cell mass no more "human" than a skin cell.
  - Some parties contend that embryos are not human persons, believing that the life of *Homo sapiens* only begins when the heartbeat develops, which is during the fifth week of pregnancy, or when the brain begins developing activity, which has been detected at 54 days after conception.
  - In vitro fertilization (IVF) generates thousands of unused embryos. Many of these thousands of IVF embryos are slated for destruction. Using them for scientific research uses a resource that would otherwise be wasted.

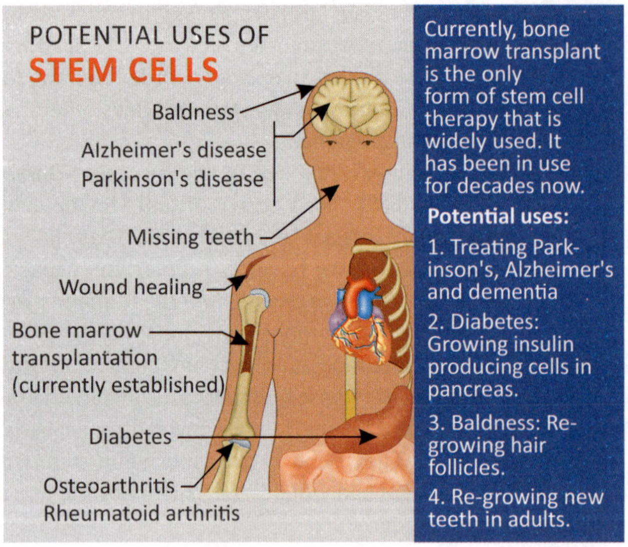

Fig. 4.9 Stem cell therapy

- While the destruction of human embryos is required to establish a stem cell line, no new embryos have to be destroyed to work with existing stem cell lines. It would be wasteful not to continue to make use of these cell lines as a resource.
- Embryonic stem cells make up a significant proportion of a developing embryo, while adult stem cells exist as minor populations within a mature individual (e.g., in every 1000 cells of the bone marrow, only one will be a usable stem cell). Thus, embryonic stem cells are likely to be easier to isolate and grow ex vivo than adult stem cells.
- Embryonic stem cells divide more rapidly than adult stem cells, potentially making it easier to generate large numbers of cells for therapeutic means. In contrast, adult stem cell might not divide fast enough to offer immediate treatment.
- Embryonic stem cells have greater plasticity, potentially allowing them to treat a wider range of diseases.
- Adult stem cells from the patient's own body might not be effective in treatment of genetic disorders. Allogeneic embryonic stem cell transplantation (i.e., from a healthy donor) may be more practical in these cases than gene therapy of a patient's own cell.
- DNA abnormalities found in adult stem cells that are caused by toxins and sunlight may make them poorly suited for treatment.
- Embryonic stem cells have the potential to cure chronic and degenerative diseases which current medicine has been unable to effectively treat.
- Viability is another standard under which embryos and foetuses have been regarded as human lives. "**Viability**" is the point at which a foetus is "potentially able to live outside the mother's womb, albeit with artificial aid." The point of viability is generally considered to be about 24–28 weeks. Embryos used in medical research for stem cells are well below development that would enable viability.

FM 4.13 – 4.15: Core – Written/Viva Voce

- Describe social aspects of medicolegal cases with respect to victims of assault, rape, attempted suicide, homicide, domestic violence, dowry-related cases.
- Describe and discuss the challenges in managing medicolegal cases including development of skills in relationship management – human behaviour, communication skills, conflict resolution techniques.
- Describe the principles of handling pressure – definition, types, causes, sources and skills for managing the pressure while dealing with medicolegal cases by the doctor.

These issues have been dealt with under various other Competencies, and involve attitudinal, ethical and communication (AETCOM) domains. They can be learnt/ taught in the form of role play based on various kinds of scenarios.

FM 4.16: Core – Written/Viva Voce

- Describe and discuss Bioethics.

- **Bioethics** is the study of the ethical issues emerging from advances in biology, medicine and technologies. It proposes the discussion about moral discernment in society and it is often related to medical policy and practice, but also to broader questions such as environment and well-being.
- The field of bioethics addresses a broad area of human inquiry:
  - abortion
  - euthanasia
  - surrogacy
  - organ donation
  - right to refuse medical care for religious or cultural reasons.
- The scope of bioethics is bound to expand with biotechnology, including cloning, gene therapy, life extension, human genetic engineering, etc.

Principles

- One of the first areas addressed by modern bioethicists was that of **human experimentation**. The National Commission for the Protection of Human Subjects of Biomedical and Behavioral Research was initially established in 1974 to identify the basic ethical principles that should underlie the conduct of biomedical and behavioral research involving human subjects. However, the fundamental principles announced in the **Belmont Report (1979)** – namely, respect for persons, beneficence and justice – have influenced the thinking of bioethicists across a wide range of issues. Others have added non-maleficence, human dignity, and the sanctity of life to this list of cardinal values.

- The four main moral commitments are respect for **autonomy**, **beneficence**, **non-maleficence** and **justice**. Using these four principles and thinking about what the physicians' specific concern is for their scope of practice can help physicians make moral decisions. Many bioethicists, especially medical scholars, accord the highest priority to autonomy. They believe that each patient should determine which course of action they consider most in line with their beliefs. In other words, the patient should always have the freedom to choose their own treatment.
  - **Medical ethics** tends to be understood narrowly as applied professional ethics; whereas **Bioethics** has a more expansive application, touching upon the philosophy of science and issues of biotechnology.
  - The two fields often overlap, and the distinction is more so a matter of style than professional consensus. Medical ethics shares many principles with other branches of healthcare ethics, such as nursing ethics.
  - A bioethicist assists the health care and research community in examining moral issues involved in our understanding of life and death, and resolving ethical dilemmas in medicine and science.
    - Examples of this would be the topic of equality in medicine, the intersection of cultural practices and medical care, ethical distribution of healthcare resources in pandemics and issues of bioterrorism.
  - Bioethicists come from a wide variety of backgrounds and have training in a diverse array of disciplines. The field contains individuals trained in philosophy, medically trained clinician ethicists, lawyers, political scientists, religious scholars and theologians.
  - Leading journals in the medical field include The Journal of Medicine and Philosophy, the American Journal of Bioethics, the Journal of Medical Ethics, etc.
- Many religious communities have their histories of inquiry into bioethical issues and have developed rules and guidelines on how to deal with these issues from within the viewpoint of their respective faiths.
  - The Jewish, Christian and Muslim faiths have each developed a considerable body of literature on these matters. In the case of many non-Western cultures, a strict separation of religion from philosophy does not exist.
  - Buddhist bioethics, in general, is characterized by a naturalistic outlook that leads to a rationalistic, pragmatic approach.
  - In India, there are many leading bioethicists speaking from the Hindu tradition.
- Bioethics is today taught in courses at the undergraduate and graduate level in different academic disciplines or programmes, such as Philosophy, Medicine, Law, Social Sciences. It has become a requirement for professional accreditation in many health professional programmes (Medicine, Nursing, Rehabilitation), to have obligatory training in ethics (e.g., professional ethics, medical ethics, clinical ethics, nursing ethics).

FM 4.17: Core – Written/Viva Voce
- Describe and discuss Ethical Principles: Respect for autonomy, non-malfeasance, beneficence and justice.

Discussed under FM 4.1 *(page 277)* **and** FM 4.2. *(page 278)*

FM 4.18: Core – Written/Viva Voce
- Describe and discuss Medical Negligence including:
  - Civil and Criminal negligence
  - Contributory negligence
  - Corporate negligence & Products liability
  - Vicarious liability
  - Res ipsa loquitor
  - Prevention of medical negligence
  - Defence in medical negligence litigations

PROFESSIONAL NEGLIGENCE

(MEDICAL NEGLIGENCE; MEDICAL MALPRACTICE)

- **"Negligence" can be defined as doing something which a reasonable man would not do, or the omission to do something which a reasonable man would do.**
- In the medical context, negligence may result either from the doctor's lack of knowledge and skill, or from failure by the doctor in exercising due care in the performance of a procedure.
- Every medical practitioner is required to possess reasonable medical knowledge, and to exercise reasonable skill and care in the treatment of his patients. It does not imply that he should possess the highest degree of skill or knowledge. He is only expected to possess such skill and knowledge as possessed by ordinary competent men practicing medicine at that time under similar circumstances and conditions.
- He must therefore merely follow the prevalent standard procedures, and methods of diagnosis and treatment. No doctor is expected to possess all currently available medical knowledge, nor is he expected to be able to apply all known diagnostic and therapeutic techniques. But, a doctor of a particular standing as regards grade and experience, is expected to have a standard knowledge and capability commensurate with his professional status.
  - Thus, a house surgeon is not expected to possess the same skills as a consultant surgeon, but at the same time he is expected to provide a level of medical care which is within his competence.
- **Professional Negligence** is completely different from **Professional Misconduct (Infamous Conduct)**. **Table 4.2** outlines salient differences.

Elements of Negligence

- The elements of a negligent action generally comprise the following:
  - Existence of a **duty of care**.

Table 4.2 Differences between Professional Negligence and Professional Misconduct (Infamous Conduct)

Sl. No.	Feature	Professional Negligence	Professional Misconduct
1	Nature of offence	Absence of care and skill during treatment of patient	Violation of Code of Medical Ethics
2	Duty of care to patient	Should be present	Need not be present
3	Damage to patient	Should be present	Need not be present
4	Offence is tried in	Civil or Criminal Court	State Medical Council
5	Punishment	Payment of compensation and/or imprisonment	Warning or erasure of name from medical register
6	Appeal	Can be made to higher court	Can be made to State and Central Govt

- Failure to exercise such duty of care (**dereliction**).
- Causation of **damage** to the patient on account of dereliction.
- Reasonable **foreseeability of damage**.

- Professional negligence of doctors leading to **death of the patient** is punishable under **Sec 304-A** of the **Indian Penal Code**. According to this section. "*Whoever causes death of any person by any rash and negligent act not amounting to culpable homicide, shall be punished with imprisonment for a term which may extend to 2 years, with or without fine*".

Duty of Care

- A doctor charged with negligence must be shown to have been under a **duty of care** to the person complaining of negligence. If the doctor was not under a duty of care to the complainant, he cannot be charged for the negligence even though his conduct has caused damage to the complaining party.
- This relationship may be formed easily, and by no means depends on any formal acceptance of a patient by a doctor. Even in an acute emergency, once a doctor approaches an ill or injured person with the object of assisting him, a completely valid relationship is built, notwithstanding the fact that the patient may be unconscious and quite unaware of the doctor's presence.
- The fact that no payment is offered or expected makes no difference to the duty of care.
- However, when a doctor acts as a "Good Samaritan" and helps an injured person in a roadside accident, he will not be bound by duty of care.
- Again, when a doctor examines a patient for some purpose other than providing advice and treatment, no contractual obligation is established, and therefore no duty of care exists, e.g., medicolegal examination for disability, drunkenness, etc.

Dereliction of Duty

- Failure of a doctor to honour his duty that is owed to his patient is referred to as "**dereliction**."
- Such breach of duty may be an ***act of commission*** or an ***act of omission***. For example,
  - mistaken ligation of ureter during hysterectomy constitutes an act of commission,
  - failure to give anti-tetanus prophylaxis when it is required, is an act of omission.
- Breach of duty of care and skill is said to occur whenever a doctor fails to reach a standard of proficiency expected from him, i.e., his action will be compared to that of others with the same qualifications and expertise. Thus, a fresh medical graduate is not expected to have the same proficiency of skill as a senior specialist.
- Again, a doctor will not be held guilty of negligence, if he acts in accordance with accepted prevalent practice considered appropriate by a responsible body of medical opinion, even though other doctors adopt a different practice.
- However, with advances in knowledge, what is deemed negligent today may have been accepted practice yesterday. So, it is important for a doctor to constantly update his knowledge, failing which he may face litigation for negligence sooner or later.
- A doctor is not legally liable for genuine errors of judgement either relating to diagnosis or treatment, as long as he applies a reasonable standard of skill and care in arriving at that decision.

Damage

- '**Damage**' refers to the injury or disability suffered by the patient. The failure to exercise a duty of care must lead to actual damage in order to be actionable. However negligent the doctor might be, a patient cannot sue him for negligence, if no damage has occurred.
- It should be proved that the breach of duty was the real cause of damage complained of, and such a damage was reasonably foreseeable.
- Errors of judgement either in diagnosis or treatment, will not constitute negligence as long as it is proved that the doctor had exercised minimum reasonable standards of skill and care.

- The term '**damages**' refers to monetary compensation that is intended to restore the injured patient as far as possible, to the state he was in before he suffered from a negligent act. Though money cannot be expected to restore a wrongly amputated limb, it could help to compensate for the loss of wages in the case of a patient who can no longer pursue his trade. Damages are categorised into the following types:
  - ***General***: Awarded for more subjective effects of injury, such as pain and suffering, loss of enjoyment of life, loss of function, etc.
  - ***Special***: Those which can be more exactly computed, e.g., cost of treatment, loss of future income, expense of care for a badly disabled person, etc.
- The highest compensation awarded so far in a criminal medical negligence case in India is that of the death of **Anuradha Saha (Fig. 4.10)**, a US-based child psychologist, who died in AMRI Hospital, Kolkata on 28th May 1998. On 24th Oct 2013, the Supreme Court of India ordered the hospital to pay compensation for medical negligence that led to her death. The total amount (with interest) came to Rs. 11.41 crore (which translates to US$1.86 million in 2013 when the case was decided by the court).

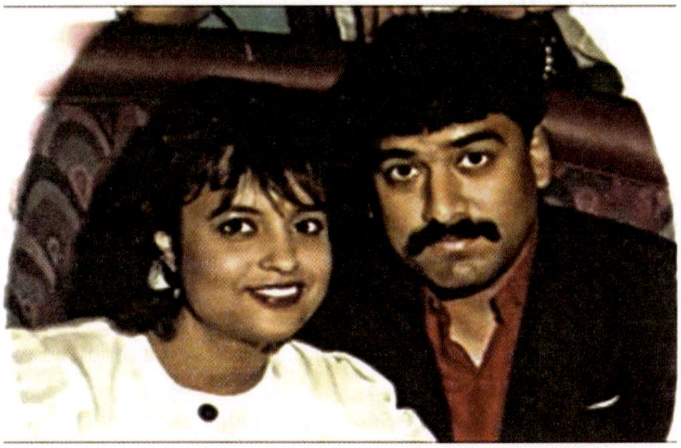

Fig. 4.10 Anuradha Saha with her NRI husband Dr Kunal Saha

Reasonable Foreseeability of Damage

- It is not every failure to exercise a duty of care that renders the doctor liable. The damage has to be foreseeable. One would have to take into consideration whether a reasonably competent doctor under the same circumstances would have foreseen the injury or not. If not, the doctor would not be liable for negligence.
  - For example, dyspepsia (impaired digestion) may be an early symptom of serious illness such as gall bladder disease, peptic ulcer or stomach carcinoma, but often no organic lesion is found in the early stages. Before the doctor orders special (and expensive) investigations such as sonography, barium studies, endoscopy, mucosal biopsy, etc., he may advise a detailed study of stool to exclude parasitic infestation. It is possible that stomach cancer may be missed or diagnosed late, but is certainly not negligence in this case, as the doctor's approach is based on sound judgement.
- A doctor will be considered negligent in the following circumstances:
  - If the doctor's professional performance falls below the standard of a reasonably competent medical practitioner.
  - If there is overt evidence of negligence in diagnosis, treatment procedure (including administration of medicines), surgical operation, etc.
  - Evidence of failure in undertaking all reasonable precautions.

Types of Negligence

Civil Negligence

- The question of **Civil Negligence** arises in the following situations:
  - When a patient or his/her relative files a suit in a Civil Court for getting compensation from the doctor claiming that he/she suffered injury due to negligence.
  - When a doctor files a suit in a Civil Court to claim his fees from the patient or relatives who are refusing to pay on the grounds of professional negligence.
- Examples of Civil Negligence:
  - Failure to obtain informed consent for a medical procedure.
  - Failure to examine a patient himself after agreeing to treat, but instead getting it done by a colleague.
  - Failure to call for relevant investigations.
  - Making a wrong diagnosis due to lack of care or skill.
  - Failure to warn the patient of side effects of a drug that has been prescribed.
  - Discharging a patient prematurely before full cure or recovery.

Criminal Negligence

- The question of **Criminal Negligence** arises in the following situations:
  - When a doctor shows gross absence of skill or care during treatment resulting in serious injury or death.
  - When a doctor shows gross lack of competence, or gross inattention or inaction, gross recklessness or wanton indifference to the patient's safety.
- Examples of Criminal Negligence:
  - Amputation of wrong limb.
  - Surgery on the wrong patient.
  - Leaving behind instruments, swabs, etc., in the abdomen after surgery.
  - Administration of injurious drugs in the eye leading to loss of vision.
  - Death on the operating table due to gross lack of competence or skill, or due to the surgery having been performed under the influence of alcohol or other intoxicant drugs.

The differences between Civil Negligence and Criminal Negligence are listed in **Table 4.3**.

Table 4.3 Differences between Civil Negligence and Criminal Negligence

Sl. No.	Feature	Civil Negligence	Criminal Negligence
1	**Nature of offence**	No specific violation of law	There is violation of a specific criminal law
2	**Nature of negligence**	Basic absence of care or skill	Gross lack of skill, care or competence
3	**Conduct of physician**	Should be comparable to an accepted standard of professional conduct	May not be possible to compare
4	**Consent from patient**	If obtained, can be a good defence	Not a defence; can be prosecuted
5	**Nature of litigation**	Between two parties (patient and doctor)	Between the State and the doctor
6	**Tried in**	Civil Court	Criminal Court
7	**Nature of evidence**	Strong evidence is sufficient	Evidence must be so strong that the guilt is proved beyond reasonable doubt
8	**Punishment**	Liable to pay minor damages (compensation)	Payment of hefty compensation with or without imprisonment

Res Ipsa Loquitur

- This expression (***res ipsa loquitur***) when translated from Latin means "***the thing speaks for itself***".
- It is a situation where the facts of the case itself are sufficient to justify the conclusion that most probably the defendant (doctor) was negligent, and the negligence caused the injury. In other words, it is a reasonable conclusion from the circumstances, that it was undoubtedly the doctor's fault.
- The plaintiff (patient) does not have to prove that the act was negligent as it could be nothing else. It is for the doctor to prove if he can, that the negligence was not his doing.
- Examples:
  - Amputation of wrong limb or digit.
  - Leaving a swab or instrument in the patient after operation.
  - Operating on the wrong part.

Contributory Negligence

- **Contributory negligence** refers to any unreasonable conduct or negligence on the part of the patient which has contributed to the causation of damage alleged, although the doctor has also been negligent.
- This may occur when, for example, the patient interferes with his dressings and induces infection, or removes a plaster cast or bandage, or more commonly, fails to attend the follow-up clinic.
- In claiming that there was contributory negligence, the burden of proof will be on the doctor to show that it has happened.
- If it is proved, the compensation payable will be reduced.

Corporate Negligence

- Sometimes, a patient's care is affected by malfunctioning equipment, inadequate accommodation, incompetent staff, etc. In these cases, if harm results to the patient, the hospital becomes liable for negligence. This is referred to as **corporate negligence**.

Products Liability

- Sometimes, injury or death of a patient may result from:
  - The use of faulty, defective or negligently designed medical or surgical equipment.
  - The use of a drug that is adulterated, contaminated or of inferior quality.
  - The lack of accurate guidelines in the use of any equipment or drug.
- In such cases, the manufacturer concerned becomes liable for harm resulting to the patient. This is referred to as **products liability**.
- However, the manufacturer will not be liable in the following situations:
  - If the doctor or hospital misused an equipment or medical product.
  - If the instrument was functioning well at the time of supply, and was not defective.
  - If the instrument malfunctioned due to improper use, or due to wear and tear, and was not serviced regularly, or replaced in time.

Vicarious Liability

- As per law, a person may become liable to pay damages for an act of negligence committed by his servants or agents in the course of their employment or agency. This is called **vicarious responsibility** or **vicarious liability**, or as the Latin phrase goes "***respondeat superior***", meaning *let the superior be responsible*, or ***let the master answer***.

- For a person to become vicariously liable for the act of another, it must be proved that
  - The negligent act was done in the course of carrying out his duties.
  - The person was his servant or agent.
- Examples:
  - A surgeon may be vicariously liable for the negligent act of his assistant when he is in charge and directing the operation. However, the action of an anaesthetist is not imputed to the surgeon, unless the surgeon issues specific orders to the anaesthetist.
  - A medical officer may be vicariously liable, if a house surgeon posted under him commits a negligent act under his supervision.

Preventive Measures against Negligence

1. **Do not criticise another doctor**: A physician must remember that one of the most common causes of negligence arises out of criticising adversely, the professional conduct of another physician, without knowing the full facts. It has been observed that quite often patients go from doctor to doctor asking for an opinion regarding investigations or treatment adopted by another who is either a family physician or the medical officer at the place of work. The patient is perhaps just seeking psychological reassurance, but a casual remark by any doctor can create complications by shaking the patient's confidence in the doctor whom he has originally consulted.
2. **Employ qualified staff and associate with good partners**: The doctor must always remember that he is responsible for the acts of omission/commission of his assistants, non-technical staff and partners in profession during the course of treating the patient. Therefore, selection must be done very carefully, and only those who are properly qualified should be employed.
3. **Update your knowledge**: A doctor must keep abreast with the latest developments with regard to his profession and its practice.
4. **Keep accurate and complete records**: Human memory can fail, but accurate and detailed medical records will never fail a physician in his hour of need, even after a considerable lapse of time.
   a. The doctor must keep up-to-date records, complete, with respect to:
      i. History – including negative and positive information.
      ii. Present illness – in the patient's own words as far as possible.
      iii. Physical examination – both subjective complaints and objective findings.
      iv. Course of investigations – advised, executed and their results.
      v. Impressions about the case – before and after diagnostic procedures, and the diagnosis.
      vi. Treatment adopted – a complete day-to-day record.
      vii. Any consultation advised or references made to specialists.
      viii. Any refusal on the part of the patient regarding treatment, or diagnostic investigations, etc., or discontinuing treatment against the physician's advice, should be recorded and the signature of the patient obtained against the statements.
5. **Take valid consent**: Consent of the patient must be obtained before starting an examination, diagnostic or investigative procedure, or the treatment. Failure to obtain valid consent before commencing of such measures may make a doctor liable for assault and battery. For the consent to be valid, it must be ***informed***, with the patient being informed of the relevant facts regarding the procedures being adopted or to be adopted, including the risks involved. It is better to obtain written consent for certain special procedures of diagnostic and therapeutic value.
6. **Ensure reasonable skill and care**: A doctor should take all due care, and use reasonable skill within his knowledge. When in doubt, it is good to take a second opinion or consult a specialist, and adopt the necessary diagnostic procedures available. While ensuring reasonable skill and care, do not guarantee results even in an implied manner. A doctor must ensure that all the instruments used by him are maintained well, and sterilized whenever necessary. He should treat his patient as long as it is necessary, and not withdraw from the case without prior notice to the patient. If more than one doctor is involved in treating a case, good communication is essential and of benefit, both to the patient and to the doctor.
7. **Guard against therapeutic hazards**: Before commencement of treatment, the doctor should enquire about the past history of the patient for any adverse drug reactions. Though he may have taken enough precautions to inject a test dose, he should be prepared in advance to handle a case of adverse drug reaction.

Defences against Negligence

1. **No duty** was owed to the plaintiff.
2. Duty was discharged according to **prevailing standards of care**.
3. There was only an **error of judgement**, and no negligence was involved.
4. There was **contributory negligence** on the part of the patient (this provides only partial defence).
5. The case was filed **beyond the statute of limitation**: A suit for damages for negligence against a doctor must be filed within 2 years from the date of the alleged incident.
   a. However, if there was a breach of duty to provide care as per a specific contract, the suit can be filed up to 3 years from the date of the incident.
6. It was a case of **therapeutic misadventure**:
   a. This is applicable in those situations where a diagnostic procedure or treatment carries inherent risks of complications.

b. The employment of some investigative procedures or therapeutic measures by a doctor involving considerable risk and compulsion, in the absence of an alternative option, will not provide grounds for medical negligence, unless the doctor failed to draw the attention of the patient to the risk at the time of obtaining consent.
c. Examples:
   i. Hypersensitivity reactions to common drugs.
   ii. Adverse reaction to an antidote given for poisoning.
   iii. Blood transfusion reaction.
   iv. Hazards from a radiological procedure.

7. **Res judicata** (dealt with in Section 300 of CrPC): If a question of negligence against a doctor has already been decided by a Court in a dispute between the doctor and his patient, the patient will not be allowed to contest the same question in another case between himself and the doctor on the same set of facts in a different court. Only appeal is allowed.

FM 4.19: Core – Written/Viva Voce
- Define Consent.
  - Describe different types of consent and ingredients of informed consent.
  - Describe the rules of consent and importance of consent in relation to age, emergency situation, mental illness and alcohol intoxication.

CONSENT

Definition

- **Consent has been defined to mean "voluntary agreement, compliance, or permission for a specified act or purpose".**
- **The Indian Contracts Act**, *Section 13*, states "two or more persons are said to consent when they agree upon the same thing in the same sense."
- To be legally valid, the consent that is given must be intelligent and informed, i.e., the consent must be given after understanding what it is given for, and the knowledge of risks involved.
- Medical practitioners must always remember to obtain explicit consent from a patient before examining or treating him. If they treat or operate on a patient without express authority to do so, such treatment or operation will be deemed to be intentional interference with the patient's body without legal sanction. This in turn amounts to assault and battery for which the patient will be entitled to recover damages.

Types

- Consent may be either **expressed** or **implied**.
  - **Expressed consent*** may be ***written*** or ***verbal***.
  - **Implied consent** is indicated by the demeanour and behaviour of the patient, and is adequate for routine general examinations, but when special examinations such as vaginal examination, rectal examination, etc., are required, expressed consent must be obtained.
  - For more complicated diagnostic procedures like endoscopy, or for surgical procedures, written consent is essential. In hospitals, expressed consent (verbal or written) should preferably be obtained in the presence of a disinterested third party such as a nurse or a receptionist.
  - As far as possible, consent must be obtained after explaining the nature and consequences of the treatment procedure being contemplated. This is termed ***informed consent***.
    - **Ingredients of Informed Consent**: Since every adult human being has the right to decide as to what is best for his own body, a doctor prescribing a particular diagnostic or therapeutic procedure must necessarily disclose all the risks associated with the procedure to the patient so as to enable him to decide whether to undergo the same or not. The following points must be borne in mind:
      - All relevant information about the ailment and treatment options must be outlined.
      - Significant risks associated with every medical procedure being contemplated must be disclosed.
      - The patient must be informed about all available alternative treatment options.
      - Everything that is told to the patient must be explained in simple language that is comprehensible to him.
      - Failure to take informed consent can expose a doctor to legal action, if anything goes wrong during a particular procedure.
      - However, in some cases, a doctor is permitted to withhold some information if he is convinced that disclosure of the same can be counter-productive to the patient's own health, or that it can cause psychological harm. This is referred to as **therapeutic privilege**.
      - Even if informed consent has been obtained in a given case, it can be deemed invalid if the doctor exceeds his brief, for instance, carrying out a different procedure from what was originally contemplated, or extending the scope of operation beyond what was told to the patient.
      - However, the courts have invariably recognized the possibility that complete diagnosis of an internal ailment may not be certain until the incision has been made and the organ is laid bare. So, when a surgeon is confronted with an unanticipated condition for which immediate action is required, he is justified in extending the operation and doing whatever is necessary to save the life of the patient. This is referred to as the **extension doctrine**.

**Note*: *Often incorrectly referred to as "Express consent".*

Rules & Principles

- The consent given by any person must necessarily be voluntary and free. Consent obtained by force, fear or fraud is invalid. Though for routine examinations and treatment, a broad-based consent (***blanket consent***) may suffice, for special operative procedures, specific informed consent in written form is necessary.
- Consent may not be deemed necessary in the following situations:
  - The patient is in coma and needs emergency treatment.
  - The patient is a child admitted as an emergency case, and the parents are not immediately accessible.
  - When a medicolegal case is referred by a court of law for examination.
- Consent is to be obtained from the following persons for examination and treatment:
  - Conscious, mentally sound adults.
  - Children above 12 years of age.
  - The spouse of a person who is to undergo sterilization, termination of pregnancy, etc., (not always essential legally).
  - The parent or guardian of a child who is less than 12 years of age.
  - Permission of ***loco-parentis*** (e.g., headmaster of a residential school) may be obtained when it is an emergency situation, and the consent of the parents concerned is not easily obtainable.
- Utmost care must be taken to preserve the sentiments of patients with regard to their religious beliefs, even if these appear to be a little unusual. A prime example is the religious group referred to as **"Jehovah's Witnesses,"** which was founded in the late 19th century in Pennsylvania, USA, a few members of which exist in India also. These individuals believe that all hopes for eternal life will be forfeited, if blood transfusion is accepted from another person. In fact, even autologous transfusion is not acceptable to strict adherents, since they believe that once the blood has left the body it is rendered unclean. While the courts have allowed such refusal of treatment on the part of adults, they have indicated in some cases that the policy may be different in the case of children.
- Mentally unsound persons are not capable of giving valid consent. The legal guardian must provide the same.
- A person under the influence of alcohol cannot give valid consent for any invasive medical procedure. The parent, spouse or legal guardian has to be involved. For medicolegal certification of drunkenness, the accompanying policeman must be entrusted with providing consent for the examination. However, the findings and conclusion must be reserved until after the person has recovered from the effects of intoxication, following which it must be explained to him that it would be in his interests to consent to divulge the results of his examination to the authorities concerned. Failure to comply can be presumed to be evidence of guilt which can go against him in legal proceedings.
- Consent obtained for an illegal procedure is necessarily invalid.
- Before volunteering to participate in any research programme or clinical trial, a person is entitled to know the exact methods of experimentation, aims of the experiment, and risks associated with it. It is also desirable for the person to know whether he is permitted to withdraw from the experiment at any stage.

FM 4.20: Core – Written/Viva Voce
- Describe:
  - Therapeutic privilege
  - Malingering
  - Therapeutic misadventure
  - Professional secrecy
  - Human experimentation

Therapeutic privilege is explained under FM 4.19 *(page 308)*; **Therapeutic misadventure under** FM 4.18 *(page 303)*; **Human experimentation under** FM 4.25–FM 4.27. *(page 314 to 319)*

MALINGERING

(FEIGNING, SHAMMING, FABRICATION)

- **Malingering** is the fabrication or exaggeration or pretence of physical or psychological symptoms designed to achieve a desired outcome, such as relief from duty or work, or to falsely accuse another person of assault.
- Malingering is categorized as distinct from other forms of excessive illness behaviour such as **somatization disorder** and **factitious disorder**.
  - **Somatization disorder** is a mental/ behavioural disorder characterized by recurring, multiple, clinically significant complaints about somatic symptoms. It is often associated with depression, anxiety, etc., and was formerly referred to as **hypochondriasis**.
  - **Factitious disorder** is a condition in which a person, without a malingering motive, acts as if he has an illness by deliberately producing, pretending, or exaggerating symptoms, purely to attain (for himself or for another) a patient's role. People with a factitious disorder may produce symptoms by contaminating urine samples, taking hallucinogens, injecting infective material to produce abscesses, etc.
    - Factitious disorder imposed on oneself is called **Munchausen syndrome**, while factitious disorder imposed on another person is called **Munchausen syndrome by proxy**.
- Failure to detect actual cases of malingering can impose an economic burden on health care systems, workers' compensation programmes and disability programmes. False accusations of malingering often harm genuine patients or claimants.
- A malingerer who wishes to frame another person on a false charge of assault, sometimes produces or fabricates injuries on his own body to substantiate his claim. This may be in the form of superficial cuts or an **"artificial**

bruise" caused by the application of irritant plant juices (e.g., Calotropis).

- **Feigned insanity** is a form of malingering indulged in by a sane individual to convince authorities that he is actually insane in order to escape the consequences of a serious crime such as murder. As per Indian laws, an insane criminal cannot be punished as he is deemed to be without "***mens rea***" or "***criminal mind***" and hence cannot be held responsible for his actions. He must be sent to a psychiatric facility for treatment, and incarcerated there for as long as required.
  - The Structured Inventory of Malingered Symptomatology (SIMS) is a 75-item true-false questionnaire intended to measure malingering in relation to psychiatric symptoms, cognitive impairment or neurological disorders.

PROFESSIONAL SECRECY

- During the course of treatment, a patient may reveal matters of a personal nature to his doctor. The doctor is obliged to maintain the secrecy of all such information, except when he is required by law to divulge it, or when the patient has consented for the disclosure.
- The doctor is liable for damages, if he discloses without valid grounds, any such information which the patient may reasonably claim as secret or confidential.
- The following examples can serve as guidelines:
  - A doctor should not disclose any secret information about his patient or his private life, which he learns in the course of his examination, to a third party.
  - Without the consent of the patient, no information about his illness, or any matter about his family can be disclosed, even to the patient's spouse or employer.
  - In the case of domestic servants, even if the master pays the fees of the doctor towards the treatment of the servant, the doctor should not disclose any information to the master about the nature of the illness, without the patient's consent.
  - Information about the nature of illness of a minor child, mentally ill person or intoxicated patient, may be disclosed to the guardian of the patient. But, in the case of a mentally sound major patient, nothing should be disclosed to his parents or any other relative without his consent.
  - While treating a minor inmate of a hostel or a boarding house, the doctor may disclose relevant information about the patient to the warden or superintendent. But if the patient is a major, he cannot do so without the consent of the patient, unless the matter poses risk to the other inmates of the hostel.
  - In the course of treatment of a **convicted prisoner** in a jail, the matter relating to his illness may be conveyed to the jailor or the superintendent of the jail. But, in the case of a **prisoner under trial** or a **person in police custody**, this cannot be done without his consent.
  - When a person approaches a medical practitioner for a medical certificate or a report, it may be taken as implied that he has given consent for the disclosure of all information about his illness. Hence, in such a situation, disclosure of relevant information about the person, will not amount to breach of trust.
  - While reporting a case in any scientific journal, the doctor should take care that the identity of the patient is not disclosed.

Privileged Communication

- From the foregoing, it is clear that every doctor must observe professional secrecy as far as possible. However, there are certain circumstances in which a doctor is bound by law to divulge information, even if it is of a confidential nature. This is referred to as **privileged communication**. In other words, it is an exception to the usual policy of professional secrecy.
- **Privileged communication** is therefore defined as "a statement made by a person who has an interest to protect, or a legal/social/moral duty to perform to another person having a corresponding interest, even though such communication may under normal conditions, amount to defamation or slander.
- For instance, a medical practitioner cannot claim professional secrecy in those cases where he has a statutory duty to notify births, deaths, infectious diseases, etc., to the public health authorities.
- On certain occasions, he has a moral duty to protect the interests of the community or the public, and in doing so, if he divulges the secrets of his patient obtained in the course of his professional examination and treatment, he will be absolved from legal liabilities.
- In all such cases, the communication (if made bonafide and without malice), will be deemed to be privileged by the circumstances. However, it should be made only to persons directly concerned, otherwise he may be penalised.
- The following examples are self-explanatory:
  - A medical practitioner has a duty to inform the warden of a hostel, if any boarder is suffering from venereal or other communicable or infectious disease.
  - He must inform the railway authority if he finds that a particular engine driver is colour blind, and he does not wish to change his employment, although he is persuaded to do so.

FM 4.21: Core – Written/Viva Voce
- Describe:
  - Products liability
  - Medical Indemnity Insurance

Products liability is explained under FM 4.18 *(page 303)*; and **Medical Indemnity Insurance** under FM 4.8. *(page 289)*

FM 4.22: Core – Written/Viva Voce
- Explain Oath
  - Hippocrates, Charaka and Sushruta
  - Procedure of administration of Oath

OATH

- Traditionally, an **oath** is a statement made by a religious person as a sign of possessing true belief.
- Nowadays, even when there is no notion of sanctity involved, certain promises said out loud for ceremonial or juridical purpose are referred to as **oaths**.
- Medical professionals are expected to take an oath before or at the time of graduating, swearing to practice their profession honestly and sincerely. **Hippocratic Oath** and **Charaka Shapath** are examples of such medical oaths.
- The Hippocratic Oath has been traditionally administered to medical students in India when they transition from preclinical to clinical subjects, during what is known as the **White Coat Ceremony**.
    - The National Medical Commission (NMC) made the suggestion of using the **Charak Shapath** rather than the Hippocratic Oath in one of its meetings with all medical college representatives; the minutes of the meeting stated: "No Hippocratic Oath. During white coat ceremony (with parents) the oath will be 'Maharishi Charak Shapath' present in NMC website."
    - However, several medical practitioners individually and collectively protested against the proposal, and it is now not mandatory.

Hippocrates

- **Hippocrates** was a Greek physician of the classical period who is considered one of the most outstanding figures in the history of medicine. He is traditionally referred to as the "**Father of Medicine**" in recognition of his lasting contributions to the field, such as the use of prognosis and clinical observation, the systematic categorization of diseases, or the formulation of humoral theory.
- The Hippocratic school of medicine revolutionized ancient Greek medicine, establishing it as a discipline distinct from other fields with which it had traditionally been associated (theurgy and philosophy), thus establishing medicine as a profession.
- Hippocrates is commonly portrayed as the paragon of the ancient physician and credited with coining the **Hippocratic Oath**, which is still relevant and in use today. He is also credited with greatly advancing the systematic study of clinical medicine, summing up the medical knowledge of previous schools and prescribing practices for physicians through the **Hippocratic Corpus** and other works.

Hippocratic Oath

- The **Hippocratic Oath** is an oath of ethics historically taken by physicians.
- The oath is the earliest expression of medical ethics in the Western world, establishing several principles of medical ethics which remain of paramount significance today. Swearing a modified form of the oath remains a rite of passage for medical graduates in many countries, and is a requirement enshrined in legal statutes of various jurisdictions, such that violations of the oath may carry criminal or other liability beyond the oath's symbolic nature.
- The original oath was written in Greek, between the 5th and 3rd centuries BC.
- English translation:
    - I swear by Apollo Healer, by Asclepius, by Hygieia, by Panacea, and by all the gods and goddesses, making them my witnesses, that I will carry out, according to my ability and judgment, this oath and this indenture.
    - To hold my teacher in this art equal to my own parents; to make him partner in my livelihood; when he is in need of money to share mine with him; to consider his family as my own brothers, and to teach them this art, if they want to learn it, without fee or indenture; to impart precept, oral instruction, and all other instruction to my own sons, the sons of my teacher, and to indentured pupils who have taken the Healer's oath, but to nobody else.
    - I will use those dietary regimens which will benefit my patients according to my greatest ability and judgment, and I will do no harm or injustice to them. Neither will I administer a poison to anybody when asked to do so, nor will I suggest such a course. Similarly, I will not give to a woman a pessary to cause abortion. But, I will keep pure and holy both my life and my art. I will not use the knife, not even, verily, on sufferers from stone, but I will give place to such as are craftsmen therein.
    - Into whatsoever houses I enter, I will enter to help the sick, and I will abstain from all intentional wrong-doing and harm, especially from abusing the bodies of man or woman, bond or free. And whatsoever I shall see or hear in the course of my profession, as well as outside my profession in my intercourse with them, if it be what should not be published abroad, I will never divulge, holding such things to be holy secrets.
    - Now if I carry out this oath, and break it not, may I gain for ever reputation among all men for my life and for my art; but if I break it and forswear myself, may the opposite befall me.

Charaka

- **Charaka** was one of the principal contributors to Ayurveda, a system of medicine and lifestyle developed in Ancient India. He is known as an editor of the medical treatise entitled **Charaka Samhita**, one of the foundational texts of classical Indian medicine and Ayurveda, included under Brhat-Trayi.
- Charaka most probably lived somewhere between 100 BCE and 150-200 CE.
- The following statements are attributed to Charaka:
    - A physician who fails to enter the body of a patient with the lamp of knowledge and understanding can never treat diseases. He should first study all the factors, including environment, which influence a patient's disease, and then prescribe treatment. It is more important to prevent the occurrence of disease than to seek a cure.

- A body functions because it contains three **dosha** or principles, namely movement (**vata**), transformation (**pitta**) and lubrication and stability (**kapha**). The doshas correspond to the Western classification of humors, **wind**, **bile** and **phlegm**. These doshas are produced when **dhatus** (blood, flesh and marrow) act upon the food eaten. For the same quantity of food eaten, one body, however, produces dosha in an amount different from another body. That is why one body is different from another.
- Illness is caused when the balance among the three doshas in a human body are disturbed. To restore the balance he prescribed medicinal drugs. Although he was aware of germs in the body, he did not give them primary importance.

- Charaka studied the anatomy of the human body and various organs. He identified 360 as the total number of bones, including teeth, present in the human body. He was right when he considered heart to be a controlling centre. He claimed that the heart was connected to the entire body through 13 main channels. Apart from these channels, there were countless other ones of varying sizes which supplied not only nutrients to various tissues but also provided passage to waste products. He also claimed that any obstruction in the main channels led to a disease or deformity in the body.
- **Agnivesa**, under the guidance of the ancient physician **Atreya**, composed an encyclopedic medical compendium in the 8th century BCE, the **Agnivesha Samhitā**. The work received little attention. The Agnivesha Samhitā was revised by Charaka and renamed the **Charaka Samhitā**. In this form it became well known.
  - The **Charaka Samhita** is one of the two foundational texts of Ayurveda, the other being the **Sushruta Samhita**.

Charaka Shapath

- **Charaka shapath** (or **Charaka oath**) is a certain passage of text in **Charaka Samhita**, a Sanskrit text on Ayurveda, believed to have been composed between 100 BCE and 200 CE. The passage is written in the form of a set of instructions by a teacher to prospective students of the science of medicine.
- According to **Charaka Samhita**, the unconditional agreement to abide by these instructions is a necessary precondition to be eligible to be taught in the science of medicine. The passage gives explicit instructions on the necessity of practicing asceticism during student life, student–teacher relationship, the importance of committing oneself fully and completely for the well-being of the patient, whom to treat, how to behave with women and several other related issues.
- The original text of Charaka Shapath is in the Sanskrit language in the Devanagari script. The English translation of the same is reproduced below:
  - The teacher then should instruct the disciple in the presence of the sacred fire, brahmanas and physicians (saying) – "Thou shalt lead the life of a bachelor (Brahmachari), grow thy hair and beard, speak only the truth, eat no meat, eat only pure articles of food, be free from envy and carry no arms. There shall be nothing that thou oughtest not do at my behest except hating the king or causing another's death or committing an act of great unrighteousness or acts leading to calamity."
  - Thou shall dedicate thyself to me and regard me as thy chief. Thou shalt be subject to me and conduct thyself for ever for my welfare and pleasure. Thou shalt serve and dwell with me like a son or a slave or a supplicant. Thou shalt behave and act without arrogance and with care and attention, and with undistracted mind, humility, constant reflection and with ungrudging obedience. Acting either at my behest or otherwise, thou shalt conduct thyself for the achievement of thy teacher's purpose alone to the best of thy abilities.
  - If thou desirest success, wealth and fame as a physician and heaven after death, thou shalt pray for the welfare of all creatures beginning with the cows and brahmanas.
  - Day and night, however thou mayest be engaged, thou shalt endeavour for the relief of patients with all thy heart and soul. Thou shalt not desert or injure thy patient even for the sake of thy life or thy living. Thou shalt not commit adultery even in thought. Even so, thou shalt not covet other's possessions. Thou shalt be modest in thy attire and appearance. Thou shouldst not be a drunkard or a sinful man nor shouldst thou associate with the abettors of crimes. Thou shouldst speak words that are gentle, pure and righteous, pleasing, worthy, true, wholesome and moderate. Thy behaviour must be in consideration of time and place and heedful of past experience. Thou shalt act always with a view to the acquisition of knowledge and the fullness of equipment.
  - No persons, who are hated of the king, or who are haters of the king or who are hated of the public, shall receive treatment. Similarly, those that are very unnatural, wicked and miserable character and conduct, those who have not vindicated their honour and those that are on the point of death, and similarly women who are unattended by their husbands or guardians shall not receive treatment.
  - No offering of meat by a woman without the behest of her husband or guardian shall be accepted by thee. While entering the patient's house, thou shalt be accompanied by a man who is known to the patient and who has his permission to enter and thou shalt be well-clad and bent of head, self-possessed, and conduct thyself after repeated consideration. Thou shalt thus properly make thy entry. Having entered, thy speech, mind, intellect and senses shall be entirely devoted to no other thought than that of being helpful to the patient and things concerning him only. The peculiar customs of

the patient's household shall not be made public. Even knowing that the patient's span of life has come to a close, it shall not be mentioned by thee there where if so done it would cause shock to the patient or to others.

- Though of knowledge one should not boast very much of one's knowledge. Most people are offended by boastfulness of even those who are otherwise good and authoritative.
- There is no limit at all to the "Science of Life". So, thou shouldst apply thyself to it with diligence. This is how thou shouldst act. Again thou shouldst learn the skill of practice from another without carping. The entire world is a teacher to the intelligent and the foe to the unintelligent. Hence, knowing this well, thou shouldst listen and act according to the words of instruction of even an unfriendly person, when they are worthy and such as bring fame to you and long life, and are capable of giving you strength and prosperity."
- Thereafter the teacher should say this - "Thou shouldst conduct properly with gods, the sacred fire, the twice-born, the guru, the aged, the adepts and the preceptors. If thou hast conducted thyself well with them, the fire, the fragrances, the tastes, the precious stones, the grains and the gods become well disposed towards thee. If thou shouldst conduct thyself otherwise, they become unfavourable to thee."
- To the teacher that has thus spoken, the disciple should say "Even so". If he behaves as instructed, he deserves to be taught, else, he does not deserve to be taught.
    - The teacher who teaches the worthy disciples will obtain all the auspicious fruits of teaching, those described and even others not described here and obtains all auspicious qualities for himself as well as for his disciples. Thus has been described the method of instruction.

Sushruta

- **Sushruta**, or **Susŕuta** was an ancient Indian physician, and the world's first surgeon known as "**Father of Surgery**", "**Father of Plastic Surgery**" and "**Father of Brain Surgery**" for inventing and developing surgical procedures.
- His work on the subject, the **Sushruta Samhita** (Sushruta's Compendium) is considered one of the oldest texts in the world on plastic surgery, and is highly regarded as one of the Great Trilogy of Ayurvedic Medicine, the Brihat-Trayi; the other two being the **Charaka Samhita**, which preceded it, and the **Astanga Hridaya**, which followed it.
- The Sushruta Samhita is one of the most important surviving ancient treatises on medicine and is considered a foundational text of Ayurveda. The treatise addresses all aspects of general medicine, but the impressive chapters on surgery have led to the false impression that this is its main topic. The translator GD Singhal dubbed Sushruta "the father of surgery" on account of these detailed accounts of surgery.
- Sushruta attracted a number of disciples who were known as Saushrutas and were required to study for 6 years

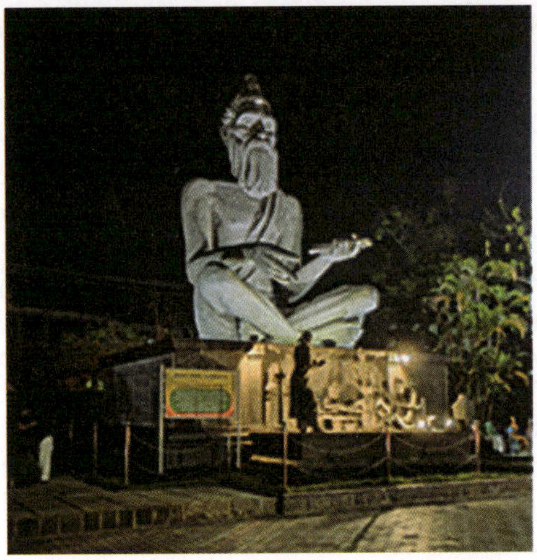

Fig. 4.11 Sculpture of Sushruta – Amrita Hospital, Cochin

before they even began hands-on training in surgery. Before starting their training, they had to take a solemn oath to devote themselves to healing and to do no harm to others; which can be compared to the Hippocratic Oath. After the students had been accepted by Sushruta, he would instruct them in surgical procedures by having them practice cutting on vegetables or dead animals to perfect the length and depth of an incision. Once students had proven themselves capable with vegetation, animal corpses, or with soft or rotting wood – and had carefully observed actual procedures on patients – they were then allowed to per form their own surgeries. These students were trained by their master in every aspect of the medical arts, including anatomy.

- Sushruta wrote the **Sushruta Samhita** as an instruction manual for physicians to treat their patients holistically. Disease, he claimed (following the precepts of Charaka), was caused by imbalance in the body, and it was the physician's duty to help others maintain balance or to restore it if it had been lost. To this end, anyone who was engaged in the practice of medicine had to be balanced themselves.
- The highlight of Sushruta's surgical prowess was the surgery of nasal reconstruction or **rhinoplasty** (repairing the disfigured nose with a flap of skin from the forehead) that he used to reconstruct noses that were amputated as a punishment for crime. The technique is practised almost unchanged to this day, the pedicled forehead flap being named the **Indian flap**.

> **FM 4.23: Core – Written/Viva Voce**
> - Describe the modified Declaration of Geneva and its relevance.

DECLARATION OF GENEVA

- The **Declaration of Geneva** was adopted by the General Assembly of the World Medical Association at Geneva in

1948, amended in 1968, 1983 and 1994, editorially revised in 2005 and 2006, and amended in 2017.

- It is a declaration of a physician's dedication to the humanitarian goals of medicine, a declaration that was especially important in view of the medical crimes which had just been committed in German-occupied Europe. The Declaration of Geneva was intended as a revision of the **Hippocratic Oath** to a formulation of that oath's moral truths that could be comprehended and acknowledged in a modern way. Unlike the case of the Oath of Hippocrates, the World Medical Association calls the statement a "**pledge**".
- The **Modified Declaration of Geneva (2017)**, as currently published by the World Medical Association reads as follows:
  - As a member of the medical profession,
    - I solemnly pledge to dedicate my life to the service of humanity;
    - The health and well-being of my patient will be my first consideration;
    - I will respect the autonomy and dignity of my patient;
    - I will maintain the utmost respect for human life;
    - I will not permit considerations of age, disease or disability, creed, ethnic origin, gender, nationality, political affiliation, race, sexual orientation, social standing or any other factor to intervene between my duty and my patient;
    - I will respect the secrets that are confided in me, even after the patient has died;
    - I will practice my profession with conscience and dignity and in accordance with good medical practice;
    - I will foster the honour and noble traditions of the medical profession;
    - I will give to my teachers, colleagues and students the respect and gratitude that is their due;
    - I will share my medical knowledge for the benefit of the patient and the advancement of healthcare;
    - I will attend to my own health, well-being and abilities in order to provide care of the highest standard;
    - I will not use my medical knowledge to violate human rights and civil liberties, even under threat;
    - I make these promises solemnly, freely and upon my honour.
- The **Modified Declaration of Geneva** acknowledges respect for human rights of patients, the value of sharing knowledge with the community and profession, and the right and obligation of physicians to care for themselves, and to maintain their abilities for the benefit of society.

> FM 4.24: Core – Written/Viva Voce
> - Enumerate rights, privileges and duties of a Registered Medical Practitioner.
> - Discuss doctor–patient relationship: Professional secrecy and Privileged communication.

Rights, privileges and duties of a Registered Medical Practitioner are dealt with under FM 4.5 *(page 284)* and FM 4.6 *(page 287)*, while Professional secrecy and Privileged Communications are discussed under FM 4.20 *(page 309)*.

> FM 4.25: Non-Core – Written/Viva Voce
> - Clinical research & ethics.
> - Discuss human experimentation including clinical trials.

- Ethics in clinical research focuses largely on identifying and implementing the acceptable conditions for exposure of some individuals to risks and burdens, for the benefit of society at large. Ethical guidelines for clinical research were formulated only after discovery of inhumane behaviour with participants during research experiments.
- The **Nuremberg Code** was the first international code laying ethical principles for clinical research.
- With increasing research all over, World Health Organization formulated guidelines in the form of **Declaration of Helsinki** in **1964**.
- The US laid down its guidelines for ethical principles in the **Belmont Report** after discovery of the Tuskegee's Syphilis study.
- The Indian Council of Medical Research has laid down the '**Ethical Guidelines for Biomedical Research on Human Subjects**' in the year **2000** which were revised in **2006**. It comprises of 12 general principles to be followed by all biomedical researchers working in the country.
- Ethics Committees represent the bridge between the researcher and the ethical guidelines of the country. The basic responsibility of an Ethics Committee is to ensure an independent, competent and timely review of all ethical aspects of the project proposals received in order to safeguard the dignity, rights, safety and well-being of all research participants. A well-documented informed consent process is the hallmark of any ethical research work. Informed consent respects individual's autonomy, to participate or not to participate in research. Concepts of vulnerable populations, therapeutic misconception and post-trial access hold special importance in ethical conduct of research, especially in developing countries like India, where most of the research participants are uneducated and economically backward.

All this is discussed in greater detail under **FM 4.26, FM 4.27** and **FM 4.30**.

HUMAN EXPERIMENTATION AND CLINICAL TRIALS

- **Human experimentation** or **human subject research** refers to systematic scientific investigation that can be either **interventional** (a "***trial***") or **observational** (no "test article"), and involves human beings as research subjects, commonly known as test subjects.
- Human subject research can be either **medical (clinical) research** or **non-medical** (e.g., social science) research.

Systematic investigation incorporates both the collection and analysis of data in order to answer a specific question.

- **Medical human subject research** often involves analysis of biological specimens, epidemiological and behavioural studies and medical chart review studies.
- A specific, and especially heavily regulated, type of medical human subject research is the "**clinical trial**", in which drugs, vaccines and medical devices are evaluated.
- On the other hand, **human subject research in the social sciences** often involves **surveys** which consist of questions to a particular group of people. Survey methodology includes questionnaires, interviews, and focus groups.

Clinical Trials

- **Clinical trials** are experiments or observations done in clinical research. Such prospective biomedical or behavioral research studies on human participants are designed to answer specific questions about biomedical or behavioural interventions, including new treatments (such as novel vaccines, drugs, dietary choices, dietary supplements and medical devices), and known interventions that warrant further study and comparison.
- Clinical trials generate data on dosage, safety and efficacy.
- They are conducted only after they have received health authority/ethics committee approval in the country where approval of the therapy is sought. These authorities are responsible for vetting the risk/benefit ratio of the trial—their approval does not mean the therapy is 'safe' or effective, only that the trial may be conducted.
- Depending on product type and development stage, investigators initially enroll volunteers or patients into small pilot studies, and subsequently conduct progressively larger scale comparative studies.
- Clinical trials can vary in size and cost, and they can involve a single research centre or multiple centres, in one country or in multiple countries.
- Clinical study design aims to ensure the scientific validity and reproducibility of the results.
- Costs for clinical trials can range from thousands to millions of dollars per approved drug. The sponsor may be a governmental organization or a pharmaceutical, biotechnology or medical device company.
- Certain functions necessary to the trial, such as monitoring and lab work, may be managed by an outsourced partner, such as a contract research organization or a central laboratory.
- **Trials of Drugs**
  - Some clinical trials involve healthy subjects with no pre-existing medical conditions. Other clinical trials pertain to people with specific health conditions who are willing to try an experimental treatment. Pilot experiments are conducted to gain insights for design of the clinical trial to follow.
  - There are two goals to testing medical treatments:
    - to learn whether they work well enough, called "efficacy" or "effectiveness"; and
    - to learn whether they are safe enough, called "safety".

    Neither is an absolute criterion; both safety and efficacy are evaluated relative to how the treatment is intended to be used, what other treatments are available, and the severity of the disease or condition. The benefits must outweigh the risks. For example, many drugs to treat cancer have severe side effects that would not be acceptable for an over-the-counter pain medication, yet the cancer drugs have been approved since they are used under a physician's care and are used for a life-threatening condition.
  - People over 55 (or a similar cut-off age) are often excluded from trials because their greater health issues and drug use complicate data interpretation, and because they have different physiological capacity than younger people. Children and people with unrelated medical conditions are also frequently excluded. Pregnant women are often excluded due to potential risks to the foetus.
  - The sponsor designs the trial in coordination with a panel of expert clinical investigators, including what alternative or existing treatments to compare to the new drug, and what type(s) of patients might benefit. If the sponsor cannot obtain enough test subjects at one location investigators at other locations are recruited to join the study.
  - During the trial, investigators recruit subjects with the predetermined characteristics, administer the treatment(s) and collect data on the subjects' health for a defined time period. Data include measurements such as vital signs, concentration of the study drug in the blood or tissues, changes to symptoms, and whether improvement or worsening of the condition targeted by the study drug occurs. The researchers send the data to the trial sponsor, who then analyzes the pooled data using statistical tests.
  - Except for small, single-location trials, the design and objectives are specified in a document called a clinical trial protocol. The protocol is the trial's "operating manual" and ensures all researchers perform the trial in the same way on similar subjects and that the data is comparable across all subjects.
  - The most common clinical trials evaluate new pharmaceutical products, medical devices, biologics, psychological therapies or other interventions.
- **Trials of Devices**
  - Similarly to drugs, manufacturers of medical devices are also required to conduct clinical trials for premarket approval.
  - Device trials may compare a new device to an established therapy, or may compare similar devices to each other. An example of the former in the field of vascular

surgery is the Open versus Endovascular Repair (OVER trial) for the treatment of abdominal aortic aneurysm, which compared the older open aortic repair technique to the newer endovascular aneurysm repair device. An example of the latter are clinical trials on mechanical devices used in the management of adult female urinary incontinence.

- **Trials of Procedures**
  - Similarly to drugs, medical or surgical procedures may be subjected to clinical trials, such as case-controlled studies for surgical interventions.

Types of Clinical Trial

- Clinical trials may be classified by the **research objective** created by the investigators.
  - In an **observational study**, the investigators observe the subjects and measure their outcomes. The researchers do not actively manage the study.
  - In an **interventional study**, the investigators give the research subjects an experimental drug, surgical procedure, use of a medical device, diagnostic or other intervention to compare the treated subjects with those receiving no treatment or the standard treatment. Then, the researchers assess how the subjects' health changes.
- Trials may also be classified by their **purpose**.
  - **Prevention trials** look for ways to prevent disease in people who have never had the disease or to prevent a disease from returning. These approaches may include drugs, vitamins or other micronutrients, vaccines, or lifestyle changes.
  - **Screening trials** test for ways to identify certain diseases or health conditions.
  - **Diagnostic trials** are conducted to find better tests or procedures for diagnosing a particular disease or condition.
  - **Treatment trials** test experimental drugs, new combinations of drugs, or new approaches to surgery or radiation therapy.
  - **Quality of life trials (Supportive care trials)** evaluate how to improve comfort and quality of care for people with a chronic illness.
  - **Genetic trials** are conducted to assess the prediction accuracy of genetic disorders making a person more or less likely to develop a disease.
  - **Epidemiological trials** have the goal of identifying the general causes, patterns or control of diseases in large numbers of people.
  - **Compassionate use trials (expanded access trials)** provide partially tested, unapproved therapeutics to a small number of patients who have no other realistic options. Usually, this involves a disease for which no effective therapy has been approved, or a patient who has already failed all standard treatments and whose health is too compromised to qualify for participation in randomized clinical trials.
  - **Fixed trials** consider existing data only during the trial's design, do not modify the trial after it begins, and do not assess the results until the study is completed.
  - **Adaptive clinical trials** use existing data to design the trial, and then use interim results to modify the trial as it proceeds. Modifications include dosage, sample size, drug undergoing trial, patient selection criteria and "cocktail" mix.

Phases of Clinical Trial

- Clinical trials involving new drugs are commonly classified into **5 phases**, i.e., **Phases 0–4 (Table 4.4)**. Each phase of the drug approval process is treated as a separate clinical trial. The drug development process will normally proceed through phases I–IV over many years, frequently involving a decade or longer. If the drug successfully passes through phases I, II and III, it will usually be approved by the national regulatory authority for use in the general population. Phase IV trials are performed after the newly approved drug, diagnostic or device is marketed, providing assessment about risks, benefits or best uses.

Trial Design

- A fundamental distinction in evidence-based practice is between **observational studies** and **randomized controlled trials**.
- Types of observational studies in epidemiology, such as the **cohort study** and the **case–control study**, provide less compelling evidence than the **randomized controlled trial**.
- In observational studies, the investigators retrospectively assess associations between the treatments given to participants and their health status, with potential for considerable errors in design and interpretation.
- A randomized controlled trial can provide compelling evidence that the study treatment causes an effect on human health.
- Currently, some Phase II and most Phase III drug trials are designed as randomized, double-blind and placebo-controlled.
  - **Randomized**: Each study subject is randomly assigned to receive either the study treatment or a placebo.
  - **Blind**: The subjects involved in the study do not know which study treatment they receive. If the study is **double-blind**, the researchers also do not know which treatment a subject receives. This intent is to prevent researchers from treating the two groups differently. A form of double-blind study called a "**double-dummy**" design allows additional insurance against bias. In this kind of study, all patients are given both placebo and active doses in alternating periods.
  - **Placebo-controlled**: The use of a placebo (fake treatment) allows the researchers to isolate the effect of the study treatment from the placebo effect.
- Clinical studies having small numbers of subjects may be "sponsored" by single researchers or a small group of researchers, and are designed to test simple questions or feasibility to expand the research for a more comprehensive randomized controlled trial

Table 4.4 Phases of Clinical Trial

Phase	Aim	Notes
Phase 0	Pharmacodynamics and pharmacokinetics in humans	Phase 0 trials are optional first-in-human trials. Single sub-therapeutic doses of the study drug or treatment are given to a small number of subjects (typically 10–15) to gather preliminary data on the agent's pharmacodynamics (what the drug does to the body) and pharmacokinetics (what the body does to the drugs). For a test drug, the trial documents the absorption, distribution, metabolism and clearance (excretion) of the drug, and the drug's interactions within the body, to confirm that these appear to be as expected.
Phase I	Screening for safety	Often are first-in-person trials. Testing within a small group of people (typically 20–80) to evaluate safety, determine safe dosage ranges, and identify side effects.
Phase II	Establishing the preliminary efficacy of the drug in a "treatment group", usually against a placebo control group	Phase IIa is specifically designed to assess dosing requirements (how much drug should be given), while a Phase IIb trial is designed to determine efficacy, and studies how well the drug works at the prescribed dose(s), establishing a therapeutic dose range.
Phase III	Final confirmation of safety and efficacy	Testing with large groups of people (typically 1000–3000) to confirm its efficacy, evaluate its effectiveness, monitor side effects, compare it to commonly used treatments, and collect information that will allow it to be used safely.
Phase IV	Safety studies during sales	Post-marketing studies delineate risks, benefits and optimal use. As such, they are ongoing during the drug's lifetime of active medical use.

FM 4.26: Core – Written/Viva Voce
- Discuss the constitution and functions of ethical committees.

CONSTITUTION & FUNCTIONS OF ETHICS COMMITTEES

- An **Ethics Committee (EC)** is a body responsible for ensuring that medical experimentation and human subject research are carried out in an ethical manner in accordance with national and international law.
- In **1964**, the World Medical Association published a code of research ethics, the **Declaration of Helsinki**. The convening of Ethics Committees to approve research protocols in human experiments was first written into international guidelines in the first revision to the Declaration of Helsinki (**Helsinki II, 1975**). The **Belmont Report** issued in **1979** further emphasized the need for review of all clinical research by such committees, which came to be known as Ethics Committees.
- In India, the requirement for an Ethics Committee to oversee clinical research was first made in the Indian Council of Medical Research (ICMR) Policy Statement for Ethics published in 1980, and then again in the original version of the Schedule Y issued in 1988.
- Then, came the Indian Good Clinical Practices (GCP) in 2001, the watershed Amended Schedule Y in 2005, and the **ICMR's Ethical Guidelines for Biomedical Research on Human Participants** in **2006**.
- Schedule Y (2005) detailed for the first time regulatory requirements of an EC. The ICMR guidelines released by the same Ministry (Health and Family Welfare) a year later described in more detail the composition, roles and responsibilities of an EC.

Constitution of Ethics Committee

- The Ethics Committee shall have a minimum of 7 and maximum of 15 members from medical, non-medical, scientific and non-scientific areas with at least: (i) one lay person; (ii) one woman member; (iii) one legal expert; (iv) one independent member from any other related field such as social scientist, or representative of nongovernmental voluntary agency, or philosopher or ethicist or theologian.
- One member of the Ethics Committee who is not affiliated with the institute or organization shall be the Chairperson, and shall be appointed by such institute or organization, and one member who is affiliated with the institute or organization shall be appointed as Member Secretary of the Ethics Committee by such Institute or organization.
- The Ethics Committee shall consist of at least fifty percent of its members who are not affiliated with the institute or organization in which such committee is constituted.
- The committee shall include at least one member whose primary area of interest or specialisation is non-scientific,

and at least one member who is independent of the institution.

- The Ethics committee can have as its members, individuals from other Institutions or Communities, if required.
- Members should be conversant with the provisions of **New Drug and Clinical Trials Rules, 2019**, Good Clinical Practice Guidelines for Clinical Trials in India, and other regulatory requirements to safeguard the rights, safety and well-being of the trial subjects.
- The members representing medical scientists and clinicians shall possess at least postgraduate qualification in their respective area of specialization, adequate experience in the respective fields, and requisite knowledge and clarity about their role and responsibility as committee members.
- As far as possible, based on the requirement of research area such as HIV, genetic disorder, etc., specific patient group may also be represented in the Ethics Committee.
- The Ethics Committee may associate such experts who are not its members, in its deliberations but such experts shall not have voting rights, if any.
- No member of an Ethics Committee, having a conflict of interest, shall be involved in the oversight of the clinical trial or bioavailability or bioequivalence study protocol being reviewed by it, and all members shall sign a declaration to the effect that there is no conflict of interest.
- While considering an application which involves a conflict of interest of any member of the Ethics Committee, such member may voluntarily withdraw from the Ethics Committee review meeting, by expressing the same in writing, to the Chairperson.
- No clinical trial or bioavailability or bioequivalence protocol shall be reviewed by an Ethics Committee in a meeting, unless at least five of its members as detailed below are present in the meeting, namely: (i) medical scientist (preferably a pharmacologist); (ii) clinician; (iii) legal expert; (iv) social scientist, or representative of non-governmental voluntary agency, or philosopher, or ethicist, or theologian, or a similar person; (v) lay person.

Functions of Ethics Committee

- The Ethics Committee shall review and accord approval to a Clinical trial, Bioavailability and Bioequivalence study protocol, and other related documents, as the case may be, in the format specified in the Third Schedule of New Drugs and Clinical Trials Rules, 2019, and oversee the conduct of clinical trial to safeguard the rights, safety and wellbeing of trial subjects in accordance with these rules, Good Clinical Practices Guidelines, and other applicable regulations.
- Where a clinical trial site does not have its own Ethics Committee, clinical trial at that site may be initiated after obtaining approval of the protocol from the Ethics Committee of another trial site; or an independent Ethics Committee for clinical trial constituted in accordance with the provisions, provided that the approving Ethics Committee for clinical trial shall be located within the same city, or within a radius of 50 km of the clinical trial site.
- The Ethics Committee shall indicate the reasons that weighed with it while rejecting or asking for a change or notification in the protocol in writing, and a copy of such reasons shall also be made available to the Central Licencing Authority.
- The Ethics Committee shall make, at appropriate intervals, an on-going review of the trials for which they have reviewed the protocol. Such a review may be based on the periodic study progress reports furnished by the investigators, or monitoring and internal audit reports furnished by the sponsor, or by visiting the study sites.
- Where any serious adverse event (SAE) occurs to a trial subject or to study subject during clinical trial or bioavailability or bioequivalence study, the Ethics Committee shall analyse the relevant documents pertaining to such event and forward its report to the Central Licencing Authority and comply with the provisions of Chapter VI, New Drugs and Clinical Trials Rules, 2019.
- The Ethics Committee shall undertake proper causality assessment of SAEs with the help of subject experts wherever required, for deciding relatedness and quantum of compensation.
- Where at any stage of a clinical trial, it comes to a conclusion that the trial is likely to compromise the right, safety or wellbeing of the trial subject, the Ethics Committee may order discontinuation or suspension of the clinical trial, and the same shall be intimated to the head of the institution conducting the clinical trial and the Central Licencing Authority.
- The Ethics Committee shall comply with the requirements or conditions specified under the Drugs & Cosmetics Act, 1940 and New Drugs and Clinical Trials Rues, 2019, as also the directives of the Central Licencing Authority, with the approval of the Central Government, to safeguard the rights of clinical trial subject, or bioavailability or bioequivalence study subject.
- The Ethics Committee shall review and approve the suitability of the investigator and trial site for the proposed trial.
- The Ethics Committee shall maintain data, record, registers and other documents related to the functioning and review of clinical trial or bioavailability study or bioequivalence study, as the case may be, for a period of 5 years after completion of such clinical trial.
- Funding mechanism for the Ethics Committee to support their operations should be designed and approved to ensure that the committee and their members have no financial incentive to approve or reject particular study.
- Standard Operating Procedures (SOPs) for funding of the Ethics Committee in order to support their operations, must be maintained. The records of income and expenditure of Ethics Committee shall be maintained for review and inspection.
- The Ethics Committee shall allow any officer authorized by the Central Licensing Authority to enter, with or without prior notice, to inspect the premises, any record, or any

documents related to clinical trial, furnish information to any query raised by such authorized person, in relation to the conduct of clinical trial, and to verify compliance with the requirements of these rules, Good Clinical Practices Guidelines, and other applicable regulations for safeguarding the rights, safety and well-being of trial subjects.

- Where Central Licencing Authority is of the opinion that the Ethics Committee fails to comply with any provision of the Drugs and Cosmetics Act, 1940 and New Drugs & Clinical Trials Rules, 2019, it may issue show cause notice to such Ethics Committee specifying therein such non-compliances and the period within which reply shall be furnished by such Ethics Committee. After consideration of the facts and reply given by the Ethics Committee, the Central Licencing Authority may take one or more actions specified under provision of Rule 14, Chapter III of New Drugs and Clinical Trials Rules, 2019.

FM 4.27: Non-Core – Written/Viva Voce
- Describe and discuss ethical guidelines for biomedical research on human subjects and animals.

and

FM 4.30: Core – Written/Viva Voce
- Demonstrate ability to conduct research in pursuance to guidelines or research ethics.

ETHICAL GUIDELINES FOR BIOMEDICAL & HEALTH RESEARCH INVOLVING ANIMALS

- Those involved in experimentation on animals must follow all the existing regulations and guidelines contained in:
  - **Prevention of Cruelty to Animals Act, 1960**, amended in 1982.
  - **Breeding and Experimentation Rules, 1998**, amended in 2001 and 2006.
  - **Guidelines for Care and Use of Animals in Scientific Research, 1982**, amended in 2000.
  - **ICMR Guidelines on Humane Care and Use of Laboratory Animals, 2006**.
  - **Committee for the Purpose of Control and Supervision of Experiments on Animals (CPSCSEA) Guidelines for Laboratory Animal Facilities, 2003**.
  - **Guidelines for Rehabilitation of Animals used in Research, 2010**.

NATIONAL ETHICAL GUIDELINES FOR BIOMEDICAL & HEALTH RESEARCH INVOLVING HUMAN PARTICIPANTS, 2017

- The **Indian Council of Medical Research (ICMR)** issued a **Policy Statement** on **Ethical Considerations Involved in Research on Human Subjects** in **1980**.
- Due to rapid advances in biomedical science and technology, new ethical dimensions emerged which necessitated further updates of these guidelines. Subsequently, the **Ethical Guidelines for Biomedical Research on Human Subjects** was released in **2000**, followed by the revised **Ethical Guidelines for Biomedical Research on Human Participants in 2006**.
- Emerging ethical issues necessitated further revision of the earlier guidelines and release of the current **National Ethical Guidelines for Biomedical and Health Research Involving Human Participants, 2017**.

General Principles

1. ***Principle of Essentiality***:
   - Only after due consideration of all alternatives in the light of existing knowledge, the use of human participants is to be considered to be essential for the proposed research. This should be duly vetted by an ethics committee (EC) independent of the proposed research.
2. ***Principle of Voluntariness***:
   - Respect for the right of the participant to agree or not to agree to participate in research, or to withdraw from research at any time, is paramount.
   - Informed consent is mandatory.
3. ***Principle of Non-exploitation***:
   - Research participants must be equitably selected so that the benefits and burdens of the research are distributed fairly and without arbitrariness or discrimination.
   - Sufficient safeguards to protect vulnerable groups should be ensured.
4. ***Principle of Social Responsibility***:
   - The research must be planned and conducted in such a way as to avoid creation or deepening of social and historic divisions, or in any way disturb social harmony in community relationships.
5. ***Principle of Ensuring Privacy and Confidentiality***:
   - It is essential to maintain privacy of the potential participant, her/his identity and records are kept confidential, and access is limited to only those authorized.
   - However, under certain circumstances (suicidal ideation, homicidal tendency, HIV positive status, when required by court of law, etc.) privacy of the information can be breached in consultation with the EC for valid scientific or legal reasons, as the right to life of an individual supersedes the right to privacy of the research participant.
6. ***Principle of Risk Minimization***:
   - Due care is to be taken by all stakeholders (including researchers, ECs, sponsors, regulators) at all stages of the research to ensure that the risks are minimized and appropriate care and compensation is given if any harm occurs.
7. ***Principle of Professional Competence***:
   - The research must be planned, conducted, evaluated and monitored throughout by persons who are competent, and have the appropriate and relevant qualifications, experience and/or training.
8. ***Principle of Maximization of Benefit***:
   - Due care is to be taken to design and conduct the research in such a way as to directly or indirectly maxi-

mize the benefits to the research participants and/or to the society.

9. ***Principle of Institutional Arrangements***:
   - Institutions (where the research is being conducted), must have policies for appropriate research governance and take the responsibility to facilitate research by providing required infrastructure, manpower, funds and training opportunities.
10. ***Principle of Transparency and Accountability***:
    - The research plan and outcomes emanating from the research must be brought into the public domain through registries, reports and scientific and other publications while safeguarding the right to privacy of the participants.
    - Stakeholders involved in research should disclose any existing conflict of interest and manage it appropriately.
    - The research should be conducted in a fair, honest, impartial and transparent manner to guarantee accountability.
    - Related records, data and notes should be retained for the required period for possible external scrutiny/ audit.
11. ***Principle of Totality of Responsibility***:
    - All stakeholders involved in the research are responsible for their actions. The professional, social and moral responsibilities compliant with ethical guidelines and related regulations are binding on all stakeholders directly or indirectly.
12. ***Principle of Environmental Protection***:
    - Researchers are accountable for ensuring protection of the environment and resources at all stages of the research, in compliance with existing guidelines and regulations.

General Ethical Issues

1. ***Benefit–Risk Assessment***:
   - Benefits to the individual, community or society refer to any sort of favourable outcome of the research, whether direct or indirect. The social and scientific value of research should justify the risk, which is the probability of causing discomfort or harm anticipated as physical, psychological, social, economic or legal.
   - The researcher, sponsor and **Ethics Committee (EC)** should attempt to maximize benefits and minimize risks to participants, so that risks are balanced to lead to potential benefits at individual, societal and/or community levels.
   - The EC should assess the inherent benefits and risks, ensure a favourable balance of benefits and risks, evaluate plans for minimizing the risk and discomfort, and decide on the merit of the research before approving it.
   - The EC should also assess any altered risks in the study at the time of continuing review.
   - The type of EC review based on risk involved in the research, is categorized as given in **Table 4.5**.

Table 4.5 Categories of Risk

Type of Risk	Definition/Description
Less than Minimal risk	Probability of harm or discomfort anticipated in the research is nil or not expected. For example, research on anonymous or non-identified data/samples, data available in the public domain, meta-analysis, etc.
Minimal risk	Probability of harm or discomfort anticipated in the research is not greater than that ordinarily encountered in routine daily life activities of an average healthy individual or general population or during the performance of routine tests where occurrence of serious harm or an adverse event (AE) is unlikely. Examples include research involving routine questioning or history taking, observing, physical examination, chest X-ray, obtaining body fluids without invasive intervention, such as hair, saliva or urine samples, etc.
Minor increase over Minimal risk or Low risk	Increment in probability of harm or discomfort is only a little more than the minimal risk threshold. This may present in situations such as routine research on children and adolescents; research on persons incapable of giving consent; delaying or withholding a proven intervention or standard of care in a control or placebo group during randomized trials; use of minimally invasive procedures that might cause no more than brief pain or tenderness, small bruises or scars, or very slight, temporary distress, such as drawing a small sample of blood for testing; trying a new diagnostic technique in pregnant and breastfeeding women, etc. Such research should have a social value. Use of personal identifiable data in research also imposes indirect risks. Social risks, psychological harm and discomfort may also fall in this category.
More than Minimal risk or High risk	Probability of harm or discomfort anticipated in the research is invasive and greater than minimal risk. Examples include research involving any interventional study using a drug, device or invasive procedure such as lumbar puncture, lung or liver biopsy, endoscopic procedure, intravenous sedation for diagnostic procedures, etc.

2. ***Informed Consent Process***:
   - Informed consent protects the individual's autonomy to freely choose whether or not to participate in the research.
   - The process involves three components:
     - providing relevant information to potential participants
     - ensuring the information is comprehended by them
     - assuring voluntariness of participation.
   - Informed consent should explain medical terminology in simple terms and be in a language that the participant understands.
   - The informed consent document (ICD), which includes patient/participant information sheet (PIS) and informed consent form (ICF) should have the required elements, and should be reviewed and approved by the EC before enrolment of participants. For all biomedical and health research involving human participants, it is the primary responsibility of the researcher to obtain the written, informed consent of the prospective participant or legally acceptable/authorized representative (LAR). In case of an individual who is not capable of giving informed consent, the consent of the LAR should be obtained. If a participant or LAR is illiterate, a literate impartial witness should also be present during the informed consent process.
   - In certain circumstances, audio-visual recording of the informed consent process may be required, e.g., in certain clinical trials as notified by CDSCO (Central Drugs Standard Control Organisation).
   - Verbal/Oral consent/Waiver of consent/Re-consent may be obtained under certain conditions after due consideration and approval by the EC.
3. ***Privacy and Confidentiality***:
   - Privacy is the right of an individual to control or influence the information that can be collected and stored and by whom and to whom that information may be disclosed or shared.
   - Confidentiality is the obligation of the researcher/research team/organization to the participant to safeguard the entrusted information. It includes the obligation to protect information from unauthorized access, use, disclosure, modification, loss or theft. The researcher should safeguard the confidentiality of research related data of participants and the community.
   - Potential limitations to ensure strict confidentiality must be explained to the participant. Researchers must inform prospective participants that although every effort will be made to protect privacy and ensure confidentiality, it may not be possible to do so under certain circumstances.
   - Any publication arising out of research should uphold the privacy of the individuals by ensuring that photographs or other information that may reveal the individual's identity are not published. A specific re-consent would be required for publication, if this was not previously obtained.
   - Some information may be sensitive and should be protected to avoid stigmatization and/or discrimination (e.g., HIV status; sexual orientation such as lesbian, gay, bisexual and transgender (LGBT); genetic information or any other sensitive information).
   - While conducting research with stored biological samples or medical data, coding or anonymization of personal information is important, and access to both samples and records should be limited.
   - Data of individual participants/community may be disclosed in certain circumstances with the permission of the EC such as specific orders of a court of law, threat to a person's or community's life, public health risk that would supersede personal rights to privacy, serious adverse events (SAEs) that are required to be communicated to an appropriate regulatory authority, etc.
4. ***Distributive Justice***:
   - Efforts must be made to ensure that individuals or communities invited for research are selected in such a way that the benefits and burdens of research are equitably distributed.
   - Vulnerable individuals/groups should not be included in research to solely benefit others who are better-off than themselves.
   - Research should not lead to social, racial or ethnic inequalities.
   - Plans for benefit sharing in all types of research with participants, donors of biological materials or data should be included in the study, especially if there is a potential for commercialization. This should be decided a priori in consultation with the stakeholders and reviewed by the EC.
5. ***Payment for Participation***:
   - If applicable, participants may be reimbursed for expenses incurred relating to their participation in research, such as travel related expenses. Participants may also be paid for inconvenience incurred, time spent and other incidental expenses in either cash or kind or both, as deemed necessary (e.g., loss of wages and food supplies).
   - Participants should not be made to pay for any expenses incurred beyond routine clinical care and which are research related including investigations, patient work up, any interventions or associated treatment. This is applicable to all participants, including those in comparator/control groups. If there are provisions, participants may also receive additional medical services at no cost.
   - When the LAR is giving consent on behalf of a participant, payment should not become an undue inducement and to be reviewed carefully by the EC. Reimbursement may be offered for travel and other incidental expenses incurred due to participation of the child/ward in the research.

- ECs must review and approve the payments (in cash or kind or both) and free services and the processes involved, and also determine that this does not amount to undue inducement.

6. ***Compensation for Research-related Harm***:
   - Research participants who suffer direct physical, psychological, social, legal or economic harm as a result of their participation are entitled, after due assessment, to financial or other assistance to compensate them equitably for any temporary or permanent impairment or disability. In case of death, participant's dependents are entitled to financial compensation. The research proposal should have an in-built provision for mitigating research related harm.
   - The researcher is responsible for reporting all Serious Adverse Events (SAEs) to the EC within 24 hours of knowledge. This may be done via email or fax communication (including on non-working days). A report on how the SAE was related to the research must also be submitted within 14 days.
   - The EC is responsible for reviewing the relatedness of the SAE to the research, as reported by the researcher, and determining the quantum and type of assistance to be provided to the participants.
   - For clinical trials under the purview of CDSCO, the timeline and procedures as notified from time to time may be followed.
   - All research participants who suffer harm, whether related or not, should be offered appropriate medical care, psycho-social support, referrals, clinical facilities, etc.
   - Medical management should be free, if the harm is related to the research.
   - Compensation should be given to any participant when the injury is related to the research. This is applicable to participants in any of the arms of research, such as intervention, control and standard of care.
   - While deliberating on the quantum of compensation for participants who have suffered research-related injury, the EC should consider aspects including the type of research (interventional, observational, etc.), extent of injury (temporary/permanent, short/long term), loss of wages, etc.
   - For other sponsored research, it is the responsibility of the sponsor (whether a pharmaceutical company, government or non-governmental organization, national or international donor agency/institution) to include insurance coverage or provision for possible compensation for research related injury or harm within the budget.
   - It is the responsibility of the host institution to provide compensation or cover for insurance for research related injury or harm to be paid as decided by the EC. The institution should create a mechanism to be able to provide for compensation, such as a corpus fund.
   - In the applications for research grants to funding agencies, the researcher should keep a budgetary provision for insurance coverage and/or compensation depending upon the type of research, anticipated risks and proposed number of participants.
7. ***Ancillary Care***:
   - Participants may be offered free medical care for non-research-related conditions or incidental findings, if these occur during the course of participation in the research, provided such compensation does not amount to undue inducement as determined by the EC.
8. ***Conflict of Interest***:
   - Conflict of interest (COI) is a set of conditions where professional judgement concerning a primary interest such as participants welfare or the validity of research tends to be unduly influenced by a secondary interest, financial or non-financial (personal, academic or political). COI can be at the level of researchers, EC members, institutions or sponsors. If COI is inherent in the research, it is important to declare this at the outset and establish appropriate mechanisms to manage it.
   - Research institutions must develop and implement policies and procedures to identify, mitigate conflicts of interest and educate their staff about such conflicts.
   - Researchers must ensure that the documents submitted to the EC include a disclosure of interests that may affect the research.
9. ***Selection of Vulnerable and Special Groups as Research Participants***:
   - Vulnerable groups and individuals may have an increased likelihood of incurring additional harm as they may be relatively (or absolutely) incapable of protecting their own interests.
   - Characteristics that make individuals vulnerable are legal status – children; clinical conditions – cognitive impairment, unconsciousness; or situational conditions – including but not limited to being economically or socially disadvantaged (e.g., certain ethnic or religious groups, individuals/communities which have hierarchical relationships, institutionalized persons, humanitarian emergencies, language barriers and cultural differences).
   - In general, such participants should be included in research only when the research is directly answering the health needs or requirements of the group. On the other hand, vulnerable populations also have an equal right to be included in research so that benefits accruing from the research apply to them as well. This needs careful consideration by researchers as well as the EC.
   - The EC should determine vulnerability and ensure that additional safeguards and monitoring mechanisms are established. It should also advise the researcher in this regard.
10. ***Community Engagement***:
    - Community can be defined as a social group of people of any size sharing the same geographical location, beliefs, culture, age, gender, profession, lifestyle, disease,

etc. The community should be meaningfully engaged before, during and after the research to mitigate culturally sensitive issues and ensure greater responsiveness to their health needs and requirements.

- A Community Advisory Board/Group (CAB/CAG) can act as an interface between the community (from which participants are to be drawn), the researchers and the concerned EC. Members of the CAB should be such that they do not coerce the members of the community to participate in the research and also protect the rights and serve the requirements of the group.
- Members of the community can also be represented in the EC either as members or special invitees.
- Community engagement does not replace individual informed consent. It ensures that the community's health needs and expectations are addressed, informed consent is appropriate, and access to research benefits are provided through research that is designed and implemented in the best interests of science and the community.
- After the study is completed, the researcher may communicate with the community representative, local institution or the government department from where the data was collected to help in dissemination of the results to the entire community.

11. ***Post-Research Access and Benefit Sharing***:
    - The benefits accruing from research should be made accessible to individuals, communities and populations whenever relevant. Sometimes more than the benefit to the individual participant, the community may be given benefit in an indirect way by improving their living conditions, establishing counselling centres, clinics or schools and providing education on good health practices.
    - Efforts should be made to communicate the findings of the research study to the individuals/communities wherever relevant.
    - The research team should make plans wherever applicable for post-research access and sharing of academic or intervention benefits with the participants, including those in the control group.
    - Post-research access arrangements or other care must be described in the study protocol, so that the EC may consider such arrangements during its review.
    - If an investigational drug is to be given to a participant post-trial, appropriate regulatory approvals should be in place.

FM 4.28: Core – Written/Viva Voce

- Demonstrate respect to laws relating to medical practice and ethical code of conduct prescribed by Medical Council of India and rules and regulations prescribed by it from time to time.

and

FM 4.29: Core – Written/Viva Voce

- Demonstrate ability to communicate appropriately with media, public and doctors.

Laws relating to medical practice and ethical code of conduct prescribed by Medical Council of India and rules and regulations prescribed by it from time to time have been dealt with under FM 4.2 *(page no. 278)* **and FM 4.6** *(page no. 287)*, **while the importance of communicating appropriately with media, public and doctors, have been discussed under FM 4.10** *(page no. 296)*.

FM 4.30: Core – Written/Viva Voce

- Demonstrate ability to conduct research in pursuance to guidelines or research ethics.

Research guidelines and research ethics have been dealt with under FM 4.25 *(page no. 314)*, **FM 4.26** *(page no. 317)* **and FM 4.27** *(page no. 319)*, **which should be consulted and followed while carrying out medical research.**

Topic 5

FORENSIC PSYCHIATRY

(Number of Competencies – 6: FM 5.1 to 5.6)

FM 5.1: Core – Written/Viva Voce

- Classify common mental illnesses including post-traumatic stress disorder (PTSD)

CLASSIFICATION OF PSYCHIATRIC DISORDERS (MENTAL ILLNESS)

- There are two internationally recognised methods of classifying psychiatric disorders – **DSM-5** and **ICD-11**.
  - DSM-5:
    - It is an essentially American system, and is an abbreviation of **Diagnostic and Statistical Manual of Mental Disorders, 5th edition, 2013**.
    - It is a classification prepared and regularly updated by the American Psychiatric Association (APA). DSM-5 was published on May 18, 2013, superseding the DSM-4-TR, which was published in 2000.
    - In most respects DSM-5 is not greatly changed from DSM-4-TR. Notable changes include dropping Asperger syndrome as a distinct classification; loss of subtype classifications for variant forms of schizophrenia; dropping the "bereavement exclusion" for depressive disorders; a revised treatment and naming of "gender identity disorder" to "gender dysphoria", and removing the A2 criterion for "post-traumatic stress disorder (PTSD)" because its requirement for specific emotional reactions to trauma did not apply to combat veterans and first responders with PTSD.
  - ICD-11:
    - It stands for **International Classification of Diseases, 11th edition, 2022**. The title of the ICD is formally the **International Statistical Classification of Diseases and Related Health Problems**, although the original title, International Classification of Diseases, is still informally the name by which it is usually known.
    - It officially came into effect on 1st Jan 2022.
    - This classification has been prepared by the WHO, and is periodically updated.
    - Chapter 'F' of the ICD deals with psychiatric disorders.

The ICD-11 classification will be followed in this book, as it has wider acceptance all over the world.

Mental and Behaviour Disorders (ICD-11)

This is the latest classification of psychiatric (mental) disorders and supersedes all earlier methods of classifying such disorders. The latter must not be taught to students, and must not feature in examinations.

1. **Neurodevelopmental Disorders**:
   a. Disorders of acquisition and execution of specific intellectual, language, motor and social functions have been included here.
   b. The most notable change is the renaming of "**mental retardation**" and "**disorders of psychological development**" of ICD-10 as **"disorders of intellectual development"**, in an effort to decrease the associated stigma.
      i. This provides a comprehensive set of behavioural indicators, and intellectual functioning domains, organized according to age groups (early childhood, childhood/adolescence and adulthood) and four levels of severity (mild, moderate, severe, profound).
   c. **Attention deficit hyperactivity disorder (ADHD)** has been added in this group and replaced the term "**hyperkinetic disorder**."
2. **Schizophrenia and Other Primary Psychotic Disorders**:
   a. The term "primary" has been incorporated here to exclude the cases of affective or induced psychosis, and including only those cases in which psychosis is the core feature.
   b. Other changes include elimination of subtypes of schizophrenia due to their lack of predictive validity or utility in treatment selection.
3. **Mood Disorders**:
   a. Persistent mood disorders in ICD-10, consisting of dysthymia and cyclothymia, have been eliminated, and included in depressive disorders and bipolar disorders accordingly.
4. **Anxiety and Fear-related Disorders**:
   a. Disorders primarily presenting with anxiety or fear were regrouped here.
5. **Obsessive Compulsive and Related Disorders (OCRD)**:
   a. The OCRD group was introduced for differentiating from other anxiety disorders on the basis of presence of core feature of unwanted thoughts and related repetitive behaviours.
   b. The group includes:
      i. **Body dysmorphic disorder**

   ii. **Olfactory reference disorder**
   iii. **Hypochondriasis (illness anxiety disorder)** and
   iv. **Hoarding disorder**.
   c. The subgroup of **body-focused repetitive behaviour disorders**, including **trichotillomania (hair-pulling disorder)** and **excoriation (skin-picking) disorder**, was introduced as both share the core feature of repetitive behaviour without the cognitive aspect of other OCRDs.
   d. **Tourette syndrome** is cross-listed in this group because of its frequent co-occurrence with **obsessive compulsive disorder (OCD)**.
6. **Disorders Specifically Associated with Stress**:
   a. Reactive and disinhibited attachment disorders of childhood are reclassified to this group owing to the lifespan approach.
   b. **Post traumatic stress disorder (PTSD)**, **Prolonged grief disorder** and **Adjustment disorder** have been added here.
7. **Dissociative Disorders**:
   a. The term "conversion" in ICD-10 is eliminated from the group title.
   b. **Dissociative neurological symptom disorder** is presented as a single disorder with 12 subtypes.
   c. Dissociative fugue is not counted as a separate disorder but kept as a qualifier for **dissociative amnesia**.
   d. The ICD-10 "possession trance disorder" is separated into **trance disorder** (typically involves the repetition of a small repertoire of simpler behaviours) and **possession trance disorder** (a greater range of more complex behaviours).
   e. **Dissociative identity disorder** in ICD-11 corresponds to the concept of ICD-10 **multiple personality disorder**.
8. **Feeding and Eating Disorders**:
   a. **Avoidant restrictive food intake disorder (ARFID)** and **Binge eating disorder** are included here.
   b. In the diagnosis of **Anorexia nervosa**, requirement for the presence of a widespread endocrine disorder has been eliminated.
   c. **Bulimia nervosa** can be diagnosed regardless of the current weight, until the body mass index is not very low, and even if there are only "subjective" binges in the absence of "objective" binges.
9. Elimination Disorders.
10. **Disorders of Bodily Distress and Bodily Experience**:
   a. The group includes two disorders: **Bodily distress disorder** (represents ICD-10 concepts of somatoform disorders and neurasthenia) and **Body integrity dysphoria**.
11. **Disorders due to Substance Use and Addictive Behaviours**:
   a. The major conceptual change entertained in substance use disorders is the addition of "**single episode of harmful substance use**," which provides an opportunity for early intervention and prevention of escalation of use or harm, whereas the diagnoses of "**harmful pattern of substance use**" and "**substance dependence**" suggest the need for intensive interventions.
   b. Importantly, the so-called behavioural addictions namely **Gambling disorder** ("pathological gambling" in ICD-10) and **Gaming disorder** were introduced in this grouping.
12. **Impulse Control Disorders**:
   a. The group includes **kleptomania** and **pyromania**.
   b. Significant changes include the introduction of **Intermittent explosive disorder** and **Compulsive sexual behaviour disorder**, which reclassifies ICD-10 excessive sexual drive.
13. **Disruptive Behaviour and Dissocial Disorders**:
   a. The group includes **Oppositional defiant disorder** and **Conduct dissocial disorder**.
14. **Personality Disorders**:
   a. The crucial change entertained in ICD-11 was the addition of qualifiers – mild, moderate or severe – based on the pervasiveness of disturbances in the functioning of self, interpersonal dysfunction; severity and chronicity of emotional, cognitive and behavioural manifestations; and the extent of psychosocial impairment.
   b. A new category "**personality difficulty**" has been added, which refers to those individuals where deviant traits are present, but not up to the severity amounting to be labelled as a disorder.
15. **Paraphilic Disorders**:
   a. Paraphilic disorders replace the ICD-10 grouping of "disorders of sexual preference". More focus is placed on the fact that behaviours are inflicted on non-consenting others; resultantly, private behaviours, such as "**Sadomasochism**", "**Fetishism**" and "**Transvestism**", have been eliminated, as they are found to be not relevant to public health.
   b. However, disorders like **Asphyxophilia**, although being a solitary private behaviour, is retained in this group under "other paraphilic disorders."
16. **Factitious Disorders**:
   a. The new grouping of factitious disorders includes **Factitious disorder imposed on self** and **Factitious disorder imposed on another**.
   b. **Malingering** is not classified as a mental, behavioural or neurodevelopmental disorder, but appears in the chapter on "factors influencing health status or contact with health services".
17. **Neurocognitive Disorders**:
   a. This group includes **Delirium**, **Mild neurocognitive disorder** (called "mild cognitive disorder" in ICD-10), **Amnestic disorder** and **Dementia**.
   b. Dementia is classified as mild, moderate or severe.

POST-TRAUMATIC STRESS DISORDER (PTSD)

- A mental and behavioural disorder that can develop because of exposure to a traumatic event, such as sexual assault, warfare, traffic accident, child abuse, domestic violence, etc.
- Symptoms may include:
  - Disturbing thoughts, feelings or dreams related to the event

- Mental or physical distress to trauma-related cues
- Attempts to avoid trauma-related cues
- Alterations in the way the person thinks and feels, and
- An increase in the fight-or-flight response.

- These symptoms last for more than a month after the event.
- A person with PTSD is at a higher risk of suicide and intentional self-harm.
- It is more common in women than men.
- People who experience interpersonal violence such as rape, kidnap, stalking, physical abuse by an intimate partner, childhood sexual abuse, etc., are more likely to develop PTSD than those who experience non-assault based trauma, such as accidents and natural disasters.
- Those who experience prolonged trauma, such as slavery, concentration camps or chronic domestic abuse, may develop **Complex post-traumatic stress disorder (C-PTSD)**. C-PTSD is similar to PTSD but has a distinct effect on a person's emotional regulation and core identity.
- The main treatment for patients with PTSD comprises
  - Counselling (psychotherapy)
  - Antidepressants

FM 5.2: Core – Written/Viva Voce
- **Define, classify and describe with examples:**
  - Delusion
  - Hallucination
  - Illusion
  - Lucid interval
  - Obsession

SYMPTOMS OF MENTAL ILLNESS

Delusion

- It is a disturbance of thought.
- It is a false belief in something which is not a fact, and which persists even after its falsity has been clearly demonstrated.
- Types*:
  - **Delusion of Grandeur**: The patient imagines that he is rich or famous, when he is actually poor or inconsequential.
  - **Delusion of Poverty**: Imagines he is poor when in fact he is wealthy.
  - **Delusion of Persecution**: Imagines that other people are out to harm him.
  - **Delusion of Reference**: Imagines that people or events relate or refer to him in some special way.
  - **Delusion of Influence (control)**: Imagines that his thoughts or actions are controlled by some external agency.
  - **Delusion of Infidelity**: Imagines that the spouse is unfaithful.
  - **Delusion of Self-accusation (self-reproach)**: Keeps blaming himself for trivial incidents that happened in the past.
  - **Nihilistic Delusion**: The patient is convinced that nothing exists around him in the real sense of the term.
  - **Erotomania (Clerambault-Kandinsky complex)**: Usually seen in women. The patient is convinced that a particular individual (invariably an employer or superior) is in love with her.
  - **Pseudologia phantastica**:
    - A variation of this is the ***Munchausen syndrome***, in which a person is convinced that he is seriously ill, and goes from doctor to doctor, hospital to hospital, in a vain attempt to diagnose his non-existent illness. It is a psychiatric factitious disorder more than a form of delusion, wherein those affected feign disease, illness or psychological trauma to draw attention, sympathy or reassurance to themselves. It is also known as ***hospital addiction syndrome***, ***thick chart syndrome*** or ***hospital hopper syndrome***. True Munchausen syndrome fits within the subclass of factitious disorder with predominantly physical signs and symptoms, but they also have a history of recurrent hospitalization, travelling, and dramatic, untrue, and extremely improbable tales of their past experiences.
    - Munchausen syndrome is related to ***Munchausen syndrome by proxy (MSbP/MSP)***, which refers to the abuse of another person, typically a child, in order to seek attention or sympathy for the abuser.

Hallucination

- It is a disturbance of perception.
- It is a false sensory perception without any real, external stimulus.
- Types**:
  - **Auditory**: The patient hears imaginary voices.
  - **Visual**: The patient sees non-existent shapes (*unformed images*), or people or animals (*formed images*).
  - **Olfactory**: Perceiving non-existent odours.
  - **Gustatory**: Perceiving a bad taste in the mouth constantly without apparent cause.
  - **Tactile (haptic)**: This may take the form of imaginary sensations over the skin (***formication***), or in a limb that has been amputated (***phantom limb***).
  - **Lilliputian (micropsia)**: Perceiving objects to be much smaller than they are.
  - **Synesthesia**: A stimulus perceived by a sensory organ other than the one that should actually perceive it, e.g., visualising music, hearing different colours, etc.

Illusion

- It is a disturbance of perception.

Can be remembered by the mnemonic **GRIN PEPPSI: Grandeur, Reference, Influence, Nihilistic, Persecution, Erotomania, Poverty, Pseudologia phantastica, Self accusation, Infidelity.*

***Can be remembered by the mnemonic **VAGOLTS**: Visual, Auditory, Gustatory, Olfactory, Lilliputian, Tactile, Synesthesia*

- It is a misinterpretation of a real external stimulus, e.g., perceiving a rope as a snake.
  - A sane person may also make such mistakes, but quickly realizes that he is wrong.

Obsession

- It is a disturbance of thought.
- A single idea or thought is constantly entertained by the patient, which is irrational, but persists in spite of all efforts to drive it from his mind.
- Examples:
  - Checking and re-checking (repeatedly) whether a door has been bolted or not.
  - Washing hands every few minutes.
  - Peeping under the bed for intruders every now and then, at bedtime.
  - Arranging and rearranging objects on a table constantly.

Lucid Interval

- In forensic medicine (or more precisely, forensic psychiatry), the term **"Lucid Interval"** is said to refer to the period of complete resolution of symptoms in a patient with mental disease that is usually unpredictable and temporary in nature. The cause is unknown, but it is an extremely rare entity, and some psychiatrists question the very existence of such a condition.
  - If such a condition can be proved to be the case in a crime committed by an otherwise mentally ill person, he is liable to be held accountable (culpable) for the crime, and can be punished.
- In emergency medicine, the term **"Lucid Interval"** refers to the period of consciousness between two episodes of unconsciousness in blunt force injury to the head. The first episode is due to **concussion**, while the second (and virtually fatal) period of unconsciousness is due to an **extradural haemorrhage** compressing the brain relentlessly. Unless the pressure is released and the clot evacuated surgically, death can result.

> **FM 5.3: Core – Written/Viva Voce**
> - Describe Civil Responsibility and Criminal Responsibility of a mentally ill person

MENTAL ILLNESS AND RESPONSIBILITY

- The term **responsibility** in the legal sense refers to the liability of a sane person for his actions (or omissions), and consequent **culpability** (liability for punishment) if such be contrary to law.
- The law presumes every individual to be sane, unless proved otherwise.

Civil Responsibility

1. **Marriage**:
   a. If it is proved that at the time of marriage, one of the parties (spouses) was mentally ill, then such marriage is declared as ***null and void***, i.e., as per law the marriage never took place even if consummation had been accomplished.
   b. Mental illness developing later in the course of married life, which was not present at the time of marriage, may constitute sufficient grounds for ***divorce***, but not for ***nullity***.
2. **Business contract**:
   a. As per the **Indian Contract Act** of **1872**, if it is proved that at the time of signing a contract one of the two parties was mentally ill, then the contract becomes legally invalid.
   b. However, mental illness developing subsequent to a legal agreement will not necessarily invalidate the contract.
   c. Also, if at the time of signing, the fact that one of the signatories to the contract was mentally ill was not known to the other party, then the contract may not be declared invalid.
   d. For the purposes of a contract, a person is said to be of sound mind if at the time of making the contract, he is capable of understanding it, and of forming a rational judgement.
3. **Management of property**:
   a. If a person who owns property becomes mentally ill and is incapable of managing his affairs with sound judgement, any relative or friend can approach the court for a judicial inquisition. If it is proved that the person is mentally ill in the course of such inquisition, then the court can appoint a Guardian or Manager depending on the circumstances.
4. **Capacity to depose as witness**:
   a. As per **section 118** of the **Indian Evidence Act**, a mentally ill person is not competent to give evidence if he is incapable of understanding the questions put to him, or giving rational answers to them.
   b. However, such a person can give evidence during a **lucid interval**, depending on the discretion of the judge.
5. **Testamentary capacity**:
   a. **"Testamentary capacity"** refers to the ability of a person to make a valid **"Will."**
   b. Mental capacity is a broader construct and refers to decision-making in several areas of life. **Testamentary capacity (TC)** is considered a part of overall mental capacity. An individual with sound mental capacity is expected to have the ability to make a **testament (Will)**, i.e., **Testamentary capacity**.
   c. A "**Will**" is a legal declaration or a document of a person's written wishes regarding the disposal of all of his or her movable or immovable property and all worldly possessions (all of which are together called "*Estate*") after death.
      - According to the Indian Succession Act, 1925, "A Will is a legal declaration of the testator's intention, concerning his property which he desires to be carried into effect after his death."

d. If the individual has not made a Will, the disposition or distribution of his/her estate is done as per the prevailing **laws of succession**.
e. The essential requirements for making a valid Will are laid out in **Box 5.1**.

Box 5.1—Testamentary Capacity

Important Points

1. A Will can be made by anyone who is of sound mind, and is not a minor.
2. A mentally unsound person can make a Will during an interval (Lucid interval), when he is of sound mind.
3. Deaf, dumb or blind people can execute a Will, if they understand its nature and consequences, and are able to communicate their wishes clearly.
4. No person can make a Will, if he is in a condition of mind, where he is unsure of what he is doing, whether due to intoxication, illness, or any other reason.
5. A Will is a voluntary act on the testator's part and is made on the testator's own free will and without any undue influence.
6. A Will becomes enforceable only after the death of the person who has made it.
7. The Will may be made with the help or legal assistance of a solicitor. However, this is not a legal requirement, and one can choose to compose a Will without any legal aid.
8. The Will has to be a written document, except for Muslims, in which case, it may be oral. It may be made either on plain paper or stamp paper, but no particular form has been prescribed by law for the purpose. The testator has to sign or affix thumb impression in the Will clearly and legibly on every page of the Will, and at the end of the Will.
9. Registration of the Will – After making the Will, it may be registered after paying the stamp duty under Section 18 of the Indian Registration Act, 1908. Under the act, this registration is optional, and the Will is perfectly valid without being registered. However, a registered Will is always of more value than an unregistered Will. The testator has to personally present the executed Will along with the witnesses after payment of the required registration fee. The endorsement of the registrar is sufficient to prove the fact of the execution of the Will.
10. A Will can be revoked or altered by the testator any number of times before his death.
11. Only the last Will executed by the testator is taken into consideration for disposal of the property.
12. The Will should include the list of the properties owned by the testator. Before making the Will, the testator should know the nature and extent of his property and be aware of his legal heirs, i.e., potential beneficiaries.
13. The testator may also mention that the Will covers the properties not known by the testator at the time of making the Will.
14. The testator can also bequeath properties, incomes and interests that he may acquire after the execution of the Will.
15. The Will must be attested and signed by two or more witnesses, who have to sign the Will simultaneously and in the presence of the testator. The witnesses, who have signed on the Will, cannot be beneficiaries or be married to the recipients of the Will. While the witnesses must attest and sign the Will, it is not legally necessary for them to see and be aware of the contents of the Will.
16. The Will should also identify an executor responsible for executing the Will after the testator's death.
17. Secrecy of the Will: Once the Will is made, it should be kept secret, though the testator may inform that he has made a Will to any person he considers trustworthy.
18. Safe custody of the Will: The Will could be kept in a secure location, such as a bank or a solicitor's office. A registered will can be preserved at the registrar's office in a sealed cover with the testator's and agent's names on it.
19. After the death of a person, his property may be disposed of as follows:
    a. If no Will is made, according to the prevailing laws of succession, i.e., intestate.
    b. If a Will is made, according to the content of the Will, i.e., testamentary.

Criminal Responsibility

- The entire concept of criminal responsibility revolves around the principle of **mens rea** or **guilty mind**.
- This is itself a component of a legal dictum (in Latin): "***Actus reus non facit reum nisi mens sit rea***".* When translated, it reads: "*The physical act alone does not make a person guilty; the mental component in the form of evil intent (guilty mind) is equally important*".
- Since a mentally ill person cannot comprehend the nature of his own actions, or that they may be contrary to law, he is exempted from criminal responsibility.
- However, mental illness per se is not enough to render a person innocent (of his criminal action). He must satisfy certain conditions which are laid out in law. In India, **Section 84** of the **Indian Penal Code** outlines the guidelines applicable to criminal responsibility of mentally ill individuals. This is an offshoot of the **McNaughten Rule** which came into force in the UK in the 19th century.
- **Daniel McNaughten**** was a psychotic suffering from delusions of persecution, who was convinced that his problems would end only with the demise of the then Prime Minister of Britain, Sir Robert Peel. In January 1843, he lay in wait for the Prime Minister, and when he encountered him, fired at him with his revolver. But because of mistaken identity, the Secretary to the Prime Minister, Edward Drummond was assassinated, and Sir Robert Peel escaped.

*__Source__: *Jonathan Law, Elizabeth A Martin. A Dictionary of Law. 7th edn. Oxford University Press; 2014.*

__Note__: *Also spelt* ***M'Naghten, McNaughtan* *or* ***McNaughton***.

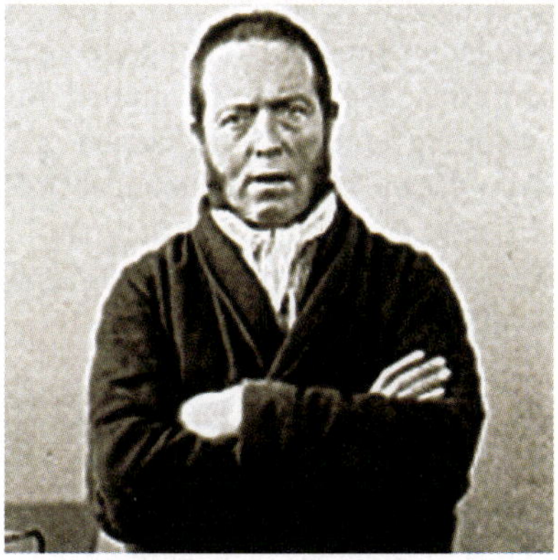

Daniel McNaughten
(Photographed by Henry Hering, 1856)

McNaughten was arrested and tried, but the jury after testification by 9 physicians, found him "not guilty by reason of mental illness". The people were outraged, as also Queen Victoria and Sir Robert Peel himself. As a result, 15 prominent judges were invited by the House of Lords. They were asked to respond to a series of questions on criminal responsibility. The answers were subsequently condensed and put forth as the **McNaughten Rule**.

After his acquittal, McNaughten was transferred from the prison to the State Criminal Lunatic Asylum at Bethlem Hospital. Apart from one hunger strike, which ended with force-feeding, McNaughten's 21 years at Bethlem appear to have been uneventful.

In 1864, he was transferred to the newly opened Broadmoor Asylum. He had developed diabetes and heart problems in Bethlem; by the time he was transferred to Broadmoor his health was declining and he died on 3rd May 1865.

Section 84 (Indian Penal Code)

- **Nothing is an offence which is done by a person, who, at the time of doing it, by reason of unsoundness of mind, is incapable of knowing the nature of the act, or that he is doing what is either wrong or contrary to law.**
- In order to apply Sec 84 in a given case, it has to be clearly established that at the time of committing the offence, the accused was labouring under a defect of reason which had been caused by unsoundness of mind, with the result that he was rendered incapable of knowing the nature of the act, or that he was doing what was wrong or contrary to law.
- A plea of mental illness at the time of the trial will not help the accused. Two things have to be therefore, clearly established, i.e.,
  - that at the time of committing the crime the accused was of unsound mind, and
  - that the unsoundness of mind was of a degree and nature which rendered the accused incapable of knowing the nature of the act, or that he was doing what was either wrong or contrary to law.
- It is important to note that "**legal mental illness**" is not the same as "**medical mental illness**". While the latter follows the classification laid down in psychiatry, "legal mental illness" is mainly with reference to mental deficiency and psychotic conditions. It does not recognise most of the neuroses and personality disorders as evidence of mental illness.
- It is also important to remember that it is the state of mind of the accused at the time of the commission of the offence that matters, and not at any other time before or after the event.
- The burden of proving mental illness is cast upon the accused, and he must prove that at the time of the incident he was by reason of unsoundness of mind incapable of judging the nature of his act (**Sec 105, Indian Evidence Act**).
- Every man is presumed to be sane and to possess sufficient degree of reason to be responsible for his crime unless the contrary is proved.
- One major defect in the **McNaughten Rule** (which in turn is reflected in Sec 84 IPC), is that emotional aspects relating to unsoundness of mind are not given due weightage. Hence, some of the major psychiatric disorders, especially neurotic disorders, are not given any importance.
- This aspect has been attempted to be rectified in Western countries such as the UK and the USA, by way of new guidelines:
  - **Durham Rule (1954)** – or "Product Test" was adopted by the United States Court of Appeals for the District of Columbia Circuit in 1954, and states that "... an accused is not criminally responsible, if his unlawful act was the product of mental disease or defect". This rule was however later overturned in 1972, as it places too much emphasis on "mental disease or defect," and thus on testimony by psychiatrists, and is said to be quite ambiguous.
  - **Currens Rule (1961)** – Outlined by Judge Biggs in the case of Currens vs United States, but lost favour with the courts, since it was too liberal a view.
  - **American Law Institute's Test (1962)**:
    - This rule (also called the **Model Penal Code**) was formulated in **1962**, and is used as a test of criminal responsibility in most criminal cases in the United States today.
    - The **ALI Test** says that an individual accused of a crime is not criminally responsible, if at the time of such conduct as a result of mental disease or defect, the person lacks substantial capacity either to appreciate the wrongfulness of the conduct, or to conform such conduct to the requirements of law.
    - The ALI test also requires that the mental disease or defect be a medical diagnosis. In this way, it manages to incorporate elements of all three of its predecessors: the knowledge of right and wrong required by McNaughten, the prerequisite of lack of control in the Currens Rule, and the diagnosis of mental disease and defect required by Durham.

Role of the Medical Officer in Criminal Cases with Mental Illness Plea

- In a criminal case where mental illness is pleaded as a defence, the opinion of a psychiatrist is necessary to prove its existence in the accused. If he is requested by the authorities to examine the accused and furnish his opinion, he must proceed cautiously and meticulously.
- Some helpful pointers to an insane crime include the following:
  - History of mental disease in the family of the accused.
  - Lack of motive in the commission of the offence.
  - Lack of premeditation/pre-planning.
  - Absence of accomplices.
  - No attempt to destroy evidence, or to flee from the scene of crime.
  - Ghastly or bizarre nature of crime.

FM 5.4: Core – Written/Viva Voce
- Differentiate between true insanity and feigned insanity

FEIGNED INSANITY

- Since the law provides for exempting a criminal from punishment if he was insane at the time of the offence (though he may be incarcerated in a psychiatric hospital for treatment), it is not uncommon for an offender to plead insanity as a defence, especially in cases of murder. Such a defence may be put forth even though the culprit is actually sane, so that he may escape stiff punishment such as life imprisonment or death. In order to substantiate his claim, the person may pretend to be insane by manifesting fabricated signs and symptoms. This is referred to as **feigned insanity**.
- The court or the police may then request for the opinion of a psychiatrist to clarify the issue. When called upon to do so, the psychiatrist must meticulously examine the individual and pay special attention to certain clues which could indicate pretence ("feigning or shamming or malingering"). Some of these are mentioned in **Table 5.1**.
- Some **practical clues** to indicate that an individual is feigning insanity include the following:
  - The first step is to do a thorough review of the suspect's history. Mental illness does not develop overnight, so it is important to know if the person has been hospitalized or treated for similar symptoms.
  - The investigator must also review the crime-scene report. If the suspect has hidden the weapon, washed off his fingerprints, or taken other steps to elude the police, it is a sign of clear thinking—not mental illness.

Table 5.1 Differences between True and Feigned Insanity

S. No	Feature	True Insanity	Feigned Insanity
1	Onset	Usually gradual	Sudden
2	Motive	Absent	Present (to escape punishment for a serious crime)
3	Predisposing factors	Present (e.g., familial tendency)	Absent
4	Facial expressions	Either normal or exaggerated abnormal	Consistent with the nature of mental illness
5	Presence of symptoms	Irrespective of his conduct being observed or not	Usually shows signs of insanity only when he thinks he is being observed, while symptoms are absent when he thinks that he is alone, or not being watched
6	Nature of symptoms	Consistent or expected for the type of mental illness he is suffering from	Inconsistent, exaggerated or bizarre
7	Capacity to endure exertion	Present (e.g., can be hyperactive, or go without sleep for a number of days)	Absent
8	Personal hygiene & habits	Often appears dirty or ill dressed	Usually appears neat
9	Skin, hair, nails	Often uncared for	Usually has clean skin, combed hair, trimmed nails
10	Repeated medical examination	Does not mind	Resents frequent medical or psychiatric examination for fear of being caught

- It is recommended to conduct long, rambling interviews—the longer the better, because after a few hours, some suspects begin to lose track of their symptoms or grow weary of the pretence.
- Most malingerers are not aware as to how a mentally disturbed individual is expected to behave, so they may present a confusing or even bizarre picture – a Bollywood version of insanity!
- Malingerers often exaggerate their symptoms and ignore common, subtle signs such as the blunting of a mentally ill patient's emotions. Some fakers say one thing and do another. They might feign confusion to the psychiatrist but later converse easily with cell-mates, or claim to be paranoid while sitting at ease. Some combine symptoms from different conditions, such as hallucinations of schizophrenia and suicidal ideations of a depressive.
- Today, there are standardized tests that trip up malingerers. A preliminary, 10-minute test, called **M-FAST** (Miller Forensic Assessment of Symptoms Test), presents a series of 25 questions that intermix phony and real symptoms. It is almost impossible to pick the right combinations if the suspect is not mentally ill. A more thorough series of questions called **SIRS** (Structured Interview of Reported Symptoms) is used subsequently.
- There is even a test for faking amnesia, which is among the most common of feigned mental illnesses. Contrary to popular belief, people with amnesia do not completely lose their ability to remember things. Therefore, forensic psychologists give a memory test that is so easy that even a person with amnesia could pass it. They show a series of letters, numbers and shapes for a few seconds and then ask him to draw them on a blank sheet of paper. Even people with amnesia caused by brain damage can reproduce most of the symbols. If the suspect says he cannot remember anything, he is most probably a malingerer.

> FM 5.5: Core – Written/Viva Voce
> - Describe & discuss Delirium tremens

DELIRIUM TREMENS (DTs; "THE HORRORS"; "THE SHAKES")

- It is one of the five withdrawal reactions encountered in chronic alcoholism.
- ***Onset***: 3–5 days.
- ***Mechanism***:
  - Delirium tremens is caused by the effect of alcohol on GABA receptors. Constant consumption of alcoholic beverages (and the consequent chronic sedation) causes a counter-regulatory response in the brain in an attempt to regain homeostasis. This causes down-regulation of these receptors, as well as an up-regulation in the production of excitatory neurotransmitters, primarily glutamate, and also noradrenaline, dopamine, adrenaline, and serotonin, all of which further the drinker's tolerance to alcohol. When alcohol is no longer consumed, these down-regulated $GABA_A$ receptor complexes are so insensitive to GABA that the typical amount of GABA produced has little effect; compounded with the fact that GABA normally inhibits action potential formation, there are not as many receptors for GABA to bind to—meaning that sympathetic activation is unopposed. This is also known as an '**adrenergic storm**'.
  - This is made worse by excitatory neurotransmitter up-regulation, so not only is sympathetic nervous system over-activity unopposed by GABA, there is also more of the serotonin, noradrenaline, dopamine, adrenaline and particularly glutamate. Excitatory NMDA receptors are also up-regulated, contributing to the delirium and neurotoxicity (by excito-toxicity) of withdrawal.
- ***Features***:
  - There is a dramatic onset of disordered mental activity characterised by clouding of consciousness, disorientation and loss of recent memory.
  - There are vivid hallucinations which are usually visual, but sometimes auditory in nature.
  - There is severe agitation with restlessness and shouting, tremor, and truncal ataxia. Insomnia is prolonged.
  - Autonomic disturbances include sweating, fever, tachycardia, hypertension and dilated pupils.
  - Dehydration and electrolyte disturbances are characteristic.
  - Blood testing shows leucocytosis and impaired liver function.
- ***Treatment***:
  - Well lit, reassuring environment.
  - For agitation – Diazepam 10 mg IV initially, and then 5 mg every 5 minutes until full control, followed by 5–10 mg orally 3 times daily. In severe cases, low levels of antipsychotics, such as haloperidol, or stronger benzodiazepines like temazepam or midazolam can be given until symptoms subside.
  - Thiamine in the usual dose.
  - Correction of fluid and electrolyte imbalance.
  - In cases of benzodiazepine resistance, patients can be given a second GABAergic drug. Phenobarbitone, given in combination with benzodiazepine, in IV doses of 130 mg, is a reasonable choice. Caution is required to avoid stacking doses of phenobarbitone, as the onset of clinical effect takes approximately 20–40 minutes. Alternatively, propofol in standard doses may be administered. Although propofol has a rapid onset, it is difficult to titrate. The main drawback to the use of these drugs is their narrow therapeutic-toxic index, with the potential for profound respiratory depression. This is especially true of propofol, which should generally only be used in the setting of mechanical ventilation.
  - Acamprosate is often used to augment treatment, and is then carried on into long term use to reduce the risk of relapse.

- ***Forensic Significance***:
  - It is a withdrawal reaction to alcohol, and is seen in chronic alcoholics who are suddenly deprived of liquor.
  - It is a form of acute psychosis and is classified as a psychiatric condition in ICD-11.

FM 5.6: Non-Core – Written/Viva Voce
- Describe the Indian Mental Health Act, 1987 with special reference to admission, care and discharge of a mentally ill person.

MENTAL HEALTH ACT, 1987

- The **Mental Health Act** (**MHA**), **1987**, came into effect only in **April 1993**, in all the states and union territories of India. It replaced the **Indian Lunacy Act** of **1912**, which had earlier replaced the **Indian Lunatic Asylums Act** of **1858**.
- The **Mental Health Care Act 2017** was passed on 07th April 2017, and has some revolutionary changes (**Box 5.2**).
  - The Act uses the term 'mentally ill person' instead of the more offensive 'lunatic', and 'mentally ill prisoner' instead of 'criminal lunatic'. Also the term 'psychiatric hospital' is used in place of 'mental hospital.'
  - A **mentally ill person** is defined by the Act as ***a person who is in need of treatment by reason of any mental disorder other than mental retardation***.

Box 5.2—Mental Health Care Act, 2017

The Mental Health Care Act, 2017 was passed on 07th April 2017. It supersedes the previously existing Mental Health Act, 1987.

Changes from the Mental Health Act, 1987:
- The Mental Healthcare Act, 2017 aims at decriminalising "attempt to commit suicide" by seeking to ensure that the individuals who have attempted suicide are offered opportunities for rehabilitation from the government as opposed to being tried or punished for the attempt.
- It looks to empower persons suffering from mental illness, thus marking a departure from the Mental Health Act, 1987. The 2017 Act recognises the agency of people with mental illness, allowing them to make decisions regarding their health, given that they have the appropriate knowledge to do so.
- The Act aims to safeguard the rights of the people with mental illness, along with access to healthcare and treatment without discrimination from the government. Additionally, insurers are now bound to make provisions for medical insurance for the treatment of mental illness on the same basis as is available for the treatment of physical ailments.
- It includes provisions for the registration of mental health related institutions and for the regulation of the sector. These measures include the necessity of setting up mental health establishments across the country to ensure that no person with mental illness will have to travel far for treatment, as well as the creation of a mental health review board which will act as a regulatory body.
- The Act has restricted the usage of electroconvulsive therapy (ECT) to be used only in cases of emergency, and along with muscle relaxants and anaesthesia. Further, ECT has additionally been prohibited to be used as viable therapy for minors.
- The responsibilities of other agencies such as the police with respect to people with mental illness have been outlined in the Act.

ADMISSION, CARE AND DISCHARGE OF A MENTALLY ILL PERSON (as per MHA 2017)*

- **Admission of person with mental illness as independent patient in mental health establishment**:
  - Refers to the admission of a person who has the capacity to understand treatment decisions.
  - Any person, who is not a minor and who considers himself to have a mental illness and desires to be admitted to any mental health establishment for treatment, may request the medical officer in charge of the establishment to be admitted as an independent patient.
  - On receipt of such request, the medical officer in charge of the establishment shall admit the person, if he is satisfied that—
    - the person has a mental illness of a severity requiring admission to a mental health establishment.
    - the person is likely to benefit from admission and treatment.
    - the person has understood the nature and purpose of admission, and has made the request for admission of his own free will, without any duress or undue influence.
  - An independent patient shall not be given treatment without his informed consent.
  - The mental health establishment shall admit an independent patient on his own request, and shall not require the consent or presence of a relative or care-giver for admitting the person.
  - An independent patient may get himself discharged from the mental health establishment without the consent of the medical officer in charge of such establishment.
- **Admission of minor**:
  - The nominated representative of the minor shall apply to the medical officer in charge of a mental health establishment for admission of the minor to the establishment.
  - Upon receipt of such an application, the medical officer in charge of the mental health establishment may admit

*__Note__: *The procedures described under the older version of the Act (MHA - 1987) are no more relevant, and must not be taught to students, nor feature in examinations.*

such a minor to the establishment, if two psychiatrists (or one psychiatrist and one mental health professional, or one psychiatrist and one medical practitioner), have independently examined the minor on the day of admission or in the preceding 7 days, and both independently conclude that—
  - the minor has a mental illness of a severity requiring admission to a mental health establishment;
  - admission shall be in the best interests of the minor, with regard to his health, well-being or safety;
  - the mental healthcare needs of the minor cannot be fulfilled unless he is admitted.
- A minor so admitted shall be accommodated separately from adults, in an environment that takes into account his age and developmental needs.
- The nominated representative shall stay with the minor in the mental health establishment for the entire duration of the admission of the minor.
- In the case of minor girls, where the nominated representative is male, a female attendant shall be appointed, and shall stay in the establishment for the entire duration of her admission.
- Any admission of a minor to a mental health establishment shall be informed by the medical officer in charge to the concerned Board within a period of 72 hours.
- The concerned Board shall carry out a mandatory review within a period of 7 days of being informed of admission of a minor continuing beyond 30 days, and every subsequent 30 days.

■ **Discharge of independent patients**:
- The medical officer in charge of a mental health establishment shall discharge from the establishment any person admitted as an independent patient immediately on request made by such person.
- Where a **minor** has been admitted and attains the age of 18 years during his stay in the mental health establishment, the medical officer in charge shall re-classify him as an **independent patient**.
- A mental health professional may prevent discharge of a person admitted as an independent person for a period of 24 hours so as to allow his assessment necessary for admission, if he is of the opinion that—
  - such person is unable to understand the nature and purpose of his decisions, and requires substantial support from his nominated representative; or
  - has recently threatened or attempted to cause bodily harm to himself; or
  - has recently behaved violently towards another person, or is causing another person to fear bodily harm from him.

■ **Admission of person with mental illness with high support needs, up to 30 days (Supported admission)**:
- The medical officer in charge of a mental health establishment shall admit every such person to the establishment, upon application by the nominated representative of the person, if—
  - the person has been independently examined on the day of admission or in the preceding 7 days, by one psychiatrist and the other being a mental health professional or a medical practitioner, and both independently conclude that the person has a mental illness of such severity that the person—
    - can cause bodily harm to himself; or
    - behave violently towards another person or
    - is showing an inability to care for himself to a degree that places the individual at risk of harm to himself;
    - is ineligible to receive care and treatment as an independent patient because the person is unable to make treatment decisions independently, and needs very high support from his nominated representative.
- The admission of a person with mental illness to a mental health establishment under this section shall be limited to a period of 30 days.
- On the expiry of the period of 30 days, the person may continue to remain in the mental health establishment as an independent patient, and the medical officer in charge shall inform the person of his admission status under this Act, including his right to leave the mental health establishment.
- The medical officer in charge of a mental health establishment shall report to the concerned Board—
  - within 3 days, the admissions of a woman or a minor;
  - within 7 days the admission of any person not being a woman or minor.
- The concerned Board shall review the decision of the medical officer in charge, and give its findings thereon within 7 days of receipt of request for such review, which shall be binding on all the concerned parties.
- In case a person with mental illness admitted under this section has been discharged, such person shall not be readmitted under this section within a period of 7 days thereafter.
- If the medical officer in charge of the mental health establishment is of the opinion that the person with mental illness admitted under this section requires further treatment beyond the period of 30 days, then he shall be duty bound to refer the matter to be examined by two psychiatrists for his admission beyond 30 days.

■ **Admission of person with mental illness with high support needs, beyond 30 days (Supported admission beyond 30 days)**:
- The medical officer in charge of a mental health establishment, upon application by the nominated representative of a person with mental illness, shall continue admission of such person with mental illness, if—

  - two psychiatrists have independently examined the person with mental illness in the preceding 7 days and both independently conclude that the person has a mental illness of such severity that he can harm himself or others, or is unable to take care of himself.
- The medical officer in charge shall report all admissions or readmission under this section, within a period of 7 days of such admission or readmission, to the concerned Board.
- The Board shall, within a period of 21 days from the date of last admission or readmission of person, permit such admission or readmission, or order discharge of such person.
- The admission of a person with mental illness to a mental health establishment under this section shall be limited to a period up to 90 days in the first instance.
- If the period of 90 days is exceeded, it may be extended for a further period up to 120 days, and thereafter for a period of 180 days.
- If the Board refuses to permit admission or readmission, or on the expiry of the extended periods, such person shall be discharged from such mental health establishment.

- **Emergency treatment**:
  - Any medical treatment, including treatment for mental illness, may be provided by any registered medical practitioner to a person with mental illness either at a health establishment or in the community, subject to the informed consent of the nominated representative, and where it is immediately necessary to prevent—
    - death or irreversible harm to the health of the person; or
    - the person inflicting serious harm to himself or to others; or
    - the person causing serious damage to property belonging to himself or to others.
  - The emergency treatment referred to in this section shall be limited to 72 hours, or till the person with mental illness has been assessed at a mental health establishment.
- **Restraints and seclusion**:
  - A person with mental illness shall not be subjected to seclusion or solitary confinement, and, where necessary, physical restraint may only be used when,—
    - it is the only means available to prevent imminent and immediate harm to person concerned or to others;
    - it is authorised by the psychiatrist in charge of the person's treatment at the mental health establishment.
  - The restraint shall not be used as a form of punishment or deterrent in any circumstance.
  - The nominated representative of the person with mental illness shall be informed about every instance of restraint within a period of 24 hours.

Topic 6

FORENSIC LABORATORY INVESTIGATIONS IN MEDICOLEGAL PRACTICE

(Number of Competencies – 3: FM 6.1 to 6.3)

FM 6.1 - 6.2: Core – Written/Viva Voce

- Describe different types of specimens and tissues to be collected both in the living and dead: Body fluids (blood, urine, semen, faeces, saliva), skin, nails, tooth pulp, vaginal smear, viscera, skull, specimens for:
  - Histopathological examination
  - Blood grouping
  - HLA typing
  - DNA fingerprinting
- Describe Locard's Exchange Principle
- Describe the methods of sample collection, preservation, labelling, dispatch and interpretation of reports.

and

FM 6.3: Core – Viva Voce/Objective Structured Practical Examination (OSPE)

- Demonstrate professionalism while sending biological or trace evidence to Forensic Science Laboratory, specifying the required tests to be carried out, objectives of preservation of evidence sent for examination, and personal discussions on interpretation of findings.

COLLECTION, PACKING, PRESERVATION AND DESPATCH OF SPECIMENS & TISSUES FOR ANALYSIS IN THE LIVING AND THE DEAD

- A wide range of samples may need to be taken before, during or after the examination of a living or dead victim, for relevant investigations and analysis.
- The nature of such ancillary investigations will depend upon the nature of the crime, or death, as well as the history of the case, request of the investigating officer and the suspicions of the pathologist.

Collection, Packing, Preservation and Despatch of Specimens from Crime Scene

Collection

The principal methods of collection of trace material from a crime scene include

- ***Handpicking***: Gross and macroscopic items large enough to be seen visually should be recovered by hand or by the use of tweezers. As far as possible, gloves must be worn.
- ***Tape lifting***: This is an effective method of collecting material such as hairs and fibres from a variety of surfaces, especially garments (**Fig. 6.1**) and motor vehicle seats. Transparent adhesive tape of no more than 7.5 cm length is applied to the surface and then placed over a clean piece of glass or rigid plastic, which is then put inside a clean, labelled plastic bag. Care should be taken not to tape too much material on a single tape piece.
  - Fingerprints can also be tape-lifted from surfaces (**Fig 6.2**).
- ***Swabbing***: Dry swabs are used to collect minute particles, while swabs moistened with distilled or injection water can be used to collect body fluids (**Fig. 6.3**).
- ***Sweeping***: This method is particularly useful for collecting material from inaccessible sites, or where there is a mass of material to be collected. The best implement for sweeping is a paintbrush approximately 2.5 cm wide. It is imperative that a clean brush is used each time.
- ***Vacuuming***:
  - Collection of minute particles from garments, motor vehicles and other large objects is best facilitated by vacuuming.
  - Specialized nozzles (custom-made from stainless steel) must be employed.
  - Ordinary vacuum cleaners must not be used.
  - Material is collected on to a clean filter paper or cotton material resting on the perforated plate located in the central compartment.
  - When not in use, the nozzle should be cleaned and stored in a sealed plastic bag.

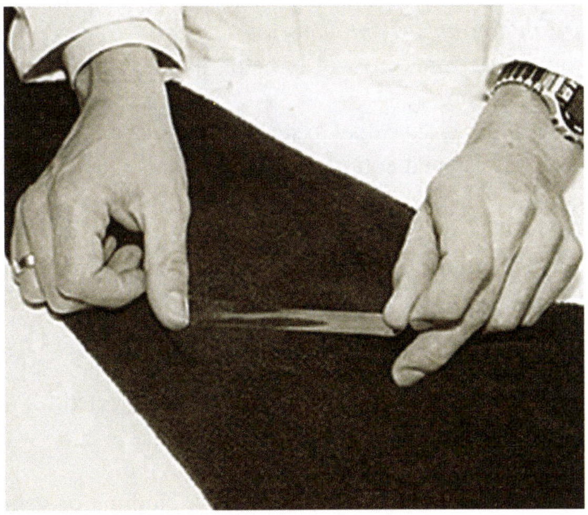

Fig. 6.1 Recovering fibre debris from a garment using clear adhesive tape

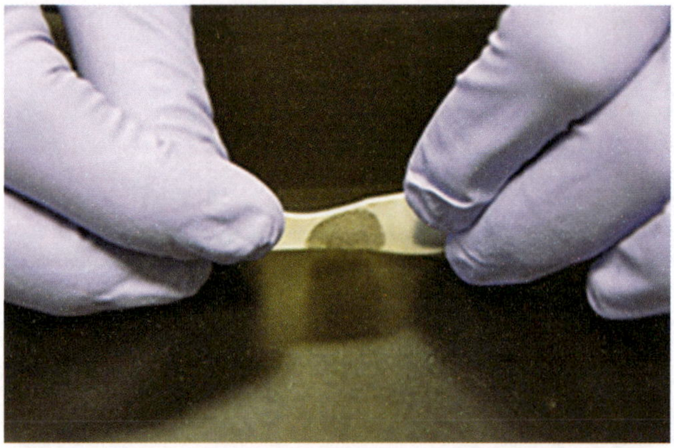

Fig. 6.2 Recovering fingerprint from a surface

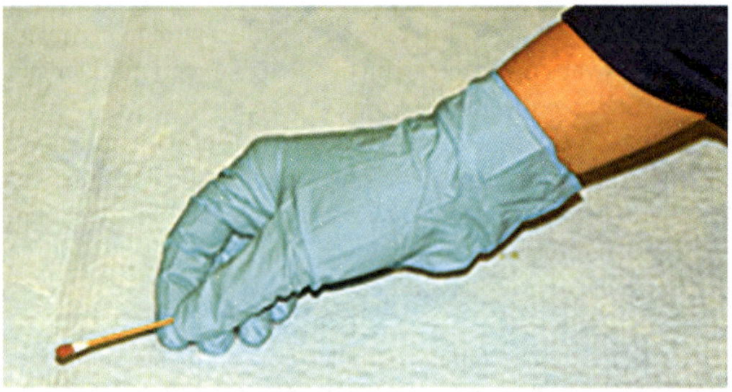

Fig. 6.3 Swabbing a blood stain at a crime scene

Packing and Despatching

Procedures for packing and despatching are the same as for any specimen in medicolegal cases. A summary is given below:

1. **Blood**:
   a. *On absorbent material*:
      i. Cut material, air dry and pack separately.
      ii. Include control sample. Pack large items in paper, while small samples can be placed in plastic vials.
   b. *On non-absorbent material*:
      i. ***Wet***: Suck up with pipette, or soak small piece of cotton.
      ii. ***Dry***: Use scalpel to scrape off the stain, or rub with moistened cotton. Include controls. Pack in plastic or glass vials.
2. **Saliva**:
   a. ***Wet***: Collect on clean white gauze. Air dry and pack.
   b. ***Dry***: Use moistened swab. Pack in plastic container.
3. **Semen**:
   a. Stains can be photographed.
   b. Items bearing seminal stains must be collected, air dried and packed. Pack in paper bags.
4. **Paint**:
   a. If possible, collect the item (tool, clothing or vehicle) containing the evidence.
   b. Collect paint chips separately. Pack in folded paper inserted inside envelope, plastic bag or plastic container.
5. **Hairs and Fibres**:
   a. If hairs or fibres are present on a movable item, collect the item.
   b. If it is a fixed object, use plastic tweezers or adhesive tape to collect the hairs or fibres.
   c. Pack in folded paper inserted inside envelope, plastic bag or plastic container.
6. **Clothing**:
   a. Photograph, note and describe.
   b. Remove clothing from body over clean white paper, air dry and pack.
   c. Pack trace material from clothing separately.
   d. Pack in paper bags. Each item must be placed in a separate bag.
7. **Ammunition**:
   a. Projectiles, cartridges, shot or wads, must be wrapped in tissue paper or small plastic bags.
   b. Each item is placed in a separate plastic or cardboard container.
   c. It is advisable not to mark ammunition. Label the container instead.
   d. Wash projectiles and air dry, if removed from the body. Pack each item separately in plastic or cardboard container.
8. **Cigarette butts**:
   a. Collect with plastic tweezers, air dry and pack.
   b. Look for trace evidence: Lipstick, fingerprints, etc. Pack each butt separately in plastic or glass vials.

All packed evidentiary items must be labelled and sealed, preferably in an Evidence Bag (Fig. 6.4).

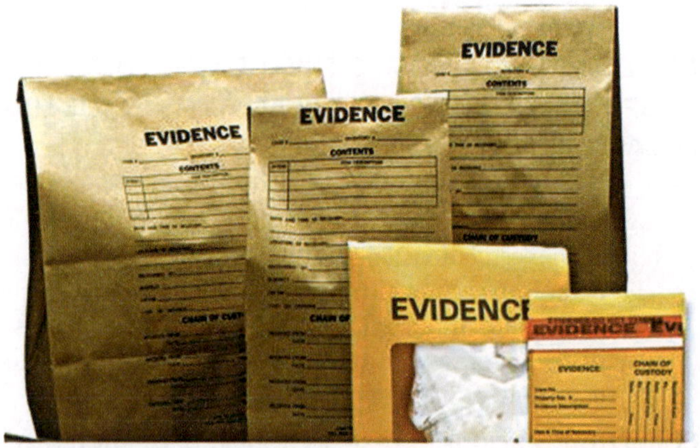

Fig. 6.4 Types of Evidence Bag

Collection, Packing, Preservation and Despatch of Specimens from Autopsied Body

Microbiology

- Though more common in clinical autopsies than in forensic work, culture samples for bacteriological, virological or even mycological study may be needed.
- Plain swabs, or swabs immersed in an appropriate transport medium can be employed for sampling a wide variety of sites at autopsy.

- Tissue samples may be collected in sterile containers, and this is the usual method for virological culture of lung and brain.
- If blood culture is required to be done, it is best to take blood with a sterile needle and syringe from a large blood vessel such as the femoral vein, before starting the autopsy. Alternatively, blood can be taken from a freshly opened heart chamber using sterile instruments.
- In all autopsy investigations, unless cultures are performed soon after death, there is often widespread contamination by organisms that travel rapidly through the dead tissues, especially from the gastrointestinal tract. It requires the expertise of a qualified microbiologist to opine as to what is significant, with reference to the subsequent growth in the laboratory.

Toxicology

- Collection of specimens should be done carefully, if reliable analytical results are expected.
- Blood, urine, stomach contents, intestinal contents, organs (liver, kidney), CSF, bile and ocular fluid may be required.
- The containers in which they are collected must be chemically clean.
- The pathologist should submit a form with the samples indicating the nature of analysis required, the personal details of the deceased person, a brief history with details of suspected toxic substances, and a statement as to whether the subject was known to suffer from any infective conditions, including hepatitis or AIDS.

Described in detail under FM 8.5 *(page no. 385)*.

Histopathology

- In most autopsies, the pathologist will need to carry out a histological examination on a range of tissues, even if only to exclude some occult natural disease.
- It is customary to retain samples of liver, spleen, kidney, heart, lung, thyroid, adrenal, pancreas, muscle and brain for this purpose.
- Where there are indications to examine other parts of the body, these may be retained in addition to the routine tissues.
- The required tissue is placed in sufficient quantity of **formalin**, and allowed to fix for several days before processing. The volume of fixative should be six times the total volume of tissue.
- There are several specialised procedures in use at present, such as histochemistry, fluorescent microscopy and immuno-histochemical examination, if evidence of early myocardial infarction is being sought. However, even light microscopy can be helpful in many cases.

Collection, Packing, Preservation and Despatch of Specimens from Living Victim of Assault/Sexual Assault

Assault

- All material evidence collected during the general and local examinations must enter a chain of evidence by proper sealing and labelling, with the name, case number, date and time of collection, and the name and designation of the examining physician, and despatched to the nearest Forensic Science Laboratory through the police constable concerned.
- **A checklist** of the said material evidence, for ready reference, is as follows:
  - **Clothing** that is torn, blood stained or soiled.
  - **Foreign debris**: Hair, fibres and fresh/ dried secretions on the surface of the body.
  - **Fingernail scrapings**.
  - **Blood** for grouping, and presence and levels of ethanol and/or other intoxicating agents.
  - **Urine** for the presence and levels of ethanol and/or other intoxicating agents.

Sexual Assault (Fig. 6.5)

- **Clothing** that is torn, blood stained or soiled.
- **Foreign debris**: Hair, fibres and fresh/ dried secretions on the surface of the body.
- **Fingernail scrapings**.
- **Combings** from pubic hair, and **clippings** of the victim's pubic hair for comparison.
- **Washings** from the posterior fornix and vagina, for histochemical and histological examination for the detection of the constituents of seminal fluid.
- **Vaginal swabs**
  - For the detection of *Mycobacterium smegmatis*, and for the presence of sexually transmitted disease (by Gram's staining and culture of secretions).
  - Inspection of a **wet mount** slide of vaginal swabs under light microscope (for sperms): The presence of motile sperm in the vaginal pool is the best indication of recent ejaculation. The absence of motile sperm, however, does not negate the possibility of recent ejaculation as sperm may become non-motile within hours of entering the vaginal environment. Place a drop of normal saline or buffered nutrient medium on the slide to preserve the motility of the sperm. A glucose fortified solution of balanced salts, such as Ringer's, Tyrode's, or Dulbecco's at normal osmolality, pH 7.2–7.4 is recommended. Prepared solutions of media designed to enhance sperm survival during microscopic examinations are commercially available. Select one of the swabs collected from the vaginal pool and roll the swab back and forth in the drop to transfer cellular debris to the medium. Place a cover slip on the slide. Examine the wet mount slide within 5–10 minutes using a biological microscope at 400 power, or by using a phase contrast or other "optically staining" microscope to determine whether or not motile or non-motile sperms are present.
- **Blood** for grouping, baseline serology for sexually transmitted disease, and presence and levels of ethanol and/or other intoxicating agents.
- **Urine** for the presence and levels of ethanol and/or other intoxicating agents, and pregnancy tests.

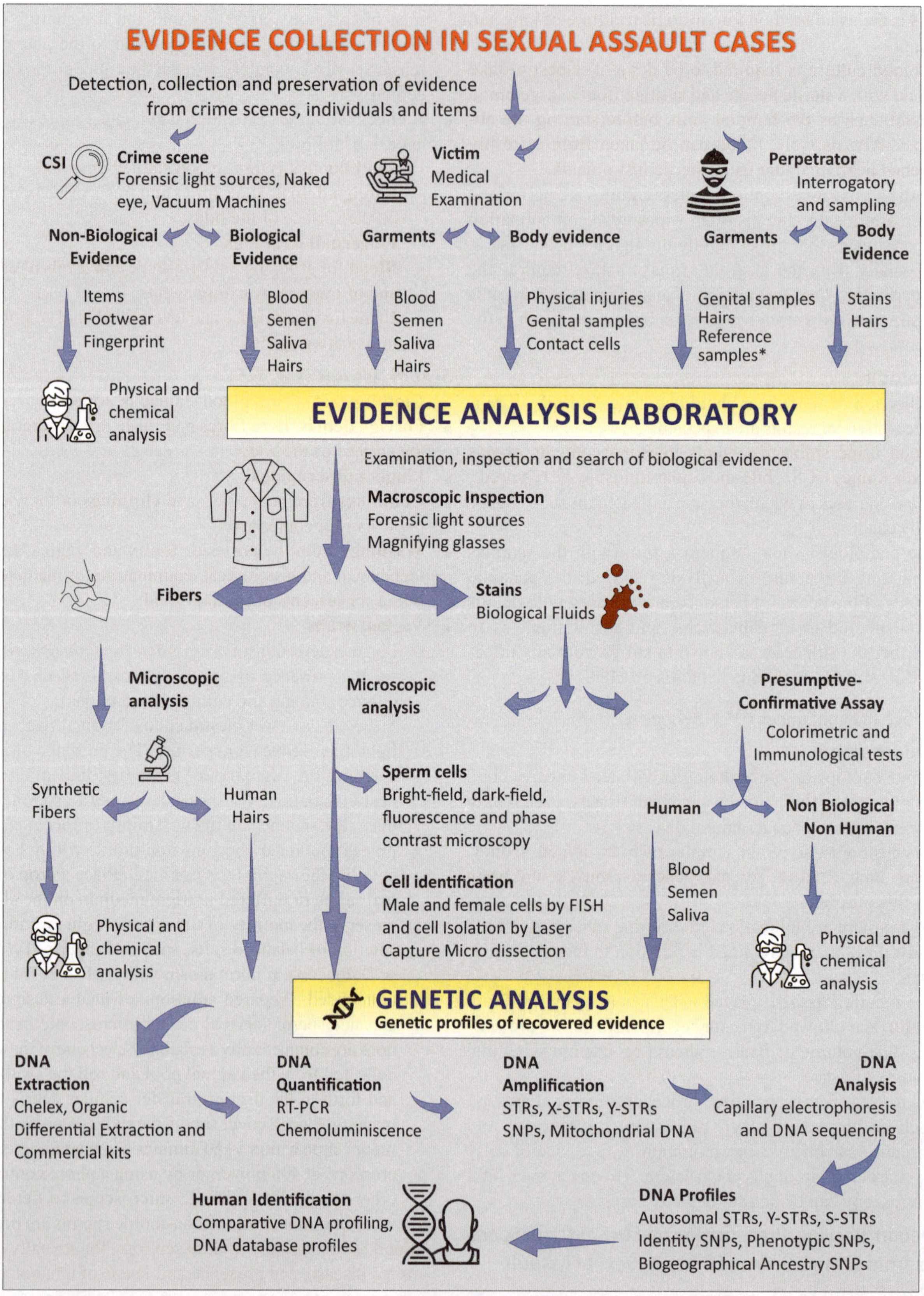

Fig. 6.5 Evidence collection in sexual assault cases

- In addition to clinical implications, presence of ethanol and/or drugs in the patient's blood or urine or vomitus may have legal significance. The assailant may have used drugs to subdue the victim (**drug-facilitated sexual assault**). The victim may have lost the ability to make rational decisions, or to offer resistance, or she may have lost consciousness, or may have no recollection of events. There may not be any physical or genital injuries in such cases. Drugs such as marijuana (cannabis), cocaine, methamphetamine, benzodiazepines and gammahydroxybutyrate (GHB) can be detected through testing blood and urine samples.

LOCARD'S PRINCIPLE OF EXCHANGE

- **Edmond Locard** (1877–1966; French Forensic Scientist) stated "***Whenever two objects come into contact with each other, there is a mutual transfer of material from one object to the other***."
- The above famous quote underlines the main principle of Forensic Science, which constitutes the basis of all crime detection.

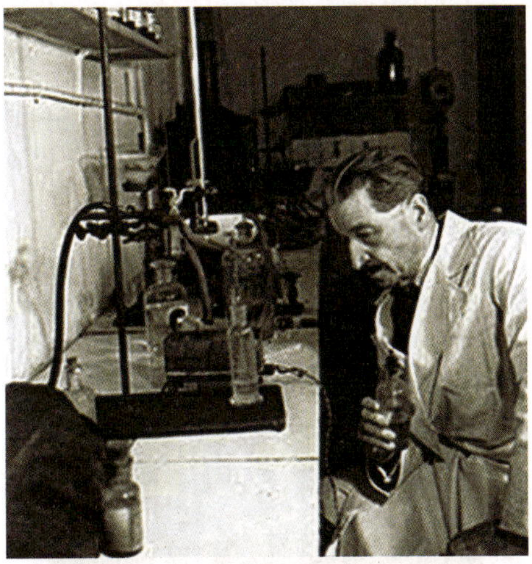

Fig. 6.6 Edmond Locard

COLLECTION, PACKING, PRESERVATION AND DESPATCH OF TRACE EVIDENCE: BIOLOGICAL MATERIALS

- Since awareness among criminals has increased regarding scientific investigation of crime, the forensic scientist is left only with microtraces of evidence in many modern day offences. That is why in recent times, several technologically advanced instruments and methods have been developed, to detect such microtraces of evidence.
- Biological materials, such as blood and other body fluids – semen, saliva, sweat, etc., are well-known examples of trace evidence which are commonly encountered in scenes of violent crime. A clever criminal may try to clear the scene of crime in an attempt to obliterate such evidence, so much so that only microtraces may be left behind.
- The routine use of ultraviolet light can help in detecting stains of various origins such as blood, semen, saliva, pus, milk, etc., as they all fluoresce under UV light. But, confirmation requires the performance of sophisticated tests.

Identification of Blood and Bloodstains

- Testing for the presence of blood is perhaps the most important step in the examination of a stain associated with a violent crime. Unless this issue is resolved, it may be futile to proceed with further analysis.
- Identification of blood is based upon the presence of blood cells or compounds characteristic of blood, such as:
  - Erythrocytes (RBC) and leukocytes (WBC)
  - Blood serum proteins
  - Haemoglobin and its derivatives.

Microscopy

- The observation of a fresh bloodstain under the microscope would reveal the presence of erythrocytes and leukocytes.
- Apart from identification of blood, microscopic examination may also reveal other information such as the species origin, sex of the individual (on the basis of Davidson body, *page no. 123*), and evidence of disease, e.g., sickle-shaped erythrocytes indicate sickle cell anaemia.

Chemical Tests

A. Presumptive Tests

1. **Luminol Test**
   - This is essentially a **crime scene test**, and is more of a screening nature than a confirmatory test.
   - In case bloodstains are rendered invisible by washing of the crime scene (in an attempt to obliterate the stains), the suspected area can be sprayed with **luminol**, which would make the entire area glow in the dark, if blood is present (**Fig. 6.7**).
   - **Luminol**, i.e., **3-aminophthalylhydrazide**, is a colourless substance which reacts with blood in the presence of an oxidant to form a product which luminesces in the dark. It reacts with iron found in haemoglobin.
   - To exhibit its luminescence, the luminol must first be activated with an oxidant. Usually, a solution of hydrogen peroxide (H_2O_2) and a hydroxide salt in water is

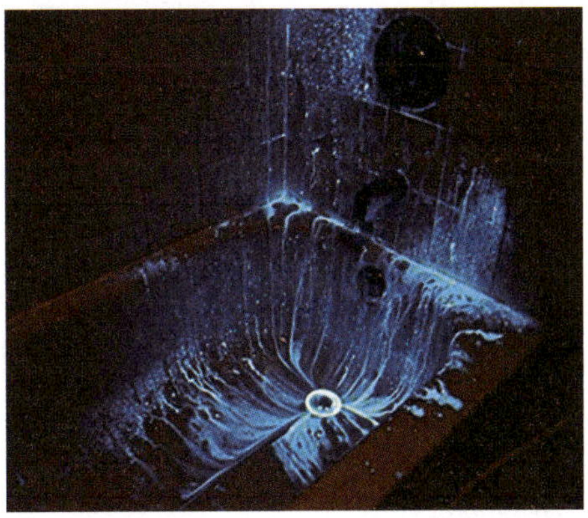

Fig. 6.7 Blood stains in a bath tub as revealed by the luminol test

used as the activator. The investigator prepares a solution of luminol and the activator, and sprays it throughout the area under investigation. The iron present in any blood in the area catalyzes the chemical reaction that leads to the luminescence revealing the location of the blood.

- The amount of catalyst necessary for the reaction to occur is very small relative to the amount of luminol, allowing the detection of even trace amounts of blood.
- The glow lasts for about 30 seconds and is **blue** in colour. Detecting the glow requires a fairly dark room. Any glow detected may be documented by a long exposure photograph.
- ***Drawbacks***:
  - Luminol chemiluminescence can also be triggered by copper or copper-containing alloys, and certain bleaches; and, as a result, if a crime scene is thoroughly cleaned with a bleach solution, residual bleach will cause the entire crime scene to produce the typical blue glow, effectively camouflaging any organic evidence, such as blood.
  - Luminol also reacts with urine, faecal matter and animal blood in almost the same manner as human blood.

2. **Visible blood stains** are usually tested by the following tests, all of which make use of the peroxidase-like activity of the haem group of haemoglobin, which in the presence of an oxidant like hydrogen peroxide oxidises a colourless material, such as phenolphthalein, benzidine, o-toluidine etc., to a coloured one. The colours produced by various reagents are listed in **Table 6.1**.

a. **Benzidine Test (Adler's Test)**

i. Benzidine is widely used in spite of its carcinogenicity, since the reagent is easy to prepare, and the test is easy to perform and is highly sensitive.

ii. Though this test is highly sensitive to minute traces of haemoglobin and its derivatives, it is not specific to blood, since certain chemical oxidants and catalysts (such as copper and nickel salts, rust, paint, etc.), peroxidase present in plant sources (such as apple, potato, onion, tomato, cabbage, etc.) and other body fluids (such as saliva, CSF, pus, etc.) also give false positive reaction.

iii. In general, a negative result provided by the Benzidine test is said to indicate the absence of blood in the stain.

iv. ***Method***:
- The suspected stain is treated with glacial acetic acid and ether.
- This is then decanted and treated with hydrogen peroxide and a solution of benzidine in acetic acid.
- The presence of blood is indicated by a **bluish** colour (**Fig. 6.8**) turning to **purple**.

v. ***Drawbacks***:
- The test will give a false positive result in the presence of vegetable peroxidases such as those in horseradish, broccoli, cauliflower, etc., as well as several other vegetables, fruits and chemicals (*see above*).
- Animal blood gives the same result.

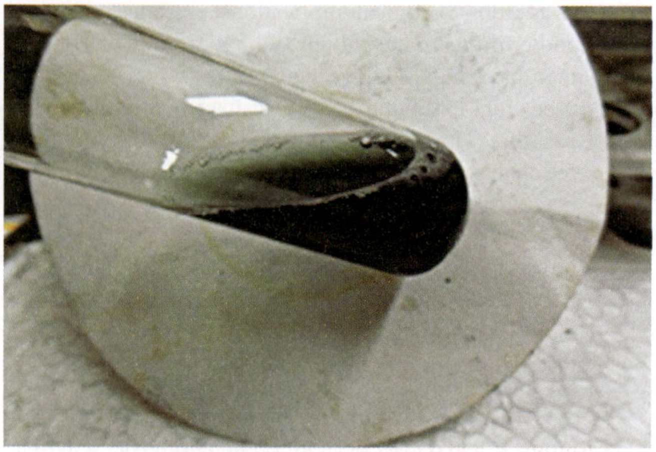

Fig. 6.8 Positive Benzidine test

b. **Phenolphthalein Test (Kastle-Meyer Test)**

i. A drop of phenolphthalein reagent is added to the sample, and after a few seconds, a drop of hydrogen peroxide is added. If the sample turns **pink** rapidly, it is said to be presumptive for blood (**Fig. 6.9**).

ii. ***Drawbacks***:
- Waiting for over 30 seconds will result in the sample turning pink even in the absence of blood, as natural oxidation will occur in the air.
- The same drawbacks of benzidine test also apply to this test.

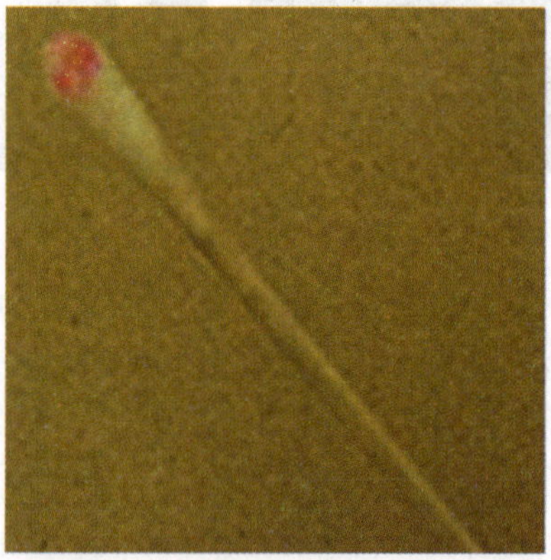

Fig. 6.9 Swab testing positive with phenolphthalein test (Kastle-Meyer test)

c. **O-Toluidine Test**

i. Same principle as the above mentioned tests.

ii. O-Toluidine reagent is used.

iii. A positive test is indicated by the development of a **green** to **blue** colour.

iv. The same drawbacks of benzidine test also apply to this test.

d. **Leucomalachite Green Test**
   i. Same principle as the above mentioned tests.
   ii. The reagent is the dye leucomalachite green dissolved in water along with sodium perborate ($NaBO_3$).
   iii. A **bluish green** colour indicates a positive result.
   iv. The same drawbacks of benzidine test also apply to this test.

B. Confirmatory Tests*

1. **Crystal Tests**: All the crystal tests are based upon the formation of haemoglobin-derived crystals such as haematin, haemin, haemochromogen, etc.
   a. **Teichmann Test (Haemin Crystal Test)**
      i. Place material to be tested on a microscope slide and cover with a cover slip. Let the reagent flow under the cover slip. Warm the slide gently on a hot plate at 65°C for 10–20 seconds. Allow to cool and observe under microscope at 100×. The appearance of **brown rhomboid crystals** of ferroprotoporphyrin chloride is a positive reaction for haem (**Fig. 6.10**).
      ii. Overheating, presence of rust or any other substance which degrades haemoglobin or haematin to haematoporphyrin will interfere with crystal formation.
         - **Teichmann's reagent**: Add KCl, KBr and KI (about 0.1 g each) in 100 mL of glacial acetic acid.
   b. **Takayama Test (Haemochromogen Crystal Test)**
      i. Place the material to be tested on a microscope slide and cover with a cover slip. Add a drop of Takayama reagent and allow to flow under the cover slip. Warm slide gently on a hot plate at 65°C for 10–20 seconds.
      Allow to cool and observe under microscope at 100×. The appearance of **pink needle shaped crystals** of pyridine haemochromogen (pyridine-ferroprotoporphyrin) is positive reaction for haem and confirms the presence of haemoglobin (**Fig. 6.11**).
         - **Takayama reagent**:
            - Saturated solution of glucose 3 mL
            - Pyridine solution 3 mL
            - 10% NaOH (sodium hydroxide solution)
            - 3 mL glacial acetic acid 7 mL

Both these tests are highly specific for blood, and require as little as 0.001 mL of blood or 0.1 mg of haemoglobin.

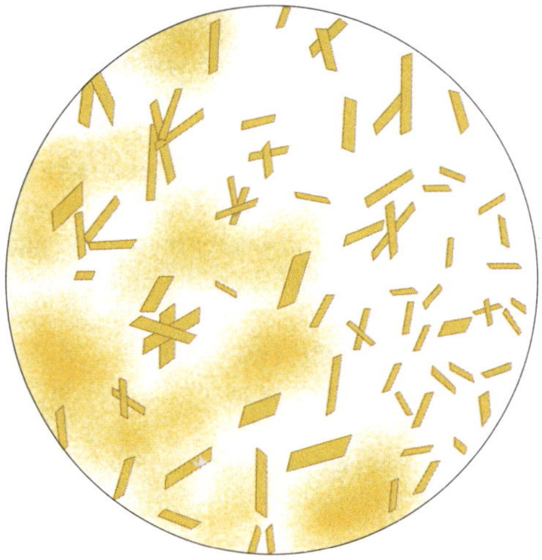

Fig. 6.10 Teichmann (haemin crystal) test

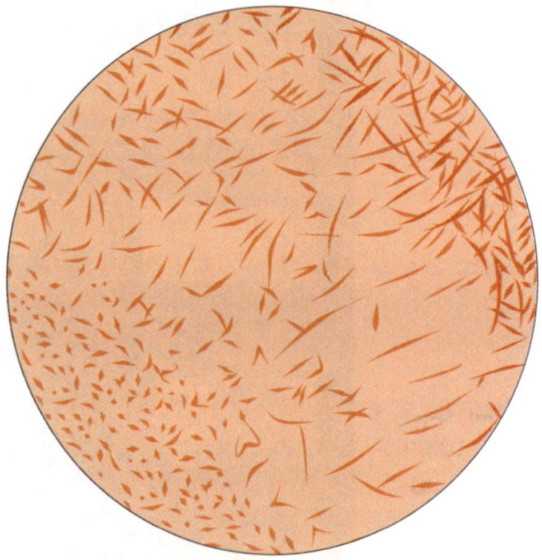

Fig. 6.11 Takayama (haemochromogen crystal) test

2. **Absorption Spectroscopy**:
   - **This is said to be the most sensitive and reliable test for detecting the presence of blood in recent or old stains.**

Table 6.1 Colours Produced by Various Tests

S. No.	Name of Test	Colour (Positive Test)
1	Benzidine Test (Adler's Test)	Blue to Purple
2	Phenolphthalein Test (Kastle-Meyer Test)	Pink
3	O-Toluidine Test	Green to Blue
4	Leucomalachite Green Test	Bluish Green

**Source*: *Gupta AK, Sodhi GS, Rarh V, Mishra M, Kumar R, Rao MS. Forensic Science. Paper 12: Forensic Biology and Serology. Module 14: Examination of Blood. SGTB Khalsa College, University of Delhi.*

- **Haemoglobin** and its derivatives exhibit characteristic bands of absorption at specific wavelengths which can be observed by spectroscopy (**Fig. 6.12**).
- The suspected blood stain is dissolved in water or normal saline, and is placed in a test tube which is then kept between the spectroscope and the source of light.
- Haemoglobin and its derivatives show a common absorption band at 400–425 nm (**Soret band**), apart from one or more bands at their characteristic wavelengths. Hence, the presence of two or more absorption bands in the spectroscope confirms the presence of blood in the stain:
    - ***Oxyhaemoglobin***: Two bands between Fraunhofer lines D and E, the one nearer D being about half the width of the other.
    - ***Reduced haemoglobin***: One broad band between D and E.
    - ***Carboxyhaemoglobin***: Similar to oxyhaemoglobin, but remains unchanged after addition of ammonium sulphide, while the former becomes reduced haemoglobin.
    - ***Methaemoglobin***: Similar to oxyhaemoglobin, with a third band between C and D, and a fourth between E and F.
- **Porphyrin compounds** and their derivatives from other animal and vegetable sources may share a common band with haemoglobin and its derivatives. Hence, a single absorption spectrum should never be relied upon for confirming the presence of blood.

3. **Electrophoresis**:
    - Haemoglobin and its derivatives are made up of conjugated proteins and carry a specific charge, which at a particular pH, can be separated by induction of an electric field on a suitable medium like agarose gel.

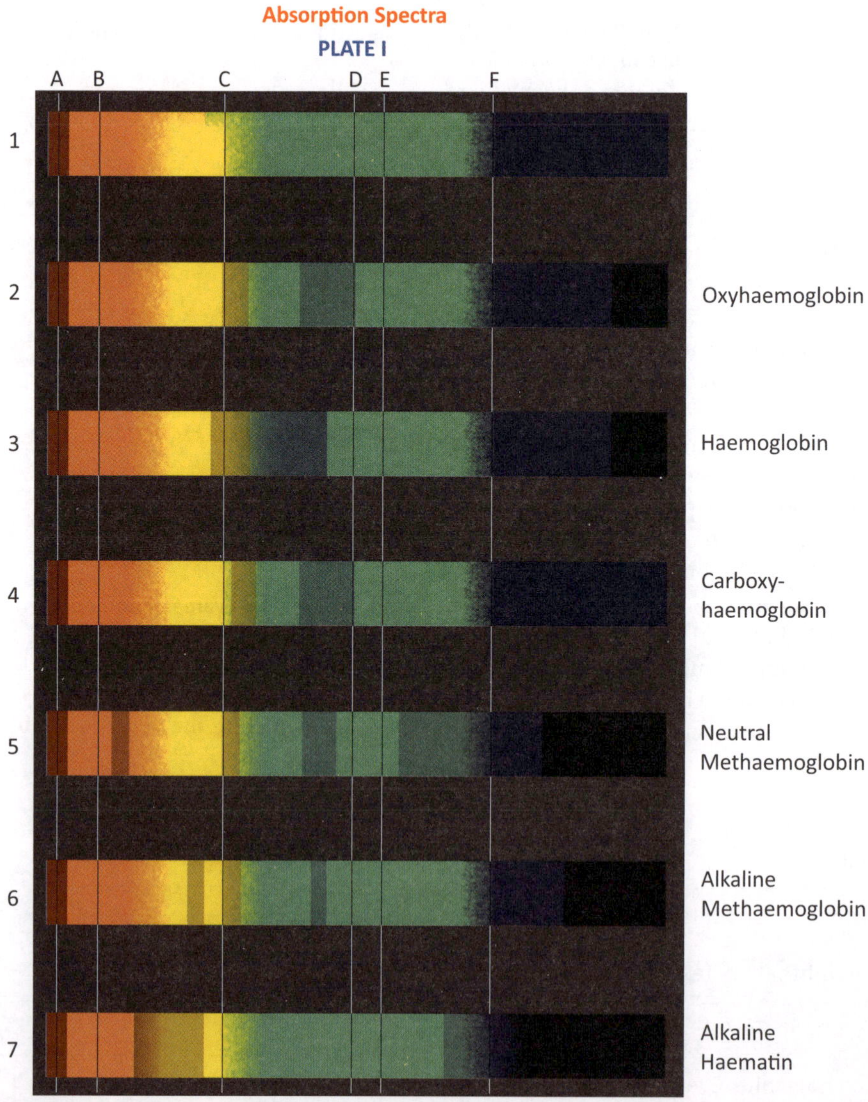

Fig. 6.12 Absorption spectroscopy for blood stain

- The distance travelled by each is characteristic for that particular substance, and can be detected on the gel medium by spraying any one of the common colour reagents (benzidine, leucomalachite green, etc.).
- The false positives given by the colour tests are obviated in this procedure, since such substances either carry no charge, or possess a different charge other than haemoglobin and its derivatives, and hence would not be separated by electrophoresis. This makes the method a reliable confirmatory test for blood.

4. **Immunoelectrophoresis**:
   - Immunoelectrophoresis further enhances the reliability of the above method by combining immmunodiffusion with electrophoresis.
   - In this procedure, the extract of the stain is subjected to electrophoresis and then the slide is placed in a well which contains antiserum.
   - The antiserum diffuses into the gel, and there is migration of serum proteins towards the diffusing antiserum forming a white line of precipitation of Ag–Ab complex, whereas haemoglobin and its derivatives remain at the point of origin giving a pinkish ring around the sample well.
   - The white precipitin line of Ag–Ab reaction, and the pink ring of haemoglobin or its derivatives, constitute double confirmation for the presence of blood.
5. **Chromatography**:
   - The principle of this method is the separation and migration of haemoglobin and its derivatives in a suitable stationary phase such as silica gel, alumina, etc. (or paper, in paper chromatography), with respect to a particular solvent system.
   - The distance travelled by Hb and derivatives in relation to that particular solvent system (termed as the Rf value) is a highly characteristic feature aiding in their identification.
   - The separated derivatives can be detected on the TLC (thin layer chromatography) plate by either UV radiation or the use of appropriate colour reagent.

Determination of Species Origin

- After identifying the stain as blood, the next step is to find out the species, as to whether it is human or animal.
- Many immunological tests are used to determine this. When the antigen derived from a particular species is injected into the body of another, the latter recognises it as a foreign body, and produces antibody (antiserum). This antiserum forms an antigen–antibody (Ag–Ab) complex with the antigen, both in vivo and in vitro. The white precipitin formed by the Ag–Ab complex in vitro, forms the basis for the following tests employed in the determination of species (**Fig. 6.13**): ring test, immunodiffusion, immunoelectrophoresis, crossed-over electrophoresis, etc. All these are grouped under the collective term **precipitin test**. Antihuman sera prepared from horses (H type), and rabbits (R type), are generally used to determine the blood of human origin.
- The classical **precipitin test** is the double gel diffusion (double immunodiffusion) technique of Ouchterlony.
  - Thomas G Ouchterlony, a Swedish bacteriologist, developed the double immunodiffusion technique in 1948 that, when used in forensics, determines whether a bloodstain is human or animal.
  - The technique involves cutting cylindrical wells into a purified preparation of agar gel in a Petri dish. The wells are filled with antibody or antigen and the dish is allowed to incubate.
  - Homologous antigen and antibody diffuse toward each other from the individual wells to a point in the agar where optimum concentration of each is reached. Subsequently, a precipitin line will form within 18–24 hours somewhere between the two wells.
  - If challenges are mixed together in a single well and allowed to diffuse out into the agar towards the serum test well, multiple precipitin bands are seen.
  - Non-specific reactants diffuse past each other, forming no precipitate.
  - However, the **Ouchterlony method** is rarely done today due to the time and expertise required, and the need for reagent sensitivity and selectivity validation. Today, **immunoassay tests** are used that rely on immunological principles similar to the Ouchterlony test. Results are accurate, more sensitive and visible within 10 minutes; the test apparatus is portable and simple to use, requiring no prior experience to conduct and interpret the results.

Determination of Blood Group

- The common blood groups such as ABO, MNS and Rh systems are determined in a bloodstain by one of the following methods:
  - Latte's crust method
  - Absorption-elution technique
  - Absorption-inhibition
  - Latex method
- Whereas absorption-elution technique is suitable for small stains, the absorption-inhibition technique is less susceptible to interferences.
- The various blood group systems (ABO, Rh, MNS, Kell, Duffy, Lutheran, Kidd, etc.), polymorphisms exhibited by serum proteins (Hp, Gc, Ag, Gm1, Gm2, KM, etc.) and red cell enzymes (PGM, GPT, ADA, AK, GLO-I, etc.) can help in individualising blood stains to great extent. HLA typing and DNA fingerprinting can accomplish this beyond any doubt.
- Disputed maternity and paternity: The blood group systems and the polymorphisms of serum proteins, red cell enzymes, and HLA and DNA typing mentioned above, are all inherited from the parents and follow Mendelian laws of inheritance. This fact enables the forensic scientist to determine the parentage of a child in disputed cases.
- **Table 6.2** mentions salient principles with reference to inheritance of blood groups.

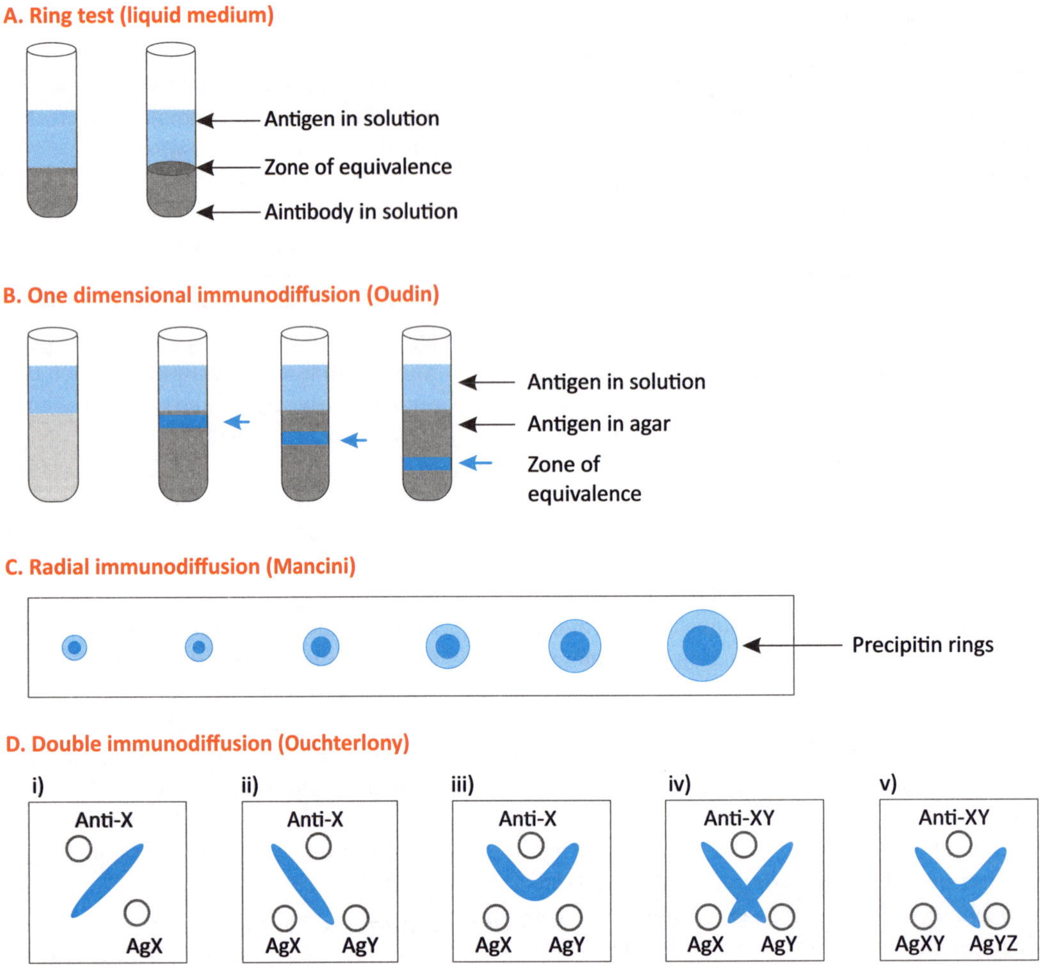

Fig. 6.13 Precipitin test

Table 6.2 Inheritance of Blood Groups

MOTHER'S BLOOD TYPE \ FATHER'S BLOOD TYPE	A	B	AB	O
A	A or O	A, B, AB, or O	A, B, AB	A or O
B	A, B, AB or O	B or O	A, B, or AB	B or O
AB	A, B, or AB	A, B or AB	A, B or AB	A or B
O	A or O	B or O	A or AB	O

(Cells: CHILD'S BLOOD TYPE)

Determination of Other Information from Blood or Bloodstains

- Apart from being an identification marker, a bloodstain can also give information regarding the following:
  - **Source of Blood**:
    - Foetal blood can be distinguished from adult blood by electrophoretic determination of HbF or alpha-fetoprotein (AFP).
    - Blood of pregnancy and abortion/parturition can be differentiated by the presence of chorionic gonadotropin (in the earlier stages), or heat-stable alkaline phosphatase (in the later stages). Detection of certain types of alkaline phosphatase and placental lactogen (from 15th week of pregnancy), would enable the identification of placental blood.
    - Menstrual blood is detected on the basis of absence of fibrin content in it.
    - Arterial and venous blood can be differentiated to some extent on the basis of amount of blood loss and spurting characteristics. Arterial blood loss is generally copious in nature, bright red in colour, and shows spurting due to high pressure and velocity, whereas venous blood is dark in colour, and oozes out gradually, as a result of which there is no evidence of spurting.
    - Blood which has effused during life can be peeled off in scales upon drying, due to the presence of fibrin, whereas blood which has flowed after death tends to break up into a powder on drying.
  - **Direction of Fall of Blood (Blood Spatter Analysis)**:
    - Modern origin of the study of blood spatter analysis began in the 1950s.
    - A trail of blood stains, or splashes of blood on walls or furniture may be encountered in a scene of crime. It is important to determine the height and direction of fall of blood in such cases (**Figs. 6.14 & 6.15**).
      - If blood falls vertically from a relatively low height (not exceeding a few centimetres), the drops are round and sharply delineated.
      - If height is increased above 30 cm, the spots show prickly edges, the projections growing finer and larger in number with increase in height.
      - Splashes of blood striking a surface obliquely may appear like spears or exclamation marks, depending upon the velocity and angle of fall; the pointed end indicates the direction of motion. This is especially important in assessing the relative positions of victim and assailant.
      - While blood spatter analysis has a solid foundation in science and can be a useful tool for inves-

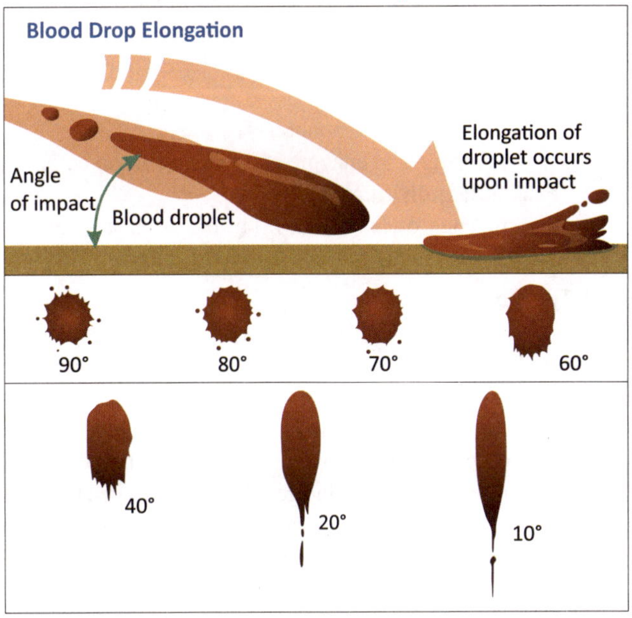

Fig. 6.15 Blood spatter pattern depending on angle of impact

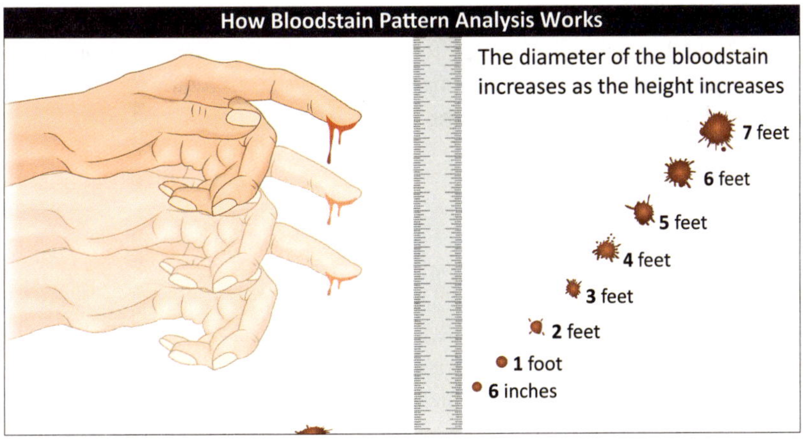

Fig. 6.14 Blood spatter pattern depending on height

tigators, the reliability of courtroom testimony by bloodstain pattern analysts has come under fire in recent years. Care needs to be taken to ensure that the bloodstain pattern analyst has appropriate credentials and training as well as uses appropriate methods. Even with proper training and methods, there are still many times where reputable analysts disagree on their findings, which calls into question the reliability of their conclusions and its value as evidence in court.

- **Age of Bloodstains**
  - Several points can help in dating bloodstains:
    - Progressive decrease in solubility of bloodstain in various aqueous solutions, with age.
    - Change in colour from red to brown due to oxidation of haemoglobin to methaemoglobin.
    - Measuring colour changes by colourimetry and spectrophotometry.
    - Immunoelectrophoresis.
    - Changes in enzyme activities of blood cells.
- **Sex of the Individual**
  - Presence of Davidson body or Y chromosome in WBCs, can help in sexing blood stains.

HLA Typing

- HLA antigens are highly polymorphic and therefore considered useful for personal identification in forensic medicine, before the advent of DNA typing.
- The gene complex of Human Leukocyte Antigen (HLA) is located on chromosome 6p21, which is the most complicated dominant polymorphic genetic system. The HLA system has 108 genotypes. It was considered the best human genetic marker till the late 1980s, and was applied to forensic paternity testing, and individual identification.
- The HLA system is no more used in the classical manner as described in some textbooks of forensic medicine. It is sometimes applied to DNA typing, but is almost never undertaken alone for forensic purposes.
- Today, HLA typing or HLA matching (as it is referred to currently) is mainly used for organ transplantation: the tissues of a prospective donor and recipient are tested for compatibility prior to transplantation. Mismatched donor and recipient tissues can lead to rejection of the tissues.

Forensic DNA Analysis

Described in detail under FM 7.1 *(page no. 349)*.

Identification of Semen and Seminal Stains

- Identification of semen is particularly useful in the investigation of sex crimes.
  - Semen is a suspension of spermatozoa in seminal plasma which is a pool of different secretions by different structures and glands such as vas deferens, seminal vesicles, prostate gland and mucous glands.
  - Seminal plasma consists of a very high concentration of citric acid, fructose, zinc, phosphoryl choline, spermine and spermidine, acid phosphatase, y-seminal protein, etc. Identification of seminal stain is based on the detection of any of these constituents.
- Invisible stains can be detected by examining the material in question under UV light. Seminal stains fluoresce bluish-white in colour on a dark background. This is true of other body fluids also such as blood, saliva, pus, milk, etc. Since certain fabric whiteners also fluoresce under UV light, it might not be reliable, if the stain is present on cloth, and has to be subjected to other tests characteristic of semen.

Chemical Tests

- The seminal stain is extracted by soaking a small bit of the stained material in sufficient quantity of sodium acetate buffer (pH 4.5). The extract is subjected to various tests:
  - **Acid Phosphatase Test**
    - Acid phosphatase is a prostatic gland secretion found in very high concentration in semen when compared with other body fluids.
      - Semen recovered from vagina retains recognisable amounts of acid phosphatase up to 36 hours.
      - Dried stains which are not decomposed, retain acid phosphatase activity for weeks or months, whereas heating the specimen above 60°C destroys the activity.
    - Acid Phosphatase test is a presumptive test for semen. It may be performed directly on a cut out portion of a stain, an extract of a stain, or a "wipe" of the stained material. A wipe may be made using a piece of filter paper, thread or swab. Wet the wipe with water, then rub over the stained area while still wet.
      - **Procedure**:
        - Apply a drop of the Alpha-Naphthyl Phosphate reagent; wait 60 seconds. If a purple colour occurs at this point, the testing results should indicate "inconclusive."
        - Apply a drop of the Fast Blue B reagent. An immediate purple colour is a positive reaction.
    - However, many other organisms and materials, such as bacteria, snake venom, almonds, cauliflower, etc., contain acid phosphatase, which can interfere with the screening of seminal fluid or stain. Hence, a qualitative acid test is insufficient to prove semen in the absence of other independent tests.
    - It has recently been reported that acid phosphatase of semen can be separated and identified from other acid phosphatases by polyacrylamide gel electrophoresis (PAGE) which can be used to confirm the presence of semen in the stains.
  - **Zinc Test**
    - The concentration of zinc in semen is unusually high (140 mg/mL in contrast to 1.2 mg/mL for normal blood serum). Zinc, a secretion of prostatic gland, is supposed to maintain microbiological sterility.
    - Reagents which give brightly coloured products in the presence of zinc are used to distinguish semen

from other body fluids. Laboratory-based methods use atomic absorption spectrometer for quantitative detection of zinc in semen.
   - Acid phosphatase degrades slowly in moist samples, whereas zinc does not, making it a more useful parameter in the case of older specimens.
- **Florence Iodine Crystal Test**
   - Semen contains phosphoryl choline, a secretion of seminal vesicles, which on standing liberates free choline. Choline reacts with **Florence iodine reagent*** to form rhomboidal brownish crystals of choline iodide.
- **Barberio's Test**
   - Semen contains spermine, a prostatic gland secretion, which reacts with picric acid to form needle-shaped yellowish crystals of spermine picrate.

Microscopy

- The presence of semen in a stain can be considered a certainty only if spermatozoa or sperm heads are detected microscopically.
   - A smear of the seminal extract on a microscope slide is stained with haemotoxylin or Ziehl-Neelsen's stain, and viewed through an oil immersion microscope.
   - Phase contrast microscopy gives better results.
   - The most reliable confirmation for the presence of semen is said to be the positive visual identification of spermatozoa using the Christmas tree stain (**Fig. 6.16**).
      - Christmas tree staining stains the heads and tails of sperm in a characteristic manner, making it a reliable method for improving identification. Essentially, a Nuclear Fast Red stain solution is used to stain the heads of sperm red and the part of the tip, known as the acrosomal cap, pink. A Picro Indigo Carmine stain solution is used to stain the tails blue and green.
- Microscopic visualisation of spermatozoa is still considered to be confirmatory of semen, but can show false-negative results for a variety of reasons, such as azoospermia, vasectomy or old age. In such cases, the stain can be reported to be semen, if it gives positive results with a combination of Florence test, human precipitin test and acid-phosphatase test.

Immunological Method

- Human seminal plasma (HSP) contains specific antigens which are absorbed to the spermatozoal surface and are called as sperm-coating antigens. They can be detected both on the sperm cells and in the ejaculated fluid.
- The following antigens have been identified: the specific antigen **P-30** (also called **prostate specific antigen**) produced by the epithelial cells of the prostatic gland, **MHS-5**, originating from the epithelial cells of seminal vesicles, and an antigen corresponding to **Mab 4E6**. Antibodies specific to these antigens can be detected by various immunological tests such as immunodiffusion, ELISA, etc. An immunoassay is often used to test for P-30.

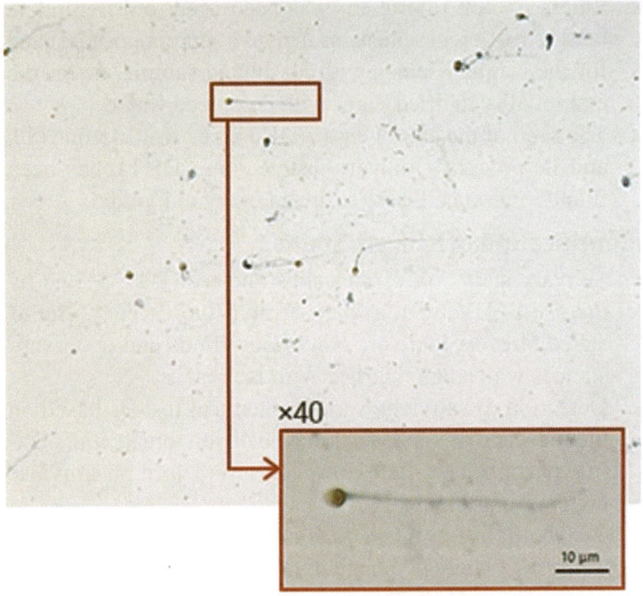

Fig. 6.16 Christmas tree stain: spermatozoa

- These HSP antigens have been reported to be present in the semen of aspermic persons as well, making them a very reliable confirmatory test for semen.
- **RSID-Semen Strip Test**: The RSID-Semen test provides sensitivity as well as specificity to human semen. It deals with identification of human semenogelin in a membrane strip for the detection of semen. Similar in format to a pregnancy test strip, the RSID-semen test identifies the presence of the seminal vesicle-specific antigen, or semenogelin. This antigen is unique to semen, and therefore, there is no cross reactivity with other bodily fluids in males and females or with semen from other mammals. This test can also identify semen even if the stain was stored under less favourable conditions which have been shown to affect other tests such as the Acid Phosphatase test.

Determination of Species

- Semen originating from various animal species as well as humans, can be differentiated by a number of immunological methods based on the precipitin reaction (same as for blood, *vide supra*).
- LDH isoenzyme pattern, presence of Y-body in the sperm, and human seminal plasma-specific antigens, are also highly characteristic of human semen.

Individualization of Seminal Stain

- ABO grouping, PGM, AK, HLA, LDH, GLO, etc., can all be demonstrated in the semen of secretors.
- With the advent of DNA fingerprinting, conclusive identity of the perpetrator can be fixed.

**Florence iodine reagent*: *Potassium iodide, 1.65 g; iodine, 2.54 g; distilled water, 30 mL.*

- Single photon fluorimetry has been used to differentiate between different semens, as it gives a superimposable band for the original semen with its diluted sample, or for the extract of such dried stains with deionized water.
- The ratio of the androgens (T:DHT), i.e., testosterone (T), and its precursor dihydro-testosterone (DHT), has been found to be specific for each and every individual.

Identification of Salivary Stains

- Salivary stains on various substrates can be detected by the use of UV light, as they exhibit fluorescence. But as stated already, there are other body fluids and other substances which can interfere with the results.
- Detection of saliva by various chemical tests is based on the presence of amylase, thiocyanate ion, nitrite ion, alkaline phosphatase, etc. However, tests based on **amylase** are most commonly used.
    - Qualitative amylase tests are used for screening purposes, whereas quantitative tests are reliable in confirming a salivary stain, since amylase is present in maximum concentration in saliva as compared to other body fluids.
    - Several types of amylase isoenzymes have been identified exhibiting genetic variations and hence can be used for individualisation.
- Further individualisation methods include ABO grouping, red cell enzyme and serum protein polymorphisms in secretors, and DNA fingerprinting.
- **Medicolegal Importance**:
    - ***Circumstantial evidence*** – The presence of saliva in cigarette butts, beedi, or sputum, at the scene of a crime can link the perpetrator to the crime.
    - ***Sexual offences*** – The presence of saliva in a bite mark (if present), can help to identify the offender. Saliva is a non-invasive specimen which can be obtained with ease from anyone to test for ***drugs of abuse***.

Topic 7

EMERGING TECHNOLOGIES IN FORENSIC MEDICINE

(Number of Competencies – 1: FM 7.1)

FM 7.1: Non-Core – Written/Viva Voce
- Enumerate the indications and describe the principles and appropriate use for:
  - DNA profiling
  - Facial reconstruction
  - Polygraph (Lie detector)
  - Narcoanalysis
  - Brain mapping
  - Digital autopsy
  - Virtual autopsy
  - Imaging technologies

Teachers and students, please note: Entire Topic 7 is categorised as 'Non-Core' in the new CBME curriculum. But its practical relevance is of paramount importance.

DNA PROFILING

Introduction

- **DNA profiling** or **DNA typing** (previously referred to as "DNA fingerprinting" or "Genetic typing") is one of the most important advances in the field of forensic sciences in recent years.
- The first application of DNA typing in forensic science was done by **Dr Alec Jeffreys** of Leicester University, who was called in by police to apply his new technique (called DNA fingerprinting by him at that time) to help solve two murders in Leicestershire, UK (**Box 7.1**).
- DNA profiling is a procedure wherein DNA extracted from a biological sample obtained from an individual is analyzed. The DNA is processed to generate a pattern for each person that is generally termed as a '**DNA profile**.' This profile is unique for each person excepting that derived from identical twins.

Principles

Chromosomes and Genes

- A **chromosome** contains two complementary strands of **deoxyribonucleic acid** or **DNA**. These are long **polymers** of **nucleic acids** (**nucleotides**) each consisting of
  - Phosphate
  - Deoxyribose, and
  - One of four "bases" which consist of:
    - Adenine
    - Thymine
    - Guanine
    - Cytosine (A, T, C and G)
    - These always form base pairs based on hydrogen bonds between complementary bases: A-T or C-G. (The two strands are termed **anti-parallel**, in that they "run" in opposite directions.)
    - RNA differs from DNA in that the sugar consists of **ribose** rather than deoxyribose, and the base **uracil (U)** is present instead of thymine.
- Genes are the parts of chromosomes containing stretches of DNA which actually code for proteins. **A gene could be thought of as a discrete unit of information influencing inherited characteristics**.

Box 7.1—The Dawn of DNA Profiling

On 21st Nov 1983, a 15-year-old girl (Lynda Mann) of Narborough, Leicestershire, UK, took a shortcut on her way home from babysitting, instead of taking her normal route home. She did not return and her parents and neighbours spent the night searching for her. The next morning, she was found raped and strangled on a deserted footpath known locally as the Black Pad. Using forensic science techniques available at the time, police linked a semen sample taken from her body to a person with type A blood and an enzyme profile that matched only 10% of males. With no other leads or evidence, the case was left open.

On 31st July 1986, a second 15-year-old girl, Dawn Ashworth, left her home in the nearby village of Enderby of Leicestershire, to visit a friend's house. Her parents expected her to return at 9:30 pm; when she failed to do so they called police to report her missing. Two days later, her body was found in a wooded area near a footpath called Ten Pound Lane. She had been beaten, savagely raped and strangled. The modus operandi matched that of the first attack, and semen samples revealed the same blood type.

An initial suspect was Richard Buckland, a local 17-year-old with learning difficulties who, while innocent of both crimes, revealed knowledge of Ashworth's body, and admitted to the Ashworth crime under questioning, denying the first murder.

In 1985, Alec Jeffreys, a genetics researcher at the University of Leicester, developed DNA profiling along with Peter Gill and Dave Werrett of the Forensic Science Service (FSS). Using this technique, Jeffreys compared semen samples from both murder victims against a blood sample from Buckland and conclusively proved that both girls were killed by the same man but not by Buckland. Buckland became the first person in history to have his innocence established by DNA fingerprinting.

contd.

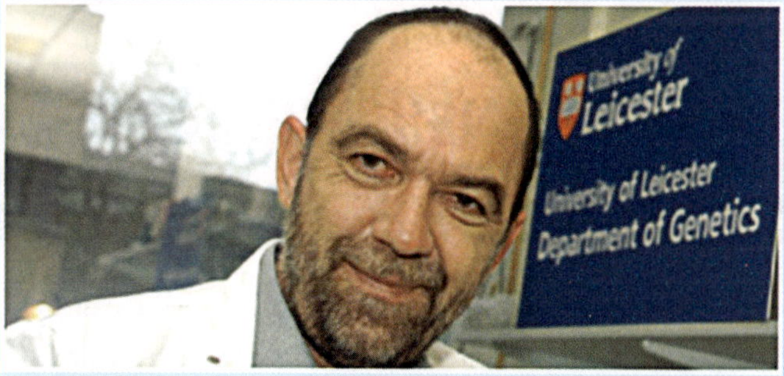

Sir Alec Jeffreys

Leicestershire Constabulary and the FSS then undertook an investigation in which more than 5500 local men were asked to volunteer blood or saliva samples. This took 6 months, but no matches were found. On 1st Aug 1987, a worker at Hampshires Bakery in Leicester, Ian Kelly, revealed to fellow workers in a local pub that he had taken the blood test while masquerading as another worker in the same bakery: Colin Pitchfork. The latter had told Kelly that he wanted to avoid being harassed by police because of prior convictions for indecent exposure. A woman who overheard the conversation reported it to police.

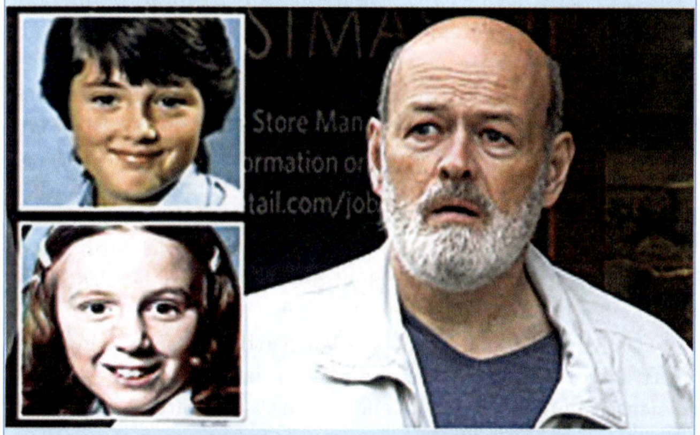

Colin Pitchfork (right) and his two victims (left – Dawn and Lynda)

On 19th Sept 1987, Pitchfork was arrested. During questioning, Pitchfork admitted to exposing himself to more than 1000 women, a compulsion that began in his early teens. He later progressed to sexual assault, and then to strangling his victims. Pitchfork said this was in order to protect his identity. The Court rejected this, viewing the motivation for the strangulations as 'perverted sadism'. During his interviews with the police he admitted his crimes, but lied about the level and nature of the violence he had inflicted on his victims. He pleaded guilty to the two rapes and murders in addition to another incident of sexual assault, and was sentenced to life imprisonment. A psychiatric report prepared for the Court described Pitchfork as possessing a psychopathic personality disorder, accompanied with a serious psycho-sexual pathology.

Genetic Polymorphism

- Within a species, one chromosome of a given type is very similar to another, but at some places (**loci**) on the chromosome, there may be some variability in the DNA sequence between chromosomes.
- These (physical) differences can lead to the (genetic) phenomenon of **polymorphic alleles**.
- **Alleles are detectable variations occurring at a single genetic locus, with the possibility that individual chromosomes may differ in the allele each has at a given locus.**
- Alleles are detected using **genetic markers**.
- Where allelic variation is frequently found (at least 10% of chromosomes have an allele other than the most commonly occurring one), it is known as a **polymorphism**.
- The term **genetic marker** can be used very broadly to apply to any observable variation which results from a variation at a single genetic locus.
  - This may be a serological marker such as ABO blood group, or a **DNA marker**:
    - The four main types of **DNA marker** are:
      - Restriction Fragment Length Polymorphisms (RFLPs)
      - Variable Number of Tandem Repeats (VNTRs)
      - Short Tandem Repeats (STRs) and
      - Single Nucleotide Polymorphisms (SNPs).

The Scientific Basis of DNA Typing

- DNA typing is founded based on a number of genetic and molecular principles. Basic to the understanding of the complexity of DNA typing is the concept of the cell.
  - A cell is the building unit of an organism made up of its component parts, one of which is the **nucleus** that functions as its command centre. As the command centre of the cell, the nucleus houses the **DNA** or **deoxyribonucleic acid** that codes for genetic information responsible for all cellular processes.
  - Several DNA molecules comprise **genes** which in turn are located in minute bodies called **chromosomes**. In humans, there are 23 pairs of chromosomes within a cell thus making up a total of 46 chromosomes.
  - Some chromosomal regions contain repeating units of the same type of DNA molecule which may or may not code for a specific protein. The number of repeating units in individuals may vary.
  - Today, chromosomal regions with short tandem repeating DNA units (known as **Short Tandem Repeats** or **STRs**) are most often used as markers for human identification in forensic casework.
- DNA can also be found in another part of the cell called the **mitochondrion**. Unlike nuclear DNA with two copies per cell, multiple copies of mitochondrial DNA (up to 100,000 copies) are present per human cell. Because of this, **mitochondrial DNA analysis** is the method of choice when dealing with environmentally challenged samples, e.g., identification of mass disaster victims, exhumed human remains, etc.
- There are at least **four** different forensic techniques of DNA typing:
  - **RFLP—Restriction Fragment Length Polymorphism,**

the oldest technique, essentially involves radioactive fragmentation and examiner comparison.
- **STR—Short Tandem Repeats**, a PCR-based method which uses markers for short, repeating segments of microvariant allele patterns, as short as three to seven base pairs, usually involving computer expert systems, although visual detection is also possible.
- **Mitochondrial DNA Analysis**—A type of PCR used on samples subjected to extreme environmental conditions, and since mitochondrial DNA is inherited solely from the mother, it has also been used in cases of disputed maternity.
- **Rapid DNA ID Microchip-Based Genetic Detectors**—These are field-ready laptop analysis units capable of being used at crime scenes, displaying profiles onsite, or electronically uploading to a CODIS database.

Most laboratories use the twin techniques of RFLP and PCR-STR as part of their double result requirement.

From the year 2000, however, for forensic purposes, STR Typing alone is the recommended method, which must involve the study of at least 13 core loci.

RFLP DNA Typing

- This method is of historical importance only as most laboratories have switched over to STR Typing for forensic purposes.
- The first step in RFLP DNA typing is extraction of the DNA from the sample, be it blood, saliva, semen or some other biological sample.
- The purified DNA is then cut into fragments by **restriction enzymes**.
  - Take the pattern GCGC, and imagine it occurs more than once in the DNA.
  - The number of times it occurs is unique to the individual. The restriction enzyme chops the DNA in two at every place where the GCGC pattern occurs. For example:
    - Person 1: **GCGC**ATGTT**GCGC**AAGA**GCGC**
    - Person 2: **GCGC**ATTGAATGCAAGTA**GCGC**

    In this example, Person 1 has the repeat sequence three times, while Person 2 has it twice. The restriction enzyme will cut between the first G and the first C. Thus,
    - Person 1: CGCATGTTCGCAAGAG – 2 small fragments
    - Person 2: CGCATTGAATGCAAGTAG – 1 large fragment
- The restriction fragments have negative charge and can be separated by a technique called **gel electrophoresis**, which separates the pieces of DNA based on their size.
- The samples of DNA that have been treated with restriction enzymes are placed in separate lanes on a slab of electrophoretic gel across which is placed an electric field.
  - The fragments migrate toward the positive electrode, the smaller fragments moving faster than the larger fragments, thus separating the DNA samples into distinct bands.
  - The bands can be visualised using **autoradiography** or **luminescent dyes**.
- This approach to DNA typing requires quite large samples of biological material in order to obtain reasonable results.
- The entire procedure of RFLP-based forensic DNA typing is laid out pictorially in **Fig. 7.1**.

DNA Typing Using STRs

- Tandemly repeated DNA sequences are widespread throughout the human genome and show sufficient variability among individuals in a population to have become important in several fields including human identity testing.
- These tandemly repeated regions of DNA are typically classified into several groups depending on the size of the repeat region.
  - **Minisatellites (variable number of tandem repeats, VNTRs)** have core repeats with 9–80 base pairs (bp).
  - **Microsatellites (short tandem repeats, STRs)** contain 2–5 bp repeats. The forensic DNA community has moved primarily towards tetranucleotide repeats, which may be amplified using the polymerase chain reaction (PCR) with greater accuracy than dinucleotide repeats.
- The variety of alleles present in a population is such that a high degree of discrimination among individuals in the population may be obtained when multiple STR loci are examined.
- **PCR-based STRs** have several advantages over conventional Southern blotting techniques of the larger variable number tandem repeats (VNTRs).
  - Discrete alleles from STR systems may be obtained due to their smaller size, which puts them in the size range where DNA fragments differing by a single basepair in size may be differentiated.
  - Smaller quantities of DNA, including degraded DNA, may be typed using STRs. Thus, the quantity and integrity of the DNA sample is less of an issue with PCR-based typing methods than with conventional RFLP methods.
- With **PCR (polymerase chain reaction)**, a chemical solution is added to the sample and boiled to remove the DNA, which is then combined with short fragments of known DNA, called **primers**, and other chemicals that stimulate replication by means of a reaction called the polymerase chain reaction.
  - To perform a PCR reaction, a small quantity of the target DNA is added to a test tube with a buffered solution containing:
    - DNA polymerase,
    - Oligonucleotide primers,
    - Four deoxynucleotide building blocks of DNA and
    - Cofactor $MgCl_2$.
  - The PCR mixture is taken through replication cycles consisting of:

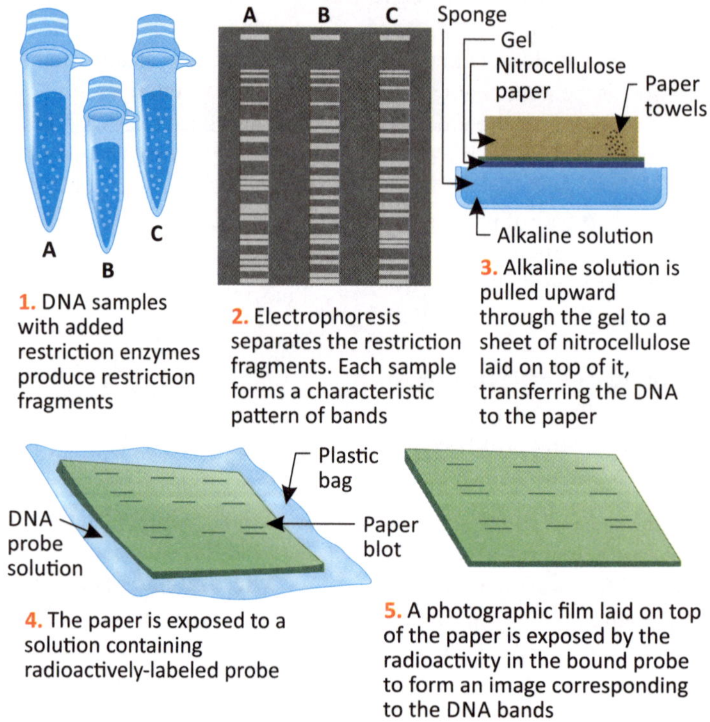

Fig. 7.1 RFLP technique

    - one to several minutes at 94–96°C, during which the DNA is denatured into single strands,
    - one to several minutes at 50–65°C, during which the primers hybridize or "anneal" (by way of hydrogen bonds) to their complementary sequences on either side of the target sequence,
    - one to several minutes at 72°C, during which the polymerase binds and extends a complementary DNA strand from each primer.
  - As amplification proceeds, the DNA sequence between the primers doubles after each cycle. Following 30 such cycles, a theoretical amplification factor of one billion is attained.
  - PCR techniques offer the advantage of requiring only trace amounts of DNA, and they can be done very quickly.
- There are hundreds of STR systems that have been mapped throughout the human genome. Several dozen have been investigated for application to human identity testing. These STR loci are found on almost every chromosome in the genome. Tetranucleotide repeats have been most popular among forensic scientists due to their fidelity in PCR amplification although some tri- and pentanucleotide repeats are also used.
- For forensic purposes, 13 selected loci are used, as stipulated by the FBI, USA (**Combined DNA Indexing System or CODIS**).
- The STR profiling kit that is currently used in the United Kingdom and many other parts of the world is the **AMPFISTR® SGM Plus™ PCR Amplification kit. The SGM (Second Generation Multiplex)** decreases the probability of a chance match from 1×10^{-8}, to **one in trillions** for unrelated individuals!
- The entire procedure of STR-based forensic DNA typing is laid out pictorially in **Fig. 7.2**.

Applications of DNA Profiling*

- Establishment of **paternity and maternity**.
- Establishment of **biological relationship** for immigration purpose, kidney transplantation, etc.
- Detection of cases of **child swapping**.
- Identification of rapist in **rape cases** including gang rape cases.
- Identification of victim/perpetrator in **murder cases**.
- Identification of **mutilated remains**, as in cases of murder, bomb blasts, mass disasters.
- Identification of bodies in **exhumation** cases.
- All cases of **wildlife identification**.
- Determination of **pedigree** for seed or livestock breeds.
- Detection of **bacteria and other organisms** that may pollute air, water, soil and food.
- Authentication of **consumables** such as wine.

*****Note***: *Important applications can be remembered by the mnemonic*: ***3M-PER*** *which stands for Murder, Mutilated remains, Maternity dispute, Paternity dispute, Exhumation, Rape.*

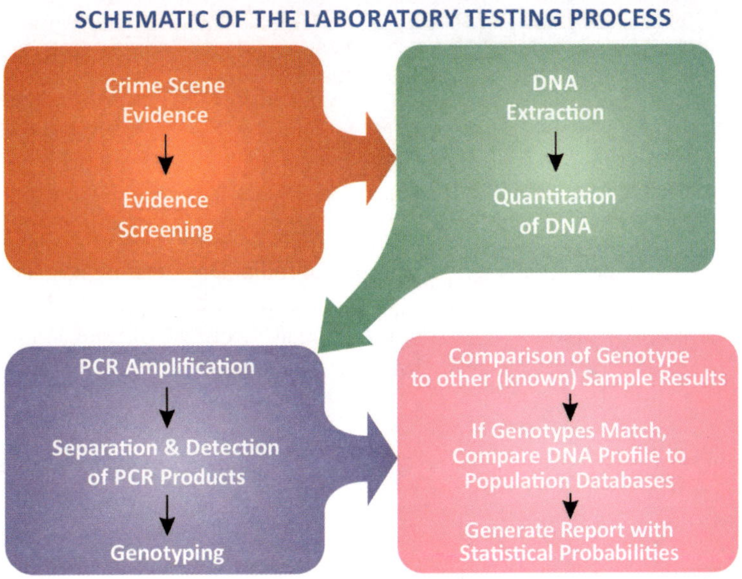

Fig. 7.2 STR typing technique

Indian Scenario

- In India, initially the use of DNA testing in paternity cases far outnumbered criminal cases. But today, use of DNA typing in criminal cases is quite routine and is undertaken in such cases frequently.
- It all began with the very first case in **1988** in **Kerala** (**Kunhiraman vs Manoj**, final verdict delivered on 27 Feb, 1991), which was a paternity dispute case (**Box 7.2**), and since then the technique has rapidly gained acceptance among police and judiciary in relation to a wide variety of offences.
- The scientist who introduced the technology of DNA typing in India is **Dr Lalji Singh** (1947–2017), former Director of the Centre for Cellular and Molecular Biology (CCMB), Hyderabad.
- Usually during court trials involving DNA typing evidence, emphasis is laid on **population genetics**, i.e., how the probability has been calculated that a particular suspect's DNA profile matches with that of the DNA evidence. Often the labs carrying out DNA typing calculate the odds of one in millions or billions against a random match. For example, the chance that the semen stains present on a victim's undergarment originating from someone other than the suspect whose DNA typing matches, would be one in 82 billion. Naturally, such high odds indicate that the suspect alone must be the culprit. The chance that the suspect's DNA coincidentally matches with the crime sample depends on how frequently the particular pattern of genetic variants revealed in his or her DNA profile occurs in the general population. Obviously, if all the three billion nucleotides of the suspect's DNA were compared, then there would be no doubt about the interpretation of a match. Methods available today, reduce the possibility of random matches by examining more and more specific physical sites on DNA. Well established and highly proficient DNA typing laboratories such as the **Centre for DNA Fingerprinting and Diagnostics** (**CDFD**), **Hyderabad**, or the **Central Forensic Science Laboratory** (**CFSL**), **Kolkata**, usually maintain databases of the markers used. As more and more such loci are included, the odds against the chance match would become even higher.
- Another point being debated hotly today is the creation of a **national database**, i.e., mapping the DNA pattern of every single individual. That way, when a rape is committed, there is no need to look for a suspect. All that needs to be done is to take the semen sample and elucidate its DNA pattern, and check it against the national database to find out whom it belongs to.

Box 7.2—Kunhiraman Case – The First Forensic DNA Case of India

DNA typing started its journey through the Indian legal system in 1988. It is a matter of pride that in India, the first use of DNA evidence in a paternity trial was in Kerala in 1988 during the maintenance case of Manoj, i.e., from the very next year of its first admission in the United States. This very first trial resulted in the admissibility of the technique in Indian courts.

The facts in connection with the case were that the petitioner's mother Vilasini and the counter-petitioner **Kunhiraman** were neighbours. **Vilasini** was working as an agent in an insurance company. As a part of her job, she went to the house of Kunhiraman for canvassing him to take a policy of the company, and he readily obliged. She later stated that Kunhiraman took great interest in her and offered to help her by canvassing policies for her from others. In connection with such insurance work, when one day Vilasini went to meet Kunhiraman, he was alone in the house, and he forced her to have sex with him on the promise that he would marry her. This sexual relationship became regular and when she became pregnant, Kunhiraman denied all the

contd.

facts and changed his attitude towards marrying her. After the birth of her child, Manoj, Vilasini filed a maintenance suit under Section 125 of the Code of Criminal Procedure before the Chief Judicial Magistrate, Thalassery. In the absence of a legal marriage between Vilasini and Kunhiraman, the court found it difficult to apply Section 12 of the Indian Evidence Act in order to fix the legitimacy of the child. The court was of the opinion that the legitimacy of Manoj and the responsibility of Kunhiraman as the father of Manoj could be established only through scientific evidence. For that, the court ordered for the novel scientific technique of DNA typing to be done for determining the paternity of Manoj.

Manoj, Vilasini and Kunhiraman proceeded to the Centre for Cellular and Molecular Biology (CCMB), Hyderabad for giving their blood samples for conducting DNA typing. After conducting the test, the CCMB reported that Kunhiraman and Vilasini were the biological parents of Manoj. Senior scientist **Dr Lalji Singh** gave his opinion supported by adequate scientific explanation detailing the procedure of conducting the test. But when the case came for trial, Kunhiraman raised objection by stating that though the DNA test conducted in Western countries was fool-proof, the DNA test conducted by CCMB was not fool-proof because the process and techniques developed in CCMB were slightly different and did not have the same reliability. Therefore, the court permitted the parties to examine the expert witnesses for determining the reliability of the report of the CCMB.

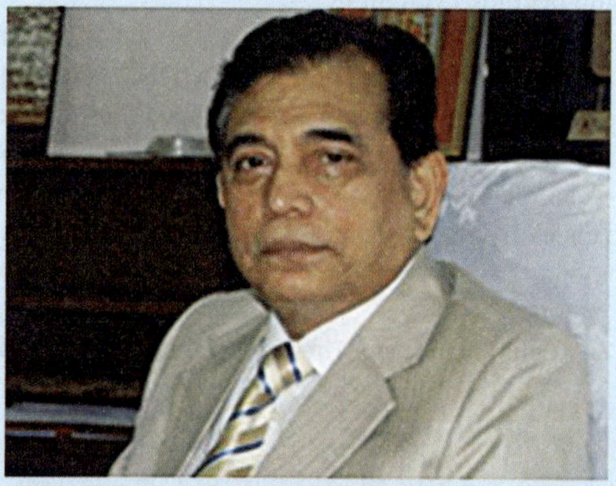

Dr Lalji Singh

Dr Lalji Singh was examined, and in his chief examination he stated that the process that he had followed in this case was recognized and the papers published by him on the subject were also recognized. Regarding his experience, he stated that he had experience in molecular biology since 1976 and he had worked for 13 years in the University of Edinburgh. When he was cross examined, he admitted that there were certain differences between the method propounded by CCMB and the DNA Fingerprinting technique conducted in other countries. The court examined other expert witnesses who corroborated Dr Singh's statement and pronounced judgement accepting the technique's admissibility.

Kunhiraman was declared to be the biological father of Manoj and was asked to pay maintenance costs to Vilasini for rearing Manoj. On appealing the verdict, the High Court of Kerala confirmed the findings of the lower court and ruled that the result of DNA test could be taken as conclusive in deciding paternity. The unique work of Dr Lalji Singh in this and other cases, prompted the Government of India's Department of Biotechnology (DBT) to form an autonomous institution **'Centre for DNA Fingerprinting and Diagnostics (CDFD)'** in 1995, in Hyderabad.

- In India, DNA testing has caught on very well. While the underlying principles of DNA typing cannot be questioned, legal scrutiny of the technique can only revolve around questions relating to the collection, forwarding and authentication of the samples.
  - Therefore, it is imperative to follow strict guidelines as a standard procedure when samples are being collected or forwarded. Unfortunately, most medical officers in India are unclear as to the exact method of collection and forwarding of crime samples for DNA analysis.
  - One of the prerequisites for successful DNA typing is an efficient method of collection of these samples from the scene of crime, and submitting them (along with control samples), to the DNA typing laboratory with minimum delay. The infallibility of DNA analysis depends mostly on the skill, ability and integrity shown by police officers and medical officers.
  - Since DNA typing is highly sophisticated and the results are unassailable, the scientists (DNA analysts) should be provided with the samples in the prescribed manner, so that they can process the samples and give their opinion based on the results they obtain, in the most befitting manner.
- Obviously, a technology that is so powerful and so sensitive must be used extremely cautiously, since for example, if a DNA scientist sneezes while working, his DNA could contaminate the sample being examined. So there is this tremendous need to avoid contamination. Whether laboratory practices in India are up to that or not can only be tested by having proficiency tests put in place. These are areas of current concern.

Collection and Forwarding of Forensic Samples for DNA Typing

Collection of Samples

A. **Liquid Blood Samples**:

1. In cases where blood samples have to be sent as evidence samples (e.g., paternity or maternity disputes) or as control samples (e.g., criminal cases), 2–5 mL of intravenously drawn blood should be collected into sterile, leak-proof screw-capped tubes containing heparin or EDTA as an anticoagulant.
2. The sample should be mixed thoroughly, but slowly, with the anticoagulant, and then the tube should be placed in a container filled with ice (e.g., a thermos flask), if it is to be transported immediately.
3. The sample tube should be labelled properly, displaying clearly the source of the blood sample, the name of

the doctor collecting the blood sample, time and date of collection and other details, such as the forwarding authority, etc.

4. If there is going to be some delay before the sample can be transported, it should be stored in a refrigerator.
5. In case, it appears to the medical officer who has carried out the blood collection that the person is suffering from an apparent genetic disorder, this fact should be mentioned in the forwarding note/letter of advice. This would help the DNA analyst to interpret the results correctly.
6. An identification card should be completed and sent along with each blood sample.

B. **Semen Samples/Vaginal Swabs**:

1. In criminal cases involving rape, or rape-murder, DNA typing can conclusively help in the identification of the culprit, provided suspects/accused persons are available for obtaining their blood samples for subsequent comparison with that of the DNA profile of the seminal stain/swab.
2. In rape cases, the role of the police officer is of utmost importance because any delay in getting the medical examination of the victim done could lead to loss of valuable evidentiary material, i.e., the seminal fluid/stain. The investigating officer should get the medical examination of the victim done by a medical officer without unnecessary delay.
3. Sterile cotton ear buds can be used as swabs.
4. After collection, the swabs should be completely air-dried, placed in dry sterile tubes, sealed and labelled.
5. Other relevant information about the sample should be enclosed separately, and sent along with the sample.
6. In gang rape cases, more than two vaginal swabs should be collected and sent in separate individual tubes.
7. The genital parts of the victim should be swabbed with wet cotton swabs, i.e., moistened with sterile water (for instance, water for injection available in medical stores can be used for this purpose).
8. These tubes should be packed in separate vials and sent to the DNA laboratory.
9. The clothes worn by the victim at the time of the offence also should be air-dried, packed in dry paper and sent to the laboratory.
10. No attempt should be made to dry the samples by either a hair drier, or by placing them under direct sunlight.
11. In cases of delay in despatching the samples to the laboratory, the vaginal swabs should be stored at 4°C either in a refrigerator, or a cold room of a hospital.
12. Cloth materials if any, may be stored at room temperature and sent along with the vaginal swabs.
13. Microscope slides smeared with vaginal swabs should be packed individually and sent at room temperature to the laboratory. The medical officer or chemical examiner concerned should not use colouring dye or stain on smeared slides because that would hamper the DNA analysis.
14. Blood samples of the accused should be collected as already described.

C. **Stains from Automobile/Scene of Crime/Large Material Objects**:

1. Body fluid stains on automobiles or large objects could be swabbed with cotton buds moistened with sterile water. Ampoules containing water for injection could be used for moistening.
2. The cotton buds should be air-dried, placed in a clean bottle and sent to the DNA laboratory at room temperature.

D. **Blood/Semen from Individuals Under Field Conditions**:

1. Blood/Semen from individuals should be collected into

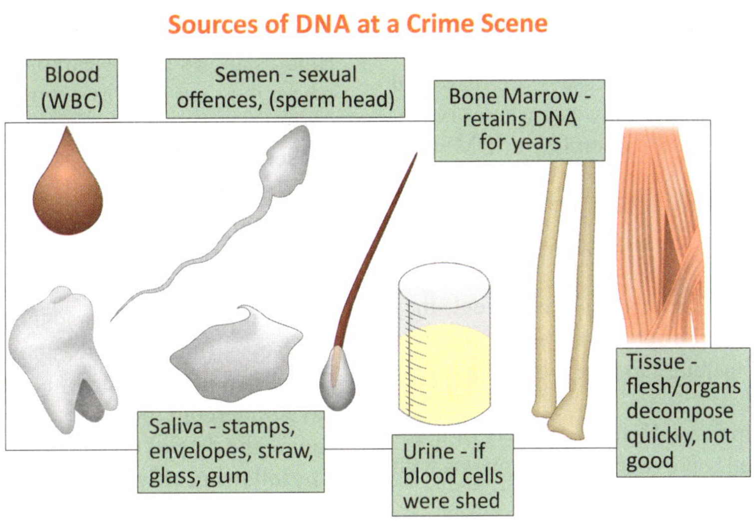

Fig. 7.3 Usual forensic samples for DNA typing

a sterile tube or container, and the same should be spread on a sterile bandage cloth folded several times so as to make it absorb all the fluid.

2. This should be air-dried under shade and not under direct sunlight.
3. After complete drying, it should be placed in a clean envelope, sealed, labelled and sent to the DNA laboratory at room temperature.

E. **Viscera Samples**:

1. Cases occur wherein mutilated bodies are recovered whose identification is difficult to establish by conventional forensic methods. In such cases, DNA typing can help to establish the source of the mutilated body with relative or absolute certainty.
2. Of the various body tissues, **muscle is the most ideal source for extracting DNA**. Therefore, muscle samples of approximately 100 mg in weight can be dissected out using sterile scalpel blades and scissors, and placed in a sterile glass or polypropylene tube containing normal saline (0.9% NS Injection IP) as a preservative. The saline solution prepared conventionally in mortuaries is not recommended because of inconsistencies in salt concentration. In hospitals or research institutions, where dimethyl sulphoxide (DMSO) is available, a 20% solution of DMSO saturated with sodium chloride can be prepared, which is a better preservative.
3. In cases where several pieces of body are found, it is recommended that sufficient number may be collected individually and sent as separate exhibits, so that the identity of the mutilated body can be established more precisely. This is especially true in the case of mass disasters/air crashes/bomb blasts, etc., where several bodies get mutilated and mixed up.
4. The sample tubes containing the tissues should be properly sealed and made leak-proof, so that the preservative does not leak from the bottle during transportation to the laboratory.
5. With regard to foetal tissue, it is recommended that associated maternal and placental tissues are dissected out, and only the foetus (preferably as a whole) is sent in normal saline (0.9% NS Injection IP), or DMSO as mentioned above.
6. The jar containing the foetus should be placed in a thermocol box containing ice, and sent to the DNA laboratory.
7. In exhumation cases, if dry tissues are present, they should be placed in a sterile bottle without preservative and sent at room temperature to the laboratory.

F. **Bones, Teeth, Hair**:

1. DNA typing can help to establish the identity of mutilated bodies, exhumed bodies and skeletal remains with a remarkable degree of certainty.
2. Bones, especially long and intact bones such as **humerus or femur, are most suitable for DNA typing analysis**.
3. In criminal cases where skulls are recovered (with teeth), molar teeth should be detached from the upper and lower jaw bones and sent to the laboratory for analysis. If molar teeth are not available, any other teeth present could be sent for analysis.
4. Bones should be packed in clean paper/cloth and placed in a polyethylene cover, sealed and sent to the laboratory at room temperature.
5. Ice or preservatives need not be used for transportation of bones. Also, there is no necessity to wash the bones before they are packed.
6. Teeth should be placed in a clean polyethylene cover and sent to the laboratory for analysis. **Teeth along with the skull, which have been subjected to superimposition test, are not useful for DNA analysis**. Therefore, a few teeth should be removed from the upper and lower jaws of the skull before they are subjected to superimposition test.
7. Hair samples should be packed in clean paper, sealed and sent at room temperature. If possible, hair with roots should be sent for analysis.
8. No preservatives should be used for storing hair.
9. At autopsy, the medical officer should always look for loose hair in the palms of a murdered person, which in some cases could be useful for identification of the culprit.

G. **Fingernail Scrapings**:

1. Fingernail scrapings in cases of rape or murder constitute a very good source of DNA of the assailant. Therefore, caution should be exercised while collecting these scrapings at the time of autopsy.
2. The palms of the victim should be placed over a clean polyethylene sheet and examined. Using a sterile sewing needle or a toothpick, the inner portions of the fingernails must be scraped gently.
3. All the material that falls on to the polyethylene sheet should be collected and sent to the laboratory without any preservative.

Authentication and Forwarding

1. Blood samples in a case of paternity dispute, and in a case where they are used as control samples for identification purposes need to be collected in the presence of a judicial officer. By doing so, questions relating to authenticity of the samples will not arise.
2. The samples should be sealed, and a specimen of the seal on paper or cloth should accompany the samples for verification at the laboratory.
3. The identification card and the forwarding note need to be completely filled, certified and sent along with the samples.
4. Blood samples should not be collected from persons who have undergone blood transfusion within 3 months preceding the date of collection.
5. **The following officials are authorised to forward a case to the DNA laboratory**:
   a. Judicial First Class Magistrate, or Subordinate Judge, or District & Sessions Judge.

b. Station House Officer of a police station, or any police officer above the rank of Sub-Inspector.
c. Medical Officer of the rank of Asst. Civil Surgeon or above, of a Government Hospital.
d. Officers of the Collectorate holding executive powers.

Status of DNA Typing as a Forensic Tool

Advantages

1. It is the most conclusive method of identification of individuals (along with digital fingerprints).
2. Since DNA is very stable, the technique can be applied even on very old (aged) stains or specimens.
3. Extremely small quantities of body fluid or tissue is sufficient for analysis.

Disadvantages

1. DNA typing cannot differentiate between identical twins. However, newer modifications have been developed to overcome this.
2. It is relatively expensive, when compared to most other methods of establishing identity.
3. Interpretation of results requires a great deal of expertise and experience.
4. While DNA evidence has been questioned in a few cases, and even discredited in some, it has never been because of the soundness of the underlying principles being doubted, but because of other reasons such as improper collection or preservation of samples, or laboratory errors, etc.
   a. One such case that attacked DNA evidence with considerable success was the sensational case involving the famous American footballer **OJ Simpson** (**Box 7.3**). The case has been adapted into a highly acclaimed TV Mini Series titled 'The People v. O.J. Simpson: American Crime Story'.

Box 7.3—The OJ Simpson Case

The OJ Simpson murder case was a criminal trial held in California, USA. The trial spanned from Nov 2, 1994 to Oct 3, 1995. Orenthal James Simpson (born July 9, 1947), a retired American football player was tried on two counts of murder after the deaths of his ex-wife, Nicole Brown Simpson, and her friend Ronald Lyle Goldman, in June 1994.

Brown and Simpson were married on Feb 2, 1985, 5 years after his retirement from professional football. The couple had two children. The marriage lasted 7 years, during which Simpson was repeatedly accused of spousal abuse. Brown filed for divorce on Feb 25, 1992 citing "irreconcilable differences".

At 12:10 a.m. on June 13, 1994, Nicole Brown and Ronald Goldman were found murdered outside Brown's apartment block in Los Angeles. Evidence found at the scene led police to suspect that OJ Simpson was the murderer. Nicole Brown had been stabbed multiple times in the head and neck and had defensive wounds on her hands.

Lawyers convinced the police to allow Simpson to turn himself in at 11 a.m. on June 17, 1994. Over 1000 reporters waited for Simpson at the police station, but he failed to appear. At 2 p.m., the Los Angeles Police Department issued an all-points bulletin. At around 6:20 p.m., a motorist in Orange County saw Simpson riding in his white Ford Bronco, driven by his friend Al Cowlings, and notified police. At 6:45 p.m., a police officer saw the Bronco going north on the highway. When the officer approached with sirens blaring, Cowlings yelled that Simpson was in the back seat and had a gun to his own head. The officer backed off, but followed the vehicle with up to 20 police cars participating in the chase. Over 20 helicopters joined the chase!

Police detective Tom Lange had Simpson's cell number and called him repeatedly. Lange pleaded with Simpson to "throw the gun out the window" for the sake of his mother and his children. Thousands of spectators and on-lookers packed overpasses along the procession's journey waiting for the white Bronco. They and millions of others watched the chase on television. The chase ended at 8:00 p.m. at Simpson's home. Simpson was allowed to go inside to speak to his mother. A few minutes later, he surrendered to authorities.

On June 20, Simpson was arraigned and pleaded not guilty to both murders. Following the preliminary hearing, the case was moved to downtown Los Angeles. Televised by Court TV, the trial began on Jan 24, 1995. The prosecution spent the opening weeks of the trial presenting evidence that Simpson had a history of physically abusing Nicole. Even with no murder weapon and no witnesses to the murders, the prosecution felt they had a very strong case. From the physical evidence collected, the prosecution claimed that Simpson drove to Nicole Brown's house on the evening of June 12 with the intention of killing her. They maintained that Nicole opened the front door after responding to a knock, when Simpson grabbed her before she could scream and attacked her with a knife. Forensic evidence suggested that Ron Goldman arrived at the front gate sometime during the assault, and the assailant apparently attacked him and stabbed him repeatedly in the neck and chest.

According to the prosecution, Simpson left a "trail of blood" from the condo to the alley behind it; there was also testimony that drops of Simpson's blood were found on the driveway near the gate to his house on Rockingham Drive. Simpson was last seen in public at 9:36 p.m. that evening, and was not seen again until 10:54 p.m., when he came out of the front door of his house to a waiting limousine hired to take him to the airport to fly to a convention in Chicago. It had been established that the murders took place between 10:15 and 10:40 p.m.

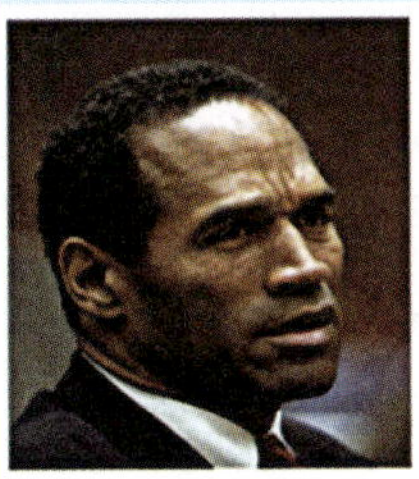

O J SIMPSON

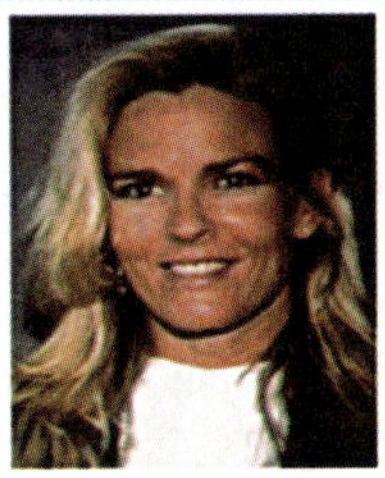

NICOLE BROWN SIMPSON

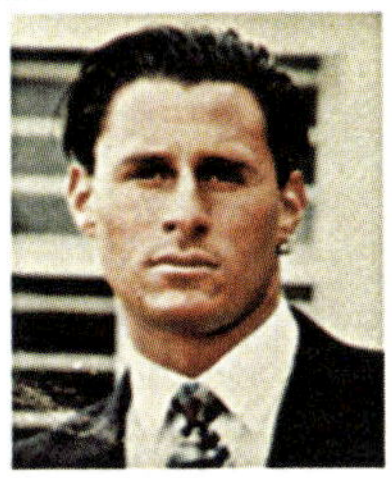

RON GOLDMAN

According to his testimony, limousine driver Allan Park arrived at Simpson's estate at 10:24 p.m. He did not see Simpson's white Bronco parked at the curb. Park began to buzz the intercom at the gate at 10:40, getting no response. He saw that the house was dark with no lights on, save for a dim light coming from Simpson's bedroom. At about 10.50, Park testified that he saw "a tall black man" of Simpson's height and build enter the front door of the house from the driveway area, after which lights went on and Simpson finally answered Park's call, explaining that he had overslept and would open the front gate soon. He then opened the gate by remote control to let Park drive in to the estate grounds, and came out of his house through the front door a few minutes later. Park helped Simpson put his belongings in the trunk of the limo for the ride to the airport. Park remarked in his testimony that Simpson looked agitated.

The prosecution used several tactics to show Simpson's culpability. DNA analysis of blood found on a pair of Simpson's socks found in his bedroom identified it as Nicole Brown's. DNA analysis of the blood found in, on and near Simpson's Bronco revealed traces of Simpson's, Brown's and Goldman's blood. DNA analysis of bloody socks found in Simpson's bedroom proved this was Brown's blood. A few strands of African-American hair were found on Goldman's shirt. DNA analysis of blood on the left-hand glove, found outside Brown's home, was proven to be a mixture of Simpson's, Brown's and Goldman's. The gloves contained particles of hair consistent with Goldman's hair and a cap contained carpet fibres consistent with fibres from Simpson's Bronco. The left-hand glove found at Nicole Brown's home and the right-hand glove found at Simpson's home proved to be a match.

However, the District Attorney's Office and the Medical Examiner's Office could not explain why 1.5 cm^3 of blood were missing from the original 8 cm^3 taken from Simpson and placed into evidence. Much of the incriminating evidence: bloody glove, bloody socks, blood in and on the Bronco, was discovered by Police Detective Mark Fuhrman, who was later charged with perjury for making some false claims.

The bloody shoe prints at the crime scene were identified by an FBI shoe expert as having been made by a pair of extremely rare and expensive Bruno Magli shoes. The large size (12) prints matched Simpson's shoe size.

Evidence collected by LAPD criminalist Dennis Fung came under criticism. He admitted to "having missed a few drops of blood on a fence near the bodies", but on the stand he said that he "returned several weeks afterwards to collect them". Fung also admitted that he had not used rubber gloves when collecting some of the evidence.

The DNA evidence: Samples from bloody shoe prints leading away from the bodies and from the back gate of the condominium were tested for DNA profiles, which matched. Dennis Fung testified that this DNA evidence put Simpson at Nicole Brown's townhouse at the time of the murders. But during cross-examination, most of the DNA evidence was questioned. Blood evidence had been tested at two separate laboratories, each conducting different tests. Despite that safeguard, it emerged during the cross-examination of Fung and the other laboratory scientists that the police scientist Andrea Mazzola (who collected blood samples from Simpson to compare with evidence from the crime scene) was a trainee who carried the vial of Simpson's blood around in her lab coat pocket for nearly a day before handing it over as an exhibit! What should have been the prosecution's strong point became their weak link amid accusations that bungling police technicians handled the blood samples with such a degree of incompetence as to render the delivery of accurate and reliable DNA results almost impossible.

One dark leather glove was found at the crime scene, its match found near the guest house behind Simpson's estate. Brown had bought Simpson two pairs of this type of glove in 1990. Both gloves, according to the prosecution, contained DNA evidence from Simpson, Brown and Goldman, with the glove at Simpson's house also containing a long strand of blonde hair similar to Brown's. On June 15, 1995, defense attorney Johnnie Cochran goaded assistant prosecutor Christopher Darden into asking Simpson to put on the leather glove that was found at the scene of the crime. The leather glove seemed too tight for Simpson to put on easily. The prosecution stated their belief that the glove shrank from having been soaked in blood and later testing. A photo was presented during the trial showing Simpson wearing the same type of glove that was found at the crime scene.

Prosecutors claimed that the presence of Simpson's blood at the crime scene was the result of blood dripping from cuts on the middle finger of his left hand. Police noted his wounds on June 13, 1994, and asserted that these were suffered during the fatal attack on Ron Goldman. However, the defense noted that none of the gloves found had any cuts. Plus, both prosecution and defense witnesses testified to not seeing any cuts or wounds of any kind on Simpson's hands in the hours after the murders took place. The defense also alleged that Fuhrman may have planted the glove at Simpson's house after taking it from the crime scene, and that the analysis finding that the hair could be Brown's could not be reliable.

On 03 Oct 1995, the jury returned a verdict of 'not guilty'. An estimated 100 million people worldwide stopped what they were doing to watch or listen to the announcement. Many were shocked at the verdict.

In 1997, the parents of Ron Goldman brought a civil suit against Simpson for wrongful death, and Brown's estate, represented by her father, also brought a suit against Simpson. The jury in the civil trial awarded Brown and Simpson's children, Sydney and Justin, $12.6 million from their father as recipients of their mother's estate. The victims' families were awarded $33.5 million in compensatory and punitive damages.

In Sept 2007, Simpson was arrested in Las Vegas, Nevada, and charged with numerous felonies, including armed robbery and kidnapping in another case. In 2008, he was found guilty and sentenced to 33 years imprisonment, with a minimum of 9 years without parole. He is currently serving his sentence at the Lovelock Correctional Center in Nevada.

FORENSIC FACIAL RECONSTRUCTION (FORENSIC FACIAL APPROXIMATION, FORENSIC SCULPTING)

- This is the process of **recreating the face of an individual** (whose identity is often not known) from their skeletal remains through an amalgamation of artistry, forensic science, anthropology, osteology and anatomy. It is one of the most subjective – as well as one of the most controversial – techniques in the field of **forensic anthropology**. Despite this controversy, facial reconstruction has proved successful frequently enough that research and methodological developments continue to be advanced.

- **Types**:
  - **Two-dimensional reconstruction**:
    - Two-dimensional facial reconstructions are based on antemortem photographs, and the skull. Occasionally skull radiographs are used, but this is not ideal since many cranial structures are not visible or at the correct scale.
    - This method usually requires the collaboration of an artist and a forensic anthropologist.
    - A commonly used method of 2D facial reconstruction was pioneered by Karen T Taylor of Austin, Texas during the 1980s. **Taylor's method** involves adhering tissue depth markers on an unidentified skull at various anthropological landmarks, then photographing the skull. Life-size or one-to-one frontal and lateral photographic prints are then used as a foundation for facial drawings done on transparent vellum (**Fig. 7.4**).

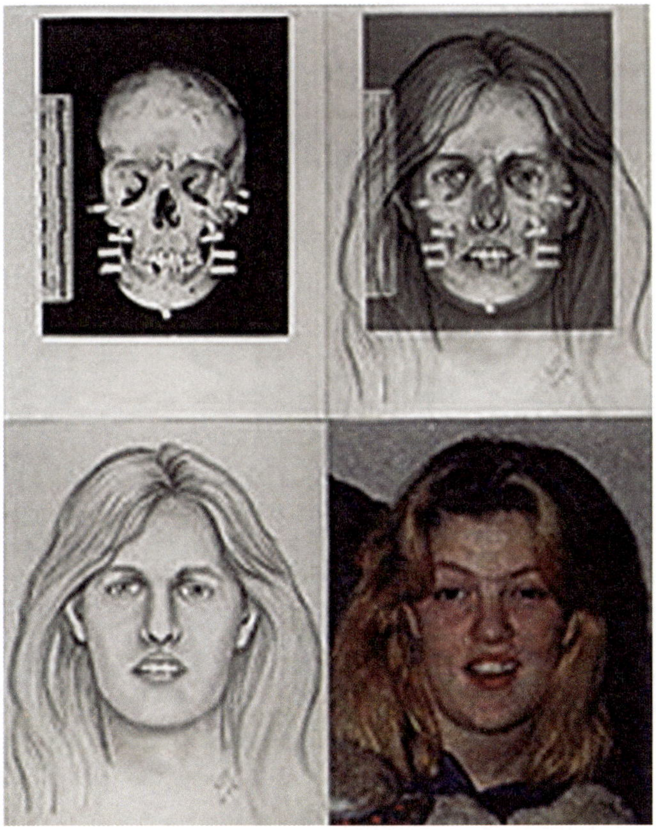

Fig. 7.4 An example of 2D facial reconstruction conducted by Karen Taylor, and subsequent identification of the victim, April Dawn Lacy

    - Recently developed, the F.A.C.E. and C.A.R.E.S. computer software programs quickly produce two-dimensional facial approximations that can be edited and manipulated with relative ease. These programs may help speed the reconstruction process and allow subtle variations to be applied to the drawing, though they may produce more generic images than hand-drawn artwork.
  - **Three-dimensional reconstruction**: Three-dimensional facial reconstructions are either:
    - Sculptures (made from casts of cranial remains) created with modelling clay and other materials or
    - High-resolution, three-dimensional computer images. Like 2D reconstructions, three-dimensional reconstructions usually require both an artist and a forensic anthropologist. Computer programs create three-dimensional reconstructions by manipulating scanned photographs of the unidentified cranial remains, stock photographs of facial features and other available reconstructions. These computer approximations are usually most effective in victim identification because they do not appear too artificial. This method has been adapted by the National Center for Missing & Exploited Children, which uses this method often to show approximations of an unidentified decedent to release to the public in hopes to identify the subject.
- One of the most sensational cases solved by forensic facial reconstruction of an absconding criminal who had killed his entire family and then disappeared for 18 years, by utilizing the procedure of an age-progressed clay bust, sculpted by forensic artist **Frank Bender**, is that of **John Emil List** (1925–2008) (**Box 7.4**).

Box 7.4—The Boogeyman of Westfield: John Emil List

John Emil List was an American mass murderer and long-time fugitive. On 09 Nov 1971, List murdered his entire immediate family at their home in Westfield New Jersey, USA, using his own semi-automatic handgun and his father's revolver. While his children were at school, he shot his wife Helen, 47, and then his mother Alma. As his daughter Patricia, 16, and younger son Frederick, 13, arrived home from school, List shot each of them in the back of the head. After making himself lunch, List drove to his bank to close his bank accounts, and then to Westfield High School to watch his elder son John Frederick, 15, play in a soccer game. After driving him home, List shot him repeatedly.

List placed the bodies of his wife and children on sleeping bags in the mansion's ballroom. He left his mother's body in her apartment in the attic. In a letter to his pastor, found on the desk in his study, List claimed that he saw too much evil in the world, and he had killed his family to save their souls. He then cleaned the various crime scenes, removed his own picture from all family photographs in the house, tuned a radio to a religious station, and departed.

contd.

The murders were not discovered until Dec 7, nearly a month later, due in part to the family's reclusive tendencies, and in part to notes sent by List to the children's schools and part-time jobs claiming that the children would be visiting their ailing maternal grandmother in North Carolina for a few weeks. List also stopped milk, mail and newspaper deliveries. Neighbours noticed that all of the mansion's rooms were illuminated day and night, with no apparent activity within the house. After light bulbs began burning out one by one, they called the police. Officers entered through an unlocked window leading to the basement and discovered the family's bodies.

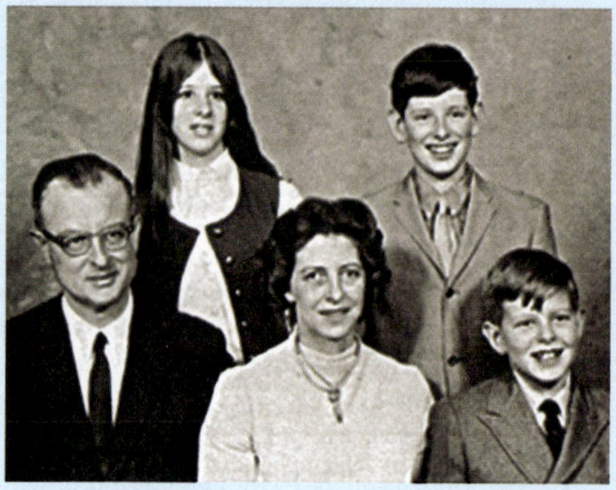

John Emil List (extreme left) with his family

A nationwide manhunt was launched. Police investigated hundreds of leads without success. All reliable photographs of List had been destroyed. The family car was found parked at the airport in New York City, but police found no evidence that List had boarded a flight.

The FBI later discovered that List had travelled by train from New Jersey to Michigan and then to Colorado. He settled in Denver in early 1972 and took an accounting job under the name Robert Peter "Bob" Clark. From 1979 to 1986, he was the comptroller at a paper box manufacturer outside Denver. He joined a Lutheran congregation, and at one religious gathering, met an Army clerk named Delores Miller whom he married in 1985. In Feb 1988, the couple moved to a house in Virginia, where List, still using the name Bob Clark, resumed work as an accountant at a small accounting firm.

In May 1989, the 18-year-old crime was recounted on a television program America's Most Wanted during its first year on the air. The segment featured an age-progressed clay bust, sculpted by forensic artist **Frank Bender**, which turned out to bear a close resemblance to List's actual appearance. On June 1, less than 2 weeks after the broadcast, List was arrested at the accounting firm after a Denver neighbour recognized the description and alerted authorities. List continued to stand by his alias for several months, even after his 1989 extradition to New Jersey; finally, faced with irrefutable evidence – including a fingerprint match with List's military records, as well as evidence found at the crime scene – he confessed his true identity on February 16, 1990.

At trial, List testified that his financial difficulties reached crisis level in 1971 when he was laid off with the closure of the Jersey City bank. To avoid sharing this humiliating development with his family, List engaged in the same routine and dress as when employed, leaving home each morning on schedule and spending the day at job interviews or at the Westfield train station, reading newspapers until it was time to come home. As the year progressed, the family's financial problems became more strained. He was also dealing with his wife's alcoholism and her untreated tertiary syphilis, contracted from her first husband and concealed for 18 years. Though her health progressively deteriorated, she said nothing to List or her physicians until 1969, when a thorough workup revealed the condition.

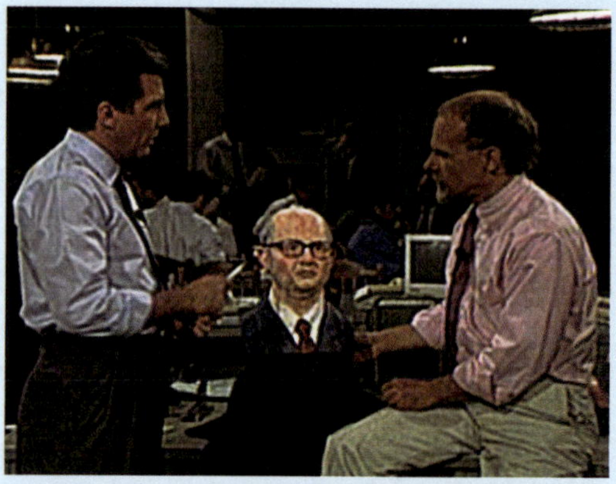

Frank Bender (R) with his bust of Emil List

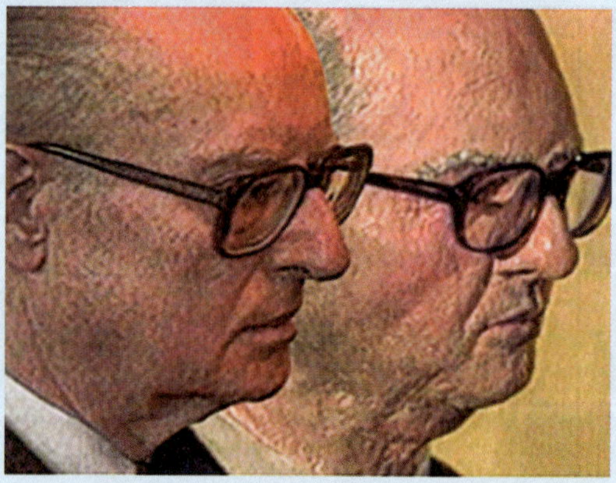

Comparison of the bust (R) with actual photo (L)

A court-appointed psychiatrist testified that List suffered from obsessive-compulsive personality disorder, and that he saw only two solutions to his situation: accept welfare, or kill his family and send their souls to heaven. Welfare was an unacceptable option, he reasoned, because it would expose him and his family to ridicule and violate his authoritarian father's teachings regarding the care and protection of family members.

On April 12, 1990, List was convicted of five counts of first degree murder, and sentenced to five terms of life imprisonment, to be served consecutively, the maximum permissible penalty at the time.

List died of complications from pneumonia aged 82 on March 21, 2008, while in prison.

In reporting his death, the New Jersey Star-Ledger referred to him as "The Boogeyman of Westfield".

SCIENTIFIC METHODS OF SUSPECT INTERROGATION

Introduction

- **Interrogation** or **questioning** is a method employed by the police for getting information from a suspect, witness or victim after a crime has been committed.
- There are multiple **methods of interrogation** including:
  - **Interviewing**
  - **Torture**
  - **Sleep deprivation** (which acts by increasing suggestibility)
  - **Hypnotism**
  - **Mind-altering drugs (Narcoanalysis)**
  - **Polygraph (Lie detector)**
  - **Brain fingerprinting**
  - **Brain mapping**
- Methods of torture and their legal and ethical aspects have been dealt with in **Topic 3** [**Torture** – **FM 3.30** *(page no. 273)* and **3.31** *(page no. 275)*].
- Police interview methods such as **Reid Technique** are not within the scope of this book, and so will not be discussed.
- In this chapter, only the scientific methods of interrogation will be discussed, though some of these are actually more in the realm of pseudo-science than pure science.

Polygraph (Lie Detector)

- A **polygraph** (popularly known as a **lie detector**) is an instrument that measures and records several physiological responses such as **blood pressure**, **pulse**, **respiration**, **breathing rhythms**, **body temperature** and **skin conductivity**, while the subject is asked and answers a series of questions, on the theory that false answers will produce distinctive measurements (**Fig. 7.5**). In other words, the polygraph measures physiological changes caused by the sympathetic nervous system during questioning.
- This method of interrogation is sometimes referred to as **psychophysiological detection of deception (PDD)**.

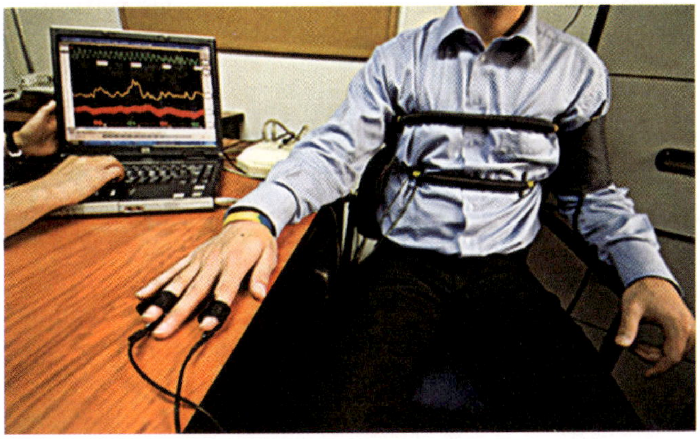

Fig. 7.5 Polygraph

The Beginning

- A device recording both blood pressure and galvanic skin response was invented in 1921 by **Dr John A Larson** of the University of California, and first applied in law enforcement work by the Berkeley Police Department. Further work on this device was done by **Leonarde Keeler**.
- **William Marston** (1893–1947), who used blood pressure and galvanic skin response to examine German Prisoners of War, however, is the self proclaimed "**father of the polygraph**" despite his predecessors' contributions. In 1938, he published a book, *The Lie Detector Test*, wherein he documented the theory and use of the device.

The Technique

- Today, there are two types of instrumentation: **analogue** and **computerized**. In many countries, the computerized instrumentation is preferred.
- A typical polygraph test starts with a **pre-test interview** to gain some preliminary information which will later be used for "Control Questions," or CQ. The tester will then explain how the polygraph is supposed to work, emphasizing that it can detect lies, and that it is important to answer truthfully. This is followed by the **actual test**:
  - Some of the questions asked are "**Irrelevant**" or **IR** ("Is your name Gopal?"), others are "probable-lie" **Control Questions** or **CQ** that most people will lie about ("Have you ever stolen money?") and the remainder are the "**Relevant Questions**," or **RQ**, that the tester is really interested in.
  - The different types of questions alternate. The test is passed if the physiological responses during the probable-lie control questions (CQ) are larger than those during the relevant questions (RQ).
- An alternative is the **Guilty Knowledge Test** (**GKT**), or the **Concealed Information Test** (**CIT**):
  - The test is usually conducted by a tester with no knowledge of the crime or circumstances in question. The administrator tests the participant on their knowledge of the crime that would not be known to an innocent person. For example: "Was the crime committed with a knife or a gun?"
  - The questions are in multiple choice and the participant is rated on how they react to the correct answer. If they react strongly to the guilty information, then proponents of the test believe that it is likely that they know facts relevant to the case.
  - This method is considered more valid by supporters of the test because it contains many safeguards to avoid the risk of the administrator influencing the results.

Reliability

- Some studies of polygraph validity have achieved rates of 80–95% accuracy in criminal cases. Despite such claims, critics argue that rather than a "test," the method amounts to an inherently unstandardizable interrogation technique whose accuracy cannot be established.
- A 1997 survey of 421 psychologists estimated the test's average accuracy at only 61%, a little better than chance.
- In 2001, William G Iacono, Distinguished Professor of Psychology and Neuroscience at the University of Minnesota published a paper in which he stated that "Although this

technique may be useful as an investigative aid and tool to induce confessions, it does not pass muster as a scientifically credible test."

- Polygraph evidence is not admissible in court in most countries of the world, including India.
- The **Frye standard (Frye test, 'general acceptance test')** is a test to determine the admissibility of scientific evidence. It provides that expert opinion based on a scientific technique is admissible only where the technique is generally accepted as reliable in the relevant scientific community This standard comes from Frye v. United States (1923), a case that discussed the admissibility of polygraph test as evidence. The Court in Frye held that expert testimony must be based on scientific methods that are sufficiently established and accepted. The Judge in this case expressed reservations about (a precursor of the current) polygraph test.

Narcoanalysis

- **Narcoanalysis Test** or **Narco Test** refers to the practice of administering barbiturates or certain other chemical substances, most often pentothal sodium (thiopentone sodium), to lower a subject's inhibitions, in the hope that the subject will more freely share information and feelings.
- The term "Narcoanalysis" was coined by Horseley. Narcoanalysis first reached the mainstream in 1922, when Robert House, a Texas obstetrician, used the drug scopolamine on two prisoners. Since then narco testing has become largely discredited in most democratic states, including the United States and Britain. There is a vast body of literature calling into question its ability to yield legal truth. Additionally, narcoanalysis has serious legal and ethical implications.

The Technique

- Experts inject the suspect or witness with **short acting barbiturates** like pentothal sodium (thiopentone sodium) or sodium amytal (amylobarbitone) under the controlled circumstances of the laboratory. Rarely, other drugs such as **scopolamine** may be used.
- The dose is dependent on the person's sex, age, health and physical condition.

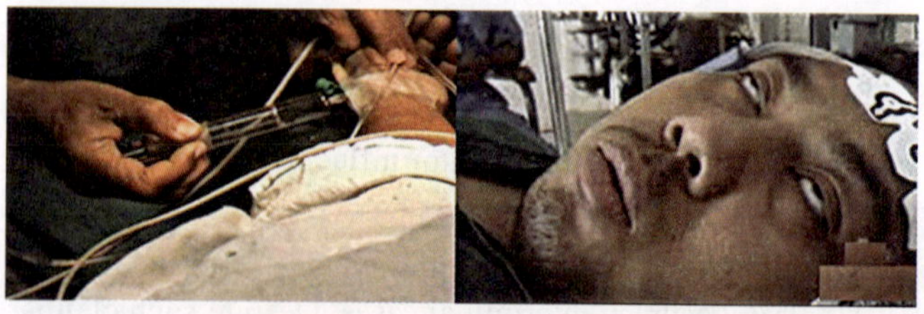

Fig. 7.6 Narcoanalysis in progress

- The subject who is put in a state of hypnotism is not in a position to speak up on his own, but can answer simple questions, after giving some suggestions.

Reliability

- In most Western countries, narcoanalysis is not admissible in court as evidence.
- Studies have shown that it is possible to lie under narcoanalysis, while conversely, an innocent person may inadvertently implicate himself in a crime.
- Unfortunately, India still continues to use narcoanalysis, though the result of such a test cannot be used as evidence in the court of law, since it violates the fundamental right against self-incrimination (Article 20(3) of the Constitution of India).
- However, on 05th May 2010, the Supreme Court in the case 'Smt Selvi vs State of Karnataka' held that narcoanalysis, polygraph and brain imaging tests can be allowed after obtaining consent of the accused. When they are conducted with consent, the material so obtained is regarded as evidence during trial of cases according to Section 27 of the Indian Evidence Act.

Imaging Technologies in Suspect Interrogation

*Brain Fingerprinting**

- **Brain Fingerprinting** is a controversial forensic science technique that determines whether specific information is stored in a subject's brain by measuring electrical brainwave responses to words, phrases or pictures that are presented on a computer screen.
- Brain fingerprinting was invented by **Lawrence Farwell**. The theory is that the brain processes known, relevant information differently than it processes unknown or irrelevant information. The brain's processing of known information, such as the details of a crime stored in the brain, is revealed by a specific pattern in the **EEG (electroencephalograph)**.
- Farwell's brain fingerprinting originally used the well known **P300 brain response** to detect the brain's recognition of the known information.
  - P300 is emitted from an individual's brain beginning approximately 300 milliseconds after it is confronted with a stimulus of special significance, e.g., a rare vs. a common stimulus, or a stimulus the subject is asked to count.
  - The application of this in brain fingerprinting is to detect the P300 as a response to stimuli related to the crime or other investigated situation, e.g., a murder weapon, victim's face or knowledge of the internal workings of a terrorist cell.

*Note: *Often confused with Brain Mapping, which is completely different: Kacker P. Understanding the differences between Brain Fingerprinting and Brain Electrical Oscillations Signature (BEOS) Profiling Systems used for forensic psychological investigation. Int J Forensic Sci. 2022;7:000249.*

- Because it is based on EEG signals, the system does not require the subject to issue verbal responses to questions or stimuli.

- Later Farwell discovered the **MERMER ("Memory and Encoding Related Multifaceted Electroencephalographic Response")**, which includes the P300 and additional features and is reported to provide a higher level of accuracy than the P300 alone.
- The person to be tested wears a special headband with electronic sensors that measure the EEG from two or more locations on the scalp (**Fig. 7.7**). The subject views stimuli consisting of words, phrases or pictures presented on a computer screen. Stimuli are of three types:
    - **Irrelevant stimuli**, that are irrelevant to the investigated situation and to the test subject.
    - **Target stimuli**, that are relevant to the investigated situation and are known to the subject.
    - **Probe stimuli**, that are relevant to the investigated situation and that the subject denies knowing. Probes contain information that is known only to the perpetrator and investigators, and not to the general public or to an innocent suspect who was not at the scene of the crime. Before the test, the scientist identifies the targets to the subject, and makes sure that he/she knows these relevant stimuli. The scientist also makes sure that the subject does not know the probes for any reason unrelated to the crime, and that the subject denies knowing the probes. The subject is told why the probes are significant, but is not told which items are the probes, and which are irrelevant.
    - By comparing the responses to the different types of stimuli, the brain fingerprinting system mathematically computes a determination of "***information present***" (the subject knows the crime-relevant information contained in the probe stimuli) or "***information absent***" (the subject does not know the information) and a statistical confidence for the determination. This determination is mathematically computed, and does not involve the subjective judgment of the scientist.

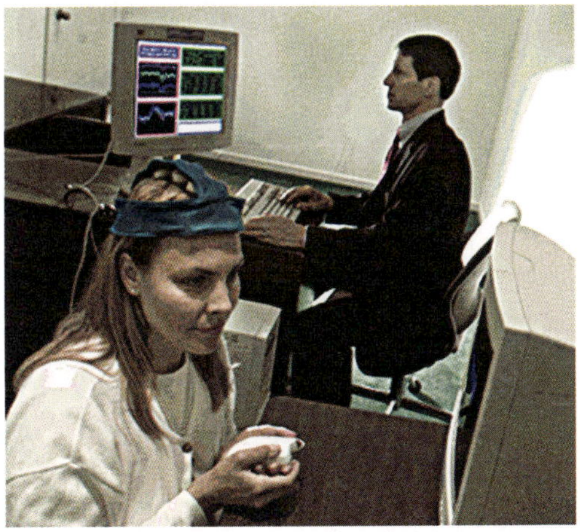

Fig. 7.7 Farwell performing the technique of brain fingerprinting on a female subject

Reliability

- In peer-reviewed publications Farwell and colleagues report over 99% accuracy in laboratory research and real-life field applications.
- Brain fingerprinting has been applied in a number of high-profile criminal cases, including helping to catch serial killer JB Grinder, and to exonerate innocent convict Terry Harrington, after he had been falsely convicted of murder.
- Brain fingerprinting has been ruled admissible in American courts.
- The situation is unclear in India. In the controversial **Sister Abhaya murder case**, the Ernakulam Chief Judicial Magistrate Court had asked the Central Bureau of Investigation to make use of all modern investigation techniques, including brain fingerprinting, lending judicial credibility to the technique.
- Brain fingerprinting technique has been criticized on a number of fronts. Although independent scientists who have used the same or similar methods as Farwell's brain fingerprinting have achieved similar, highly accurate results, different methods have yielded different results.
- For example, Peter Rosenfeld used P300-based tests incorporating fundamentally different methods, resulting in as low as chance accuracy, as well as susceptibility to errors, and criticized brain fingerprinting based on the premise that the shortcomings of his alternative technique should apply to all other techniques in which the P300 is among the brain responses measured.

Brain Mapping

- **Brain Mapping** is a higher form of **neuroimaging**, producing brain images supplemented by the result of additional (imaging or non-imaging) data processing or analysis. For example, maps projecting (measures of) behaviour onto brain regions, such as:
    - **Brain Electrical Oscillation Signature Profiling (BEOSP or BEOS)** and
    - **Functional Magnetic Resonance Imaging (fMRI)**.

Brain Electrical Oscillation Signature Profiling (BEOSP; BEOS)

- The methodology was developed by **Dr CR Mukundan**, a neuroscientist, and former Professor of Clinical Psychology at the National Institute of Mental Health and Neurosciences (Bangalore).
- **Principle**:
    - The human brain receives millions of arrays of signals in different modalities, all through the waking periods. These signals are classified and stored in terms of their relationship perceived as function of experience and available knowledge base of an individual, as well as new relationship produced through sequential processing. The process of encoding happens primarily when the individual directly participates in an activity or experiences it.

- It is considered **secondary encoding**, when the information is obtained from a secondary source viz. books, conversations, hearsay, etc. in which there is no primary experiential component and the brain deals mainly with conceptual aspects.
- **Primary encoding** is deep-seated and has specific source memory in terms of time and space of occurrence of experience, as the individual himself/herself has shared or participated in the experience/act/event at a certain time in his/her life at a certain place.
- It is found that when the brain of an individual is activated by a piece of information of an event in which he/she has taken part, the brain of the individual will respond differently from that of a person who has received the same information from secondary sources (***non-experiential***).
- BEOSP is based on this principle, thereby intending to demonstrate that the suspect who has primary encoded information of somebody who has participated in the alleged event will show responses indicating firsthand (personally acquired) knowledge of the event.

- **Procedure**:
  - Pretest interview with the suspect.
  - The suspect is acquainted with BEOSP test procedure.
  - Informed consent is obtained.
  - Ideally, no questions are to be asked while conducting the test; rather, the subject is simply provided with the probable events/scenarios in the aftermath of which, the results are analyzed to verify if the brain produces any experiential knowledge, which is essentially the recognition of events disclosed (**Fig. 7.8**). This way, all fundamental rights are protected, as neither there are any questions that are being asked or any answers reciprocated.
  - While BEOSP may be considered as an improved form of Brain Fingerprinting (BF), there are actually so many differences that they are in reality separate entities (outlined in **Table 7.1**).

Functional Magnetic Resonance Imaging (fMRI)

- It is a type of **specialized MRI scan**, and measures the haemodynamic response related to neural activity in the brain or spinal cord of humans. It is one of the most re-

Table 7.1 Differences between Brain Fingerprinting and Brain Electrical Oscillation Signature Profiling*

S. No	Feature/Parameter	Brain Fingerprinting (BF)	Brain Electrical Oscillation Signature (BEOS)
1	*Basis*	Event Related Potential (ERP) via Electroencephalogram (EEG)	Electroencephalogram (EEG)
2	*Measurement*	Recognition of P300 and MERMER	Memory of an event
3	*Detection*	Knowledge about crime when presented with images of victim, weapon, location, etc.	Experiential knowledge (whether person is involved in the crime as a perpetrator, victim or eye witness)
4	*Differentiating capacity between eye witness, victim, and perpetrator*	Cannot differentiate	Differentiates well
5	*Area of brain recorded*	Two or more areas using electrodes	Entire brain using 32 electrodes
6	*Level of sophistication*	Meant only for screening suspects	Meant for screening, as well as estimating the nature and extent of involvement of the person in the crime
7	*Stimulus*	Text and visual stimuli	Auditory probes
8	*Presentation*	Series of pictures/images	Only auditory mode
9	*Display*	P300 and MERMER recognition	Encoded information pertaining to experiential knowledge
10	*Requirement of physical evidence*	Necessary to prepare stimuli	Not essential

****Source***: *Kacker P. Understanding the differences between Brain Fingerprinting and Brain Electrical Oscillations Signature (BEOS) Profiling systems used for forensic psychological investigation. Int J Forensic Sci. 2022;7:000249.*

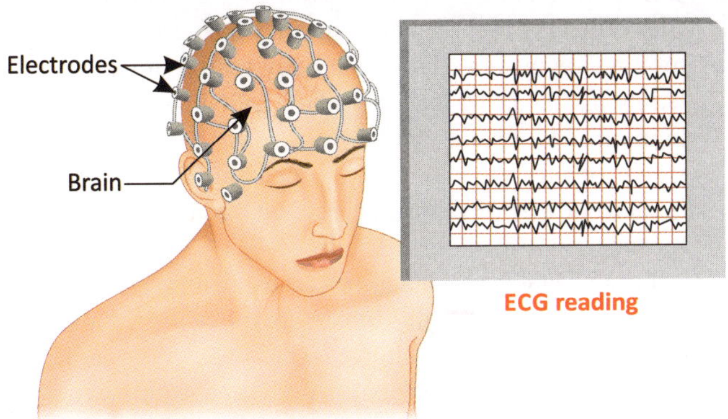

Fig. 7.8 Brain Electrical Oscillation Signature Profiling (BEOSP or BEOS)

cently developed forms of neuroimaging, and has the advantages of low invasiveness, lack of radiation exposure and relatively wide availability.

- Changes in blood flow and blood oxygenation in the brain (haemodynamics) are closely linked to neural activity.
  - When nerve cells are active they increase their consumption of energy from glucose and switch to less energetically effective, but more rapid aerobic glycolysis.
  - The local response to this oxygen utilization is an increase in blood flow to regions of increased neural activity, occurring after a delay of approximately 1–5 seconds. This haemodynamic response rises to a peak over 4–5 seconds, before falling back to baseline.
  - This leads to local changes in the relative concentration of oxyhaemoglobin and deoxyhaemoglobin, and changes in local cerebral blood flow.
- **Blood-oxygen-level dependent** or **BOLD** is the MRI contrast of blood deoxyhaemoglobin, and is critical for functional brain imaging with MRI.
  - Neurons do not have internal reserves of energy in the form of glucose and oxygen, so their firing requires more energy to be delivered quickly. Through a process called the haemodynamic response, blood releases oxygen to them at a greater rate than to inactive neurons.
  - The magnetic resonance (MR) signal of blood is slightly different depending on the level of oxygenation. Higher BOLD signal intensities arise from increases in the concentration of oxygenated haemoglobin, since the blood magnetic susceptibility now more closely matches the tissue magnetic susceptibility.
  - By collecting data in an MRI scanner, one can assess changes in BOLD contrast. These changes can be either positive or negative depending upon the relative changes in both cerebral blood flow (CBF) and oxygen consumption. Increases in CBF that outstrip changes in oxygen consumption will lead to increased BOLD signal, and vice versa.
  - The signal difference is very small, but given many repetitions of a thought, action or experience, statistical methods can be used to determine the areas of the brain which reliably show more of this difference as a result, and therefore which areas of the brain are active during that thought, action or experience.
- BOLD effects are measured using rapid volumetric acquisition of images with contrast. Such images are usually taken every 1–4 seconds, and the voxels in the resulting image typically represent cubes of tissue about 2–4 mm on each side in humans.
- Subjects participating in an fMRI experiment are asked to lie still, and are usually restrained with soft pads to prevent small motions from disturbing measurements. An fMRI experiment usually lasts between 15 minutes and 2 hours. Depending on the purpose of study, subjects may view images, hear sounds, smell odours, perform cognitive tasks, press a few buttons or perform other tasks.
- Upon completion of the experiment, the computer takes the slice images from the MRI and uses mathematical transformations and reconstruction algorithms to render the images, and then correct for distortion, subject movement, etc.
- The final image illustrates areas of activity during the experiment as coloured patterns overlaid upon the original high resolution scan (**Fig. 7.9**). Researchers can also render the combined activation slice images into 3D images which can be rotated to any angle.

Reliability

- This technology is in its early stages of development, but many of its proponents hope to replace older lie detection techniques with fMRI in the near future.

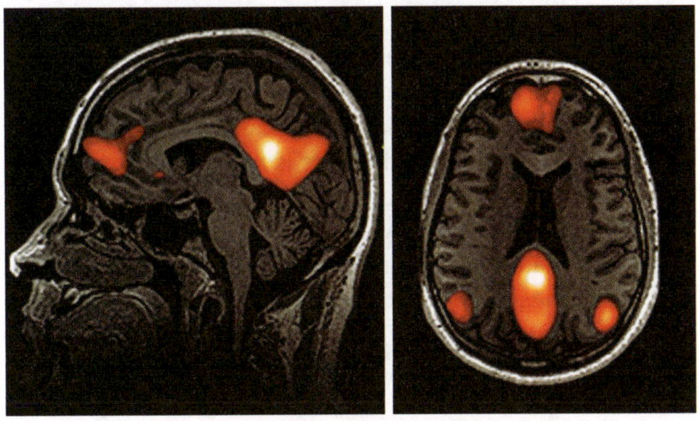

Fig. 7.9 fMRI images showing areas of activity

IMAGING TECHNOLOGIES IN FORENSIC PATHOLOGY

Digital Autopsy & Virtual Autopsy (Virtopsy)

- A digital autopsy is a **non-invasive autopsy** in which digital imaging technology, such as **Computerized Tomography (CT)** or **Magnetic Resonance Imaging (MRI)** is used to develop three-dimensional images for a virtual exploration of a human body.
- Digital autopsy, simply, means conducting autopsy in computerized environment by digital tools. The first step of digitizing starts with the medical imaging modalities that

Pillay – Textbook of Forensic Medicine & Toxicology

provide the raw data images from the deceased. The most common modalities are CT scan and MRI scan.

- The term cannot be found before 1985 in the literature. However, there are many other similar terms: **Postmortem CT scanning** for individual organs, **Virtual Autopsy** and **Virtopsy**.
- Digital Autopsy tries to answer the same investigative questions without actual dissection as in a conventional autopsy. The main concept of Digital Autopsy came into existence to overcome some problems during conventional autopsies without losing the objectivity of post-mortem examination. The main problems in conventional autopsy are:
  - It is impossible to preserve the body after dissection and gather the findings with non-destructive and contamination-free procedures.
  - Data acquisition in some body regions are difficult, particularly in cases of decomposition.
  - Observer-independent documentation of the evidence is not possible.
  - Data acquisition of the body with respect for the deceased, next of kin and religious obligations, is difficult.
  - Slow and incomplete data acquisition in disasters.
- Digital Autopsy serves as a technical solution for the above mentioned problems. Employing medical imaging modalities enables examination of the deceased visually without any destructive, contaminating and non-preservative procedures like dissection. Moreover, using these images with software processing in visualization is the second step toward acquiring data from difficult regions from anatomical perspective and dignity of the body. Digital bodies in the system can be examined multiple times and reported not only in text but also in a variety of available media (photo, movie, etc.). In addition, quick evaluation of bodies and body parts in massive disasters is possible in comparison to the time-consuming procedure of conventional autopsy.
- **Limitations in Digital Autopsy**:
  - The main constraint is the data that is provided by medical imaging modalities are based on X-Ray and Magnetic fields (CT and MRI) that limits the view to what can be recorded by these technologies. A very obvious difference is the real colour of internal body organs and their changes in the deceased, in comparison to what is simulated in the visualization software.
  - The novelty of this technological solution has not given enough time for studies on the consistency of reports among different professionals on the same cases.
  - Moreover, there are very few articles about the validity of Digital Autopsy.

Technology

- CT and MRI scanning are the most common imaging modalities employed for Digital Autopsy.
- CT Angiography has also been used to provide imaging data in some situations.
- The work output of these modalities are standard image files (DICOM files). Each image may have a thickness of 5 mm, which means after whole body scan (human average height of 175 cm) it would produce 3500 images (slices) of human body. Using volume rendering these two dimensional images are assembled to make a 3D projection of human body. The 3D model is painted through RGBA transfer function to a colourful model.
- All visualization and image processing features for manipulating and navigating this 3D model make digital tools for conducting a Digital Autopsy. These features enable the pathologist to explore the entire body, and examine regions and organs of interest from different angles. Image processing algorithms help them to virtually remove layers of body tissues like skin, muscle and bones.
- Moreover, low density objects like air, and high density objects like metallic foreign bodies can be marked and viewed in the three dimensional body. For instance, organs with air (inside) like sinuses or intestines can be separated from other parts, or any remnants of bullet in body due to gunshot injuries.
- The findings can be reported digitally in a multimedia report. This report includes all textual results accompanied by images and recorded movie of Digital Autopsy during examination. This report can be used not only for submission to the court, but can also be displayed in the court.

Acceptance

- Most countries have not yet adopted this technology, except on an experimental basis.
- Currently digital autopsy is being used in Switzerland, USA, UK, Malaysia (**Box 7.5**) and Japan.

Box 7.5—Digital Autopsy: Malaysian Initiative

Witty Charman, a Malaysian company is pioneering virtual autopsy technology in various countries. Founded in 2017 by **Dr (Major) Pramod Bagali**, Witty Charman specializes in providing advanced medical visualization applications focused on Forensic Imaging. The company has developed **WittyViz®**, a software solution that provides a seamless digital solution that overcomes the hassles of classical postmortem examination.

Inbuilt digital tools aid the forensic pathologist to view and analyse internal findings, including traumatic lesions such as fractures and stab wound tracks, and pathological lesions such as consolidated lungs, abscesses, tumours, calcifications, inflamed organs, etc. "Volume of Interest dissection" helps to examine internally, and visualise organs like the heart, lungs, kidneys, as well as skeletal and muscular systems, brain, neck structures and even small structures such as the ocular lens.

Virtual Autopsy workflow starts with placing the body from the incident (crime/accident) scene into radiolucent body bags, in the mortuary. Whole body scan is done by a Multi-slice CT Scanner, following appropriate scan protocols.

contd.

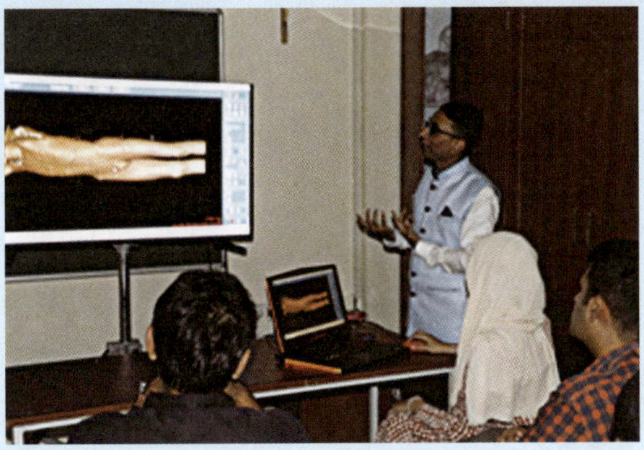

Dr Pramod Bagali conducting Virtual Autopsy demonstration at St John's Medical College, Bengaluru in 2022

2D DICOM images are obtained by usual collimation with a slice thickness of 0.5–0.625 mm, which are reconstructed by high performance computation, into a three-dimensional virtual body that could be analysed by the forensic pathologist through WittyViz® software.

The UI (User interface) of **WittyViz®** aids in selecting multiple views with ease, such as sagittal, coronal, axial (CSI, Cross-Sectional Imaging). It has Forensic Decision Support System (ForDSS) to help opinion making. In addition, all findings along with visuals and snapshot videos can be integrated and included in the final autopsy report that can be presented in the court of law. Some of the findings which are difficult to view through classical autopsy such as air embolism, vertebral column injuries, complete skeletal survey in case of a fall from height, calcium scoring of coronary arteries, etc., can be accomplished in virtual autopsy.

Section 2

TOXICOLOGY

Topic 8

GENERAL TOXICOLOGY

(Number of Competencies – 10: FM 8.1 to 8.10)

FM 8.1: Core – Written/Viva Voce
- Describe the History of Toxicology

HISTORY OF TOXICOLOGY

I. Before the Advent of Poison Control Centres

- The history of toxicology dates back several thousand years. Early poisons were almost exclusively derived from toxic plants and venomous animals, as well as a few minerals. They were used mainly for hunting purposes.
    - Some were used as "**ordeal poisons**,"* e.g., physostigmine from *Physostigma venenosum* (Calabar bean) and amygdalin from peach pits.
    - Arrow and dart poisons were quite popular for hunting animals. Common **arrow poisons** included strophanthin, aconitine, extracts from *Helleborus* (a cardiotoxic plant) and snake venom.
- The word "**toxicology**" is derived from New Latin, by combining the forms "toxico-" + "-logy", which in turn come from the Ancient Greek words "toxikos" (which means "poisonous", and "logos" (which means "subject matter").
- One of the earliest classifications of poisons was done by the Greek physician **Dioscorides** (**AD 40-80**) who placed all poisons in three groups – animal, vegetable and mineral.
- Experimental toxicology began with **Nicander** (**204-135 BC**), another Greek physician who experimented with animal poisons using condemned criminals as subjects.
- An early treatise on plant poisons is *De Historia Plantarum*, by **Theophrastus** (**370-286 BC**).
- The ancient Indian text *Rig Veda* (**12th century BC**) also describes several plant toxins.
- The Greeks often used plant toxins for purposes of judicial execution. **Socrates** (**470-399 BC**) was executed by the administration of hemlock.
- Among mineral poisons, one of the earliest known elements was lead which was discovered as early as 3500 BC. Aside from its extensive use in plumbing, lead was also utilised in the production of vessels and containers, which led to widespread chronic health problems. During the Roman period, lead acetate was widely used as a sweetening agent for wine resulting in a high incidence of plumbism, particularly among members of the aristocracy. In fact, the decline of the Roman empire is attributed to the debilitating effects of this scourge.
- Homicidal poisoning has also had a lurid past. One of the earliest laws against the murderous use of poisons was the *Lex Cornelia* passed in Rome in **81 BC**. It is interesting to note that the severity of punishment upon conviction was discriminatory. Members of high social status were only divested of their property or exiled, while those of a lower rank were cast into arenas of wild beasts!
- After the fall of the Roman empire, there was a lull in the development of Toxicology until **1198**, when **Moses Maimonides** published his classic work *Treatise on Poisons and Their Antidotes*. Then came the Renaissance toxicologists – **Paracelsus (1493–1541)** (**Fig. 8.1**), **Ambroise Pare** (**1510–1590**) (**Fig. 8.2**) & **William Piso** (**1611–1678**).
- Paracelsus' study on the dose–response relationship is generally considered as the first time that a scientific approach was made in the field of toxicology.
- Unfortunately, during this very period, poisoning as a method of homicide became increasingly popular in several parts of Europe, particularly Italy and France, where schools actually existed for teaching the art of poisoning!
    - Among the notorious poisoners in Italy, one name that stands out is that of Madame Guilia Toffana who killed more than 600 people with a solution of white arsenic which came to be called *aqua toffana.*
    - In France, two of the most infamous poisoners were Marchioness de Brinvilliers and Catherine Deshayes. The former was executed in 1676, while the latter who was responsible for the deaths of more than 2000 infants was burned alive in 1680. She also specialised in getting several women rid themselves of their husbands for the nefarious purpose of inheriting property. Deshayes developed an effective concoction made up

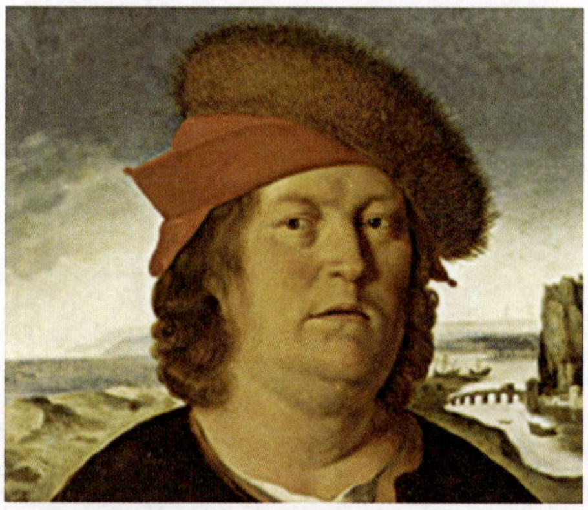

Fig. 8.1 Paracelsus *(Philippus Aureolus Theophrastus Bombastus von Hohenheim)*

****Note***: *Ingestion of these substances was believed to be lethal to the guilty and harmless to the innocent.*

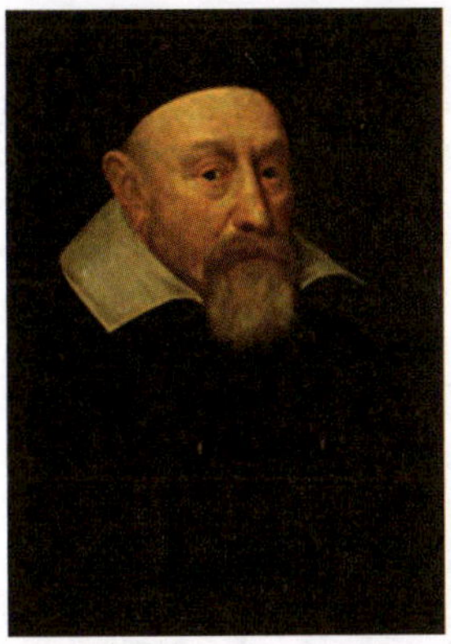

Fig. 8.2 Ambroise Pare

of arsenic, aconite, belladonna and opium, which came to be called *le poudre de succession* or "the powder of succession"!

- The actual development of toxicology as a distinct speciality began in the 18th and 19th centuries with the pioneering work of **Bonaventure Orfila (1787–1853) (Fig. 8.3)**, who is generally considered the "Father of Modern Toxicology". He advocated the practice of autopsy followed by chemical analysis of viscera to prove that poisoning had taken place. His treatise *Traite des Poisons* published in 1814 laid the foundations of forensic toxicology.
  - In 1829, one of his students, **Robert Christison (1797–1882)** published a condensed English version titled "A Treatise on Poisons."
  - The first published work on clinical toxicology was "A Practical Treatise on Poisons" written by **O Costill**, and published in **1848**.

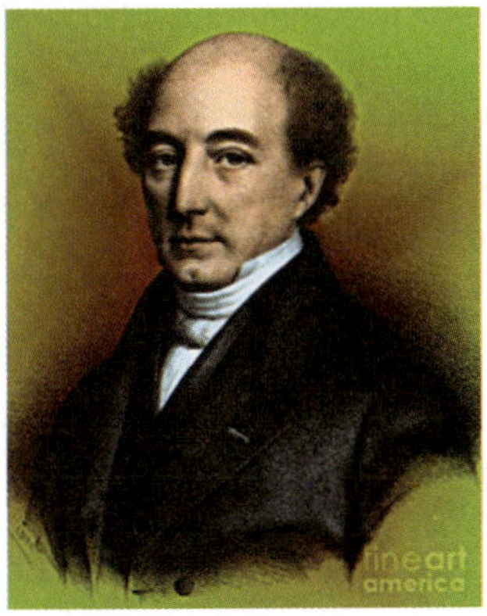

Fig. 8.3 Mathieu Joseph Bonaventure Orfila

II. After the Advent of Poison Control Centres

- After World War II, the role of Poison Control Centres began to be increasingly recognised in the prevention and treatment of poisoning, as well as in disseminating authentic information on toxicological issues to medical professionals and the general public. Since then toxicology has made significant strides in developing into an advanced speciality and is in fact among the fastest growing medical disciplines in the West today.
- Progress has unfortunately been much slower in India and other Third World countries, but is now picking up with the establishment of more and more dedicated professional organizations, such as the **Indian Society of Toxicology** which was started in 2004 and has hundreds of members drawn from various fields. The Society has also been publishing a peer reviewed journal that features research articles on toxicology mainly from the Indian sub-continent.
- Arising out of a growing concern over the rising global incidence of poisoning, coupled with a lack of public awareness about its seriousness, **Poisons Information Services** made their first appearance in the Netherlands in 1949.
- In 1961, a telephone answering service was introduced in England, which gave information to medical practitioners and others about toxicological information on a variety of household, agricultural and pharmaceutical substances.
- On 2nd Sept 1963, a National Poisons Information Service was started at Guy's Hospital, London.
- The same year, the Illinois Chapter of the American Academy of Paediatrics opened an Information Centre in Chicago, USA.
- Since then, all around the world similar centres have come up, performing the important functions of generating public awareness on poisoning, and providing much needed toxicological diagnostic and therapeutic assistance to doctors. Today, there are hundreds of certified Centres all over the world, providing information within a matter of seconds through the use of toxicology databases (POISINDEX, TOXBASE, TOXINZ) on thousands of poisonous products.
- India made a belated entry with the establishment of the **National Poisons Information Centre** at the **All India Institute of Medical Sciences, New Delhi**, in Dec 1994. A second Centre was subsequently opened at the **National Institute of Occupational Health, Ahmedabad**.
- Many more **Regional Centres** have come up in cities such as **Cochin**, **Chennai**, **Kolkata**, **Manipal**, **Vellore**, etc., and efforts are under way to establish similar centres in other parts of the country.
  - The author has established a full-fledged Centre at **Cochin** (in **Amrita Institute of Medical Sciences**) with poison information and analytical services (**Box 8.1**).

> **FM 8.2: Core – Written/Viva Voce**
> - Define the following terms:
>   - Toxicology
>   - Forensic Toxicology
>   - Clinical Toxicology
>   - Poison

DEFINITIONS

I. Toxicology

- **Toxicology** (*or more specifically* ***Medical Toxicology***) is the science dealing with the:
  - Properties
  - Action

Box 8.1—The AIMS Poison Control Centre, Cochin, Kerala, India

A full-fledged Poison Control Centre with poison information service and analytical laboratory was started at **Amrita Institute of Medical Sciences, Cochin, Kerala**, in July 2003. The Centre today offers extensive facilities relating to poisons and poisoning to all hospitals, govt doctors, private practitioners, as well as the lay public of Kerala State (and neighbouring regions). It is for the first time that such a department exclusively devoted to toxicology has been started in a hospital in the entire country. In less than a year since its inception, the department was officially listed in the World Health Organization Directory of Poison Control Centres. There are only a few other such recognized Centres in the entire country.

The Department has state-of-the-art software packages that have detailed information on more than 1 million poisons and drugs encountered worldwide.

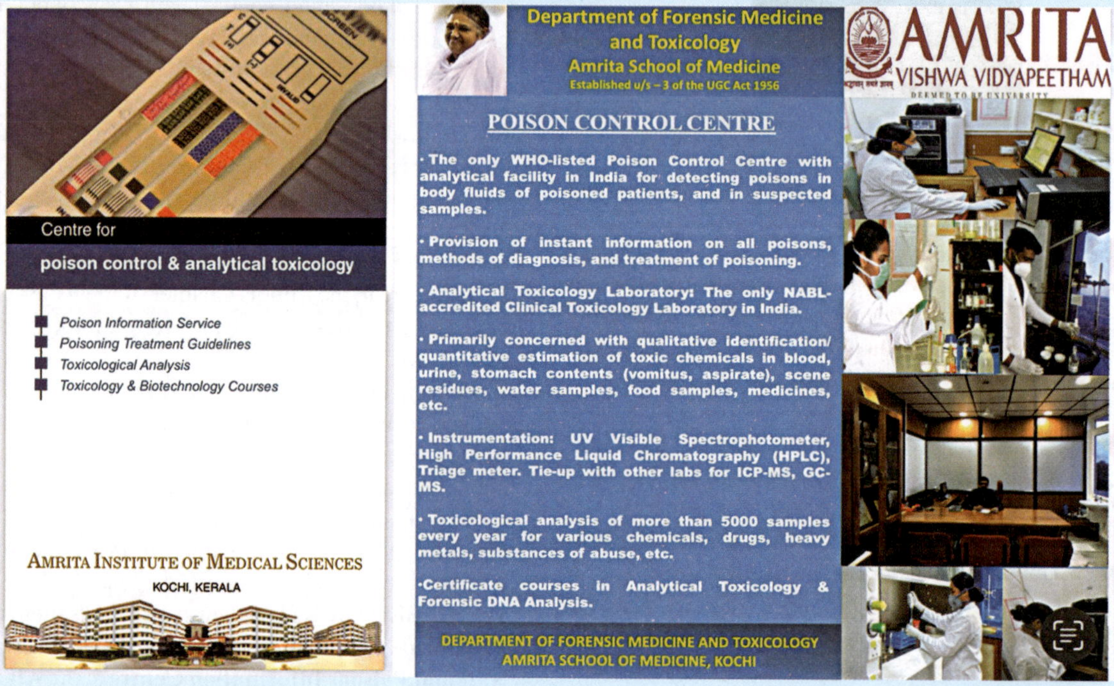
Centre for
poison control & analytical toxicology
Poison Information Service
Poisoning Treatment Guidelines
Toxicological Analysis
Toxicology & Biotechnology Courses
AMRITA INSTITUTE OF MEDICAL SCIENCES
KOCHI, KERALA
Department of Forensic Medicine and Toxicology
Amrita School of Medicine
Established u/s – 3 of the UGC Act 1956
AMRITA
VISHWA VIDYAPEETHAM
POISON CONTROL CENTRE
· The only WHO-listed Poison Control Centre with analytical facility in India for detecting poisons in body fluids of poisoned patients, and in suspected samples.
· Provision of instant information on all poisons, methods of diagnosis, and treatment of poisoning.
· Analytical Toxicology Laboratory: The only NABL-accredited Clinical Toxicology Laboratory in India.
· Primarily concerned with qualitative identification/quantitative estimation of toxic chemicals in blood, urine, stomach contents (vomitus, aspirate), scene residues, water samples, food samples, medicines, etc.
· Instrumentation: UV Visible Spectrophotometer, High Performance Liquid Chromatography (HPLC), Triage meter. Tie-up with other labs for ICP-MS, GC-MS.
· Toxicological analysis of more than 5000 samples every year for various chemicals, drugs, heavy metals, substances of abuse, etc.
·Certificate courses in Analytical Toxicology & Forensic DNA Analysis.
DEPARTMENT OF FORENSIC MEDICINE AND TOXICOLOGY
AMRITA SCHOOL OF MEDICINE, KOCHI

Facilities offered:

- Toxicological analysis of blood, urine or stomach contents (vomitus, aspirate or washing) for evidence of any poisonous substance or drug.
- Screening of urine for substances of abuse.
- Toxicological analysis of water samples for pesticides and chemicals.
- Toxicological analysis of medicinal and other commercial products for toxic adulterants or contaminants.
- Toxicological screening for common chemicals and poisons in chronic, undiagnosed ailments (skin disease, respiratory illnesses, gastrointestinal disorders, neurological disorders).
- Advanced treatment facility at AIMS for all kinds of cases of poisoning (due to chemicals, drugs, plant products, animal bites or stings, food poisons, etc.).
- Instant access to detailed information on poisons and poisoning through telephone, email, postal mail, etc.
- Free expert guidance on diagnosis and treatment of all kinds of poisoning.

How to contact the Centre:
Visit the official website – *https://www.amritahospitals.org/Facilities/Toxicology-and-Poison-Control*

  - Toxicity
  - Lethal dose
  - Estimation of and
  - Treatment of poisoning.*
- It is sub-divided into:
  - **Clinical Toxicology**
  - **Forensic Toxicology**

II. Clinical Toxicology

- **Clinical Toxicology** deals with the diagnosis and treatment of poisoning caused by chemicals, drugs and toxins. It can be sub-divided into:
  - **Emergency Toxicology**: Deals with the immediate management and stabilization of patients who are seriously poisoned. It includes decontamination measures such

**Note*: *Toxicology* is the science dealing with the *'PATLET'* of poisons. *PATLET* is an acronym (abbreviation that can be read off like a word) that stands for *P*roperties, *A*ction, *T*oxicity, *L*ethal dose, *E*stimation of and *T*reatment of poisons/poisoning.*

as administration of activated charcoal, performance of stomach wash, alkaline diuresis, whole bowel irrigation, etc.

- **Critical Care Toxicology**: Deals with management of seriously poisoned, stabilized patients in a critical care unit. It includes the use of antidotal therapy, symptomatic treatment and supportive measures.

III. Forensic Toxicology

- **Forensic Toxicology** is the branch of toxicology that deals with the medicolegal investigation of poisoning and drug use. It can be sub-divided into:
    - **Postmortem (or Autopsy) Toxicology**: Deals with determination of the cause and manner of death from poisoning, and includes the analysis of biological specimens taken from the dead body to identify the presence and concentration of drug or poison. A wide range of biological specimens may be analyzed including blood, urine, gastric contents, hair, various organ tissues and more.
    - **Human Performance Toxicology**: Estimation of dose-response relationship between a drug present in the body and the effects on the body. This branch of forensic toxicology is responsible for devising and implementing laws such as driving under the influence of alcohol or drugs.
    - **Analytical Toxicology**: Deals with:
        - Detection of poisons in body fluids of living victims of poisoning.
        - Detection of poisons in body fluids and viscera of dead victims of poisoning.
        - Detection of evidence of substance abuse among living or dead individuals.

IV. Poison

- **Paracelsus** (16th century Swiss alchemist) stated famously: "*There is no such thing as a non-poison. Every substance is a poison. It all depends on the dose and mode of administration.*" But that will not do as a definition for the examinations (sessional or university)! The standard definition of a **poison** is as follows:
    - A **poison** is any substance which:
        - when introduced into the living body
        - or brought into contact with any part thereof
        - will produce ill effects or death
        - by its local or systemic action or both.
- Poisons act by inducing
    - **Local effect**, i.e., exerting effects on the part they come in contact with, e.g., corrosives (*skin, mucosa)*, atropine (*eye*).
    - **Systemic effect**, i.e., exerting effects on one or more organ systems after absorption, e.g., opiates (*CNS)*, digitalis (*heart*).
    - **Combined effect**, i.e., both local and systemic effects, e.g., carbolic acid, phosphorus.
- A poison can be any of the following:
    - **Chemical** (inorganic substance like phosphorus, halogen, alcohol, heavy metal, toxic gas, etc.)
    - **Toxin** (organic substance like toxic principle of a poisonous plant, venom of a venomous creature, etc.)
    - **Drug** (substance used for therapeutic purpose, or abused for recreational purpose)
- Today, most toxicologists prefer to use the term '**Xenobiotic**' instead of 'Poison'.

> **FM 8.3: Core – Written/Viva Voce**
> - **Describe**:
>   - Various types of poisons
>   - Toxicokinetics
>   - Toxicodynamics
>   - Diagnosis of poisoning in the living and dead

CLASSIFICATION OF POISONS

Indian Society of Toxicology's Classification of Poisons (IST Classification of Poisons)

- **Corrosives**:
    - **Acids**:
        - **Inorganic (Mineral) Acids**: Sulphuric, Nitric, Hydrochloric
        - **Organic Acids**: Acetic, Acetylsalicylic, Carbolic, Oxalic
    - **Alkalies**:
        - Ammonia
        - Salts of Sodium, Calcium, Potassium
- **Non-Corrosive Chemicals**:
    - **Heavy Metals**:
        - Arsenic, Lead, Mercury, Copper, Iron, Thallium
    - **Non-metallic Chemicals**:
        - Phosphorus, Halogens (Chlorine, Iodine)
- **Organic Poisons (Toxins)**:
    - **Irritant Plants**:
        - Castor, Calotropis, Abrus, Capsicum
    - **Venomous Bites and Stings**:
        - Snake Bite, Spider Bite, Scorpion Sting, Bee Sting, Wasp Sting
- **Neurotoxic Poisons**:
    - **Cerebral**:
        - **Somniferous (Narcotics)**: Opium & Opiates (Opioids)
        - **Inebriants (Intoxicants)**: Alcohols (Ethanol, Methanol, Isopropanol), Chloral Hydrate, Benzodiazepines
        - **Deliriants**: Datura
        - **Stimulants**: Caffeine, Amphetamines, Cocaine
        - **Psychotropics (Mind Altering Drugs)**:
            - **Antidepressants**: Tricyclics, MAOIs, etc.
            - **Neuroleptics (Antipsychotics)**: Chlorpromazine, Haloperidol, etc.
            - **Hallucinogens (Psychedelics)**: Cannabis, LSD, Phencyclidine
    - **Spinal**:
        - **Stimulant**: Strychnine
        - **Depressant**: Gelsemine
    - **Peripherally acting**: Hemlock, Curare

- **Cardiovascular Poisons:**
  - **Antihypertensives**
  - **Anti-arrhythmics**
  - **Anticoagulants**
  - **Cardiotoxic Poisons:** Aconite, Oleander, Odallum
- **Asphyxiant Gases (Toxic Inhalants):**
  - **Simple Asphyxiants:** Carbon Dioxide, Nitrogen, Hydrocarbon Gases (Methane)
  - **Respiratory Irritants:** Ammonia, Chlorine, Formaldehyde, Methyl Isocyanate
  - **Systemic Asphyxiants:** Carbon Monoxide, Cyanide, Smoke
- **Agrochemicals:**
  - **Pesticides:**
    - **Insecticides:** Organophosphates, Carbamates, Chlorinated Hydrocarbons (Organochlorines), Neonicotinoids
    - **Insect Repellents:** Pyrethroids, Naphthalene
    - **Rodenticides:** Zinc Phosphide, Bromadiolone
    - **Herbicides:** Paraquat, Glyphosate
  - **Fumigants:** Aluminium Phosphide
  - **Fertilizers**
- **Pharmaceuticals:**
  - **Hepatotoxic Drugs:** Paracetamol
  - **Nephrotoxic Drugs:** NSAIDs
  - **Anti-infective Drugs:** Antibacterials, Antivirals, Antifungals
  - **Sedative-hypnotic Drugs:** Barbiturates
  - **Anaesthetic Drugs:**
    - **General Anaesthetics:** Nitrous Oxide, Chloroform, Halothane
    - **Local Anaesthetics:** Lignocaine
  - **Anticonvulsant Drugs:** Phenobarbitone, Phenytoin
- **Miscellaneous Poisons:**
  - **Food Poisons:** Microbes, Mushrooms, Plants, Fish, Chemicals
  - **Substances of Abuse:** Stimulants, Depressants, Hallucinogens
  - **Household Poisons:** Kerosene, Cleaning Agents, Cosmetics
  - **Riot Control Agents:** Tear Gases (Riot Control Agents), War Gases
  - **Radioactive Agents**

TOXICOKINETICS

- **Toxicokinetics** deals with what the body does with a substance (toxic chemical, or a drug given in toxic doses).
- Four processes are involved in toxicokinetics* (**Fig. 8.4**):
  - **Absorption**: The substance enters the body.
  - **Distribution**: The substance moves from the site of entry to other areas of the body.
  - **Metabolism**: The body breaks down the substance into metabolites.
  - **Excretion**: The substance or its metabolites are excreted out of the body.
- In short, after the substance is absorbed, it is distributed through the blood, lymph circulation and extracellular fluids into organs or other storage sites, and may be metabolized. Then, the substance or its metabolites are eliminated through the body's waste products.

TOXICODYNAMICS

- **Toxicodynamics** deals with the dynamic interactions of a xenobiotic with a living organism and the resultant biological effects. The functional or structural alterations caused in targeted cells eventually lead to toxic effects.
- The site of action can be binding proteins, ion channels, DNA or a variety of other receptors. When a xenobiotic enters an organism, it can interact with these receptors and produce structural or functional alterations.
- Xenobiotics have been grouped together according to their chemical properties by way of:
  - **Quantitative structure-activity relationships (QSARs)**, which allows prediction of toxic action based on these properties.
  - **Endocrine disrupting chemicals (EDCs)**.
  - **Carcinogens**, which may be genotoxic or non-genotoxic.
- The process of toxicodynamics can be useful for application in environmental risk assessment by implementing toxicokinetic-toxicodynamic (TKTD) models. TKTD models include phenomena such as time-varying exposure, carry-over toxicity, organism recovery time, effects of mixtures and extrapolation to untested chemicals and species.

DIAGNOSIS OF POISONING

I. In the Living

- A poisoning case can present to a doctor or hospital in any one of a number of ways. Broadly, there are four types of presentation:
  i. **Fulminant**: Produced by a massive dose. Death occurs very rapidly, sometimes without preceding symptoms, the patient appearing to collapse suddenly.
  ii. **Acute**: Produced by a single dose or several small doses taken in a short period. Onset of symptoms is abrupt.
  iii. **Chronic**: Produced by small doses taken over a long period. Onset is insidious.
  iv. **Subacute**: Characterised by a mixture of features of acute and chronic poisoning.
- The majority of poisoned patients presenting to the casualty (emergency) department are victims of acute exposure. Most of them are usually coherent enough to tell the doctor what the problem is, and indeed what they have taken or been exposed to. However, in an unconscious or uncooperative patient the diagnosis will have to be made on the basis of circumstantial or third party evidence. It is important to interrogate the persons accompanying the patient

*__Note__: *Can be remembered by the mnemonic:* ***ADME***.

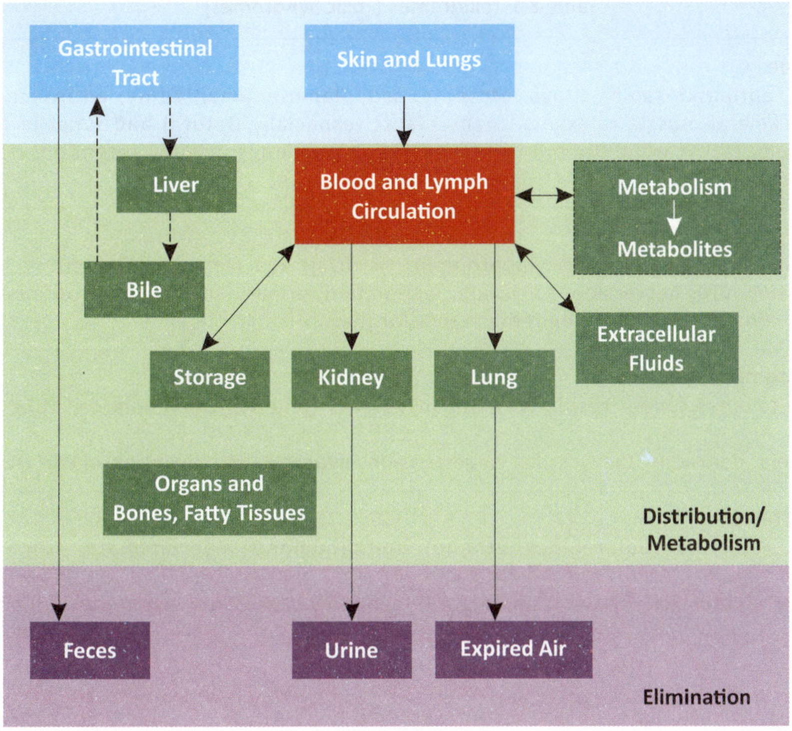

Fig. 8.4 Toxicokinetics

(relatives, friends, ambulance personnel, etc.), and to contact his or her family doctor as soon as possible. In spite of all this, unfortunately, in a significant proportion of cases the diagnosis remains uncertain. This is because unlike in other clinical conditions arising out of natural disease, there are only a very few syndromes (**toxidromes**)* characterised by specific signs and symptoms (**Table 8.1**).

- In most cases, the poisoned patient presents with one or more of the following non-specific features:
  i. Impairment of consciousness
  ii. Respiratory/Cardiovascular depression
  iii. Dehydration due to vomiting/diarrhea
  iv. Hypothermia
  v. Convulsions
  vi. Cardiac arrhythmias
- However, there are some valuable clues afforded on detailed clinical examination which can help narrow down the differential diagnosis. Most of these will be dealt with in a subsequent section (**Topic 8.8**), but a few are discussed here for the sake of convenience.
  i. **Ocular clues**: Several drugs/poisons affect the pupils of the eyes producing either miosis or mydriasis. A few produce nystagmus. These have been laid out in **Table 8.2**. Normally, both the pupils are equal in size, 3–4 mm under typical conditions, round and react directly as well as consensually to increased light intensity by constricting. Other ophthalmological manifestations along with their respective causes are mentioned in **Table 8.3**.
- **Olfactory clues**: Some poisons have distinctive odours which may be perceived in the vicinity of a poisoned patient, especially in the breath. Some important examples are mentioned in **Table 8.4**.
- **Dermal clues**: Some poisons have characteristic dermal manifestations in acute toxicity, while certain others demonstrate skin signs on chronic exposure (**Table 8.5**). Several therapeutic drugs produce irritant dermatitis even in non-toxic doses, e.g., most antibiotics, INH, phenothiazines, sulphonamides, thiazides, NSAIDs, etc.

II. In the Dead

- **Clues**:
  - Sudden, unexpected death
  - Death associated with vomiting, abdominal pain, diarrhoea
  - Unexplained death of a child or healthy adult
  - Death associated with convulsions in a non-epileptic victim
  - Slow death associated with neurological problems, nausea, weakness, hair loss.
- **Autopsy signs**:
  - Evidence of vomitus, stools, etc., on or around the dead body

Note*: *Some toxicologists prefer to restrict the term "toxidrome**" to a group of signs and symptoms that is consistently encountered in relation to a specific toxin, e.g., paracetamol, salicylates, methanol, carbon monoxide, etc.*

Table 8.1 Toxidromes (Toxic Syndromes)

Anticholinergic syndrome: ***Causes***: Antihistamines, antiparkinsonian drugs, atropine, scopolamine, amantadine, antipsychotic drugs, antidepressants, antispasmodics, skeletal muscle relaxants, many plants (especially Datura) and fungi (e.g., Amanita muscaria). ***Symptomatology***: Delirium, tachycardia, dry hot skin, mydriasis, myoclonus, urinary retention, decreased bowel sounds, convulsions, arrhythmias.
Cholinergic syndrome: ***Causes***: Organophosphates, carbamates, parasympathomimetic drugs and some mushrooms. ***Symptomatology***: Confusion, CNS depression, salivation, lacrimation, urinary and faecal incontinence, vomiting, sweating, fasciculations, seizures, miosis, pulmonary oedema, tachy/bradycardia.
Sympathomimetic syndrome: ***Causes***: Cocaine, amphetamines, upper respiratory decongestants (phenylpropanolamine, ephedrine and pseudoephedrine). ***Symptomatology***: Paranoia, delusions, tachycardia, hypertension, hyperpyrexia, sweating, mydriasis, seizures, arrhythmias.
Sedative-hypnotic syndrome: ***Causes***: Opiates, barbiturates, benzodiazepines, ethanol, methaqualone, meprobamate, ethchlorvynol, glutethimide, clonidine. ***Symptomatology***: Miosis, hypotension, bradycardia, hypothermia, CNS depression, hyporeflexia, coma, convulsions (rarely).
Opioid syndrome: ***Causes***: Morphine, codeine, pethidine (meperidine), pentazocine, buprenorphine, propoxyphene, tramadol, butorphanol, dextromethorphan, diphenoxylate, loperamide, heroin, fentanyl. **Symptomatology**: Miosis, hypotension, bradycardia, bradypnoea, hypothermia, CNS depression, hyporeflexia, decreased peristalsis, mild diaphoresis, urinary retention (occasionally), coma, convulsions (rarely).
Salicylate syndrome: ***Causes***: Salicylic acid, methyl salicylate, homosalate (homomenthyl salicylate), trolamine salicylate, acetyl salicylic acid, sodium salicylate, sodium aminosalicylate, bismuth subsalicylate, mesalamine (5-aminosalicylic acid), olsalazine (sodium azodisalicylate), sulphasalazine (salicylazosulphapyridine), diflunisal, benorylate (4-acetamidophenyl-o-acetylsalicylate). ***Symptomatology***: Tachycardia, tachypnoea, hyperthermia, sweating, delirium, decreased peristalsis, tinnitus, convulsions.
Hallucinogen syndrome: ***Causes***: LSD (lysergic acid diethylamide), phencyclidine, ketamine, designer drugs: [MDA (adam), MDEA (eve), MDMA (ecstasy), α-methyl fentanyl], tryptamines (dimethyl tryptamine, psilocin, psilocybin), mescaline, cannabinols. **Symptomatology**: Tachycardia, hypertension, hyperthermia, agitation, psychotic behaviour, miosis or mydriasis, hallucinations.
Serotonin syndrome: ***Causes***: Drugs that inhibit serotonin breakdown (non-selective MAOIs, e.g., phenelzine, moclobemide, clorgyline, isocarboxacid), drugs that block serotonin reuptake (SSRIs, e.g., fluoxetine, citalopram, paroxetine, fluvoxamine & sertraline; as well as cocaine, dextromethorphan, pethidine, pentazocine, clomipramine, trazodone, venlafaxine), serotonin precursors or agonists (LSD, tryptophan), drugs that enhance serotonin release (cocaine, amphetamines, lithium, mirtazepine, buspirone). ***Symptomatology***: Tachycardia, hypertension, hyperthermia, tachypnoea, agitation, confusion, mydriasis, sweating, flushed skin and mucosae, tremor, myoclonus, hyper-reflexia, rigidity, trismus.
Ethanol withdrawal syndrome: ***Cause***: Withdrawal reaction in an alcoholic ***Symptomatology***: Tachycardia, hypertension, hyperthermia, tachypnoea, agitation, confusion, disorientation, mydriasis, sweating, diarrhoea, tremor, convulsions.
Opioid withdrawal syndrome: ***Cause***: Withdrawal reaction in an opiate/opioid addict. ***Symptomatology***: Tachycardia, hypertension, fever, anxiety, mydriasis, sweating, vomiting, diarrhoea, rhinorrhoea, piloerection.

- Froth at mouth or nose
- Bluish face or extremities
- Unusual smell in the vicinity of corpse
- Peculiar staining of clothes or skin
- Signs of forcible feeding, injection marks
- Alteration of decomposition process

Table 8.2 Drugs/Poisons Producing Pupillary Changes

Miosis	Mydriasis	Nystagmus
Barbiturates	Alcohol (constricted in coma)	Alcohol
Benzodiazepines	Amphetamines	Barbiturates
Caffeine	Antihistamines	Carbamazepine
Carbamates	Carbon monoxide	Phencyclidine
Carbolic acid (Phenol)	Cocaine	Phenytoin
Clonidine	Cyanide	
Methyl dopa	Datura (Atropine)	
Nicotine	Ephedrine	
Opiates		
Organophosphates		
Parasympatho-mimetics		

Table 8.3 Toxic Ophthalmological Manifestations

Feature	Cause
Diplopia	*Barbiturates, cannabis, ethanol, opiates, phenytoin, tetracycline, vitamin A*
Blurred vision	*Alcohol, anticholinergics, botulism, ethanol, lithium, MAOIs, methanol*
Altered colour perception	*Cannabis, CO, digitalis, hydrocarbons, ibuprofen, nalidixic acid*
Corneal deposits	*Chloroquine, vitamin D*
Oculogyric crisis	*Phenothiazines, butyrophenones, metoclopramide*
Optic neuritis	*Chloroquine, digitalis, disulfiram, ergot, heavy metals, methanol, penicillamine, quinine*

Table 8.4 Diagnostic Odours

Odour	Substance
Acetone (apple-like)	*Chloroform, ethanol, isopropanol, lacquer*
Acrid (pear-like)	*Chloral hydrate, paraldehyde*
Bitter almond	*Cyanide*
Burnt rope	*Marijuana (Cannabis)*
Coal gas	*Carbon monoxide (CO)*
Disinfectant (hospital odour)	*Carbolic acid, creosote*
Garlicky	*Arsenic,dimethylsulphoxide, organophosphates, phosphorus, selenium, tellurium, thallium*
Mothballs	*Camphor, naphthalene*
Musty (fishy)	*Aluminium phosphide, zinc phosphide*
Rotten egg	*Carbon di sulphide, disulfiram, hydrogen sulphide, mercaptans, N-acetylcysteine*
Shoe polish	*Nitrobenzene*
Vinegar	*Acetic acid*
Wintergreen	*Methyl salicylate*

FM 8.4: Core – Written/Viva Voce

- **Describe:**
  - Laws in relation to poisons, including NDPS Act
  - Medicolegal aspects of poisons

INDIAN LAWS ON DRUGS/POISONS

1. **The Poisons Act (1919)**: This Act was amended in **1958** and repealed in **1960**. It deals with the import of poisonous substances into India, license issuance for possession of certain specified poisons, and restrictions in the sale of such substances (mostly chemicals) as poisons, over which control is to be exercised.
2. **Drugs and Cosmetics Act (1940)**: This Act was amended in 1964, and more recently in 2008, and is today referred to as the **Drugs and Cosmetics Amendment Act (2008)**. It deals with the import, manufacture, distribution, and sale of all kinds of drugs (allopathic, ayurvedic, unani, siddha, etc) and cosmetics. As per the Act, every patented or proprietary medicinal preparation should display on the label of the container, either the exact formula or a list of the ingredients. The amended Act has enhanced the scale of punishment for various offences, including sale of spuri-

Table 8.5 Dermal Manifestations of Poisoning

ACUTE		CHRONIC	
Poison/Drug	**Feature**	**Poison/Drug**	**Feature**
Datura, atropine	Dry, hot skin	*Heroin, barbiturates, morphine, phencyclidine*	Needle marks
Organophosphates, salicylates, arsenic, LSD, dinitrophenol	Profuse sweating	*Bromides, iodides, coaltar products, phenytoin*	Acne, brown colour
Carbon monoxide (CO)	Cherry pink colour	*Arsenic*	Rain drop pigmentation, hyperkeratosis, exfoliative dermatitis
Cyanide	Brick red colour	*Chlorinated hydrocarbons*	Eczematous dermatitis
Barbiturates, CO, imipramine, methadone, nitrazepam	Blisters	*Chloroquine, busulfan, clofazimine, phenothiazines, phenytoin*	Dark pigmentation
Warfarin	Petechiae and purpuric spots	*Bromides, iodides, oral contraceptives, penicillin, salicylates, tetracycline*	Erythema nodosum
Clonidine, ergot, niacin, sympathomimetics, theophylline	Flushing		

ous drugs, adulteration of drugs and cosmetics, toxic contamination, etc.

3. **Drugs and Cosmetics Rules (1945)**: This is an offshoot of the **Drugs and Cosmetics Act** of **1940**, and is concerned mainly with the standard and quality of drugs, apart from exercising control over the manufacture, sale and distribution, of drugs and cosmetics.* These rules were amended twice in the recent past, and are now referred to as **Drugs and Cosmetics (2nd Amendment) Rules, 2005**. All types of drugs used in therapeutics have been included: *allopathic*, *homeopathic*, *ayurvedic*, *unani* and *siddha*. All drugs and cosmetics are required to be labelled and packed appropriately. To advise the Central and State Governments on technical matters relating to drug control, the following Boards have been set up: the **Drugs Technical Advisory Board**, the **Ayurvedic** and **Unani Technical Advisory Boards**, and the **Drugs Consultative Committee**.

   In order to facilitate the analysis or testing of drug samples to assess their quality, the **Central Drugs Laboratory** was established in 1962. Individual states have set up **Drug Control Laboratories**. Stringent punishments have been laid down for manufacture, stocking or sale of substandard or spurious drugs.

The Drugs and Cosmetics Rules have classified drugs into various *Schedules* (**Box 8.2**).

Box 8.2—Salient Schedules under Drugs and Cosmetic Rules (1945)

Schedule C: Contains various biological products related to pharmacotherapeutics and their regulation.
Schedule E: Contains various poisons used in pharmacotherapeutics and their regulation.
Schedule F: Contains regulations and standards for running a blood bank.
Schedule F-I: Contains regulations and standards for vaccines.
Schedule F-II: Contains regulations and standards for surgical dressings.
Schedule F-F: Contains regulations and standards for ophthalmic ointments and solutions.
Schedule G: Hormonal and related preparations. The drug label must display the text *"Caution: It is dangerous to take this preparation except under medical supervision"* prominently.
Schedule H: Prescription drugs. The drug label must display the texts *"Rx"* and *"Schedule H drug. Warning: To be sold by retail on the prescription of a Registered Medical Practitioner only"* prominently. It can only be supplied to licensed parties. It cannot be sold without a prescription and only the amount specified in the prescription should be sold. The time and

contd.

**Note*: *A cosmetic is defined as any substance that is intended to be rubbed, poured, sprinkled, sprayed on, or introduced into the human body, or over any part thereof, for cleaning, beautifying, promoting attractiveness, or altering physical appearance of any person.*

date of prescription must be noted. If a Schedule H drug also comes under the purview of Narcotic Drugs and Psychotropic Substances Act, 1985, it must carry the texts "NRx" and *"Schedule H drug. Warning: To be sold by retail on the prescription of a Registered Medical Practitioner only"* on the label prominently.

Schedule J: Contains a list of various diseases and conditions that cannot be treated under any drug currently in market. No drug may legally claim to treat these diseases.

Schedule O: Contains various regulations and requirements for disinfectant fluids.

Schedule P: Contains regulations regarding life period and storage of various drugs.

Schedule P-I: Contains regulations regarding retail package size of various drugs.

Schedule Q: Contains a list of permitted dyes and pigments in soap and cosmetics.

Schedule R: Contains various regulations and requirements for condoms and other mechanical contraceptives.

Schedule S: Lists various cosmetics and toiletries, and directs the manufacturers of cosmetics to conform to the latest Bureau of Indian Standards requirements.

Schedule T: Contains various regulations and requirements for manufacture of Ayurvedic, Siddha and Unani products.

Schedule U: Contains various regulations and requirements for record keeping.

Schedule V: Contains standards for drug patents.

Schedule X: Prescription drugs not listed under Schedule H. All the regulations of Schedule H apply. The retailer must keep a copy of the prescription for two years. The drugs must be kept under lock and key.

Schedule Y: Contains requirements and guidelines for clinical trials.

4. **The Pharmacy Act (1948)**: The objective of this Act is to allow only registered pharmacists to compound, prepare, mix or dispense any medicine on the prescription of a registered medical practitioner. Under this Act, the **Pharmacy Council of India** has been constituted which regulates the study of pharmacy throughout the country. Individual states have **State Pharmacy Councils** for registration of pharmacists.
5. **The Drugs Control Act (1950)**: This Act regulates the supply and distribution of drugs, and also guides the manufacturer or dealer in fixing the maximum price for every drug.
6. **The Drugs and Magic Remedies (Objectionable Advertisement) Act (1954)**: The objective of this Act is to ensure that ethical standards are maintained when drugs are advertised by the manufacturers. Advertisements which offend decency or morality can be banned under this Act. Also, those which claim magical powers for certain drugs, e.g., enhancement of potency, cure for incurable diseases, etc. Magical remedies include the use of talismans or charms such as "*mantras*", "*kavachas*", etc.
7. **Narcotic Drugs and Psychotropic Substances Act (1985)**:
   a. The **Narcotic Drugs and Psychotropic Substances Act (NDPS Act)** was enacted in India to implement the provisions of the *Convention on Psychotropic Substances* (1971), and the *Convention Against Illicit Traffic in Narcotic Drugs and Psychotropic Substances* (1988), both held in Vienna.
   b. This Act repeals and renders obsolete three previous Acts – the **Opium Act (1857)**, the **Opium Act (1878)**, and the **Dangerous Drugs Act (1930)**. The NDPS Act has been amended thrice – in 1988, 2001 and 2014.
   c. The term "**narcotic**" in the legal sense is quite different from that used in the medical context which denotes a sleep-inducing agent.
      i. Legally, a narcotic drug could be an opiate (a true narcotic), cannabis (a non-narcotic) or cocaine (the very antithesis of a narcotic, since it is a stimulant).
   d. The term "**psychotropic substance**" is with reference to mind-altering drugs such as LSD, phencyclidine, amphetamines, barbiturates, methaqualone, benzodiazepines, mescaline, psilocybine and designer drugs (MDMA, DMT, etc.).
   e. The **NDPS Act** imposes complete prohibition on the cultivation of coca, poppy and cannabis plants, and the manufacture, sale, purchase, use, or transport of any narcotic drug or psychotropic substance except for medical or scientific purposes.
   f. Anyone who contravenes the NDPS Act will face punishment based on the quantity of the banned substance:
      - Where the contravention involves a *small quantity*, with rigorous imprisonment for a term which may extend to 1 year, or with a fine which may extend to Rs. 10,000, or both.
      - Where the contravention involves a quantity lesser than *commercial quantity* but greater than a *small quantity*, with rigorous imprisonment for a term which may extend to 10 years and with fine which may extend to Rs. 1 lakh.
      - Where the contravention involves a *commercial quantity*, with rigorous imprisonment for a term which shall not be less than 10 years but which may extend to 20 years and also a fine which shall not be less than Rs. 1 lakh, which may extend to Rs. 2 lakh.
      - As to what constitutes 'small quantity' or 'commercial quantity' with reference to some of the common drugs is mentioned in **Table 8.6**.
   g. There is also sufficient scope under the **NDPS Act** for enhanced punishment for repeat offences especially after previous convictions, which includes the imposition of even the **death penalty**. The minimum quantity of drug seized in the subsequent offence should be as per **Table 8.7**, if death penalty is to be imposed.
   h. To constitute an offence the first time around, the minimum quantity seized should be equal to or over 250 mg for heroin, 5 g for hashish or charas, 5 g for opium, 125 mg for cocaine and 500 g for ganja.
   i. A new Chapter, Chapter V-A, was introduced into the Act in May 1989 to provide for the investigation, freezing, seizure and forfeiture of property derived from or acquired through illicit trafficking in narcotic drugs and psychotropic substances.

Table 8.6 Drugs/Small quantity/Commercial quantity

Drug	Small quantity	Commercial quantity
Amphetamine	2 g (0.071 oz)	50 g (1.8 oz)
Charas	100 g (3.5 oz)	1 kg (2.2 lb)
Cocaine	2 g (0.071 oz)	100 g (3.5 oz)
Ganja	1 kg (2.2 lb)	20 kg (44 lb)
Heroin	5 g (0.18 oz)	250 g (8.8 oz)
LSD	2 mg (0.031 g)	100 mg (1.5 g)
Methadone	2 g (0.071 oz)	50 g (1.8 oz)
Morphine	5 g (0.18 oz)	250 g (8.8 oz)
Opium	25 g (0.88 oz)	2.5 kg (5.5 lb)

Table 8.7 Minimum quantity of seizure (in repeat offence) for imposition of death penalty

Narcotic drug/Psychotropic substance	Quantity (kg)
1. Opium	10
2. Morphine	1
3. Heroin	1
4. Codeine	1
5. Thebaine	1
6. Cocaine	0.5
7. Hashish	20
8. Any mixture of the above drugs	1.5
9. LSD (Lysergic acid diethyl amide)	0.5
10. THC (Tetra hydro cannabinol)	0.5
11. Amphetamines	1.5
12. Methaqualone	1.5
13. Salts and preparations of above (**9–12**)	1.5

j. In addition to persons directly involved in trafficking narcotic drugs and psychotropic substances, any person who finances trafficking, or harbours a person involved in trafficking, or abets, or is a party to a criminal conspiracy, including a criminal conspiracy to commit an offence outside India is also liable to the same scale of punishments.

k. However, immunity from prosecution is given to addicts volunteering for detoxification. **Section 64-A** of the **NDPS Act** states that any addict who is not charged with any offence punishable under **Sections 15–25,*** or **Section 27-A,**** and who voluntarily seeks to undergo medical treatment for detoxification or de-addiction from a hospital or an institution maintained or recognised by the government or a local authority, and undergoes such treatment shall not be liable to prosecution under **Section 27** of the Act (once in his lifetime).

l. Further, the Act makes a distinction between possession for personal consumption and trafficking, the punishment for the former being limited to 1 year only.

m. The Central Government of India constituted a **Narcotics Control Bureau**, in 1986 with its headquarters at New Delhi, and zonal offices at Mumbai, Calcutta, Chennai and Varanasi. In 1988, the Central Government constituted the **Narcotic Drugs and Psychotropic Substances Consultative Committee**, consisting of a chairman (the minister of finance/minister of state in the ministry of finance), and 18 members from diverse fields who would among other functions, conduct periodic review of the **NDPS Act**.

n. While the **NDPS Act** generally prohibits the cultivation of poppy, cannabis and coca plants, it does not impose a total ban. Restricted cultivation of these plants is allowed under strict control for scientific or medical use. Prior sanction in the form of license is necessary from the Central Government for this purpose. For instance, poppy can be cultivated only in certain specified tracts in the states of ***Rajasthan***, ***Uttar Pradesh*** and ***Madhya Pradesh****** during a specified period (the 'opium year' commencing on the first day of Oct every year, and ending on the 30th day of Sept the following year).

o. In 1993, the Govt of India promulgated the **NDPS (Regulation of Controlled Substances) Order**, to regulate the manufacture, distribution, etc., of any substance declared to be a "**Controlled Substance**".
   i. In exercise of its powers under the Act, the Central Govt has so far notified acetic anhydride (which is used in the processing of opium into heroin), N-acetylanthranilic acid (which is used in the illicit manufacture of methaqualone) and ephedrine & pseudoephedrine (which are used in the illicit manufacture of amphetamines) as "**controlled substances**".

**Note*: *Relate to illegal cultivation or import/export of narcotic drugs and psychotropic substances.*
***Note*: *Relates to financing illicit drug trafficking, or harbouring offenders.*
****Note*: *Easy to remember, just think of* ***RUM!***

p. The **Narcotic Drugs and Psychotropic Substances (Amendment) Act, 2014** amended the NDPS Act to relax restrictions placed by the Act on Essential Narcotic Drugs (morphine, fentanyl and methadone), making them more accessible for use in pain relief and palliative care.
   i. The Amendment also removed the NDPS Act's imposition of a mandatory death sentence in case of a repeat conviction for trafficking large quantities of drugs, giving courts the discretion to use the alternative sentence of 30 years imprisonment for repeat offences.
   ii. However, the Amendment increased the punishment for "small quantity" offences from a maximum of 6 months to 1 year imprisonment.

MEDICOLEGAL ASPECTS OF POISONS/POISONING

I. Toxicology and the Criminal Law

a. The following **Sections** of the **Indian Penal Code (IPC)** deal directly with offences involving poisons:
   i. **284**: This section deals with **negligent conduct in relation to poisons**, and states, "*Whoever does with any poisonous substance any act in any manner so rash or negligent as to endanger human life, or to be likely to cause hurt or injury to any person from such poisonous substance, shall be punished with imprisonment (up to 6 months), or fine (up to Rs.1000), or both.*" The gist of this offence is culpable negligence with respect to poisonous substances. The fact that a person has the custody of any dangerous substance suffices itself to impose upon him the duty of being careful.
   ii. **328**: Like Section 284, this section deals specifically with poisons, but with **malicious intent**. It states, "*Whoever administers to any person any poison, or any drug with intent to cause hurt to such person, shall be punished with imprisonment (up to 10 years), and shall also be liable to fine.*"
   iii. Apart from these sections, there are other non-specific sections of the **IPC** which can also be applied in cases of poisoning, e.g.,
      - **299** (culpable homicide with help of a poison)
      - **300** (culpable homicide amounting to murder with help of a poison)
      - **302** (punishment for murder)
      - **324** (causing hurt with help of a poison)
      - **326** (causing grievous hurt with help of a poison) and
      - **326A** (acid throwing or vitriolage).

II. Homicidal Poisoning

- Most cases of poisoning are either accidental or suicidal. As a mode of criminal homicide, poisoning is, compared to guns, knives, blunt objects, and ligatures, rare. But, forensic doctors believe that homicidal poisoning is more common than crime statistics suggest. Nobody can say for certain as to how many people are being murdered by poison because most of these deaths are classified as natural. In many of these cases, there are no specific external signs of poisoning. Because of this, unfortunately, in most instances, medicolegal autopsy is not undertaken. The victim may be embalmed, buried or cremated. Suspicions may be raised only by circumstantial evidence, e.g., when a surviving spouse receives a large life insurance payment, and a short while later, remarries. The only evidence of a homicidal poisoning is the poison itself. If the toxic substance is not identified or detected in the course of an autopsy, the killer could very well get away with his or her crime. Exhumations are rare.
- In addition, at the time of an autopsy, unless a specific poison is suspected, the chance of random discovery is unlikely. For example, **arsenic**, which is readily available, tasteless, and can be administered in a series of small doses that cause a period of illness before death, if used as a weapon of homicide can be virtually a foolproof method of committing murder. Other common poisons used in the commission of homicide include **cyanide, strychnine, morphine and other opiates/sedatives, heavy metals, various pesticides**, etc.
- Deaths by homicidal poisoning that do not raise suspicions, and therefore are almost always misdiagnosed as natural, have frequently involved hospital patients who are elderly, or already ill. The death of an old or gravely ill hospital patient is, almost by definition, a natural death. This is why physicians, nurses and other healthcare workers who kill ("**angels of death**") have gotten away with killing so many people (**Box 8.3** details one such sensational case of a medical practitioner who is alleged to have killed more than 200 patients deliberately).

Box 8.3—Harold Shipman: Dr Death

Dr Harold "Fred" Shipman was a general practitioner in Hyde, Greater Manchester, UK, who had a very successful practice, especially among elderly women of the small community where his clinic was located. On the morning of June 24, 1998, the 52-year-old bearded doctor made a house call on one of his patients. She was Kathleen Grundy, a sprightly lady of 82, who had been his patient for quite some time. Dr Shipman examined her and advised an injection, which she agreed to. The doctor then left, and returned to his clinic. A few hours later, Mrs Grundy was found dead, curled up on the settee in her home, by some friends who had come visiting. They immediately notified her daughter, Angela Woodruff. By the time she arrived, Dr Shipman had already certified that her mother had died of "old age." He said that her complaint earlier that morning, of indigestion, may have been actually a masked case of heart trouble. He assured Angela that there was no need of an autopsy.

Two weeks after Mrs Grundy was buried, Angela received intimation from a firm of solicitors, who informed her that her mother had made out a will leaving the entire estate (worth £386,000) to Dr Shipman. Angela was shocked and

contd.

surprised, for it was she who had always represented her mother in legal matters, since she herself was a solicitor. She asked to see her mother's will, a copy of which was immediately faxed to her. Her surprise only deepened when she saw how shabbily it had been typed, as she knew her mother to be meticulous and neat in whatever she did. Moreover, the signature looked like it had been forged. The will had been signed by two witnesses, neither of whom were known to her. Angela Woodruff went to the police.

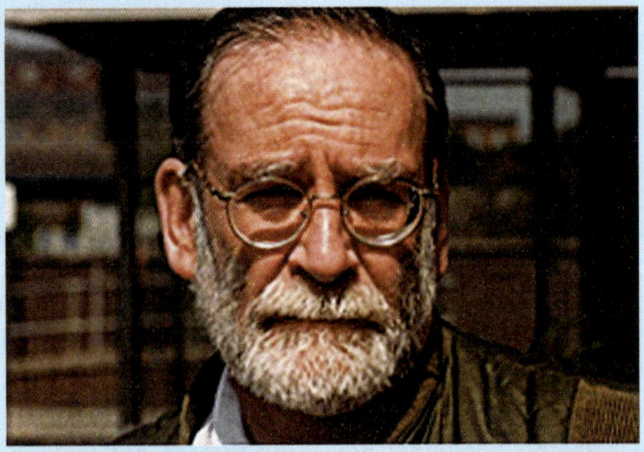

Harold Shipman

The police recorded Angela's complaint, and began an investigation. No one could have imagined the startling facts that slowly came to light over the subsequent days as the investigation progressed. The police learned to their consternation that Dr Shipman had been on a death certifying spree, involving at least 19 of his elderly patients, who had all died at home within a span of 6 months, ostensibly of old age. On each of the occasions, Dr Shipman had made a house call just prior to the death. The police decided to exhume Mrs Grundy's body, the latest victim. Forensic examination revealed nothing out of the ordinary, but samples of viscera were sent for toxicological evaluation. The report came as strongly positive for morphine, at levels that were consistent with overdose.

Dr Shipman was summoned to the police station for questioning on September 07. He said that it was possible Mrs Grundy had become addicted to morphine and had overdosed on it inadvertently. He even brought forth Mrs Grundy's medical file, but his interrogators noted that many of the entries appeared to have been made at a date subsequent to the main report. When the news of the investigation leaked to the general public, after an initial period of shock and disbelief, scores of people began to turn up at the police station, most of them relatives of elderly patients who had died under Dr Shipman's care, complaining of similar mysterious circumstances surrounding the deaths.

In the meanwhile, forensic evidence proved that Mrs Grundy could not have been taking drugs on her own. A sample of her hair showed that there was no prior history of morphine intake. Several more bodies had been exhumed by now, and all revealed the presence of large doses of morphine. The police now charged Dr Shipman with murder in 8 of these cases, where the evidence of foul play was overwhelming. On October 5, 1999, he was tried in the Sessions court, the case lasting for 57 days, during which the testimony of more than 120 prosecution witnesses was taken down. On 31st January, 2000, the jury announced that they found the accused guilty of all charges. Dr Shipman was sentenced to 15 life sentences!

In June 2001, a public enquiry into Dr Shipman's medical career was opened, which revealed that the good doctor had himself been an addict on opiates right from the time he had begun his general practice. In fact, he had faced disciplinary action from the General Medical Council. On July 19, 2002, the High Court in Manchester delivered decisions in a staggering 494 cases, which revealed that Dr Shipman had killed not just a handful, but at least 215 patients! Despite all this, the doctor himself continued to plead his innocence from his prison cell, and never confessed to any of the murders.

On 13th January 2004, Dr Shipman hanged himself in his prison cell using a bedsheet.

- Normally, homicide by poison is not an impulsive, opportunistic crime. But in the hospital, or in a home for the elderly, it is a crime of opportunity. The killer has easy access to the poison and the victim. There is no need for preparation and planning. Moreover, there may not be any motive for the homicide because many of these individuals possess personality disorders that compel them, out of generalized rage, boredom or the impulse to play God, to kill. As killers they are cold-blooded, careful and vain, making them hard to catch. When too many patients have died on their watch, and they come under suspicion, they are either terminated, or quit on their own. The tendency, among healthcare administrators, is to deny the obvious, and pass the problem on to someone else.
- Over the years, dozens of such "**angels of death**" have been caught, but only after large numbers of patients have been murdered. Given the nature of the crime, and the limited role forensic science plays in these cases, it is reasonable to assume that these angel of death convictions represent the mere tip of a rather large homicidal iceberg.
- Aside from such serial homicidal poisonings, isolated homicides by the use of poisons are not uncommon, and may be much more than the statistics reveal.

Role of the Medical Officer in Suspected Homicidal Poisoning

- Look for clues to poisoning:
  - Common symptoms in multiple individuals
  - Sudden collapse of an otherwise healthy individual
  - Nausea
  - Vomiting
  - Hair-loss
  - Shortness of breath
  - Metabolic acidosis
  - Unusual signs/symptoms, e.g., Mees lines in arsenic poisoning
  - Change in mental status over time

Role of Forensic Scientist/Police Officer in Suspected Homicidal Poisoning

- Secure the crime scene
- Document the crime scene:
  - Photograph
  - Survey
  - Video
  - Describe
- Examine the crime scene:
  - Wastebasket
  - Drawers
  - Under furniture
  - Storage
- Look for other crime scene clues:
  - Odours
  - Cleaned-up scene
  - Staging
  - Vomiting, bleeding
  - Residues
  - Containers
  - Paraphernalia
  - Caustic or toxic chemicals
- Autopsy clues:
  - Injection marks
  - Residue in the GI tract
  - Oesophageal burns
  - Hair loss
  - No anatomic cause of death
  - Frothing from mouth/nose; pulmonary oedema
- Other clues:
  - Suspicious behaviour by family members/caregivers
  - Delay in reporting symptoms
  - Insistence on no autopsy
  - Insistence on rapid cremation
  - Attempts to guide/mislead the investigation
  - Knowledge of, or access to poisons
  - Recent large insurance policies

III. Stupefying Poisons

- The term **stupefying** means "*dulling the senses or mental faculties of an individual so as to incapacitate him/her*".
  - This is usually done with an ulterior motive, for instance to rob a traveller, kidnap an individual, rape a woman, etc.
  - There are many chemicals and toxins which when administered to an unsuspecting individual can accomplish stupefaction. Common examples include **alcohol** (**ethanol**), **datura alkaloids** (**atropine, scopolamine**), **chloral hydrate, opiates, benzodiazepines, barbiturates, antidepressants**, **hallucinogens**, etc.
- In **India**, the commonest group of drugs used for stupefaction comprise the **datura (belladonna) alkaloids**, as the plant from which these alkaloids are obtained grows wild all over the country (Datura or Thorn Apple). Extract from the seeds is most often used for this purpose, usually mixed with food or drink. Sometimes, the extract may be mixed with tobacco and given to a smoker or tobacco user. Ingestion or inhalation results in drowsiness (occasionally agitation), confusion, disorientation, vertigo, etc. An individual in this state is helpless to ward off robbery, or a physical or sexual attack. **Please note**: Datura is not mentioned as a separate entry in the new curriculum. However it is discussed briefly in Annexure III owing to its importance.
- Even though datura alkaloids are still commonly encountered, increasingly, perpetrators are moving on to more sophisticated agents such as **pharmaceuticals (opiates, benzodiazepines, barbiturates, antidepressants) or substances of abuse (hallucinogens such as phencyclidine, ketamine)**.
  - One such case of stupefaction (involving the use of a benzodiazepine) handled by the Poison Control Centre of Amrita Institute of Medical Sciences is outlined in **Box 8.4**.

Box 8.4—The "Good" Samaritan

On 3rd March 2006, there was heavy rush at cinemas in Cochin (Kerala), as a new film had just been released. A middle aged male (SRN), from the nearby town of Aluva, was waiting at one of the theatres where the film was released. He had just finished his business for the day and was about to return to Aluva when he felt he deserved a little bit of relaxation. Unfortunately, the theatre displayed the sign "House Full" at its entrance.

As SRN was waiting disconsolately, undecided as to whether to return home, a stranger approached him, and said that he had an extra ticket for the film, since his friend had not turned up. He offered the ticket at no extra cost to SRN, who grabbed this unexpected act of kindness. Both of them went inside the theatre, and as the movie began and progressed, the stranger became more and more friendly. At intermission, the friendly stranger even went to the extent of buying and offering SRN a soft drink. SRN accepted. But minutes after the intermission, he began to feel uneasy, dizzy and disoriented. The friendly stranger was very concerned and suggested that they discontinue watching the film, and instead go to a nearby hospital. SRN had no choice but to agree as he was feeling quite unwell by this time with dizziness, disorientation and nausea. The stranger took him in an autorickshaw to the nearby Government District Hospital.

On arrival, SRN was minus his wristwatch, gold ring and wallet, though he was himself not aware about this at all. The stranger had him admitted in the Casualty and promptly disappeared. SRN became stuporous. The attending doctors were puzzled as they could make out no signs of illness, and routine investigations were normal. Vital parameters were stable.

At this stage, one of the medical officers suspected some foul play in the form of stupefaction having been perpetrated by the stranger who had brought him. Samples of urine and blood were collected and sent to the Poison Control Centre at Amrita Institute of Medical Sciences nearby. On receipt of the samples, the laboratory attached to the PCC

contd.

shortlisted possible agents: anticholinergics, antihistamines, benzodiazepines, barbiturates and opioids. The result: flurazepam.

This was communicated to the doctors at the hospital where SRN was admitted, and one dose of the antidote (flumazenil) was administered. Immediately thereafter, the victim recovered and became well enough to be discharged early the next morning. He could not however recall the details of the stranger who had stupefied and robbed him when the police interrogated him. The perpetrator was never caught.

- A variation of "stupefaction" is "**date rape**". This is a drug-facilitated sexual assault where-in a victim consuming alcohol or taking drugs is subjected to forcible sex, and is unable to offer resistance because of the incapacitation induced by alcohol and/or drugs.
  - The alcohol or drugs may be knowingly or unknowingly consumed by the victim. In other words, a perpetrator may intentionally drug a victim in order to commit rape, or he takes advantage of someone who is already drunk or "high".
  - Common "date rape" drugs include **street drugs (e.g., cocaine, cannabis, designer amphetamines such as "ecstacy"), prescription drugs (e.g., antidepressants, tranquilizers) or over-the-counter medications (e.g., cough syrups containing codeine)**. When these drugs are mixed with alcohol, their effects are enhanced, which makes the victim particularly vulnerable to physical or sexual attack.
  - Though **flunitrazepam (Rohypnol)** is often cited as a "date rape drug" because of its high potency, strong effects and the ability to cause strong amnesia during its duration of action, investigations into its actual use as a date rape drug have contradicted popular belief. Research has shown that flunitrazepam is used in fewer than 1% of sexual assaults where intentional drugging was suspected. The Advisory Council on the Misuse of Drugs in the UK put out a report on drug-facilitated sexual assault in 2007, which stated: "There is no reason to believe that flunitrazepam has unique properties as a weapon in drug facilitated sexual assault."
  - **Ketamine** and **GHB (gamma hydroxy butyrate)** are also commonly represented in the media as date-rape drugs. This is because they have central nervous system activity and are hard to detect. However, there is little evidence to support that they are widely used to facilitate sexual assault.

IV. Medicolegal Problems Involving Consent

a. The consent of a patient is necessary for all diagnostic and therapeutic procedures, particularly those which are invasive or risky in nature.* Undertaking such procedures without consent having been obtained first can amount to an assault in the legal sense, even if done for the benefit of the patient, unless extenuating circumstances exist.

b. A patient who has deliberately consumed a poisonous substance or overdosed on a therapeutic drug, is likely to be uncooperative and may resist all efforts at treating him. The attending physician may then be uncertain as to the legal implications of forcing treatment on the patient who may even threaten the doctor with a law suit, if therapeutic procedures are forcefully carried out. It is however a fact that a patient who attempts suicide has lost the right to refuse treatment, and no court has so far upheld a patient's complaint of "forced treatment" in such circumstances. It is also true that in many such cases of toxic ingestions, the patient can be declared "not rational" enough to refuse treatment on account of depression or disturbance of mental functions which can be deemed to impair judgement. On the other hand, a physician may become liable for negligence, if he does not do what is medically indicated.

c. There are times however, such as in a wildly agitated or extremely uncooperative patient, when overzealous attempts to remove a poison or drug overdose may place the patient at greater risk of physical harm than the ingestion itself. In such cases, the patient should be observed or partially restrained until cooperation or lethargy ensues. But, if the patient has ingested an imminently life threatening poison, then no effort should be spared in restraining the patient physically or even pharmacologically if necessary, in order to eliminate the toxin before it exerts its harmful effect.

d. In the case of a comatose patient, consent must be obtained from the next of kin. However, if it is an emergency and consent is being refused on unreasonable grounds, the physician can go ahead with the necessary treatment even in the absence of consent. In such cases, the court will always uphold his decision, if it comes to a legal action, since it was made in good faith with the wellbeing of the patient as the prime consideration.

e. Special problems arise when medical examination is requested to be done on a person who is alleged to be drunk, in order to ascertain as to whether the allegation is true. This may be with reference to offences such as disorderly behaviour in public, rash driving or commission of assault. Even if the individual concerned consents to examination, the question arises as to how valid it is, since if at the conclusion of the examination the doctor is of the opinion that the individual was intoxicated, then such consent becomes invalid because of the legal presumption that a person under the influence of alcohol is not in a fit enough mental state (**Section 90 IPC**).

f. It is pertinent to note that if an accused person has been arrested and then brought for examination, where it can be reasonably believed that such examination can afford valuable evidence as to the commission of an offence, it is not necessary for consent to be obtained from the individual.

***Note**: *If the patient happens to be a child under the age of 12 years, or a mentally unsound person, the consent of the parent or guardian should be taken.*

Medical examination can be carried out in such cases on the basis of a request made by a police officer not below the rank of a Sub-Inspector (**Section 53 CrPC**). Even "reasonable" force can be used to accomplish the examination, which can also include the collection of blood or urine sample for analysis. However, if the person to be examined is a woman, the examination should preferably be conducted by or under the supervision of a lady doctor for the sake of maintaining propriety, even if it is not legally mandatory. In case a lady doctor is not immediately available, a (disinterested) female witness can be arranged, e.g., nurse. It is also important to understand that employment of "reasonable force" for conducting a medicolegal examination is not the task of the medical officer, but that of the police.

FM 8.5: Core – Written/Viva Voce/Objective Structured Practical Examination (OSPE)
- Describe:
  - Medicolegal autopsy in cases of poisoning
  - Preservation and dispatch of viscera for chemical analysis

MEDICOLEGAL AUTOPSY IN A CASE OF POISONING

Poisoning cases being invariably medicolegal in nature, if the patient dies an inquest will have to be done, followed by postmortem examination by a forensic pathologist. This is for the purpose of ascertaining the circumstances in which poisoning occurred, and to establish the exact cause and manner of death.

The general procedure of examination is the same as for any medicolegal autopsy, with particular attention being paid to those aspects which can afford a clue to the detection of and identification of the poison involved. The following is a summary of the important points to be noted.

I. External Examination

a. **Stains** or **marks** of vomit, faecal matter, etc., on the clothing, or on the body.
b. There may be evidence of **corrosion** in the form of discoloration and sloughing especially around the mouth, in caustic ingestion (acid/alkali).
c. Presence of **jaundice** suggests a hepatotoxic poison, or one which causes haemolytic anaemia.
d. **Odour**: Several poisons have characteristic odour which may be perceptible in the vicinity of the mouth (**Table 8.4**).
e. **Colour of postmortem lividity***: Certain poisons impart characteristic colouration, for example:

i. Carbon monoxide	: Cherry pink (**Fig. 8.5**)
ii. Cyanide	: Brick red
iii. Hydrogen sulphide	: Greenish blue
iv. Phosphorus	: Brown
v. Nitrobenzene, aniline, potassium chloride	: Brownish red

Such colouration may be evident in tissues and blood also, e.g., the brick red colour of cyanide.
f. **Putrefactive changes**: Some poisons are said to retard the rate of decomposition of a dead body, e.g., arsenic, organophosphates.
g. **Injection marks**: Especially likely in a victim who had been a drug addict in life.

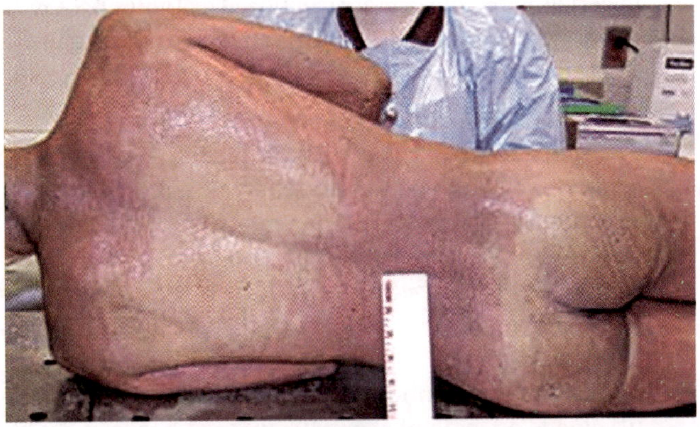

Fig. 8.5 Cherry pink colour of postmortem lividity – Death due to carbon monoxide

II. Internal Examination

a. **Odour**: It is preferable to open the cranial cavity first, since poisons impart a faint odour to the brain which may be difficult to perceive in the presence of overpowering odours from the thorax or abdomen if they have been opened earlier. Examples of such poisons include alcohol, chloroform, cresol, cyanide and phenol.
b. **Evidence of inflammation**: Ingested poisons may cause softening, reddening, corrosion or even perforation of the gastrointestinal tract. Sometimes the poisonous substance in the form of tablets, powder, plant parts or fluid may still be present. There may be associated odour.
c. **The state of the other organ systems**:
   i. Liver and kidneys are invariably congested. In some cases, there is evidence (gross or microscopic) of degenerative changes or even necrosis.
   ii. Brain may be congested or oedematous, particularly in the case of neurotoxic poisons. Petechiae in the white matter are often seen with asphyxiant poisons, which also produce pulmonary oedema with consequent froth in the airways.
   iii. The heart may demonstrate petechiae or degenerative changes in the case of cardiotoxic poisons. Subendocardial haemorrhages are said to be characteristic (though not pathognomonic) of acute arsenic poisoning.

Preservation and Dispatch of Viscera for Chemical Analysis

- In every case of death due to poisoning, an attempt must be made to demonstrate the presence of poison by

**Note: Normal colour is purplish*

standardised analytical methods. For this purpose, the pathologist conducting the autopsy must collect certain of the viscera and body fluids, and despatch them through the police to the nearest ***Forensic Science Laboratory***.

- While submitting the samples for analysis, it must be ensured that the correct quantity has been preserved in appropriate preservative in suitable, sealed containers. The materials to be collected are mentioned in **Tables 8.8A & B**, while the recommended preservatives are mentioned in **Table 8.9**.

*Sample Collection and Preservation**

- The stomach is cut between double ligatures at the cardiac and pyloric ends, and transferred to a clean tray. It is slit open along the greater curvature and the contents examined. The stomach is then placed along with its contents in a clean, wide-mouthed glass bottle of 1 litre capacity. It is preferable to preserve the contents separately in a different container.
- Similarly, the uppermost part of the small intestine is identified, and a length of about 30 cm is cut between double ligatures at either end, and transferred to a tray. It is then slit open and placed along with its contents into the same container as the stomach. However, the contents can be preserved separately.
- The liver is removed from the body in the usual manner, and about 300 g portion is cut and preserved in another container of 1 L capacity. It is desirable to include the gall bladder, since some drugs are concentrated in the bile, such as paracetamol, barbiturates and opiates. The liver should always be sliced into pieces before placing it in the container, so that the preservative can exert its action more thoroughly.
- The kidneys are dissected out of the body and one half of each is sliced and placed in the same container as the liver. Preserving one kidney alone may not be advisable, since it may happen to be dysfunctional.
- It is important that the blood collected for analysis should never be withdrawn directly from the heart or scooped out of the thoracic or abdominal cavities, since some poisons such as alcohol and barbiturates can diffuse passively after death from the stomach or intestines into adjacent organs or cavities leading to erroneous results. Blood should always be collected into a clean syringe from a peripheral vein such as those in the neck or the limbs. The femoral vein is most suitable for withdrawing a blood sample and can easily be approached percutaneously. About 10–20 mL is withdrawn and transferred to a clean vial or bottle which should be capped tightly and sealed with molten wax to minimise evaporation of volatile poisons.
  - In putrefying bodies, it may be difficult to obtain blood from peripheral veins, besides the fact that the results of analysis may be vitiated by postmortem generation of alcohol as a result of decomposition. In such cases, it may be preferable to use cerebrospinal fluid or vitreous humor for analysis. Some investigators suggest that if alcohol is detected in blood but not in urine and vitreous humor, it should be assumed that postmortem synthesis of alcohol has occurred.
- Urine can be collected by puncturing the bladder with a needle and syringe, and aspirating about 30–50 mL. However, if there is very little urine it may be necessary to make a small incision on the anterior bladder wall and scoop out the urine with a spoon, or aspirate it with a syringe or pipette. Care should be taken to ensure that the urine obtained is not contaminated with blood. Collected sample should be transferred into a clean vial/bottle and sealed in the same way as described for the blood sample.
- In some cases, additional viscera or body fluids may have to be preserved depending on the nature of the poison (**Table 8.8B**).
  - Cerebrospinal fluid is difficult to obtain by lumbar puncture at autopsy. It is easier to collect it by cisternal puncture. As an alternative, CSF can be aspirated anteriorly after evisceration by introducing a needle into the spinal theca via the spinal foramina between the 1st and 2nd lumbar vertebrae.
  - Vitreous humor can be useful in some cases of poisoning.
  - If lung is to be preserved for analysis (in inhaled poisons and solvent abuse), it is preferable to place it inside a nylon bag and then heat-seal the bag.
- If all the specimens collected for chemical analysis can be despatched to the laboratory immediately and analysis can be done within 24 hrs, no preservative need to be added to any of the specimens. However, this is almost never possible in reality, and so either the samples should be sent in an insulated ice box with sufficient crushed ice, or suitable preservative must be added to all the containers before despatching (**Table 8.9**).
- It is important to label all the containers with details as to the postmortem number, crime number (if any), name of the deceased (if known), police station to which the case belongs, the date of collection, the exact nature and quantity of the specimen, the nature of preservative, and the name, designation, and signature of the pathologist.
- A sample of the preservative used should be sent separately so that it can be analysed as to its purity and presence of contaminants, if any.
- All containers should be properly packed and sealed with sealing wax.

Source*: *Based on the recommendations of the* ***National Committee for Revised Guidelines of Sample Preservation and Analysis in Medico-legal Cases (1999)**, chaired by the author: Pillay VV, Murty OP, Dikshit PC, Mehrotra VK, Fimate L, Dutta VK, Verma SK, Shanthakumar B. Report of the National Committee for Revised Guidelines of Sample Preservation and Analysis in Medico-legal Cases. J Forensic Med Toxicol. 1999;16:44–54.*

Table 8.8A Routine Viscera and Body Fluids to be Preserved in Suspected Poisoning

S. No	Specimen	Quantity
1	Stomach	Entire
2	Stomach contents	Entire (preferable)
3	Small intestine (upper part)	30 cm (entire length in infants)
4	Small intestine contents	Up to 100 g
5	Liver (portion containing gall bladder)	200–300 g (entire liver in infants)
6	Kidney	One half of each kidney (both kidneys in infants)
7	Urine	30–50 mL
8	Blood	10–20 mL

Table 8.8B Special Viscera and Body Fluids to be Preserved in Suspected Poisoning
(*all or any of these should be preserved in addition to routine viscera, in certain cases of poisoning*)

S. No	Specimen	Quantity	Poison
1	Cerebrospinal fluid	As much as can be withdrawn	Alcohol
2	Brain	Half (one cerebral hemisphere)	Alcohol, anaesthetics, carbon monoxide, cyanide, opiates, strychnine
3	Spinal cord	Entire length	Gelsemine, strychnine
4	Lung	One	Inhaled poisons
5	Skin (with underlying tissues)	Affected portion	Corrosives, injected poisons
6	Long bone (preferably femur)	10 cm length	Heavy metals
7	Scalp hair (plucked)	15–20 strands	Heavy metals

Table 8.9 Preservatives for Viscera and Body Fluids

S. No	Specimen	Preservative
1	Viscera (except lung)	Rectified spirit* or Saturated saline
2	Blood	For every 10 mL, use 100 mg sodium fluoride + 30 mg potassium oxalate**
3	Urine	For every 10 mL, use 100 mg sodium fluoride or 1 mL of conc. HCl

**Not to be used in poisoning due to alcohol, chloroform, formaldehyde, paraldehyde, acetic acid, formic acid, phosphorus, phenol.*
***In cases of oxalic acid and ethylene glycol poisoning, do not preserve blood in potassium oxalate.*
For carbon monoxide and other gaseous/volatile poisons, use glass or plastic tube and ensure that there is very little headspace after filling.

FM 8.6: Core – Written/Viva Voce/Objective Structured Clinical Examination (OSCE)

- Describe:
  - General symptoms
  - Principles of diagnosis
  - Management of common poisons encountered in India

PRINCIPLES OF DIAGNOSIS AND MANAGEMENT OF POISONING

I. Stabilization

a. *Assessment*

i. **Airway and Breathing**:

1. Symptoms of airway obstruction include dyspnoea, air hunger and hoarseness. Signs comprise stridor, intercostal and substernal retractions, cyanosis, sweating and tachypnoea.
2. Normal oxygen delivery requires adequate haemoglobin oxygen saturation, adequate haemoglobin levels, normal oxygen unloading mechanisms and an adequate cardiac output. Increasing metabolic acidosis in the presence of a normal PaO_2 suggests a toxin or condition that either decreases oxygen carrying capacity (e.g., carbon monoxide, methaemoglobinaemia), or reduces tissue oxygen (e.g., cyanide, hydrogen sulphide).
3. The immediate need for assisted ventilation has to be assessed clinically, but the efficiency of ventilation can only be gauged by measuring the blood gases. Retention of carbon dioxide ($PaCO_2 > 45$ mm Hg or 6 kPa), and hypoxia ($PaO_2 < 70$ mm Hg or 9.3 kPa) in spite of oxygen being given by a face mask are indications for assisted ventilation.
4. A simple method of assessing respiratory status consists of determining the minute volume by a **Wright spirometer**. If this is more than 4 L/min, there is no need for ventilation. However, it must be borne in mind that ventilatory function can fluctuate and may deteriorate suddenly. **Table 8.10** lists some substances which are known to cause respiratory depression. Some drugs stimulate the respiratory centre: amphetamines, atropine, cocaine and salicylates. Some drugs are associated with non-cardiogenic pulmonary oedema, characterised by severe hypoxaemia, bilateral infiltrates on chest X-ray and normal pulmonary capillary wedge pressure (**Table 8.11**).
5. Some drugs cause or exacerbate asthma. The most important among them include NSAIDs, antibiotics like penicillins, cephalosporins, tetracycline and nitrofurantoin, cholinergic drugs, chemotherapeutic drugs and some diuretics.

ii. **Circulation**:

1. Several drugs produce changes in pulse rate and blood pressure (**Table 8.12**), while others induce cardiac arrhythmias and heart block (**Table 8.13**).

Table 8.10 Toxic Respiratory Depression

Failure of Respiratory Centre	Failure of Respiratory Muscles
Antidepressants	*Neuromuscular blocking agents*
Antipsychotics	*Nicotine*
Ethanol	*Organophosphates*
Opiates	*Shellfish poisoning*
Sedatives	*Snake bite (Cobra)*
	Strychnine

Table 8.11 Agents Causing Non-cardiogenic Pulmonary Oedema

Amphetamines	*Non-steroidal anti-inflammatory drugs*
Anticoagulants	*Opiates (especially heroin)*
Aspirated oil, talc	*Oxygen toxicity*
Beta-blockers	*Radiation*
Calcium channel blockers	*Salicylates*
Carbon monoxide	*Sulphonamides*
Cocaine	*Thiazide diuretics*
Cytotoxic and immunosuppressive drugs	*Tricyclic antidepressants*
Irritant gases	

iii. **Depression of Central Nervous System**:

1. This is generally defined as an unarousable lack of awareness with a rating of less than 8 on the **Glasgow Coma Scale** (**Annexure II**). However, the European Association of Poison Centres and Clinical Toxicologists (EAPCCT) is of the opinion that this scale while being very useful for trauma patients is inappropriate for acute poisoning. For those clinicians accustomed to applying the GCS to all patients with altered mental status, assigning a score to the overdosed or poisoned patient may provide a useful measure for assessing changes in neurologic status, but in this situation, the GCS should never be used for prognostic purposes, because complete recovery from properly managed toxic-metabolic coma despite a low GCS is the rule rather than the exception.
2. There are numerous causes for coma of which one of the most important is acute poisoning. A number of substances can induce coma (**Table 8.14**), and it will require a great deal of astuteness and expertise to pinpoint the poison. Before proceeding to an elaborate ex-

Table 8.12 Drugs Associated with Disturbances in Pulse Rate and Blood Pressure

Tachycardia & Normotension	Tachycardia & Hypotension	Tachycardia & Hypertension	Bradycardia & Hypotension	Bradycardia & Hypertension
Antihistamines, caffeine, cannabis, lomotil, thyroxine	*Carbon monoxide, cyanide, phenothiazines, theophylline*	*Amphetamines, cocaine, phencyclidine, phenylpropanolamine*	*Clonidine, levodopa, MAOIs, organophosphates, opiates, tricyclic antidepressants*	*Phenylpropanolamine*

Table 8.13 Drug/Toxin Induced Arrhythmias

Sinus Bradycardia or A-V Block	Sinus Tachycardia
Alpha adrenergic drugs, beta blockers,carbamates, cardiac glycosides, organophosphates, tricyclic antidepressants	*Amphetamines, anticholinergics, antihistamines, carbon monoxide, cocaine, phencyclidine, phenothiazines, theophylline, tricyclic antidepressants*

ercise in diagnosis however, it may be desirable to first ascertain for sure that the patient is really comatose and not just pretending (**psychogenic** or **hysterical coma**). This is often encountered in cases of "*suicide gesture*" in contrast to "*attempted suicide*." The former is an attention drawing gambit, where there is no real intention of ending one's life. The telltale fluttering eyelids, the patient who is half-walked, half-dragged in by relatives, an elaborate suicide note, a phone call to a friend or relative informing them of the act, pill bottles strewn about, all may point to such a suicide gesture. In addition, the signs and symptoms manifested by the patient usually are out of proportion to the ingestion itself.

b. *Management*

i. **Respiratory Insufficiency**:

1. First establish an open airway:
2. Remove dentures (if any).
3. Use the chin lift and jaw thrust, to clear the airway obstructed by the tongue falling back.
4. Remove saliva, vomitus, blood, etc., from the oral cavity by suction or finger-sweep method.
5. Place the patient in a semi-prone (lateral) position.
6. If required, insert an endotracheal tube.
7. If ventilation is not adequate, begin artificial respiration with **Ambu bag**.
8. Oxygen therapy: This is done to raise the PaO_2 to at least 45–55 mm Hg (6.0–7.3 kPa). Begin with 28% oxygen mask. Depending on the response as assessed by periodic arterial gas analysis, either continue with 28% or progress to 35%. If the condition is relentlessly deteriorating, consider **mechanical ventilation**.

ii. **Circulatory Failure**:

1. Correct acidaemia, if present.
2. Elevate foot end of the bed (*Trendelenberg position*).
3. Insert a large bore peripheral IV line (16 gauge or larger), and administer a fluid challenge of 200 mL of saline (10 mL/kg in children). Observe for improvement in blood pressure over 10 min. Repeat the fluid bolus if BP fails to normalise and assess for signs of fluid overload. Haemodynamic monitoring should be considered in those adult patients who do not respond to 2 L of infusion and short term low-dose vasopressors such as dopamine and norepinephrine.
4. Obtain an ECG in hypotensive patients and note rate, rhythm, arrhythmias and conduction delays.*
5. In patients who do not respond to initial fluid challenges, monitor central venous pressure and hourly urinary output. Patients with severe hypotension may need more sophisticated haemodynamic monitoring (pulmonary artery catheter and intra-arterial pressure monitoring).
6. Vasopressors of choice include dopamine and norepinephrine (noradrenaline). The doses are as follows:
   - Dopamine – Add 200 mg (1 ampoule usually) to 250 mL of 5% dextrose in water to make a solution of 800 μg/mL. Begin with 1–5 μg/kg/min (maximum being 15–30 μg/kg/min), and titrate the dose to maintain systolic BP between 90 and 100 mm Hg. Monitor BP every 15 min.
   - Norepinephrine – Add 8 mg (2 ampoules usually) to 500 mL of 5% dextrose solution to make a concentration of 16 μg/mL. Start at 0.5–1 mL/min and titrate to a clinical response. Monitor BP every 5–10 min until a clear trend is established.

iii. **ECG Changes and Cardiac Arrhythmias**:

1. Obtain an ECG, institute continuous cardiac monitoring and administer oxygen. Evaluate for hypoxia, acidosis and electrolyte disturbances (especially hypokalaemia, hypocalcaemia and hypomagnesaemia).
2. ***Abnormal P wave***:
   - Occurs with xenobiotics that depress automaticity of the sinus node, causing sinus arrest and nodal or ventricular escape rhythms (e.g., calcium channel blockers).
   - P wave is absent in rhythms with sinus arrest, e.g., cardioactive steroids and cholinergic agents.

**Note*: *PR > 0.2 sec, QRS > 0.1 sec or QT interval > 50% of PR interval.*

Table 8.14 Toxic Causes of Coma

1. Hypoxia A. ***Displacement of oxygen in blood and tissues*** - Carbon monoxide - Agents causing methaemoglobinaemia - Acetanilid - Aniline dyes - Chlorates - Dinitrophenol - Nitrites B. ***Displacement of oxygen in the atmosphere*** - Carbon dioxide - Butane - Propane - Methane
2. Acidosis - Ethylene glycol - Isopropanol - Methanol - Paraldehyde - Salicylates
3. Depression of CNS - Alcohols: ethanol, methanol, isopropanol - Anticonvulsants - Antidepressants - Antihistamines - Barbiturates - Benzodiazepines - Bromides - Chloral hydrate - Opiates - Phenothiazines
4. Hypoglycaemia - Ethanol - Hypoglycaemic drugs - Insulin - Isoniazid - Salicylates
5. Enzyme inhibition - Cyanide - Heavy metals - Organophosphates
6. Post-ictal - Amphetamines - Cocaine - Chlorinated hydrocarbons - Hallucinogens - Withdrawal from alcohol, sedatives, etc.
7. Other causes - Food poisoning: Botulism, mushrooms, shellfish, etc. - Snake bite

- A notched P wave suggests delayed conduction across the atrial septum and is characteristic of quinidine poisoning.
- P waves decrease in amplitude as hyperkalaemia becomes more severe until they become indistinguishable from the baseline (**Fig. 3.2**).

3. ***Abnormal PR interval***:
   - Xenobiotics that decrease interatrial or AV nodal conduction cause marked lengthening of the PR segment until such conduction completely ceases. At this point, the P wave no longer relates to the QRS complex; this is AV dissociation, or complete heart block. Some xenobiotics suppress AV nodal conduction by blocking calcium channels in nodal cells, as does magnesium.
   - Although the therapeutic use of digoxin, as well as early cardioactive steroid poisoning, causes PR prolongation through vagotonic effects, direct electrophysiologic effects account for the bradycardia of poisoning.
4. ***Abnormal QRS complex***:
   - Seen with xenobiotics that block fast sodium channels, e.g., cyclic antidepressants, quinidine and other type IA and IC antiarrhythmic agents, phenothiazines, amantadine, diphenhydramine, carbamazepine and cocaine.
   - An apparent increase in QRS duration and morphology, which is actually an elevation or distortion of the J point called a **J wave** or an **Osborn wave**, is a common finding in patients with hypothermia.
   - Hypermagnesemia is also associated with a widening of the QRS duration, and a slight narrowing of the QRS complex may occur with hypomagnesaemia.
   - Significant elevation in the serum concentrations of potassium may also cause widening and distortion of the QRS complex.
5. ***Abnormal ST segment***:
   - Displacement of the ST segment from its baseline typically characterizes myocardial ischaemia or infarction. The subsequent appearance of a **Q wave** is diagnostic of myocardial infarction (**Fig. 3.4**). Patients who are poisoned by xenobiotics that cause vasoconstriction, such as cocaine, are particularly prone to develop focal myocardial ischaemia and infarction.
   - However, any poisoning that results in profound hypotension or hypoxia may also result in ECG changes of ischaemia and injury.
   - Hypercalcaemia causes shortening of the ST segment through enhanced calcium influx during the plateau phase of the cardiac cycle speeding the onset of repolarization. Xenobiotic-induced hypercalcaemia may result from exposure to antacids (milk alkali syndrome), diuretics (e.g., hydrochlorothiazide), cholecalciferol (vitamin D), vitamin A and other retinoids.
   - Hypocalcaemia causes prolongation of the ST segment.

6. ***Abnormal T Wave***:
   - Isolated peaked T waves are usually evidence of early hyperkalaemia. Hyperkalaemia initially causes tall, tented T waves with normal QRS, QTc and P wave. As the measured potassium rises to 6.5–8 mEq/L, the P wave diminishes in amplitude and the PR and QRS intervals prolong. ECG changes of hyperkalaemia may occur following chronic exposure to potassium-sparing diuretics, ACE inhibitors or potassium supplements.
   - Hypokalaemia typically reduces the amplitude of the T wave and, ultimately, causes the appearance of prominent **U waves**.
7. ***Abnormal QT interval***:
   - Xenobiotics that cause sodium channel blockade prolong the QT duration, as also those that cause potassium channel blockade.
   - Hypocalcaemia is caused by a number of xenobiotics, including fluoride, calcitonin, ethylene glycol, phosphates and mithramycin.
   - Arsenic poisoning may also cause prolongation of the QTc and torsades de pointes.
8. ***Tachyarrhythmias***:
   - Sympathomimetic agents such as cocaine and amphetamines increase sympathetic tone, producing sinus tachycardia and enhancing AV nodal conduction.
   - Xenobiotics that antagonize acetylcholine released from the vagus nerve onto the sinus node enhance the rate of firing, producing sinus tachycardia, e.g., belladonna alkaloids, antihistamines and tricyclic antidepressants.
   - Whether a result of excessive circulating catecholamines observed with cocaine and sympathomimetics, myocardial sensitization secondary to halogenated hydrocarbons or thyroid hormone, or increased second messenger activity secondary to theophylline, the extreme inotropic and chronotropic effects cause arrhythmias.
   - Xenobiotics that produce focal myocardial ischaemia, such as cocaine or ephedrine, can lead to malignant ventricular arrhythmias.
   - Bidirectional ventricular tachycardia is associated with severe cardioactive steroid toxicity and aconitine.
9. ***Bradyarrhythmias***:
   - Sinus bradycardia with an otherwise normal ECG is characteristic of xenobiotics that reduce central nervous system outflow, e.g., benzodiazepines, ethanol and clonidine.
   - Calcium channel blockers, beta blockers and cardioactive steroids are the leading causes of sinus bradycardia and conduction disturbances.

Management Issues:

- Lignocaine and amiodarone are generally first line agents for stable monomorphic ventricular tachycardia, particularly in patients with underlying impaired cardiac function.
- Sotalol is an alternative for stable monomorphic ventricular tachycardia.
- Amiodarone and sotalol should be used with caution if a substance that prolongs the QT interval and/or causes torsades de pointes is involved in the overdose.
- Unstable rhythms require cardioversion.
- Atropine may be used when severe bradycardia is present and PVCs are thought to represent an escape complex.

iv. **CNS Depression**:

1. All patients with depressed mental status should receive 100% oxygen in a mask (high flow: 8–10 L/min).
2. Formerly, in every case where the identity of the poison was unknown, the following 3 antidotes (**Coma Cocktail**) were recommended to be administered:
   - *Dextrose* – 100 mL of 50% soln.
   - *Thiamine* (Vitamin B_1) – 100 mg
   - *Naloxone* – 2 mg

   —All given IV

   The rationale for the **coma cocktail** was that a significant proportion of poisoned comatose patients in whom the identity of the poison is unknown, comprise cases of overdose from opiates, alcohol and hypoglycaemic agents. Even if a particular case is not due to any of these causes, administration of these antidotes is relatively harmless.
3. However, owing to increasing dissatisfaction among toxicologists with regard to the actual benefit of the **Coma Cocktail**, the current view is that it has very limited place in practice.
4. Analeptics such as caffeine, picrotoxin, doxapram, nikethamide, etc., which were also previously advocated as "restorative remedies" to stimulate respiration in comatose patients must never be used, since they offer no substantial benefit, and instead can lead to intractable seizures and agitation.

II. Evaluation

a. *Hypothermia*

i. Some common drugs which produce hypothermia are mentioned in **Table 8.15**.

ii. It is essential to use a low reading rectal thermometer. Electronic thermometers with flexible probes are best which can also be used to record oesophageal and bladder temperatures.

iii. **Treatment**:

1. *Rewarming*:
   - For mild cases, a warm water bath (115°F) is sufficient until core temperature rises to 92°F, when the patient is placed in a bed with warm blankets. Rate of rewarming should not exceed 5°F per hour.
   - Heating the inspired air is recommended by some as very effective in raising the core temperature.

- Others advocate gastric lavage with warmed fluids, or peritoneal lavage with warmed dialysate.
- In addition, it may be necessary to correct other associated anomalies, such as hypotension, hypoventilation, acidosis and hypokalaemia.

b. *Hyperthermia*

i. Oral temperature above 102°F is referred to as hyperthermia. If it exceeds 106°F (which is very rare), there is imminent danger of encephalopathy.

ii. In a few individuals, there is a genetic susceptibility to hyperthermia, especially on exposure to skeletal muscle relaxants, inhalation anaesthetics and even local anaesthetics – **malignant hyperthermia**.
   1. This should be distinguished from **neuroleptic malignant syndrome**, which is also characterised by high fever apart from other neurological signs, but is the result of adverse reaction to antipsychotic or neuroleptic drugs, and has no genetic basis.

iii. **Table 8.16** lists some of the important toxicological causes of hyperthermia along with postulated mechanism.

iv. Complications include coagulopathy, rhabdomyolysis, renal failure and tachyarrhythmias.

v. **Treatment**:
   1. Remove all clothes, and pack the neck and groin with ice.
   2. Immersion in cold water bath (77°F) is very effective but dangerous in the elderly and in heart patients.
   3. Stop cooling measures when core temperature falls below 102°F, and nurse the patient in bed in a cool room.
   4. Administration of dantrolene may be beneficial in some cases.
   5. Do not use antipyretic drugs like paracetamol. They are ineffective.

Table 8.15 Drugs Producing Hypothermia

▪ Alcohols
▪ Barbiturates
▪ Benzodiazepines
▪ Carbon monoxide
▪ Hypoglycaemics
▪ Opiates
▪ Sedative-hypnotics

c. *Acid–Base Disorders*

i. Serum electrolytes to evaluate for metabolic acidosis should be obtained, if there is any possibility of mixed ingestion or uncertain history. The diagnosis of these acid–base disorders is based on arterial blood gas, pH, $PaCO_2$, bicarbonate and serum electrolyte disturbances.

ii. It must be first determined as to which abnormalities are primary and which are compensatory, based on the pH (**Table 8.17**). If the pH is less than 7.40, respiratory or metabolic alkalosis is primary.

iii. In the case of metabolic acidosis, it is necessary to calculate the **anion gap**. The anion gap is calculated as follows:

$$(Na^+ + K^+) - (HCO_3^- + Cl^-)$$

Normally, this translates as

$$140 - (24 + 104) = 12 \text{ mmol/L} \quad (\textit{range: 12–16 mmol/L})$$

If the anion gap is greater than 20 mmol/L, a metabolic acidosis is present regardless of the pH or serum bicarbonate concentration. Several poisons are associated with increased anion gap (**Gap acidosis**), while others do not alter it (**Non-gap acidosis**). The common causes for the various acid–base disorders are mentioned in **Table 8.18**.

iv. **Treatment** of metabolic acidosis: The drug of choice is sodium bicarbonate (**Box 8.5**). It is widely considered to be the best antidote for acidosis of almost any aetiology.

d. *Convulsions (Seizures)*

i. There are several drugs and poisons which cause convulsions (**Table 8.19**). Improper treatment or mismanagement can lead to status epilepticus which is a life-threatening condition.

ii. **Treatment**:
   1. Administer oxygen by nasal cannula or mask.
   2. Position patient's head for optimal airway patency.
   3. Establish IV line.
   4. Begin drug therapy with benzodiazepines. Either lorazepam (0.1 mg/kg) at a rate of 2 mg/min, or diazepam (0.2 mg/kg) at a rate of 5 mg/min can be administered IV. If status persists, administer 15–20 mg/kg phenytoin at 50 mg/min (adults) or 1 mg/kg/min (children), by IV.*

Table 8.16 Agents Inducing Hyperthermia

Muscular Hyperactivity	Increased Metabolic Rate	Impaired Thermoregulation
▪ *Amphetamines* ▪ *Antidepressants* ▪ *Cocaine* ▪ *MAO Inhibitors* ▪ *Phencyclidine* ▪ *Strychnine* ▪ *Withdrawal (alcohol/opiates)*	▪ *Dinitrophenol* ▪ *Salicylates* ▪ *Thyroid hormones*	▪ *Anticholinergics* ▪ *Antihistamines* ▪ *Antipsychotics* ▪ *Ephedrine* ▪ *Phenylpropanolamine* ▪ *Phenothiazines*

**Note*: *Phenytoin is incompatible with glucose containing solutions. The IV should be purged with normal saline before phenytoin infusion.*

Table 8.17 Acid–Base Disorders

Disorder	Parameter	Value	Interpretation
Respiratory alkalosis	▪ pH ▪ $PaCO_2$ ▪ HCO_3	▪ 7.50 ▪ 29 mm Hg ▪ 22 mmol/L	▪ Alkalaemia ▪ Respiratory alkalosis ▪ Normal
Respiratory acidosis	▪ pH ▪ $PaCO_2$ ▪ HCO_3	▪ 7.25 ▪ 60 mm Hg ▪ 26 mmol/L	▪ Acidaemia ▪ Respiratory acidosis ▪ Normal
Metabolic alkalosis	▪ pH ▪ $PaCO_2$ ▪ HCO_3	▪ 7.50 ▪ 48 mm Hg ▪ 36 mmol/L	▪ Alkalaemia ▪ Respiratory compensation ▪ Alkalosis
Metabolic acidosis	▪ pH ▪ $PaCO_2$ ▪ HCO_3	▪ 7.20 ▪ 21 mm Hg ▪ 8 mmol/L	▪ Acidaemia ▪ Respiratory compensation ▪ Acidosis

Table 8.18 Causes of Acid–Base Disorders

Type of disorder	Causes	
Respiratory alkalosis	Anxiety, hypoxia, lung diseases, CNS disease, pregnancy, sepsis, hepatic encephalopathy, drugs – *salicylates, catecholamines, progestone, etc.*	
Respiratory acidosis	CNS depression, airway obstruction, neuromuscular disorders (myopathies, neuropathies), severe pneumonia or pulmonary oedema, impaired lung motion (haemothorax, pneumothorax)	
Metabolic alkalosis	**Normal or high urinary chloride** Cushing's disease, Conn's syndrome, steroid administration diuretic administration, alkali overdose	**Low urinary chloride** Vomiting, past use of diuretics, post-hypercapnia
Metabolic acidosis	**Non-Gap** Diarrhoea, renal tubular acidosis, carbonic anhydrase inhibitors, aldosterone inhibitors, post-hypocapnia, bromism, iodism, and secondary to hyperkalaemia, hypercalcaemia	**Gap*** Methanol Uraemia Diabetes Paraldehyde, phenformin Idiopathic lactic acidosis, iron, isoniazid Ethanol, ethylene glycol Salicylates, solvents, starvation.
***Note**: *The important causes can be remembered by the acronym – MUDPIES.*		

Box 8.5—Sodium Bicarbonate

Uses:

1. Salicylate overdose (to alkalinize urine)
2. Tricyclic antidepressant overdose (to alkalinize blood)
3. Correction of metabolic acidosis (especially in methanol and ethylene glycol poisoning)
4. Adjuvant in poisoning with barbiturates, phenothiazines, cocaine and carbamazepine
5. Drug or toxin-induced myoglobinuria
6. As stomach wash for iron poisoning
7. Possible use in lactic acidosis, diabetic keto-acidosis, and cardiac resuscitation

Formulation:

50 mL ampoules of 8.4% and 7.5% solution containing 50 and 44.6 mEq of sodium bicarbonate, respectively.

Dose:

Add 2–3 ampoules of 8.4% $NaHCO_3$ to 1 L of 5% dextrose in water, infused IV over 3–4 hrs.
In children, add 1–2 mEq $NaHCO_3$/kg in 15 mL/kg 5% dextrose on 0.45% normal saline over 3–4 hrs.
Check urine pH in 1 hr. It should be at least 7.5–8. Maintain alkalinization with continuous infusion of 100–150 mEq in 1 L of 5% dextrose in water at 150–200 mL/hr.
Half of this dose suffices for a child.

Table 8.19 Toxic Causes of Convulsions

During Toxicity		During Withdrawal
▪ *Amphetamines* ▪ *Anticholinergics* ▪ *Antidepressants* ▪ *Antihistamines* ▪ *Caffeine* ▪ *Camphor* ▪ *Carbon monoxide* ▪ *Chlorinated hydrocarbons* ▪ *Cholinergics*	▪ *Cocaine* ▪ *Cyanide* ▪ *Heavy metals* ▪ *Isoniazid* ▪ *Organophosphates* ▪ *Strychnine* ▪ *Sympathomimetics* ▪ *Xanthines (theophylline)*	▪ *Barbiturates* ▪ *Benzodiazepines* ▪ *Ethanol* ▪ *Methaqualone* ▪ *Opiates*

5. If status still persists, administer 20 mg/kg phenobarbitone IV at 100 mg/min. If this measure also fails, give anaesthetic doses of phenobarbitone, pentobarbitone, thiopentone or halothane. In such cases obviously, ventilatory assistance and vasopressors become mandatory.
6. Monitor ECG, hydration and electrolyte balance. Watch out for hypoglycaemia and cerebral oedema.

Please note: Strychnine is not mentioned as a separate entry in the new curriculum. However it is discussed briefly in Annexure IV owing to its importance.

e. *Agitation*

i. Several drugs and poisons are associated with increased aggression which may sometimes progress to psychosis and violent behaviour (**Table 8.20**). This is especially likely, if there are other predisposing factors, such as existing mental disorder, hypoglycaemia, hypoxia, head injury and even anaemia and vitamin deficiencies.
   1. **Delirium** is the term which is often used to denote such acute psychotic episodes, and is characterised by disorientation, irrational fears, hyperexcitability, hallucinations and violence.
   2. **Dementia** refers to a more gradual decline in mental processes mainly resulting in confusion and memory loss, and though it is often organic in nature due to degenerative diseases, there are some drugs which can cause this especially on chronic exposure. Elderly patients are more vulnerable. Dementia due to drugs is usually reversible.

ii. **Treatment**: Delirium is managed by chlorpromazine, diazepam, or haloperidol. Caution is however necessary, since sedation which is inevitable with these preparations may sometimes result in more harm than benefit.

f. *Electrolyte Disturbances*

i. **Hyperkalaemia** (i.e., potassium level more than 5.5 mEq/L):
   1. The causes include digitalis, $beta_2$ antagonists, potassium sparing diuretics, NSAIDs, fluoride, heparin, succinylcholine and drugs producing acidosis.
   2. Manifestations include abdominal pain, diarrhoea, myalgia, and weakness. ECG changes are important – tall, peaked T waves, ST segment depression, prolonged PR interval and QRS prolongation. In severe cases, there is ventricular fibrillation.
   3. ***Treatment***: Glucose, insulin infusion, sodium bicarbonate and calcium gluconate. Haemodialysis and exchange resins may be required.

ii. **Hypokalaemia** (i.e., potassium level less than 3.5 mEq/L):
   1. The causes include $beta_2$ agonists, theophylline, insulin, chloroquine, caffeine, dextrose, loop diuretics, thiazide diuretics, oral hypoglycaemics, salicylates, sympathomimetics, drug-induced gastroenteritis and metabolic acidosis.
   2. Manifestations include muscle weakness, paralytic ileus and ECG changes – flat or inverted T waves, prominent U waves, ST segment depression. In severe cases there is A-V block and ventricular fibrillation.
   3. ***Treatment***: Oral or IV potassium.

iii. **Hypernatraemia** (i.e., sodium level more than 150 mEq/L):
   1. The causes include colchicine, lithium, propoxyphene, rifampicin, phenytoin, alcohol, mannitol, sorbitol, sodium salts, excessive water loss, IV saline solutions and salt emetics.
   2. ***Treatment***: Water restriction with or without loop diuretics.

iv. **Hyponatraemia** (i.e., sodium level less than 130 mEq/L):
   1. The causes include carbamazepine, chlorpropamide, NSAIDs, amitryptiline, biguanides, sulphonylureas,

Table 8.20 Drugs Associated with Agitation and Psychosis

During Toxicity		During Withdrawal
▪ *Amphetamines* ▪ *Anticholinergics* ▪ *Antidepressants* ▪ *Benzodiazepines (paradoxical agitation)* ▪ *Cannabis* ▪ *Cocaine*	▪ *Corticosteroids* ▪ *Datura (atropine)* ▪ *Digitalis* ▪ *Ethanol* ▪ *Hallucinogens*	▪ *Barbiturates* ▪ *Ethanol* ▪ *Opiates*

captopril and other ACE inhibitors, lithium, imipramine, oxytocin and excessive water intake.
2. *Treatment*: Hypertonic saline.

v. **Hypocalcaemia** (i.e., calcium level less than 4 mEq/L):
1. The causes include hydrogen fluoride, oxalates, aminoglycosides, ethanol, phenobarbitone, phenytoin, theophylline and ethylene glycol.
2. *Treatment*: Calcium gluconate IV (10% soln, 10 mL at a time, slowly).

vi. **Hypercalcaemia**: Drug-induced hypercalcaemia is uncommon.

> **FM 8.7: Core – Written/Viva Voce/ Objective Structured Clinical Examination (OSCE)**
> - Describe simple bedside tests to detect poisoning/drug overdose in a patient's body fluids.

In a given case of poisoning, it may be sufficient to know just the nature of poison (**qualitative analysis**), or there may be a need for identification as well as estimation of its concentration in the body (**quantitative analysis**).

QUALITATIVE ASSAYS IN TOXICOLOGY

Bedside Tests

I. *Colour Tests*

a. **Trinder's test**:
- Add 100 mL of ***Trinder's reagent*** (40 g mercuric chloride in 850 mL water and 120 mL HCl mixed with 40 g ferric nitrate diluted to 1 L with warm water), to 2 mL urine.
- Mix for 5 sec.
  - A **violet** or **purple colour** indicates the presence of **salicylates**.

b. **Ferric chloride test**:
- Add 1 mL of 5% ferric chloride soln to 2 mL urine.
  - A **purple colour** indicates the presence of **phenol, phenothiazines, phenylbutazone, oxyphenbutazone** or **salicylates**.

c. **FPN test**:
- Add 1 mL of FPN reagent (5 mL ferric chloride, 45 mL perchloric acid and 50 mL nitric acid), to 1 mL of urine or stomach contents and mix for 5 sec.
  - Colours **pink, red or violet** may indicate the presence of **phenothiazines**.
  - **Tricyclics** may give **green** or **blue colour**.

d. **O-cresol test**:
- Add 0.5 mL conc HCl to 0.5 mL urine or stomach contents.
- Heat in a boiling water bath for 10 min, and cool.
- Add 1 mL of O-cresol soln to 0.2 mL of the hydrolysate, followed by 2 mL ammonium hydroxide.
- Mix for 5 sec.
  - A **blue** or **blue-black colour** indicates the presence of **paracetamol** or **phenacetin**.

e. **Dichromate test**:
- Add equal volumes of 10% sodium dichromate in 50% sulphuric acid to the urine sample.
  - Development of **green colour** indicates the presence of **ethanol**.

f. **Marquis test**:
- Add 3 mL conc sulphuric acid and 3 drops formalin to the gastric fluid.
  - A **purple colour** which gradually turns **blue**, indicates the presence of **opium or its derivatives**.

g. **Lee Jones test**:
- Add a few crystals of ferrous sulphate and 5 drops of 2% sodium hydroxide to 5 mL gastric fluid.
- Boil and cool.
- Add 10 drops of 10% HCl.
  - A **greenish blue colour** indicates **cyanide**.
  - **Purple colour** indicates **salicylates**.

h. **Reinsch test**:
- 20 mL of stomach contents or urine is placed in a conical flask along with 10 mL HCl and a small strip of copper. This is gently heated for an hour in a boiling water bath inside a fume cupboard. The copper is then removed and examined.
  - A **silvery deposit** indicates **mercury** poisoning.
  - **Black deposit** indicates **arsenic** or **bismuth**.
  - **Purplish black deposit** indicates **antimony**.

i. **Meixner test**:
- This test can be done on either stool or gastric sample.
- Dilute the sample with methanol, centrifuge and filter it.
- Add a drop or two to a piece of newspaper.
- Encircle the spot with a pencil and dry it.
- Add a few drops of concentrated HCl to the spot.
  - If a **blue colour** forms within a few minutes, it is indicative of the presence of **amatoxin** (present in most toxic mushrooms).

j. **Forrest test**:
- Add 1 mL Forrest reagent (25 mL potassium dichromate, 25 mL sulphuric acid, 25 mL perchloric acid and 25 mL nitric acid) to 0.5 mL of the sample, and mix for 5 sec.
  - A **yellow-green colour** deepening to **blue** indicates the presence of **imipramine or related compounds**.

k. **Fujiwara test**:
- To three 10 mL tubes, add respectively, 1 mL portions of (a) the sample, (b) purified water and (c) trichloroacetic acid.
- Add 1 mL sodium hydroxide and 1 mL pyridine to each tube, mix carefully and heat in a boiling water bath for 2 min.
  - An intense **red/purple colour** in the top layer of tube (a) as in tube (c) indicates the presence of trichloro compounds such as **chloral hydrate, chloroform** and **trichloro ethylene**.
  - Tube (b) should show no colouration.

II. *Other Tests*

a. **Isonitrile test**:
- Mix a small amount of gastric contents with 10 mL water and add 1 mL purified aniline, followed by 2 mL 20% sodium hydroxide.
- Heat gently for a few minutes.
  - A **foul odour** (***skunk odour***) will be perceived if one of the following poisons is present: **carbon tetrachloride, chloral hydrate, chloroform, methyl bromide** or any other **chlorinated hydrocarbon**.

b. **Tensilon test (Edrophonium challenge test)**:
- When 10 mg edrophonium is given IV in a case of sudden paralysis, there will be **dramatic recovery**, if it is due to **myasthenia gravis**, while a case of poisoning (e.g., botulism) will not show any improvement.

c. **Melzer's test**:
- This is a test done to confirm whether a given mushroom is toxic (especially ***Amanita phalloides***).
- The spores obtained from the mushroom are stained with 1 drop of Melzer's reagent (20 mL water, 1.5 g potassium iodide, 0.5 g iodine and 20 g chloral hydrate), and viewed under a microscope.
- Spores of *A. phalloides* and a few other deadly mushrooms will show a bluish black colour ("**amyloid reaction**").
- However, a negative reaction does not mean that the mushroom is non-toxic.

> **FM 8.8: Core – Written/Viva Voce/ Objective Structured Clinical Examination (OSCE)**
> - **Describe basic methodologies in treatment of poisoning**:
>   - Decontamination
>   - Supportive therapy
>   - Antidote therapy
>   - Procedures of enhanced elimination.

DECONTAMINATION IN POISONING

I. Eye

a. Irrigate copiously for at least 15–20 min with normal saline or water.
b. Do not use acid or alkaline irrigating solutions.
c. As a first-aid measure at home, a victim of chemical burns should be instructed to place his face under running water or in a shower while holding the eyelids open.
d. During transportation to hospital the face should be immersed in a basin of water (while ensuring that the patient does not inhale water!).

II. Skin

Cutaneous absorption is a common occurrence, especially with reference to industrial and agricultural substances such as phenol, hydrocyanic acid, aniline, organic metallic compounds, phosphorus and most of the pesticides. The following measures can be undertaken to minimise absorption:

a. Exposed persons should rinse with cold water and then wash thoroughly with soap. Repeat the rinse with cold water.
b. Corroded areas should be irrigated copiously with water or saline for at least 15 min.
c. Remove all contaminated clothes. It is preferable to strip the patient completely and provide fresh clothes, or cover with clean bedsheet.
d. Some chemical exposures require special treatment:
   - Phenolic burns should be treated by application of polyethylene.
   - Phosphorus burns should be treated with copper sulphate solution.
   - For hydrofluoric acid burns, use of intradermal or intra-arterial calcium gluconate decreases tissue necrosis.
   - For tar, bitumen or asphalt burns, first irrigate the affected skin with cold water and then clean and apply solvents such as kerosene, petrol, ethanol or acetone. However, since these substances can not only be locally cytotoxic, but also be absorbed through the skin, it is preferable to use mineral oil, petrolatum or antibacterial ointments in a petrolatum base.

III. Gut

The various methods of poison removal from the gastro-intestinal tract include:
- Emesis
- Gastric lavage
- Catharsis
- Activated charcoal
- Whole bowel irrigation

a. *Emesis*

Not recommended any more.*

- **Emesis (induction of vomiting)** was previously recommended as a good first-aid measure for ingested poisons. And most physicians advocated the administration of **syrup of ipecacuanha** (or **ipecac syrup**) in the first hour or so of the incident. However, the initial enthusiasm associated with emesis as a first aid measure, and the use of ipecac, has declined substantially in recent years owing to doubts being raised as to the actual efficacy and safety. **The current consensus is that syrup of ipecac or any other emetic must NOT be used, except in justifiable circumstances.**
- **Syrup of Ipecac**:
  - Source: Root of a small shrub (*Cephaelis ipecacuanha* or *Carapichea ipecacuanha*) (**Fig. 8.6**) which grows well in W. Bengal.
  - Active principles: Cephaeline, emetine and traces of psychotrine.
  - Mode of action:
    - Local activation of peripheral sensory receptors in the GI tract.

****Source***: *Avau B, Borra V, Vanhove AC, Vandekerckhove P, De Paepe P, De Buck E. First aid interventions by laypeople for acute oral poisoning. Cochrane Database Syst Rev. 2018;12:CD013230.*

- Central stimulation of the chemoreceptor trigger zone with subsequent activation of the vomiting centre.
- Dose:
  - 30 mL (adult), or 15 mL (child), followed by 250–500 mL of water.
  - The patient should be sitting up.
  - If vomiting does not occur within 30 min, repeat the same dose once more.

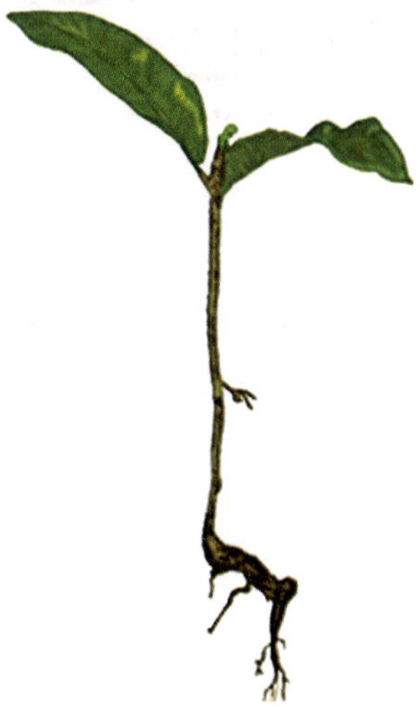

Fig. 8.6 Cephaelis ipecacuanha

- Contraindications:
  - Convulsions, or ingestion of a convulsant poison
  - Impaired gag reflex
  - Coma
  - Foreign body ingestion
  - Corrosive ingestion
  - Ingestion of petroleum distillates
  - All poisons which are themselves emetic in nature
- Complications:
  - Cardiotoxicity (bradycardia, atrial fibrillation, myocarditis)
  - Aspiration pneumonia
  - Oesophageal mucosal or Mallory Weiss tears (due to protracted vomiting)

- **Other Emetics**
  - Another method of inducing emesis that was advocated in the past, involved the use of **apomorphine**. Given subcutaneously, it causes vomiting within 3–5 min by acting directly on the chemoreceptor trigger zone. **It is not recommended any more, and is in fact unavailable.**
  - **Stimulation of the posterior pharynx** with a finger or a blunt object was also recommended previously, to induce vomiting, by provoking the gag reflex. Unfortunately, such mechanically induced evacuation is often unsuccessful and incomplete, with mean volume of vomitus about one third of that obtained by the other two methods. **Hence, this method is also not recommended any more.**
- **Obsolete Emetics: These are chemicals that must NEVER be used as they are hazardous.**
  - The use of **warm saline** or **mustard water** as an emetic is not only dangerous (resulting often in severe hypernatraemia), but also impractical since many patients, especially children refuse (fortunately) to drink this type of concoction and much valuable time is lost coaxing them to do so. One tablespoon of salt contains at least 250 mEq of sodium, and if absorbed can raise the serum level by 25 mEq/L in for instance, a 3-year-old child.* It is high time that the use of salt water as an emetic be deleted once and for all from every textbook on poisoning.
  - **Copper sulphate** induces emesis more often than common salt, but significant elevations of serum copper can occur leading to renal and hepatic damage. It is also a gastrointestinal corrosive.
  - **Zinc sulphate** is similar in toxicity to copper sulphate, and has in addition a very narrow margin of safety.

b. *Gastric Lavage (Stomach Wash)*

- The American Academy of Clinical Toxicology (AACT), and the European Association of Poison Centres and Clinical Toxicology (EAPCCT) have published position papers directed to the use of gastric lavage, which emphasise that **gastric lavage should NOT be employed routinely in the management of poisoned patients**. There is no certain evidence that its use improves outcome, while the fact that it can cause significant morbidity (and sometimes mortality) is indisputable. **Lavage should be considered only if a patient has ingested a life-threatening amount of a poison and presents to the hospital within 1–2 hrs of ingestion.**

  But in India, very often caution is thrown to the wind and the average physician in an average hospital embarks on gastric lavage with gusto the moment a poisoned patient is brought in. A sad commentary on the existing lack of awareness and a reluctance to change old convictions in spite of mounting evidence against the routine employment of such "established procedures."
- ***Indications***:
  - Gastric lavage is recommended mainly for patients who have ingested a life-threatening dose, or
  - Who exhibit significant morbidity and present within 1–2 hrs of ingestion. Lavage beyond this period may be appropriate only in the presence of gastric concretions, delayed gastric emptying or sustained release preparations. Some authorities still recommend lavage up to 6–12 hrs post-ingestion in the case of salicylates, tricyclics, carbamazepine and barbiturates.
- ***Precautions***:
  - Never undertake lavage in a patient who has ingested a non-toxic agent, or a non-toxic amount of a toxic agent.

**Note*: *"Salt is only an occasionally successful emetic, but a frequently successful poison."*

- Never use lavage as a deterrent to subsequent ingestions. Such a notion is barbaric, besides being incorrect.
- ***Contraindications***:
  - *Relative*: Haemorrhagic diathesis, oesophageal varices, recent surgery, advanced pregnancy, ingestion of alkali, coma.
  - *Absolute*: Marked hypothermia, prior significant vomiting, unprotected airway in coma, and ingestion of acid or convulsant or petroleum distillate, and sharp substances.
- ***Procedure***:
  - Explain the exact procedure to the patient and obtain his consent. If refused, it is better not to undertake lavage because it will amount to an assault, besides increasing the risk of complications due to active non-cooperation.
  - Endotracheal intubation must be done prior to lavage in the comatose patient.
  - Place the patient head down on his left lateral side (20° tilt on the table).
  - Mark the length of tube to be inserted (50 cm for an adult, 25 cm for a child).*
  - The ideal tube for lavage is the **lavacuator** (clear plastic or gastric hose).
  - In India however, the **Ewald tube** is most often used which is a soft rubber tube with a funnel at one end (**Fig. 8.7**). Whatever tube is used, make sure that the inner diameter corresponds to at least 36–40 French size.** A nasogastric tube used for gastric aspiration is inadequate and should never be used. In a child, the diameter should be at least 22–28 French (**Ryle's tube** may be sufficient) (**Fig. 8.8**).
  - The preferred route of insertion is oral. Passing the tube nasally can damage the nasal mucosa considerably and lead to severe epistaxis. Lubricate the inserting end of the tube with vaseline or glycerine, and pass it to the desired extent. Use a mouth gag so that the patient will not bite on the tube.
  - Once the tube has been inserted, its position should be checked either by air insufflation while listening over the stomach, or by aspiration with pH testing of the aspirate (acidic, if properly positioned).
  - Lavage is carried out using small aliquots (quantities) of liquid. In an adult, 200–300 mL aliquots of warm (38°C) saline or plain water are used. In a child, 10–15 mL/kg body weight of warm saline is used each time. Water should preferably be avoided in young children because of the risk of inducing hyponatraemia and water intoxication. It is advisable to hold back the first aliquot of washing for chemical analysis.

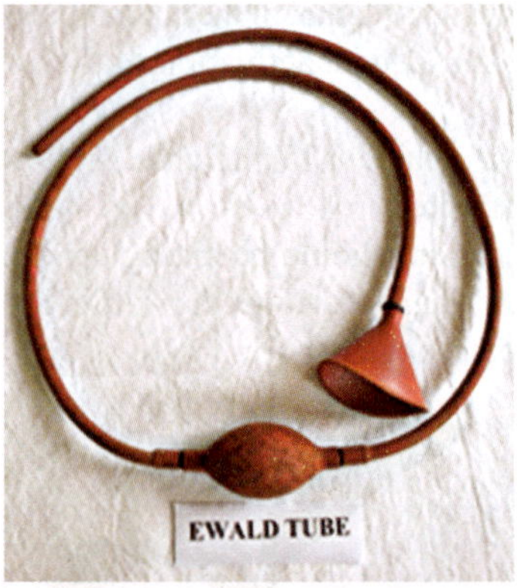

Fig. 8.7 Ewald tube (*Courtesy*: *Dr Anu Sasidharan*)

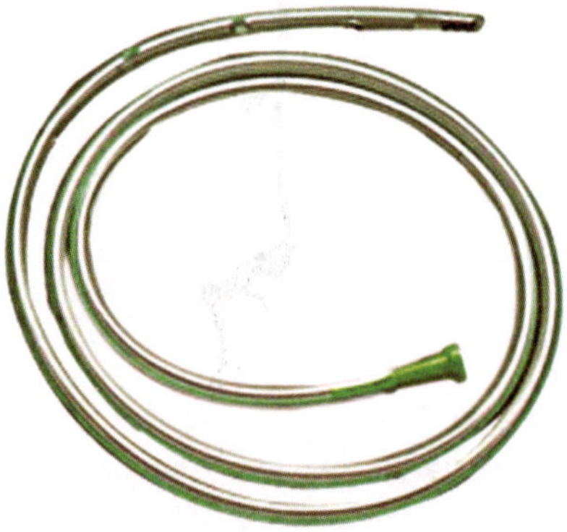

Fig. 8.8 Ryle's tube

  - In certain specific types of poisoning, special solutions may be used in place of water or saline (**Table 8.21**).
  - Lavage should be continued until no further particulate matter is seen, and the efferent lavage solution is clear. At the end of lavage, pour a slurry of activated charcoal in water (1 g/kg), and an appropriate dose of an ionic cathartic into the stomach, and then remove the tube.
- ***Complications***:
  - Aspiration pneumonia.
  - Laryngospasm.
  - Sinus bradycardia and ST elevation on the ECG.
  - Perforation of stomach or oesophagus (rare).

c. *Catharsis*

- Catharsis is a very appropriate term when used in connection with poisoning, since it means purification. It is achieved by purging the gastrointestinal tract (particularly the bowel) of all poisonous material.
- The two main groups of cathartics used in toxicology include:
  - **Ionic or Saline**:
    - These cathartics alter physico-chemical forces within the intestinal lumen leading to osmotic reten-

**Note*: *Alternatively, mark off the length corresponding to the distance between the xiphoid process and the bridge of the nose of the patient.*

***Note*: *Each unit on the French scale equals 0.3 mm.*

Table 8.21 Solutions for Gastric Lavage

Poison	Solution
Most poisons (known or unknown)	Water or Saline
Oxidizable poisons (alkaloids, salicylates, etc.)	Potassium permanganate (1:5000 or 1:10,000)
Cyanides	Sodium thiosulphate (25%)
Carbolic acid (phenols)	Castor oil and warm water (1:2)
Oxalates	Calcium gluconate
Iron	Desferrioxamine (2 g in 1 L of water)

tion of fluid which activates motility reflexes and enhances expulsion.

- Recommended cathartics: Magnesium citrate, Magnesium sulphate, Sodium sulphate.

- **Saccharides**:
  - Sorbitol (D-glucitol) is the cathartic of choice in adults because of better efficacy than saline cathartics, but must not be used as far as possible in young children owing to risk of fluid and electrolyte imbalance (especially hypernatraemia).

- ***Efficacy of catharsis***: While cathartics do reduce the transit time of drugs in the gastrointestinal tract, there is no real evidence that it improves morbidity or mortality in cases of poisoning.
- ***Contraindications***:
  - Corrosives
  - Existing electrolyte imbalance
  - Paralytic ileus
  - Severe diarrhoea
  - Recent bowel surgery
  - Abdominal trauma
  - Renal failure

d. *Activated (Medicinal) Charcoal*

- A number of studies have documented clearly the efficacy of activated charcoal as the sole decontamination measure in ingested poisoning, while emesis and lavage are increasingly being associated with relative futility.
- Activated charcoal is a fine, black, colourless, tasteless powder made from burning wood, coconut shell, bone, sucrose or rice starch, followed by treatment with an activating agent (steam, carbon dioxide, etc.) (**Fig. 8.9**). The resulting particles are extremely small, but have an extremely large surface area (**Fig. 8.10**). Each gram of activated charcoal works out to a surface area of 1000 square metres.
- ***Mode of action***: Decreases the absorption of various poisons by adsorbing them on to its surface. Activated charcoal is effective to varying extent, depending on the nature of substance ingested (**Table 8.22**).
- ***Dose***: 1 g/kg body weight (usually 50–100 g in an adult, 10–30 g in a child).
- ***Procedure***:
  - Activated charcoal is most effective when administered within 1 hr of ingestion.
  - Add four to eight times the quantity of water to the calculated dose of activated charcoal, and mix to produce a slurry or suspension. This is administered to the patient after emesis or lavage, or as sole intervention. The slurry should be shaken well before administration.
- **Multiple-dose Activated Charcoal (MDAC)**: The use of repeated doses (150–200 g of activated charcoal) is very effective in the elimination of certain drugs (theophylline, phenobarbitone, quinine, digitoxin, phenylbutazone, salicylates, carbamazepine), through a nasogastric tube over 4–8 hrs.
- ***Disadvantages***
  - Unpleasant taste (*it is gritty or sand-like in consistency, and has an unappetising look, being black in colour*).
  - Provocation of vomiting.
  - Constipation/Diarrhoea.
  - Pulmonary aspiration.

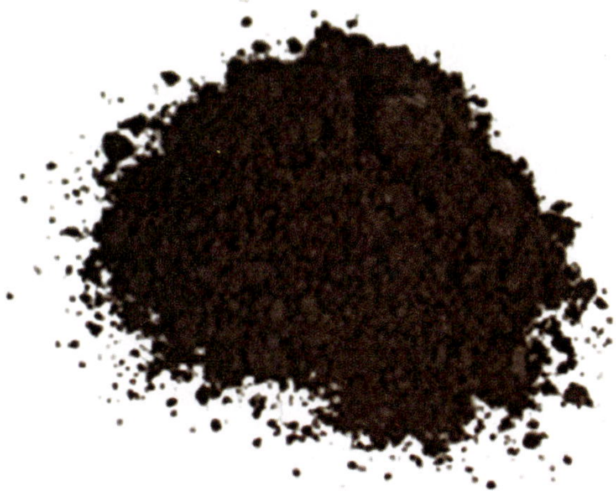

Fig. 8.9 Activated charcoal

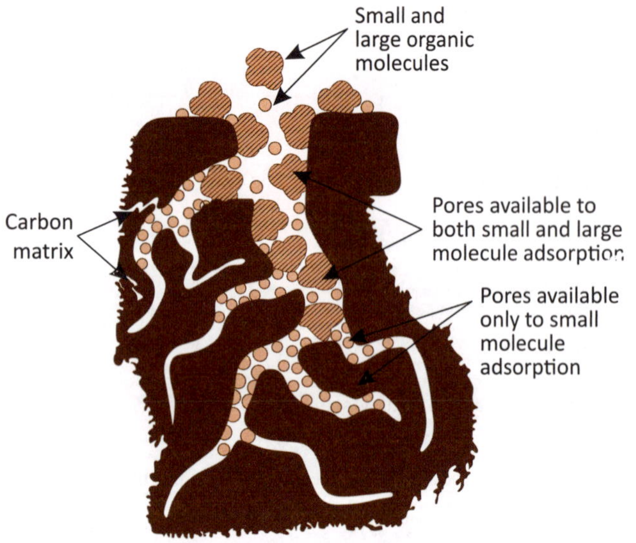

Fig. 8.10 Section of activated charcoal particle

- Intestinal obstruction (especially with multiple-dose activated charcoal).
- ***Contraindications***:
  - Absent bowel sounds or proven ileus.
  - Small bowel obstruction.
  - Caustic ingestion.
  - Ingestion of petroleum distillates.

e. ***Whole Bowel Irrigation (Whole Gut Lavage)***

- Recommended for late presenting overdoses when several hours have elapsed since ingestion.
- Involves the instillation of large volumes of a suitable solution into the stomach in a nasogastric tube over a period of 2–6 hrs producing voluminous diarrhoea.
- ***Solutions used***:
  - **PEG-ELS** (i.e., polyethylene glycol and electrolytes lavage solution combined together, which is an isosmolar electrolyte solution).
  - **PEG-3350** (high-molecular weight polyethylene glycol).
- ***Indications***:
  - Ingestion of large amounts of toxic drugs in patients presenting late (>4 hrs post-exposure).
  - Overdose with sustained-release preparations.
  - Ingestion of substances not adsorbed by activated charcoal, particularly heavy metals.
  - Ingestion of foreign bodies such as miniature disc batteries (button cells), cocaine filled packets (**body packer syndrome**), etc.
  - Ingestion of slowly dissolving substances – iron tablets, paint chips, bezoars, concretions, etc.
- ***Procedure***:
  - Insert a nasogastric tube into the stomach and instil the solution at room temperature, at a rate of 2 L/hr in adults, and 0.5 L/hr in children. The patient should preferably be seated in a commode. The use of metoclopramide IV (10 mg in adults, 0.1–0.3 mg/kg in children) can minimise the incidence of vomiting. The procedure should be continued until the rectal effluent is clear, which usually occurs in about 2–6 hrs.
- ***Complications***:
  - Vomiting
  - Abdominal distension and cramps
  - Anal irritation.
- ***Contraindications***:
  - Gastrointestinal pathology such as obstruction, ileus, haemorrhage or perforation.

PROCEDURES OF ELIMINATION OF POISON IN POISONING CASES

1. **Alkaline Diuresis**
2. **Extracorporeal Techniques**

Table 8.22 Adsorption of Toxins to Activated Charcoal

Well Adsorbed		Moderately Adsorbed	Poorly Adsorbed
Aflatoxins	Cimetidine	Antidiabetic drugs	Alcohols
Amphetamines	Dapsone	Kerosene	Boric acid
Antidepressants	Digitalis	Paracetamol	Carbamates
Antiepileptics	NSAIDs	Phenol	Corrosives
Antihistamines	Opiates	Salicylates	Cyanide
Atropine	Phenothiazines		Ethylene glycol
Barbiturates	Quinine		Heavy metals
Benzodiazepines	Strychnine		Hydrocarbons
Beta blockers	Tetracycline		Lithium
Chloroquine	Theophylline		Organophosphates

- Haemodialysis
- Haemoperfusion
- Peritoneal Dialysis
- Haemofiltration
- Plasmapheresis
- Plasma Perfusion
- Cardiopulmonary Bypass
- Extracorporeal Membrane Oxygenation (ECMO)
- Intravenous Lipid Emulsion (ILE) Therapy

A. Alkaline Diuresis

- Most useful in the case of Salicylates, Barbiturates, Formate and Methotrexate (SBFM). These weak acids are ionized at alkaline urine pH and tubular reabsorption is thereby greatly reduced.
- Alkalinization is achieved by the IV administration of sodium bicarbonate, 1–2 mEq/kg infused over 3–4 hrs. The goal is to increase urinary pH to 7–8.
- Administration of carbonic anhydrase inhibitors such as acetazolamide is not recommended. Although it enhances elimination, metabolic acidosis will ensue unless ample sodium bicarbonate is also administered.
- **Acid diuresis is no longer recommended for any drug or poison, including amphetamines, strychnine, quinine or phencyclidine**.

B. Extracorporeal Techniques

1. *Haemodialysis* (Fig. 8.11)

- ***Principle***: Involves diffusion of solutes across a semipermeable membrane.
- Haemodialysis utilizes counter-current flow, where the dialysate flows in the opposite direction to blood flow in the extracorporeal circuit. Counter-current flow maintains the concentration gradient across the membrane at a maximum and increases the efficiency of the dialysis.
- Fluid removal (ultrafiltration) is achieved by altering the hydrostatic pressure of the dialysate compartment, causing free water and some dissolved solutes to move across the membrane along a created pressure gradient.
- All drugs are not dialysable, and so it must be ensured before embarking on this procedure that the following conditions are satisfied:
  - The substance should be such that it can diffuse easily through a dialysis membrane.
  - A significant proportion of the substance should be present in plasma water.
  - The pharmacological effect should be directly related to the blood concentration.
- Extensive plasma protein binding, insolubility in water and high-molecular weight are the three most important factors in making haemodialysis ineffective.
- ***Procedure***:
  - The three basic components of haemodialysis are the *blood delivery system*, the *dialyser* itself and the *composition and method of delivery of the dialysate*. For acute haemodialysis, catheters are placed in a peripheral vein and passed into the inferior vena cava. Blood from one is pumped to the dialyser (usually by a roller pump) through lines that contain equipment to measure flow and pressure within the system. Blood returns through the second catheter. The femoral vein is preferable, but subclavian, internal jugular or other peripheral veins are also acceptable, though they have slightly higher rates of such complications as pneumothorax and arterial puncture.
  - The original dialysers were of the **coil type**. Later, the flat plate or **kiil type** of dialyser was developed. The most recent type which is becoming increasingly popular is the **hollow fibre**, in which the membrane is spun

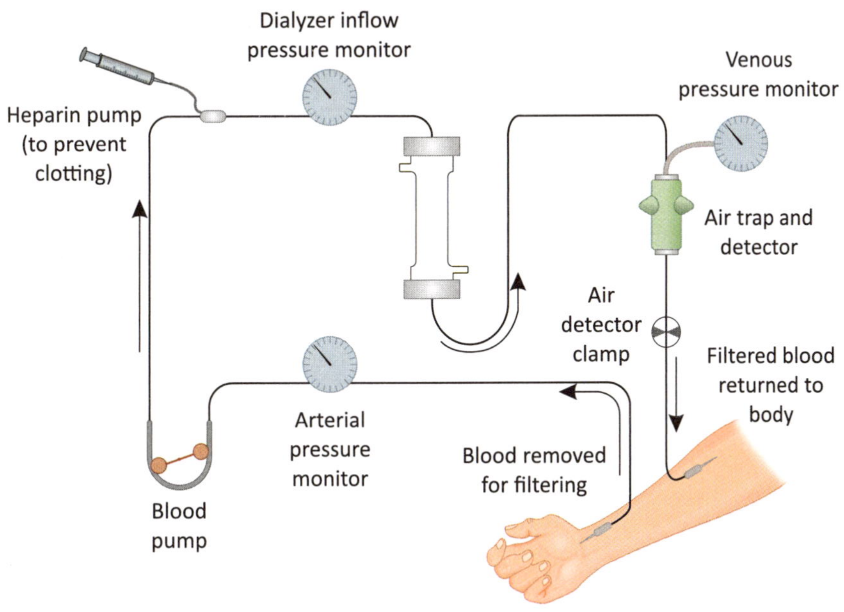

Fig. 8.11 Haemodialysis

into fine capillaries. Almost all dialyzers in use today are of the hollow-fibre variety.

- In poisoned patients, haemodialysis is usually performed for 4–8 hrs. Assuming that the patient's serum potassium concentration is normal, a standard bicarbonate-based dialysate with a potassium concentration of 3 or 4 mEq/L and a calcium concentration of 3 mEq/L, flowing at 600–800 mL/min, is sufficient.

- ***Indications***
  - **Best Indications:**
    - Methanol
    - Ethylene glycol
    - After chelation in heavy metal poisoning with renal failure
  - **Very Good Indications:**
    - Lithium
    - Phenobarbitone
    - Salicylates
    - Theophylline
  - **Fairly Good Indications:**
    - Amphetamines
    - Barbiturates (short acting)
    - Bromides
    - Chloral hydrate
    - Ethanol
    - Isopropanol
    - Isoniazid
    - Paraldehyde
    - Strychnine
- ***Complications:***
  - Infection
  - Thrombosis
  - Hypotension
  - Air embolism
  - Bleeding (due to use of heparin as a systemic anticoagulant).

2. ***Haemoperfusion*** **(Fig. 8.12)**

- In general, if a xenobiotic is adsorbed by activated charcoal, charcoal haemoperfusion clearance will exceed that of haemodialysis.
- ***Procedure:***
  - Blood is pumped through a cartridge containing a very large surface area of adsorbent (resin or activated charcoal). The adsorbent is coated with a very thin layer of polymer membrane such as cellulose acetate.
  - An arteriovenous shunt or a double-lumen venous catheter is inserted into the patient's vascular tree. The haemoperfusion column and lines are primed with heparinized saline in accordance with the manufacturer's instructions and connected to the shunt or catheter. On commencement of perfusion, a bolus of heparin is injected into the arterial line and heparinization is continued by administering an infusion of heparinized saline.

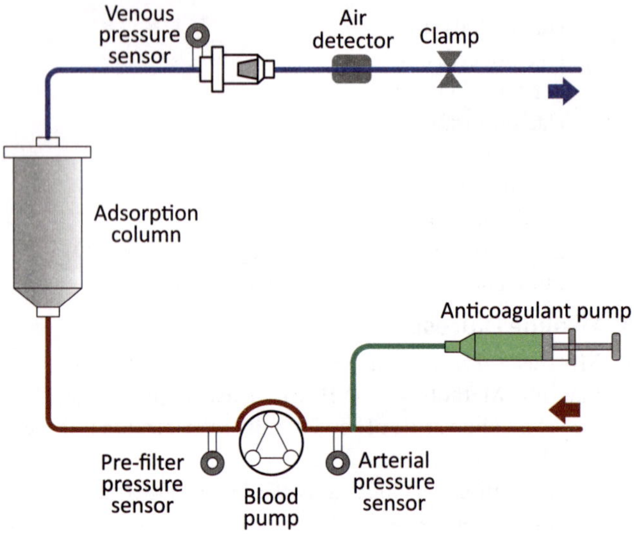

Fig. 8.12 Haemoperfusion

  - Haemoperfusion is usually performed for 4–6 hrs at flow rates of 250–400 mL/min. The characteristics of xenobiotics that make them amenable to haemoperfusion differ from those for haemodialysis in the important respect that haemoperfusion is not limited by plasma protein binding.
  - ***Indications:***
    - Haemoperfusion is the preferred method to enhance the elimination of carbamazepine, phenobarbitone, phenytoin and theophylline.
  - **Complications:**
    - Bleeding (because of heparinization)
    - Air embolism
    - Infection
    - Thrombocytopenia
    - Hypocalcaemia
    - Hypotension

Table 8.23 Toxins Removed by Haemoperfusion (*more efficiently than haemodialysis*)

▪ Amanitin	▪ Paracetamol
▪ Barbiturates	▪ Paraquat
▪ Carbon tetrachloride	▪ Phenols
▪ Chloral hydrate	▪ Phenylbutazone
▪ Chlorpromazine	▪ Promethazine
▪ Dapsone	▪ Propoxyphene
▪ Diazepam	▪ Quinidine, quinine
▪ Digoxin	▪ Salicylates
▪ Diphenhydramine	▪ Theophylline
▪ Organophosphates	▪ Valproic acid

3. ***Peritoneal Dialysis*** **(Fig. 8.13)**

- Although widely available, peritoneal dialysis today is almost never recommended for detoxification. In general, it is only 10–25% as effective as haemodialysis, and often only slightly more effective than forced diuresis. It is also time consuming, requiring 24 hrs for successful completion as compared to the 2–4-hr cycles of haemodialysis and haemoperfusion. The only advantages are that it does not require anticoagulation and uses minimal equipment.
    - ***Procedure***: Peritoneal dialysis works on the same principle as haemodialysis, allowing the diffusion of toxins from mesenteric capillaries across the peritoneal membrane into the dialysate dwelling in the peritoneal cavity. It involves the placing of a stylet catheter at the bedside under local anaesthesia, or the surgical insertion of a Tenckhoff catheter in the abdomen. Dialysate fluid is instilled, and 1–2 L is exchanged each hour.
    - ***Complications***:
        - Pain
        - Haemorrhage (from vascular laceration)
        - Perforation of viscera
        - Bacterial peritonitis
        - Arrhythmias
        - Volume depletion/Overload
        - Electrolyte imbalance

4. ***Haemofiltration***

- Haemofiltration is performed similar to haemodialysis except that the blood is pumped through a haemofilter. An arteriovenous pressure difference induces a convective transport of solutes through a hollow fibre flat sheet membrane. This allows a substantial flow of plasma water, and a high permeability to compounds with molecular weight less than 40,000. The procedure can be done intermittently at high ultrafiltrate rates of up to 6 L/hr, or continuously at rates of 100 mL/hr (**Continuous Arterio-Venous Haemofiltration**, or **CAVH**) (**Fig. 8.14**). The latter is preferred in the treatment of poisoning.
    - CAVH is useful in poisoning with aminoglycoside antibiotics, lithium, methanol, ethanol and ethylene glycol.

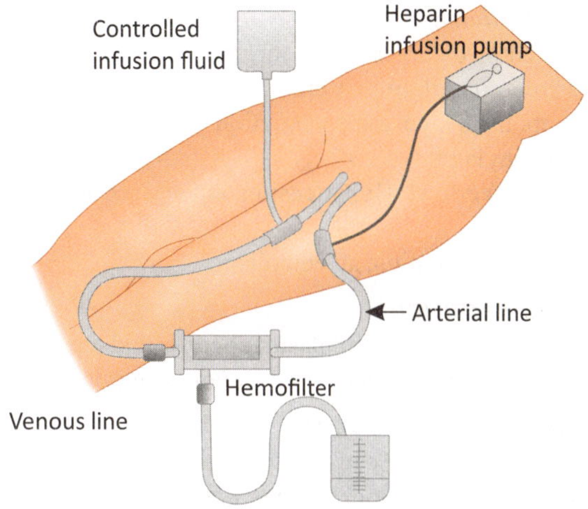

Fig. 8.14 Continuous arterio-venous haemofiltration

5. ***Haemodiafiltration***

- This is a combination of haemofiltration with haemodialysis. It has been undertaken very rarely, and nothing much is known as to its actual advantages, if any.

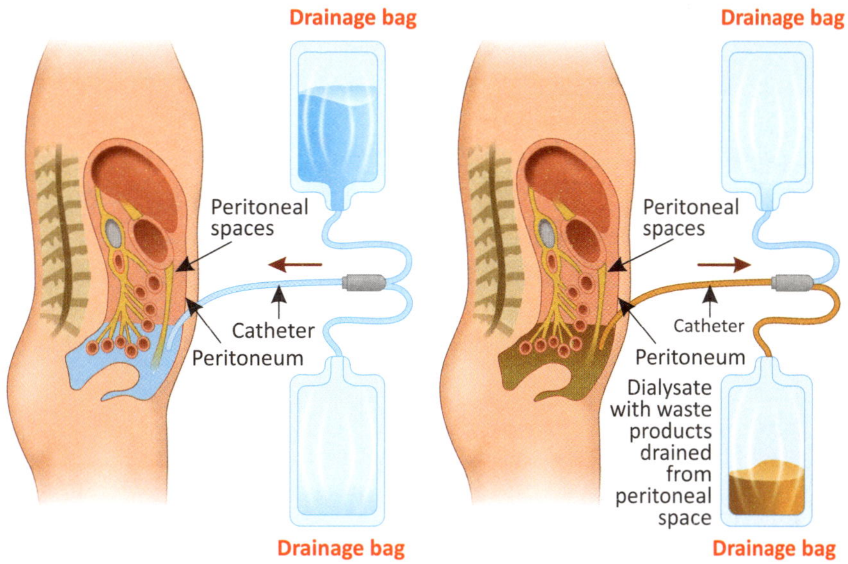

Fig. 8.13 Peritoneal dialysis

6. ***Plasmapheresis* (Fig. 8.15)**

- Plasmapheresis is a technique of separating cellular blood components from plasma. The cells are re-suspended in either colloids, albumin or fresh frozen plasma, and then re-infused.
- It is very effective in eliminating toxic substances but exacts a heavy toll: a part of the patient's plasma proteins is sacrificed in the process.
- Plasmapheresis has been used in cases of overdose with theophylline, carbamazepine, amanita, mercury, hemlock, etc., but serious complications greatly limit its utility.
- ***Complications***:
    - Bleeding disorders: DIC, thrombocytopenia
    - Hypercoagulation: Cerebral thrombosis, pulmonary embolism, myocardial infarction
    - Anaphylaxis
    - Fluid overload: Hypertension, congestive heart failure
    - Infection
    - Vessel perforation, air embolism.

7. ***Plasma Perfusion***

- This is a combination of plasmapheresis and haemoperfusion, and has rarely been used in poisoning.

8. ***Cardiopulmonary Bypass***

- This is another rarely used experimental procedure in the treatment of poisoning, and has been shown to be useful in certain cases of overdose involving cardiac depressants such as verapamil and lidocaine.

9. ***Extracorporeal Membrane Oxygenation (ECMO)*** **(Fig. 8.16)**

- Extracorporeal Membrane Oxygenation (ECMO) is an extracorporeal technique of providing prolonged cardiac and respiratory support to persons whose heart and lungs are unable to provide an adequate amount of gas exchange or perfusion to sustain life. The technology for ECMO is largely derived from cardiopulmonary bypass, which provides shorter-term support with arrested native circulation.
- The device used is a membrane oxygenator, also known as an artificial lung.
- ECMO works by temporarily drawing blood from the body to allow artificial oxygenation of the red blood cells and removal of carbon dioxide. Generally, it is used either post-cardiopulmonary bypass or in late-stage treatment of a person with profound heart and/or lung failure, although it is now seeing use as a treatment for cardiac arrest in certain centres, allowing treatment of the underlying cause of arrest while circulation and oxygenation are supported.
- Poisoning may lead to respiratory failure, shock, cardiac arrest or death. ECMO may be used to provide circulatory

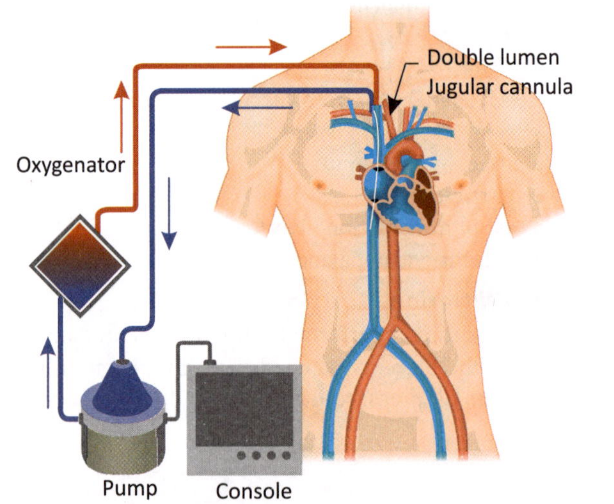

Fig. 8.16 Extracorporeal membrane oxygenation

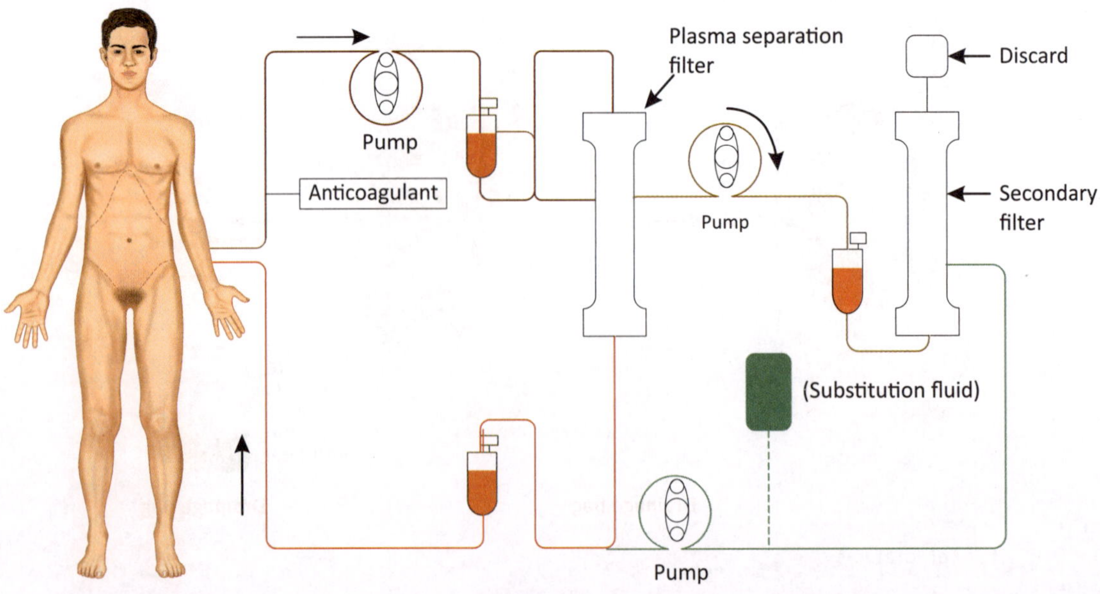

Fig. 8.15 Plasmapheresis

support, termed venoarterial (VA) ECMO; or respiratory support, termed venovenous (VV) ECMO.

- The use of ECMO in poisoned patients is significantly increasing over time. Poisoned patients treated with ECMO have reduced mortality as compared to those treated without ECMO with similar severity of illness and after adjusted analyses, regardless of the type of ingestion.
- ***Indications***
  - Poisoned patients with refractory cardiogenic shock.
  - Poisoned patients with ARDS/Severe respiratory failure.

10. *Intravenous Lipid Emulsion (ILE) Therapy*

- Intravenous lipid emulsion (ILE) therapy (also known as lipid resuscitation therapy, LRT) is the current recommended treatment for local anaesthetic systemic toxicity (LAST) by professional societies such as the American Society of Regional Anesthesia (ASRA).
- ILE therapy also extrapolates to other lipophilic agents. It has been emerging in emergency rooms and critical care units as potential rescue therapy for many other acute toxicities and poisonings. Researchers have investigated drug classes, including tricyclic antidepressants, calcium channel blockers, beta-blockers, antipsychotics, insecticides and organophosphates. Specific drugs also studied include bupropion, lamotrigine, cocaine and diphenhydramine.
- ***Procedure***:
  - For adults, a rapid 100 mL bolus of 20% lipid emulsion followed by another 200 mL infusion over 20 min is the recommended course.
  - The recommended dosing limit is approximately 12 mL/kg.
  - There are many commercially available 20% IV lipid emulsion preparations. The most prevalent formulations have 100% long-chain fatty acids derived from soybean oil.
- ***Monitoring***:
  - Due to the potential for allergic reactions, monitoring for signs and symptoms, such as dyspnoea, cyanosis or fever, is essential.
  - As lipaemia may occur with ILE, patients require assessment for hypertriglyceridaemia and symptoms of pancreatitis.
  - Lipase levels, liver enzyme tests and bilirubin levels are necessary, if there is a suspicion of acute pancreatitis or acute cholecystitis.

ANTIDOTAL THERAPY OF POISONING

In the majority of cases of acute poisoning, all that is required is **intensive supportive therapy** with attention to all the details mentioned in the preceding pages of this chapter. Specific antidotes are rarely necessary, besides the fact that only a few genuine antidotes exist in actual practice, though there is no denying the dramatic results that can be achieved with some of them in appropriate circumstances. Proper antidotal therapy can be life-saving in some situations.

Antidotes work in any one of a number of ways. Common modes of action are as follows:

1. **Inert complex formation**: Some antidotes interact with the poison to form an inert complex which is then excreted from the body, e.g., chelating agents for heavy metals, Prussian Blue for thallium, specific antibody fragments for digoxin, dicobalt edetate for cyanide, etc.
2. **Accelerated detoxification**: Some antidotes accelerate the detoxification of a poison, e.g., thiosulphate accelerates the conversion of cyanide to non-toxic thiocyanate, acetylcysteine acts as a glutathione substitute which combines with hepatotoxic paracetamol metabolites and detoxifies them.
3. **Reduced toxic conversion**: The best example of this mode of action is provided by ethanol which inhibits the metabolism of methanol to toxic metabolites by competing for the same enzyme (alcohol dehydrogenase).
4. **Receptor site competition**: Some antidotes displace the poison from specific receptor sites, thereby antagonising the effects completely. The best example is provided by naloxone, which antagonizes the effects of opiates at stereo-specific opioid receptor sites.
5. **Receptor site blockade**: This mode of action is best exemplified by atropine which blocks the effects of anticholinesterase agents such as organophosphates at muscarinic receptor sites.
6. **Toxic effect bypass**: An example of this type of antidotal action is provided by the use of 100% oxygen in cyanide poisoning.

Table 8.24 represents a list of **genuine antidotes** recommended in toxicological practice today. In addition, there are certain therapeutic agents which are not antidotes as per the accepted definition, but which through their importance and sometimes specific role in the treatment of poisons, border on the concept of "antidotes." **Table 8.25** represents a list of such **adjunctival antidotes**.

Table 8.26 is a list of substances that were formerly considered as antidotes, but are today considered **obsolete** or **hazardous**, and must not be administered.

> **FM 8.9: Core – Written/Viva Voce**
> - Describe the procedure of:
>   - Intimation of suspicious cases or actual cases of foul play to the police
>   - Maintenance of records
>   - Preservation and despatch of relevant samples for laboratory analysis.

INTIMATION OF SUSPECTED/ACTUAL CASES OF FOUL PLAY TO THE POLICE

1. All suspected homicidal cases must be informed to the police.
2. Attempted suicide has been de-criminalised under the Mental Healthcare Act of 2017, and though Section 309 IPC (attempt to commit suicide) has not yet been taken out of the Indian Penal Code, the attending physician can exercise discretion as to whether the police must be informed

or not. If it is a young child, or a mentally ill person, it is necessary to inform the police. If death occurs, the police must mandatorily be informed.

3. All food poisoning cases emerging from public eateries, hostels, etc., must be informed to the public health authorities.

MEDICOLEGAL DUTIES OF A DOCTOR IN SUSPECTED/ACTUAL POISONING

1. A hospital **cannot deny emergency medical care** to any victim under Article 21 of the Indian Constitution. It cannot deny treatment on the pretext of lack of facilities, and has to provide at least emergency care and then transfer the patient safely (via their ambulance) to the nearest facility. This includes government and private hospitals; it also includes private clinics and nursing homes. They cannot deny a patient emergency treatment on the basis that he/she is unable to pay the required fees, or that there is no close relative to sign for consent issues (consent is overridden in an emergency).
2. If a case of poisoning is indubitably accidental or suicidal in nature, the attending doctor is under no legal obligation to notify the police in case he is working in a private hospital. But if the patient dies, the police has to be informed. Death certificate must not be issued.
3. Doctors working in government hospitals are required to report every case of poisoning regardless of the nature, to the police. But, it is not clear whether this is the actual legal position, or whether it is an 'urban legend'.
4. All cases of homicidal poisoning (definite or suspected) must be compulsorily reported to the police as per Section **39** of the **Criminal Procedure Code (CrPC)**. Failure to do

Table 8.24 Genuine Antidotes

Antidote	Main Indication	Other Applications
Amyl nitrite	Cyanide	Hydrogen sulphide
Antivenom (Snake – Polyvalent)	Snakebite due to common cobra, common krait, Russells viper and saw-scaled viper	Related species of snakes
Ascorbic acid	Organic peroxides (Osmium)	–
Atropine	Organophosphate and carbamate insecticides	Other cholinergic agents
Aurintricarboxylic acid (ATA)	Beryllium	–
Botulinum antitoxin	Botulism	–
Calcium salts (gluconate, chloride)	Oxalates, fluorides, ethylene glycol	Calcium antagonists, hypomagnesaemia
L-Carnitine	Valproic acid	
Desferrioxamine	Iron, aluminium	–
Diazepam	Chloroquine	Organophosphate insecticides
Dicobalt edetate	Cyanide	–
Digoxin specific antibody fragments (Digibind, Digifab)	Digitalis glycosides	Other cardioactive steroids
Dimercaprol	Arsenic	Copper, gold, mercury
4-Dimethylaminophenol (4-DMAP)	Cyanide	Hydrogen sulphide
EDTA (ethylenediamine tetra acetate; calcium disodium edetate or versenate)	Lead	
Ethanol	Methanol, ethylene glycol	–

contd.

Flumazenil	Benzodiazepines	–
Folinic acid (Leucovorin)	Methotrexate, methanol	–
Glucagon	Beta blockers	Calcium channel blockers
Glucose	Insulin	–
Hydroxocobalamine	Cyanide	–
Isoprenaline	Beta blockers	–
Magnesium sulphate (inj)	Cardioactive steroids, hydrofluoric acid	Hypomagnesaemia
Methylene blue	Methaemoglobinaemia	–
4-Methylpyrazole (Fomepizole)	Ethylene glycol, methanol	Disulfiram, coprin
N-Acetylcysteine	Paracetamol	Amanitin, Other causes of liver failure
N-Acetylpenicillamine	Mercury	–
Naloxone	Opiates	Clonidine
Neostigmine	Peripheral anticholinergics	–
Octreotide	Oral hypoglycaemics	
Oximes	Organophosphates	–
Oxygen	Cyanide, carbon monoxide, hydrogen sulphide	–
Oxygen (Hyperbaric)	Carbon monoxide	Cyanide, hydrogen sulphide, carbon tetrachloride
Penicillamine	Copper	Gold, lead, mercury
Pentetic acid (DTPA)	Radioactive metals	–
Phentolamine	Alpha adrenergics	MAOI interactions, cocaine, adrenaline(epinephrine), ergot alkaloids
Physostigmine	Central anticholinergics	–
Phytomenadione (Vitamin K_1)	Coumarin derivatives (esp warfarin)	Anticoagulant rodenticides (bromadiolone)
Potassium ferric hexacyanoferrate (Prussian Blue)	Thallium	–
Propranolol	Beta adrenergics	–
Protamine sulphate	Heparin	–
Pyridoxine (Vit B_6)	Isoniazid	Ethylene glycol, gyrometrine, hydrazine
Sodium nitrite	Cyanide	Hydrogen sulphide
Sodium thiosulphate	Cyanide	Bromate, chlorate, iodine
Succimer (DMSA)	Lead, mercury	Arsenic
Unithiol (DMPS)	Arsenic	Copper, nickel, lead, cadmium, mercury

Table 8.25 Adjunctival Antidotes

Agent	Indication
Activated charcoal	For most poisons (*Refer **Table 8.22***)
Corticosteroids	Acute allergic reaction, laryngeal oedema
Diazepam	Poisons causing convulsions
Epinephrine (Adrenaline)	Anaphylactic shock, cardiac arrest
Furosemide	Fluid retention, left ventricular failure
Glucose	Poisons causing hypoglycaemia
Haloperidol	Poisons causing psychotic states
Heparin	Hypercoagulability
Lidocaine (Lignocaine)	Ventricular arrhythmias
Mannitol	Cerebral oedema, fluid retention
Salbutamol	Bronchoconstriction
Sodium bicarbonate	Metabolic acidosis

Table 8.26 Obsolete Antidotes

Agent	Indication
Copper sulphate	Phosphorus
Cysteamine	Paracetamol
Diethyldithiocarbamate	Thallium
Fructose	Ethanol
Levallorphan	Opiates
Nalorphine	Opiates
Silibinin	Amanitin
Tocopherol	Paraquat
Universal antidote	Ingested poisons

so will make him culpable under Section **176** of the **Indian Penal Code (IPC)**.

5. If the police require information on any case of poisoning which is either suicidal or homicidal in nature, the attending doctor has to divulge it. There is no scope for professional secrecy in such matters (**175 CrPC**). If information is witheld or wrong information is provided, the doctor becomes culpable under Sections **202** and **193 IPC**, respectively.
6. Every effort must be made by the attending doctor to collect and preserve evidence suggestive of poisoning. Deliberate omission to do so can attract punishment under Section **201 IPC**.
7. Collect vomitus, faeces, stomach washings, contaminated food, incriminating substance, etc., and despatch the same for chemical analysis to the nearest *Forensic Science Laboratory*. **Stomach wash is not mandatory, and must be done only if the attending physician is convinced that it will be of benefit to the patient**. Police manuals must not be used as a basis to decide whether to perform stomach wash or not in a case of poisoning, even if it is homicidal in nature. The life and health of a patient is supreme, and nothing must be done that can be potentially harmful, only because it is mentioned in a police manual. If the attending physician is of the opinion that performing an invasive, hazardous procedure such as stomach wash is not going to be beneficial to the patient in a particular case, he must NOT undertake it only to satisfy the police or the court.
8. If a poisoned patient is conscious but on the verge of death, record a dying declaration relating to the circumstances. It is preferable to call a magistrate for this purpose, but if death appears imminent, or if there is likelihood of delay in the arrival of the magistrate, the attending doctor must himself record the declaration as per Section **32**, Clause **1**, of the **Indian Evidence Act (IEA)**. Even when a declaration is taken down by a magistrate, the presence of a doctor is desirable to certify that the dying victim was in possession of his senses, and there was no clouding of judgement or coherence which is sometimes encountered in the final moments before death.
9. If a patient dies before the exact diagnosis could be made out, or he was brought dead to the hospital, the duty doctor must notify the police who will in all probability order an autopsy to be done. Death certificate must not be issued.
10. Relevant viscera/body fluids must be preserved for chemical analysis during the autopsy of a suspected poisoning victim (*refer **Topic 8.5**, page no. 385*).
11. Detailed written records should be made with respect to every case of poisoning and kept in safe custody. The minimum period of preservation of medicolegal case records in a hospital is controversial. Kerala Government has mandated that all medicolegal case records in Govt hospitals must be preserved for a minimum period of 15 years (except drunkenness cases in which case the minimum period is 10 years).*

Source: As per GO.(MS.) No. 06/2014/H&FWD dated 03.01.2014, issued by Health and Family Welfare Dept, Govt of Kerala.*

12. As per clause 1.3 of **Code of Medical Ethics Regulations 2002** (amended 2016) issued by the National Medical Commission, the following points must be borne in mind relating to maintenance of medical records:
    a. Every physician shall maintain the medical records pertaining to his/her indoor patients for a period of 3 years from the date of commencement of the treatment in a standard proforma.
    b. If any request is made for medical records either by the patients/authorised attendant or legal authorities involved, the same may be duly acknowledged and documents shall be issued within a period of 72 hrs.
    c. A Registered Medical Practitioner shall maintain a Register of Medical Certificates giving full details of certificates issued. When issuing a medical certificate he/she shall always enter the identification marks of the patient and keep a copy of the certificate. He/She shall not omit to record the signature and/or thumb mark, address and at least one identification mark of the patient on the medical certificate or report.
    d. Efforts shall be made to computerize medical records for quick retrieval.
13. If a doctor comes across a case of food poisoning from a public eatery (canteen, café, restaurant, etc.), he must notify the **public health authority** concerned.
14. All snakebite cases, as well as other types of envenomations, must be made medicolegal, and if death occurs, the police must be informed. This is because in many Indian states, compensation is paid to the next of kin. Also, some cases may actually be due to foul play (**Box 8.5**).

Box 8.5—Uthra Murder Case: Homicide with Snake

Uthra was a disabled young housewife who had been married for 2 years, and was the mother of a 1-year-old son. At the time of the incident, Uthra was recovering from a previous Russell's viper bite, sustained on 2nd March 2020, 2 months ago at her husband's home near Adoor (Kerala), and she was making a slow recovery in her parents' home. She was found unconscious in her bedroom when her mother came to call her on the morning of 07th May. It appeared that she had been bitten by yet another snake during the previous night! Uthra died soon thereafter. A large Indian cobra was found in the bedroom that she shared with her husband (Sooraj Kumar).

According to Uthra's mother, her daughter and Sooraj went to bed after dinner. The next morning Sooraj, usually a late riser, woke up unusually early and went outside. However, Uthra did not wake up at her usual time. Her mother went into her room and found Uthra unconscious. Later, the room was searched, and the cobra was discovered and killed.

One week after his daughter's death, Uthra's father, contacted police, stating that he suspected foul play in his daughter's death. Uthra had already informed her parents about Sooraj Kumar's expertise in handling venomous snakes. Approximately 2 months prior to her death from the cobra bite, Uthra had been bitten by a Russell's viper. The combination of the two incidents caused police to suspect Sooraj Kumar's involvement in this case.

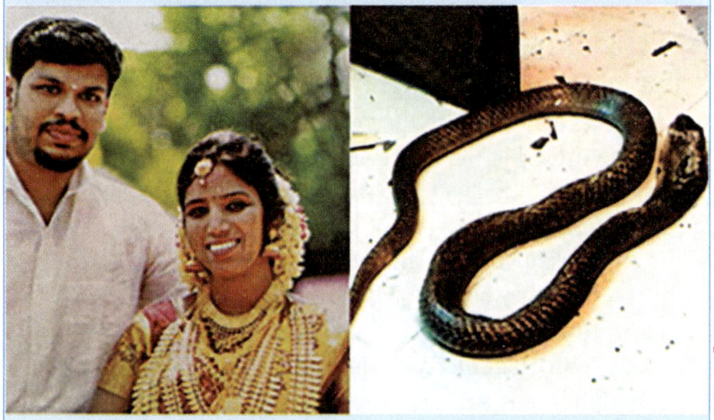

Fig. 8.17: (From left) Sooraj; Uthra; Killed cobra

The police arrested Sooraj, as the prime suspect, and a snake catcher Suresh Kumar, as a second suspect in the case. On 12th July 2020, Sooraj made a public confession about the murder. He stated that he bought two snakes from Suresh Kumar. According to the police, Sooraj admitted that he gave sleeping pills to his wife in order to sedate her before releasing the snake. He confessed that he had starved the cobra for 11 days to ensure that the cobra would bite his wife. The snake "was kept in a bottle without being fed".

Sooraj was booked under various sections of the Indian Penal Code for murder and destruction of evidence.

During the course of the investigation, it was discovered that gold from Uthra's bank locker had been removed on 2nd March, the date of her first snakebite. In early June 2020, Uthra's father-in-law was arrested, on charges of destroying evidence and hiding 38 sovereign of gold jewellery. In Aug 2020, both the mother and sister of Sooraj, were also arrested on charges of conspiracy, domestic violence and destruction of evidence. Although Suresh Kumar was originally one of the accused, he became an approver subsequently.

Sooraj was found guilty of using a live snake to kill his wife. On 13th Oct 2021, he was sentenced to 17 years imprisonment plus two consecutive life sentences, and an additional penalty of 5 lakh rupees.

FM 8.10: Core – Written/Viva Voce
- Describe:
  - The General Principles of Analytical Toxicology
- Give a brief description of analytical methods available for toxicological analysis:
  - Chromatography:
    - Thin Layer Chromatography
    - Gas Chromatography
    - Liquid Chromatography
  - Atomic Absorption Spectroscopy

GENERAL PRINCIPLES OF ANALYTICAL TOXICOLOGY

- An analytical (toxicology) laboratory has become a vital adjunct to the proper management of poisoned patients.

However, it is to be noted that the cornerstone of the management of such patients – *intensive supportive therapy* – is mostly independent of the kind of poison implicated, and hence routine employment of expensive analytical techniques should be avoided. The attending physician must be judicious in calling for necessary investigations, and exercise discretion in the choice of tests to be done.

- At the time that the IV catheter is inserted, blood samples for glucose, electrolytes, BUN, a CBC and any indicated toxicologic analysis can be drawn.
- If the patient has an altered mental status, the attending physician may be tempted to send blood and urine specimens to identify any CNS depressants or drugs of abuse, along with other medications, but the indiscriminate ordering of these tests rarely provides clinically useful information.
- For the potentially suicidal patient, a paracetamol concentration should be routinely requested, along with tests affecting the management of any specific xenobiotic such as carbon monoxide, lithium, theophylline, iron, salicylates, and digoxin (or other cardioactive steroids), as suggested by history, physical examination or bedside diagnostic tests.
- In the vast majority of cases, the blood tests that are most useful in diagnosing toxicologic emergencies are not the toxicologic assays but the "non-toxicological" routine metabolic profile tests such as BUN, glucose, electrolytes and ABGs or venous blood gases (VBGs).
- Potential indications for seeking the help of a toxicology laboratory are as follows:
    - **P**rognosis – to assess the outcome of a case of poisoning
    - **R**esearch – into toxicokinetics and mechanisms of toxicity
    - **O**rder – from court, or law enforcement officer
    - **M**onitoring – of treatment measures and their efficacy
    - **I**dentification – of the nature of poison
    - **S**everity – to assess the seriousness of a given case
    - **E**xclusion – or confirmation of toxic exposure

All the **7** indications mentioned can be remembered by the mnemonic **PROMISE**.

- Treatment of a poisoning case can be categorised into **4** groups with respect to toxicological evaluations:
    - ***Toxicity correlates very well with serum levels, and specific drug therapy can be instituted***, e.g., digoxin, ethylene glycol, lithium, methanol, paracetamol, salicylates, theophylline.
    - ***Toxicity correlates closely with serum level, but only non-specific care is required***, e.g., barbiturates, ethanol, phenytoin.
    - ***Toxicologic testing only serves to confirm fairly clear-cut clinical parameters of poisoning***, e.g., cyanide, narcotics, organophosphates, tricyclics.
    - ***Toxicity correlates poorly with serum level, and only non-specific care is required***, e.g., amphetamines, benzodiazepines, cocaine, neuroleptics.
- In fact, most poisoned patients can be treated successfully without any contribution from the laboratory other than routine clinical biochemistry and haematology. This is particularly true when there is no doubt about the poison involved, and when the results of a quantitative analysis would not significantly affect therapy.
- In those cases where an analytical toxicological investigation is deemed beneficial, an orderly progression is desirable in the performance of necessary tests and their interpretation **(Table 8.27)**.

COMMON ANALYTICAL METHODS FOR TOXICOLOGICAL ANALYSIS

A. Thin Layer Chromatography (TLC) (Fig. 8.18)

- This is a **qualitative technique** which involves the movement by capillary action of a liquid phase (usually an organic solvent) through a thin, uniform layer of stationary phase (usually silica gel) held on a rigid support (usually a glass, aluminium or plastic sheet).
- Compounds are separated by partition between the **mobile** and **stationary phases**.
- A very thin layer of silica gel or aluminium oxide is applied to a glass plate 20 cm × 20 cm × 0.5 cm, and vertical lines are drawn 1.5 cm apart to allow individual runways for each sample.
- Purified tissue extracts dissolved in 0.5 mL of methanol are serially spotted with a micropipette and dried in a small circle in the lower centre of a runway 1.5 cm from the bottom.
- Other samples are similarly spotted in other runways.
- A horizontal line (stop point) is drawn 10 or 15 cm above these starting points.
- A TLC tank is filled with suitable developing solvents to a depth of about 1 cm from the bottom. The plate properly

Table 8.27 Phases of Analytical Toxicological Investigation

Pre-analytical Phase	Analytical Phase
1. Obtain details of current admission, including circumstantial evidence of poisoning, and results of biochemical and haematological investigations. 2. Obtain patient's medical history, and decide the priorities for analysis.	1. Interpret the results and discuss them with the clinician looking after the patient. 2. Perform additional analyses, if indicated.

spotted is then dipped into the solvent, the lid is firmly closed and the atmosphere is allowed to saturate with vapour.

- When the solvent front just touches the 10 cm horizontal mark, quickly remove the plate and examine under UV light (at 254 nm and 366 nm) for characteristic fluorescence or absorbance.
- This can also be done after spraying the plate with appropriate reagents to bring out characteristic colour spots. This widens the scope of the analysis and increases the confidence of identification.
- Calculate the Rf value:

$$\text{Rf value is the ratio of } \frac{\text{Solute front}}{\text{Solvent front}} \times 100$$

- TLC is a simple, inexpensive technique which is widely used.
- It takes only about 2 hrs from beginning to completion.
- It is also a very versatile method, since the order of separation of compounds can be altered simply by changing the nature of the developing agent.
- However, interpretation of the plates can prove difficult and calls for a trained eye with considerable experience in recognising colours, spot shapes and metabolite patterns.
- It is also well known that TLC can produce false positive results because of interference between xenobiotics. It is always desirable to confirm results by more sophisticated methods, especially in forensic cases.

B. Ultraviolet Spectrophotometry (Fig. 8.19)

- This **quantitative technique** is based on the principle that many drugs when in solution will absorb UV radiation. The degree of absorption depends on the chemical structure of the drug, its concentration in the solution and the wavelength of the UVR.
- The functioning of this instrument is relatively straightforward. A beam of light from a visible and/or UV light source is separated into its component wavelengths by a prism or diffraction grating.
- The monochromator can select from the light source an ultraviolet ray of any given wavelength ranging from 200 to 340 nm.

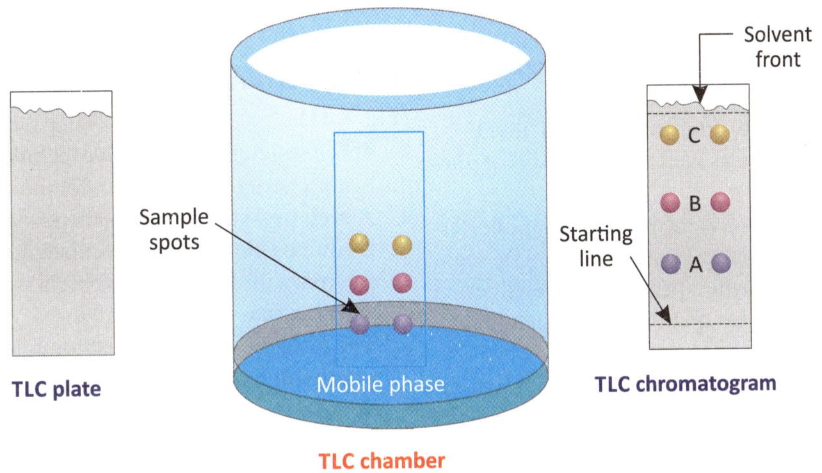

Fig. 8.18 Thin layer chromatography (TLC)

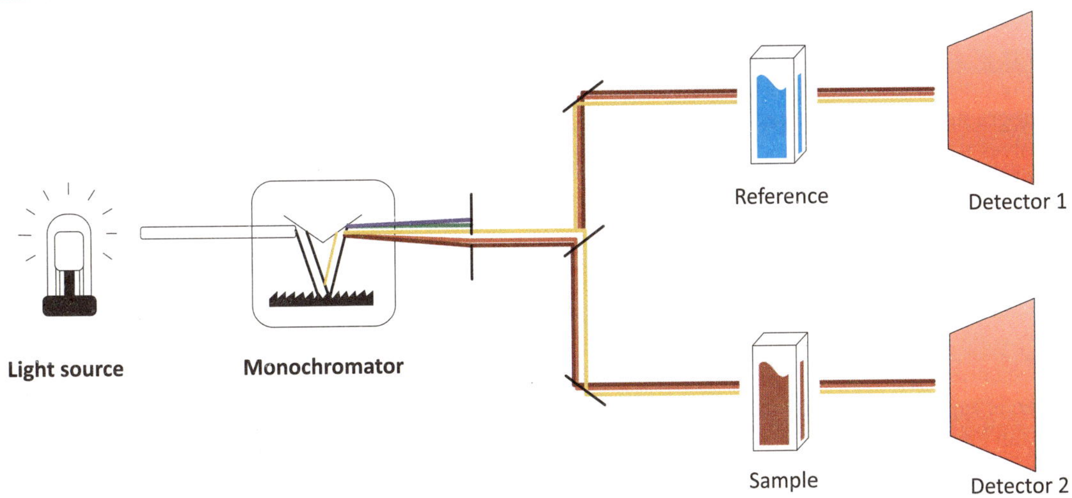

Fig. 8.19 UV-Visible Spectrophotometer

- The sample extract in aqueous medium is placed in a transparent quartz cuvette in the path of the radiation.
- Each monochromatic (single wavelength) beam in turn is split into two equal intensity beams by a half-mirrored device.
  - One beam, the sample beam passes through a small transparent container (cuvette) containing a solution of the compound being studied in a transparent solvent.
  - The other beam, the reference, passes through an identical cuvette containing only the solvent.
  - The intensities of these light beams are then measured by electronic detectors and compared.
- The amount of UV radiation which passes through the solution is measured by the photocell. By steady rotation of the monochromator, it is possible to pass sequentially UV rays of all wavelength from 200 to 340 nm through the extract.
- The photocell monitors the amount of radiation absorbed at each wavelength and this is transcribed on to a recorder chart.
- The shape of the spectrum, the wavelength at which absorption is at a maximum, and any changes brought about by changing the pH of the extract are all used as an aid to characterise the agent present.
- This technique is ideal to quantitate **blood levels** of **paracetamol** and **salicylates**, as well as **urine levels** of **phenothiazines**.
- A major disadvantage of UVS is the possibility of interference in multiple drug overdose. In such a case, UV scanning can produce a composite spectrum of bewildering complexity from which neither qualitative nor quantitative information can be derived.
- Conventional spectrophotometric methods are known for producing false positive results which can be disastrous in medicolegal cases.

C. Gas Chromatography (GC) (Fig. 8.20)

- This is a more sophisticated **quantitative technique** and has found great favour with analytical toxicologists since it offers a way of simultaneously separating, identifying, and measuring drugs and other organic poisons.
- Gas chromatography – specifically gas–liquid chromatography – involves a sample being vapourised and injected onto the head of the chromatographic column.
- The sample is transported through the column by the flow of inert, gaseous mobile phase.
- The column itself contains a liquid stationary phase which is adsorbed onto the surface of an inert solid.
- The liquid or solid specimen dissolved in a solvent is injected into the chromatograph.
- The specimen is vapourised by heat and is carried through a **column** by an inert **carrier gas** (usually nitrogen).
- The column is packed with a substance like carbowax or adiponitrile which is capable of changing the migration time of the specimen as it traverses the column.
- A **detector** recognises the presence of the chemical and graphically plots its emergence as a function of time. The **retention time** and **peak area** for a chemical compared to known standard are used to identify and to quantitate its presence. There are many detectors which can be used in gas chromatography. Different detectors will give different types of selectivity.
- The most common means of detecting the compounds is by **flame ionization**. On leaving the column, the inert gas is mixed with hydrogen and either air or oxygen, and the mixture is ignited to give a continuous jet of flame. It is decomposed into electrically charged fragments which are collected at an electrode. This results in an electrical signal which is amplified and transmitted to a pen recorder operating at a constant chart speed. This peak is transcribed each time a compound emerges from the column.
- **Flame ionization detectors (FIDs)** are mass sensitive rather than concentration sensitive; this gives the advantage that changes in mobile phase flow rate do not affect the detector's response.
- GC is most commonly employed to **quantitate blood levels of volatile liquids such as ethanol, ethylene glycol and methanol.**

D. High Performance Liquid Chromatography (HPLC) (Fig. 8.21)

- This is a similar **quantitative technique** as GC, except that it is not restricted to volatile compounds.
- A **high pressure** (1000–6000 pound per square inch) pump facilitates movement of the specimen through the columns packed with chromatographic adsorbents, e.g., silica gel and alumina.
- The effluent stream passes through a **detector**, usually an **ultraviolet spectrophotometer**, and the appearance of a drug in the solvent is signalled by a recorder peak in the same way as in GC. Again, the size of the peak is proportional to the concentration of drug in the sample.
- HPLC can be used to **separate and analyse complex mixtures**.
- In order to identify any compound by HPLC a **detector** must first be selected. Once the detector is selected and is set to optimal detection settings, a separation assay must be developed. The parameters of this assay should be such that a clean peak of the known sample is observed from the chromatograph. The identifying peak should have a reasonable retention time and should be well separated from extraneous peaks at the detection levels at which the assay will be performed.
- Identifying a compound by HPLC is accomplished by researching the literature and by trial and error. A sample of a known compound must be utilized in order to assure identification of the unknown compound. Identification of compounds can be assured by combining two or more detection methods.
- **Quantification** of compounds by HPLC is the process of determining the unknown concentration of a compound in

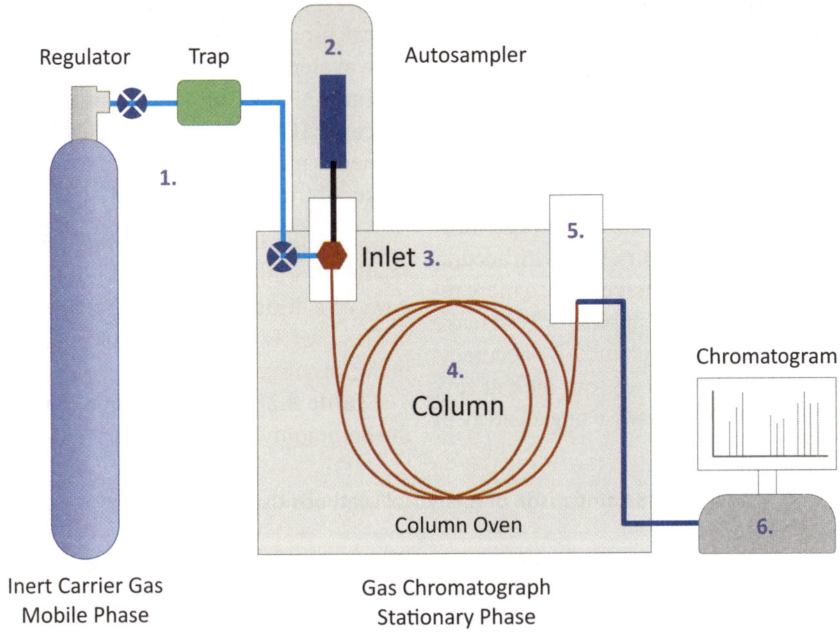

Fig. 8.20 Gas chromatography

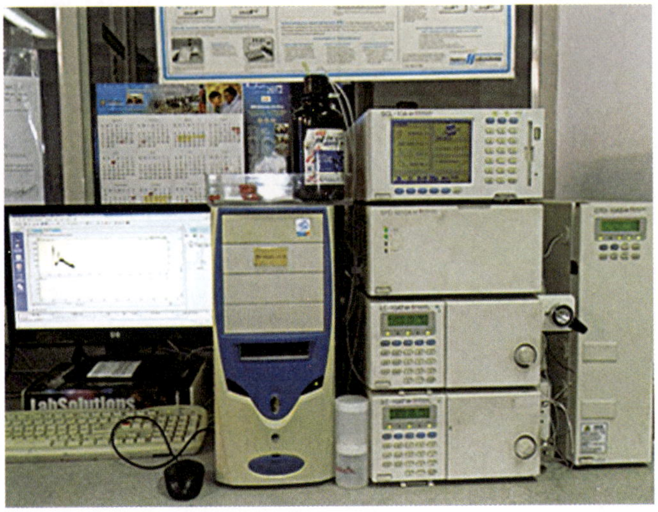

Fig. 8.21 HPLC System (*Courtesy*: *Dr Ramakrishnan UK*)

a known solution. It involves injecting a series of known concentrations of the standard compound solution onto the HPLC for detection. The chromatograph of these known concentrations will give a series of peaks that correlate to the concentration of the compound injected.

Note:

- If a **Mass Spectrometer** is combined with **Gas Chromatography (GC–MS)**, it is considered to be the **best technique for quantitative analysis of a wide variety of chemicals**, but its expense (capital as well as operational costs) greatly restricts its use.
- A **Mass Spectrometer** can also be connected to a **Liquid Chromatograph** (**LC–MS**) for detection of **non-volatile compounds**.
- **Tandem Mass Spectrometry** consists of double mass spectrometers connected to gas chromatograph (**GC–MS–MS**) or liquid chromatograph (**LC–MS–MS**). These are very costly and sophisticated instruments that can refine chemical analysis to almost flawless degree.

E. Atomic Absorption Spectrophotometry (AAS) (Fig. 8.22)

- This is one of the **best methods** for detecting **heavy metals** (arsenic, lead, mercury, thallium, etc.) in blood and other body fluid samples.
- The blood sample is introduced into a high temperature **oxyacetylene flame** situated in the path of a beam of **radiation**. The organic matrix is combusted and the metal forms a cloud of atoms which absorbs a fraction of the radiation in proportion to the concentration of metal in the sample.
- Light of a suitable wavelength for a particular element is shone through the flame, and some of this light is absorbed by the atoms of the sample. The amount of light absorbed is proportional to the concentration of the element in the solution, and hence in the original object.

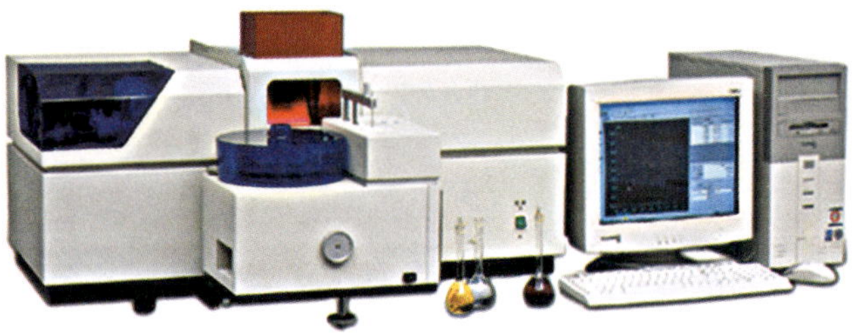

Fig. 8.22 Atomic absorption spectrophotometer

- Measurements are made separately for each element of interest in turn to achieve a complete analysis of an object, and thus the technique is relatively **slow** to use.
- However, it is **very sensitive** and it can measure trace elements down to the part per million level, as well as being able to measure elements present in minor and major amounts.
- **Flame AAS** technique is the oldest method, and can measure parts-per-million element concentrations with accuracies in the 1–3% range. **Graphite furnace AAS**, a more recent development, uses much smaller samples, and can make parts-per-billion measurements with about 20% accuracy. The newest technique, **diode laser AAS**, can look at several elements in a sample simultaneously using an array of lasers that emit various wavelengths of light. A mathematical process is then used to separate the mixture of light wavelengths that reaches the detector.
- **Inductively Coupled Plasma Atomic Emission Spectroscopy (ICP-AES)** is a new development that allows simultaneous multi-element analysis. Several metals can be measured from a single sample.

Other methodologies used in analytical toxicology include **Radio Immuno Assay** (**RIA**) and **Enzyme Mediated Immuno Assay Technique** (**EMIT**). These methods are not mentioned in the new CBME-based MBBS curriculum, and hence are not being discussed here.

Table 8.28 gives the comparative status of efficiency of the commonly used laboratory techniques in toxicology.

Table 8.28 Comparison of Analytical Methods Used in Toxicology

Method	Specificity	Sensitivity	Speed
Thin Layer Chromatography	+ +	+ +	+ +
Gas-Liquid Chromatography	+ + +	+ + +	+
High Performance Liquid Chromatography	+ + +	+ + +	+
Spectrophotometry	+	+ +	+ + +
Gas Chromatography–Mass Spectrometry	+ + + +	+ + + +	+
Immunology (RIA, EMIT)	+ + +	+ + +	+ + + +

Topic 9

CHEMICAL TOXICOLOGY

(Number of Competencies – 6: FM 9.1 to 9.6)

Teachers and students, please note:

- Topics 9–13 deal with specific categories of poisons with regard to clinical features, diagnosis and management, upon exposure to them. It is to be noted that except for Topic 13, the ***new curriculum does not mention medicolegal aspects at all!*** So, it is a moot point whether students can be assessed on these aspects.
- However, as the editor feels it is important, this book lists medicolegal aspects too (under 'Forensic Issues') for all the poisons.
- Also, there is always a possibility of a revised (corrected) curriculum being released incorporating medicolegal aspects, anytime in the future. So, it is better to be prepared!

FM 9.1: Core – Written/Viva Voce/ Objective Structured Clinical Examination (OSCE)

- Describe general principles and basic methodologies in treatment of poisoning: decontamination, supportive therapy, antidote therapy, procedures of enhanced elimination with regard to:
  - Caustics
    - Inorganic – Sulphuric, nitric and hydrochloric acids
    - Organic – Carbolic acid (phenol), oxalic and acetyl salicylic acid

CAUSTICS

- The term **caustic*** is often mistakenly presumed to denote an alkali, while actually it has a much broader meaning and refers to any substance which is **corrosive** and burning in nature. Obviously this would include apart from alkalis, the more important group comprising acids (inorganic and organic).
- **Table 9.1** lists the common caustic substances encountered in toxicological practice.

A. Acids

- Acids are hydrogen containing substances that on dissociation in water produce hydronium ions. They are potent desiccants with the ability to produce coagulation necrosis of tissues on contact.**
- When a strong acid (especially inorganic) is dissolved in a solvent, an exothermic reaction ensues resulting in the emanation of heat which is referred to as the **heat of solution**. This should be differentiated from the **heat of neutralisation** which occurs when an acid is neutralised by any alkali (or vice versa). It is also an exothermic reaction.
- While generally speaking, the lower the pH of an acid the higher is its corrosive effect, it is not the pH alone which is the determinant of severity. For instance, lemon juice which has a very low pH of 2 is not corrosive in nature at all! More important determinants include molarity, concentration, and complexing affinity for hydroxyl ions.

I. *Inorganic Acids*

1. Sulphuric Acid (Sulfuric Acid)

Table 9.1 Common Caustics (Corrosives)

Acids		Alkalis	Others
Inorganic (Mineral)	**Organic**		
Boric	Acetic	Ammonia	Hydrogen peroxide
Chromic	Carbolic	Calcium hydroxide	Iodine
Hydrochloric	Citric	Potassium carbonate	Potassium permanganate
Nitric	Formic	Potassium hydroxide	Quaternary ammonium compounds
Phosphoric	Oxalic	Sodium carbonate	
Sulphuric		Sodium hydroxide	

****Note***: *Derived from the Greek word "Kaustikos" which means "capable of burning."*

*****Note***: *Hydrofluoric acid is a prominent exception, since it produces liquefactive necrosis.*

Synonyms

- Oil of vitriol; Oleum; Battery acid; Hydrogen sulphate

Molecular Formula

- H_2SO_4

Physical Appearance

- **Sulphuric acid** is a heavy, oily, colourless, odourless, non-fuming liquid (**Fig. 9.1**).
  - Pure sulphuric acid does not occur naturally due to its strong affinity to water vapour; it is **hygroscopic** and readily absorbs water vapour from the air.
- When mixed with water, sulphuric acid reacts violently, giving off intense heat.
- There are two main forms:
  - Commercial concentrated sulphuric acid is usually a 93–98% solution in water.
  - **Fuming sulphuric acid** is a solution of sulphur trioxide in sulphuric acid. It is also called "**Oleum**" or "**Disulphuric acid**".

Uses/Sources

- Storage batteries utilise sulphuric acid as an electrolyte.
- Sulphuric acid is also used in the leather, fur, food processing, wool and uranium industries, for gas drying and as a laboratory reagent.
- Sulphuric acid can be formed in smog from the photochemical oxidation of sulphur dioxide to sulphur trioxide and subsequent reaction with water. It is a major component of acid rain.

Usual Fatal Dose

- 20–30 mL of conc. sulphuric acid.

Toxicokinetics

- Systemic absorption of sulphuric acid is negligible.

Mode of Action

- Produces coagulation necrosis of tissues on contact.

Clinical Features

1. Burning pain from the mouth to the stomach. Abdominal pain is often severe. Paradoxically, patients with severe acid injury may lack abdominal pain or even abdominal tenderness.
2. Intense thirst. However, attempts at drinking water usually provoke retching.
3. Vomiting: The vomitus is brownish or blackish in colour due to altered blood (**coffee ground vomit**), and may contain shreds of the charred wall of the stomach.
4. If there is coincidental damage to the larynx during swallowing or due to regurtitation, there may be dysphonia, dysphagia and dyspnoea.
5. Tongue is usually swollen, and blackish or brownish in colour. Teeth become chalky white. There may be constant drooling of saliva which is indicative of oesophageal injury.
6. There is often acid spillage while swallowing with consequent corrosion of the skin of the face (especially around the mouth) (**Fig. 9.2**), neck and chest. Burnt skin appears dark brown or black.
7. Features of generalised shock are usually apparent.
8. Renal failure and decreased urine output can occur after several hours of uncorrected circulatory collapse.
9. Because it is a strong acid, exposure to sulphuric acid may produce metabolic acidosis, particularly following ingestion. Acidosis may be due to severe tissue burns and shock, as well as absorption of acid.
10. Rarely, corrosion of duodenum (or even further down the small intestine) may occur (**Fig. 9.3**). If perforation of stomach occurs, a severe form of chemical peritonitis can result.
11. If the patient recovers, there are usually long-term sequelae such as stricture formation which may lead to pyloric obstruction, antral stenosis or an hour glass deformity of the stomach. The oesophagus may also be involved resulting in stenosis. There are indications of increased propensity for carcinomas.

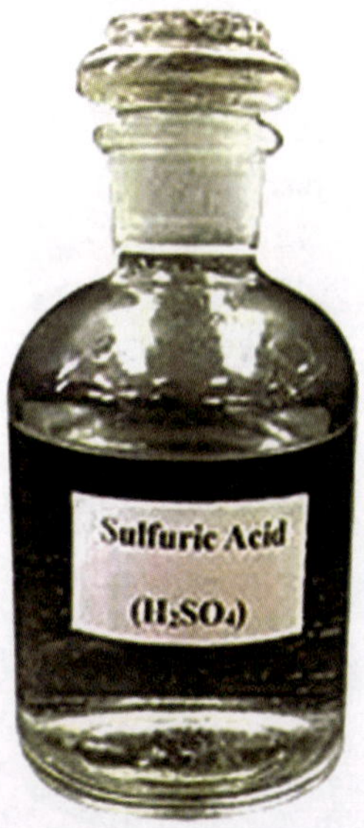

Fig. 9.1 Sulphuric acid

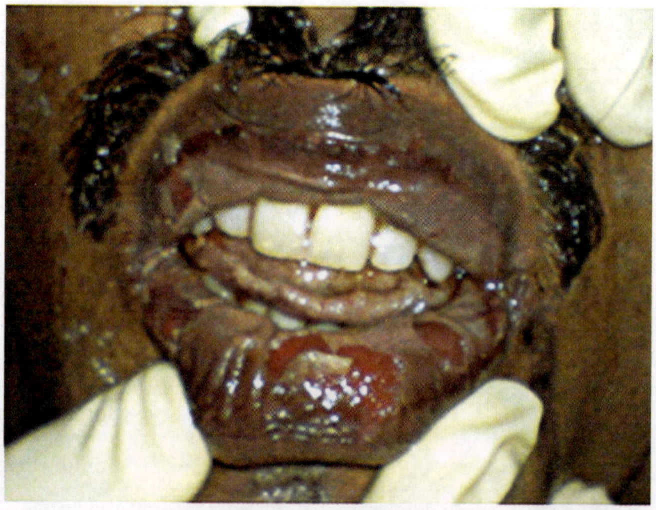

Fig. 9.2 Erosion and ulceration of lips – Sulphuric acid ingestion (*Courtesy*: *Dr Prateek Rastogi*)

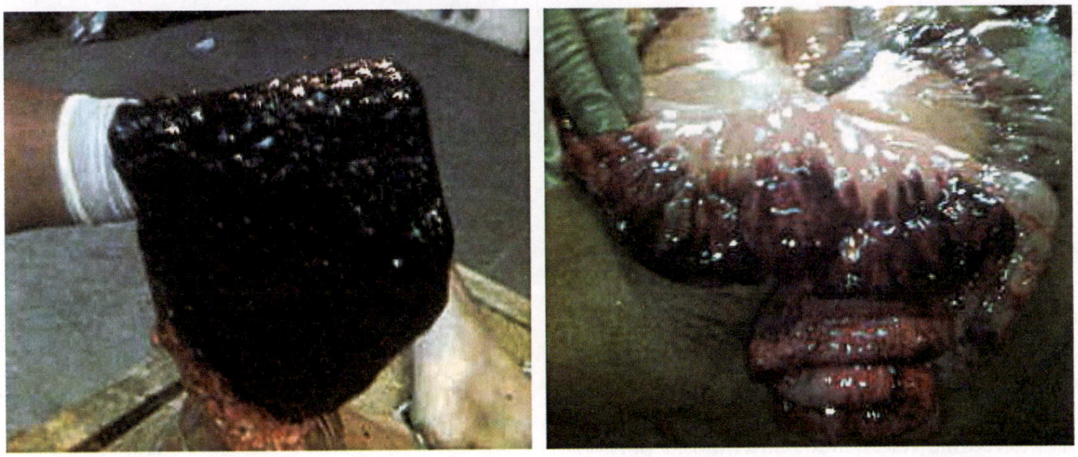

Fig. 9.3 Corrosion of stomach and intestine – Sulphuric acid ingestion *(Courtesy: Dr Puneet Arora)*

12. Contact with the eyes can cause severe injury including conjunctivitis, periorbital oedema, corneal oedema and ulceration, necrotising keratitis and iridocyclitis.
13. ***Chronic Exposure***:
    a. Occupational exposure to sulphuric acid mist can cause erosion of teeth over a period of time, as also increased incidence of upper respiratory infections.
    b. Case reports suggest that chronic exposure to sulphuric acid fumes may be linked to carcinoma of the vocal cords, as well as nasopharyngeal and laryngeal cancer.

Diagnosis

- **Litmus test**: The pH of the saliva can be tested with a litmus paper to determine whether the chemical ingested is an acid or an alkali (turns red in acid, and blue in alkaline solution).*
- Fresh stains in clothing may be tested by adding a few drops of sodium carbonate. Production of effervescence (bubbles) is indicative of an acid stain.
- If vomitus or stomach contents are available, add 10% barium chloride. A heavy white precipitate forms which is insoluble on adding 1 mL nitric acid.

Treatment

1. Respiratory distress due to laryngeal oedema should be treated with 100% oxygen and cricothyroidotomy. Endotracheal intubation is contraindicated in the presence of laryngeal swelling.
2. Some authorities recommend administration of water or milk if the patient is seen within 30 min of ingestion (120–240 mL in an adult, 60–120 mL in a child). But, no attempt must be made at neutralisation with alkalis, since the resulting exothermic reaction can cause more harm than benefit. Studies indicate that even administration of buffering agents such as antacids can produce significant exothermic reaction.
3. Remove all contaminated clothes and irrigate exposed skin copiously with saline. Deep second degree burns may benefit from topical silver sulfadiazine.
4. Eye injury should be dealt with by retraction of eyelids and prolonged irrigation for at least 15–30 min with normal saline or lactated Ringer's solution, or tap water, if nothing else is available. Anaesthetic agents and lid retractors may be necessary. It is desirable to continue with the irrigation until normal pH of ocular secretions is restored (7.4), which can be tested with litmus paper or urine dipstick. Slit lamp examination is mandatory after decontamination, to assess the extent of corneal damage.
5. The following measures are **contraindicated**: oral feeds, induction of vomiting, stomach wash and use of activated charcoal.
6. Steroids are not beneficial for corrosive upper GI burns. Therefore, the use of corticosteroids in the management of corrosive ingestions should be abandoned as they do not prevent the development of strictures and may lead to the development of serious adverse effects.
7. Administer antibiotics only if infection occurs. Prophylactic use is not advisable unless corticosteroid therapy is being undertaken.
8. Since there is often severe pain, powerful analgesics such as morphine may have to be given.
9. The use of flexible fibreoptic endoscopy is now standard practice in the first 24–48 hrs of ingestion to assess the extent of oesophageal and gastric damage. If there are circumferential 2nd or 3rd degree burns, an exploratory laparotomy should be performed. If gastric necrosis is present, an oesophagogastrectomy may have to be done.
10. Emergency laparotomy is mandatory, if there is perforation or peritonitis.
11. If the patient recovers, there may be long-term sequelae, such as stenosis and stricture formation. Follow-up is therefore essential to look for signs of obstruction – nausea, anorexia, weight loss. Surgical procedures such as dilatation, colonic bypass and oesophagogastrostomy may have to be undertaken.

*pH > 11.5 (alkali); pH < 2.0 (acid).

Autopsy Features

- Corroded areas of skin and mucous membranes appear **brownish** or **blackish** (**Fig. 9.4**). Teeth appear **chalky white**.
- Stomach mucosa shows the consistency of **wet blotting paper**.
- There may be inflammation, necrosis or perforation of the GI tract (**Fig. 9.5**).

Forensic Issues

- Accidental poisoning may arise from mistaken identity, since sulphuric acid resembles glycerine and castor oil. It is therefore imperative that it is stored in a distinctive bottle, clearly labelled and kept in a safe place.
- Sulphuric acid is a rare choice for either suicide or homicide.
- In addition to routine viscera and body fluids, a portion of corroded skin should be cut out, placed in rectified spirit or absolute alcohol and sent for chemical analysis.

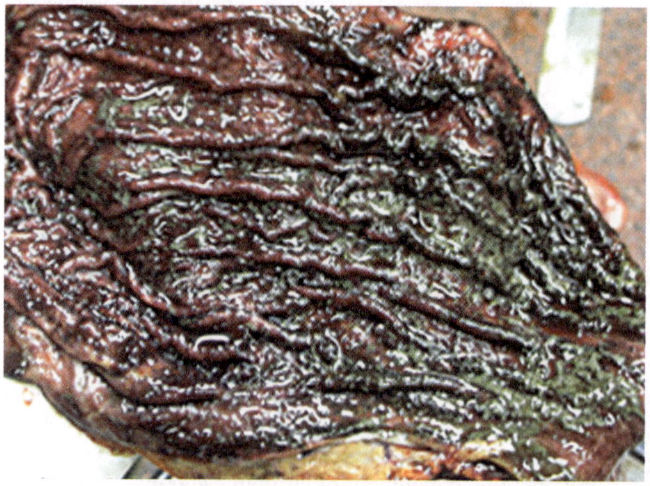

Fig. 9.4 Blackish corrosion of stomach – Sulphuric acid ingestion (*Courtesy*: *Dr Shashidhar C Mestri*)

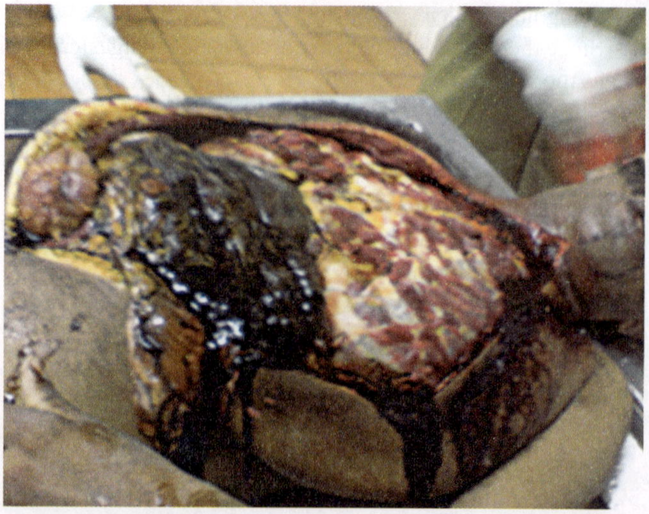

Fig. 9.5 Perforation of stomach with peritonitis – Sulphuric acid ingestion *(Courtesy: Dr Prateek Rastogi)*

- **Vitriolage**: This term refers to the throwing of an acid on to the face or body of a person in order to disfigure or blind him (**Fig. 9.6**). The motive is usually revenge or jealousy. This ghastly practice had its origins in the industrial unrest of Glasgow in the 1820s. Though sulphuric acid is commonly used (hence the term *vitriolage* which is derived from "oil of vitriol"), other acids are also employed. In fact any corrosive which is easy to hand may be used, including organic acids, alkalis and irritant plant juices.
  - Going by newspaper reports, vitriolage is a fairly common crime in India, though it is regarded as a serious offence (**grievous hurt**), and carries stiff punishment.
  - As per **The Criminal Law Amendment Act, 2013**, a new sub-section has been added in the **Indian Penal Code**, specifically to address vitriolage (acid throwing): **326A** – It states that "*Whoever causes permanent or partial damage or deformity to, or burns or maims or disfigures or disables, any part or parts of the body of a person or causes grievous hurt by throwing acid on or by administering acid to that person, or by using any other means with the intention of causing or with the knowledge that he is likely to cause such injury or hurt, shall be punished with imprisonment of either description for a term which shall not be less than ten years but which may extend to imprisonment for life, and with fine*". Provided that such fine shall be just and reasonable to meet the medical expenses of the treatment of the victim. Provided further that any fine imposed under this section shall be paid to the victim.

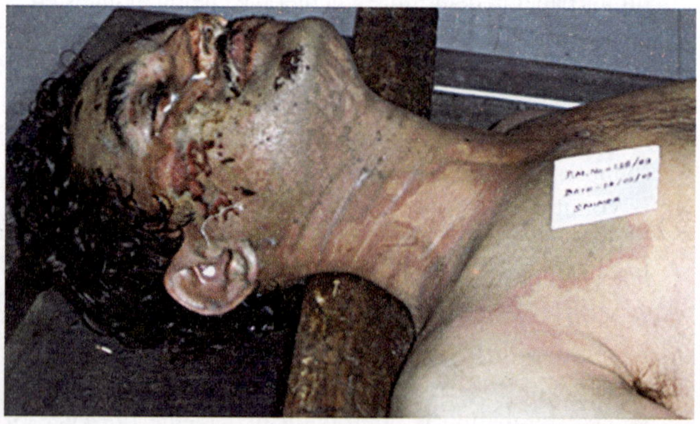

Fig. 9.6 Vitriolage (*Courtesy*: *Dr Iliyas Sheikh*)

2. Nitric Acid

Synonyms

- Aqua fortis; Azotic acid; Engraver's acid; Hydrogen nitrate; Red spirits of nitre

Molecular Formula

- HNO_3

Physical Appearance

- Nitric acid is a colourless or yellowish fuming liquid (**Fig. 9.7**) with an acrid, penetrating odour. It is essentially a solution of nitrogen dioxide (NO_2) in water and is available commercially in several forms.

Uses/Sources

- Nitric acid is formed in smog from the reaction between nitric oxide and hydrocarbons. Individuals living in heavily polluted areas may receive chronic inhalation exposure to nitric acid.
- Workers in the following professions may be exposed to nitric acid: glassblowing, engraving and electroplating, welding and fire fighting.

Usual Fatal Dose

- **20–30 mL.**

Toxicokinetics

- Systemic absorption is negligible.

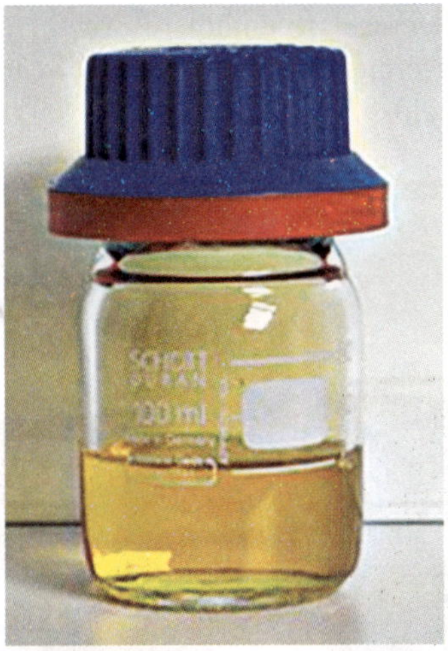

Fig. 9.7 Nitric acid

Mode of Action

- Nitric acid is a powerful oxidising agent and reacts with organic matter to produce trinitrophenol, liberating nitrogen monoxide (**xanthoproteic reaction**).
- Corrosion is less severe when compared to sulphuric acid.

Clinical Features

The general picture is the same as in the case of sulphuric acid, with the following differences:

- Corroded areas appear yellowish due to xanthoproteic reaction (**Fig. 9.8**). Stains on clothing and teeth also appear yellowish.
- More severe eructation and abdominal distension due to gas formation.
- Perforation of GI tract is less common.
- Inhalation of fumes can produce coughing, rhinorrhoea, lacrimation, dyspnoea and pulmonary oedema.

Diagnosis

1. **Litmus test**: *See page no.* 417.
2. Drop a small piece of copper into the stomach contents and heat it. Pungent, dark brown heavy fumes will emanate if nitric acid is present in sufficient concentration.

Treatment

- Same as for sulphuric acid. Respiratory distress is present more often and requires special attention.

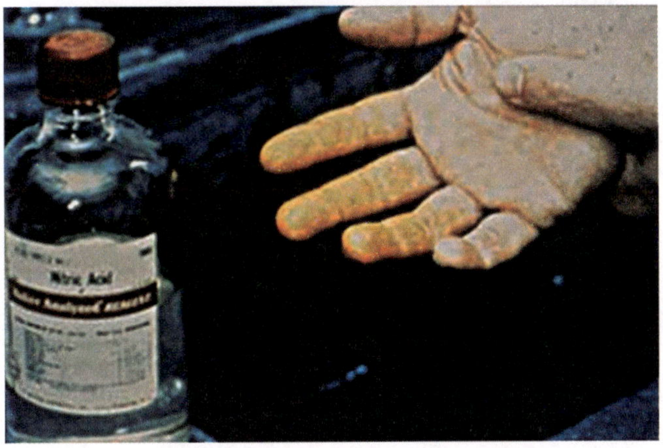

Fig. 9.8 Nitric acid - Xanthoproteic reaction

Autopsy Featurezs

1. Corroded areas of skin, teeth and mucous membranes appear **yellowish**. Stains on clothing also show yellowish discolouration.*
2. Gastrointestinal perforation is less common.

Forensic Issues

- Same as for sulphuric acid. Mistaking it for glycerine or castor oil, however is rare because it is a fuming liquid.

3. Hydrochloric Acid

Synonyms

- Muriatic acid; Spirit of salts; Aqueous hydrogen chloride; Chlorohydric acid

Molecular Formula

- HCl

Physical Appearance

- Hydrochloric acid is a colourless, fuming liquid which may acquire a yellowish tinge on exposure to air (**Fig. 9.9**). It is actually hydrogen chloride in water.

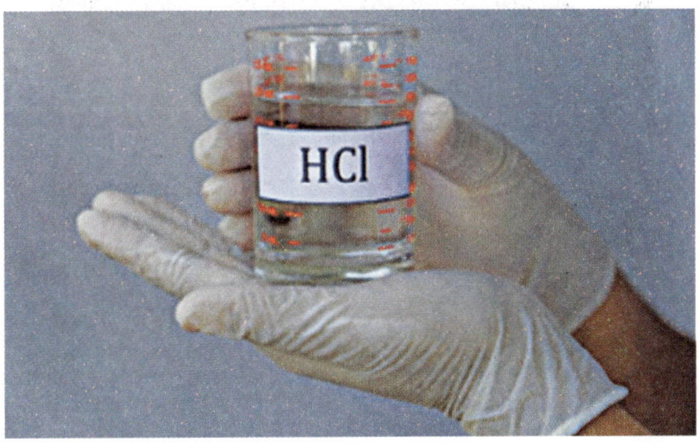

Fig. 9.9 Hydrochloric acid

****Note***: *To differentiate this from stains produced by iodine, apply ammonia solution. Iodine stains will be decolourised, while those due to nitric acid will deepen in intensity and turn to orange.*

Uses
1. Bleaching agent (<10% HCl).
2. Dyeing industry.
3. Metal refinery.
4. Metal cleaner, drain cleaner
5. Laboratory reagent

Usual Fatal Dose
- 30–40 mL.

Diagnosis
1. **Litmus test**: *See page no* 417.
2. If an open bottle of conc. ammonia solution is placed near the stomach contents or vomitus, copious white fumes of ammonium chloride will emanate. Though normal stomach contents contain hydrochloric acid, this is usually too dilute (0.2–0.5%) to vitiate the value of this test.

The rest of the information on HCL is practically the same as for H_2SO_4, except that corroded areas are more likely to be **greyish** (**Fig. 9.10**), and symptoms are generally less severe. But respiratory manifestations are more pronounced.

II. *Organic Acids*

Organic acids differ from inorganic acids in two major respects:
- They are weaker in action locally.
- They are better absorbed into the systemic circulation, and therefore have more powerful remote action.

1. Acetyl Salicylic Acid

Discussed under **Topic Pharmaceutical Toxicology – Competency** FM 10.1 *(page no. 513)*.

2. Carbolic Acid

Synonyms
- Benzenol; Hydroxybenzene; Oxybenzene; Phenic acid; **Phenol**; Phenolum; Phenyl alcohol; Phenylic acid; Phenylic alcohol; Phenyl hydrate; Phenyl hydroxide.

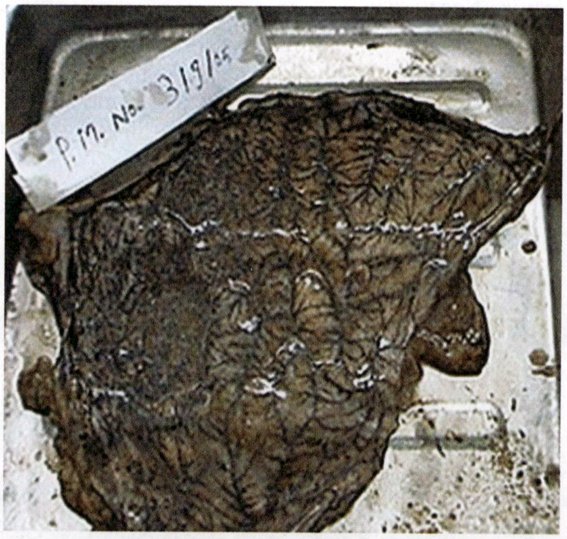

Fig. 9.10 Greyish corrosion of stomach – HCl ingestion (*Courtesy*: *Dr Iliyas Sheikh*)

Molecular Formula
- C_6H_6O; C_6H_5OH.

Physical Appearance
- Colourless, needle-like crystals which turn pink and liquefy when exposed to air. It is a coal tar derivative (creosote).
- Commercial phenol is a brownish liquid containing impurities like cresol (**Fig. 9.11**).
- Household phenol (often sold as **phenyle**) contains 5% phenol in water. It has a characteristic, aromatic odour ("**hospital odour**").
- **Derivatives**:
  - Catechol, cresols, menthol, resorcinol, thymol – *Toxic*
  - Hexyl resorcinol, naphthol – *Less Toxic*
  - Tannic acid – *Least toxic*

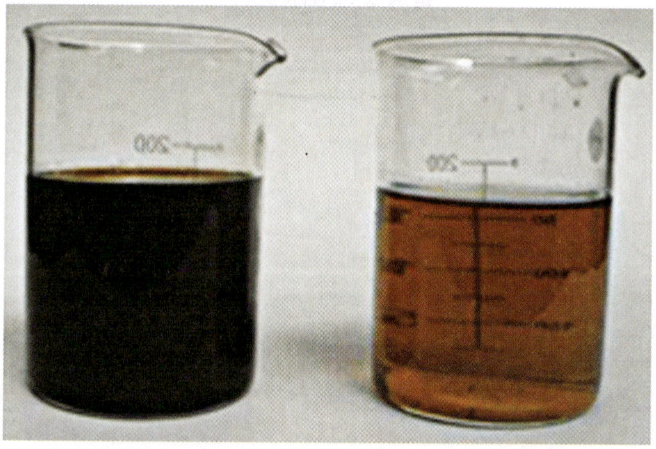

Fig. 9.11 Varieties of commercial phenol

Uses
- Carbolic acid was introduced as a disinfectant in the **19th century** by **Lemaire**, and quickly became popular ever since **Joseph Lister** (**Fig. 9.12**) advocated its use in surgery for asepsis.
- Even today, it is popular as a hospital and household disinfectant along with its related counterpart Lysol,* even though several safer and more effective alternatives have been developed including:
  - Cetrimide + Chlorhexidine (**Savlon**)
  - Chloroxylenol (**Dettol**)
- The various uses of carbolic acid are as follows:
  - **Antiseptic and disinfectant**: especially for sterilising floors, walls, furnishings, glassware, and instruments.
  - **Preservative**: Phenol is a commonly used preservative in injectable medications, e.g., glucagon, pethidine, neostigmine, quinidine and epinephrine.
  - Pharmaceuticals
  - Manufacture of plastics, explosives, fertilizer, etc.

****Note*: Protected trade mark in some countries, hence always use initial capital letter or face legal action! It consists of 50% cresol in saponified vegetable oil.*

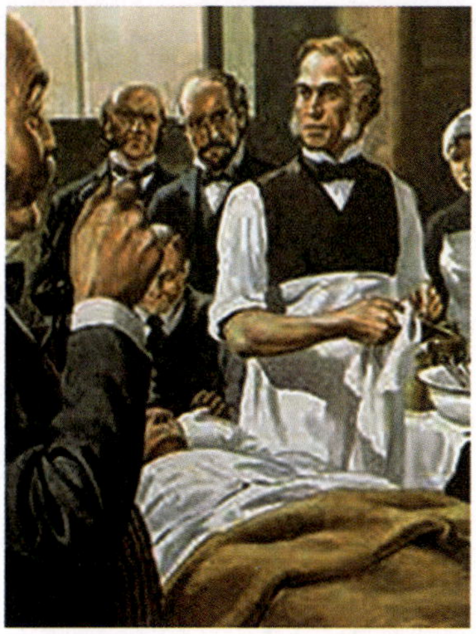

Fig. 9.12 Joseph Lister performs first antiseptic surgery (1865) by applying piece of lint dipped in carbolic acid

- **Medical uses**:
  - "Face peel" in plastic surgery.
  - Neurolysis for spasticity (by injecting phenol solution into neuromuscular junctions).
  - Phenol is still used in preparations for treatment of localized skin disorders (Castellani's paint), and as a local anaesthetic.

Usual Fatal Dose

- Probable oral lethal dose is reported at 50–500 μg/kg.
- 25–50 mL of household phenol can cause death.
- The UFD for Lysol is 60–120 mL.

Toxicokinetics

- Carbolic acid is rapidly absorbed through GI mucosa, lungs, and even intact skin.

Mode of Action

- Carbolic acid is actually a very mild corrosive, but has profound systemic effects after absorption.
  - There is CNS depression, metabolic acidosis, and renal damage.

Clinical Features

1. **Acute Poisoning**
   a. *Local*:
      i. Skin or mucosal contact results in mild corrosion with hardening and whitish discolouration. However the white eschar (especially in the skin) drops off in a few days, leaving a brown stain.
      ii. Locally there may be burning pain followed by tingling, numbness, and anaesthesia.
      iii. Eye contact causes irritation, conjunctival and corneal oedema, and blindness in severe cases.
   b. *Systemic*:
      i. GIT – Burning pain, vomiting.
      ii. CNS – Vertigo, convulsions, coma. Pupils are constricted.
      iii. RS –Tachypnoea, bronchospasm, pulmonary oedema. Adult respiratory distress syndrome and fatal respiratory failure have been reported.
      iv. CVS – Tachycardia, hypotension, cardiac arrhythmias
      v. Blood – Haemolysis, methaemoglobinaemia.
      vi. Metabolic – Hypothermia, with cold and clammy skin, metabolic acidosis.
      vii. Hepatorenal:
         - **Carboluria**: Oliguria, with scanty urine which turns greenish or brownish on exposure to air because of phenolic metabolites (hydroquinone and pyrocatechol).
         - Later there is renal and hepatic failure. Renal dysfunction and acute tubular necrosis is possible potentially requiring haemodialysis.
2. **Chronic Poisoning (*Phenol Marasmus*)**
   a. This was common in earlier days among medical personnel when phenol was routinely used as a skin disinfectant. It is characterised by anorexia, weight loss, headache, vertigo, dark urine, and greenish pigmentation of skin and sclerae (***ochronosis***) (**Fig. 9.13**).
   b. An association between occupational exposure to chlorophenol and nasal and nasopharyngeal cancers has been observed.

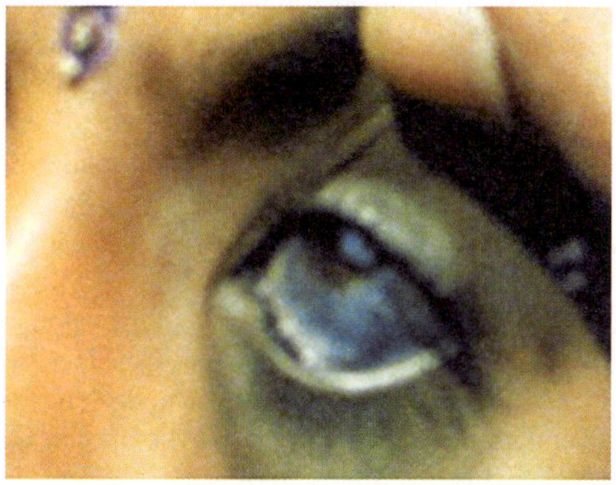

Fig. 9.13 Ochronosis – Pigmentation of sclera (*Courtesy*: *Dr Shashidhar C Mestri*)

Diagnosis

- Typical odour in the vicinity of the patient.
- Urine collected and stored in a transparent container shows a gradual change in colour to brown or green (**Table 9.2** contains a list of poisons and drugs which discolour urine).
- To 10 mL of urine, add 1 mL of 10% ferric chloride. A purple or blue colour which persists even on heating indicates phenol poisoning. Cresol is associated with green colour.
- When 10 mL of urine is boiled with **Millon's reagent**,* a red colour is produced.

*****Millon's reagent***: Dissolve 10 g mercury in 20 mL nitric acid. Dilute with an equal amount of distilled water. Allow to stand for 2 hrs. Decant.*

Table 9.2 Poisons/Drugs Which Discolour Urine

Urine Colour	Poison/Drug
Orange	Phenothiazines, Rifampicin, Warfarin, Carrots, Vitamin A
Red or Pink	Aniline, Ibuprofen, Phenytoin, Rhubarb, Beetroot
Purple	Porphyrins, Phenolphthalein
Brown	Chloroquine, Iron, Methaemoglobin, Metronidazole, Methyl dopa, Furazolidone, Nitrofurantoin, Primaquine, Sulphamethoxazole
Brownish black	Homogentisic aid, Nitrobenzene
Yellow	Fluorescin dye, Riboflavin, Trinitrophenol, Quinacrine
Greenish blue	Chlorophyll Breath Mints (Clorets®), Methylene blue, Thymol
Greenish brown	Cresol, Phenol

Treatment

1. Decontamination following surface contamination:
    - This should be performed in a well-ventilated area, preferably with its own ventilation system.
    - Contaminated clothing should be removed, double-bagged, sealed and stored safely.
    - Decontaminate open wounds first and avoid contamination of unexposed skin.
    - Any particulate matter adherent to skin should be removed and the patient washed with copious amounts of water under low pressure for at least 10–15 min.
2. The use of water (100–200 mL in an adult; 2 mL/kg in a child) as diluent in the management of corrosive ingestion may be of some symptomatic benefit.
3. The benefit of gastric decontamination is uncertain. Consider activated charcoal (50 g for adults; 1 g/kg for children). Optimal effects are within 1 hr of ingestion.
4. Treatment of methaemoglobinaemia: Consider treatment with methylthioninium chloride (methylene blue), if methaemoglobin concentration is 30% or more.
5. Control convulsions with IV diazepam (10–20 mg in adults; 0.1–0.3 mg/kg in children), lorazepam (4 mg in adults; 0.1 mg/kg in children) or midazolam (5–10 mg in adults; 0.05–0.15 mg/kg in children).
6. Correct hypotension by adequate fluid resuscitation with a crystalloid. Treat brady and tachyarrhythmias appropriately.
7. If metabolic acidosis persists despite correction of hypoxia and adequate fluid resuscitation, consider correction with IV sodium bicarbonate.
8. Features of severe tissue injury (severe abdominal pain, abdominal distension, circulatory collapse or lactic acidosis) may indicate the presence of bowel necrosis or perforation. Immediate surgical assessment is recommended urgently because early resection of necrotic tissue and intraluminal stenting has been shown to improve survival and reduce the risk of oesophageal stricture formation.
9. Both CT scan and fibreoptic endoscopy have been shown to be useful in assessing the severity of injury, risk of mortality and risk of subsequent stricture formation.

Autopsy Features

1. Distinct **odour** of phenol, especially around the mouth and in the stomach contents.
2. Corroded areas are at first white, but if death has been delayed they turn brownish **(Fig. 9.14)**.
3. Gastric mucosa is greyish white, swollen and hardened **(leathery)**, but Lysol poisoning is associated with soapy and soft mucosa.
4. Urine is greenish or brownish.

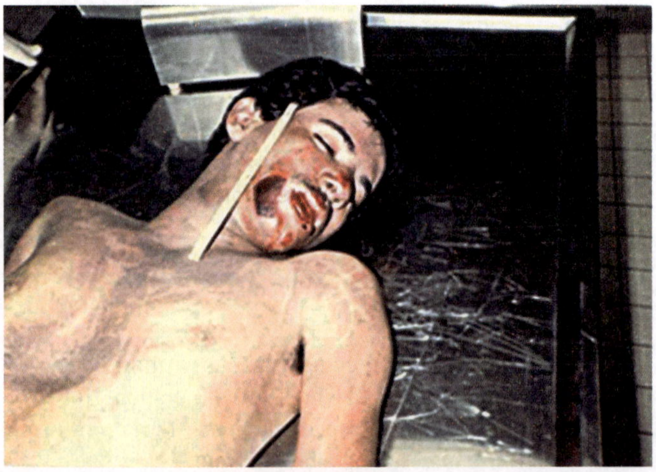

Fig. 9.14 Carbolic acid burns

Forensic Issues

- Most cases of poisoning are accidental in nature arising out of occupational exposure or therapeutic misuse.
- Formerly, suicidal ingestions were common.
- Poisoning with phenolic derivatives causes similar but usually less severe manifestations, and must be treated on the same lines as phenol.

3. Oxalic Acid

Synonyms

- Ethanediolic acid; Dicarboxylic acid; Salt of sorrel

Molecular Formula

- $C_2H_2O_4$

Physical Appearance/Derivatives

- Oxalic acid is a toxic chemical which is synthesized commercially and is also naturally present as a salt in many plants.
- It is a relatively strong acid, and forms a white precipitate.

Uses/Sources

- Oxalic acid occurs naturally in plants and vegetables such as **rhubarb** (*Rheum* species) (**Fig. 9.15**), **dumbcane** (*Dieffenbachia*) (**Fig. 9.16**) and **sorrel** (*Rumex* species) (**Fig. 9.17**). Also found in **spinach** (**Fig. 9.18**).
- Oxalic acid is used in paint, stain and varnish removers, rust and ink stain removers, and ceramics.

Usual Fatal Dose

- **15–30 g of oxalic acid**.

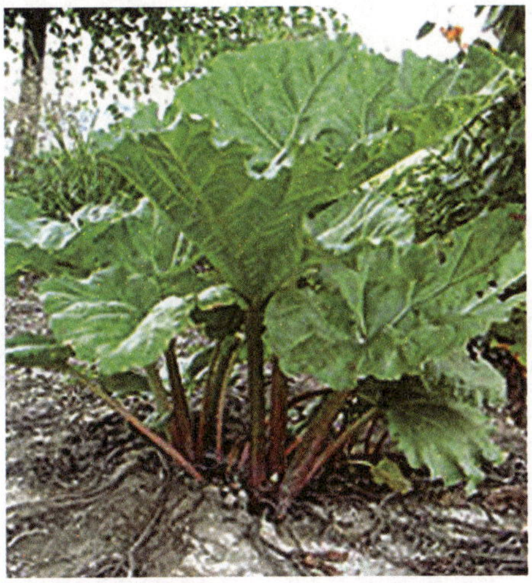

Fig. 9.15 Rhubarb

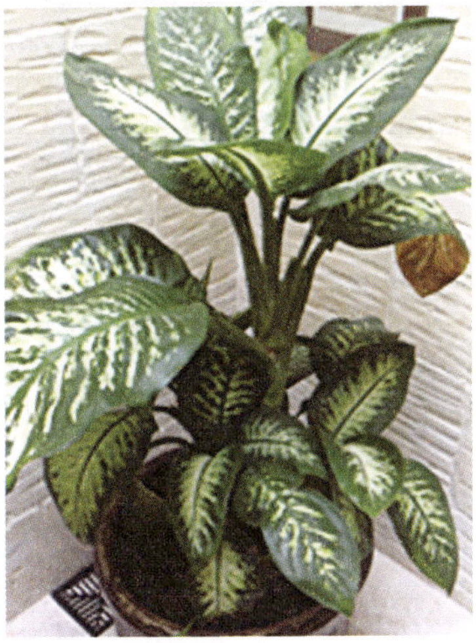

Fig. 9.16 Dumbcane

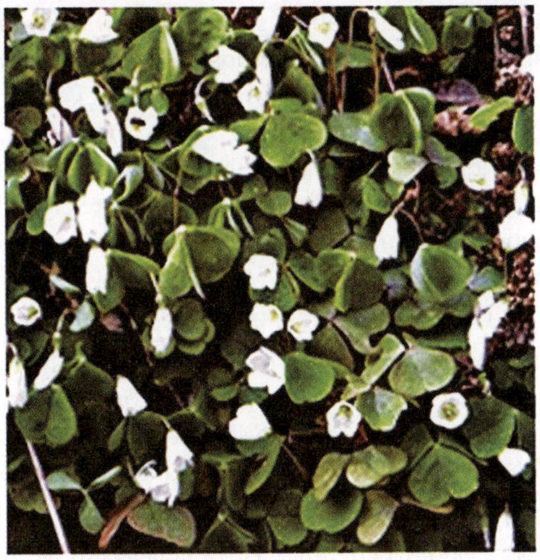

Fig. 9.17 Sorrel

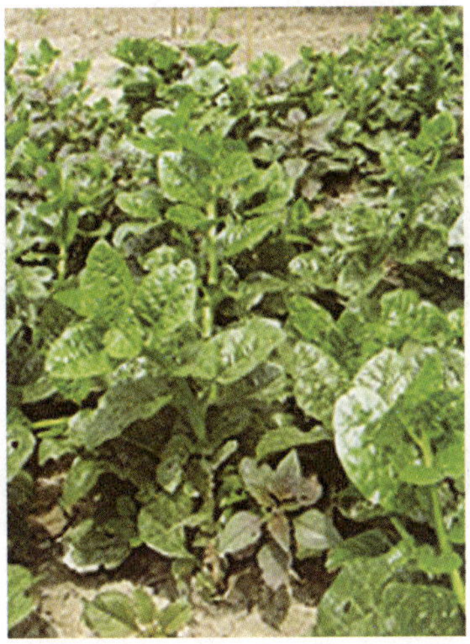

Fig. 9.18 Spinach

Mode of Action

- Liquid oxalic acid has moderate corrosive action on skin and mucosa.
- Systemic absorption leads to hypocalcaemia, since it reacts with calcium in plasma, and insoluble calcium oxalate is precipitated which accumulates in the liver, kidneys, heart, lungs and blood, and is excreted in the urine.

Clinical Features

A. **Local**:

  a. Skin exposure will produce irritation and possibly corrosive damage: whitish or yellowish corrosion (mucosa), or discolouration (skin), with underlying congestion. The corroded mucosa is often referred to as "**scalded**" in appearance.

  b. Exposures of natural oxalates have produced photosensitivity dermatitis.

B. **Systemic**:

  a. Vomiting and diarrhoea, followed by signs and symptoms of hypocalcaemia (**tetany**), characterised by tonic muscle spasms, cramping, and *accoucher's hand** (**Fig. 9.19**). There is often a positive *Trousseau's*** and *Chvostek's**** **sign** (**Figs. 9.20 & 9.21**).

b. Pupils are usually dilated.

c. Later there may be metabolic acidosis, ventricular fibrillation, and renal failure. Calcium oxalate crystals can be deposited in the liver resulting in hepatic necrosis and failure in severe cases.

Diagnosis

1. Demonstration of **urinary oxalate crystals** which may occur either as monohydrates (prism or needle-like), or dihydrates (tent or envelope shaped) (**Fig. 9.22**).
2. Oxalic acid can be measured in the urine by colourimetry.

Treatment

1. It is better not to attempt gastric lavage. Some investigators still recommend stomach wash with calcium gluconate or lactate solution.
2. Although oxalates have been shown to be adsorbed to activated charcoal in vitro, the benefit of administration is uncertain and may not be advisable following ingestion of a concentrated solution since this may interfere with endoscopic visualisation.
3. Encourage oral fluids, hydration is important to prevent the deposition of crystals. Measure blood calcium, urea, creatinine and liver function tests in all patients.
4. If the patient has proven hypocalcaemia or clinical symptoms/signs suggestive of severe hypocalcaemia (tetany, arrhythmias, QTc prolongation or convulsions), give 5–10

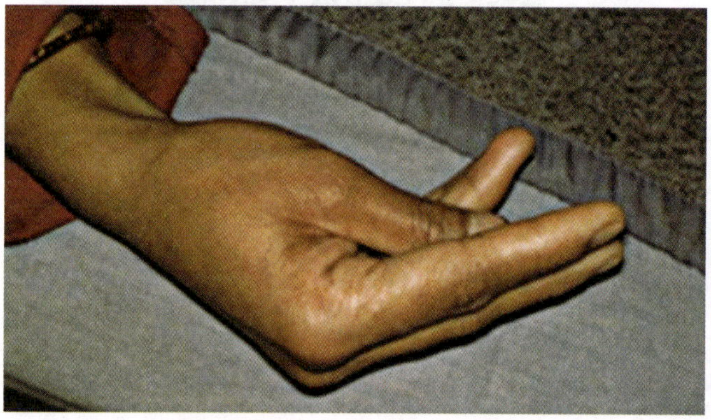

Fig. 9.19 Accoucher's hand

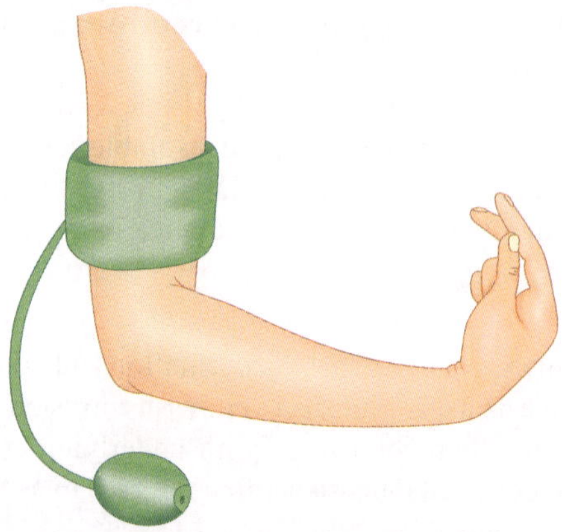

Fig. 9.20 Trousseau's sign

Eliciting Chvostek's Sign

Begin by telling the patient to relax his facial muscles. Then stand directly in front of him, and tap the facial nerve either just anterior to the earlobe and below the zygomatic arch or between the zygomatic arch and the corner of his mouth. A positive response varies from twitching of the lip at the corner of the mouth to spasm of all facial muscles, depending on the severity of hypocalcaemia.

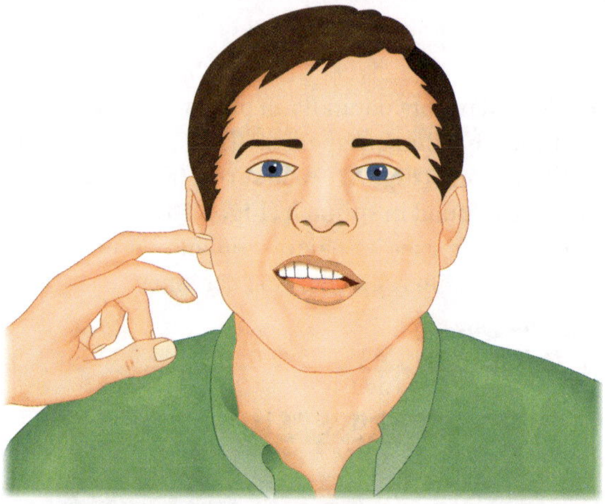

Fig. 9.21 Chvostek's sign

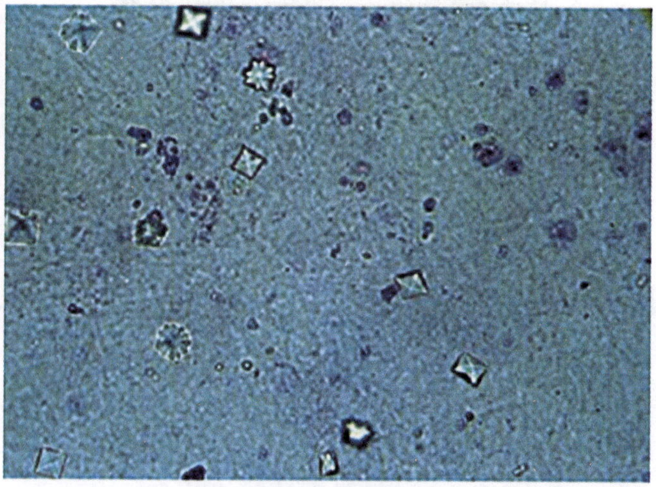

Fig. 9.22 Urinary oxalate crystals (*Courtesy: Dr S Senthilkumaran*)

Note: *Due to carpopedal spasm.*

****Note***: *Trousseau's sign: Spasm resulting from pressure applied to nerves and vessels of upper arm.*

*****Note***: *Chvostek's sign: Spasm of facial muscles following a tap on the facial nerve area.*

mL of 10% calcium chloride IV in adults. Alternatively, give 10–30 mL of 10% calcium gluconate IV. In severe hypocalcaemia, an infusion of 10% calcium gluconate may be required, e.g., 40 mL over 1 hr in an adult. For children, give 0.2 mL/kg (max 10 mL) of 10% calcium chloride IV. Alternatively, give 0.5 mL/kg of 10% calcium gluconate IV over 5 min (max 20 mL).

5. Control convulsions with IV diazepam (10–20 mg in adults; 0.1–0.3 mg/kg in children), lorazepam (4 mg in adults; 0.1 mg/kg in children) or midazolam (5–10 mg in adults; 0.05–0.15 mg/kg in children).
6. Correct hypotension by adequate fluid resuscitation with a crystalloid. Treat brady and tachyarrhythmias appropriately.
7. Haemodialysis and charcoal haemoperfusion have been used to remove oxalate in primary oxalosis.

Autopsy Features

- "Scalded" mucosa of GI tract (especially stomach). Sometimes, there is a brown or black colour due to acid haematin. Crystals of calcium oxalate may be demonstrated in scrapings of the mucosa (examine with polarising microscope).
- Whitish or yellowish discolouration of corroded areas.
- Microscopic evidence of renal damage.

Forensic Issues

- Most cases of oxalic acid or oxalate poisoning result from accidental causes, e.g., mistaking the substance for Epsom salt, sodium bicarbonate, etc.
- Accidental poisoning may also result from excessive ingestion of certain vegetables rich in oxalates, e.g., rhubarb leaves, sorrel, etc. Even tea is said to contain significant amounts of oxalate.
- Chronic consumption of oxalic acid can lead to renal calculi with consequent renal colic.
- Occasional cases of suicide and homicide with oxalic acid have been reported.

B. Alkalis

Alkalies (compounds with a pH > 7) commonly encountered in poisoning include ammonia (usually in the form of ammonium hydroxide), carbonates of sodium and potassium, and hydroxides of sodium, potassium and calcium. Sodium hypochlorite is also increasingly being implicated.

Please note that the new CBME curriculum does not mention 'Alkalis'. Hence, it is not being discussed here. Questions pertaining to Alkalis must not be asked in the examinations.

FM 9.2: Core – Written/Viva Voce/ Objective Structured Clinical Examination (OSCE)

- Describe general principles and basic methodologies in treatment of poisoning: decontamination, supportive therapy, antidote therapy, procedures of enhanced elimination with regard to:
  - Phosphorus
  - Iodine
  - Barium

PHOSPHORUS

Physical Appearance

- The name "phosphorus" is derived from Greek, meaning "light-bearing". Phosphorus was the 13th element to be discovered. For this reason, and also due to its use in explosives, poisons and nerve agents, it is sometimes referred to as the "***Devil's element***". **Fig. 9.23** displays the various forms of phosphorus along with relevant physical and chemical properties.
- There are two main varieties:
  - **White (Yellow) Phosphorus**
    - This is a whitish, waxy, crystalline solid with a **garlicky odour**.
    - On exposure to air, it is highly combustible and ignites into flame. Oxidation causes it to release whitish fumes of phosphorus pentoxide. Hence, it is generally stored under water (**Fig. 9.24**).
    - It is luminescent and glows in the dark (***phosphorescence***).
    - White phosphorus gradually changes to red phosphorus. This transformation is accelerated by light and heat, and samples of white phosphorus almost

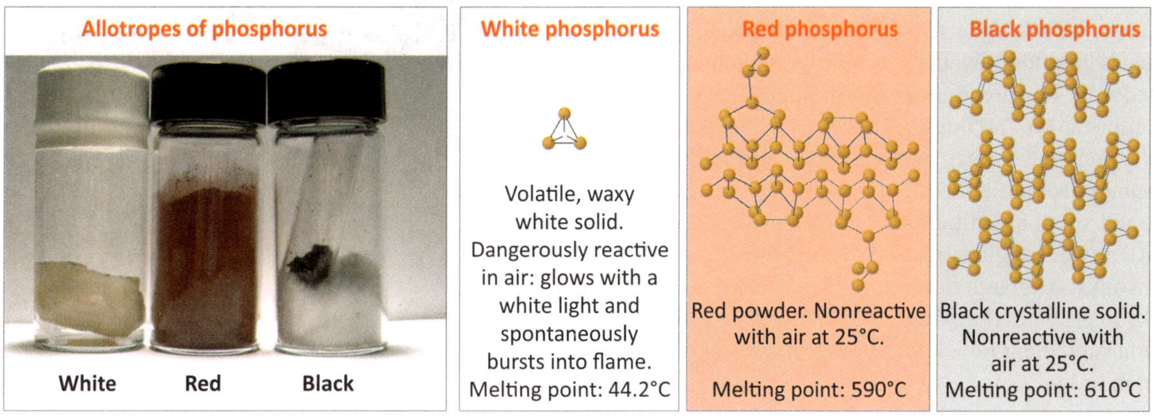

Fig. 9.23 Various forms of phosphorus

always contain some red phosphorus and accordingly appear yellow. For this reason, it is also called yellow phosphorus.

- **Red Phosphorus**
  - This is a reddish or brownish, amorphous, odourless substance. It is insoluble and relatively harmless, since it is not absorbed from the GI tract.

Derivatives and related compounds of phosphorus include **phosphoric acid**, **phosphine**,* **aluminium phosphide** and **zinc phosphide**.

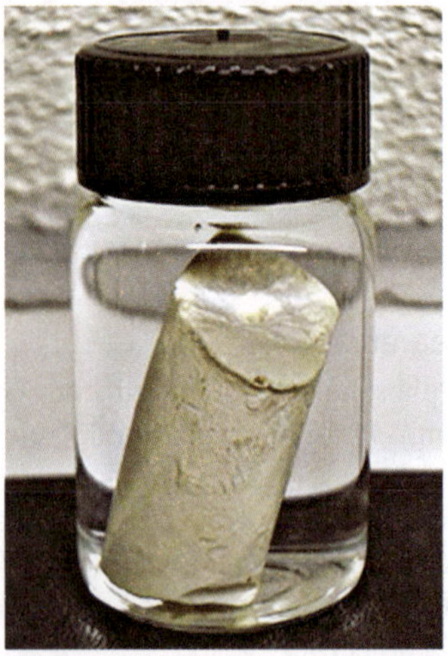

Fig. 9.24 White (yellow) phosphorus stored under water

Uses

1. **Matches**: White phosphorus was extensively used in the manufacture of friction matches during the 19th century. However, because of its propensity to produce chronic poisoning in workers of the match industry, most countries agreed at an international convention in Berne, Switzerland in 1906 to prohibit the manufacture and import of white phosphorus for the making of matches. Hence, these so-called "**lucifer matches**" (**Fig 9.25**) gradually (and fortunately) faded out. Today's "**safety match**" (**Fig. 9.26**) contains only potassium chlorate and antimony sulphide. It has to be struck against a prepared surface to ignite it, which is provided by the sides of the match box being coated with powdered glass and red phosphorus. This is in contrast to the "**strike anywhere**" match which does not need a prepared surface to ignite it. Its composition is 6% phosphorus sesquifluoride (non-toxic), 24% potassium chlorate, and small quantities of zinc oxide, red ochre (a pigment), powdered glass, glue and water.
2. **Fireworks**: Although the use of white phosphorus in fireworks is prohibited in Western countries, it is still an important ingredient in several types of fireworks manufactured in India.
3. **Military Uses**: White phosphorus is an ingredient of tracer bullets, incendiary bombs, smoke screens and air-sea rescue flares.
4. **Insecticide and Rodenticide**: There are several pastes and powders available in India which contain phosphorus (or zinc phosphide) used for killing cockroaches and rats (e.g., *Ratol*). Such pastes are usually mixed with molasses or butter and spread on bread as bait. Obviously, unintentional ingestion by children is quite possible leading to serious poisoning.
5. **Fertilizer**: The majority of phosphorus-containing compounds are produced for use as fertilizers. For this purpose, phosphate-containing minerals are converted to phosphoric acid.

Usual Fatal Dose

- **60 mg (roughly 1 mg/kg body weight)**.

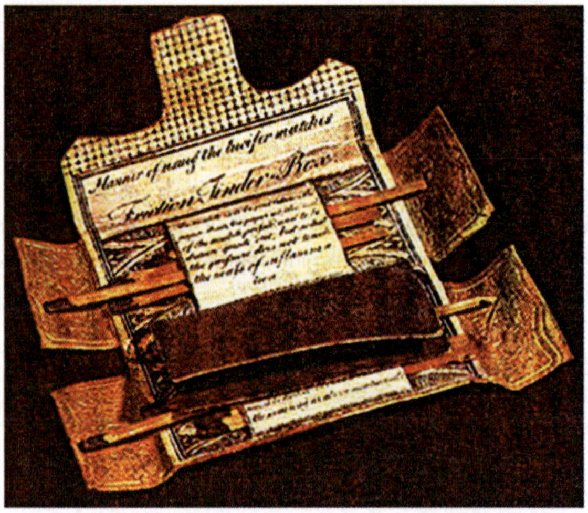

Fig. 9.25 Lucifer matches

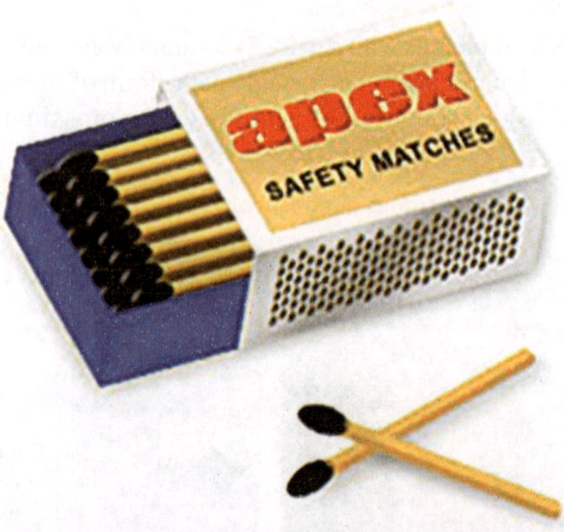

Fig. 9.26 Safety matches

**Note*: Not phosgene, which is carbonyl chloride ($COCl_2$). It is produced by high temperature decomposition of chlorinated hydrocarbons such as carbon tetrachloride.*

Mode of Action

- White phosphorus, a protoplasmic poison is a potent hepatotoxin (Table 9.3). Massive hepatic steatosis is a hallmark of white phosphorus toxicity, with a rise in hepatic triglycerides beginning within 2 hrs and peaking in 36 hrs. Hepatic necrosis may be prominent, particularly in zone 1, in distinction to most other classic hepatotoxins, such as paracetamol and carbon tetrachloride, that produce zone 3 necrosis.
- In large doses, phosphorus can cause shock and cardiovascular collapse since it is also toxic to the heart.
- Locally, it produces severe irritation of skin and mucosa.
- Rate of absorption is greatly enhanced, if phosphorus is administered in an oily vehicle. Phosphorus is fat-soluble.
- Toxicity is enhanced when yellow phosphorus is dissolved/coingested in solvents, e.g., alcohol, digestible fats and oils.

Clinical Features

A. **Fulminant Poisoning**:

a. This results from ingestion of a massive dose, i.e., more than 1–2 g.

b. The dominant clinical picture is one of peripheral vascular collapse.

c. Death usually occurs in 12–24 hrs, and signs of hepatic or renal damage are not seen.

B. **Acute Poisoning**:

a. ***First Stage*** (up to 3 days) – Local effects include severe burning pain, vomiting, diarrhoea and abdominal pain. Breath smells of garlic. Vomitus and stools may be luminous in the dark. There may be haematemesis. Faint fumes may emanate from the stools (***Smoky stool syndrome***).

b. ***Second Stage*** (up to several days after the first stage subsides) – This is an essentially symptom-free (treacherous) period, and the patient may feel well enough to be discharged from the hospital.

c. ***Third Stage*** – This is due to the systemic effects of phosphorus after it has been absorbed. There is a return of the digestive symptoms with increased severity. In addition, manifestations of **liver damage** are prominent – tender hepatomegaly, jaundice which may progress to an olive green hue, pruritis, bleeding from multiple sites and finally hepatic encephalopathy characterised by drowsiness, confusion, ataxia, flapping tremor of hands (*asterixis*), stupor and coma. At this stage there is a mousy odour to the breath (*foetor hepaticus*). Renal damage results in oliguria, haematuria, albuminuria and acute renal failure. ECG changes include tachycardia, ST and T waves changes, QTc prolongation and various arrhythmias.

d. Dermal contact with phosphorus results in acutely painful corrosion with yellow, necrotic, severely painful second or third degree chemical burns emitting garlic-like odour. Absorption from damaged skin may result in acute systemic phosphorus poisoning.

e. *Diagnosis of Acute Poisoning*:

i. Garlicky odour of breath and vomitus.

ii. Fuming or luminous vomitus and stools.

iii. Evidence of hepatic and renal failure.

iv. Hypokalaemia, hyperchloraemia, hypocalcaemia and both hyperphosphataemia and hypophosphataemia have been reported.

v. Hypoprothrombinaemia and thrombocytopenia may occur following ingestion, and lead to a delayed onset of haematemesis, haematochezia, haematuria and haemorrhages into the skin and mucous membranes.

C. **Chronic Poisoning**:

a. This usually results from long term occupational exposure to the fumes of phosphorus pentoxide and results in the condition called **Phossy Jaw** (***Glass Jaw, Lucifer's Jaw***) which was first described by **Bristowe** in **1862**.

b. Main features include toothache (usually originating in a carious tooth), which because of its recurrence would be eventually extracted leading to exposure of bone followed by necrosis, sequestration and osteomyelitis of jaw (invariably the lower jaw) (**Fig. 9.27**).

Treatment

A. **Acute Poisoning**:

1. Gastric lavage with potassium permanganate has been advocated in the past, as it oxidises phosphorus into

Table 9.3 Hepatotoxic Agents

Acute Hepatocellular Injury	Cholestasis	Steatosis	Chronic Active Hepatitis
▪ Arsenic ▪ Carbon tetrachloride ▪ Ethyl alcohol ▪ Halothane ▪ Iron ▪ Isoniazid ▪ Methyldopa ▪ Paracetamol ▪ Phosphorus (White) ▪ Tetracycline	▪ Chlorpromazine ▪ Ethyl alcohol ▪ Erythromycin ▪ Nitrofurantoin ▪ Rifampicin	▪ Ethyl alcohol ▪ Phosphorus (White) ▪ Sodium valproate ▪ Tetracycline ▪ Zidovudine	▪ Isoniazid ▪ Methyl dopa ▪ Nitrofurantoin ▪ Trazodone

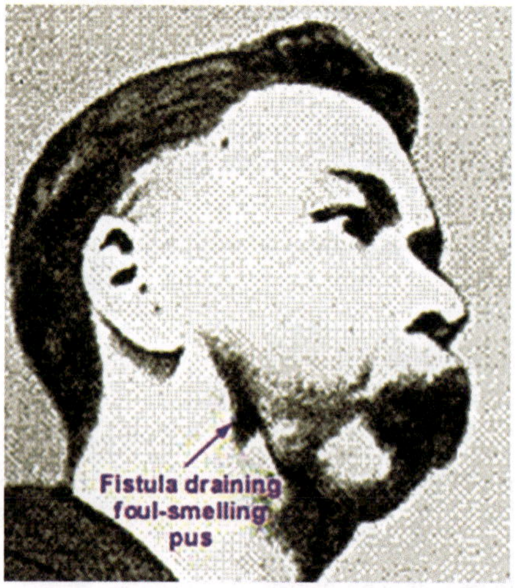

Fig. 9.27 Phossy jaw

relatively less toxic phosphoric acid and phosphates. It is not recommended anymore. Some authorities recommend administration of copper sulphate solution (250 g in a glass of water), which converts phosphorus to non-toxic copper phosphide. Alternatively, a 0.2% solution of copper sulphate may be used for stomach wash. It must however be noted that copper sulphate being a highly toxic substance by itself is not a desirable antidote, and in fact is placed in the international list of obsolete antidotes.

a. If stomach wash is contemplated, it is best to use saline or warm water. However, care is advised while washing out or aspirating stomach contents in a known case of phosphorus ingestion – combustion has been reported during the procedure leading to production of flame and emission of fumes!

2. Do not administer milk or any oily/fatty foods, since this will enhance the absorption of phosphorus.
3. Vitamin K by IV drip (65 mg) slowly, to combat hypoprothrombinaemia.
4. **Intravenous fluids**:
   a. Isotonic saline and sodium lactate to treat shock, dehydration and acidosis.
   b. Glucose to combat hypoglycaemia.
   c. Calcium gluconate for hypocalcaemia.
5. Whole blood/fresh frozen plasma to correct coagulation defects.
6. Steroids and inotropic support for shock.
7. Anticonvulsants for seizures.
8. N-Acetyl cysteine (NAC) may be helpful in patients with stage I phosphorus toxicity (to prevent progression of liver damage). *Regimen*: 150 mg/kg in 200 cc D5W for 15 min, then 50 mg/kg in 500 cc D5W for 4 hrs, then 100 mg/kg in 1000 cc D5W for 16 hrs.
9. Exchange transfusion may be beneficial, but haemodialysis and haemoperfusion are not useful.
10. **Treatment of dermal burns**:
    a. After initial flushing with large volumes of water to remove any residual chemical material, clean wounds with a mild disinfectant soap and water. Loose, non-viable tissue should be removed by gentle cleansing with surgical soap or formal skin debridement. Intravenous analgesia may be required.
    b. Blisters should be left intact until they rupture spontaneously or healing is well underway, unless they are extremely large or inhibit motion.
    c. Prophylactic topical antibiotic therapy with silver sulfadiazine is recommended for all burns except superficial partial thickness (first-degree) burns. For first-degree burns bacitracin may be used, but effectiveness is not documented.
    d. Analgesics such as paracetamol with codeine may be used for pain relief, if needed.
    e. Phosphorus particles in dermal burns can be visualized by employing the use of Wood's lamp. Phosphorus will fluoresce under ultraviolet light. With the exposed areas immersed in water, loose or embedded phosphorus particles that are visualized under UV light can be mechanically but delicately removed safely under water.
    f. Traditionally, copper sulphate solution has been topically applied to skin burns caused by white phosphorus. However, acute renal failure and massive haemolysis may occur if significant copper sulphate is absorbed from the burn site.
11. **Treatment of eye exposure**:
    a. Immediately irrigate the affected eye thoroughly with 0.9% saline 1000 mL.
    b. Anaesthetise the eye with a topical local anaesthetic.
    c. Irrigate for 10–15 min irrespective of initial conjunctival pH. Aim for a final conjunctival pH of 7.5–8.0. The conjunctivae may be tested with indicator paper. Retest 20 min after irrigation and use further irrigation, if necessary.
    d. Corneal damage may be detected by instillation of fluorescein and examination under the slit lamp or ophthalmoscope.

B. **Chronic Poisoning**:
   1. Removal of patient from source of exposure.
   2. Dental treatment and follow-up.

Autopsy Features

- **Garlicky odour** in the vicinity of the mouth and in the gastric contents.
- Bleeding points in the skin (subcutaneous haemorrhages).
- Luminous gastric contents.* The contents will fluoresce under UV light.
- Congestion and inflammation of affected skin and mucosa.
- Enlarged fatty liver. Later there is evidence of acute yellow atrophy with jaundice.

*__Note__: *Examine in the dark!*

- There may also be fatty degeneration of heart and kidneys.
- Viscera for chemical analysis must be preserved in saturated saline and not rectified spirit, otherwise luminosity especially of the stomach contents will be lost.

Forensic Issues

1. **Accidental Poisoning**: This used to be common in the past because of unrestricted use of phosphorus in matches and fireworks. Today, most cases of accidental poisoning result from inadvertent ingestion of cockroach or rat poison by children, or because of contamination of food by these substances.
2. **Suicidal Poisoning**: This was also previously quite common, especially in Western countries. Today, rat pastes containing phosphorus are occasionally implicated in suicidal ingestions.
3. **Homicidal Poisoning**: Formerly, phosphorus was quite frequently employed for committing murder. Several accounts are mentioned in the literature where poisoning was accomplished by mixing phosphorus in soup, jam, or rum, and administered to unsuspecting victims.

IODINE

Physical Appearance

- Blue-black, glittering crystals which constantly give off violet coloured vapour (a process called ***sublimation***) (**Fig 9.28**) with a peculiar odour.
- Iodine is an essential trace element in the human diet, necessary for the formation of thyroid hormone.

Uses

- ***Antiseptic preparations***:
  - *Lugol's iodine* (iodine with potassium iodide in water).
  - *Tincture of iodine* (iodine & potassium or sodium iodide with alcohol & water).
  - *Povidone-iodine* (iodophor, i.e., mixture of polyvinylpyrrolidone and iodine).
  - *Iodex* (iodine with methyl salicylate).
- As a component of some expectorants (e.g., potassium iodide), anti-asthmatics (e.g., iophylline), anti-arrhythmics (e.g., amiodarone), anti-amoebics (e.g., iodoquinol), antifungals (e.g., vioform), antithyroid drugs (e.g., potassium iodide) and radiographic contrast agents (e.g., diatrizoate sodium, iopanoic acid, ipodate sodium, etc.).

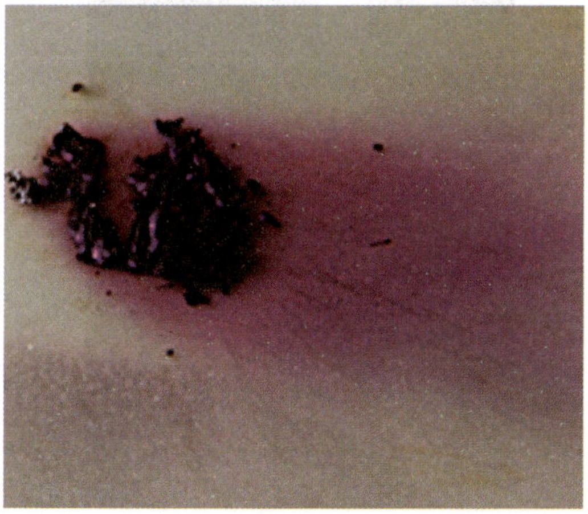

Fig. 9.28 Iodine sublimation

- As a solution for preparing patients for thyroid surgery (e.g., collosol liquid).
- Clioquinol, which is an iodinated hydroxyquinoline, is used sometimes in amoebiasis.
- Surgical scrub (7.5% povidone iodine in aqueous solution).
- Iodine is used commonly to treat drinking water to make it potable.

Usual Fatal Dose

- **2–5 g of free iodine, or 1–2 ounces of strong iodine tincture**.
  - The presence of food in the stomach inactivates iodine by converting it to iodide which is relatively innocuous.

Mode of Action

- Locally, strong iodine solution can be an intense irritant.
- Systemic toxicity is due to combination of free iodine with serum sodium bicarbonate, leading to metabolic acidosis.
- Elevated serum iodine concentrations have also been associated with hyperchloraemia, hypernatraemia and renal failure.

Clinical Features

- Initial manifestations of iodine poisoning include rhinorrhoea, conjunctivitis and cough (especially, if fumes have been inhaled).
- There is burning pain extending from the mouth to the abdomen, salivation, metallic taste, vomiting and diarrhoea. Vomitus and stools may appear yellowish (or sometimes bluish) in colour. Blue coloured emesis indicates the presence of food (starch) in the stomach and the conversion of iodine to iodide.
- Skin and mucous membranes are stained yellowish brown.
- The following features have also been reported: glottic oedema, pulmonary oedema, delirium, hallucinations, convulsions, tachycardia, hypotension, metabolic acidosis and renal failure. There may be hyperkalaemia and hypoglycaemia.
- Eye exposure can result in severe ocular burns.
- Hypersensitivity reactions including angioedema and a serum sickness-like reaction may occur following oral, topical, vaginal (douche) or IV administration of iodine.
- Iodides and iodophores (e.g., povidone-iodine) are much less toxic and usually require only supportive treatment. But, **chronic poisoning** can result from long-term therapeutic intake of iodide salts leading to **iodism** which is characterised by metallic taste, anorexia, insomnia, lymphadenopathy, parotid swelling ("***iodide mumps***"), stomatitis, pharyngitis, conjunctivitis, rhinorrhoea and skin manifestations (erythema, urticaria, acne, etc., together referred to as "***ioderma***").
- Hypothyroidism, hyperthyroidism and thyrotoxicosis have been reported secondary to iodine exposure.

Diagnosis

1. ***Specific Tests***:
   a. *Iodine*
      i. Yellowish stains of clothing, skin (**Fig. 9.29**), and mucosa (see *page no. 419* for distinguishing these stains from nitric acid stains).
      ii. Characteristic odour.
      iii. Vomitus or stomach contents when heated in a beaker will cause the iodine to sublime on a cold surface (e.g., a watch glass placed on top of the beaker with some ice).
      iv. To 10 mL of vomitus or gastric aspirate, add 1 mL of starch solution. A blue-black colour will develop.
      v. Urine test: Add 5 mL of chloroform and a few drops of nitric acid to 10 mL of urine. Allow to stand for 3 min. A pinkish-violet chloroform layer forms.
   b. *Iodides*
      i. To 10 mL of vomitus or gastric aspirate, add 1 mL of 10% silver nitrate solution and 1 mL nitric acid. Formation of a yellow precipitate which is insoluble in ammonia is characteristic of iodides.
2. ***Ancillary Tests***:
   a. Serum iodine levels are elevated, as also aminotransferase.
   b. There is also hyperbilirubinaemia, neutropenia and hypoxaemia.

Treatment

1. **Decontamination**:
   a. *Skin*: Wash thoroughly with soap and water, or 20% alcohol.
   b. *Eyes*: Irrigate with water for 15 min.
   c. *GIT*: If oesophageal injury is not present or suspected, gastric lavage can be attempted with starch solution or 5% solution of sodium thiosulphate, or even plain milk. Activated charcoal binds iodine, and can be administered.
2. Sodium bicarbonate IV for metabolic acidosis.
3. There is no specific antidote for iodine or bound iodine. Treatment is primarily supportive and includes monitoring for the development of gastroenteritis, renal failure, tachycardia, hypotension and circulatory collapse. Anaphylactic type reactions may occur as well.
4. Osmotic diuresis, chloruretic diuresis and salt loading may enhance elimination.
5. Haemodialysis and haemodiafiltration have been used to reduce iodine levels in severe toxicity.
6. *Iodism* is treated by ceasing iodide intake while enhancing the intake of sodium chloride which promotes excretion of iodides, since chloride competes with iodide at the level of the renal tubules.

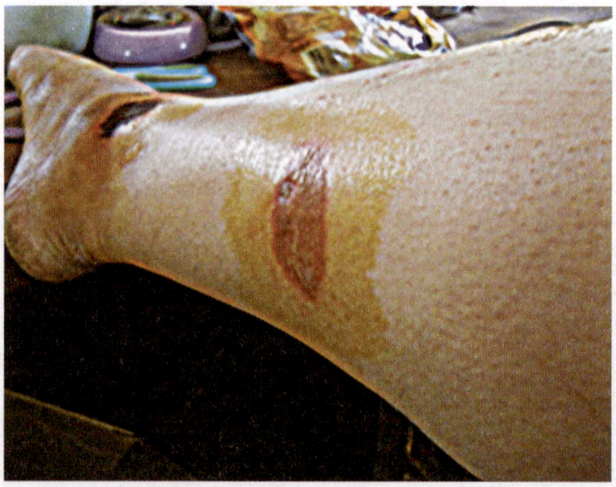

Fig. 9.29 Iodine stains around abrasions

Autopsy Features

1. Brownish or yellowish stains of skin and mucosa. The mucosal staining in the GI tract will appear bluish, if starch solution had been administered while attempting to treat the patient.
2. Characteristic odour (rarely perceptible).
3. Congestion of viscera, especially the kidneys.

Forensic Issues

- Most cases result from accidental therapeutic exposure where iodine or iodides had been administered in excess.
- Chronic poisoning can occur from prolonged therapy with iodides, or may be a result of occupational exposure.
- Iodinated radiologic contrast agents are well known to produce anaphylactic reactions.

BARIUM

Barium was discovered in **1774** by **KW Scheele**, a Swedish chemist. Important derivatives include barium sulphate, sulphide, chloride and carbonate. Most of these exist as white crystalline powders.

Uses

- Rat poison – *Barium carbonate, hydroxide* or *chloride*.
- Depilatory – *Barium sulphide*.
- Gastrointestinal X-ray – *Barium sulphate* (**"barium meal"**) (**Fig. 9.30**).

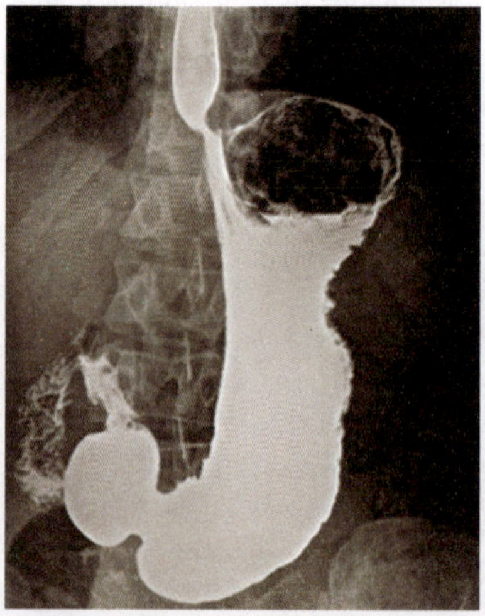

Fig. 9.30 Barium meal

- Golf balls – *Barium sulphate* (along with calcium carbonate, zinc sulphide, castor oil and fish oils).
- Barium compounds are added to fireworks to impart a green colour.

Usual Fatal Dose

- The average fatal dose of soluble barium salts is cited as 1–15 g, depending on the salt ingested.

Mode of Action

- Hypokalaemia and neuromuscular blockade.

Clinical Features

1. *GIT* – Salivation, vomiting, abdominal pain, diarrhoea.
2. *CNS* – Mydriasis, paraesthesias, depressed tendon reflexes, headache, confusion, convulsions.
3. *CVS* – Hypertension, cardiac arrhythmias.
4. *LMS* – Myoclonus, myalgia, cramps, dysarthria. In extreme cases, flaccid quadriplegia develops.
5. *RS* – Pulmonary oedema, respiratory failure.
6. Hypokalaemia, metabolic and respiratory acidosis, and renal failure are commonly reported.
7. Allergic reactions (including anaphylaxis) can occur following barium sulphate administration for radiologic purposes.
8. Barium sulphate is almost insoluble and lacks the severe toxicity characteristic of ingestion of other salts. However, rare cases of toxicity have been reported.

Diagnosis

1. X-ray of abdomen.
2. Endoscopy may be indicated if there is oropharyngeal or abdominal pain indicative of GI burns.
3. ECG
4. Serum potassium levels.
5. Blood barium level.

Treatment

1. Gastric decontamination (lavage). For lavage, 5–10 g sodium sulphate can be added to the solution. Activated charcoal is not beneficial.
2. Monitor cardiac rhythm and serum potassium. Cardiac arrhythmias usually respond to potassium administration. If not, consider lignocaine, amiodarone or procainamide.
3. IV fluids (liberally, to flush out barium by diuresis). Administer 0.45% NaCl in D5W, and a diuretic such as intravenous furosemide (1 mg/kg) to obtain a urine flow of 3–6 mL/kg/hr.
4. 30 g magnesium sulphate through a nasogastric tube. It precipitates the compound ingested into insoluble barium sulphate.
5. Treat hypokalaemia with potassium infusions (up to 250 mEq administered over 24 hrs has been effective).
6. Haemodialysis or haemodiafiltration.

Autopsy Features

1. Haemorrhagic gastritis and duodenitis.
2. Pulmonary oedema.

Forensic Issues

- Most cases are accidental, usually the result of mistaken identity, when a soluble barium salt is administered for a "barium meal" instead of the insoluble barium sulphate.
- Barium salts are sometimes also mistakenly ingested in place of Epsom salt, Glauber's salt or even common salt.
- Inhalation of a "barium meal" can produce granulomas in the lungs.
- A few cases of mass poisonings have been reported, the most remarkable being ***Pa Ping*** an endemic form of periodic paralysis which occurred in the early 1940s in the Szechuan province of China. This was due to massive contamination of table salt by barium chloride.

FM 9.3: Core – Written/Viva Voce/ Objective Structured Clinical Examination (OSCE)

- Describe general principles and basic methodologies in treatment of poisoning: decontamination, supportive therapy, antidote therapy, procedures of enhanced elimination with regard to:
  - Arsenic
  - Lead
  - Mercury
  - Copper
  - Iron
  - Cadmium
  - Thallium

ARSENIC

Arsenic is today the commonest source of acute heavy metal poisoning, and is second only to **lead** in the incidence of chronic toxicity.

Physical Appearance

- Though arsenic is classified as a **heavy metal**, it is actually a **metalloid**, i.e., it is an element which resembles a metal in some respects, and is by itself not very toxic. However, almost all the salts are toxic to varying degree.
- Arsenic (**Fig. 9.31**) is a silver-grey, crystalline and metallic-looking element.
- **Table 9.4** lists the physical properties and uses of elemental arsenic and some of its salts.

Usual Fatal Dose

- **200–300 mg for arsenic trioxide**.
- In general, the pentavalent form of arsenic (*arsenate or arsenic V*) is less toxic than the trivalent form (*arsenite or arsenic III*) because it is less water soluble. The most toxic form is arsine gas (25–30 ppm can be lethal in 30 min).

Toxicokinetics and Mode of Action

- Arsenic is absorbed through all portals of entry including oral, inhalational and cutaneous routes.
- After absorption it is redistributed to the liver, lungs, intestinal wall and spleen, where it binds to the sulphydryl groups of tissue proteins. Arsenic replaces phosphorus in the bone where it may remain for years. It gets deposited also in hair.

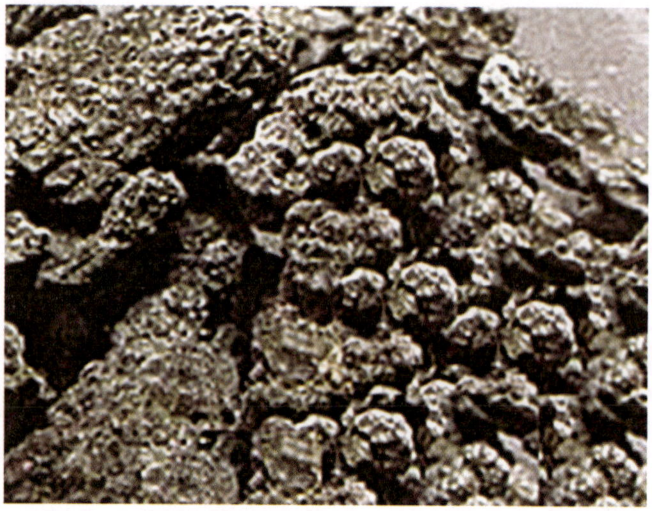

Fig. 9.31 Arsenic

- The main route of elimination is the kidney.
- The primary mode of action of trivalent arsenicals is inhibition of the pyruvate dehydrogenase (PDH) complex. They bind the sulphydryl groups of dihydrolipoamide, blocking lipoamide regeneration. Acetyl-CoA is a central molecule in metabolism, and the resulting decrease leads to several deleterious effects: decreased citric acid cycle activity and thus decreased adenosine triphosphate (ATP) production, disruption of oxidative phosphorylation leads to production of hydrogen peroxide and oxygen radicals, decreased gluconeogenesis which worsens hypoglycaemia.
- Trivalent arsenic also inhibits glutathione synthetase, G6PD (required to produce NADPH), and glutathione reductase. These inhibitions result in decreased levels of reduced glutathione, which is required to facilitate arsenic metabolism, protect RBCs from oxidative damage, maintain haemoglobin in the ferrous state and scavenge organic peroxides.
- Pentavalent arsenicals resemble phosphate chemically and structurally, and can uncouple oxidative phosphorylation by substituting for inorganic phosphate (P_i) in the glycolysis reaction.
- Effects on RBCs include decreased membrane fluidity and ATP depletion. Chronic arsenic exposure is associated with vascular disease.
- Proposed mechanisms by which arsenic induces cancer include DNA damage induced by a dimethyl sulphide.

Table 9.4 Inorganic and Organic Arsenicals

Chemical Name	Synonyms	Physical Properties	Uses
Elemental arsenic	Metallic arsenic, grey arsenic	Grey, brittle, metallic-looking substance	In alloys
Arsine	Arsenic trihydride	Colourless gas with garlicky odour	Lead plating, soldering, galvanising
Trimethyl arsine	Gosio gas	Colourless gas	Present in sewage
Arsenic trioxide	Arsenic oxide, white arsenic	White powder	Manufacture of glass, insecticide, rodenticide
Arsenic trichloride	Butter of arsenic	Yellowish, oily liquid	Pottery
Lead arsenate	Acid lead arsenate	Heavy, white powder	Insecticide
Sulphides of arsenic	Red realgar (*disulphide*) Yellow orpiment (*trisulphide*)	Red powder Yellow powder	Depilatory Depilatory & colour pigment
Copper arsenite	Scheele's green	Greenish powder	Colouring agent for toys
Copper acetoarsenite	Paris or Emerald green	Greenish powder	Insecticide
Organic arsenicals (*carbarsone, tryparsamide, glycobiarsol, melarsoprol, etc.*)	–	–	Melarsoprol is used to treat West African (Gambian) and East African (Rhodesian) trypanosomiasis. Other organic arsenicals are not used in therapeutics any more.

***Note**: Arsenic compounds are also used in paints, and in the tanning industry.*

- Pigmentary changes also occur, and hyperpigmentation is attributed to increased melanin.

Clinical Features

- Mentioned in **Table 9.5**.
- ***Aldrich-Mees' lines*** (often shortened to ***Mees' lines***) are characteristic of arsenic poisoning (acute as well as chronic) (**Fig. 9.32**).
- **Dermal pigmentation** is consistently seen in chronic arsenic poisoning (**Fig. 9.33**), as also **hyperkeratosis of palms and soles** (**Fig. 9.34**).

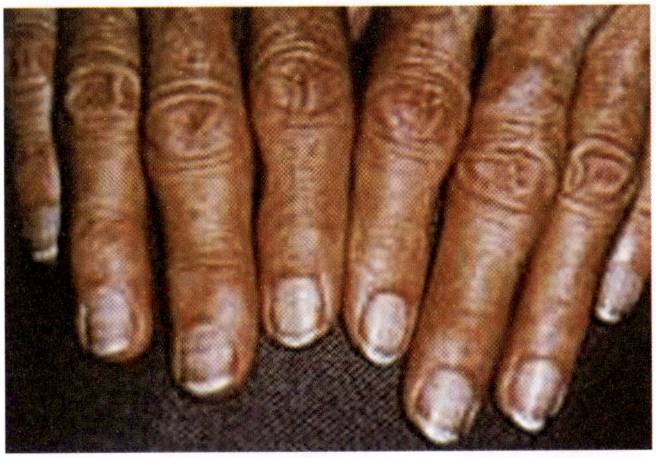

Fig. 9.32 Aldrich-Mees lines

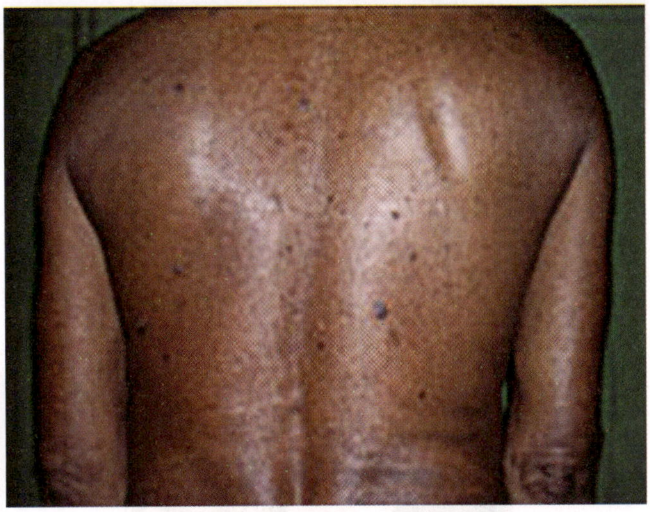

Fig. 9.33 Raindrop pigmentation – Arsenic poisoning

Diagnosis

One of the best analytical methods for the detection of arsenic in biological samples is atomic absorption spectroscopy.

1. **Urine level**:
   a. If the 24-hr excretion of arsenic exceeds 100 µg (regardless of urine volume), it is indicative of toxicity. Urine should be collected in metal-free polyethylene containers; acid-rinsed containers are not necessary.

Table 9.5 Arsenic Poisoning

System	Acute	Chronic
Dermal	Hair loss, transverse bands of opacity in nails (*Mees' lines*)*	Melanosis (neck, eyelids), Bowen's disease, hyperkeratosis, skin pigmentation (*rain drop pattern*), skin cancer
Ocular	Conjunctivitis, lacrimation	Dimness of vision
GIT	Abdominal pain, metallic taste, dysphagia, vomiting, rice—water diarrhoea.** Garlicky odour in the breath.	Anorexia, vomiting, diarrhoea, weight loss
Airways	Irritation of upper airways	Chronic laryngitis, bronchitis
Liver	Fatty degeneration	Hepatomegaly, jaundice, cirrhosis
Kidney	Oliguria, uraemia	Nephritic changes
Neurological	Hyperpyrexia, convulsions, coma	Encephalopathy, polyneuritis, tremor, ataxia, difficulty in walking
Blood	–	Anaemia, leucopenia, thrombocytopenia, basophilic stippling, pancytopenia
Cardiac	Tachycardia, hypotension, cardiac arrhythmias***	Hypertension, myocarditis

**After 2 weeks.*
***May mimic cholera.*
****ECG changes include myocardial depression, ST-T wave changes, prolonged QT interval, ventricular tachycardia.*

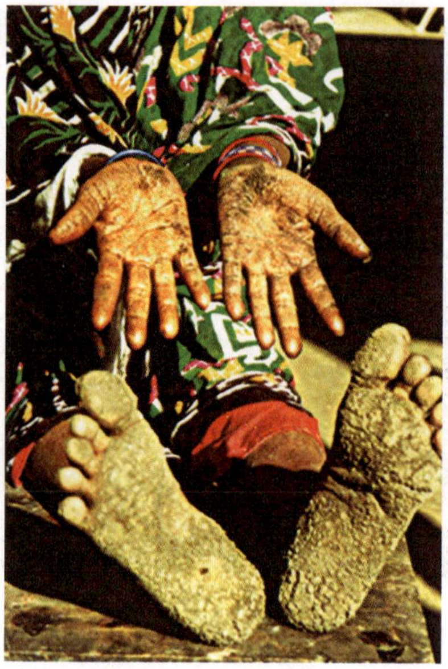

Fig. 9.34 Arsenic keratosis (palms & soles)

b. Ingestion of seafood can interfere with interpretation since considerable concentrations of organic arsenicals such as *arsenobetaine* and *arsenocholine* may be present in shellfish*, cod, haddock, etc., although it is not associated with toxic effects. In such cases, the analysis must be repeated after 2 days of "no fish" diet.

2. **Blood level**:
   a. This is less reliable than urine level because of short half-life of arsenic in the blood. However, a blood level of arsenic less than 5 µg/100 mL (0.665 µmol/L) is generally considered in the normal range.
3. **Hair level**
   a. Arsenic can be detected in the proximal portions of hair within 30 hrs of ingestion.
4. **Radiography**
   a. Since arsenic is radiopaque, abdominal X-ray may reveal its presence in the gastrointestinal tract in acute poisoning.
   b. **Table 9.6** presents a list of **radiopaque poisons** commonly encountered in practice.
5. **Additional Investigations**
   a. Monitor CBC, serum electrolytes, urinalysis (for proteinuria, haematuria or pyuria), liver and renal function tests.
   b. Obtain an ECG and institute continuous cardiac monitoring in symptomatic patients.

Table 9.6 Radiopaque Poisons

- Carbon tetrachloride
- Chloral hydrate
- Heavy metals
- Iodides
- Methotrexate
- Phenothiazines
- Salicylates
- Sustained release capsules

***Mnemonic**: CCHIMPSS*

Treatment

1. **Supportive measures**:
   a. Gastric lavage (acute poisoning), intravenous fluids, cardiac monitoring, etc. Activated charcoal is unlikely to be of benefit.
   b. Commence intravenous fluids in patients with diarrhoea and vomiting. Correct electrolyte disturbances and consider need for blood transfusion, if haemorrhagic gastroenteritis is present. Careful attention to fluid balance is important because cerebral and pulmonary oedema may be present.
   c. Drugs that prolong the QTc, such as the class IA, class IC, and class III antiarrhythmics, should be avoided. Consider magnesium sulphate when the QT-heart rate nomogram indicates a risk of torsade de pointes, especially if other risk factors are present. Magnesium sulphate is administered IV over 10–15 min: adults 2 g, children 25–50 mg/kg.

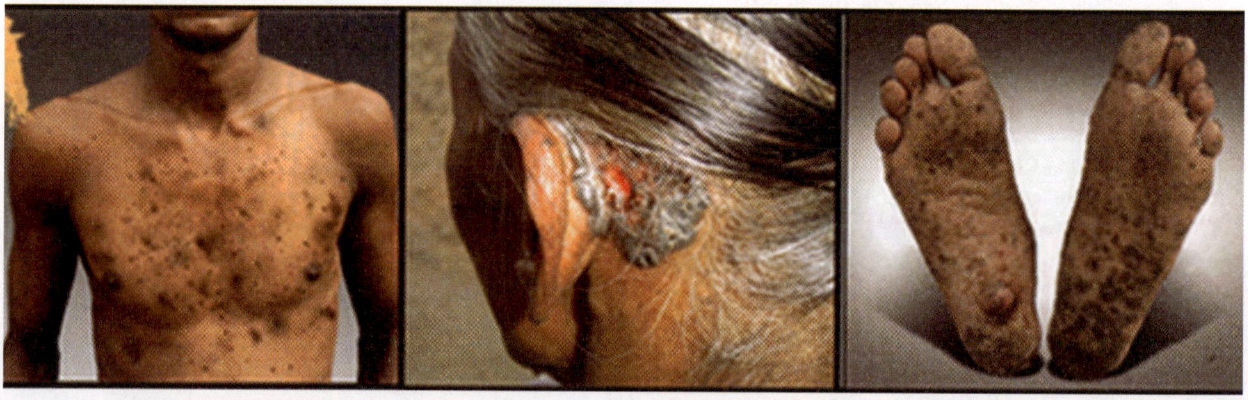

Fig. 9.35 Various dermatologic lesions – Arsenic poisoning

****Note***: *Oyster, mussel, prawns, shrimps, crab, etc.*

d. Glucose concentrations and glycogen stores should be maintained parenterally with dextrose and hyperalimentation solutions, or with enteral feedings.

e. If radiopaque material is visualized in the gastrointestinal tract, whole-bowel irrigation can be administered until the radiopaque material is no longer seen on repeat abdominal radiograph.

f. In cases of chronic toxicity, patients should be removed from the arsenic source and gastric decontamination should be performed, if there is evidence of arsenic in the gastrointestinal tract.

2. **Chelation therapy**:

a. This can be done with **BAL** (**British Anti Lewisite** or **dimercaprol**), penicillamine, DMSA (Dimercapto succinic acid) or DMPS (Dimercapto propane sulphonic acid).

b. The usual agent employed is **BAL** at a dose of 3–5 mg/kg intramuscularly every 4–6 hrs until the urinary arsenic excretion dips below 50 μg/24 hrs. BAL is administered intramuscularly in peanut oil; the injections are painful and can lead to sterile skin abscesses. Usual duration of therapy is 7–10 days.

c. In patients who are not allergic to penicillin, penicillamine can be given orally at a dose of 100 mg/kg/day, 6th hourly for 5 days.

d. DMSA and DMPS said to be superior to BAL and penicillamine, are currently not available in India.

i. DMPS, Intravenous: IV DMPS should be given, at least initially, in a dose of 30 mg/kg/day for 5 days, which may be repeated, if necessary after 5–7 days.

ii. **DMSA**: 30 mg/kg/day (3 divided doses) orally for 5 days, repeated after 5–7 days, if necessary.

3. **Haemodialysis** or **haemodiafiltration** may be required for the clinical management of patients with established renal failure.

Autopsy Features

1. Gastrointestinal congestion is a noteworthy feature in acute arsenic poisoning and varies from a mere reddening of mucosa (***red velvet***) to frank haemorrhagic gastritis. Focal haemorrhages giving rise to a ***flea bitten*** appearance is said to be characteristic. The intestines may be inflamed and may contain "***rice water***" contents.
2. Subendocardial haemorrhages are often seen in the heart.*
3. There may be evidence of fatty degeneration of heart, liver and kidneys.
4. Chronic arsenic poisoning may present features of non-specific gastrointestinal inflammation, as well as renal and hepatic damage, at autopsy.
5. It is conventional to preserve apart from the routine viscera and body fluids, a piece of long bone (preferably femur), a bunch of pulled scalp hair, a wedge of muscle and a small portion of skin (from the back of the trunk) for chemical analysis. The gruesome practice of pulling out finger and toe nails is best dispensed with.

Forensic Issues

- Arsenic has had an outstanding reputation as an **ideal homicidal poison**, especially in the West, particularly United Kingdom in the Victorian era. Several celebrated murders are said to have been accomplished with the help of arsenic during this period. One of the most shocking cases was that of French Emperor **Napoleon Bonaparte**, though in a 2008 publication, it is mentioned that researchers analysed samples of Napoleon's hair from throughout his life, as well as samples from his family and other contemporaries, and found that all samples had high levels of arsenic (approximately 100 times higher than the current average). According to these researchers, Napoleon's body was already contaminated with arsenic as a boy, and the high arsenic concentration in his hair was not caused by intentional poisoning; people were constantly exposed to arsenic from glues and dyes throughout their lives. They dismissed allegations of arsenic poisoning, suggesting peptic ulcer and gastric cancer as the probable cause of death.

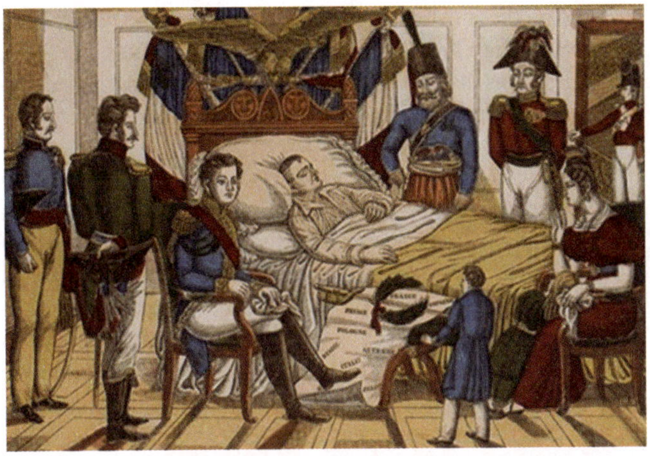

Fig. 9.36 A painting of Emperor Napoleon in his death bed

- Arsenic trioxide being almost tasteless and colourless in solution can be administered without arousing the suspicion of a victim. The main obstacle is relative insolubility. But the solubility can be greatly enhanced, if hot solutions are used such as coffee, tea, cocoa, porridge or gruel and soups. The only problem is that on cooling, much of the dissolved arsenic will separate out to yield a gritty deposit.
- On chronic successful administration to a victim, arsenic produces insidious but relentlessly progressive symptoms which are likely to be mistaken even by a medical practitioner for natural causes such as neurological disease, alcoholism, tuberculosis and hepatic or renal afflictions, while acute poisoning may be confused with gastroenteritis or cholera.

**Note: While this is a constant feature in arsenic poisoning, it may also be encountered in head injury, raised intracranial pressure, sudden loss of blood due to injury resulting in abrupt hypotension and obstetric complications.*

- However, the popularity of arsenic has declined in recent times because of various factors – legal restrictions on its sale, availability of sophisticated methods which can detect even minute quantities in a dead body, and of course the emergence of better poisons to accomplish nefarious deeds! Today most cases of arsenic poisoning are accidental, though murders are still reported from time to time.
- Accidental poisoning may be the result of industrial or occupational exposure, or it may be due to consumption of contaminated water or food.
  - Methylation of inorganic arsenic is a naturally occurring detoxification process for arsenic and results in the accumulation of organoarsenic compounds (e.g., arsenobetaine) in some fish and vegetables.
  - In the past, certain allopathic drugs used to contain arsenic and iatrogenic poisoning was not uncommon.
  - Today ayurvedic preparations constitute the main hazard, some of which can contain substantial concentrations of arsenic that can produce chronic poisoning on prolonged use.
- Organic arsenic compounds were used as chemical weapons during World War I as either Adamsite or Lewisite.
- Today, the most outstanding source of chronic accidental poisoning in India is consumption of well water. There are indications that sizeable populations of several Asian countries are exposed to arsenic tainted water, particularly tube well water.
  - A devastating health crisis (***endemic hydroarsenicism***) began to unfold in **West Bengal** in the early **1980s** due to exposure to arsenic laced well water. High levels of arsenic have been demonstrated which probably leached from natural underground sources into thousands of village wells affecting more than 250,000 people who display overt manifestations (especially related to the skin) such as hyperkeratosis, pigmentation and skin cancer, while more than 1 million who are continuing to drink the tainted water may develop lesions over a period of time. Analysis of water from more than 200,000 tube wells demonstrated arsenic content above the WHO permissible limit of 0.01 mg/L in many samples.

LEAD

Lead is the commonest metal involved in chronic poisoning. It was one of the first metals known to man and has been widely used during the last 2000 years for domestic, industrial and therapeutic purposes. Lead is abundant in soil, being distributed throughout the earth's crust.

Physical Appearances and Uses

- Elemental lead exists as a lustrous, heavy, silvery-grey metal that assumes a bluish tint, as it tarnishes in air (**Fig. 9.37**). It is quite soft and malleable.
- Several of its salts occur as variously coloured powders or liquids and are used widely in industry.
  - Lead acetate (*sugar of lead*) has been used in therapeutics.*
  - Lead carbonate (*white lead*) is still used in paints.
  - Lead oxide (*litharge*) is essential for glazing of pottery and enamel ware.
  - Tetraethyl lead is mixed with petrol as an antiknock to prevent detonation in internal combustion engines. Among cosmetics, lead tetroxide is the most common compound in *vermilion* ("*sindoor*") applied by married Hindu women to the parting of their scalp hair (**Fig. 9.38**), while lead sulphide is used widely as an eye cosmetic ("*surma*" *or* "*kohl*") (**Fig. 9.39**) by various communities in India.** Sometimes mercuric sulphide is used as "*sindoor*," while antimony sulphide is used as "*surma*."

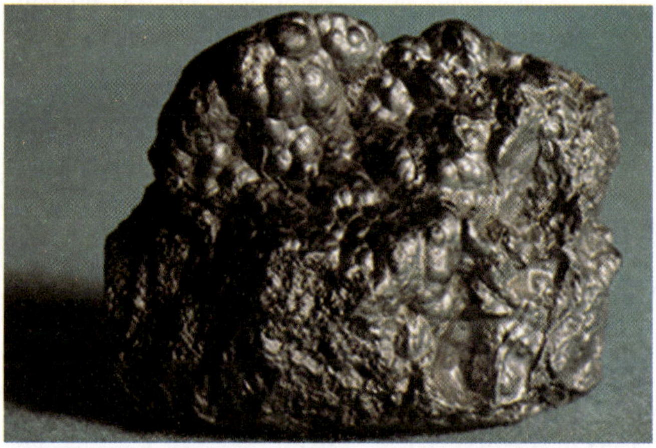

Fig. 9.37 Elemental Lead

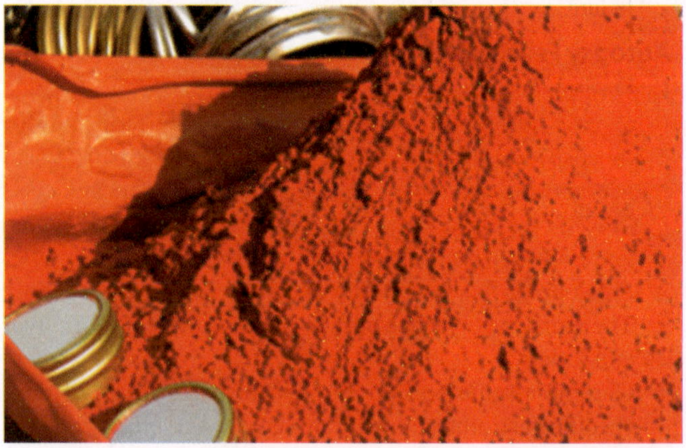

Fig. 9.38 Sindoor (Vermilion)

****Note***: *It has a sweetish astringent taste, and so was also used to sweeten wine in the olden days, leading to chronic poisoning in wine drinkers ("Dry gripes").*

*****Note***: *Surma or Kohl is an eye cosmetic that is widely used in South Asia, the Middle East, North Africa and parts of West Africa to darken the eyelids and as mascara for the eyelashes. It is worn mostly by women, but also by some men and children. In addition, mothers apply kohl to their infants' eyes soon after birth. Some do this to "strengthen the child's eyes", and others believe it could prevent the child from being cursed by the "evil eye".*

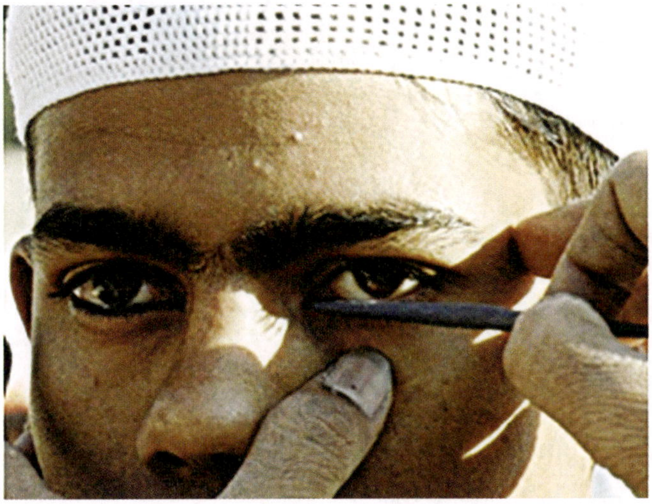

Fig. 9.39 Surma (Kohl)

Usual Fatal Dose

This is not really relevant to lead, since acute poisoning is very rare. The average lethal dose is said to be **10 g/70 kg for most lead salts**, while it is **100 mg/kg for tetraethyl lead**.

Toxicokinetics

- Lead is absorbed through all portals of entry. Occupational exposure results mainly from inhalation, while in other situations the mode of intake is ingestion.
- Following absorption, it is stored in the bones as phosphate and carbonate. In children, about 70% of total body lead is skeletal, while in adults over 95% is in osseous tissues. Lead is drawn to those areas of the skeleton which are growing most rapidly. These include the radius, tibia and femur, which are the most metabolically active. The hypermineralisation is reflected in the form of densities which are the classic "***lead lines***" observed on X-ray (**Fig 9.40**). The width of the lead lines is related to the duration of exposure. Significant amounts of skeletal lead are released from bone into the blood stream periodically resulting in symptoms of toxicity.

Mode of Action

- Lead combines with sulphydryl enzymes leading to their dysfunction.
- It decreases haem synthesis by inactivating the enzymes involved such as *aminolaevulinic acid dehydrase*, *aminolaevulinic acid synthetase*, *coproporphyrinogen oxidase* (or *decarboxylase*) and *ferrochelatase*. This results in anaemia.*
- It increases haemolysis as a result of which immature red cells are released into circulation such as reticulocytes and ***basophilic stippled cells*** (the result of aggregation of ribonucleic acid due to inhibition of the enzyme pyrimidine-5′-nucleotidase which normally eliminates degraded RNA) (**Fig. 9.41**).
- In the CNS, lead causes oedema and has a direct cytotoxic effect leading to decreased nerve conduction, increased psychomotor activity, lower IQ and behavioural/learning disorders. Children are especially susceptible.
- Lead also has deleterious effects on the CVS (hypertension and myocarditis), kidney (nephritis) and reproductive organs (infertility).
- In addition, lead can decrease uric acid renal excretion, thereby raising blood urate levels and predisposing to gout (***saturnine gout***).
- Acute intoxication can cause haematuria, aminoaciduria, glycosuria and hyperphosphaturia (***Fanconi syndrome***).
- Traditionally, the accepted upper level for blood lead (BL) has been 80 μg/100 mL, but this was reduced recently to 35 μg/100 mL. There is substantial evidence to show that blood lead concentrations of 30–40 μg/100 mL have adverse

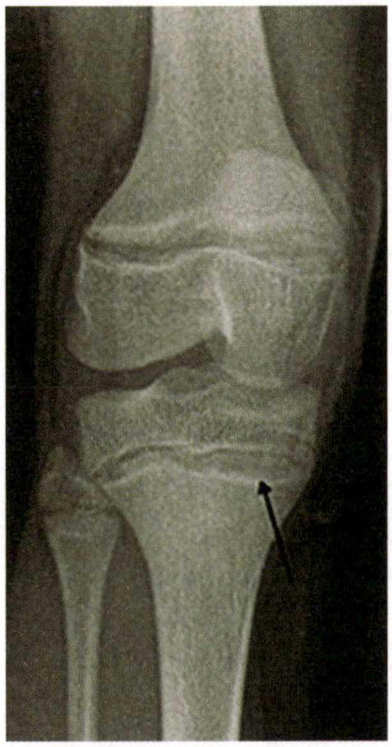

Fig. 9.40 Lead line (*arrowed*)

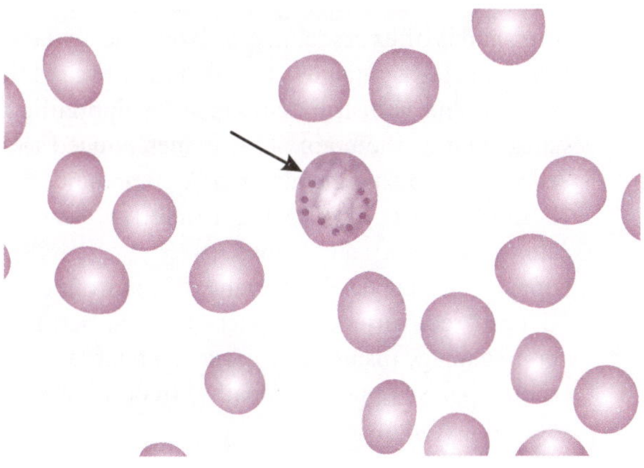

Fig. 9.41 Basophilic stippled cell (*arrowed*)

****Note***: *Aminolaevulinic acid (ALA) & coproporphyrin levels rise in the urine and can be used as "markers" to diagnose lead poisoning.*

effects on the nervous system, haematopoietic system, renal system and reproductive system. Hence, the current trend is to consider even levels as low as 10 µg/100 mL as unacceptable.

Clinical Features

1. **Acute Poisoning**:
   i. This is rare. Many reported cases of acute poisoning may actually be exacerbations of chronic lead poisoning when significant quantities of lead are suddenly released into the bloodstream from bone.
   ii. Symptoms include metallic taste, abdominal pain, constipation or diarrhoea (stools may be blackish due to lead sulphide), vomiting, hyperactivity or lethargy, ataxia, behavioural changes, convulsions and coma.
2. **Chronic Poisoning (*Plumbism* or *Saturnism*)**:
   a. *Mild Toxicity (BL 40–60 µg/100 mL)*:
      i. Myalgia
      ii. Paraesthesia
      iii. Fatigue
      iv. Irritability
      v. Abdominal discomfort
   b. *Moderate Toxicity (BL 60–100 µg/100 mL)* :
      i. Arthralgia (especially nocturnal)
      ii. Muscular exhaustibility
      iii. Tremor
      iv. Headache
      v. Diffuse abdominal pain
      vi. Anorexia, metallic taste, vomiting
      vii. Constipation
      viii. Weight loss
      ix. Hypertension
   c. *Severe Toxicity (BL more than 100 µg/100 mL)* :
      i. ***Lead palsy*** – Wrist drop (**Fig. 9.42**) or foot drop.
      ii. A bluish black ***lead line*** on gums (***Burton's line***) (**Fig. 9.43**).*
      iii. ***Lead colic*** – Intermittent severe abdominal cramps. There may be tenderness around the umbilicus.
      iv. ***Lead encephalopathy*** – It is more common in children and is often associated with organic lead toxicity, especially tetraethyl lead or TEL which is lipid soluble and is distributed widely in lipophilic tissues such as the brain. TEL is metabolised to triethyl lead which is the major toxic compound. There is sudden onset of vomiting, irritability, headache, ataxia, vertigo, convulsions, psychotic manifestations, coma and death. Mortality rate is around 25%. Even if recovery occurs, there is often permanent brain damage manifesting as mental retardation, cerebral palsy, optic neuropathy, hyperkinesis and periodic convulsions.

      Facial pallor, especially circum-oral is said to be a characteristic feature of chronic lead poisoning and is due to vasospasm, though anaemia may contribute to a significant extent. The anaemia that is encountered in plumbism is similar to that due to iron deficiency, i.e., it is hypochromic and microcytic in type; but anaemia due to the latter is neither associated with reticulocytosis, nor are basophilic stippled cells seen.

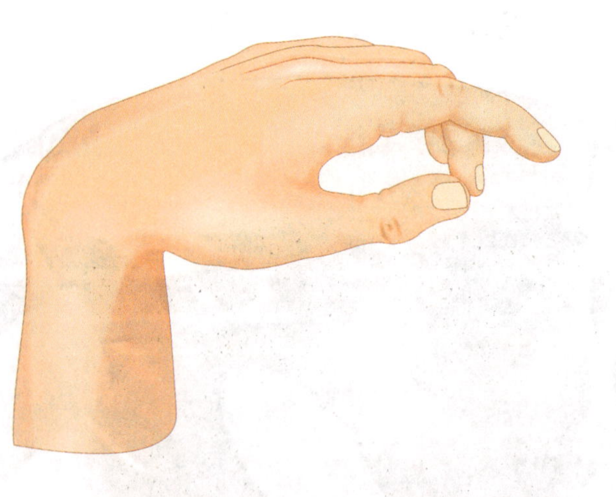

Fig. 9.42 Wrist drop

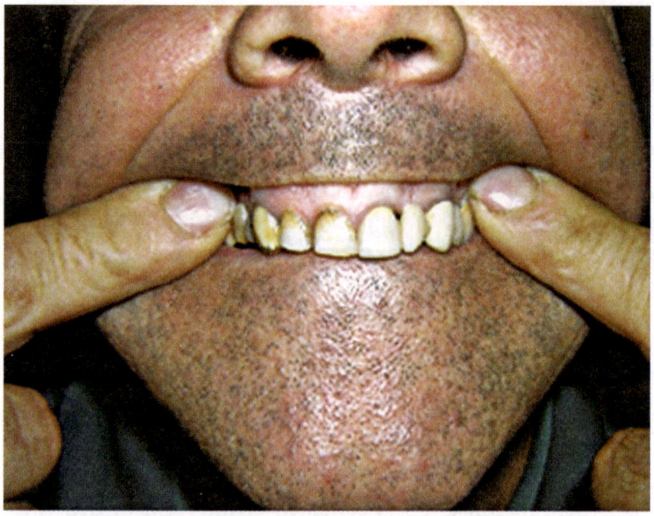

Fig. 9.43 Burton's line

3. **Organic Lead Poisoning**:
   a. Clinical symptoms of tetraethyl lead (TEL) toxicity are usually nonspecific initially, and include insomnia and emotional instability. Nausea, vomiting and anorexia may occur. There may be tremor and increased deep-tendon reflexes.
   b. In more severe cases, these symptoms progress to encephalopathy with delusions, hallucinations, and hyperactivity, which may resolve or deteriorate to coma

****Note***: *It may also be seen around the anal margin, and is due to bacterial action on blood lead precipitating insoluble lead sulphide. A similar dark line is sometimes seen in poisoning due to mercury, iron, thallium, silver or bismuth.*

and, occasionally, death. Severe cases may also develop hepatic and renal injury.

Diagnosis

Laboratory Tests for Lead

a. **Blood**

i. *Complete blood count and Peripheral smear* – General and non-specific findings include low haematocrit and haemoglobin values with normal total and differential cell counts. Hypochromia and basophilic stippling are strongly suggestive of lead intoxication, but their absence does not rule out lead poisoning. It must be borne in mind that such stippled RBCs may also be seen in arsenic and zinc poisoning.

ii. *FEP and ZNp levels* (>50 µg/100 mL) – Elevated FEP (free erythrocyte protoporphyrin) and ZnP (zinc protoporphyrin) levels indicate impairment of the haem biosynthetic pathway and may result from lead poisoning or iron deficiency. In order to confirm whether it is due to the former, the BL (blood lead) must be estimated. Today ZnP levels are more commonly studied than FEP.

iii. ***Blood lead level* (*BL*)** – Blood lead levels reflect recent exposure or exposure over a period of up to 3–5 weeks. In individuals with high or chronic past exposure, BL usually under-represents the total body burden because most lead is stored in the bone and may be found at normal levels in the blood. However, during stressful circumstances, patients with a high-body burden may have elevated BL because of the release of lead stored in bones.

- The recommended methods of estimating blood lead level (BL) include atomic absorption spectroscopy (AAS), electrothermal atomic absorption spectroscopy (EAAS), anodic stripping voltametry (ASV), inductively coupled plasma atomic emission spectroscopy (ICP-AES) and X-ray fluorescence spectroscopy.
- In recent years, **inductively coupled plasma mass spectrometry (ICP-MS)** has become the technique of choice, owing to superior specificity and sensitivity. It provides highly accurate and rapid results.

b. **Urine**:

i. The concentration of ALA in urine is widely used as a measure of lead toxicity in workers who are exposed occupationally. For this purpose, colourimetric methods were employed previously, but today fluorometry (after separation by HPLC) is preferred.

- *Urine lead level*: If this is above 150 µg/L, it is a significant finding, but it is unfortunately not very reliable.
- *Calcium disodium EDTA mobilisation test*: This test is done mainly in children to find out whether a child whose BL is between 25 and 45 µg/100 mL will respond to chelation therapy with a brisk lead diuresis. *Procedure* – First the patient is asked to empty the bladder. Then $CaNa_2EDTA$ is given at a dose of 500 mg/m^2 in 5% dextrose infused over 1 hr. All urine must be collected with lead-free equipment over the next 8 hrs. To obtain the total lead excretion (µg), the concentration of lead in the urine (µg/mL) is multiplied by total urinary volume (mL). Total urinary excretion of lead (µg) is divided by the amount of $CaNa_2EDTA$ given (mg) to obtain the lead excretion ratio:

$$\frac{\text{Lead excreted } (\mu g)}{CaNa_2EDTA \text{ given (mg)}}$$

The test is considered positive, if the lead excretion ratio is more than 0.6. Such a child should undergo a 5-day course of chelation.

- *Urine porphyrin level*: Patients with lead poisoning usually excrete elevated levels of porphyrins in the urine.

c. **Bone**:

i. X-ray fluorescence technique is brief and non-invasive and carries low risk. It is based on the specific atomic property of lead to emit characteristic X-rays upon stimulation induced by external irradiation. The stimulated radiation is monitored externally by a solid state detector and can be expressed in terms of lead concentration in the bone.

ii. Many investigators now recommend such an "in vivo analysis" of bone lead concentration as superior to the more cumbersome *$CaNa_2EDTA$ chelation provocative test*.

d. **Radiology**:

i. Radiological examination of the abdomen may show radiopaque foreign material, if the material has been ingested during the preceding 24–36 hrs.

ii. The significant finding in bone is the appearance of dense transverse bands or ***lead lines*** extending across the metaphyses of the long bones, and along margins of flat bones such as the iliac crest. It usually takes 4–8 weeks of heavy exposure for dense bands to develop.

Treatment

A. ***Severe acute poisoning with encephalopathy***:

This is a medical emergency and the following measures must be undertaken immediately:

1. BAL 4 mg/kg immediately.
2. *Cranial CT scan*: To rule out cerebral oedema. If there is cerebral oedema, it can be managed by the following measures:

   i. Controlled hyperventilation, maintaining an arterial CO_2 tension of 25–30 mm Hg.

   ii. Diuretics:

      a. Mannitol 20%: 1–1.5 g/kg by infusion over 10–20 min.

      b. Glycerol: 0.3–1 g/kg orally.

iii. Corticosteroids:
Dexamethasone: *Low dose*, 16 mg/day in divided doses.
Dexamethasone: *High dose*, 1–2 mg/kg/day in divided doses.
iv. Barbiturates: Pentobarbitone, 30 mg/kg/day by IV infusion.

3. *KUB*: To rule out lead chips in GI tract.
4. *For seizures*: Treat seizures with IV diazepam (up to 10 mg).
5. *Foley catheterisation*: to monitor urinary specific gravity, sediment, lead level.
6. $CaNa_2EDTA$ 75 mg/kg/day IV infusion.
7. After the initial dose of BAL, repeat the same dose at 4 hourly intervals until blood lead level falls below 40 µg/100 mL. Then, reduce BAL to 12 mg/kg/day in three divided doses.
8. Reduce $CaNa_2EDTA$ to 50 mg/kg/day as condition improves.
9. Continue the above regimen until patient is asymptomatic and can tolerate oral chelation with D-penicillamine or DMSA.

B. ***Severe poisoning without encephalopathy*** (*BL more than 70 µg/100 mL*):
1. BAL 12/mg/kg/day.
2. EDTA 50 mg/kg/day.
3. Discontinue BAL when the BL falls below 40 µg/100 mL, but continue EDTA for 5 more days.
4. Change to oral chelation subsequently which may have to be continued until the BL falls below 15 µg/100 mL, or 3 months have been completed.

C. ***Moderate poisoning*** (*BL between 45 and 70 µg/100 mL*):
1. EDTA 50 mg/kg/day.
2. When blood lead falls below 40 µg/100 mL, begin oral chelation.

D. ***Mild poisoning*** (*BL 20–45 µg/100 mL*): D-Penicillamine 30 mg/kg/day in three divided doses. Double this after 1 week. Double again (to full dose) after 1 week. Continue this until the BL falls to less than 15 µg/100 mL, or 3 months have been completed.

E. In recent times, a new chelating agent called ***Succimer*** has been introduced in the management of lead poisoning, and is said to be more efficacious and less toxic.
i. **Succimer** (*2,3-Dimercaptosuccinic acid, DMSA*): It is available abroad as microspheres in hard gelatin capsules. The capsules which contain 1000 mg of succimer can be opened prior to use and the contents mixed with juice. A 5-day course of 30 mg/kg/day in adults or 1050 mg/m^2/day in children is safe and effective in treating lead intoxication. If there is rebound in lead level, a 14-day course (20 mg/kg/day in adults, or 700 mg/m^2/day in children) should follow the 5-day regimen.

F. Supportive measures.

Autopsy Features

1. Pale skin, conjunctivae and mucosa (*anaemia*).
2. Emaciation.
3. Burtonian line.
4. Lead lines on X-ray.
5. Pathological lesions or changes are sometimes found in kidneys, liver, male gonads, nervous system, blood vessels.

Forensic Issues

- Hippocrates is credited with the earliest description of chronic lead poisoning when he associated persistent abdominal colic in a man, with his occupation of extracting metals (around 370 BC).
- The ancient Romans were however the first to experience the metal's adverse effects on a massive scale mainly because of chronic poisoning through lead acetate which was used to sweeten wine in those days. Chemical analyses of the bones of Roman rulers have demonstrated high lead content and the madness of some of the Roman aristocracy (*Nero, Caligula*), may actually have been the result of lead poisoning.
- Lead-laced wine and lead-based cosmetics caused havoc among the English in the 18th and 19th centuries which included even members of the royalty. The many ailments suffered by Queen Anne including her disastrous obstetric history are said to be because of lead poisoning.
- In 1763, Benjamin Franklin reported on ***dry gripes*** (abdominal colic), and ***dangles*** (wrist drop), which afflicted painters and typesetters, as well as the *gripes* due to rum distillation in leaden condensing coils.
- In 1863, Charles Dickens described graphically the plight of lead mill workers in "The Uncommercial Traveller."
- Today chronic lead poisoning is said to be the most important environmental health problem, particularly among young children. Children are especially susceptible to lead poisoning because of their increased absorption of lead from the GIT when compared with the adult. The child with **pica** is in enhanced danger because of the tendency in such a case to lick lead-based paints off walls, furniture, toys, pencils, etc. The increasing antisocial behaviour of street urchins and slum dwelling children in congested and polluted cities may also be the offshoot of chronic lead poisoning, since studies have demonstrated a high incidence of plumbism in juvenile boys with delinquent behaviour.
- Blood levels of some vulnerable populations (e.g., traffic police) have come down significantly ever since unleaded petrol was introduced in India in the 1990s.
- Another important step taken to minimise the incidence of plumbism was to ban lead-based household paints. However, industrial paints for cars, machinery, bridges, highway stripes, etc., still contain lead.
- Though today lead pipes are hardly used for supplying drinking water in most parts of India, the latter even now constitutes an important source of lead poisoning. Contamination can occur through atmospheric lead or indus

trial wastes, or from the soldered joints in the water distribution system.

- The most sizeable chunk of plumbism occurs from occupational exposure among workers exposed to lead such as miners, plumbers, battery makers, plastic manufacturers, garage workers, etc.

MERCURY

Synonyms

Quick silver; Liquid silver

Physical Appearance

- Metallic or **elemental mercury** (Hg^0) is a heavy, silvery liquid (**Fig. 9.44**) which is *per se* non-toxic, but vapourises at room temperature to give off a toxic vapour: mercuric mercury.* Volatilisation is greatly enhanced by heating.
- **Salts of mercury** may be inorganic or organic in nature.
  - Inorganic salts are of two types – mercuric (bivalent, i.e., Hg^{2+}) and mercurous (monovalent, i.e., Hg^{+}).
    - Common mercuric salts include **mercuric chloride** (***corrosive sublimate***) which is a white crystalline corrosive powder, **mercuric oxide** which is a red crystalline powder and **mercuric sulphide** (***vermilion*** or ***sindoor***) which is a red crystalline powder.
    - The most important mercurous salt is **mercurous chloride** (*calomel*) which is fibrous and heavy.
- **Organic mercurials** (organomercury compounds) are generally more toxic and comprise mainly ethylmercury, **methyl mercury** and phenylmercury. Mercurochrome is also an organic mercurial and exists as iridescent green scales.
  - **The most toxic compound of mercury is methyl mercury**.

Uses

Listed in **Table 9.7**.

Sources of Exposure

- Breaking of mercury light bulbs, heating of mercury-gold amalgams in order to extract gold, use of mercury-containing paint and vacuuming of carpet contaminated with mercury.

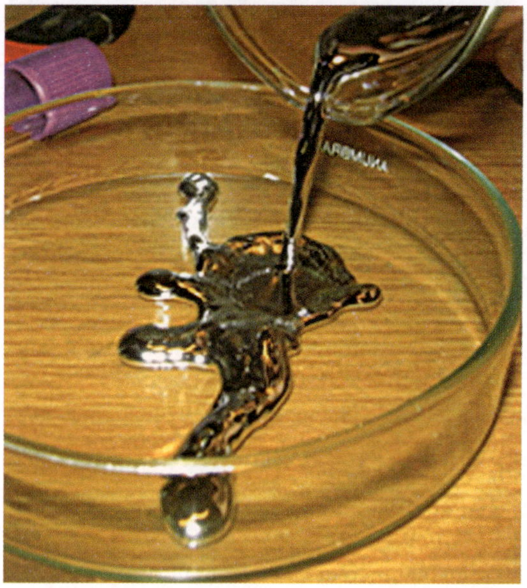

Fig. 9.44 Elemental mercury

- Ingestion or handling of liquid mercury following breakage of thermometers or other mercury-containing devices.
- Insertion or removal of dental amalgam restorations can generate mercury vapour or respirable particulates. Bruxism, chewing and tooth brushing may increase amalgam release of mercury vapour.
- Dietary exposure to mercury (in the form of methyl mercury) from consumption of fish and shellfish.

Usual Fatal Dose

- Amount of **ingested mercury** that would be fatal to a man is estimated at **100 g**.
- **Mercuric chloride: 0.5–1 g.**
- **Mercurous chloride: 1.5–2 g.**

Toxicokinetics

1. ***Absorption and Distribution***:
   a. Elemental mercury is absorbed primarily via inhalation of vapour. As elemental mercury is negligibly absorbed

Table 9.7 Uses of Mercury Compounds

Industry	Medicine & Dentistry	Miscellaneous
1. Barometer, thermometer, etc.	1. Antiseptic & disinfectant	1. Embalming
2. Dry cell batteries	2. Dental amalgam	2. Fingerprint powder
3. Mercury switches	3. Diuretic	3. Grain preservative
4. Explosives & fireworks	4. Purgative	4. Paints
5. Felt hats	5. Pesticides	
6. Mercury vapour lamps		

**The fact that mercury vapourises constantly was demonstrated for the first time by Michael Faraday who suspended a gold leaf above and out of contact with mercury. It gradually turned into an amalgam.*

from the gut, it is usually considered nontoxic when ingested.

b. Main route of absorption for inorganic mercury salts is the GI tract. The degree of dermal absorption varies according to the concentration of mercury, skin integrity and the lipid solubility of the vehicle.

c. Organic mercury compounds are also primarily absorbed from the GI tract. Dermal and inhalational absorption of organic mercury compounds can also occur.

d. After it is absorbed, mercury distributes widely to all tissues, predominantly the kidneys, liver, spleen and central nervous system (CNS).

e. With regard to organic mercurials, methylmercury readily distributes across all tissues, including the blood-brain barrier and placenta. The greatest methylmercury concentrations are found in the kidneys and liver.

2. ***Elimination***:
   a. Elemental mercury/inorganic mercury salts: Mercuric ions are excreted through the kidney by both glomerular filtration and tubular secretion, and in the GI tract by transfer across gut mesenteric vessels into faeces.
   b. Organic mercury compounds: Elimination is predominantly faecal.

Mode of Action

- The disruption of normal cell physiology by mercury is believed to arise from its avid covalent binding to sulphur, replacing the hydrogen ion in the body's widespread sulphydryl groups.
- Mercury also reacts with phosphoryl, carboxyl and amide groups, resulting in dysfunction of enzymes, transport mechanisms, membranes and structural proteins.
- Mercury gets deposited in all tissues, and therefore the clinical manifestations of mercury toxicity involve multiple organ systems with variable features and intensity.
- Organic mercury disrupts neuronal cell function and development, and also affects the renal, cardiovascular and immune systems. These effects cause a number of multifactorial conditions including hypertension, cardiovascular disease and stroke.
- Atrophy of the cerebellar hemispheres, postcentral gyri and calcarine area of the brain on MRI in organic mercury-poisoned patients, correlate with clinical findings of ataxia, sensory neuropathy and visual field constriction, respectively.

Clinical Features

A. *Poisoning with Elemental Mercury & Inorganic Salts*

1. **Acute Poisoning**

i. **Inhalation**:
   a. This usually occurs while heating metal in a closed room, or following gold refining in an enclosed area.
   b. Symptoms include dyspnoea, cough, fever, headache, chills, GI disturbances, metallic taste and blurring of vision. Stomatitis, swelling of the salivary glands and gingivitis may develop within a few days. Teeth may become loose due to gum inflammation.
   c. In severe cases there may be non-cardiogenic pulmonary oedema, dyspnoea, convulsions, etc.
   d. Sometimes manifestations similar to ***Kawasaki disease (mucocutaneous lymph node syndrome)*** are seen especially in children, which may be mistaken for scarlet fever: conjunctival congestion, fever, reddened palms and soles, deep red oral mucosa with "strawberry tongue" (**Fig. 9.45**), skin rash (**Fig. 9.46**) and cervical lymphadenopathy.

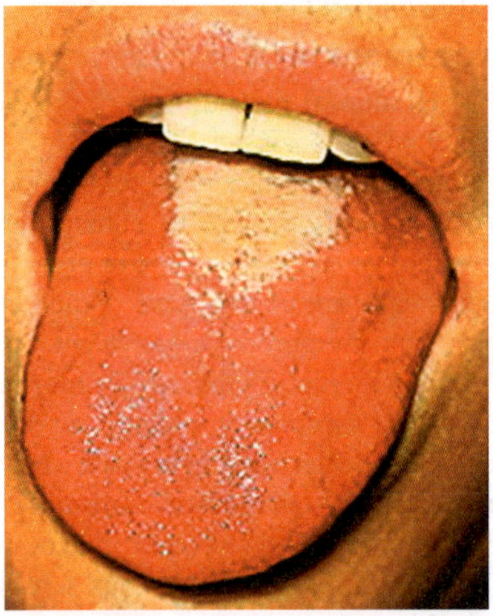

Fig. 9.45 Strawberry tongue – Kawasaki disease

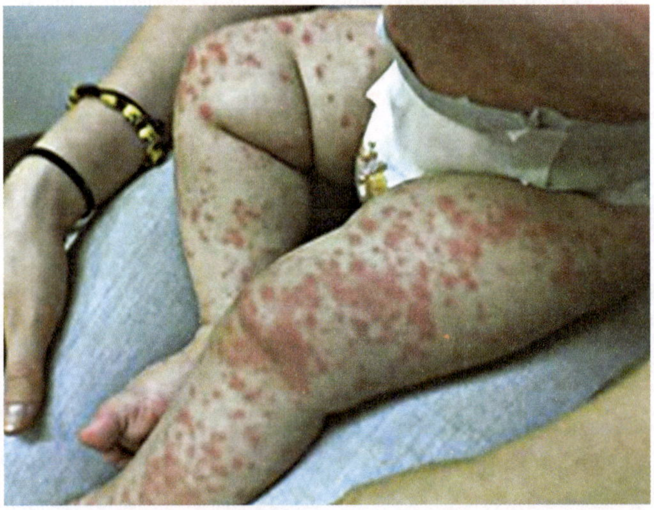

Fig. 9.46 Skin rash – Mucocutaneous lymph node syndrome

ii. **Ingestion**:
   a. Small quantities of elemental mercury usually cause no harm on ingestion. Sometimes even a relatively large amount may pass out of the body uneventfully (egged on by a mild laxative!). It is however advisable to take X-rays to monitor the progress of the elemental mercury through the GI tract.
   b. Ingestion of mercuric salts produces corrosion leading to abdominal pain, vomiting, diarrhoea and

shock. The mucosa of the GI tract usually appears greyish. There may be haematemesis. In severe cases there is onset of renal failure, pulmonary oedema and coma. Urine may appear pinkish.

c. Ingestion of button (or disc) batteries (**Fig. 9.47**) poses special problems since they contain a variety of caustic substances apart from mercury. These batteries are used in hearing aids, watches, calculators and some hand-held computer games. They range in size from 7 to 25 mm and can easily be swallowed by children. Each such battery contains a heavy metal (usually mercury) along with a variety of caustic alkalies, especially sodium or potassium hydroxide.

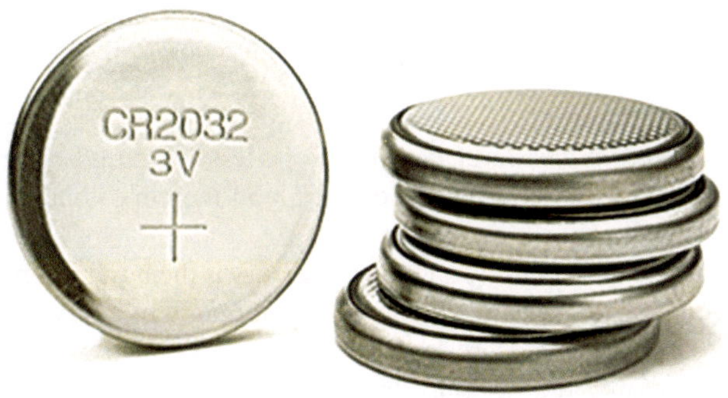

Fig. 9.47 Button (disc) batteries

d. In the majority of cases of button battery ingestion, there are no serious consequences, and the object usually passes out in the stools quite uneventfully over a period of 1–4 days. However, if the contents of the battery leak out during transit, there can be production of burns by the caustic alkalies, and a theoretical risk of mercury poisoning (so far unreported).

iii. **Injection**:

a. Subcutaneous or intramuscular injections of elemental mercury may cause abscess formation with ulceration, extruding tiny droplets of mercury.

b. Intravenous injection can result in ***mercurialism*** characterised by thrombophlebitis, granuloma formation and pulmonary embolism. Repeated haemoptysis is a characteristic feature.

c. Intra-arterial injection can result in peripheral embolisation with ischaemia, and sometimes frank gangrene. There may also be abscess formation and ulceration. X-ray usually reveals multiple, tiny spheres in the veins draining the entry site. Mercury globules may also be seen in various organs.

2. **Chronic Poisoning (Hydragyrism)**:

i. **Inhalation**:

a. *Tremor*: It is one of the classical and most consistent manifestations of chronic mercury poisoning and is sometimes referred to as the ***Danbury tremor***. It begins in the hands and is of a coarse, intentional type, interspersed with jerky movements. Later, it progresses to the lips, tongue, arms and legs. The advanced condition is referred to as ***Hatter's shakes***,* when the tremor becomes so severe that daily activities involving some delicacy of movement become grossly impaired, e.g., shaving, writing, holding a tumbler or spoon, etc. The most severe form of the condition is referred to as ***concussio mercurialis***, when literally no activity is possible. Even years after exposure to mercury has ceased, tremor may persist.

b. Ataxia, reeling gait.

c. Metallic taste (**Table 9.8**), anorexia, nausea, increased salivation.

Table 9.8 Poisons/Drugs Producing Metallic Taste

Heavy metals: Arsenic, lead, mercury, copper, iron, lithium
Acetaldehyde
Ciguatoxin
Disulfiram
Metoclopramide
Metronidazole

d. Gingivitis, halitosis, blue line on gums (similar to the *Burtonian line* of plumbism).

e. Erythematous macular or papular rashes are common with mercury vapour poisoning.

f. ***Erethism***: Another classic manifestation, it refers to a cluster of psychiatric symptoms including abnormal shyness, loss of self-confidence, depression, irritability, amnesia, excitability, progressing in later stages to delirium with hallucinations, or suicidal melancholia, or manic depressive psychosis (***mad hatter***).**

g. ***Mercuria lentis***: Characterised by the brown reflex of anterior lens capsule of the eye. There may be fine punctate opacities. Visual blurring is often present, and sometimes there is concentric constriction of visual fields ("tunnel vision"). Diagnosis is made by slit lamp examination.

h. Renal damage results in membranous glomerulonephritis with hyaline casts and fatty casts in the urine.

i. Hepatic dysfunction and failure.

j. Occasionally, chronic inhalation of mercury produces the ***asthenic vegetative syndrome***, characterised by neurasthenic symptoms, increased uptake of radio-iodine by the thyroid with goitre for-

*__Note__: *So called because the condition was first described among felt hat workers.*

**__Note__: *Derived from a character of the same name in Lewis Carroll's "Alice's Adventures in Wonderland" published in 1865.*

mation, tachycardia, labile pulse, gingivitis and dermographia (urticaria due to allergic reaction).

ii. **Ingestion**:
   a. Colitis.
   b. Melanosis coli.
   c. Dementia.
   d. Tremor.
   e. Renal failure.
   f. ***Acrodynia*** (***Pink disease***) (**Fig. 9.48**): This is seen mainly in children. Formerly most cases were related to chronic use of teething powders containing mercurous chloride. But, almost any form of chronic mercury exposure can cause this condition including inhalation of elemental mercury vapour. The onset is usually insidious with anorexia, insomnia, profuse sweating, skin rash and photophobia. The hands and feet become *p*uffy, *p*inkish, *p*ainful, *p*araesthetic, *p*erspiring and *p*eeling (*the child pees!*). Teeth may be shed, with ulceration of gums. Today the incidence of childhood acrodynia is uncommon since the use of mercurial teething powders and diaper rinses has been abandoned.

B. *Poisoning with Organic Mercurials*

1. Most cases of human poisoning from **methylmercury** due to ingestion of contaminated foods (especially fish) over a long period. In such patients, there is often a latent period of several weeks before the development of systemic, predominantly neurological, features (**Minamata disease**) (**Box 9.1**):

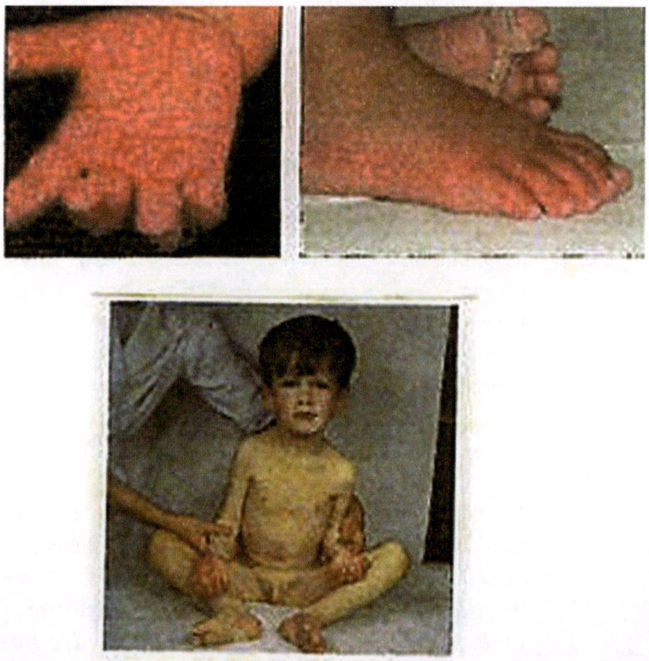

Fig. 9.48 Pink disease (Acrodynia)

   i. These include tremor, drowsiness, dizziness, cerebellar ataxia, dysarthria, hyperreflexia, muscle weakness, memory loss, headache, irritability, confusion, personality changes, insomnia, hearing impairment, blurred vision, diplopia, optic atrophy, constriction of the visual fields leading to blindness in severe cases, seizures and coma.
   ii. Fatalities have occurred.
   iii. There may be pain and paraesthesiae around the mouth and in the limbs, the latter indicative of a peripheral neuropathy.
2. Gastrointestinal features include nausea, vomiting, diarrhoea, gingivitis, hypersalivation, abdominal pain and anorexia.
3. Chronic exposure to methylmercury has been associated with an increased incidence of liver cancer, cirrhosis, renal disease and cerebral haemorrhage.

Diagnosis

1. X-ray.
2. *Blood mercury level*: Normal level is less than 3 μg/L. Symptoms of toxicity may occur at blood mercury concentrations of 5 μg/L or greater.
3. *Urine mercury level*: Urinary mercury is the best biological marker for chronic elemental or inorganic mercury exposure. Urinary mercury concentrations are also useful for assessing the response to chelation therapy. The average normal morning urine mercury is 1.9 μg/g creatinine (1.1 nmol/mmol), range 0–7.6 μg/g (0–4.3 nmol/mmol). A 24-hr urine collection is recommended. Because organic mercury is eliminated via the faecal route, urine mercury levels are not useful in methylmercury poisoning.
4. *Hair analysis*: External contamination can however vitiate the results.
5. Neutron activation procedure for urinary mercury analysis is reported by the WHO as the most accurate and sensitive method. Atomic absorption, gas chromatography and reverse-phase HPLC are other methods which can be used.

Box 9.1—The Environmental Curse of Mercury

Organic Mercury Compounds

Important **organic mercury compounds (organic mercurials)** include the following: methylmercury, ethylmercury, dimethylmercury, diethylmercury and merbromin ("Mercurochrome"). Thiomersal is used as a preservative for vaccines and intravenous drugs.

Methylmercury is notoriously toxic, and was responsible for the **Minamata disease** which occurred in the city of Minamata, Japan, in 1956. It was caused by the release of methylmercury in the industrial wastewater from a chemical factory owned by the Chisso Corporation, which continued from 1932 to 1968. This highly toxic chemical bioaccumulated and biomagnified in shellfish and fish in Minamata Bay

contd

**Note*: *So called because the condition was first described among felt hat workers.*

***Note*: *Derived from a character of the same name in Lewis Carroll's "Alice's Adventures in Wonderland" published in 1865.*

and the Shiranui Sea, which, when eaten by the local population, resulted in mercury poisoning. While cat, dog, pig and human deaths continued for 36 years, Chisso Corpn did little to prevent the epidemic. The animal effects were severe enough in cats that they came to be named as having "dancing cat fever".

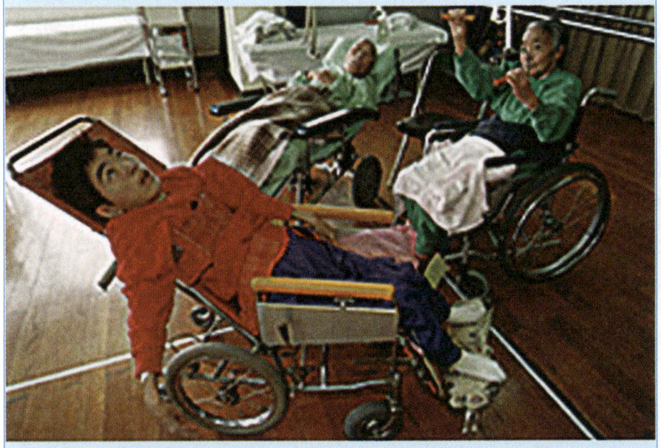

Victims of Minamata disease

Effects in humans: Ataxia, numbness in the hands and feet, general muscle weakness, loss of peripheral vision, and damage to hearing and speech. In extreme cases, insanity, paralysis, coma and death follow within weeks of the onset of symptoms. A congenital form of the disease can also affect foetuses in the womb and may cause cerebral palsy. As of March 2001, 2265 victims had been officially recognized as having Minamata disease, and had received financial compensation from Chisso Corpn.

A second outbreak of Minamata disease occurred in Niigata Prefecture in 1965.

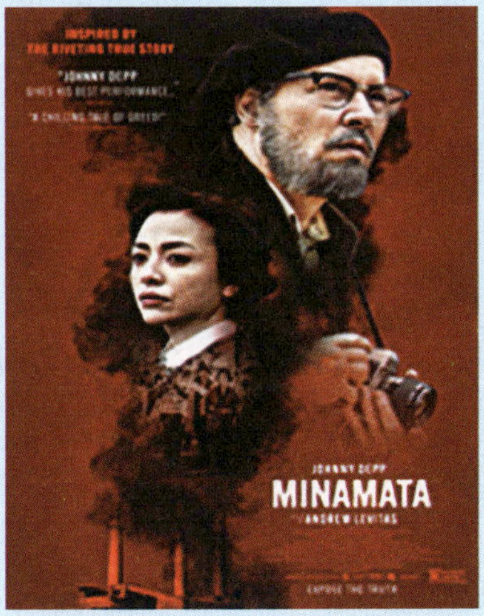

Poster of "Minamata", a 2020 film starring Johnny Depp

Elemental Mercury

Kodaikanal mercury poisoning is a case of mercury contamination in the hill station of Kodaikanal, Tamil Nadu, by Hindustan Unilever, in the process of making mercury thermometers for export around the world.

Unilever acquired the thermometer factory from cosmetics maker Pond's India Ltd. Pond's moved the factory from the United States to India in 1982 after the plant owned there by its parent company had to be dismantled following increased awareness in developed countries of polluting industries.

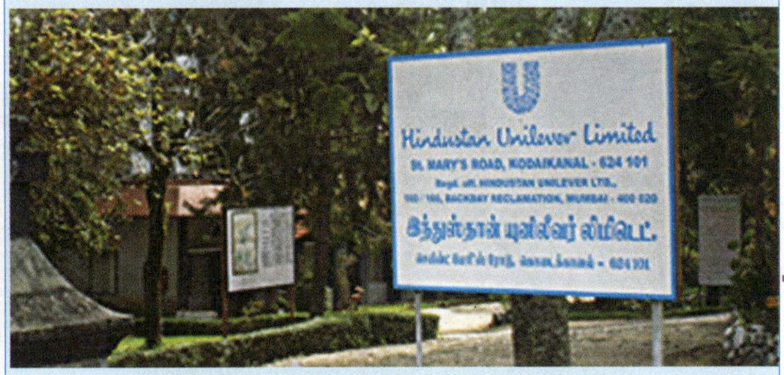

Hindustan Unilever Factory in Kodaikanal (before it was closed down)

The factory imported mercury from the United States, and exported finished thermometers to markets in Europe. Around 2001, a number of workers at the factory began complaining of kidney and related ailments. Public interest groups alleged that the company had been disposing of mercury waste without following proper protocols. In early 2001, they unearthed a pile of broken glass thermometers with remains of mercury from an area of the nearby forest, which they suspected could have come from the company. Subsequently, a public protest led by the local workers' union and international environmental organisation Greenpeace, forced the company to shut down the factory. Soon the company admitted that it did dispose of mercury contaminated waste. However, it went on to claim that there was no adverse health effect on the workers of the factory, or any impact on the environment. This was hotly contested by the public interest groups, which demanded the return of the remaining mercury waste to the United States for recycling, remediation of the factory site and address of the health complaints of the workers. They also initiated legal action against the company.

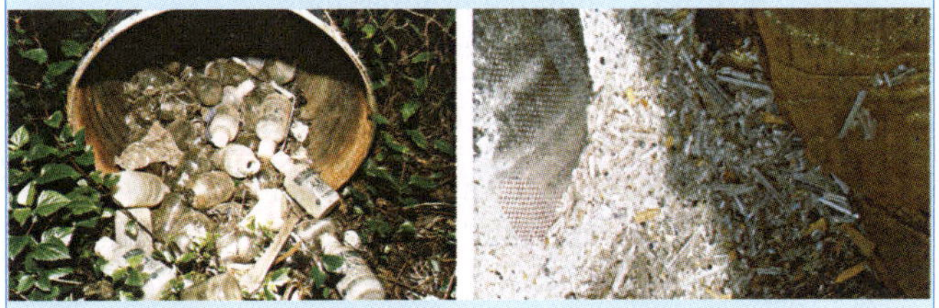

Mercury containing wastes found dumped in and around the factory

Finally, the company was forced to collect 290 tonnes of dumped mercury waste from the forest and send back to the United States for recycling in 2003. This was widely hailed by the media as 'reverse dumping'.

In March 2016, Hindustan Unilever entered into an out-of-court settlement with its ex-employees to provide "undisclosed" ex-gratia payment, in addition to long-term health and well-being benefits, to 511 of its former workers of the thermometer factory.

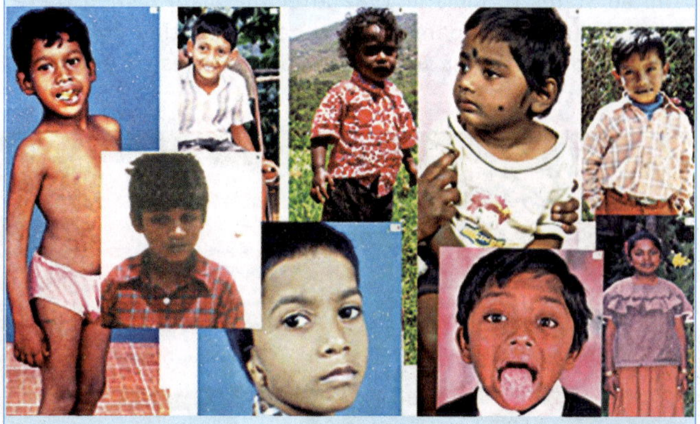

Victims of Kodaikanal Mercury Poisoning

Treatment

1. *Acute Poisoning*

a. **Metallic mercury and inorganic compounds**:

i. *Inhalation*

- Removal from source of exposure.
- Supportive measures.
- Chelation: **Dimercaprol (BAL)** can be used in the management of mercury poisoning, but its use is associated with adverse effects. It has been superseded by **DMPS** and **DMSA** which increase urine mercury excretion and decrease blood mercury concentrations.
  - BAL is given 100 mg by deep IM., every 4 hrs for 48 hrs, followed by 100 mg every 8 hrs for 8–10 days.
  - DMSA is given orally: 30 mg/kg/day (in 3 divided doses) for 5 days, repeated after 5–7 days if necessary.

ii. *Ingestion*

- In elemental mercury ingestion, take X-ray and repeat it to study the progression.
- Administer laxatives.
- Demulcents for corrosive compounds such as mercuric chloride.
- Stomach wash: It may be advisable to add egg white or 5% albumin or just plain milk to the lavage fluid to bind the mercury.
- Whole-bowel irrigation with polyethylene glycol solution may also be useful in removing residual mercury and should be considered, following its progress with serial radiographs.
- Chelation (*vide supra*).

iii. *Injection*

- If there is abscess formation, perform repeated incisions to remove the mercury. If the globules are very minute and widely distributed in the intercellular spaces, excise the affected tissue.
- Monitor the CNS and renal functions for evidence of toxicity.
- Chelation (*vide supra*).

b. **Organic Mercurials**:

i. Supportive measures.

ii. As the neurologic impairment associated with methylmercury is essentially irreversible, early recognition of poisoning and prevention of neurotoxicity are essential to a successful outcome.

iii. Chelation with succimer may prove to be the treatment of choice for methylmercury poisoning because of its apparently low toxicity and reported efficacy in animal trials.

2. *Chronic Poisoning*

The mainstay of chronic mercury poisoning is **chelation therapy** (*vide supra*).

Autopsy Features

1. In death due to acute mercury poisoning, the mucosa of the mouth, throat, oesophagus and stomach appears greyish in colour with softening and superficial corrosion. There may be haemorrhagic points.
2. If there had been survival for a few days, the large intestine may reveal ulceration.
3. Kidneys are often pale and swollen due to oedema of renal cortex. Microscopy usually demonstrates necrotic changes in the renal tubules.

Forensic Issues

- Mercury and its compounds constitute important industrial, agricultural and occupational toxic hazards.
- Mercury and mercury salts, including mercurous chloride and mercurous oxide, are prohibited for use in cosmetic products as skin-lightening agents because of their high toxicity.
- Even today calomel (mercurous chloride) is sometimes recommended as a laxative or used for other medical conditions in Indian or Chinese medicines. Prolonged use can cause colitis dementia, tremor and renal failure. Acrodynia resulting from teething powders containing calomel has fortunately become a rarity.
- The tragic consequences of chronic industrial exposure to mercury have been outlined in the foregoing sections.
- Domestic exposure though not often reported is today a distinct threat. Such exposure may result from inadvertent mercury spills (broken thermometers), or from home gold-ore processing.
- Despite the commitment of various hospitals in India to be mercury free, mercury containing-thermometers/sphygmomanometers are still preferred by health professionals leading to the possibility of accidental mercury exposure in the hospital setting.
- Another important area that must be considered in relation to chronic mercury exposure is dentistry. Dental amalgams used for fillings often contain mercury (**Fig. 9.49**). The clinical importance of volatilized metallic mercury from dental

amalgams for both the dentist and patient has been a matter of controversy for years. The current view is that dental amalgam does not cause mercury poisoning.

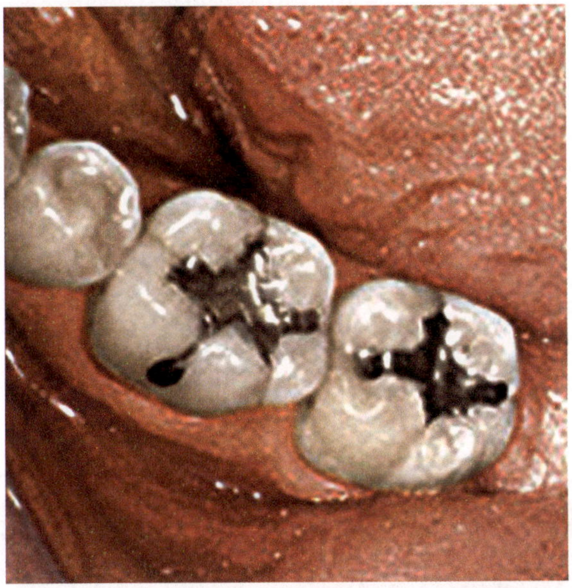

Fig. 9.49 Mercury containing dental fillings

- Food poisoning (especially involving fish) through mercury compounds is well known. There are indications that Indian sea and fresh waters may also be contaminated with mercury that can enter the food chain via seafood.
- A relatively new hazard concerns dry cell batteries used in cameras, hearing aids, torches and watches.

IRON

Physical Appearance

- Metallic iron is silvery white in colour, occurring naturally as *haematite*, *magnetite*, etc., and usually causes no problems. In fact, it is an essential element and deficiency results in anaemia. Even if there is more than the required intake daily, the excess is excreted. But in some individuals with inborn errors, even normal dietary iron can cause toxic effects due to accumulation, e.g., **haemochromatosis** (***Bronze diabetes***).
- Various iron salts are administered therapeutically in individuals with iron deficiency anaemia which can result from a wide variety of causes. Iron poisoning is related in most instances to overdose of such salts. One of the commonest is **ferrous sulphate (*green vitriol*)** which occurs as bluish green crystals (**Fig. 9.50**). Iron (ferric) oxide, i.e., rust does not cause iron poisoning.

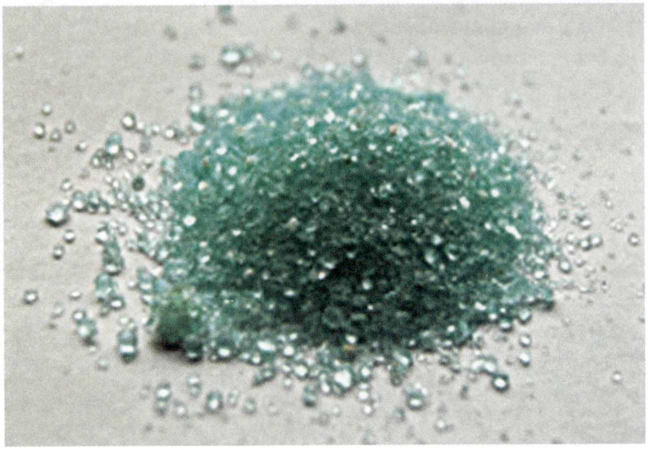

Fig. 9.50 Ferrous sulphate

Uses/Sources

1. ***Dietary Sources***:
   a. The required daily amount of iron of 10–20 mg for adults is supplied through average diet.
   b. The average daily intake for adults is 15 mg.
2. ***Uses***:
   a. *Industrial Uses*
      i. Powder metallurgy (serves as a catalyst in chemical reactions).
      ii. Iron is a component of carbon steel, cast iron and stainless steel.
      iii. Wrought iron is almost pure iron.
      iv. Iron uses include magnets, dyes, pigments and abrasives.
   b. *Biological Uses*
      i. Iron is essential to life. It is a constituent of biological pigments such as haemoglobin, cytochromes and ferrichromes.

Usual Fatal Dose

Commonly used iron salts in therapeutics along with respective iron content are mentioned in **Table 9.9**.

The **usual fatal dose** corresponds to about **200–250 mg of elemental iron per kg of body weight**. However, toxic effects

Table 9.9 Elemental Iron Content of Iron Salts

Iron Salt	Iron Content (%)	Iron Salt	Iron Content (%)
Ferrous gluconate	12	Ferrous fumarate	33
Ferric ammonium citrate	14–18	Ferrous succinate	35
Ferrous sulphate (hydrated)	20	Ferric phosphate	37
Ferric chloride (hydrated)	20	Ferrous chloride (hydrated)	28

of iron poisoning have occurred at doses of 10–20 mg/kg. Hence, just a handful of these tablets (15–20 in number), can be lethal to a young child.

Toxicokinetics

- Iron poisoning occurs when serum iron level exceeds the total iron-binding capacity (TIBC), resulting in free circulating iron in the bloodstream.
- The body cannot directly excrete iron, so body iron stores are regulated by controlling iron absorption from the GI tract. Iron absorption, which occurs predominantly in the duodenum, is determined by the body's iron requirements. In iron deficiency, iron uptake into intestinal mucosal cells may increase from a normal of 10–35% to as much as 80–95%.
- Following uptake into the intestinal mucosal cells, iron is either stored as ferritin and lost when the cell is sloughed, or released to transferrin, a serum iron-binding protein. In therapeutic doses, some of these processes become saturated, and absorption into the intestinal cell may be limited. However, in overdose the oxidative effects of iron on gastrointestinal mucosal cells lead to dysfunction of this regulatory balance, and increased passive absorption of iron occurs.

Mode of Action

Free iron causes:

- Massive post-arteriolar dilatation which results in **venous pooling**.
- Increased capillary permeability resulting in **decreased plasma volume**.
- Oxidation of ferrous to ferric iron releasing hydrogen ions. Subsequent hydration of ferric iron results in **metabolic acidosis**.
- Inhibition of mitochondrial function leading to **hepatic damage, hypoglycaemia** and **hypoprothrombinaemia**.
- Thrombin induced conversion of **fibrinogen into fibrin**.
- Direct **corrosive action** on the GI mucosa.

Clinical Features

- *Stage I* (0.5–2 hrs) includes vomiting, haematemesis, abdominal pain, diarrhoea, haematochezia, lethargy, shock, acidosis and coagulopathy. Necrosis of the GI tract occurs from the corrosive effect of iron on GI mucosa.
- *Stage II* (after *Stage I*) includes apparent recovery and may contribute to a false sense of security. Observe closely.
- *Stage III* (2–12 hrs after *Stage I*) includes profound shock, severe acidosis, cyanosis and fever.
- *Stage IV* (2–4 days) includes hepatotoxicity, convulsions, and coma. Monitor liver function tests and bilirubin. The primary site of hepatic injury is the periportal areas of the hepatic lobule.
- *Stage V* (days to weeks) includes GI scarring and strictures.

Diagnosis

1. **X-ray**: Like all other heavy metals, iron and its compounds are radiopaque. However, chewable iron tablets and liquid iron formulations are usually not visualised on X-ray.
2. **Serum iron level (Table 9.10)**: Poisoning is indicated, if this exceeds 150 μg/100 mL, and serious toxicity is usually associated with levels beyond 500–600 μg/100 mL. Peak levels are seen around 4 hrs after ingestion. Measuring the total iron binding capacity and relating it to the serum iron level is often misleading and unreliable.
3. Total leucocyte count (TLC), electrolytes, glucose, blood gas, clotting studies, liver function and renal function tests are useful estimates.
4. **Chelation challenge test**: Desferrioxamine in a dose of 25 mg/kg (max 1 g) is given IM. If the serum iron has exceeded iron binding capacity, the excess iron is chelated to desferrioxamine and the complex is excreted as a pinkish (***vin rosé***)* colour in the urine (**Fig. 9.51**). But, a negative result does not rule out iron poisoning.

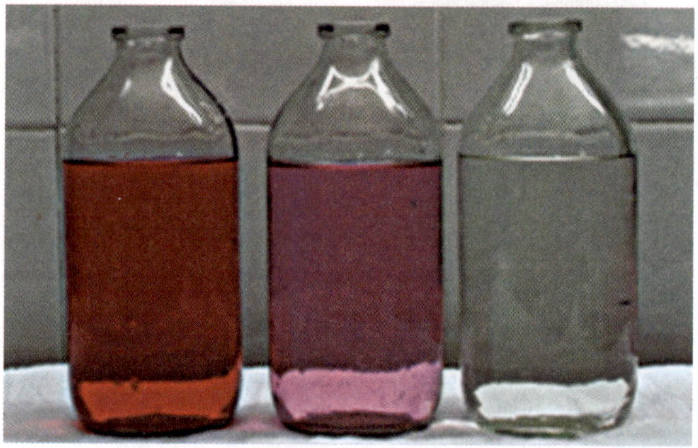

Fig. 9.51 Iron poisoning – Vin rose urine (*Courtesy: Dr S Senthilkumaran*)

5. **Qualitative desferrioxamine colour test (QDCT)**: 2 mL of gastric fluid and 2 drops of 30% hydrogen peroxide are placed in 2 plastic tubes. 0.5 mL of desferrioxamine soln is added into one tube and the resulting colour change is compared with the other tube (control). If the test is positive, a red colour will develop in the tube in which desferrioxamine was added.

Treatment

1. Stomach wash with normal saline. Desferrioxamine must not be used for lavage.

Table 9.10 Severity of Iron Poisoning

Serum Iron	Severity
Less than 3 mg/L (55 μmol/L)	Mild toxicity
3–5 mg/L (55–90 μmol/L)	Moderate toxicity
More than 5 mg/L (>90 μmol/L)	Severe toxicity

**Note*: *French for "light pink wine".*

2. Activated charcoal is ineffective.
3. Magnesium hydroxide (1%) administered orally may help reduce absorption of iron by precipitating the formation of ferrous hydroxide.
4. Whole bowel irrigation (WBI) may be helpful.
5. For patients who demonstrate persistent iron in the GI tract despite orogastric lavage and WBI, upper endoscopy or gastrotomy and surgical removal of iron tablets adherent to the gastric mucosa may be necessary and lifesaving.
6. Obtain serum iron levels, creatinine, electrolytes, blood haemoglobin concentration, blood prothrombin time, baseline liver function tests and arterial blood gases in seriously poisoned patients.
7. Correction of hypovolaemia.
8. If metabolic acidosis persists despite correction of hypoxia and adequate fluid resuscitation, consider correction with IV sodium bicarbonate. In adults, an initial dose of 50 mmol may be given and repeated as necessary, guided by arterial blood gas monitoring (aim for a pH of 7.44).
9. Control convulsions that are frequent or prolonged with IV diazepam (10–20 mg in adults; 0.1–0.3 mg/kg in children), lorazepam (4 mg in adults and 0.1 mg/kg in children) or midazolam (5–10 mg in adults; 0.05–0.15 mg/kg in children). If convulsions are unresponsive to initial treatment, second-line therapy is phenobarbitone sodium (10 mg/kg at maximum rate of 100 mg/min; maximum dose 1 g).
10. **Chelation therapy**: This is indicated in any of the following situations:
    a. More than one episode of vomiting or diarrhoea.
    b. Significant abdominal pain, hypovolaemia, or acidosis.
    c. Multiple radiopacities on abdominal radiograph.
    d. Serum iron level greater than 350 µg/100 mL.

    Chelation can be done either with **desferrioxamine** (*parenteral*) or **deferiprone** (*oral*). **Box 9.2** discusses desferrioxamine in greater depth.
11. Haemodialysis does not remove iron effectively but should be considered on a supportive basis for acute renal failure as this will facilitate removal of the iron–desferrioxamine complex. Continuous arteriovenous haemofiltration (CAVH) may be helpful in severe poisoning.
12. In toddlers with severe poisoning, exchange transfusion may help to physically remove free iron from the blood while replacing it with normal blood.
13. Liver transplantation is the only therapeutic avenue open in the presence of fulminant hepatic failure.

Box 9.2—Desferrioxamine (DFO) (Deferoxamine)

Desferrioxamine or **DFO** is the chelator of choice for iron poisoning. It is extracted from the microorganism *Streptomyces pilosus* (belonging to Actinomycetes). DFO cannot chelate iron which is bound to transferrin, and can only accomplish this when the iron is free or in transit between transferrin and ferritin in the plasma. DFO is also said to be useful in aluminium poisoning.

Indications:

Institute intravenous desferrioxamine chelation therapy if:

- Free serum iron is present,
- If patient is symptomatic and a serum iron (SI) cannot be readily obtained or
- The peak SI exceeds 350–500 µg/dL

Efficacy:

Desferrioxamine binds 8.5 mg of elemental iron per 100 mg of the chelate.

Dose:

- *IV Dose* – Continuous infusion at a rate of 15 mg/kg/hr.
- *IM Dose* – Administer 90 mg/kg, up to a maximum of 1 g/dose, every 8 hrs as needed.
- *Duration of Infusion* – Patients with moderate toxicity are generally treated for 8–12 hrs, those with severe toxicity may require deferoxamine for 24 hrs or longer.
- *Therapy Endpoint/Colour Change*: Monitor urine for characteristic pink to orange-red colour ("vin rose") indicating the excretion of ferrioxamine (chelated iron).

Adverse Effects:

- *Sepsis* – The use of desferrioxamine in iron-overdosed children has been associated with *Yersinia enterocolitica* septicaemia and mucormycosis.
- *Visual Toxicity* – It appears that continuous intravenous administration of desferrioxamine, often in the presence of low iron stores, can produce visual toxicity (decreased visual acuity, night blindness, colour blindness, retinal pigmentary abnormalities).
- *Pulmonary Toxicity* – A "pulmonary syndrome" has been associated with high dose IV (10–25 mg/kg/hr) desferrioxamine therapy for several days. Features include tachypnoea, hypoxaemia, fever, eosinophilia, urticaria and pulmonary infiltrates.
- *Hypotension* appears to be rate related. It is advisable that IV desferrioxamine be administered at a dose NOT exceeding 15 mg/kg/hr.
- *Renal Toxicity* – Elevated creatinine levels and decreased creatinine clearance.

Autopsy Features

- Elevated iron concentrations in major organs: stomach, liver, brain, heart, lung, small bowel, kidney.
- Congestion, oedema, necrosis and iron deposition in the gastric and intestinal mucosa.
- Haemorrhage and congestion in the lungs.
- In ferrous sulphate poisoning, gastric contents may appear bluish green in colour.

Forensic Issues

- Acute iron poisoning has assumed grave significance in recent years and cases of accidental poisoning are being reported with alarming frequency in young children. Since most iron preparations (syrups and tablets) are brightly coloured and pleasantly flavoured, they constitute an irresistible, fatal attraction for these innocent victims. To compound the tragedy, in several instances the parents themselves are ignorant about the toxicity of these preparations and tend to dismiss them as "harmless vitamins." It is imperative that public awareness be generated about the treacherous lethality of iron preparations. Introduction of childproof containers would be very effective in minimising inadvertent ingestions by children as demonstrated by the Western experience.

- Iron poisoning can also occur after ingestion of other iron salts, such as ferric chloride, used in industry.
- Parenteral iron, such as iron dextran, administered intravenously to patients with renal failure and chronic anaemia, also can result in toxicity, especially anaphylactoid reactions.
- Newer parenteral formulations, including iron sucrose and sodium ferrous gluconate, appear to be safer.

COPPER

Physical Appearance

- Copper is a lustrous, ductile, malleable, odourless solid with a distinct golden-red or reddish-brown colour (**Fig. 9.52**).
- It is an essential trace element, being the third most abundant trace element in the body, and is an important catalyst for haem synthesis and iron absorption.
- The main mechanism of copper toxicity is oxidative stress caused by reactive intermediates produced during redox reactions involving copper ions. Copper salts such as **copper sulphate (blue vitriol)** (**Fig. 9.53**), are strong irritants to skin and mucous membranes (**Table 9.11**).
- An X-linked copper disorder known as **Menkes "kinky-hair" syndrome** has been reported, in which intestinal copper uptake is impaired. It is characterized by mental retardation, thermoregulatory dysfunction, hypopigmentation, connective tissue abnormalities, pili torti (kinky hair), brain degeneration and death in the first few years of life.

Uses

- *Elemental Copper*:
  - Copper has excellent electrical conductivity, corrosion resistance, malleability and ductility, which make it very useful as an industrial metal.
  - Copper is useful in electroplated coatings and undercoatings for products made from nickel, chromium and zinc, and in cooking utensils.
  - Copper is also made into corrosion-resistant plumbing pipes, used in materials for building construction, and has applications in industrial machinery and in automobiles.
  - Copper's contraceptive effects (as a spermatocide) are exploited for intrauterine devices.
- *Copper Compounds*:
  - Copper oxide is used as a catalyst and a pigment for ceramic, glass, enamel and porcelain.
  - Copper acetate and Copper carbonate are used as paint pigment, insecticide and fungicide.
  - Copper chloride is used as a disinfectant, in metallurgy, for the preservation of wood pulp and in water purification.
  - Copper nitrate is used in pharmaceutical preparations, and in paints, varnishes and enamels.
  - **Copper sulphate** is used as a fungicide, molluscicide and wood preservative, for water treatment as a bactericide and algaecide, and in some fertilizers. It is also used medicinally as an emetic, and in intrauterine contraceptive devices.
- *Copper Alloys*:
  - **Brass** is an alloy of copper and zinc.
  - **Bronze** contains copper alloyed with tin.

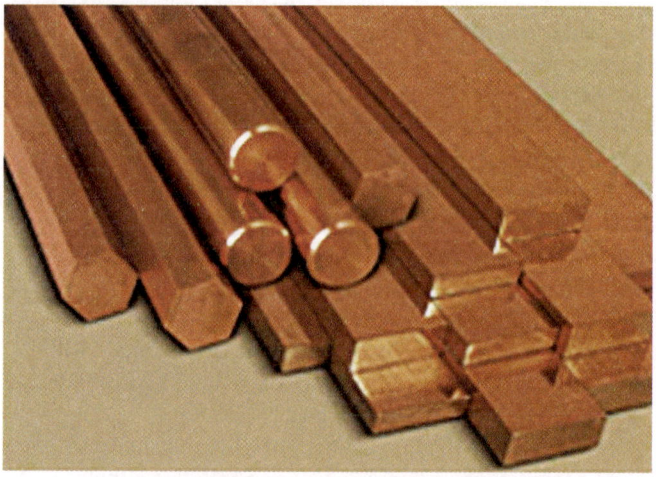

Fig. 9.52 Metallic copper

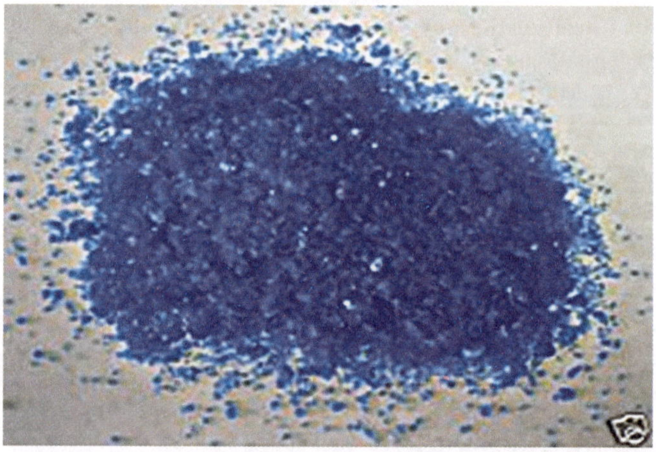

Fig. 9.53 Copper sulphate

Table 9.11 Toxic Salts of Copper

Chemical Name	Common Name
Copper acetoarsenite	Paris green
Copper arsenite	Scheele's green
Copper carbonate (native)	Mountain green
Copper carbonate (with chalk)	Brunswick green
Copper subacetate	Verdigris
Copper sulphate	Blue vitriol

- **Gun metal** contains copper, tin and zinc.
- **Sterling silver** and **white gold** also contain copper.

Usual Fatal Dose

10–20 g of copper sulphate.

Toxicokinetics

- Daily requirement of copper is 0.8 mg/day (or 30 μg/kg). It is required for the functioning of enzymes such as catalase and peroxidase.
- Copper can be absorbed through GI mucosa, and from intact skin. Once absorbed, copper is rapidly bound to carriers such as albumin, caeruloplasmin and amino acids such as histidine for transport to the liver and other tissues.
- After being released locally in the reduced form from its carrier, copper uptake by the hepatic cells occurs via a specific uptake pump. In the hepatocyte, complex trafficking systems exist to prevent copper toxicity and to aid delivery to the appropriate enzymes.
- Some copper is released from the liver, bound primarily to caeruloplasmin, which accounts for approximately 90-95% of serum copper. Copper is oxidized directly by caeruloplasmin, thereby avoiding the generation of reactive oxygen species. Approximately 5–10% of serum copper is bound to albumin under normal conditions, but following acute poisoning, the majority of the excess copper binds to albumin. The albumin–copper complex represents the "free" or toxicologically active copper.

Mode of Action

- In acute overdose, a high fraction of the serum copper remains bound to low-affinity proteins, such as albumin, and thus is biologically active. Because copper, as a transition metal, is capable of assuming one of several different oxidation, or valence, states, it is an active participant in **redox reactions**. In particular, participation in the Fenton reaction and Haber-Weiss cycle explains the toxicologic effects of copper as a generator of oxidative stress and inhibitor of several key metabolic enzymes.
- Cupric ion **inhibits sulphydryl groups** on enzymes in important antioxidant systems, including glucose-6-phosphate dehydrogenase and glutathione reductase.
- Liver damage follows a **centrilobular** pattern of **necrosis**. Once liver necrosis occurs, typically at liver concentrations greater than 50 mg/g dry weight, massive release of copper into the blood occurs, which may be of sufficient magnitude to cause haemolysis.
- Reactive oxygen species are probably also responsible for the **nephrotoxic** effects of copper.

Clinical Features

A. **Acute Poisoning**:

1. While most cases of acute poisoning result from ingestion of copper salts, swallowing large amounts of metallic copper, for example as coins, can also (rarely) produce acute copper poisoning.
2. Copper intoxication is characterised by myalgia, abdominal pain, vomiting (bluish or greenish),* diarrhoea, acidosis, pancreatitis, methaemoglobinaemia, haemolysis, jaundice, oliguria, renal failure, seizures, delirium and coma.
3. Hepatomegaly, liver tenderness, increased levels of transaminase and jaundice may occur on the second or third day after ingestion of copper salts.
4. Haemolysis is more common than hepatotoxicity, and is especially so in those with liver damage.
5. Acute renal failure develops in 20–40% of patients with acute copper sulphate intoxication and is believed to be mainly due to intravascular haemolysis. This might also occur after ingestion of other copper salts.
6. Inhalation of copper dust or fumes can cause cough, sore throat and conjunctivitis, while copper oxide is one of the incriminating agents in metal fume fever.
7. Eye exposure to copper can result in conjunctivitis and corneal ulceration or turbidity as well as palpebral oedema. Copper or copper alloy foreign bodies lodged in the eye (***chalcosis lentis***) can result in uveitis, abscess, serious injury or loss of the eye; over time, the copper may dissolve and disseminate to the lens, cornea and iris, where it may produce a greenish-brown discolouration of the anterior capsule visible by slit-lamp microscope.
8. Dermal exposure to irritant copper salts such as copper sulphate can cause itching and eczema.

B. **Chronic Poisoning**:

1. Chronic inhalation of copper sulphate spray used as an insecticide in vineyards can cause ***vineyard sprayer's lung disease*** characterised by a histiocytic granulomatous lung. Liver damage is also common.
2. Chronic contact with swimming pool water containing algicidal copper chemicals can cause green hair discolouration.
3. Churches in some developing countries distribute "spiritual green water" to devotees which contains copper sulphate. When this is ingested, serious toxicity and even death can result.
4. Cooking in copper or brass vessels can cause copper poisoning due to **verdigris**. Copper poisoning can also result from the leaching of copper containers in which carbonated water, citrus fruit juices and other acidic beverages have been stored.
5. Chronic copper toxicity is the hallmark of **Wilson's disease**, an autosomal recessive genetic disorder in which there is deficiency of caeruloplamin. Discolouration of the peripheral part of the cornea (***Kayser-Fleischer ring***) (**Fig. 9.54**) is a pathognomonic feature of this condition charac-

**Note*: *Bile is also greenish but can be differentiated by adding ammonium hydroxide. The vomitus becomes deep blue in colour in copper poisoning, while bile will not change colour.*

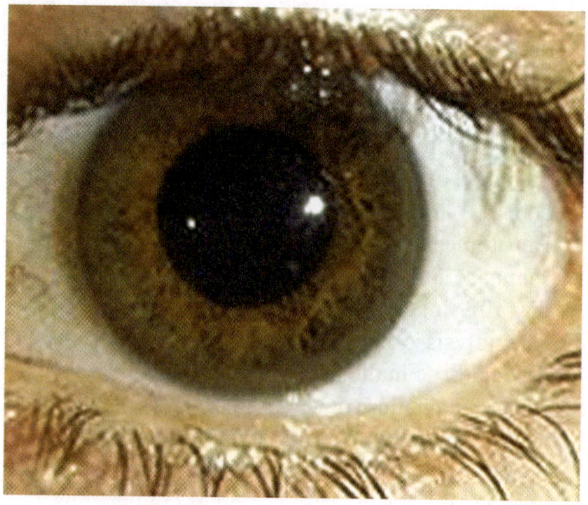

Fig. 9.54 Kayser-Fleischer ring

terized by deposition of copper in parenchymal tissue. A 'sunflower-like' discolouration of the most anterior layers of the lens has also been reported in patients with Wilson disease.

6. **Metal fume fever**, wheezing and rales have been reported in workers exposed to fine copper dust. Dyspnoea has developed after oral copper exposure.

Diagnosis

- Routine laboratory testing following acute copper salt poisoning should include an assessment for both haemolysis and hepatotoxicity.
- *Serum caeruloplasmin level*: A value of 35 mg% or less at 24 hrs is associated with serious toxicity.
- *Serum copper level*: If this is elevated beyond 1.5 mg/100 mL, there is likelihood of serious toxicity. Average normal levels are 1.09 mg/L for men, 1.2 mg/L for women.
- *Urine level:* Normal daily excretion of copper in the urine is less than 0.6 μmol/day.
- *Radiography*: Metallic copper is radiopaque. X-rays may be useful to establish diagnosis. Copper salts are not considered radiopaque.

Treatment

1. Administration of egg white or milk orally may help in detoxifying copper resulting in the formation of an albuminate.
2. Stomach wash can be done with a solution of potassium ferrocyanide. It converts the copper salt (especially copper sulphate) into insoluble cupric ferrocyanide.
3. Induction of emesis is contraindicated.*
4. Save blood for measurement of serum total copper concentration (reference range 10–21 μmol/L; 0.7–1.3 mg/L).
5. **Chelation therapy** is generally recommended in symptomatic patients.
   a. **Penicillamine**:
      i. *Usual Adult Dose:* 1000–1500 mg/day divided every 6–12 hrs, before meals.
      ii. *Usual Paediatric Dose:* Initially, 10 mg/kg/day, gradually increase to 30 mg/kg/day divided in two or three doses as tolerated.
   b. **Dimercaprol**:
      i. Most patients with copper poisoning are initially treated with intramuscular dimercaprol (British anti-Lewisite or BAL). Although BAL may be less effective, its use is appropriate in patients in whom vomiting or gastrointestinal injury prevents oral D-penicillamine administration.
      ii. *Dose:* 3–5 mg/kg/dose deep IM every 4 hrs for 2 days, every 4–6 hrs for an additional 2 days, then every 4–12 hrs for up to 7 additional days.
   c. **Calcium disodium edetate**:
      i. EDTA has been used to treat patients with acute copper sulphate intoxication but data regarding efficacy are lacking.
      ii. *Dose*: 75 mg/kg/24 hrs deep IM, or slow IV infusion given in 3–6 divided doses up to 5 days; may be repeated for a second course after a minimum of 2 days; each course should not exceed a total of 500 mg/kg body weight.
6. Symptomatic measures – Antacids and ranitidine for prevention of gastric erosions, dopamine for shock, etc.
7. Haemodialysis is said to be useful in the early stages of poisoning when the metal is still circulating in the blood stream as free copper. It is of course necessitated in patients with renal failure, and liver transplantation may be needed for patients with life-threatening hepatic failure.

Autopsy Features

1. Jaundiced skin and conjunctivae.
2. Greenish or bluish stomach contents.
3. Hepatic and renal necrosis.

Forensic Issues

- In India, the incidence of suicidal ingestion of copper sulphate was quite high till recently. Of late, there has been a decline.
- Copper contamination of drinking water due to stagnation in a copper main, or due to corrosion of copper plumbing has resulted in outbreaks of abdominal pain, diarrhoea, nausea and vomiting.

CADMIUM

- Cadmium is a bluish, lustrous and light metal (**Fig. 9.55**) which is a common contaminant of several metal ores such as lead, copper and zinc.
- Daily cadmium intake from food averages 10–25 μg/day. Shellfish such as mussels, scallops and oysters are a major source of dietary cadmium, and may contain 100–1000 μg/kg.

***Note**: *In fact copper salts (particularly copper sulphate) are strong emetics by themselves and were recommended in the past to induce vomiting in all cases of poisoning!*

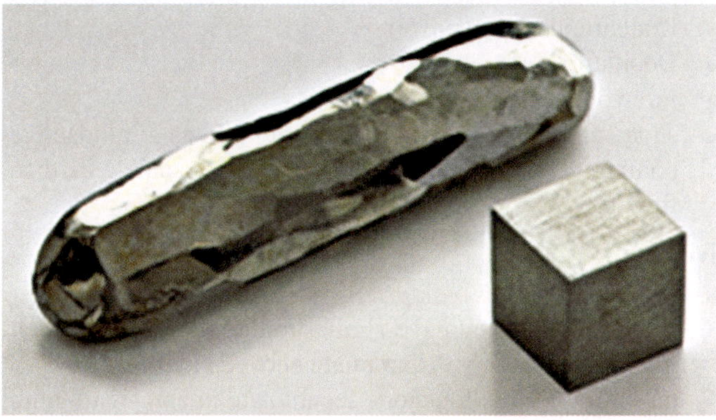

Fig. 9.55 Cadmium

- Smokers usually have twice the body burden of cadmium as non-smokers due to cadmium in cigarettes (up to 30 μg/pack) producing inhalation of 2–4 μg cadmium/pack smoked.

Uses

- Cadmium is highly resistant to corrosion and is widely used in industry (welding, electroplating).
- Batteries (nickel-cadmium).
- Shampoo: As a 1% solution for the treatment of seborrhoeic dermatitis and dandruff.

Mode of Action

- Cadmium's toxic effects may be due to the displacement or substitution of cadmium for zinc in critical metabolic processes. Cadmium interferes with the uptake, distribution and action of zinc.
- Oral or inhaled cadmium is transported to the liver, where it induces metallothionein, which binds and detoxifies cadmium. A slow release of this complex produces cadmium-methiothionein complex in all organs, particularly the kidney.
- The kidney accumulates cadmium over a lifetime. Renal damage is believed to occur once the cadmium concentration in the kidney cortex reaches or exceeds about 200 μg/g of kidney weight.
- Death has been reported following ingestion of up to 150 g of cadmium chloride.

Clinical Features

A. **Acute Poisoning**: This is rare. It can occur in two ways –
   1. *Ingestion* – Nausea, metallic taste, salivation, vomiting, abdominal pain, diarrhoea and myalgia. Sudden muscle cramps can cause the victim to cry out in pain periodically (***Itai-Itai* disease***, or ***Ouch-Ouch disease***). There is also bone demineralisation with osteomalacia and pathological fractures. Vertigo, shock, unconsciousness and convulsions have been reported. Death can occur due to dehydration or renal failure.
   2. *Inhalation* – The symptoms of acute poisoning after inhalation exposure may be delayed 12–36 hrs. These include chest pain, cough (with bloody sputum), difficulty breathing, sore throat, '***metal fume fever***' (shivering, sweating, body pains, headache) dizziness, irritability, weakness, nausea, vomiting, diarrhoea, tracheobronchitis, pneumonitis and pulmonary oedema.

B. **Chronic Poisoning**:
   1. Yellow staining of teeth (*yellow teeth line*).
   2. Vertigo.
   3. Anorexia, fatigue.
   4. Rhinitis and anosmia (due to damage to olfactory nerve).
   5. Musculoskeletal pain (due to osteopenia-osteomalacia). Long-term daily oral intake of more than 1 mg of cadmium may result in severe bone disease.
   6. Dyspnoea, emphysema.
   7. Hypochromic or normochromic anaemia.
   8. Renal damage producing microhaematuria, proteinuria, leukocyturia, urinary calculi. The most common finding in chronic cadmium poisoning is in fact proteinuria.
   9. Occupational cadmium exposure is also associated with nephrolithiasis, likely as a result of hypercalciuria.
   10. Hypertension.
   11. Cadmium is said to be carcinogenic, and increased incidence of lung, prostate, pancreas and bladder cancers in humans have been reported.

Diagnosis

1. Normal blood cadmium level in non-smokers is 0.4–1 μg/L, and in smokers 1.4–4 μg/L.
2. Urinary cadmium excretion of more than 2 μg/24 hrs or 10 μg/L is nephrotoxic.
3. *Radiography*:
   a. Chest X-ray findings after acute inhalation exposures may indicate diffuse pulmonary oedema. Later, they are those of bronchopneumonia (proliferative interstitial pneumonitis).
   b. In chronic poisoning, X-ray findings are characteristic of osteomalacia and may show multiple fractures.

Treatment

1. Chelation with **$CaNa_2EDTA$** or **DMSA (Succimer)** for acute poisoning. BAL is contraindicated since it can aggravate nephrotoxicity.
   a. Dose of **$CaNa_2EDTA$**: 75 mg/kg/24 hrs deep IM or slow IV infusion, given in 3–6 divided doses for up to 5 days.
   b. For **DMSA** (which is said to be the best chelator for cadmium), the initial dose is 10 mg/kg orally every 8 hours for 5 days. The dosing interval then is increased to every 12 hrs for the next 14 days. Repeat course may be given, if indicated by elevated blood levels. A minimum of 2 weeks between courses is recommended.
2. Haemoperfusion is ineffective due to high cadmium plasma protein and red blood cell binding.
3. Chelation for chronic cadmium toxicity is not currently recommended. There is no evidence that chelation of chroni-

****Note***: *Japanese for Ouch-Ouch!*

cally poisoned victims improves long-term outcomes. Removal from exposure and supportive treatment are the only measures recommended.

Forensic Issues

- Most cases of poisoning result from occupational or industrial exposure.
- Cadmium contamination of the environment can occur through soil, water, and food. The outbreak of ***Itai-Itai disease*** (a form of painful osteomalacia leading to pathological fractures) in Japan occurred in 1945 and continued into the 1950s; it was the result of consumption of rice grown in paddy fields which were irrigated by the local Jintzu river containing cadmium contaminated water (as a result of effluents from a nearby mine). The drinking water was also found to be contaminated.
- Certain types of soil have high cadmium content, and consumption of vegetables grown in such soil can result in elevated blood cadmium levels. This may be a factor in the aetiology of some cases of hypertension and renal failure.
- Tobacco smoke contains cadmium, and significant concentrations may be inhaled by chronic smoking, especially unfiltered cigarettes. Accumulation occurs mainly in the lung and kidney with resultant inflammatory and degenerative changes.
- Consumption of acid fruit juices stored in cadmium-plated metal ware can cause poisoning in families. Other sources of food contamination include pots and pans with cadmium-containing glazing, and vending machines for hot/cold drinks in which cadmium soldering has been done.

THALLIUM

- **Thallium** is a soft and pliable metal (**Fig. 9.56**) which is acquiring an increasingly notorious reputation as an **ideal homicidal poison**.
- Thallium (atomic number 81) is located between mercury and lead on the periodic table. Important derivatives include thallous sulphate (thallium sulphate), acetate, chloride, iodide, nitrate and carbonate. Most of these salts (particularly thallous sulphate) are odourless, tasteless and freely soluble in water.

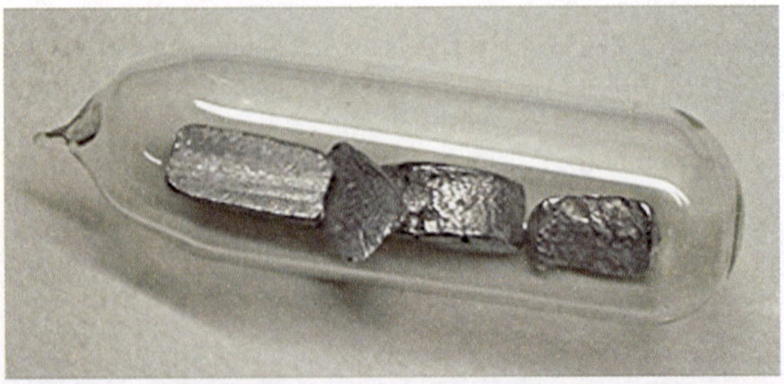

Fig. 9.56 Thallium pieces in an ampoule

Uses

- Manufacture of optical lenses (to increase refractory index)
- Dye industry
- Rodenticide (*previously*)
- Depilatory
- Fireworks
- Trace amounts of thallium salts are used as a radioactive contrast agent to image tumours and to visualize cardiac function.

Mode of Action

- Thallium behaves biologically in a manner similar to potassium because they have similar ionic radii. Because cell membranes cannot differentiate between thallium and potassium ions, thallous ions accumulate in areas with high potassium concentrations, such as central and peripheral nervous system and hepatic and muscle tissue.
- Thallium replaces potassium in the activation of potassium-dependent enzymes. As a result of both potassium substitution and interaction with thiol groups, thallium is capable of triggering automated cell death (apoptosis).
- Thallium has a high affinity for the sulphydryl groups present in many other enzymes and other proteins. It interferes with the formation of disulphide bonds, which may lead to the development of alopecia and defects in nail growth resulting in Mees lines.

Toxicokinetics

- Thallium is rapidly absorbed following all routes of exposure. Bioavailability is greatest following ingestion, and exceeds 90%.
- Thallium can be found in all organs, but highest concentrations are found in the intestine, liver, kidney, heart, brain and muscles.

Usual Fatal Dose

- Usual fatal dose is estimated to be **10–15 mg/kg**.
- Blood thallium concentrations greater than 1 mg/L are considered toxic. Normal urine values are below 5 μg/L.

Clinical Features

A. **Acute Poisoning**: A time scale of likely symptoms and signs is shown below:
   - **Less than 24 hrs**: Nausea, vomiting, GI bleeding (usually after ingestion).
   - **0–4 days**: Pancreatic and parotid damage, constipation.
   - **0–7 days**: Acne, confusion, delirium, organ failure (renal, hepatic, cardiac and respiratory failure, bone marrow damage), coma and death.
   - **0–14 days**: Peripheral sensori-motor neuropathy, ocular nerve paralysis, cardiac features (disturbances of BP and pulse).
   - **0–21 days**: Alopecia.

   Ataxia, tremor, marked tenderness of the soles, together with personality changes and severe loss of intellectual function are invariably present. A characteristic, dark pigmented band is often noticed in the scalp hair in about 3–4 days. Urine that is first voided after poisoning may show a green discolouration.

B. **Chronic Poisoning**:

- ***Alopecia*** – One of the pathognomonic signs of chronic thallium intake, it begins about 10 days after the first dose and may lead to total scalp hair loss in about a month if the intake is continued (**Fig. 9.57**). Facial and axillary hair, especially the inner one-third of the eyebrows, may be spared, but in some cases, full beards, as well as all scalp hair, are lost. Regrowth of the hair occurs if the patient survives the poisoning, but is often abnormally fine and unpigmented. **Table 9.12** lists some important substances which produce alopecia.
- ***Skin rash*** – This is in the form of a papulomacular rash which often assumes a "butterfly" distribution on the face. There may be acneiform eruptions. Acne, palmar erythema and dry scaly skin that results from damage to the sebaceous glands.
- *Dystrophy of the nails* (Mees stripes or lines)*
- Painful ascending ***peripheral sensorimotor neuropathy***. Pain and paraesthesias are most pronounced in the lower limbs, particularly the soles. Painful peripheral neuropathy and paraesthesia, primarily of the legs and feet, are among the first symptoms noted. Pain may be described as aching, tingling or burning and may be so severe as to prohibit walking. Paraesthesias may develop within 2–6 days in severe poisoning. Loss of pain, temperature, vibratory and position sense may all occur and an unsteady gait may develop.
- *Ataxia*: Ataxia can develop within 48 hrs after ingestion.
- *Other neurological manifestations* – cranial nerve palsies, optic neuropathy, choreoathetosis, tremor, encephalopathy and psychotic behaviour.
- *Ophthalmological manifestations* – Ocular features include nystagmus, ptosis and abnormalities of gaze due to involvement of the third, fourth and sixth cranial nerves. Retrobulbar neuritis, facial paralysis, decreased visual acuity, optic atrophy and defective colour vision may develop.
- *Cardiovascular & haematological manifestations* – Hypertension, cardiomyopathy, ECG changes, leukocytosis and thrombocytopenia.
- *Other symptoms & signs* – Autonomic dysfunction, testicular toxicity, hypokalaemia, renal failure and hepatic dysfunction. A bluish line in the gums may appear 3–4 weeks post-ingestion.

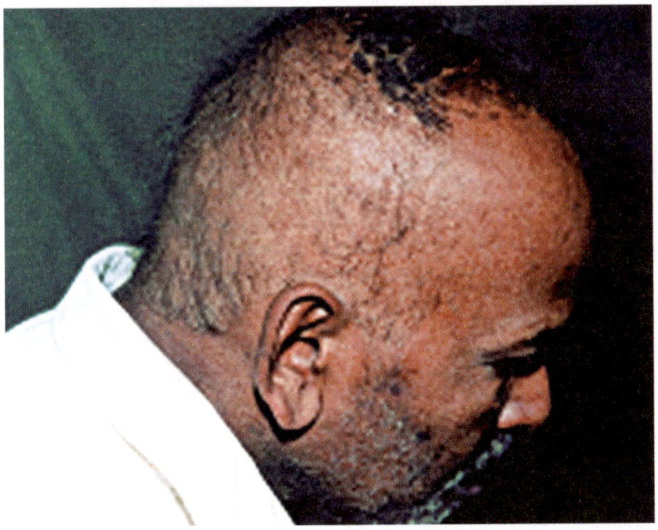

Fig. 9.57 Alopecia – Thallium poisoning

Table 9.12 Substances Producing Alopecia

▪ Allopurinol	▪ 5-Fluorouracil	▪ Oral contraceptives
▪ Androgens	▪ Gold salts	▪ Quinacrine
▪ Arsenic	▪ Lead	▪ Thallium
▪ Mercury	▪ Vincristine	▪ Vinblastine
▪ Cyclophosphamide	▪ Methotrexate	▪ Warfarin

The outstanding combination of **alopecia & skin rash, painful peripheral neuropathy** and **mental confusion with lethargy (*thallium triad*)**, in any clinical case must immediately arouse the suspicion of chronic thallium poisoning. A high level of suspicion should be kept for thallium poisoning in patients with painful ascending peripheral neuropathy and gastrointestinal symptoms, which appear much earlier than alopecia, since the prognosis is much better with early diagnosis and treatment. Pain and paraesthesias are present in lower extremities (especially the soles of the feet: '***burning feet syndrome***'), and although numbness is present in fingers and toes, there is also decreased sensation to pinprick, touch, temperature, vibration and proprioception. Motor weakness is always distal in distribution, with the lower limbs more affected than the upper limbs.

The progression of symptoms may sometimes mimic other conditions, particularly **Guillain Barre' syndrome** (Landry's paralysis or acute infectious polyneuritis), acute porphyria, psychosis or thiamine deficiency.

Sequelae, including mental retardation, psychosis, abnormal reflexes, ataxia, tremor, flaccid paraparesis, cerebellar ataxia and mental impairment have been reported. There are reports of neurological sequelae lasting more than 30 years.

Diagnosis

1. ***X-ray***: May reveal opacities in the GIT or liver.
2. Tests of contrast sensitivity and colour vision are useful in the early detection of optic neuropathy in thallium poisoning.
3. Abnormal EEG and delayed peripheral nerve conduction.

*Note: See page no. 433

4. ***Microscopic studies*** of scalp hair show thallium deposition as dark brown or black pigmentation located in the roots of hair samples. In patients with chronic exposures, several bands may be noted on the hair shaft, demonstrating multiple exposures.
5. ***Urine test***: Combine a few drops of urine with 3 drops of saturated bromine water, 3 drops of sulphosalicylic acid, 1 drop of HCl, 2 drops of a solution of 0.05 g of rhodamine B in 100 mL of conc HCl. Mix. Add 1 mL of benzene, shake, centrifuge and examine the benzene layer. A bright yellow or fluorescent red colour indicates a positive result.
6. ***Atomic absorption spectroscopy***: Measure thallium concentrations in blood in cases of suspected toxicity. Blood concentrations of more than 50 nmol/L (10 µg/L) signify significant exposure.
7. Urinary excretion of thallium in excess of 10–20 mg in 24 hrs (100 nmol/L or 20 µg/L) is considered diagnostic.
8. Whole blood thallium exceeding 100 µg/dL indicates potential poisoning.
9. ***Hypocalcaemia***: Monitor calcium levels during the acute phase.

Treatment

1. Consider gastric lavage, if a substantial amount has been ingested within 1 hr. Stomach wash can be done with **Prussian Blue** or **Berlin Blue** [*potassium ferric ferrocyanide or potassium ferric hexacyanoferrate, i.e.,* $KFe(Fe(CN)_6)$] which prevents the absorption of thallium by binding with it, exchanging potassium for thallium in its crystal lattice network.
   a. Prussian Blue is then instilled through a duodenal tube (125 mg/kg twice a day, with 50 mL of 15% mannitol).*
   b. This is continued until the urinary excretion falls below 0.5 mg/day.
2. In some Western countries, insoluble Prussian Blue is available as 0.5 g blue powder in gelatin capsules for oral administration (**Fig. 9.58**).

   Dose: Give oral Prussian Blue 250–300 mg/kg/day (approximately 10 g twice daily for an adult) or 3 g orally three times a day (*for children*: 1 g three times a day).

   Optimal duration of therapy is not established, but it is recommended that Prussian Blue administration must be continued until thallium is no longer detected in the faeces.
3. Activated charcoal is beneficial. Thallium is thought to undergo enterohepatic recirculation, and multiple dose activated charcoal may enhance its elimination. In fact, if Prussian Blue is not immediately available, repeat dose activated charcoal is mandatory. As thallium causes ileus later in the course of poisoning, an osmotic laxative must be given with each dose.
4. Forced diuresis in conjunction with potassium chloride. Potassium chloride therapy has been reported to enhance excretion of thallium, but there are conflicting reports as to its efficacy in enhancing elimination. It promotes renal excretion of thallium through the exchange of potassium for thallium, thereby releasing thallium from tissue sites into blood and enhancing urinary excretion. But, neurologic symptoms may be aggravated because of redistribution of thallium into the brain.

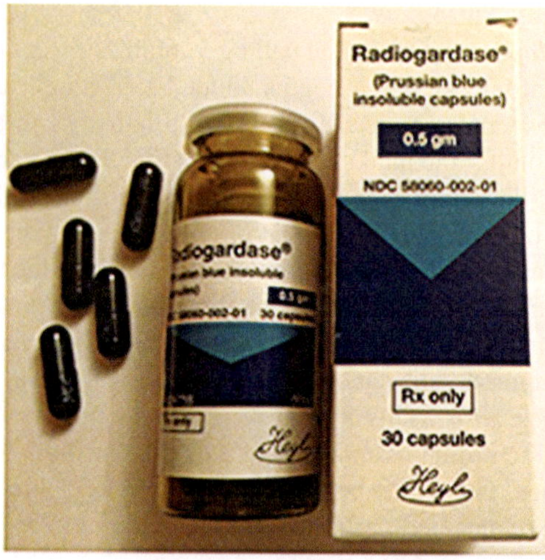

Fig. 9.58 Alopecia – Thallium poisoning

5. Haemodialysis along with haemoperfusion may be beneficial, especially in the presence of renal failure.
6. Chelating agents such as BAL, EDTA, etc., are not effective.
7. Diethyldithiocarbamate (Dithiocarb) was till recently advocated as an antidote. However, it sometimes leads to a worsening of the patient's condition and is therefore not recommended today.
8. Shaving the patient's head may reduce the psychological stress of hair loss, and improve the patient's morale.

If treatment is instituted in time, recovery from thallium poisoning is the rule, though this may take a long time. There may be residual effects such as amnesia, ataxia, tremor and foot drop.

Autopsy Features

1. Alopecia.
2. Stomatitis.
3. Fatty degeneration of heart (with "*tabby cat striation*" of the ventricles).
4. Fatty degeneration of liver.
5. Renal damage.
6. Pulmonary oedema.
7. Cerebral oedema with widespread degeneration of nerve cells and axons.

Forensic Issues

1. Accidental poisoning occurs due to industrial or occupational exposure. It can also occur inadvertently from its use as a rodenticide. Several instances of accidental poisoning have been reported in children who have consumed cockroach or rat bait containing thallium.

***Note**: *Prussian Blue can cause blue discolouration of sweat and tears.*

2. Suicides with thallium have always been rare in India, though they were relatively common abroad until the 1960s, when legislation was passed in most Western countries greatly restricting its availability for use as pesticides. In 1975, USA banned its use altogether as a rodenticide.
3. **The most disturbing aspect about thallium today is its increasing deployment by poisoners to commit murder**. There have been several celebrated cases of murder reported over a period of time, especially in Western countries.
   a. Thallium salts unfortunately possess several properties of a **"perfect" poison** – they are odourless, tasteless, freely soluble in water and produce toxic manifestations which closely resemble natural disease.
   b. The commonest salt is **thallous sulphate** which can be mixed in tea or coffee or even water, and administered to a victim without arousing suspicion. Following ingestion there is a relatively long latent period before symptoms begin to manifest (12–48 hrs), which gives the criminal time to cover his tracks.
      i. One of the most infamous cases of thallium murders is undoubtedly the **Graham Young** case of 1971. A strange illness (nicknamed the *Bovingdon Bug*) broke out among the employees of a small factory manufacturing optical instruments in Bovingdon, near London, a few months after a 23-year-old man named Graham Young joined as a storeman in April 1971 (**Fig. 9.59**). Symptoms included abdominal pain, diarrhoea, numbness in the legs, visual disturbances, and unusual hairloss. Out of the nearly 70 staff members affected, two died. Ian Anderson, the factory's medical officer suspected poisoning and believed Young to be the culprit because of his peculiar con duct and obsession with poisonous substances. The police was informed and they arrested Young on suspicion. A bottle of thallium was found on his person at the time of arrest and a search of his room revealed numerous chemicals and poisons, and an incriminating diary in which he had jotted down his modus operandi of offering thallium-contaminated tea to his co-workers, and daily observations regarding the progression of symptoms in the victims. A study of his past life revealed serious psychiatric problems. He had in fact been admitted to an asylum at Broadmoor for attempted murder of his own father, sister and a school friend at the age of 14! After being granted a conditional discharge following nearly 10 years of detention, he had joined the factory at Bovingdon in 1971 only to begin his nefarious homicidal activity all over again. Young was finally sentenced to life imprisonment after being convicted of the Bovingdon murders.
      ii. In 1991, another sensational case was reported, this time from the USA, where a distinguished University college professor (**George Trepal**) poisoned his neighbours by lacing several bottles of cola with thallium. George Trepal (**Fig. 9.60**) and his wife moved into their home in Alturas, Florida during the early 1980s. Parealyn and Peggy Carr along with their sons, Travis Carr and Duane Dubberly, were their neighbours. Unfortunately, relations between the neighbours were not cordial, and Trepal and the Carrs were involved in a number of altercations, including one incident in which Trepal threatened to kill one of the Carr children. The Carrs also received an unsigned letter threatening harm to their family if they did not leave Florida. In October 1988, Peggy Carr began to suffer from a mysterious illness. She was admitted to the hospital and remained there for several days before being discharged. After discharge, Peggy's condition worsened and she was readmitted to the hospital. Travis Carr and Duane Dubberly also exhibited similar symptoms and were transported to the hospital. The attending physician suspected thallium poisoning based on the symptoms displayed. Within 1 day, thallium poisoning was confirmed. Peggy Carr's condition worsened, and she fell into a coma. She died when life support was disconnected in March 1988. In November 1989, officials collected samples from the Carr household in an attempt to determine the origin of the thallium. The residue in several empty Coca-Cola bottles (retrieved during the collection of samples) was tested. Thallium was detected in the Coca-Cola bottles. Subsequent investigations revealed Trepal to be the main suspect, and he was charged with seven counts of poisoning. A subsequent search of Trepal's home turned up chemistry books and equipment, including information about poisons. Finally, the police found a bottle-capping machine that could be used to replace the bottle caps of Coca-Cola bottles after the cap was removed to introduce the poison into the drink. Trepal was convicted on 06 March 1991, and sentenced to death.

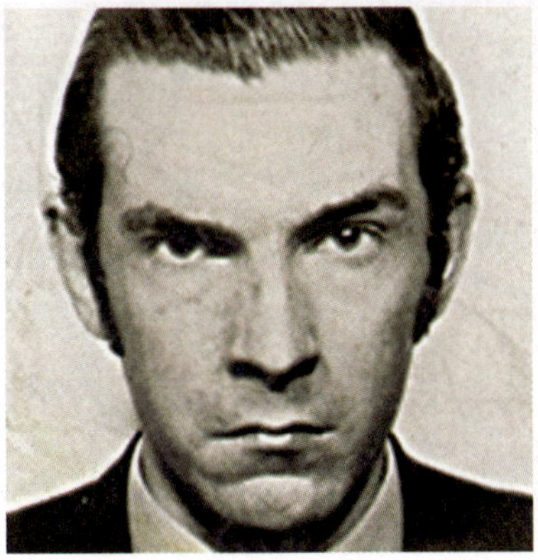

Fig. 9.59 Graham Young

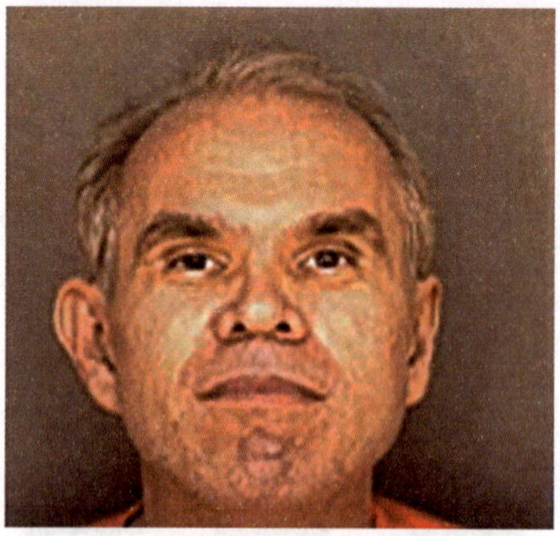

Fig. 9.60 George Trepal

> **FM 9.4: Core – Written/Viva Voce/ Objective Structured Clinical Examination (OSCE)**
> - Describe general principles and basic methodologies in treatment of poisoning: decontamination, supportive therapy, antidote therapy, procedures of enhanced elimination with regard to:
>   - Ethanol
>   - Methanol
>   - Ethylene glycol

ALCOHOLS

Alcohols are classified as Inebriants, which are substances that induce intoxication or inebriation, and comprise in addition, **barbiturates**, **benzodiazepines** and **chloral hydrate**.

ETHANOL

Synonyms

Ethyl alcohol; Grain alcohol; Spirits of wine

Molecular Formula

C_2H_5OH; C_2H_6O; CH_3CH_2OH.

Physical Appearance

- Clear, colourless liquid with a faint fruity odour and sweetish burning taste.
- It is both water soluble and lipid soluble.

Sources

1. Ethanol is produced mostly by synthetic production from ethylene. This is mainly by direct hydration process (replacing the earlier method of indirect hydration using sulphuric acid).
2. Fermentation of sugar, cellulose or starch. Such is the method used in the production of beverage alcohol.
3. Enzymatic hydrolysis of cellulose.

Beverage ethanol is produced by fermentation of a sugar (from cereal, vegetable or fruit) with yeast. If cereal is used as raw material, it has to be malted first to convert the starch to maltose, since yeast cannot ferment starch. Malt is produced by moistening barley and allowing it to sprout which is then dried, ground and added to the cereal in water resulting in the formation of ***mash***. Beer is brewed by filtering *mash* and treating the filtered liquid (***wort***) with yeast. Whisky is made by adding yeast directly to the malted *mash*. Strong alcoholic beverages are distilled after fermentation.

The ethanol content of various alcoholic beverages is expressed by volume percent or by proof,* the latter being twice the percentage of alcohol by volume. In the United Kingdom, the Customs and Excise Act of 1952, declared **proof spirits (100 proof) as those in which the weight of the spirits is 12/13 the weight of an equal volume of distilled water at 51°F**. Thus, proof spirits are **48.24% ethanol by weight**, or **57.06% by volume**. Other spirits are designated over- or underproof, with the percentage of variance noted. While this is the method followed in India also, in the United States, a proof spirit (100 proof) is one containing 50% ethanol by volume. **Table 9.13** lists the ethanol content of various alcoholic beverages.

Apart from ethanol however, these beverages also contain several congeners to varying extent, e.g., low-molecular weight alcohols such as methanol and butanol, as well as aldehydes, esters, phenols, tannins and heavy metals (lead, cobalt, iron, etc.). **Vodka is the purest form and contains no congeners**. It is virtually odourless. White rum is also relatively pure.

Uses

- *Beverage*:
  - Popular alcoholic beverages include beer, wine, whisky, gin, brandy, rum and vodka.
  - In addition, there are several indigenous preparations peculiar to particular regions, e.g., arrack, toddy and feni in India, tequila in Mexico, sake in Japan, *eau de vie* or fruit brandy in France, etc.
- Solvent for after-shaves, colognes, mouthwashes and perfumes. The alcohol content in these is variable (15–80%).
- *Medicinal*:
  - Several antihistaminic, decongestant, multivitamin and cough syrups contain varying percentage of alcohol (2–25%).
  - Ethanol has been popular in the past as an antiseptic. Surgical spirit used even today is mostly ethanol with a small quantity of methanol (90–95% and 10–5%, respectively), along with traces of castor oil and methyl salicylate.
  - Ethanol sponging is an effective remedy for hyperthermia.
  - Injection of dehydrated alcohol (absolute alcohol) in close proximity of nerves or sympathetic ganglia is said to be effective for the relief of long lasting pain in conditions such as trigeminal neuralgia.
  - Antidote for methanol and ethylene glycol.

****Note**: *The term "proof" originated long ago when sailors in the British Navy suspected that their superior officers were diluting their rum (grog) ration and demanded "proof" that this was not happening. The proof was derived by pouring a sample of grog on black gunpowder. If the gunpowder ignited on lighting a match, the rum was up to standard, 100% proof that the liquor was 50% ethanol. This became shortened to 100 proof.*

Table 9.13 Ethanol Content in Alcoholic Beverages

Beverage	Ethanol Content (vol.%)
Light Beer (*Lager and Pilsener*)	4–6
Heavy Beer (*Ale and Stout*)	6–12
Natural Wine (*Cider*)	2–8
Fortified Wine (*Sherry, Port, Vermouth*)	10–20
Whisky, Gin, Tequila, Brandy	40–45
Rum	40–60
Liqueurs (*Cognac, Crème De Menthe, Schnapps, etc.*)	15–55

- *Preservative*: Rectified spirit (90–95 % ethanol) is used as a preservative for viscera, for chemical analysis.
- Fuel.
- Ethanol is used to extract nucleic acids from whole tissue or tissue culture in virtually all biotechnology processes.

Usual Fatal Dose

- One pint (approximately 550 mL) or quart (two pints or approximately 1100 mL) of a strong distilled spirit such as whisky taken in a short span of time can be lethal.
  - Jai Singh, a 45 year-old e-rickshaw puller in Agra (Uttar Pradesh) accepted a challenge from two of his friends to consume 540 mL of country liquor in 10 min, on the evening of 8th Feb 2023. He fell unconscious, and was dead by the time, he was taken to hospital a few hours later – *Times of India, 15 Feb 2023.*
- The **usual fatal dose** corresponds to approximately **6 g of ethanol/kg body weight (adult); 3 g/kg (child)**.
- In terms of blood alcohol, a level in excess of **400–500 mg/100 mL** is usually considered to be lethal. However, there is a great deal of controversy regarding this since there are case reports of individuals succumbing to much lower BAC, while there have been reports of survival even with a BAC of over 1000 mg%.

Toxicokinetics

- Ethanol is toxic by oral, inhalation, subcutaneous, intravenous, intra-arterial, intraperitoneal and dermal routes.
- Following oral administration, ethanol is rapidly absorbed from the stomach (20%) and small intestine (80%). Maximum or peak alcohol concentration in blood is reached in 30–90 min following the last drink.
  - Many factors can delay absorption: undiluted ethanol (by provoking pylorospasm), presence of food, delayed gastric emptying due to any cause and presence of congeners in alcohol.
  - Following an equivalent dose of ethanol, women achieve a higher blood alcohol level than do men as a result of decreased gastric alcohol dehydrogenase activity. It is also a fact that liver damage occurs after consumption of relatively smaller quantities of alcohol in women as compared to men.
- Vapourised ethanol can be rapidly absorbed by inhalation leading to intoxication.
- More than 90% of ethanol ingested is metabolised in the body, and only 5–10% is excreted unchanged by the kidneys, lungs and sweat.
- Excretion of ethanol by the lungs obeys **Henry's Law**: *the ratio between the concentration of ethanol in the alveolar air and the blood is constant*. This alveolar air/blood constant (1:2100) forms the basis for reliably estimating blood alcohol concentration by breath analysis.
- Metabolism of alcohol is accomplished through three pathways in the liver:
  i. **Alcohol dehydrogenase pathway** (in the cell cytosol);
  ii. Microsomal ethanol oxidising system (MEOS, (*CYP2E1*), located on the endoplasmic reticulum);
  iii. Peroxidase-catalase system (in the hepatic peroxisomes).

  The first is the main pathway, while the third is the least important. In the alcohol dehydrogenase mediated pathway, the acetaldehyde that is formed is converted to acetic acid by aldehyde dehydrogenase, which in turn is converted to acetylcoenzyme A and enters the Krebs (citric acid) cycle, where it is metabolised to carbon dioxide and water.*

  The MEOS system becomes important when ethanol use becomes chronic.
- Adults absorb 80–90% of ingested alcohol within 1 hr and on average metabolise it at a rate of 100–125 mg/kg/hr (reducing blood concentrations by approximately 150–200 mg/L (3.26–4.35 mmol/L) per hour. Tolerant drinkers metabolise ethanol at higher rates and therefore blood concentrations fall more rapidly.
- Volume of distribution for ethanol is 0.4–0.6 L/kg. ADH is saturated at relatively low blood ethanol concentrations.

****Note***: *The ability of acetylcoenzyme A to enter the Krebs cycle is dependent on adequate thiamine stores.*

As the system is saturated, ethanol elimination changes from first-order to zero-order kinetics.

- In adults, the average rate of ethanol metabolism is 100–125 mg/kg/hr in occasional drinkers and up to 175 mg/kg/hr in habitual drinkers. As a result, the average-sized adult metabolizes 7–10 g/hr and the blood ethanol concentration falls 15–20 mg/dL/hr (3.26–4.35 mmol/L/hr). Tolerant drinkers, by recruiting CYP2E1, may increase their clearance of ethanol to 30 mg/dL/hr (6.52 mmol/L/hr).
- An important point to remember with reference to Asians is that nearly 40% of the population may harbour an inactive aldehyde dehydrogenase variant (due to a point mutation in the ALDH5 gene) which significantly reduces the capacity for acetaldehyde metabolism leading to severe flushing reactions in such individuals even with relatively small amounts of ethanol.

Mode of Action

- Till recently, it was postulated that ethanol depresses the CNS by dissolving in the cell's lipid membrane and causing disorganisation of the lipid matrix (membrane fluidisation). However this mechanism has been challenged by studies which demonstrated that such membrane fluidisation occurred only at ethanol concentrations much above the pharmacologic range, and also that the same changes can be produced by minor temperature changes which produce no signs of intoxication.
- Ethanol affects a number of membrane proteins that are involved in signalling pathways, including neurotransmitter receptors, enzymes and ion channels, and there is definitive evidence that ethanol interacts with a variety of neurotransmitters. The major effects of ethanol involve enhancing the inhibitory effects of gamma-aminobutyricacid (GABA) at $GABA_A$ receptors and blockade of the N-methyl-D-aspartate (NMDA) subtype of glutamate, an excitatory amino acid (EAA) receptor.
- Chronic ethanol administration results in tolerance, dependence and an ethanol withdrawal syndrome, mediated, in part, by desensitization or downregulation of $GABA_A$ receptors.

Pharmacological Effects of Ethanol

- **CNS**: Ethanol is a CNS depressant but produces some apparently stimulating effects initially because of depression of inhibitory control mechanisms in the brain. First, those mental processes which depend on training and previous experience are affected (memory, concentration and insight). Later the person becomes expansive, garrulous and may demonstrate emotional lability with mood swings. With severe intoxication there is general impairment of CNS function, and finally coma supervenes.
- **CVS**: In moderate doses, ethanol produces tachycardia and vasodilation of cutaneous vessels with resultant warm and flushed skin. However, no beneficial increase in coronary blood flow occurs; in fact, there may be appreciable vasoconstriction which can aggravate existing angina. In spite of this fact, recent studies have indicated that regular use of moderate amounts of ethanol is associated with reduced risk for coronary heart disease.
- **GIT**: Ethanol normally stimulates salivary and gastric secretions, but if the concentration is too high (>40%) they are inhibited, and the GI mucosa becomes congested and inflamed leading to erosive gastritis. Regular intake of excessive amounts of ethanol leads to chronic gastritis, pancreatitis and cirrhosis of liver.
- **Genito-urinary**: Ethanol induces diuresis by inhibition of antidiuretic hormone (ADH). There is a popular misconception (perpetuated in pulp fiction and films) that ethanol is an aphrodisiac. While it is true that there is often enhanced sexual inclination with (sometimes) aggressive behaviour, this is due to loss of inhibition and restraint rather than the result of sexual stimulation. Objective measurements in human beings of penile tumescence and vaginal pressure show that ethanol actually significantly decreases sexual responsiveness in both men and women. Chronic ethanol consumption can lead to impotence, sterility, testicular atrophy and gynaecomastia (because of hyperoestrogenisation, and reduced production as well as enhanced metabolic inactivation of testosterone).
- In women, there is increased predisposition to breast cancer.
- The teratogenic effects of alcohol are discussed in a subsequent section of this Topic.

Clinical Features

1. **Acute Poisoning** (***Intoxication, Inebriation***):
   a. Initially, ethanol produces excitement which progresses to loss of restraint, behavioural changes, garrulousness, slurred speech, ataxia, unsteady gait, drowsiness, stupor and finally coma (**Table 9.14**).
   b. Rarely, alcohol induces allergic reactions (usually in the form of urticaria, nasal congestion, headache, etc.), which may be severe and may even result in death.
   c. There are also reports of cardiac dysrhythmias (especially atrial fibrillation) associated with binge drinking.
   d. Through all the 5–7 stages of ethanol intoxication, a distinct **odour** is perceptible in the breath of the individual. It is however not the alcohol itself which imparts this odour, but other nonalcoholic constituents that give a particular flavour depending on the type of beverage consumed (wine, beer, whisky, etc.). It is important to remember that even after a person has completely sobered up from the effects of ethanol, the odour may persist in the breath for a considerable period of time.
   e. Ethanol is a **mydriatic**, but towards terminal stages (stages of stupor and coma), the pupils may become constricted, only to dilate once again at about the time of death. The **McEwan sign*** is highly **unreliable** and

**Pinching the skin of the face or neck, or light slapping, is supposed to dilate the constricted pupils of alcoholic coma momentarily. It is unreliable and can mislead the physician.*

Table 9.14 Acute Alcohol Poisoning (Intoxication, Inebriation)

Blood Alcohol Concentration (mg/100 mL)	Stage of Intoxication	Clinical Features
0–50	Sobriety	Near normal behaviour
50–100	Euphoria	Feeling of well being, talkativeness, increased self-confidence, decreased inhibitions, fine movements affected
100–150	Excitement	Emotional instability, impairment of memory and comprehension, increased reaction time, mild ataxia
150–200	Confusion	Disorientation, confusion, vertigo, diplopia, ataxia, slurred speech, staggering gait
200–300	Stupor	General inertia, diminished response to stimuli, inability to stand or walk, vomiting
300–500	Coma	Unconsciousness, abolished reflexes, subnormal temperature, incontinence of urine and faeces, respiratory compromise
>500	Death	Death due to respiratory failure
*The **7** stages can be remembered as a series of D's: **D**ecent, **D**elighted, **D**elirious, **D**azed, **D**ejected, **D**ead drunk, **D**ead.*		

must not be depended upon for diagnosis of alcoholic coma.

f. Hypothermia is common.

g. Hypotension and tachycardia may be present. Atrial fibrillation and atrioventricular block have been reported with acute overdose. Cardiac output may be decreased in persons with pre-existing cardiac disease.

   i. **Alcoholic cardiomyopathy** has insidious onset and can be clinically inapparent. Symptoms of alcoholic cardiomyopathy are often present for an average of 10–12 months before diagnosis, but as much as 85% of cases have not been diagnosed through routine screening, unless angiography was performed.

h. Bradypnoea may occur early, and tachypnoea may develop in cases of metabolic acidosis.

i. Poor control of eye movements, with **diplopia** and **nystagmus** may occur and alter vision and performance. Acute overdoses of ethanol have caused spontaneous (not gaze-evoked) horizontal nystagmus. Amblyopia due to peripheral neuritis has been reported in chronic alcoholics. Bilaterally decreased vision occurs. Vitamin deficiencies correlate with the ocular defects and early administration of B vitamins causes recovery in some patients.

j. Lactic or ketoacidosis may occur.

k. **Hypoglycaemia** which can result in seizures and coma is a serious complication of acute alcoholic intoxication, especially in children.

l. Medicolegally, **stages 3 and 4** of alcoholic intoxication (stages of excitement and confusion) are the most important, since most of the offences associated with drinking are committed during these two stages. It is pertinent to mention that stage 7 (death) is extremely rare in pure ethanol ingestion. In most cases, there is recovery after prolonged sleep, with some residual after effects (***hangover***), consisting of headache, irritability, lethargy, nausea and abdominal discomfort. While the last mentioned is mainly due to gastritis produced by ethanol, the other symptoms are actually the result of congeners and impurities present in alcoholic beverages which cause mild cerebral oedema. Part of the hangover may also be the result of hypoglycaemia induced by ethanol.

m. While the subject of some professional dispute, some data indicate that a small number of people may be exceptionally sensitive to ethanol, exhibiting combative and irrational behavior after ingesting non-intoxicating amounts. This has been termed **pathological intoxication** or **ethanol idiosyncratic intoxication**.

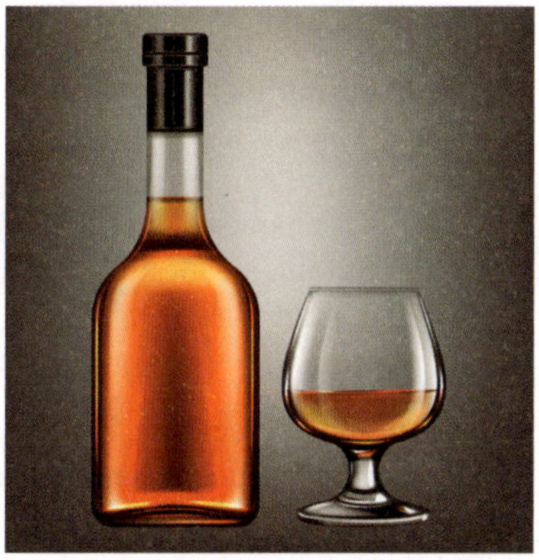
Stage 1: Sober
Stage 2: Euphoria
Stage 3: Excitement
Stage 4: Confusion
Stage 5: Stupor
Stage 6: Coma
Stage 7: Death

Fig. 9.61 Seven stages of alcohol intoxication

Pillay – Textbook of Forensic Medicine & Toxicology

n. Alcoholic intoxication (through all the stages) can mimic several conditions which can lead to errors in diagnosis. **Table 9.15** lists the differential diagnosis for acute ethanol intoxication.

Diagnosis

- *Bedside test* – Place 1 mL of unknown solution plus 1 mL of acetic acid and 1 drop of H_2SO_4 in a test tube and heat gently for 1 min. A characteristic, strong fruity odour (due to ethyl acetate) is positive for ethanol.
- *Blood alcohol level* – The blood alcohol concentration (BAC) estimated by immunoassay or gas chromatography is the commonest method employed by laboratories in India. Although accurate, the results of these tests are often delayed several hours and are not really appropriate in the clinical scenario.
- Determine serum electrolytes, glucose, ethanol. Hypoglycaemia, hypokalaemia and metabolic acidosis (lactic or ketoacidosis) may occur.
- BUN, creatinine, liver transaminases and CPK may be useful in identifying secondary effects, such as hepatotoxicity (chronic ethanol use), respiratory depression or rhabdomyolysis (if seizures are present).
- Qualitative determination of urinary ethanol is commonly included in a toxicology screen. However, urinary ethanol levels may be falsely elevated in patients with diabetes.

2. **Chronic Poisoning (*Alcoholism, Ethanolism*)**:
   a. Alcoholism is a condition in an individual who consumes large amounts of alcohol over a long period of time. It is characterised by:
      - a pathological desire for alcohol intake
      - black-outs during intoxication
      - withdrawal symptoms on ceasing alcohol intake.

Way back in the 19th century, it was recognized that chronic alcoholism could lead to personal, financial and social decline of an individual (**Fig. 9.62**).

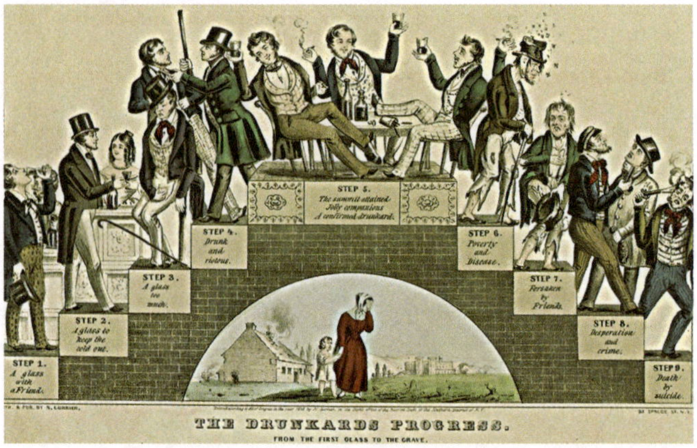

Fig. 9.62 The Drunkard's Progress (1846) By Nathaniel Currier – The Library of Congress

   b. Unfortunately, many patients are not diagnosed correctly as alcoholics by their doctors. A high index of suspicion is important, particularly in cases where there are repeated consultations for vague symptoms or minor accidents. If in doubt, a drinking history should be taken in which the patient is asked to describe a typical week's drinking.
      - Consumption should be quantified in terms of units of alcohol. One unit contains approximately 8–10 g of alcohol and is the equivalent of half a pint of beer, a single measure (30 mL) of spirits, or a glass of table wine. Current opinion suggests that drinking becomes a problem at levels above 21 units/week for men and 14 units/week for women.
   c. Laboratory tests are useful in confirming alcohol abuse. Mean corpuscular volume (MCV) or gamma-glutamyl transpeptidase (gamma GT) is raised in approximately 50% of problem drinkers.
   d. **Medical complications of alcoholism**:
      - *GIT* – Gastritis, periodic diarrhoea, increased incidence of oropharyngeal and oesophageal cancer.

Table 9.15 Differential Diagnosis of Alcoholic Intoxication

Pre-Coma	Coma
Barbiturate ingestion (and other similar drugs)	Hypoglycaemic or diabetic coma
Carbon monoxide poisoning	Coma due to hypnotics, sedatives and other drugs
Hypoglycaemia	
Head injury (post-concussional state)	
Cerebrovascular accident	
Psychotic states	
Disseminated sclerosis (or similar neurological afflictions)	

- *Liver* – Fatty liver with portal hypertension, hepatitis (**Fig. 9.63**), cirrhosis (**Fig. 9.64**), increased incidence of hepatic carcinoma.
- *Pancreas* – Acute or chronic pancreatitis, pancreatic cancer.
- *CVS* – Cardiomyopathy (**Fig. 9.65**), dysrhythmias, hypertension.
- *CNS* – Polyneuropathy, cerebellar degeneration, demyelination of corpus callosum (Marchiafava-Bignami disease), amblyopia, stroke.
- *RS* – Aspiration pneumonia, alcohol-induced asthma.
- *Endocrine* – Hypogonadism and feminisation in males, amenorrhoea, menorrhagia, and infertility in females, pseudo-Cushing syndrome.
- *Blood* – Anaemia, thrombocytopenia.
- *Skeletal muscle* – Myopathy.
- *Neuropsychiatric* – Memory disturbances (amnesia), delusions, delirium tremens, Wernicke's encephalopathy, Korsakoff's psychosis, dementia, alcoholic hallucinosis.
- *Teratogenecity* – **Foetal alcohol syndrome (FAS)** - This syndrome is characterized by facial dysmorphias (**Fig. 9.66**) and other congenital abnormalities, prenatal growth retardation and neurodevelopmental abnormalities in some children of mothers who abused ethanol during pregnancy. Main abnormalities reported include:
  - Cleft palate
  - Spina bifida
  - Ventricular & atrial septal defects
  - Tetralogy of Fallot
  - Pulmonary stenosis, and
  - Patent ductus arteriosus.
  - Attention deficits, short-term memory, sequential processing deficits and behavioural problems have been associated with FAS in school-age children.
- *Carcinogenicity* – Alcohol consumption has been associated with various cancers, including liver cancer, oesophageal cancer, breast & prostate cancer and colorectal cancer.

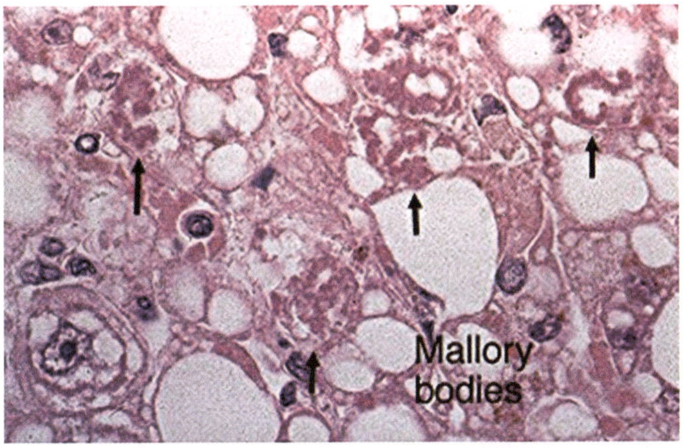

Fig. 9.63 Alcoholic hepatitis

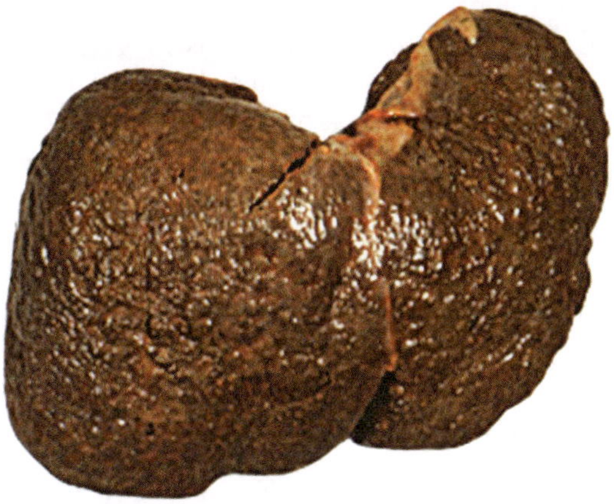

Fig. 9.64 Liver - Alcoholic cirrhosis

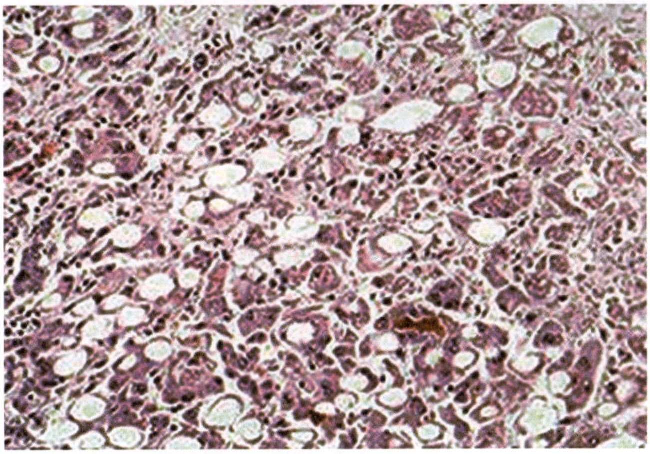

Fig. 9.65 Alcoholic cardiomyopathy

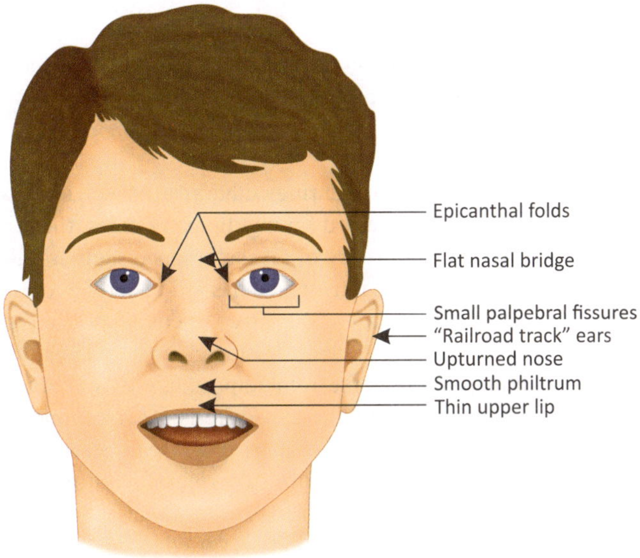

Fig. 9.66 Foetal alcohol syndrome (facial features)

e. **Withdrawal syndromes**: Sudden cessation of alcohol intake in a chronic alcoholic can provoke a withdrawal reaction which may manifest as one of seven conditions*:

i. ***Common abstinence syndrome***:
- *Onset*: 6–8 hrs after cessation of alcohol.
- *Features*: Tremor affecting hands, legs and trunk ("the shakes"), agitation, sweating, nausea, headache, insomnia.

ii. ***Alcoholic hallucinosis***:
- *Onset*: 24–36 hrs.
- *Features*: Objects appear distorted in shape, shadows seem to move, shouting or snatches of music may be heard.
- *Treatment*: Administration of phenothiazines (e.g., chlorpromazine 100 mg, 8th hourly).

iii. ***Seizures (Rum fits)***:
- *Onset*: 7–48 hrs.
- *Features*: Clonic-tonic movements, with or without loss of consciousness.

iv. ***Alcoholic ketoacidosis***:
- *Onset*: 24–72 hrs.
- *Features*: Occurs during withdrawal as well as after episodes of heavy drinking. In many cases, there is a preceding history of GI disturbance such as gastritis or pancreatitis which has led to sudden diminution of alcohol intake. To compensate for the loss of carbohydrates and depleted glycogen stores, the body mobilises fat from adipose tissue as an alternative source of energy. There is a corresponding decrease in insulin and an increased secretion of glucagon, catecholamines, growth hormone and cortisol. Fatty acids are oxidised and the final product, acetylcoenzyme A is converted to acetoacetate. This in turn is converted to beta-hydroxybutyrate because of ethanol-induced low redox state. The arterial pH may be normal due to a compensatory respiratory alkalosis and a primary metabolic alkalosis due to vomiting.
  - Clinical features include drowsiness, confusion, tachycardia, and tachypnoea, progressing to Kussmaul breathing pattern and coma.
- *Diagnosis*:
  - Blood alcohol concentration is typically not high.
  - Blood glucose may be slightly elevated.
  - There is an elevated anion-gap metabolic acidosis.
  - Serum ketones are markedly elevated.
  - Hypokalaemia and hypochloraemia are often present.
- *Treatment*:
  - IV normal saline with dextrose.
  - Potassium supplementation may be required.
  - Thiamine (50–100 mg) to prevent development of Wernicke-Korsakoff syndrome.

v. ***Delirium tremens (DTs)*** (*Latin for "shaking frenzy", also referred to as "DTs", "the horrors" or "the shakes"*)
- *Onset*: 3–5 days.
- *Mechanism*: Caused by the effect of alcohol on GABA receptors. Constant consumption of alcoholic beverages causes a counter-regulatory response in the brain in an attempt to regain homeostasis. This causes downregulation of these receptors, as well as an up-regulation in the production of excitatory neurotransmitters: glutamate, and also noradrenaline, dopamine, adrenaline and serotonin. When alcohol is no longer consumed, these down-regulated $GABA_A$ receptor complexes are so insensitive to GABA that the typical amount of GABA produced has little effect; compounded with the fact that there are not as many receptors for GABA to bind to. Thus, sympathetic activation is unopposed ('adrenergic storm').
- *Features*: There is a dramatic onset of disordered mental activity characterised by clouding of consciousness, disorientation and loss of recent memory. There are vivid hallucinations which are usually visual in nature. There is severe agitation with restlessness and shouting, tremor and truncal ataxia. Insomnia is prolonged. Autonomic disturbances include sweating, fever, tachycardia, hypertension and dilated pupils. Dehydration and electrolyte disturbances are characteristic.
- *Treatment*:
  - Well lit, reassuring environment.
  - For agitation – diazepam 10 mg IV initially, and then 5 mg every 5 minutes until full control, followed by 5 to 10 mg orally 3 times daily. In severe cases, low-levels of antipsychotics, such as haloperidol, or stronger benzodiazepines like temazepam or midazolam can be given until symptoms subside.
  - Thiamine in the usual dose.
  - Correction of fluid and electrolyte imbalance.
  - Acamprosate is often used to augment treatment, and is then carried on into long-term use to reduce the risk of relapse.

vi. ***Wernicke-Korsakoff syndrome***: This is very rare as a withdrawal phenomenon, and is actually the result of thiamine deficiency due to impoverished diet in an alcoholic. The syndrome is a combined manifestation of two disorders, **Wernicke's encephalopathy** and **Korsakoff's psychosis**, named after Carl Wernicke and

---

****Mnemonic**: CASA-DW, which stands for Common abstinence syndrome, Alcoholic hallucinosis, Seizures, Alcoholic ketoacidosis, Delirium tremens, Wernicke-Korsakoff syndrome.*

Sergei Korsakoff respectively. It involves an acute Wernicke-encephalopathy phase, followed by the development of a chronic Korsakoff's syndrome phase.

- *Pathophysiology*: Brain atrophy associated with WKS occurs in the following regions of the brain: mamillary bodies, thalamus, walls of the 3rd ventricle, floor of the 4th ventricle, cerebellum and frontal lobe.
- *Features*: Wernicke's encephalopathy* is the acute form and is characterised by drowsiness, disorientation, amnesia, ataxia, peripheral neuropathy, nystagmus and external ocular palsies. When recovery from Wernicke's encephalopathy is incomplete, a chronic amnesic syndrome develops called Korsakoff's psychosis which is characterised by impairment of memory and confabulation (falsification of memory).
- *Treatment*: For Wernicke's encephalopathy – 500 mg of thiamine hydrochloride infusion over 30 min, for 2–3 days. Following this, treatment should be continued with a 250-mg dose delivered IV or IM for 3–5 days.

vii. Studies indicate that repeated episodes of alcohol withdrawal lead to permanent dysregulation of GABA receptors. This may explain the "**kindling phenomena**" which is the clinical observation of increasing severity of alcohol withdrawal in individuals, and the development of benzodiazepine-resistant alcohol withdrawal.

Treatment

1. **Acute Poisoning** (***Intoxication, Inebriation***):
   a. Airway protection, ventilatory support.
   b. Activated charcoal is NOT useful.
   c. Stomach wash.
   d. Thiamine 100 mg IV
   e. Dextrose
   Indications – If rapidly determined bedside glucose level is less than 60 mg/100 mL, or if rapid determination is not available.
   Adult – 25 g (50 mL of 50% dextrose) IV.
   Paediatric – 1 g dextrose per kg as 25% dextrose.
   Precautions – Glucose administration should be preceded by 100 mg of thiamine IV or IM if chronic alcoholism or malnutrition is suspected, to prevent development of Wernicke's encephalopathy.
   f. Intravenous fluids.
   g. A variety of drugs have been tried to hasten the elimination of ethanol or reverse its intoxicating effects, including naloxone, physostigmine and caffeine. None of them have been proved to be truly effective.
   h. Haemodialysis can eliminate ethanol 3–4 times more rapidly than liver metabolism. May be useful in patients with excessive blood levels, impaired hepatic function and in those whose condition deteriorates in spite of maximal supportive measures.
2. **Chronic Poisoning**:
   - Treatment of withdrawal – Apart from the treatment measures outlined earlier (*vide supra*), the following drugs have also been tried with varying degrees of success:
     - Carbamazepine – It has been shown to be effective in treating alcohol withdrawal, including delirium tremens.
     - Chlormethiazole – It is one of the most popular drugs used for alcohol withdrawal abroad and is administered in a rapidly reducing dosage over 6–7 days. However, it is itself associated with a strong abuse potential.
     - Clonidine and gamma-hydroxybutyric acid have also shown promising results in the treatment of withdrawal symptoms.
     - One of the most recent entrants is **tiapride**, an atypical neuroleptic agent which is a selective dopamine D_2-receptor antagonist. But, it should be given only as an adjunct while seizures, hallucinosis, etc., are being taken care of by other drugs.
     - Chronic alcoholism has also been treated with the long acting opiate antagonist **naltrexone** which is said to reduce the craving for alcohol. **Acamprosate** is a recent entrant which is claimed to be even more effective in reducing such craving.
     - Antioxidant vitamins such as E and C have shown promising results.
   - **Aversion therapy**:
     - The main aim in the treatment of alcoholism is to gradually wean away the patient from the clutches of ethanol, once the acute manifestations of withdrawal have been taken care of. This process referred to quite loosely as **de-addiction** or **detoxification**, should be undertaken only after admission to a hospital over a period of several days, under close medical supervision.
     - The insatiable craving for alcohol that is often present must be tackled effectively, and usually requires strongly deterrent measures. Many methods have been tried in this connection, and one of the more successful ways is to administer a drug called **Disulfiram**:
       - It interferes with the oxidative metabolism of ethanol at the acetaldehyde stage, as a result of which acetaldehyde accumulates producing unpleasant symptoms** (**Table 9.16**). Aldehyde dehydrogenase and dopamine betahydroxylase are inhibited, which leads to interference of alcohol oxidation at the acetylation stage, resulting in high levels of acetaldehyde (**disulfiram–ethanol reaction**).

****Note***: *May also result from severe starvation, prolonged vomiting and diarrhoea.*

*****Note***: *There are several therapeutic drugs which react with disulfiram in diverse ways – amitryptiline, benzodiazepines, coumarin derivatives, isoniazid, metronidazole, paraldehyde, phenytoin, rifampicin & theophylline.*

- Ensure that the patient is off alcohol for a minimum period of 12 hrs before starting therapy.
- Administer disulfiram only by the oral route.
- Warn the patient explicitly that while he is on disulfiram, alcohol must not be consumed even in small quantity, since it can provoke a severe (and sometimes fatal) reaction. He must also avoid taking medicinal preparations containing alcohol.
- The usual dose of disulfiram is 250 mg/day which may have to be taken for an indefinite period of time. Such chronic use unfortunately often produces side effects like halitosis (rotten egg/garlicky odour due to sulphide metabolites), metallic taste, nausea, pruritis, headache, drowsiness, impotence, peripheral neuropathies, ataxia, depression, psychosis, optic neuritis and hepatotoxicity.
- Other than disulfiram, there are numerous other substances which evoke a similar reaction with ethanol (**Table 9.17**).

- **Supportive psychotherapy** – More than individualised psychotherapy, it is **group therapy** which is effective in the long-term management of abstinence. Groups provide an opportunity for re-socialisation and a sense of mutual commitment. Self-support organisations such as **Alcoholics Anonymous** (AA) play an important role. The AA which had its origins in the USA in 1935 now has more than 100,000 groups spread worldwide including India (**Fig. 9.67**). The only requirement for membership is a "desire to stop drinking". There is no membership fee and the organisation functions on a self-supporting basis through contributions from the members. Meetings are generally held once a week and are informal affairs conducted in a friendly atmosphere. Generally, two or three speakers share their experiences during each session relating to their addiction and recovery.

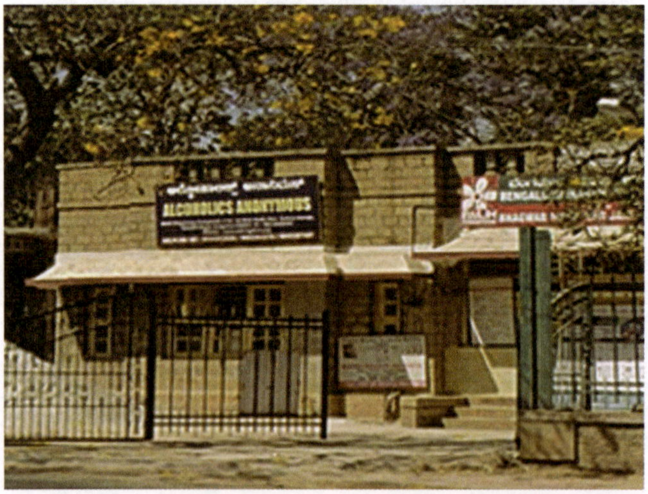

Fig. 9.67 Alcoholics Anonymous – a branch office in Karnataka

Table 9.17 Substances Producing Disulfiram-like Reaction with Ethanol

Antimicrobials ▪ Cephalosporines ▪ Metronidazole ▪ Trimethoprim-sulphamethoxazole ▪ Chloramphenicol ▪ Griseofulvin ▪ Nitrofurantoin
Other Drugs ▪ Phentolamine ▪ Oral hypoglycaemics (sulphonylureas): chlorpropamide, tolbutamide
Chemicals ▪ Carbon disulphide ▪ Carbon tetrachloride ▪ Chloral hydrate ▪ Thiram analogs (fungicides) ▪ Trichloroethylene
Mushrooms ▪ *Coprinus* mushrooms: *C. Atramentarius*

Autopsy Features

1. Congested conjunctivae.
2. Characteristic odour in the vicinity of the mouth and nose, and in the gastric contents.
3. Congestion of GI tract.
4. Pulmonary and cerebral oedema.
5. Stigmata of chronic alcoholism may be present (*fatty or cirrhotic liver, cardiomyopathy and characteristic lesions in other organs*) (**Figs. 9.68 & 9.69**).
6. **Chemical analysis of viscera and body fluids**:
   - Apart from the routine viscera and body fluids, one half of brain (one cerebral hemisphere), as well as samples of CSF and vitreous humor should be collected and preserved for chemical analysis.

Table 9.16 Disulfiram–Ethanol Reaction

GIT	CNS	CVS	Skin	RS
▪ Abdominal pain ▪ Nausea ▪ Vomiting ▪ Headache ▪ Weakness	▪ Blurred vision ▪ Confusion ▪ Vertigo ▪ Dysrhythmias ▪ Myocardial infarction	▪ Syncope ▪ Hypotension ▪ Tachycardia ▪ Pruritis	▪ Sweating ▪ Flushing ▪ Sensation of heat	▪ Tachypnoea

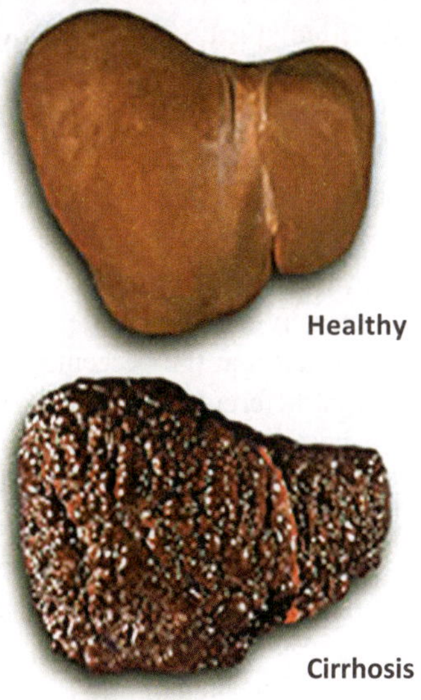

Fig. 9.68 Liver – normal (*top*) and alcoholic cirrhosis (*bottom*)

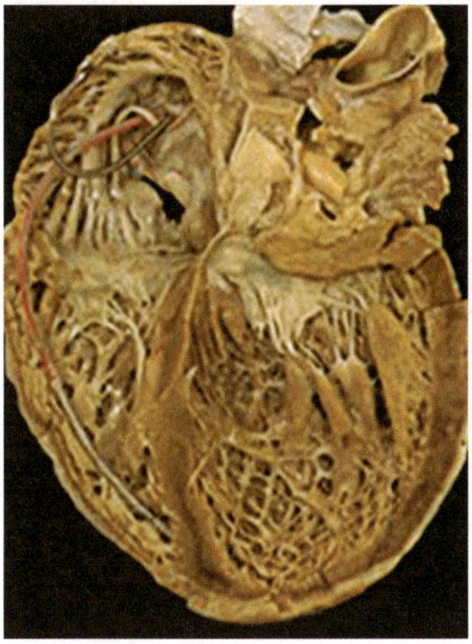

Fig. 9.69 Heart – Alcoholic cardiomyopathy

- Blood should always be collected from a peripheral vein such as femoral vein and never directly from the heart.
- Caution must be exercised in interpreting the results of chemical analysis conducted on putrefying dead bodies, since **postmortem production of ethanol** occurs in such cases due to the action of certain microorganisms. This can result in a **BAC of up to 20–30 mg/100 mL** even when no alcohol had been consumed at all prior to death. Similar erroneous results may be obtained (in the case of a non-putrefied body) in a blood sample that has not been properly preserved. In all such cases the urine should be mandatorily tested, and if no alcohol is detected it can be safely presumed that the BAC is false due to postmortem production.
- While blood is the sample of choice when relating the ethanol concentration to the degree of intoxication of the individual before death, it is necessary on occasions to resort to the use of other biological fluids and tissues, if it is not possible to obtain a satisfactory sample of blood.
  - Studies have been performed comparing the concentrations of ethanol in blood with other sources of biological material such as bone marrow, vitreous humor, bile and urine.
  - As far as urine is concerned, the concentration of alcohol would be about 25% higher than that of blood that was collected at the same time. In order to compare blood and urine alcohol, a ratio of 1:1.35 is generally considered acceptable.
    - If the postmortem urine alcohol concentration exceeds that of the blood by more than 25%, it indicates that higher blood alcohol must have existed during life, than was estimated at autopsy.
  - It is also important to remember that in a postmortem blood sample there may be volatile reducing substances if the deceased had been a diabetic, which could raise the BAC by interfering with the analysis. It has been suggested that an allowance of 20 mg/100 mL should be made in such cases.
  - Rarely, death can result from an allergic reaction to ethanol.

Forensic Issues

1. Alcohol abuse is prevalent worldwide. Efforts have been made to totally prohibit alcohol consumption in different countries without much success (with the possible exception of those countries where religious law is in force). Such attempts usually lead to illicit brewing and consumption with even more serious consequences. At present in India, **total prohibition** is in force only in the following states: **Bihar, Gujarat,* Mizoram & Nagaland**. Efforts to implement the same in some other states have met with dismal failure.
2. All over India (except where prohibition is in force), the mere consumption of alcohol and consequent drunken behaviour in themselves do not constitute any offence. Only when the drunken individual behaves in such a manner as to become a public nuisance,** or poses a threat, or actually commits an act endangering the life or property of another person, will the law take cognisance of the fact.

**Note*: *Gujarat is the only Indian state with a death penalty for the manufacture and sale of homemade liquor that results in fatalities. The legislation is titled the Bombay Prohibition (Gujarat Amendment) Act, 2009.*

Note*: ***S. 510, IPC: *Whoever in a state of intoxication appears in any public place, and there conducts himself in such a manner as to cause annoyance to any person, shall be punished with simple imprisonment for a term which may extend to 24 hrs, or with fine, or with both.*

3. **Drunkenness**:
   a. A doctor is sometimes called upon by the police to examine an individual who has been taken into custody for creating public annoyance in a state of intoxication, or for driving a vehicle under the influence of alcohol (*p. no. 470*), or for being involved in a criminal offence after drinking. In such a case, the doctor must exercise great caution before coming to a conclusion. He must first be familiar with the exact meaning of the term '**drunkenness**". An individual can be certified to be drunk only when there is evidence that "he was so much under the influence of alcohol as to have lost control of his faculties to such an extent as to render him unable to execute safely the occupation in which he was engaged at the material time."* The essence of this definition is that the doctor must search for evidence indicating that the individual concerned was ***under the influence of alcohol***. The smell of ethanol in the breath, the pulse rate, dilatation of pupils, colour of the face, etc., give no indication of the degree of intoxication. Conclusion regarding this must be arrived at after a detailed examination with special reference to the state of mind, coordination of movements, visual acuity, etc.
   b. As in every medicolegal case, before embarking on the physical examination of the individual, the doctor must first obtain his written consent. This must be tempered by the fact that if an individual really is drunk, then he is probably in no fit medical condition to give or refuse consent! In such cases, the doctor can proceed with the examination but should not divulge the results or his conclusions until the individual has sobered up and provides valid consent. However, if there is an explicit direction from a judicial court to divulge the results without delay, the doctor must comply with such direction. If an individual refuses consent and is uncooperative, the doctor can proceed with the examination without bothering about this formality, if the former has been arrested for a criminal offence and is under the custody of the police (**S. 53 (1), CrPC**). But, the requisition in such a case should have been issued by a police officer not below the rank of a Sub-Inspector. The doctor can conduct not only the physical examination, but can even collect samples of urine or blood for analysis.
   c. **Procedure of Examination: Box 9.3**.
   d. Sometimes the question is asked (when it is proved that a person had consumed alcohol), as to how much he could have drunk, i.e., the **quantity of liquor consumed**. To answer this question, two facts must be known:
      i. The BAC
      ii. The nature of alcoholic beverage taken.

      If these are known an estimate can be made as to the minimum quantity of liquor consumed by consulting **Table 9.18**. A rule of thumb is that every ounce (30 mL) of an 80° proof liquor will raise the BAC by 25 mg% (i.e., one peg of distilled spirit, or one glass of wine, or a quarter to half bottle of beer). Average elimination rate is 15–20 mg%/hr. Before employing such data however, it must be borne in mind that calculations relating ethanol consumption to BAC are the outcome of statistical generalisations and may not apply to every individual case. Moreover, they are often based on laboratory experiments which may be at variance with clinical settings. It is also a fact that the percentage of alcohol is highly variable in different brands of wine. This could mean that one person's glass of wine can contain as much as twice or even four times the alcohol of another person's glass! Similar problems are experienced with distilled spirits where "a peg" may refer to a volume of liquor which varies from 25 to 60 mL. Measures of whisky poured at home are usually double the quantity that are given as single whiskies in a public bar!
   e. As an alternative or supplement to BAC, the level of alcohol can also be estimated in the urine (UAC).
      i. Two samples of urine are required to be collected: First sample should be collected as soon as possible following the incident, the bladder being completely emptied, and the second, 25–30 min later. The difference in the alcohol concentrations in the two samples will indicate whether the subject was in the absorptive phase, or peak phase, or elimination phase.
      ii. Multiplication of blood alcohol concentration in the second sample by 0.75 (based on blood–urine alcohol ratio of 1:1.35) will give an approximate value of the blood alcohol level.
      iii. The first sample of urine voided after the individual was taken into custody by the police must not be used for analysis, since there is a likelihood of erroneous interpretation. The urine sample will contain very low concentration of alcohol even after heavy drinking if the person had started consuming alcohol when his bladder was already containing urine. On the other hand, a very high concentration will be obtained, if he had emptied his bladder and then commenced drinking heavily.
4. **Ethanol and Crime**:
   a. Brawls, assaults (sexual and non-sexual), homicides, and suicides are commonly associated with intoxication.
   b. Even if the assailant was so drunk that he had lost total control over his mental faculties and therefore was not in a position to judge whether his actions were right or wrong, he is still punishable for any criminal act committed by him (**S. 86, IPC**), unless the alcohol was administered to him without his knowledge or against his will (**S. 85, IPC**).
5. **Ethanol and Traffic Accidents**:
   a. It is well known that consumption of ethanol and consequent intoxication has adverse effects on the driver

****Source***: *Based on the report of the* ***Special Committee*** *of the* ***British Medical Association****, 1927, on drunkenness.*

Box 9.3—Scheme of Examination for Certification of Drunkenness

Objective:

To decide, whether

- The subject is under the influence of alcohol.
- His condition is due to illness or injury.
- It is safe for him to be detained in a police station, or he should be admitted to a hospital.

Consent:

Obtain informed, written consent.

Preliminary Particulars:

- Name, age, sex, occupation and residential address.
- Identification marks: Record at least two permanent marks of identification as for any medicolegal case.
- Time of commencement of examination.
- Escorts: Record the name and number of escorting police constable, and the police station to which he is attached.
- History:
  - Has he consumed alcohol? If so, at what time, and what was the nature and quantity consumed?
  - Is he in the habit of consuming alcohol regularly? If so, since how long and how frequently?
  - Does he suffer from any disease or disability?
  - Is he taking any medication or drugs? If so, what is the nature and dose?

Physical Examination:

- General appearance: State of clothing, behaviour, disposition, etc.
- Speech: Normal or slurred or overprecise.
- Breath: Odour of alcohol present or absent.
- Stance: Does he sway when standing erect with his feet together and eyes closed?
- Gait: Ask him to walk across the room and observe whether the gait is normal or staggering, straight or irregular. Ask him to stop or turn around and observe whether there is a delay in response, as well as the manner of turning (tendency to fall).
- Writing: Ask him to write or copy a few sentences in the language he is familiar with. Note the time taken, repitition/omission of words, etc.
- Eyes and visual acuity: Note whether the eyes are reddened, presence or absence of nystagmus, status of pupils and test for pupillary reaction to light.
- Vital data: Record the pulse, temperature and blood pressure.
- Reflexes: Normal or depressed.
- Muscular coordination: Test this by asking the individual to perform a few simple tests:
  - Finger-nose test
  - Buttoning/unbuttoning shirt
  - Picking up pencil/pen from the floor.
- Examine also the cardiovascular, pulmonary and alimentary systems in the usual way.
- Look for the presence of injuries. Pay particular attention to evidence of head injury.

Mental Examination:

- Memory: Test for ability to recall recent events.
- Orientation:
  - To time – Ask him to state the approximate time of day, or the day of the week.
  - To space – Ask him as to whether he is aware of his present location, the direction in which the entrance to the building lies, etc.

Laboratory Investigations:

- Collect blood and urine samples.
- With reference to the blood sample, about 5 mL drawn from a peripheral vein is usually sufficient.
- The site to be punctured should not be swabbed with surgical spirit, since it can result in a false positive test for alcohol.
- Instead, the area can be washed with soap and water prior to puncture and swabbed with spirit after the blood sample has been withdrawn.
- The collected sample of blood must be preserved in a chemically clean container with sodium fluoride as preservative (50 mg for 5 mL).
- Some doctors believe that it is desirable to add potassium oxalate (15 mg).
- Refrigeration of the sample or placing it in an icebox is a good alternative.
- For urine sample, the recommended preservative is phenyl mercuric nitrate. Alternatively, sodium fluoride (50 mg/10 mL) can be used.

contd.

Opinion:

This should be phrased in one of the following ways:

a. The individual examined has not consumed alcohol.
b. The individual examined has consumed alcohol, but is not under its influence.
c. The individual examined has consumed alcohol and is under its influence.

Opinion (a) is given, if there is no smell of alcohol in the breath and/or laboratory analysis is negative for alcohol; and all the clinical findings are normal.

Opinion (b) is given, if there is smell of alcohol in the breath and/or laboratory analysis reveals the presence of alcohol; but clinical examination reveals only normal findings.

Opinion (c) is given, if there is smell of alcohol in the breath and/or laboratory analysis reveals the presence of alcohol; and clinical examination reveals abnormal findings.

Authentication:

Signature of the medical officer, his name & designation and the time of concluding the examination.

Table 9.18 Relationship Between Liquor Consumed & Blood Alcohol

Blood Alcohol Concentration (mg%)	**Minimum Quantity of Liquor Consumed**		
	Beer (L)	***Wine*** (L)	***Distilled Spirits*** (mL)
50	0.8	0.2	70
100	1.6	0.3	130
200	3.2	0.7	275
300	4.8	0.9	410
400	6.4	1.3	550
500	8	1.6	690
600	9.6	1.9	825

of a vehicle in the form of visual blurring, motor incoordination, impairment of judgement and increased reaction time.

i. *BAC up to 50 mg%* – Driving ability of most individuals is unaffected, though there may be slight impairment in some individuals.
ii. *BAC 50–100 mg%* – Most people are affected to varying degree.
iii. *BAC 100–200 mg%* – There is severe impairment of driving ability with increased liability to accident.
iv. *BAC over 200 mg%* – There is a high likelihood of an accident.

b. Driving a vehicle on a public thoroughfare under the influence of alcohol (or any other intoxicating drug) is an offence in almost every country of the world. In India, it is an offence punishable under **Section 185** of the **Motor Vehicles Act (1988, Amended 1994)** in the form of a fine which can extend up to Rs. 2000, or imprisonment which can extend up to 6 months, or imposition of both. For a second offence committed within 3 years of the previous one, the punishment is enhanced to Rs. 3000, or 2 years, or both.

i. As per the **2019 amendment**, for the first offence, one might have to face imprisonment for 6 months and/or a traffic violation fine up to Rs. 10,000. (Before 2019, the fine for first offence was Rs. 2000.)
ii. For the second offence, one can face imprisonment up to 2 years and/or a fine of Rs. 15,000 (increased in 2019 from Rs. 3000), and all repeat offenders may also face penalties regarding their driving license.

c. Many countries permit mild degrees of intoxication, but beyond a certain statutory BAC, it becomes a culpable offence. For example, the statutory limit is 20 mg% in Poland and Sweden, 50 mg% in Finland, Norway, Netherlands, Yugoslavia, Portugal and Greece, 80 mg% in Denmark, Germany, Belgium, UK, France, Switzerland, Austria, Italy and Spain, 100 mg% in Ireland and 80–150 mg% in the different states of the USA. Some countries do not allow even traces of alcohol in the blood of a driver, e.g., Russia, Czechoslovakia, Hungary, Bulgaria, Romania and Turkey. **In India, the statutory limit has been fixed at 30 mg%**. But, the general practice is to convict only on the basis of a medical examination, i.e., when it is proved that the driver of the vehicle was under the influence.

d. **Back extrapolation of blood levels** – Calculation of a previous blood alcohol level (i.e., at the time of a driving offense) from a single subsequent level can be done, but is fraught with pitfalls and assumptions that may be inaccurate.
   i. Erroneous assumptions include necessity for the peak level to occur within 60 min of ceasing drinking.
   ii. Many conditions can affect absorption of ethanol and alter this assumption, such as amount, nature and timing of food intake, rate of ethanol consumption and race, age, sex and weight of the patient.

e. One aspect of traffic accidents that is sometimes neglected is the fact that the victim (e.g., a pedestrian who was hit) may have himself been intoxicated and could have been guilty of contributory negligence. If this fact is demonstrated on subsequent analysis, then insurance money may not be payable to him (if still alive), or his next of kin (if he has died), even though his life had been insured. Contributory negligence may also be the result of visual impairment, e.g., cataract or neurological afflictions which affect coordination or gait.

f. **Breathalyser***:
   i. In many countries including India, traffic police carry special equipment in the form of breathalysers to detect alcohol in the breath of a suspect driver (**Fig. 9.70**). It serves as an "on the spot test." Estimates of BAC based on breath analysis are legally admissible as per **Sec 185** of the **Motor Vehicles Act, 1988** (amended **1994**).
   ii. In the earliest type of breathalyser, the individual concerned was asked to blow into a plastic balloon containing a crystalline dichromate–sulphuric acid mixture. If the BAC was above a certain prescribed limit, the crystals would turn green to a predetermined distance. However today, this has been superseded by more sophisticated versions based on fuel-cell sensing, electrochemical oxidation, infrared photometry and microprocessors which accurately predict the BAC. The basic principle underlying a conventional breathalyser involves calculating the weight of alcohol which accompanies 190 mg of CO_2 in the subject's breath. This is converted to BAC using the observations that: 1) alveolar air normally contains close to 5.5% (by vol) of CO_2, i.e., 190 mg of CO_2 in 2100 mL of alveolar air at 34°C and 2) the weight of alcohol present in 1 mL of blood is equal to that present in 2100 mL of alveolar air.
   iii. Hand-held field testing devices are generally based on electrochemical platinum fuel cell analysis and, depending upon jurisdiction, may be used by officers in the field as a form of "**field sobriety test**" commonly called **PBT (preliminary breath test)** or **PAS (preliminary alcohol screening)** or as evidential devices in **POA (point of arrest)** testing.
   iv. From numerous experiments conducted it is now well established that there is an excellent correlation between the breath and blood level, and the ratio is generally 2100:1. This is based on **William Henry's law** which states that when a volatile chemical (ethanol) is dissolved in a liquid (blood) and is brought to equilibrium with air (alveolar breath), there is a fixed ratio between the concentration of the volatile compound (ethanol) in air (alveolar breath) and its concentration in the liquid (blood), and the ratio is constant at a given temperature, i.e., in this case 34°C which is the temperature at which the breath usually leaves the mouth. But, there can be some variation in the ratio between different individuals which is one of the sources of error in the use of breathalysers.
   v. Other potential sources of error include recent use of ethanol containing products, belching or regurgitation of gastric alcohol contents, inadequate expiration (in uncooperative subjects), obstructive pulmonary disease, use of metered dose inhalers and poor technique. Any number of other products found in the workplace can cause erroneous BAC results. These include compounds found in lacquer, paint remover, gasoline and cleaning fluids.

6. **Ethanol and Medical Practice**:
   a. The medical profession is considered to be one of the noble professions and it therefore behoves a doctor

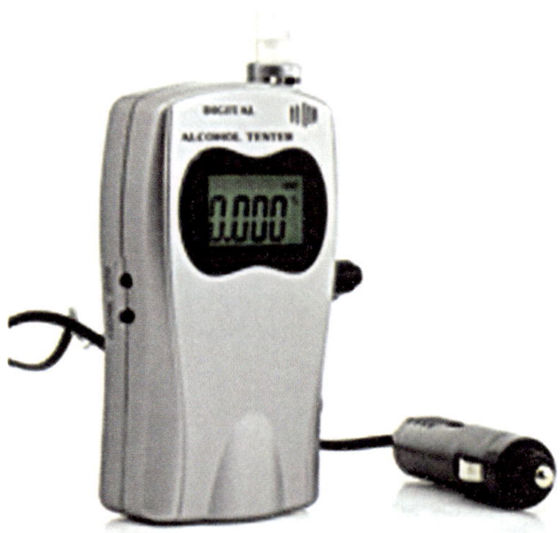

Fig. 9.70 Breath analyzer device

*__Note__: *More correctly called "breath analyzer". Breathalyzer is actually the brand name of a series of models made by one manufacturer of breath alcohol testing instruments (National Draeger), and is a registered trademark for such instruments. Other brand names include "Alcometer", "Intoximeter" and "Drunkometer".*

to conduct himself at all times with decency and decorum. Although he can use his discretion with regard to moderate consumption of alcohol when not on hospital duty, or when not dealing with patients, he can be held liable in the following situations:

i. A surgeon performing an operation under the influence of alcohol can be prosecuted under **Sec 304-A** of the **IPC**, if the patient dies during the course of surgery. The fact that he was drunk at the time of the operation is likely to be considered as strong evidence of rashness.
ii. A doctor may be sued for damages in the event of the patient suffering damage or death due to his negligent conduct. If he was intoxicated at the time he administered treatment, it would only strengthen the evidence against him.
iii. Patient management under the influence of alcohol will be considered as infamous conduct (professional misconduct), and the doctor is liable to be proceeded against by the State Medical Council. The drunken doctor runs the risk of his name being erased from the medical register.

METHANOL

Synonyms

Methyl alcohol; Methyl hydroxide; Colonial spirit; Columbian spirit; Purple lady (*slang*); Wood alcohol; Wood spirit

Molecular Formula

CH_4O or CH_3OH

Physical Appearance

- Methanol is the simplest of the primary alcohols and is a colourless, highly polar, flammable liquid.
- Pure methanol has a faintly sweet odour; crude methanol may have a repulsive, pungent odour.
- It has a bitter taste.

Uses & Sources

1. Antifreeze (10–50%)
2. Carburettor cleaner (20%)
3. **Denatured spirit (5–10%)**
   - While denatured spirit most often is a mixture of ethanol (90–95%) with methanol (5–10%), occasionally other substances may be used instead of the latter, e.g., acetone, aniline dyes, benzene, camphor, castor oil, ether, isopropanol or terpineol.
4. Embalming fluid (20%)
5. Paint remover
6. Solid canned fuels (4%)
7. Varnish & shellac (5%)
8. Windshield washing fluid (35–95%)

Usual Fatal Dose

- **70–100 mL (range 15–250 mL).**
- Serious toxicity may occur from ingestion of 0.25 mL/kg of 100% methanol. Fatalities might occur from ingestion of 0.5 mL/kg of 100% methanol.
- Most experts agree that a blood methanol concentration of 25 mg/dL is the threshold for treatment.

Mode of Action

- Methanol is rapidly absorbed through the skin, respiratory tract and gastrointestinal tract.
- Peak plasma levels are usually reached within 30–60 min following ingestion, although a long latent period (roughly 18–24 hrs) usually is seen before toxic symptoms develop.
- In the liver, methanol is metabolised to **formaldehyde** (by alcohol dehydrogenase) and then to **formic acid** (by aldehyde dehydrogenase) which is responsible for retinal toxicity as well as metabolic acidosis (**Fig. 9.71**).
- There are two pathways for metabolism of formic acid, oxidation via the catalase-peroxidase system, or metabolism by formyl-tetrahydrofolate synthetase.
- Since metabolism is slow, significant levels of methanol can be found in the body for up to 7 days after ingestion.

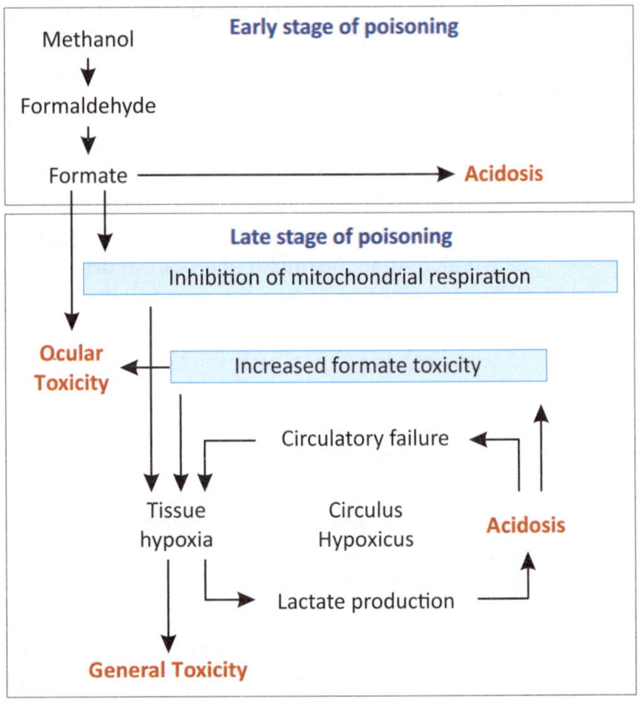

Fig. 9.71 Methanol poisoning – Mode of action

Clinical Features

- Symptoms may be delayed for 12–24 hrs (range: 1–72 hrs).
- Earliest manifestations include vertigo, headache with stiff neck (*meningismus*), nausea, vomiting and abdominal pain.
- Neurologic symptoms of methanol intoxication can mimic those of an ethanol "hangover" and may include general malaise, headache, dizziness, vertigo, neuritis and weakness.
- **Ocular toxicity** is characterised by
  - Blurred or dimmed vision ("flashes" or "snowstorm")
  - Photophobia.
  - Constricted visual fields, spots before the eyes, sharply reduced visual acuity, optic atrophy, blindness and nystagmus have all been described.

- Ophthalmologic examination usually reveals dilated pupils with sluggish light reaction. Fixed dilated pupils suggest severe poisoning.
- Fundoscopy reveals hyperaemia of optic disc followed by retinal oedema (**Fig. 9.72**). Irreversible sequelae include optic atrophy and visual field impairment. Retrobulbar degeneration in the form of necrosis of myelinated portion of optic nerve is the basis for visual loss in methanol poisoning.

- **Metabolic acidosis (high anion gap)** is usually severe. Acidosis may be delayed for 18–24 hrs, or longer with concurrent ethanol ingestion. A pH < 7.0 and bicarbonate < 10 mEq/L are not uncommon following significant intoxication. Urinary pH concomitantly may drop to 5.
- Other features include tachycardia, hypotension and hypothermia.
- Convulsions are a late feature and may be followed by coma.
- Hypomagnesaemia, hypokalaemia and hypophosphataemia have been reported.
- Occasionally, a patient develops transient ***Fanconi syndrome*** (hypouricaemia, hypophosphataemia, glycosuria and hyperchloraemic metabolic acidosis). Acute renal failure and haematuria have been reported.
- Acute necrotizing pancreatitis may result from severe methanol poisoning.
- Cause of death is usually respiratory failure, which may precede the cessation of heart beat by several minutes. In fatal methanol poisoning cases, marked sinus bradycardia may develop with widening of the pulse pressure. Further, severe hypotension, requiring fluid and vasopressor therapy, occurs terminally in severe methanol intoxications.
- The most common permanent sequelae following recovery from severe poisoning are:
  - Optic neuropathy
  - Blindness
  - Parkinsonism (due to basal ganglia necrosis)
  - Toxic encephalopathy
  - Polyneuropathy.

Diagnosis

1. **High anion gap (AG) acidosis.**
2. **Elevated osmolal gap (OG)**: The osmolal gap is the difference between the measured and calculated osmolality and is normally <10 mOsm/kg. An elevated osmolal gap (>10) suggests the presence of toxic alcohols.
3. **Hypophosphataemia.**
4. **Elevated creatine phosphokinase.**
5. **Elevated amylase.**
6. **Blood methanol level**: More than 50 mg/100 mL indicates serious poisoning.
7. A detectable **serum formic acid level** may be consistent with methanol poisoning, as methanol is metabolized to formic acid.
8. **CT Scan/MRI**: Symmetrical areas of necrosis in the putamen of the brain are a classic finding in cases of acute lethal methanol toxicity.
9. **Fundoscopy**: Fundoscopic changes are notable within only a few hours after methanol ingestion and range from retinal oedema in the perimacular region to the entire fundus. Optic disc oedema and hyperaemia are observed within 48 hrs.
10. **Electroretinography/Visual evoked response**: Characteristic findings include loss of retinal sensitivity, scotomata and decreased amplitudes on visual evoked-response testing.
11. **Optical coherence tomography (OCT)** has been found to be very useful for evaluating the severity of retinal oedema and detecting swelling of nerve fibres in patients with methanol poisoning.

Treatment

Most experts agree that a blood methanol concentration of 25 mg/dL is the threshold for treatment. An ingestion of 0.25 mL/kg of 100% methanol would theoretically result in a toxic methanol concentration.

1. Stomach wash with sodium bicarbonate.
2. Activated charcoal does not adsorb significant amounts of methanol.
3. **Antidotal therapy (Fig. 9.73)**:
   a. **Ethanol** is the specific antidote since it preferentially competes for the same enzyme (alcohol dehydrogenase) and prevents the metabolism of methanol which is then excreted unchanged in the urine. Ethanol has about 20 times the affinity for alcohol dehydrogenase compared

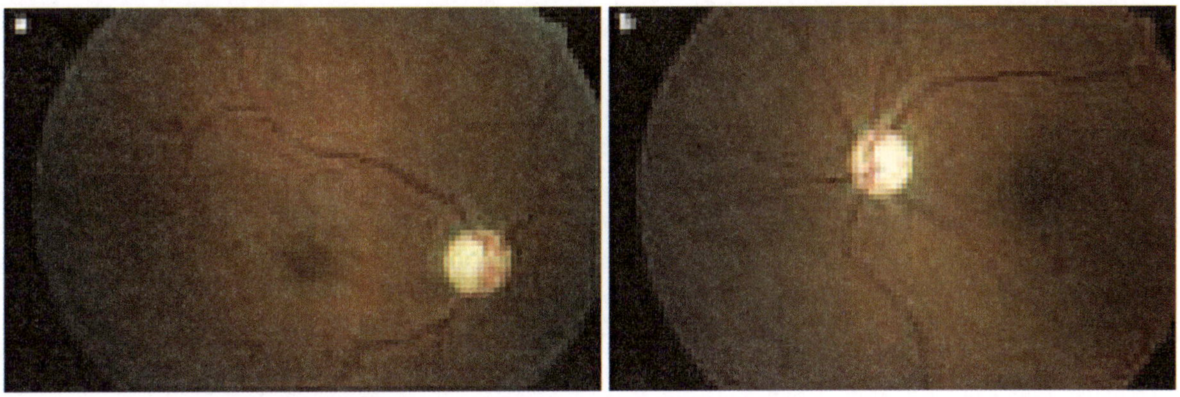

Fig. 9.72 Fundus in methanol poisoning (*Courtesy: Dr S Senthil Kumaran*)

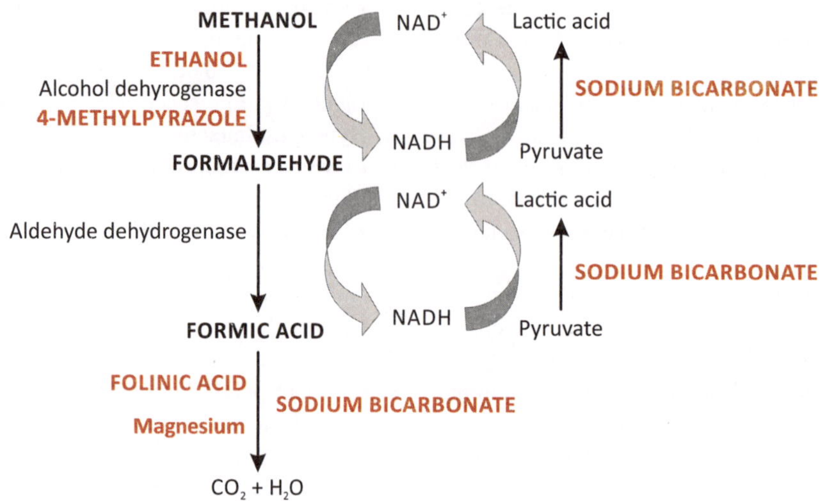

Fig. 9.73 Antidotes in methanol poisoning

to methanol. Formic acid is metabolized to carbon dioxide and water via a folate dependent system.

i *Mode of administration*:

- 10% ethanol at a dose of 10 mL/kg administered IV over 30 min, followed by 1.5 mL/kg/hr, so as to produce and maintain a blood ethanol level of 100 mg/100 mL.
- Alternatively, 1 mL/kg of 95% ethanol in fruit juice (180 mL) can be given orally over 30 min.
- If neither of these is practicable, give 125 mL of a distilled alcoholic beverage (gin, vodka, whisky or rum) orally, diluted in glucose solution or juice, and repeat as required cautiously.
- Ethanol therapy should be continued until methanol blood concentration is <10 mg/100 mL, or formate blood concentration is <1.2 mg/100 mL. Methanol-induced acidosis (pH, blood gases), clinical findings (CNS), electrolyte abnormalities (bicarbonate), serum amylase and osmolal gap should have resolved.

b. In recent times, a new antidote has been introduced viz., **4 methyl pyrazole (4MP)**, or **fomepizole** which does not cause CNS depression (unlike ethanol). The usual loading dose is 15 mg/kg, followed by doses of 10 mg/kg every 12 hrs for 4 doses, then 15 mg/kg every 12 hrs, thereafter until methanol concentrations are undetectable or have been reduced below 20 mg/dL and the patient is asymptomatic with normal pH. Administer all doses as a slow intravenous infusion over 30 min.

4. **Sodium bicarbonate IV**: 1–2 mEq/kg, titrated to correct arterial pH.
5. **Folinic acid IV**: 1–2 mg/kg, 6th hourly. It hastens the elimination of formic acid. Folinic acid or leucovorin or citrovorum factor is a biologically active form of folic acid, which is an essential water soluble vitamin.
6. For convulsions: Attempt initial control with a benzodiazepine (diazepam or lorazepam). If seizures persist or recur administer phenobarbitone.
7. **Haemodialysis** is very effective in removing methanol, formaldehyde, and formic acid. While ethanol treatment is also quite effective, it is extremely difficult to maintain therapeutic ethanol levels for long periods of time. Haemodialysis is strongly recommended in patients with acidosis or serum methanol levels of >25–50 mg/100 mL. Dialysis, once begun, should continue until the patient's clinical picture improves and the methanol level decreases below 20 mg/dL.
8. Haemoperfusion is not effective.
9. Peritoneal dialysis and continuous venovenous haemofiltration are less effective than haemodialysis but may be of some use.

Autopsy Features

1. Cyanosis is very prominent, especially in the upper parts of the body.
2. Liver and kidneys show toxic damage.
3. Lungs may reveal oedema, emphysematous changes and desquammation of alveolar epithelium.
4. Eyes show evidence of retinal oedema.
5. Viscera must be preserved in saturated solution of sodium chloride and not rectified spirit, as in the case of all alcohols. In addition to routine viscera, it is advisable to preserve one cerebral hemisphere.

Forensic Issues

- Most cases of methanol poisoning are accidental arising out of either an alcoholic (deprived of ethanol) consuming methanol containing products, or intentional adulteration of arrack resulting in mass deaths.
- The latter are referred to quaintly as "**liquor tragedies**" and are reported in Indian newspapers at depressingly regular intervals from all parts of the country. **Fig. 9.74** depicts the Indian states with highest incidence of such tragic incidents.

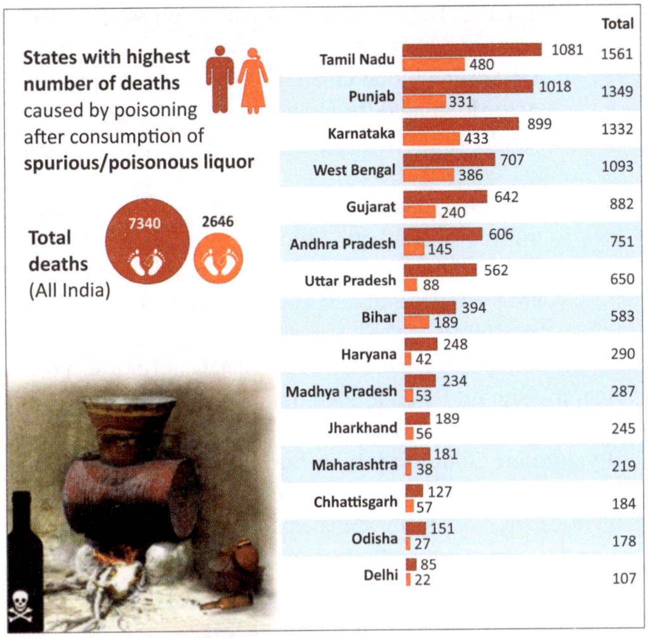

Fig. 9.74 Deaths by adulterated liquor consumption, state-wise: 2004–2014

ETHYLENE GLYCOL

Synonyms

1,2-Ethanediol; Glycol alcohol

Molecular Formula

CH_2OHCH_2OH or $C_2H_6O_2$

Physical Appearance

- Colourless, syrupy, odourless, non-volatile liquid, with a bitter-sweet or sweetish taste. In fact, ethylene glycol (like all other glycols) is referred to as a "glycol" because of its sweet taste.

Uses

1. ***Antifreeze***: Ethylene glycol lowers the freezing point of water. More than 25% of the ethylene glycol produced is used in antifreeze and coolant mixtures for motor vehicles.
2. Solvent.
3. Hydraulic brake fluid.
4. As a glycerine substitute in commercial products such as paints, lacquers, detergents and cosmetics.

Usual Fatal Dose

- **70–100 mL (1.4 mL/kg or 1.56 g/kg of 95% ethylene glycol).**
- Blood level: More than 30–50 mg/100 mL of ethylene glycol can cause serious toxicity.

Mode of Action

- Ethylene glycol is not absorbed through skin, and because of its low vapour pressure does not produce toxicity upon inhalation. It is however absorbed rapidly through the GI tract and is metabolised by alcohol dehydrogenase (more than 80%) to glycoaldehyde, glycolic acid and oxalic acid.
- The pathophysiology of the CNS, metabolic, cardiopulmonary and renal toxicity are primarily due to the formation and accumulation of **glycolic acid** (acidaemia, oxalosis and renal interstitial oedema), and to a lesser but histologically important extent, **oxalate** production and excretion.
- Unchanged ethylene glycol is thought to be responsible for the initial signs and symptoms resembling ethanol inebriation.

Clinical Features

- **First Phase** (*CNS stage*): Up to 12 hrs post-ingestion.
  - This stage is mainly due to the parent compound itself and is characterised by vomiting, inebriation, lethargy, nystagmus, ataxia, convulsions and coma.
  - Cranial nerve deficits have been observed, and may result in dysarthria, dysphagia, facial weakness, ataxia, hearing loss or absent gag reflex. The defects mainly involve cranial nerves II, V, VII, VIII, IX, X and XII.
- **Second Phase** (*CVS stage*): 12–24 hrs post-ingestion.
  - This stage is characterised by tachycardia, hypertension (sometimes hypotension), tachypnoea, congestive heart failure and circulatory collapse.
  - Severe metabolic acidosis with compensatory hyperventilation can develop with multiple organ failure in significant poisonings. Tachypnoea and Kussmaul's respiration may be the first clinical signs of developing metabolic acidosis which, if untreated, can progress and become life-threatening.
  - Cardiogenic pulmonary oedema may occur with severe poisoning.
- **Third Phase** (*Renal stage*): 24–72 hrs post-ingestion.
  - There is oliguria, flank pain, acute tubular necrosis and renal failure. Urine contains calcium oxalate or hippurate crystals. **Calcium oxalate crystals** are found as monohydrates (prism or needle-like) or dihydrates (tent or envelope-shaped) (**Fig. 9.75**). It is important to note that absence of calcium oxalate crystals does not rule out the diagnosis.

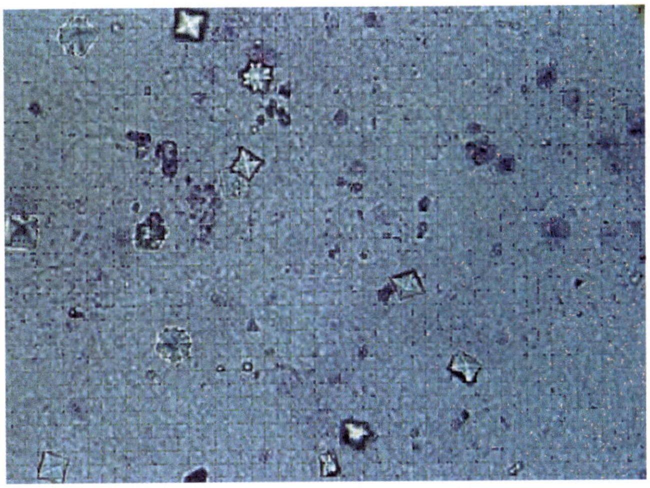

Fig. 9.75 Calcium oxalate crystals in urine (*Courtesy*: *Dr S Senthil Kumaran*)

- Haematuria and proteinuria are common.
- In surviving cases, renal function usually returns to normal, but in some cases permanent renal damage has occurred.
- **Hypocalcaemia** results in manifestations of tetany.
- Exposures to glycols have resulted in teratogenicity, specifically craniofacial and neural tube closure defects and skeletal dysplasia in animal studies.

Diagnosis

1. **High-anion gap acidosis**: Increased anion gap metabolic acidosis results from the metabolism of ethylene glycol to acidic metabolites, predominantly glycolic acid. However, it is important to remember that a normal anion gap does not preclude a diagnosis of ethylene glycol toxicity.
2. **Osmolal gap**: High.
3. **Calcium oxalate crystals** in urine.
4. **Xanthochromic CSF** with pleocytosis.
5. Determine **blood ethylene glycol concentration** on all patients. Shortly after ingestion, ethylene glycol concentrations >30–50 mg/100 mL (8.06 mmol/L) are frequently associated with severe intoxication.
6. **Glycolic acid**, the major metabolite of ethylene glycol, can be detected and measured by HPLC or GC. In forensic autopsy cases, confirmation of death due to ethylene glycol ingestion can be done by measurement of blood and urine glycolic acid levels using these methods.
7. If antifreeze has been ingested, the **urine will fluoresce** from the fluorescent dye in the product, when examined under Wood's lamp. A fluorescent dye, sodium fluorescein, is present in many commercial antifreeze products. However, fluorescent urine is not a reliable indicator of ethylene glycol ingestion, due to variations in interpretation of urine fluorescence among observers and the fact that most normal urine specimens exhibit some degree of fluorescence.

Treatment

1. **Stomach wash** and **activated charcoal** are of **doubtful benefit**. The utility of activated charcoal is limited due to ethylene glycol's rapid absorption from the GI tract and its poor binding affinity for activated charcoal.
2. **Ethanol** is the **antidote** and must be given IV (same as for methanol poisoning). It inhibits the metabolism of ethylene glycol. **4-Methyl pyrazole** (**Fomepizole**) is a better alternative.
   a. *Loading Dose* (*ethanol*):
      i. Intravenous Loading Dose
         - Administer 7.6 mL/kg IV of 10% ethanol (v/v) in dextrose 5% in water over 30 min to achieve a blood ethanol conc of above 100 mg/100 mL.
      ii. Oral Loading Dose
         - 95% ethanol: Administer 1 mL/kg orally in 6 ounces of orange juice over 30 min.
   b. *Maintenance Dose* (*ethanol*):
      i. Dosing to maintain a blood ethanol level of 100 mg/100 mL. Begin maintenance infusion as soon as the loading dose is infused.
      ii. Determine blood ethanol concentrations at the end of the loading dose and hourly thereafter until stable levels of 100–120 mg/100 mL have been achieved.
   c. *Dose* (*fomepizole*):
      i. An initial loading dose of 15 mg/kg is intravenously infused over 30 min followed by doses of 10 mg/kg every 12 hrs for 4 doses, then 15 mg/kg every 12 hrs until ethylene glycol concentrations are below 20 mg/100 mL.
3. **Haemodialysis***: Highly effective, but ethanol or fomepizole therapy should be continued during dialysis.
4. **Sodium bicarbonate** IV.
5. **Pyridoxine 50 mg** and **thiamine 100 mg** IM, 6th hourly for 2 days. Thiamine is recommended to stimulate the conversion of glyoxylate to alpha-hydroxy-beta-ketoadipate, a non-toxic metabolite. Pyridoxine is recommended to allow adequate stores of cofactor necessary for the conversion of glyoxylate to nontoxic glycine.
6. Monitor serum calcium level and replace as indicated, with **10% calcium gluconate** IV.
7. Maintenance of **good urine volume** enhances urinary elimination of ethylene glycol.

Autopsy Features

- Cerebral oedema, chemical meningoencephalitis.
- Toxic damage of liver and kidneys.
- Oxalate crystals in brain, spinal cord and kidneys.

FM 9.5: Core – Written/Viva Voce/ Objective Structured Clinical Examination (OSCE)

- Describe general principles and basic methodologies in treatment of poisoning: decontamination, supportive therapy, antidote therapy, procedures of enhanced elimination with regard to:
  - Organophosphates
  - Carbamates
  - Organochlorines
  - Pyrethroids
  - Paraquat
  - Aluminium phosphide
  - Zinc phosphide

Pesticides are compounds that are used to **kill or repel pests** which may be **insects**, **rodents**, **fungi**, **nematodes**, **mites**, **ticks**, **molluscs** and **unwanted weeds** or **herbs**.

CLASSIFICATION

1. **Insecticides**: Compounds which kill or repel ***insects*** and related species, e.g., organophosphates, carbamates, organochlorines (organochlorides), diethyltoluamide (DEET) and pyrethrum and its derivatives (pyrethroids). Two groups of new entrants comprise neo-nicotinoids and ryanoids.

****Note***: *Addition of 95% ethanol to dialysate is necessary to replace the ethanol lost during the procedure.*

2. **Rodenticides**: Compounds which kill ***rats, mice, moles*** and ***other rodents***, e.g., anticoagulants (bromadiolone), thallium, vacor, phosphorus, alpha-naphthyl-thiourea, cholecalciferol, barium carbonate, bromethalin and zinc phosphide. Aluminium phosphide is a rodent repellent used in the form of fumigant.
3. **Herbicides (Weedicides)**: Compounds which kill ***unwanted herbs*** or ***weeds***, e.g., acrolein, dalaphon, glyphosate, paraquat, diquat, atrazine and chlorophenoxy compounds.
4. **Fungicides**: Compounds which kill ***fungi*** and ***moulds***, e.g., thiocarbamates, captan, captafol, hexachlorobenzene and sodium azide.
5. **Nematicides**: Compounds which kill ***nematodes*** (i.e., ***worms***), e.g., ethylene dibromide.
6. **Acaricides**: Compounds which kill ***mites, ticks*** and ***spiders***, e.g., azobenzene, chlorobenzilate, tedion and kelthane.
7. **Molluscicides**: Compounds which kill ***molluscs*** such as ***snails*** and ***slugs***, e.g., metaldehyde.
8. **Fumigants**, e.g., Methyl bromide, phosphine, aluminium phosphide, naphthalene and hydrogen cyanide.

The pesticides listed in the new curriculum will now be discussed. There will be no discussion with regard to other pesticides, though some of these are actually as important, if not more important than the ones mentioned in the curriculum.

ORGANOPHOSPHATES (ORGANOPHOSPHORUS COMPOUNDS, OPCs)

They are among the most popular and most widely used insecticides in India.

Physical Appearance

- These compounds are available as dusts, granules or liquids.

Usual Fatal Dose

- **Based on toxicity rating***:
  - The following compounds are **extremely toxic** (*LD50: 1–50 mg/kg*), or **highly toxic** (*LD50: 51–500 mg/kg*) – Chlorfenvinphos, Chlorpyriphos, Diazinon, Dimethoate, Ediphenphos, Ethion, Fenitrothion, Fenthion, Methyl Parathion, Monocrotophos, Phorate, Phosphamidon.
  (**Mnemonic**: CC DD EE FF MM PP)
  - The following compounds are **moderately toxic** (*LD50: 501–5000 mg/kg*), or **slightly toxic** (*LD50: more than 5000 mg/kg*) – Acephate, Malathion, Temephos, Triazophos, Trichlorphon.
  (**Mnemonic**: AM TTT)

Toxicokinetics

- Organophosphorus compounds are very well absorbed from the lungs, GI tract, skin, mucous membranes and conjunctiva following inhalation, ingestion or topical contact. The difficulty in removing these compounds from the skin and clothing may explain some chronic poisonings.
- Most OP insecticides are lipophilic. Adipose tissue gradually accumulates the highest levels. Cholinergic crisis may recur in patients when unmetabolized OP agents are mobilized from fat stores.
- Peak levels of most OP insecticides are measured around 6 hours after oral ingestion in man. Although serum half-lives of these compounds range from minutes to hours, prolonged absorption or redistribution from fat stores may allow for measurement of circulating insecticide concentrations for up to 48 days.
- OP insecticides are metabolized by various mixed function oxidases in the liver and intestinal mucosa, though the exact pathways are not yet clearly understood.
- Recent studies have suggested possible relationship between human serum paraoxonase (PON) activity and susceptibility to acute and chronic effects of OP poisoning. Paraoxonase is an A-esterase that can hydrolyze the active (oxon) metabolites of some OP compounds.

Mode of Action (Figs. 9.76 & 9.77)

- Organophosphates are powerful **inhibitors of acetylcholinesterase** which is responsible for hydrolysing acetylcholine to choline and acetic acid after its release and completion of function (i.e., propagation of action potential).
- As a result, there is **accumulation of acetylcholine** with continued stimulation of local receptors and eventual paralysis of nerve or muscle.**
- Although organophosphates differ structurally from acetylcholine, they can bind to the acetylcholinesterase molecule at the active site and phosphorylate the serine moiety. When this occurs, the resultant conjugate is infinitely more stable than the acetylcholine–acetylcholinesterase conjugate, although endogenous hydrolysis does occur. Phosphorylated enzymes degrade very slowly over days to weeks, making the acetylcholinesterase essentially inactive.
- **Fig. 9.78** represents the basic formula for organophosphorus compounds. The "**X**" or "**leaving group**" determines the main characteristics of the compound and is useful in classifying organophosphates into four main groups:
  - **Group 1 compounds** contain a quaternary nitrogen at the X position, and are called ***phosphorylcholines***. These chemicals originally developed as chemical warfare agents are powerful cholinesterase inhibitors and can also directly stimulate cholinergic receptors, because of their structural resemblance to Ach. Example – echothiophate iodide.
  - **Group 2 compounds** are called ***fluorophosphates*** because they possess a fluorine molecule as the leaving group. Like group 1 compounds, these compounds are volatile and highly toxic, making them also well-suited for chemical warfare. Examples – dimefox, sarin, mipafox.

Note*: *Partly as per the **Insecticide Rules, 1971.*

***Note**: *Acetylcholine is the neurotransmitter at pre- and postganglionic parasympathetic synapses, sympathetic preganglionic synapses and at the neuromuscular junction.*

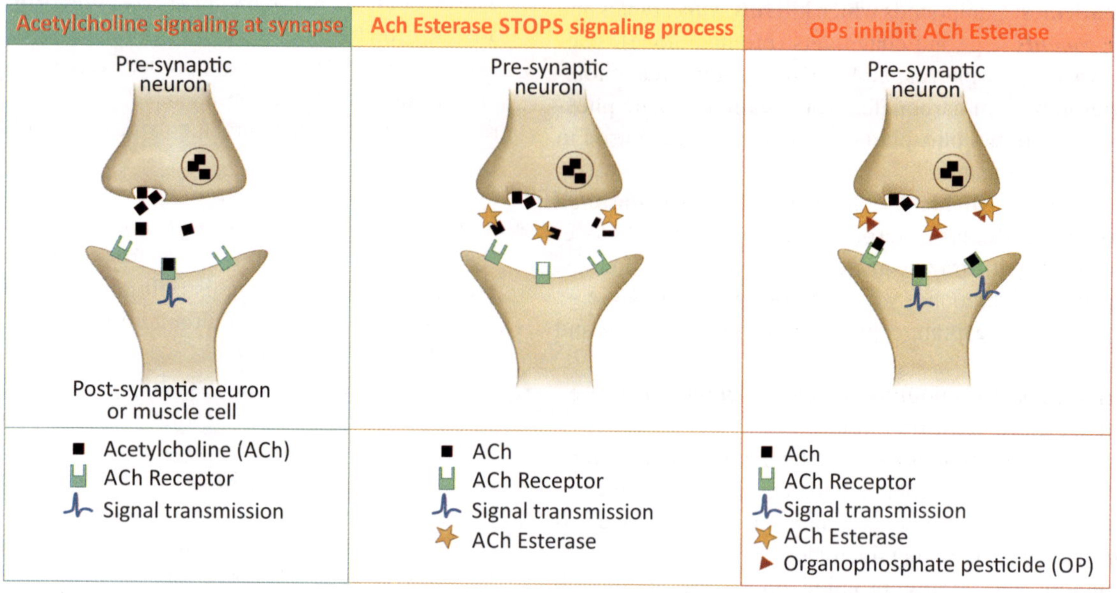

Fig. 9.76 Mode of action – Organophosphate pesticides

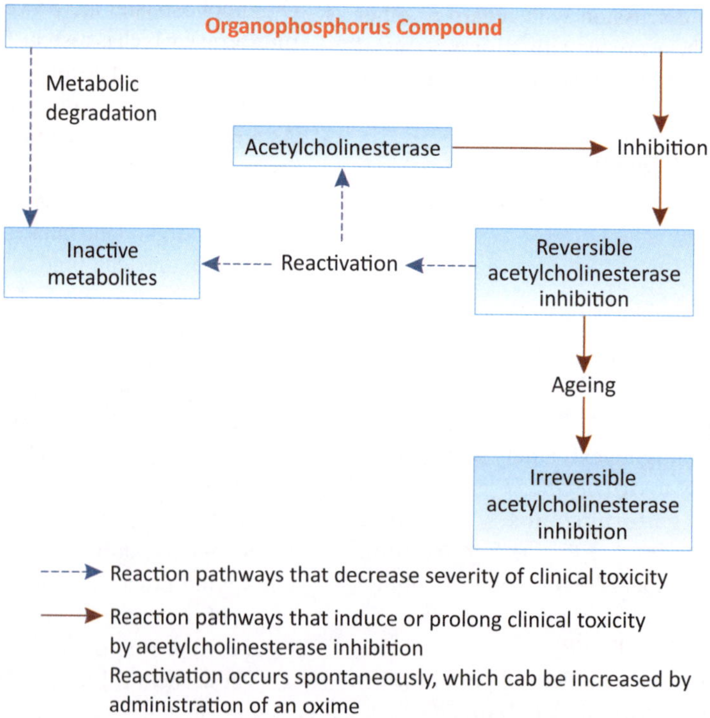

Fig. 9.77 Organophosphates: Reaction pathways

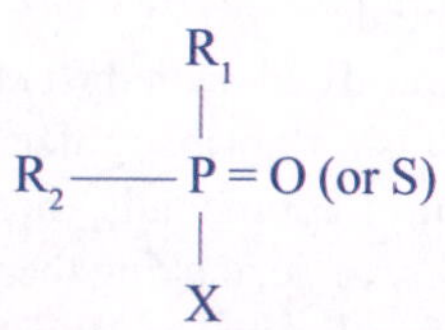

Fig. 9.78 Leaving group

- The leaving group of **Group 3 compounds** is a cyanide molecule or a halogen other than fluorine. Examples – cyanophosphates such as tabun.
- **Group 4** is the broadest and comprises various subgroups based on the configuration of the R_1 and R_2 groups, with the majority falling into the category of either a **dimethoxy** or **diethoxy compound**. Most of the insecticides in use today fall into this last class.

- Organophosphorus insecticides may be biologically active (**oxons**) or pro-poisons (**thions**) requiring activation after absorption.
- In OP poisoning, the complex becomes irreversibly bound during the next 24–72 hrs when one of the R groups leaves the phosphate molecule. This step is termed "**ageing**". As this occurs, the enzyme can no longer spontaneously hydrolyse and becomes permanently inactivated. De novo synthesis of AChE is required to replenish its supply once aging has occurred.
- Apart from acetylcholinesterase, organophosphates exert powerful inhibitory action over other carboxylic ester hydrolases such as chymotrypsin, plasma cholinesterase (pseudocholinesterase), hepatic carboxylesterase, paraoxonases and other non-specific proteases.
  - It has been proposed that **delayed peripheral neuropathy** caused by organophosphates is due to phosphorylation of some esterase(s) other than acetylcholinesterase, such as **neurotoxic esterase**, also known as **neuropathy target esterase (NTE)**. Neuropathy caused by inhibition of NTE may develop 2–4 weeks after an acute poisoning.

Clinical Features

I. **Acute Poisoning**:

a. Patients with massive ingestions can become symptomatic very quickly, sometimes within 5 min following ingestion, and deaths have occurred within 15 min of ingestion. Most victims however become symptomatic in about 8 hrs of exposure, and virtually all within 24 hrs.

b. Symptoms may last for variable periods of time, again based on the exact compound and the nature of the exposure. For example, lipophilic compounds such as dichlofenthion can cause cholinergic excess for several days following ingestion.

c. **Cholinergic Excess***:

i. ***Muscarinic Effects*** (hollow organ parasympathetic manifestations) – Common manifestations include bronchoconstriction with wheezing and dyspnoea, cough, pulmonary oedema, vomiting, diarrhoea, abdominal cramps, increased salivation, lacrimation & sweating, bradycardia, hypotension, miosis and urinary incontinence.

ii. ***Nicotinic Effects*** (autonomic ganglionic and somatic motor effects due to stimulation of nicotinic adrenal receptors and postganglionic sympathetic fibres) – Fasciculations, weakness, hypertension, tachycardia and paralysis. Mydriasis has been reported in as many as 13% of cases, presumably from nicotinic stimulation of sympathetic receptors. Muscle weakness, fatiguability and fasciculations are very common.

Cardiac arrhythmias and conduction defects have been reported in severely poisoned patients. ECG abnormalities may include sinus bradycardia or tachycardia, atrioventricular and/or intraventricular conduction delays, idioventricular rhythm, premature ventricular extrasystoles, ventricular tachycardia or fibrillations, torsades de pointes, prolongation of the PR, QRS and/or QT intervals, ST-T wave changes and atrial fibrillation.

d. **CNS Effects** – Restlessness, headache, tremor, drowsiness, delirium, slurred speech, ataxia and convulsions. Coma supervenes in the later stages. Death usually results from respiratory failure due to weakness of respiratory muscles, as well as depression of central respiratory drive. Acute lung injury (noncardiogenic pulmonary oedema) is a common manifestation of severe poisoning. Metabolic acidosis has occurred in severe poisonings.

e. A characteristic **kerosene-like odour** is often perceptible in the vicinity of the patient since the solvent used in many organophosphate insecticides is some petroleum derivative such as **aromax**. **The intensity of the odour is not an indication of the toxicity of the pesticide**.

f. The **Peradeniya Organophosphorous Poisoning (POP) Scale** is predictive of death, necessity for mechanical ventilation, and the required total atropine dose over the first 24 hrs. This scale rates 5 clinical variables, each on a 0–2 scale: miosis, muscle fasciculations, respirations, bradycardia and level of consciousness.

g. It is important to note that:

i. In a given case, there may be either tachy- or bradycardia; hypo- or hypertension.

ii. Miosis while being a characteristic feature, may not be apparent in the early stages. In fact mydriasis is very often present, and hence treatment should not be delayed if there is absence of pupillary constriction. Blurred vision may persist for several months.

iii. Ocular exposure can result in systemic toxicity. It can cause persistent miosis in spite of appropriate systemic therapy, and may necessitate topical atropine (or scopolamine) instillation.

iv. Exposure to organophosphate vapours rapidly produces symptoms of mucous membrane and upper airway irritation and bronchospasm, followed by systemic symptoms, if patients are exposed to significant concentrations.

v. While respiratory failure is the commonest cause of death, other causes may contribute including hypoxia due to seizures, hyperthermia, renal failure and hepatic failure.

vi. Because liquid preparations are usually dissolved

**Note*: *Two mnemonics which help in remembering the main manifestations are*:

1. ***DUMBELS*** – *Diarrhoea, Urination, Miosis, Bronchospasm, Emesis, Lacrimation, Salivation.*
2. ***SLUDGE** and the **Killer Bees** - Salivation, Lacrimation, Urination, Diarrhoea, Gastric distress, Emesis and Bronchospasm, Bronchorrhoea & Bradycardia.*

in a hydrocarbon, aspiration frequently results following ingestion in severe poisoning and can lead to hydrocarbon pneumonitis.

vii. Excessive adrenergic influences on metabolism cause glycogenolysis with hyperglycaemia and ketosis that may be mistaken for diabetic ketoacidosis. Hypoglycaemia can also occur, although the mechanism is unclear.

viii. Elevations of hepatic enzymes can occur following OP pesticide exposures.

h. **Sequelae**:

i. An ***Intermediate Syndrome*** sometimes occurs one to four days after poisoning due to long-lasting cholinesterase inhibition and muscle necrosis. It is termed the "intermediate syndrome" because it occurs in between the periods of acute and delayed toxicity. Redistribution of lipophilic pesticides and their metabolites from adipose tissue may be responsible, and the syndrome may resolve when the body burden of these metabolites diminish and cholinesterase levels normalize.

- Main features include muscle weakness and paralysis. The most commonly affected muscles are the facial, extraocular, palatal, respiratory and proximal limb muscles. Paralytic signs include inability to lift the neck or sit up, ophthalmoparesis, slow eye movements, facial weakness, difficulty swallowing, limb weakness (primarily proximal), areflexia, respiratory paralysis and death.
- There is speculation that intermediate syndrome may result from inadequate oxime therapy, although more recent case reports question this theory.
- Once it sets in, the intermediate syndrome will have to be managed by supportive measures, since it does not respond to oximes or atropine. However, because some reports correlating pralidoxime dose and intermediate syndrome suggest that insufficient dosing may play a part, it is recommended that pralidoxime infusion be reinstituted at 500 mg/hr when intermediate syndrome is suspected. The weakness and paralysis commonly resolve in 5–18 days.

ii. A ***Delayed Syndrome*** (now called ***Delayed Encephalopathy and Neuropathy Syndrome***) sometimes occurs 1–4 weeks after poisoning due to nerve demyelination, and is characterised by flaccid weakness and atrophy of distal limb muscles, or spasticity and ataxia.

- A mixed sensory-motor neuropathy usually begins in the legs, causing burning or tingling, then weakness. Severe cases progress to complete paralysis, impaired respiration and death.
- The nerve damage of organophosphate-induced delayed neuropathy is frequently permanent. Recovery of these patients is variable and occurs over months to years, with residual deficits common.
- This disorder appears to result from inhibition of an enzyme within nervous tissue named **neurotoxic esterase** or **neuropathy target esterase**.
- Pathologic findings demonstrate effects primarily on large distal neurons, with axonal degeneration preceding demyelination.
- Electromyograms and nerve conduction studies may be helpful in diagnosing the delayed syndrome by identifying the type of neuropathy (such as axonopathy, myelinopathy or transmission neuropathy) and differentiating it from similar presentations such as Guillain-Barre syndrome.

iii. ***Hyperamylasaemia*** is occasionally reported in cases of severe OP pesticide poisoning, and although pancreatitis may result from spasm of the sphincter of Oddi, hyperamylasaemia is most often the result of salivary gland stimulation and not the result of pancreatic dysfunction. Haemoperfusion is said to be beneficial, if this occurs.

iv. Patients poisoned with highly lipid soluble OPs such as fenthion have rarely developed ***extrapyramidal effects*** including dystonia, resting tremor, cog-wheel rigidity and choreoathetosis.

v. It is important to note that ***children may have different predominant signs of organophosphate poisoning than adults***. The major signs and symptoms include CNS depression, stupor, flaccidity, dyspnoea and coma. Other classical signs of organophosphate poisoning such as miosis, fasciculations, bradycardia, excessive salivation and lacrimation, and gastrointestinal symptoms are infrequent.

II. **Chronic Poisoning**: It usually occurs as an occupational hazard in agriculturists, especially those who are engaged in pesticide spraying of crops. Route of exposure is usually inhalation or contamination of skin. The following are the main features:

a. ***Polyneuropathy***: Paresthaesias, muscle cramps, weakness, gait disorders.

b. ***CNS Effects***: Drowsiness, confusion, irritability, anxiety.

c. ***Sheep Farmer's Disease***: Psychiatric manifestations encountered in sheep farmers involved in long-term sheep-dip operations.

d. Organophosphate poisoning has been associated with a variety of subacute or delayed onset chronic neurological, neurobehavioural or psychiatric syndromes. One author has termed these "***chronic organophosphate induced neuropsychiatric disorder***" (**COPND**). Signs and symptoms include confusion, psychosis, anxiety, drowsiness, depression, fatigue and irritability. Although no specific treatment is effective, most psychological abnormalities resolve within a year.

Diagnosis

1. **Depression of cholinesterase activity**:
   a. **Plasma cholinesterase (butyrylcholinesterase)** metabolizes various xenobiotics, including succinylcholine and cocaine. Erythrocytes contain a form of AchE (**red blood cell cholinesterase** or **RBC cholinesterase**) that is structurally similar to the enzyme found in neuronal tissue.
      i. Inhibition of either RBC cholinesterase or plasma cholinesterase serves as markers for cholinesterase inhibitor poisoning, but the extent of inhibition of these enzymes do not correlate well with the severity of poisoning.
      ii. After significant exposure, plasma cholinesterase activity usually falls first, followed rapidly by RBC cholinesterase. By the time patients present with acute symptoms, levels of both cholinesterase activities have usually fallen well below baseline values, and often have fallen below detectable limits.
      iii. Plasma cholinesterase activity usually recovers before RBC cholinesterase activity, often returning to normal within a few days.
      iv. However, plasma cholinesterase activity is less specific for exposure than is RBC cholinesterase activity. The former can be lowered significantly in patients with a number of disorders, including hereditary deficiency of the enzyme, malnutrition, hepatic parenchymal disease, chronic debilitating illnesses and iron deficiency anaemia. In fact, day-to-day variation in the activity of this enzyme in healthy individuals may be as high as 20%.
      v. RBC cholinesterase activity is more reliable because the AChE in red blood cells is true AChE. Some authors suggest that clinical OP pesticide poisoning can be said to have occurred when RBC cholinesterase activity falls to below 50% of baseline values.

   b. However, there are several pitfalls in interpreting cholinesterase laboratory values. Firstly, it is AChE inhibition in nervous tissue that causes toxicity, and RBC and plasma cholinesterase activity may not always reflect neuronal enzyme activity. Because these tests are only markers of neuronal enzyme inhibition, this variation may lead to some patients presenting highly symptomatic after minimal reductions in RBC or plasma cholinesterase, although others can be asymptomatic after losing 50% activity. It is also well known that there is a wide normal range of RBC and plasma cholinesterase activity, which allows for patients with high normal values to suffer significant falls in cholinesterase activity, yet still register near normal levels of cholinesterase activity on laboratory assay.
   c. RBC cholinesterase regenerates more slowly than AChE found in neurons. To completely replenish the RBC AChE supply, the red blood cells in circulation at the time of the OP insecticide exposure must be replaced, or pralidoxime administered. An average of 66 days may be necessary for RBC cholinesterase activity to recover following severe inhibition, and activity may take up to 120 days to return to normal.
   d. It is important to note that depressed RBC cholinesterase activity may be the result of exposures or conditions other than insecticide poisoning, such as in therapy with antimalarial agents such as chloroquine and pernicious anaemia. Genetic and circadian variations are also common, with daily fluctuations within the same individual as high as 10%. Oral contraceptives raise RBC cholinesterase activity.
   e. Blood samples for cholinesterase activity must be obtained in the appropriate blood tubes. Tubes containing fluoride will permanently inactivate the enzyme, yielding falsely low activity levels, and should not be used.
      i. Specimens for RBC cholinesterase must drawn into tubes containing a chelating anticoagulant such as ethylenediaminetetraacetic acid (EDTA) to prevent clot formation.
      ii. Plasma cholinesterase does not require an anticoagulant and can be drawn into a tube without chelators or anticoagulants. But, it is advisable to collect blood samples in an EDTA tube for measurement of both erythrocyte and plasma cholinesterase activities.
      iii. The assay should be performed as soon as possible and blood samples should preferably be taken onto ice to ensure a reliable result.

   Table 9.19 gives an overview of the benefits and disadvantages of estimating RBC and plasma cholinesterase levels in suspected OP or carbamate pesticide poisoning.
2. **P-Nitrophenol test**: P-nitrophenol is a metabolite of some organophosphates (e.g., parathion, ethion), and is excreted in the urine.
   a. **Procedure**: Steam distill 10 mL of urine and collect the distillate. Add sodium hydroxide and heat on a water bath for 10 min. Production of yellow colour indicates the presence of p-nitrophenol. The test can also be done on vomitus or stomach contents.
3. **Atropine challenge test**: An atropine sulphate challenge may be helpful in diagnosing cholinergic poisoning in a patient who presents with findings suggestive of this disorder, but in whom no history is available to suggest excessive exposure to an OP or carbamate insecticide. In an individual not exposed to significant amounts of insecticide a test dose of 1–5 mg of atropine (adult), or 0.05 mg/kg (children) should produce classic antimuscarinic findings such as mydriasis, tachycardia and dry mucous membranes. Conversely, the persistence of cholinergic signs and symptoms after an atropine challenge strongly suggests the presence of OP compound or carbamate poisoning.
4. **Electromyogram**: Repetitive nerve stimulation testing is an accurate method of quantifying AChE inhibition at the neuromuscular junction. Spontaneous repetitive potentials

Table 9.19 Comaparison of RBC and Plasma Cholinesterase Assays in OP/Carbamte Poisoning

	RBC Cholinesterase	Plasma Cholinesterase
Advantage	More reliable	Easier to measure, declines faster
Site	RBC (reflects CNS grey matter, motor end plate)	CNS white matter, plasma, liver, pancreas, heart
Regeneration (*untreated*)	1%/day	25–30% in first 7–10 days
Normalization (*untreated*)	35–49 days	28–42 days
Use	Unsuspected prior exposure with normal plasma cholinesterase	Acute exposure
False depression	Pernicious anaemia, haemoglobinopathies, antimalarial treatment, oxalate blood tubes	Liver dysfunction, malnutrition, hypersensitivity reactions, drugs (succinylcholine, codeine, morphine), pregnancy, genetic deficiency

or fasciculations following single-nerve stimulation resulting from persistent ACh at nerve terminals can be a sensitive indicator of AChE inhibition at the motor endplate, and may be useful in the early diagnosis of OP or carbamate poisoning.

5. **Thin layer chromatography (TLC)**: The presence of an organophosphate in a lavage, or vomit, or gastric aspirate sample can also be determined by TLC. The sample is extracted twice with 5 mL of petroleum ether, and the extract is washed with distilled water. It is then dried in steam compressed air, reconstituted in methanol and spotted on silica gel-coated TLC plate along with the standard and run in a mixture of petroleum ether and methanol (25:1). After the solvent has travelled a considerable distance, the plate is dried and exposed to iodine vapour. The RF is compared with that of the standard.
6. **Ancillary investigations**: There may be evidence of:
   a. Leukocytosis (with relatively normal differential count).
   b. High haematocrit.
   c. Anion gap acidosis.
   d. Hyper- or hypoglycaemia. Hypoglycaemia can be recalcitrant to treatment.
   e. Elevation of serum creatine kinase.

Treatment

Determine plasma or red blood cell cholinesterase activities. Depression in excess of 50% of baseline is generally associated with severe symptoms (*vide supra*).

1. **Decontamination***:
   a. If **skin spillage** has occurred, it is imperative that the patient be stripped and washed thoroughly with soap and water.
      - *Procedure*:
        - Shower is preferable. Make the patient stand (if he is able to) under the shower, or seated in a chair.
        - Wash with cold water for 5 min from head to toe using non-germicidal soap. Rinse hair well.
        - Repeat the wash and rinse procedure with warm water.
        - Repeat the wash and rinse procedure with hot water.
      - Treating personnel should protect themselves with water-impermeable gowns, masks with eye shields, and shoe covers. Neoprene or nitrile gloves must be used, if available. Double-gloving with standard vinyl gloves may be protective for short intervals.
      - Exposed leather clothing or products should be discarded because decontamination is very difficult once impregnation has occurred.

   b. If **ocular exposure** has occurred, copious eye irrigation should be done with normal saline or Ringer's solution. If these are not immediately available, tap water can be used.
   c. In the case of **ingestion**, stomach wash can be done, though this is often unnecessary because the patient would have usually vomited several times by the time he is brought to hospital. Activated charcoal can be administered in the usual way even though evidence is lacking as to its efficacy in OP poisoning. One dose (1 g/kg) may be sufficient.
2. **Antidotes**:
   a. **Atropine**: Atropine, a competitive antagonist of acetylcholine at the muscarinic postsynaptic membrane and in the CNS, will block the muscarinic manifestations of organophosphate poisoning.
   b. **Pralidoxime**: This is a nucleophilic oxime which helps to regenerate acetylcholinesterase at muscarinic, nico-

__Note__: Patients with clinically significant hypoxia, bradycardia and/or hypotension require oxygen and atropine before decontamination.

tinic and CNS sites. Actually, human studies have not substantiated the benefit of oxime therapy in acute organophosphate poisoning, but they are widely used. Many authors advocate the continued use of pralidoxime in the clinical setting of severe organophosphate poisoning, while some investigators have started questioning the rationale for administering oximes in OP poisoning.

The antidotes for organophosphates have been discussed together in detail in **Box 9.4**.

3. **Supportive measures**:
   a. Administer IV fluids to replace losses.
   b. Correct hypotension by adequate fluid resuscitation with a crystalloid. Treat brady and tachyarrhythmias appropriately. Vasopressors and inotropes can be initiated in an emergency through peripheral venous access.
   c. Perform a 12-lead ECG in all patients who require assessment. Repeat 12-lead ECGs are recommended, especially in symptomatic patients. Check cardiac rhythm, QRS duration and QT interval.
   d. Oxygenation/intubation/positive pressure ventilation. To minimize barotrauma and other complications, use the lowest amount of PEEP possible while maintaining adequate oxygenation.
   e. Review flexor neck strength regularly in conscious patients by asking them to lift their head off the bed and keep it there when pressure is applied to their forehead. Any sign of weakness is a sign that the patient is at risk of developing neuromuscular junction failure (**intermediate syndrome**) and acute respiratory failure. The tidal volume should be checked in such patients every 4 hrs. Values <5 mL/kg are an indication for intubation and ventilation.
   f. The following drugs are **contraindicated**: parasympathomimetics, phenothiazines, antihistamines and opiates. Do not administer succinylcholine (suxamethonium) or other cholinergic medications.
   g. For agitation/delirium: Adults can be sedated with an initial dose of oral or IV diazepam (0.1–0.3 mg/kg). Further boluses, given IV, may be administered if the patient remains severely agitated 10–15 min after the initial bolus, provided there is no impairment of respiratory function. If agitation persists despite the above measure, consider oral (5–10 mg) or parenteral (2–10 mg) haloperidol, 0.5–2 mg (oral or IV) initially in the elderly. In children, it is better to manage agitation without sedation and exclude other causes (e.g., hypoxia, infection, hypoglycaemia and raised ICP). If required, midazolam is the most appropriate drug for managing agitation in children and young people. Intravenous lorazepam is an alternative.
   h. Control convulsions that are frequent or prolonged with IV diazepam (10–20 mg in adults; 0.1–0.3 mg/kg in children), lorazepam (4 mg in adults and 0.1 mg/kg in children) or midazolam (5–10 mg in adults; 0.05–0.15 mg/kg in children). If convulsions are unresponsive to initial treatment, second-line therapy is phenobarbitone sodium (10 mg/kg at maximum rate of 100 mg/min; maximum dose 1 g). An alternative is phenytoin (loading dose 18 mg/kg IV infusion in adults and children, given via slow IV [maximum rate 50 mg/min] over 20–30 min with BP and ECG monitoring). Thiopentone sodium is the preferred antiepileptic for status epilepticus not responding to the above measures. The role of newer agents such as propofol and levetiracetam in toxicological seizures is currently unclear because of a lack of clinical or animal studies.
   i. If metabolic acidosis persists despite correction of hypoxia and adequate fluid resuscitation consider correction with IV sodium bicarbonate. In adults, an initial dose of 50 mmol may be given and repeated as necessary, guided by arterial blood gas monitoring (aim for a pH of 7.44 [Hydrogen ion concentration 36]). In children, use 8.4% sodium bicarbonate diluted in an equal volume of 5% glucose and give a "calculated" dose: dose (in mmol) = desired change in base deficit (current-target) × 0.3 × weight of child up to a maximum of 50 mmol. Administer at a rate of 1 mmol/min. Monitor electrolytes, since there is a risk of hypokalaemia and possibly hypernatraemia.
   j. Antibiotics are indicated only when there is evidence of infection.
   k. Haemoperfusion, haemodialysis and exchange transfusion have not been shown to affect outcome or duration of toxicity in controlled trials of organophosphate poisoning.
4. **Prevention of further exposure**:
   a. After the patient has recovered, he should not be reexposed to organophosphates for at least a few weeks, since he is likely to suffer serious harm from a dose that normally would be harmless, owing to alteration of body chemistry.
   b. Following acute poisoning, patients should be precluded from further organophosphate exposure until sequential RBC cholinesterase (AChE) levels have been obtained and confirm that AChE activity has reached a plateau. Plateau has been obtained when sequential determinations differ by no more than 10%. This may take 3 to 4 months following severe poisoning.
5. **Treatment of pregnant victim**:
   a. Both atropine and pralidoxime are pregnancy class C drugs, and therefore not contraindicated outright.
   b. Glycopyrrolate: Unlike atropine, glycopyrrolate usually does not readily cross the placenta and would not directly affect foetal poisoning.

Autopsy Features

1. **External**:
   1. Characteristic **odour** (garlicky or kerosene-like).
   2. **Frothing** at mouth and nose. Some compounds may

Box 9.4—Antidotes for Organophosphates

1. ***Atropine***
   a. **Mode of action**: Blocks the muscarinic manifestations of organophosphates. However, since atropine affects only the postsynaptic muscarinic receptors, it has no effect on muscle weakness or paralysis.
   b. **Diagnostic dose**: Adult – 1 mg intravenously or intramuscularly; Child – 0.25 mg (about 0.01 mg/kg) intravenously or intramuscularly.
   c. **Therapeutic dose**: 1–2 mg IV or IM (adult); 0.05 mg/kg IV (child); every 15 min until the endpoint is reached, i.e., drying up of tracheobronchial secretions. Pupillary dilatation and tachycardia are not reliable indicators of the end point. Atropine can also be administered as an IV infusion after the initial bolus dose, at a rate of 0.02–0.08 mg/kg/hr. Once the end point has been reached, the dose should be adjusted to maintain the effect for at least 24 hrs. Doubling the dose of atropine every 5–10 min until clinical improvement is evident speeds atropinisation and reduces mortality. Continuous infusions have been used for as long as 32 days in severely poisoned patients.
   d. Atropine therapy must be withdrawn slowly to prevent recurrence or rebounding of symptoms, often in the form of pulmonary oedema.
   e. **Precautions**:
      - Effects of overdosing with atropine include fever, warm dry skin, inspiratory stridor, irritability and dilated & unresponsive pupils.
      - A urinary catheter should be inserted in all atropinized patients to prevent urinary retention.
   f. **End-point**: "Atropinization" is said to have occurred when the patient exhibits dry skin and mucous membranes, decreased or absent bowel sounds, tachycardia, reduced secretions, no bronchospasm and mydriasis. Reduction or disappearance of pulmonary secretions is the most important target in atropine therapy and can be guided by following lung sounds and oxygenation. Tachycardia is not a contraindication to atropine therapy.
   g. **Adverse effects**: Atrial arrhythmias, A–V dissociation, multiple ventricular ectopics, photophobia, raised intraocular pressure, hyperpyrexia, hallucinations and delirium.
2. ***Glycopyrrolate***
   a. When antimuscarinic CNS toxicity becomes evident, yet peripheral cholinergic findings necessitate the administration of more atropine (e.g., bradycardia, bronchorrhoea, vomiting), glycopyrrolate bromide can be substituted for atropine because its quaternary ammonium structure limits CNS penetration.
   b. The initial IV dose of glycopyrrolate for adults is 1–2 mg, repeated as needed, and in children 0.025 mg/kg up to adult doses.
3. ***Pralidoxime (Pyridine-2-aldoxime methiodide; 2-PAM)***
   a. **Mode of action**:
      - It is usually given along with atropine. Although phosphorylated AChE undergoes hydrolytic regeneration at a very slow rate, this process can be markedly enhanced by using an oxime such as pralidoxime hydrochloride (2 PAM). Regeneration of AChE lowers ACh concentrations to normal levels, reversing both muscarinic and nicotinic effects.
      - Pralidoxime competes for the phosphate moiety of the organophosphorus compound and releases it from the acetylcholinesterase enzyme, thereby liberating the latter and reactivating it. Most phosphorylated AChE will usually be "aged" within 24–48 hrs of exposure. Pralidoxime is unable to rejuvenate active enzyme from the OP compound–AChE complex that has undergone aging. Therefore, pralidoxime therapy is most effective, if started early in the course of toxicity. The actual rate of aging however, varies significantly among OP compounds. While, it is advisable to begin pralidoxime therapy within 48 hrs of poisoning, it can be administered even much later with beneficial effects.
      - Pralidoxime is not equally effective in reversing cholinergic symptoms in all types of OP compound poisonings. It is particularly effective in reversing toxicity from parathion, diazinon, methyl parathion, dimethoate and dichlorvos, but dimethoxy compounds, such as malathion and methyl demeton may be more resistant to reversal.
   b. **Contraindications**: Till recently, pralidoxime was said to be contraindicated in carbamate poisoning because experiments with carbaryl (Sevin) suggested a worsening of symptoms when it was administered. However, studies have pointed out that while pralidoxime is not a necessary adjunct to atropine in carbamate overdose, it may be beneficial in some cases.
   c. **Dose**:
      - For adults: 1–2 g in 100–150 mL of 0.9% sodium chloride, given IV over 30 min. This can be repeated after 1 hr, and subsequently every 6–12 hrs, for 24–48 hrs. Alternatively, a 2.5% concentration of pralidoxime can be given as a loading dose followed by a maintenance dose. Serious intoxication may require continuous infusion of 500 mg hr in adults. Maximum dose should not exceed 12 g in a 24-hr period. Infusion over a period of several days may be necessary and is generally well tolerated. Present recommendations for adults are to begin the maintenance infusion at 250–500 mg/hr, titrating to symptoms. The WHO currently recommends an initial bolus of at least 30 mg/kg, followed by an infusion of more than 8 mg/kg/hr.

contd.

- For children: 20–40 mg/kg to a maximum of 1 g/dose given IV, and repeated every 6–12 hrs for 24–48 hrs. Alternatively, IV infusion can be resorted to, at a rate of 9–19 mg/kg/hr.

d. **Adverse effects:**
- Side effects of pralidoxime are usually minimal at normal doses. Severely poisoned patients have received 500 mg/hr for weeks without adverse effects.
- Occasional visual complaints are also reported in patients receiving pralidoxime.
- Rapid administration can cause tachycardia, laryngospasm and even cardiac or respiratory arrest.
- Other adverse effects include drowsiness, vertigo, headache and muscle weakness.
- It is generally not advised for the treatment of carbamate overdose, especially carbaryl.
- In some countries, obidoxime is used instead of pralidoxime, though it does not appear to be superior to the latter. It is apparently favoured over pralidoxime in clinical practice in Belgium, Israel, The Netherlands, Scandinavia and Germany, and is the only oxime available in Portugal.

e. **Controversies**: Some investigators have started suggesting that oximes have only a limited role in organophosphate poisoning, and successful management is possible without employing them at all, though this view is not shared by other workers in the field.

4. **Diazepam**

a. Several studies demonstrate that administering diazepam along with oximes in the treatment of OP nerve agents (sarin, soman, tabun, VX) or OP pesticides can increase survival and decrease the incidence of seizures and neuropathy.

b. **Dose**: For adults – 5–10 mg IV slowly, every 15 min, up to a maximum of 30 mg. For children – 0.25–0.4 mg/kg IV slowly, every 5–10 min, up to a maximum of 10 mg.

c. If diazepam is ineffective, phenytoin or phenobarbitone can be used instead.

impart a characteristic discolouration, e.g., greenish in dichlorvos poisoning (**Fig. 9.79**)

3. **Cyanosis** of extremities.
4. **Constricted pupils**.

2. **Internal**:
   1. Congestion of GI tract; **garlicky** or **kerosene-like odour** of contents.
   2. Pulmonary and cerebral oedema.
   3. Generalised visceral congestion.

Forensic Significance

- **Suicidal poisoning** with pesticides is a significant public health problem in countries such as India. Many of these cases occur in rural agrarian locations. Organophosphorus insecticides account for a large proportion of these cases.

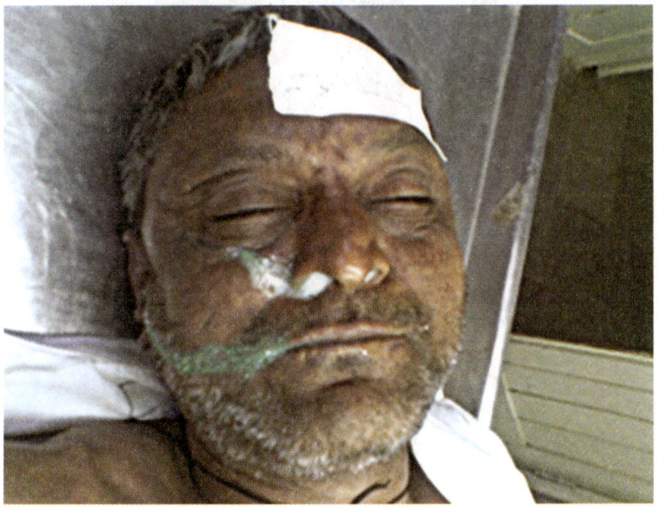

Fig. 9.79 Greenish frothy fluid oozing out of mouth and nose – Dichlorvos poisoning (*Courtesy*: *Dr Swapnil Agarwal*)

- The terrible potential for pesticides to cause **mass poisoning** was not realised in India till the **Kerala food poisoning tragedy** in **1958**. Wheat flour and sugar had been inadvertently stored in the same cabin on a ship as parathion, which leaked into the packages containing the former. Over a thousand people were poisoned subsequently due to consumption of the contaminated material and more than a hundred died. In the **1970s**, a severe convulsive epidemic broke out among several hundred people in **Uttar Pradesh** due to shocking ignorance on the part of farmers who were preserving food grains with BHC! Another (more recent) incident involved accidental spraying of BHC in concentrated form in a thickly populated area leading to similar mass morbidity.
- Unfortunately, lessons are not learnt from history and even today instances of negligent storage of food grains, sugar, vegetables and fruits along with toxic pesticides leading to large-scale **contamination** are not uncommon. Pesticide contamination of vegetables is an even bigger problem in India as compared to many other countries. In fact, the contamination of food with pesticides resulting from excessive crop spraying or improper storage is so widespread in India, that blood samples and milk samples (from lactating mothers) collected randomly from several people in one study demonstrated residual insecticide levels in most of the samples.
- There are concerns that some pesticides may have **carcinogenic potential**, especially on chronic ex-posure. Vietnam war veterans potentially exposed to chlorophenoxy herbicides were noted to have chronic liver abnormalities.

- Organophosphates which are very rapid-acting, such as tabun, sarin, soman and VX, have been developed as "**nerve gases**" for chemical warfare. Human exposure secondary to terrorist activity has occurred. The most notable case of sarin use by a terrorist group occurred in **March, 1995**, when **Sarin** was released in a **Tokyo, Japan subway system**. Estimates are that 1000 people were affected by the attack with 12 deaths (**Fig. 9.80**).

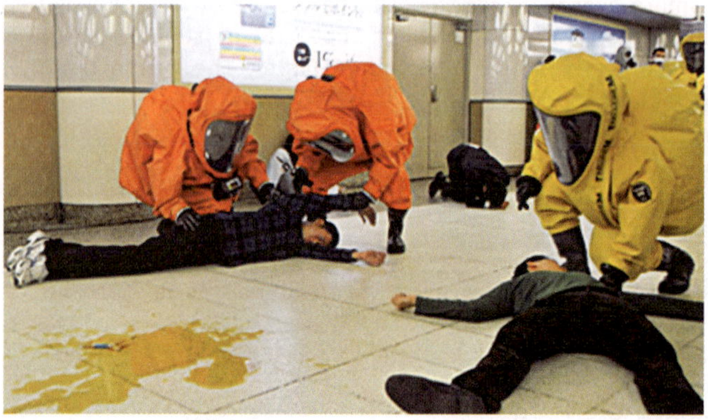

Fig. 9.80 Tokyo subway attack – 1995

CARBAMATES (CARBAMATE INSECTICIDES)

They are as popular as organophosphates in their role as insecticides (and fungicides) and share a number of similarities. Only the differentiating features will be discussed.

Usual Fatal Dose

Based on toxicity rating*:

- The following are **extremely toxic** (*LD50: 1–50 mg/kg*), or **highly toxic** (*LD50: 51–500 mg/kg*) – Aminocarb, Bendiocarb, Carbaryl, Carbofuran, Dioxacarb, Methiocarb, Propoxur.
- The following are moderately toxic (*LD50: 501–5000 mg/kg*) or slightly toxic (*LD50: more than 5000 mg/kg*) – Aldicarb, Bufencarb, Pirimicarb.

Mode of Action & Clinical Features

- Carbamates were discovered in the 19th century when it was observed that the **Calabar bean** (*Physostigma venenosum*) (**Fig. 9.81**) was being used in tribal rituals in West Africa. These beans were imported to Great Britain in 1840, where in 1864, Jobst and Hesse isolated an active alkaloid they named "**physostigmine**." In the 1930s, the synthesis of aliphatic esters of carbamic acid led to the development and introduction of **carbamate pesticides**, marketed initially as fungicides. In 1953, the Union Carbide Corporation developed and first marketed **carbaryl**, the very same insecticide that was being manufactured at the notorious plant in Bhopal, during the methyl isocyanate tragedy in 1984.
- Those cholinesterase-inhibiting (anticholinesterase) insecticides that contain phosphorus are collectively termed organophosphorus (OP) compounds, while those that contain the OC=ON linkage are termed carbamates. Most carbamate insecticides are N-methyl carbamates derived from carbamic acid.
  - **Medicinal carbamate compounds include physostigmine, pyridostigmine and neostigmine**.
  - Drugs such as meprobamate and various urethanes are also carbamate derivatives, but they do not inhibit cholinesterase.
  - **Thiocarbamate fungicides** and **herbicides** (e.g., maneb, zineb, nabam, mancozeb) also **do not inhibit AChE** and do not produce cholinergic excess.
- **Carbamates (like organophosphates) are inhibitors of acetylcholinesterase, but carbamylate the serine moiety at the active site instead of phosphorylation**. This is a **reversible** type of binding and hence symptoms are less severe and of shorter duration.
  - **Aging cannot occur** since the carbamate–AChE bond hydrolyzes spontaneously, reactivating the enzyme. As such, the duration of symptoms in carbamate poisoning is generally <24 hrs. As a result both morbidity and mortality are limited when compared to organophosphate poisoning.
  - Also, since carbamates do not penetrate the CNS to the same extent as organophosphates, CNS toxicity is likewise much less.
  - With respect to all other clinical manifestations, there is **general similarity between carbamates and organophosphates**.
- Carbamates are well absorbed across skin and mucous membranes, and by inhalation and ingestion. Peak serum levels

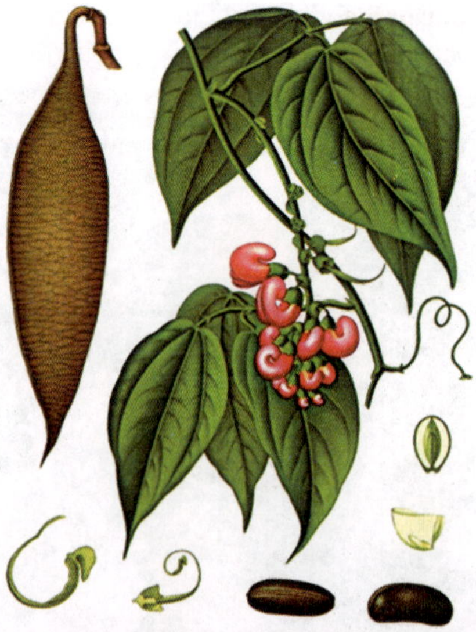

Fig. 9.81 Physostigma venenosum – Various parts of the plant

Note: Partly as per the Insecticide Rules, 1971.

of some compounds are generally achieved in 30–40 min following ingestion. Most carbamates undergo hydrolysis, hydroxylation and conjugation in the liver and intestinal wall, with 90% excreted in the urine within 3 days.

- There are two main toxicokinetic differences between carbamates and OP compounds:
  - First, carbamates do not easily cross into the central nervous system. CNS effects are thus limited, although CNS dysfunction may still occur in massive ingestion (especially aldicarb), or from hypoxia secondary to pulmonary toxicity and paralysis.
  - Second, the carbamate-cholinesterase bond does not "age" as in OP compound poisoning; thus, it is reversible with spontaneous hydrolysis occurring usually within several hours. Carbamates are rapidly metabolized.
- Miosis, a muscarinic effect, is characteristic of severe and moderately severe poisonings, but may appear late. Pupil dilation may occur as a nicotinic effect and may be present in up to 10% of patients.
- Sinus tachycardia with ST segment depression may occur early in the course of poisoning. Repolarization abnormalities may occur and are generally transient. Complete heart block has been reported.
- Dyspnoea is a common manifestation of carbamate exposure. Chest tightness, bronchospasm, increased pulmonary secretions and rales may develop secondary to muscarinic effects. Acute lung injury (pulmonary oedema) is a potential clinical manifestation of severe carbamate poisoning and is attributed to the muscarinic action of the insecticide.
- Headache, dizziness, blurred vision, tremor, paresis, mental depression, coma, delayed neuropathies, various dystonias, weakness, muscle twitching and convulsions have all been reported with carbamate poisoning.
- **Children may be more likely to develop CNS depression, convulsions and hypotonia than the typical cholinergic syndrome**. Absence of classic muscarinic effects has been reported in several children intoxicated with carbamate insecticides.
- **Delayed neuropathies are not usually associated with carbamate insecticides**. One reason for this difference is presumed to be that "aging" of the neuropathy target esterase-pesticide complex does not occur, which is a requirement for neuronal degeneration.
- EMG findings in these subjects are variable. The symptoms are similar to those seen with organophosphates.
- Behavioural toxicity following carbamate exposure is extremely rare.
- Acute pancreatitis has been reported with some carbamates, such as propoxur.

Diagnosis

- **Carbamates inhibit neuronal and RBC AChE, and plasma cholinesterase**. However, the relative rapidity with which spontaneous decarbamylation of cholinesterase takes place may result in the measurement of relatively normal RBC cholinesterase activity despite severe cholinergic symptoms, if the assay is not performed within several hours of sampling. As in the case with OP pesticide poisoning, the wide "normal" range of cholinesterase values may make interpretation of cholinesterase activity difficult at times when the patient's baseline values are unknown. Unlike OP pesticides, carbamates generally do not cause persistent depressed RBC and plasma cholinesterase activities.
- The **atropine challenge test**, as described for diagnosis of OP pesticide poisoning, can be done in carbamate poisoning also.
- Chest X-ray should be obtained in all symptomatic patients. The major cause of morbidity and mortality in carbamate insecticide poisonings is respiratory failure and associated pulmonary oedema.

Treatment

- An important differentiating point from organophosphates is that oximes are generally not recommended, while atropine can be given. Especially in carbaryl poisoning, oxime therapy can lead to the production of a carbamylated oxime which may be a more potent acetylcholinesterase inhibitor than carbaryl itself. With other carbamate insecticides (particularly aldicarb), oximes may be a useful adjunct to atropine therapy.
  - As per general consensus of toxicology experts, **pralidoxime can be used in conjunction with atropine** for specific indications as follows:
    - Life-threatening symptoms such as severe muscle weakness, fasciculations, paralysis or decreased respiratory effort.
    - Continued excessive requirements of atropine.
    - Concomitant organophosphate and carbamate exposure.
  - Fortunately, because of the rapid hydrolysis of the carbamate–AChE complex, symptoms, including weakness and paralysis, usually resolve within 24–48 hrs without pralidoxime therapy.
  - There are no reported cases of delayed poisonings following carbamate poisoning. Therefore, repeating cholinesterase tests after patients are asymptomatic is usually unnecessary.
- If there is bronchorrhoea and/or bronchospasm and/or marked hypotension, urgently give **atropine** (2.0 mg for adults and 0.02 mg/kg for children) intravenously. Further bolus doses of atropine 2 mg in an adult (0.02 mg/kg in children) should be given every 5–10 min until the chest is clear, the heart rate is >80/min and the blood pressure is adequate.
- Treat convulsions, agitation/delirium, etc., as for organophosphate insecticide poisoning.

ORGANOCHLORINES (ORGANOCHLORIDES)

- Organochlorine pesticides are one variety of **chlorinated hydrocarbons**.

- Dichlorodiphenyltrichloroethane (DDT) was one of the earliest organochlorine insecticides to be introduced into agriculture in the early 1940s. These compounds were inexpensive to manufacture, non-volatile, environmentally stable and had relatively low toxicity when compared to the other insecticides. This led to their widespread use from 1940s to 1970s. Medical and public health applications of DDT and its analogues were also found in the control of diseases such as typhus and malaria by eliminating the vector (mosquitoes).
- However, over a period of time it came to be known that these compounds were actually potent **environmental hazards** because of the following reasons: slow metabolism, lipid solubility, chemical stability and environmental persistence. This led to the severe restriction or total ban of DDT and most other organochlorine compounds in the West.
- But, the flip side to this is the tragic fact that ever since DDT was banned, less-effective replacements have placed many more millions at risk for malaria, and is responsible, at least in part, for millions of deaths from this disease. That is why DDT is still favoured by many investigators who consider it to be a highly effective mosquito control agent with a low order of acute toxicity. It is also quite inexpensive when compared to newer replacement insecticides. For these reasons, the World Health Organization (WHO) exempted DDT from its list of banned pesticides, and it is still widely used for malaria control programs in many countries, including India.
- There are **4 distinct categories** of organochlorine pesticides:
  1. **DDT & analogues** – *DDT (dichlorodiphenyltrichloroethane), methoxychlor, dicofol, chlorobenzilate*
  2. **Hexachlorocyclohexanes** – *Lindane (gamma-hexachlorocyclohexane)**
  3. **Cyclodienes and related compounds** – *Aldrin, dieldrin, dienochlor, endosulfan (thiodan), endrin, isobenzan, chlordane, heptachlor, toxaphene*
  4. **Miscellaneous compounds** – *Chlordecone, mirex*

Physical Appearance

Available as dusting powders, wettable powders, emulsions, granules and solutions.

Uses

- **Insecticide**
- Gamma benzene hexachloride is used as a **scabicide** (treatment of scabies) and a pediculocide (eradication of head lice). It is available as topical ointment, cream or lotion.

Usual Fatal Dose

- **DDT, lindane: 15–30 g**.
- **Aldrin, dieldrin, endrin: 2–6 g**.
- **Based on toxicity rating**:
  - Dieldrin is placed in the "**extremely toxic**" category (*LD50: 1–50 mg/kg*), while DDT, endosulfan and lindane are considered "**highly toxic**" (*LD50: 51–500 mg/kg*), as per the ***Insecticide Rules, 1971***.
  - In addition, the following are **extremely toxic**: endrin, aldrin, chlordane and toxaphene, while these are **highly toxic**: kepone, heptachlor, mirex.
  - The following are **least toxic**: methoxychlor, perthane, kelthane, chlorobenzilate and hexachlorobenzene.

Toxicokinetics

- All organochlorine pesticides are well-absorbed orally and by inhalation; transdermal absorption is variable, depending on the particular compound. None of these compounds is water-soluble; they are either dissolved in organic solvents or manufactured as powders for dusting.
- Most organochlorines are metabolized by the hepatic microsomal enzyme systems by dechlorination, oxidation, with subsequent conjugation.
  - However, metabolism may result in the production of a metabolite with more toxicity than the parent compound, such as heptachlor to heptachlor epoxide, chlordane to oxychlordane and aldrin to dieldrin.
- Excretion of organochlorine compounds does not follow first order kinetics. As body stores get lower, the half-life for the remaining store increases dramatically. This is probably due to complex lipoprotein binding, wherein different bound forms exhibit different dissociation characteristics. The half-lives of fat-stored compounds and poorly metabolized organochlorines such as DDT and chlordecone are measured in months or years.
- The primary route of excretion of the organohlorines is in the bile, but most also have detectable urinary metabolites. However, as with other compounds excreted in bile, most of the organohlorines have significant enterohepatic or enteroenteric recirculation.

Mode of Action

- Organochlorine compounds exert their main toxic effects in the central nervous system. They act by affecting the neuronal membrane by either **interfering with repolarization, prolonging depolarization, or impairing the maintenance of the polarized state of the neuron**. The end result is **hyperexcitability of the nervous system** and repetitive neuronal discharges.
- Many organochlorine compounds act as gamma aminobutyric acid (GABA) antagonists. This explains the efficacy of GABA agonists, such as benzodiazepines and phenobarbitone, in treating the seizures and neurotoxicity of these organochlorines.
- **Organochlorines do not depress cholinesterase enzymes**.

Clinical Features

I. **Acute Poisoning**:
   a) Tremor is often the only initial manifestation.
   b) Nausea, vomiting, hyperaesthesia and paraesthesias of the face, tongue & extremities, headache, dizziness,

****Note***: *Gamma benzene hexachloride is not the same as lindane.*

myoclonus, weakness, agitation and confusion usually follow.

c) **Seizures** generally occur after substantial exposure only. However, with regard to some organochlorine compounds, e.g., lindane, there may not be any prodromal signs or symptoms, and the first manifestation of toxicity is a generalized seizure. Seizures usually begin within 1–2 hrs of ingestion, and are often self-limited, but may recur or result in status epilepticus. If the seizures are brief and hypoxia has not occurred, recovery is usually complete. EEG abnormalities are common before, during, and following seizures.

d) **Hyperthermia** secondary to central mechanisms, increased muscle activity and/or aspiration pneumonitis is also common.

e) Hypotension occurs commonly and is due to fluid loss (following vomiting and diarrhoea) and cardiotoxicity (especially common with endosulfan).

f) Fever, aspiration pneumonitis, renal failure.

g) Severe metabolic acidosis has been reported.

h) Less common features include pulmonary oedema, ARDS, pancreatitis, disseminated intravascular coagulation, intravascular haemolysis and increased liver enzymes.

II. **Chronic Poisoning**:

a) Long-term exposure can result in cumulative toxicity with weight loss, tremor, weakness, opsoclonus, ataxia, pseudotumour cerebri, mental changes, oligospermia, and increased tendency to leukaemias, aplastic anaemia, hepatomegaly and liver cancer.

b) Chlordecone, unlike the other organochlorines, produces an insidious picture of chronic toxicity related to its extremely long persistence in the body. Between 1974 and 1975, 133 workers were heavily exposed to chlordecone for 17 months in a small factory in Hopewell, Virginia, USA. They developed a clinical syndrome which became known as the "**Hopewell epidemic**", comprising coarse tremor of the hands, a fine tremor of the head, and trembling of the entire body ("***Kepone shakes***"). Other findings included weakness, opsoclonus (rapid, irregular, dysrhythmic ocular movements), ataxia, mental changes, skin rash, weight loss and elevated liver enzymes. Idiopathic intracranial hypertension, oligospermia and decreased sperm motility were also found in some of these workers.

c) The International Agency for Research on Cancer (IARC) has listed some of these agents (e.g., DDT) as "**possibly carcinogenic to humans**".

d) The **Kasargod endosulfan tragedy** is testimony to the devastating effects of organochlorine environmental toxicity. Kasargod, at the northern end of Kerala, has the largest cashew plantation belt that covers 5600 acres in 11 village panchayats. The plantations were aerially sprayed with endosulfan from 1976, three times a year regularly till 2000, to check the menace of the tea mosquito bug. Aerial spraying of this organochlorine pesticide polluted water bodies, soil and vegetation. The after-effects of the indiscriminate use of endosulfan haunt Kasargod. Kerala's health department has identified 4600 victims and issued health cards entitling patients to free medical care. In 1979, the local community noticed stunted growth and deformed limbs among newborn calves. By 1990, the health disorders were noticed among humans. Mothers started delivering children with congenital anomalies, mental retardation, physical deformities, cerebral palsy, epilepsy and hydrocephalus (**Fig. 9.82**). Endosulfan was banned in the state of Kerala in 2001 following a recommendation by the National Institute of Occupational Health. Later, on a petition filed in the Supreme Court of India, the production, storage, sale and use of the pesticide was banned permanently all over India in 2011.

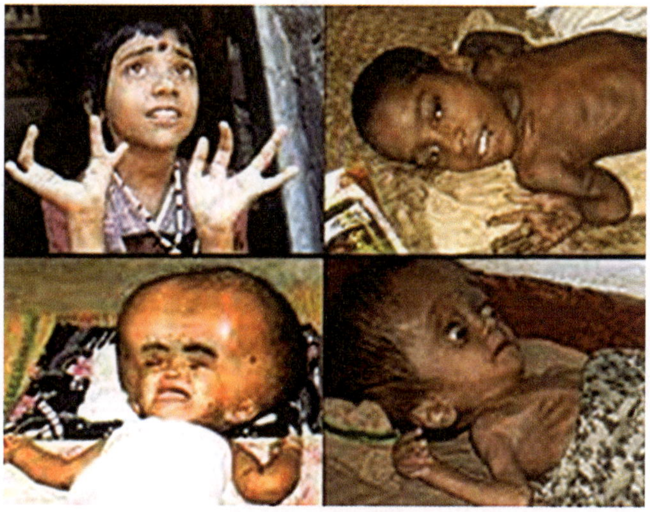

Fig. 9.82 Children afflicted with congenital anomalies – Kasargod

Diagnosis

1. Odour in the vicinity of the patient, especially in the breath may be characteristic, e.g., kerosene-like, as the commercial vehicle for many of these compounds is a petroleum distillate.
2. Abdominal radiograph may reveal the presence of certain organochlorines which are radiopaque.
3. Perform a 12-lead ECG in all patients. Check cardiac rhythm, QRS duration and QT interval.
4. Organochlorines can be detected in serum, adipose tissue, and urine by gas chromatography.

Treatment

1. **Decontamination** – The same measures as detailed under organophosphate poisoning must be undertaken.
   a. Move patient from the toxic environment to fresh air. Monitor for respiratory distress. If cough or difficulty in breathing develops, evaluate for hypoxia, respiratory tract irritation, bronchitis or pneumonitis. Administer

100% humidified supplemental oxygen, perform endotracheal intubation and provide assisted ventilation as required. Administer inhaled beta adrenergic agonists if bronchospasm develops.

b. Activated charcoal (AC) can be used after or instead of gastric lavage, when lavage is not indicated. However, the ability of AC to adsorb the various organohlorines is not adequately studied, and mixtures containing petroleum distillates would preclude the use of AC.

c. Exposed skin and eyes should be flushed with copious amounts of water. Remove contaminated clothing and jewellery; wash skin, hair and nails vigorously with repeated soap washings. Leather absorbs pesticides; all contaminated leather should be discarded.

2. Do NOT give oils by mouth. They tend to increase intestinal absorption of these lipophilic toxicants.
3. Control convulsions that are frequent or prolonged with IV diazepam (10-20 mg in adults; 0.1-0.3 mg/kg in children), lorazepam (4 mg in adults and 0.1 mg/kg in children), or midazolam (5-10 mg in adults; 0.05-0.15 mg/kg in children). If convulsions are unresponsive to initial treatment, second-line therapy is phenobarbitone sodium (10 mg/kg at maximum rate of 100 mg/min; maximum dose 1 g). An alternative is phenytoin (loading dose 18 mg/kg IV infusion in adults and children, given via slow IV [maximum rate 50 mg/min] over 20-30 min with BP and ECG monitoring). Thiopentone sodium is the preferred antiepileptic for status epilepticus not responding to the above measures.
4. **Cholestyramine, a non-absorbable bile acid binding anion exchange resin is effective in enhancing the faecal excretion of organochlorine compounds**. It is administered at a dose of 16 g/day for several days. It can be mixed with fruit juice and given orally (4 g, 6th hourly).
5. There is some evidence that **sucrose polyester (olestra**, a nonabsorbed synthetic dietary oil substitute) can increase excretion of a wide variety of fat-soluble organic chlorine chemicals. This would be an inexpensive and more palatable alternative to cholestyramine to increase excretion in patients with increased body burdens from chronic toxicity.
6. Mild to moderate hyperthermia may respond to conventional cooling measures. When rising body temperature exceeds 39°C, core temperature monitoring should be considered (rectal probe) and urgent cooling measures should be employed according to local protocols. Sedation should be employed where it can be safely performed (diazepam 10-20 mg in adults; 0.25 mg/kg in children). Cooling methods include:
   a. Ice-baths (may achieve rapid cooling but caution in elderly/comorbidities).
   b. Internal/invasive measures – cold fluid lavage (gastric, bladder, peritoneal), intravascular cooling techniques.
   c. Ice packs to groin and axillae.
   d. Mist and fan techniques.
   e. External cooling devices.
   f. Dantrolene may be considered where there is muscular hyperactivity (1 mg/kg IV to a maximum of 10 mg/kg).
7. If rhabdomyolysis is present (CK activity > 5× the upper limit of the normal range), renal failure can develop, particularly if the CK activity is >5000 IU/L.
   a. Give volume replacement as soon as possible and consider the need for urine alkalinization. In an adult give 225 mmol of 8.4% sodium bicarbonate (in a child 3–5 mmol/kg) over 1 hr to increase the urine pH to >7.5; further doses of bicarbonate will be required to maintain pH > 7.5.
   b. Haemodiafiltration can effectively remove myoglobin from the circulation; haemodiafiltration combined with urine alkalinization is more effective than urine alkalinization alone.
   c. Haemodialysis/Haemodiafiltration/Haemofiltration may be required, if acute renal failure develops or severe hyperkalaemia is present.
8. **Supportive measures** – special attention must be paid to the airway and breathing, and adequate circulation should be maintained.
9. Some organochloride insecticides such as endosulfan are cardiotoxic. Check serum potassium, magnesium and calcium concentrations and replace as necessary to keep within the high normal range. Check ABGs and correct any hypoxia or acidosis. Consider magnesium sulphate when the QT-heart rate nomogram indicates a risk of torsade de pointes, especially if other risk factors are present.
10. If metabolic acidosis persists despite correction of hypoxia and adequate fluid resuscitation consider correction with IV sodium bicarbonate. In adults, an initial dose of 50 mmol may be given and repeated as necessary, guided by arterial blood gas monitoring (aim for a pH of 7.44 [Hydrogen ion concentration 36]). In children, use 8.4% sodium bicarbonate diluted in an equal volume of 5% glucose and give a "calculated" dose: dose (in mmol) = desired change in base deficit (current-target) × 0.3 × weight of child up to a maximum of 50 mmol. Administer at a rate of 1 mmol/min.

PYRETHRINS & PYRETHROIDS

- **Pyrethrins** are active extracts of the **Chrysanthemum plant** (*Chrysanthemum cinerariaefolium*) (**Fig. 9.83**), and include **pyrethrum** and **piperonyl butoxide**.
- **Pyrethroids** are synthetic analogues and number over 1000 varieties which are used as insecticides to incapacitate or "knock out" insects. Most mammals are resistant since they can rapidly metabolise and detoxify these agents.

Uses

- These compounds are used as **insect repellants** and **insecticides** in household sprays, mosquito coils and mats.
- They are also used to prevent pest infestation in granaries, and in agriculture as pesticides.
- They are sold as **liquids**, **sprays**, **dusts**, **powders**, **mats** and **coils**.
- **Pyrethrum** extract is effective for treating **pediculosis** of the head, body and pubic area.

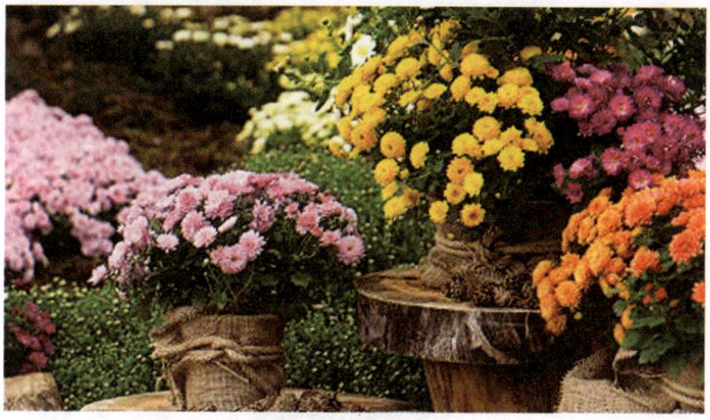

Fig. 9.83 Chrysanthemum

Usual Fatal Dose

- Pyrethrum is said to have an LD50 of over 1 g/kg, while the approximate acute toxic dose of lambda cyhalothrin in rats is much less (80 mg/kg body weight).
- Most cases of toxicity in clinical practice are however the result of allergic reactions.

Mode of Action

- Structurally, pyrethroids are of 2 types:
  - **Type I pyrethroids** do not contain a cyano group, e.g., permethrin.
  - **Type II pyrethroids** contain a cyano group, e.g., deltamethrin, cypermethrin, fenpropathrin, fenvalerate, etc.
- Like DDT, pyrethroids **prolong the inactivation of the sodium channel** by binding to it in the open state. Type II agents are more potent in this regard, and also act by **inhibiting GABA-mediated inhibitory chloride channels**. Low toxicity in mammals is probably due to rapid metabolic breakdown in the liver.
- Two types of **allergens** present in crude pyrethrum oleoresin have been identified: **glycoproteins** or **glycopeptides**, and the **sesquiterpene lactones**, principally ***pyrethrosin***. Refined pyrethrins and synthetic pyrethroids are said to have little or no allergenic effect.

Clinical Features

1. **Skin contact**: Localized paraesthesia, dermatitis, blistering. Symptoms usually resolve within 24 hrs without specific treatment.
2. **Eye contact**: Eye exposures may result in lacrimation, conjunctivitis and mydriasis. There may be mild to severe corneal damage that generally resolves with conservative care.
3. **Inhalation**: Rhinorrhoea, sore throat, wheezing, dyspnoea. Asthma or reactive airways disease syndrome can occur following inhalation exposures, as also hypersensitivity pneumonitis with chest pain, cough, dyspnoea and bronchospasm.
4. **Ingestion** (large doses): Paraesthesias, nausea, vomiting, vertigo, fasciculations, hyperthermia, altered mental status, seizures, pulmonary oedema, coma. Hypotension and tachycardia, associated with anaphylaxis, may occur.
5. Some pyrethroids are **possible carcinogens** on long-term exposure.

Diagnosis

1. Blood cholinesterase levels are normal.
2. ECG changes include ST wave and T wave changes, QT prolongation, sinus tachycardia, ventricular ectopics.
3. Thin layer chromatography can help detect pyrethroids in body fluid samples, and is a cheap and simple method.

Treatment

1. **Skin contact** – Decontaminate with soap and water.
2. **Eye contact** – Irrigate with normal saline or water for 10–15 min.
3. **Systemic poisoning**:
   a. Allergic reactions may be treated with antihistamines (e.g., diphenhydramine 50 mg orally) with or without inhaled beta agonists, corticosteroids (e.g., methyl prednisolone 1–2 mg/kg intravenously every 6–8 hrs) or adrenaline (1:10,000 solution, 3–5 mL diluted in 10 mL 0.9% saline slow intravenous push over 5–10 min).
   b. Treatment of severe anaphylaxis also includes oxygen supplementation, aggressive airway management, adrenaline, ECG monitoring and IV fluids.
   c. Gastric decontamination:
      i. Do not undertake gastric lavage because some formulations contain solvents and lavage may increase the risk of aspiration pneumonia.
      ii. Activated charcoal is beneficial. However, if the pyrethrin is formulated in a petroleum base, the risk of hydrocarbon pneumonitis may exceed the toxic hazard of the insecticide.
      iii. *Gastric decontamination is therefore generally not recommended.*
   d. Oils and fats (including milk) promote the intestinal absorption of pyrethroids and should be avoided.
   e. Oxygen and ventilatory assistance must be administered as indicated.
   f. Perform a *12-lead ECG* in all patients who require assessment. Check cardiac rhythm, QRS duration and QT interval. Check ABGs and correct any hypoxia or acidosis.
   g. *Bronchospasm* is treated with standard broncho-dilators. Administer $beta_2$ adrenergic agonists. Consider systemic corticosteroids in patients with significant bronchospasm, e.g., prednisone 60 mg/day (adult) or 1–2 mg/kg/day (child).
   h. *For agitation/delirium*: Adults can be sedated with an initial dose of oral or IV diazepam (0.1–0.3 mg/kg). If agitation persists, consider oral (5–10 mg) or parenteral (2–10 mg) haloperidol, 0.5–2 mg (oral or IV) initially in the elderly. In children, it is better to manage agitation without sedation and exclude other causes (e.g., hypoxia, infection, hypoglycaemia and raised ICP). If required, midazolam is the most appropriate drug for managing agitation in children and young people.

i. Control *convulsions* that are frequent or prolonged with IV diazepam (10–20 mg in adults; 0.1–0.3 mg/kg in children), lorazepam (4 mg in adults and 0.1 mg/kg in children) or midazolam (5–10 mg in adults; 0.05–0.15 mg/kg in children). If convulsions are unresponsive to initial treatment, second-line therapy is phenobarbitone sodium (10 mg/kg at maximum rate of 100 mg/min; maximum dose 1 g). An alternative is phenytoin (loading dose 18 mg/kg IV infusion in adults and children, given via slow IV [maximum rate 50 mg/min] over 20–30 min with BP and ECG monitoring). Thiopentone sodium is the preferred antiepileptic for status epilepticus not responding to the above measures.

j. If *hypotensive* give 500–2000 mL crystalloid initially (20 mL/kg in children) and titrate to desired effect (stabilization of vital signs, mentation, urine output); adults may require up to 6–10 L/24 hrs.

k. **Atropine and oximes are contraindicated**, but some investigators recommend the former for drying up secretions.

l. *Cutaneous paraesthesias* are said to respond to topical applications of **vitamin E**.

PARAQUAT

- **Paraquat** is a widely used **herbicide**, which belongs to the bipyridyl group.
- It is available either in granular form or as water soluble concentrate which is an odourless brown liquid. In India, most of the concentrates of paraquat are available as 10-20% solutions, and therefore 10 mL of a 20% solution can contain about 2 g of paraquat. The aqueous concentrates often contain appropriate adjuvant agents and sometimes deterrent adjuvants (such as an emetic agent) to prevent or mitigate unintentional ingestion. Such preparations are usually coloured blue or green (**Fig. 9.84**). If no blue dye is added, the concentrate may look like dark brown cola (**Fig. 9.85**), for which it can be mistaken, especially if decanted into a soft drink bottle.
- Paraquat was withdrawn from sale in countries belonging to the European Union in 2005 (amateur formulations) and 2008 (professional formulations).

Toxicokinetics

- Absorption through inhalation, skin contact or eye contact is minimal, though prolonged contact can be hazardous.
- On ingestion, paraquat solution is much more rapidly absorbed than the granular form.
- More than 90% of an absorbed dose is excreted by the kidneys as the parent compound within 12–24 hrs.
- Paraquat is distributed into all organs. **Highest concentrations are found in kidney and lung; paraquat also accumulates in muscle tissue**, which may represent a reservoir, explaining prolonged detection of plasma or urine paraquat weeks or months following ingestion.

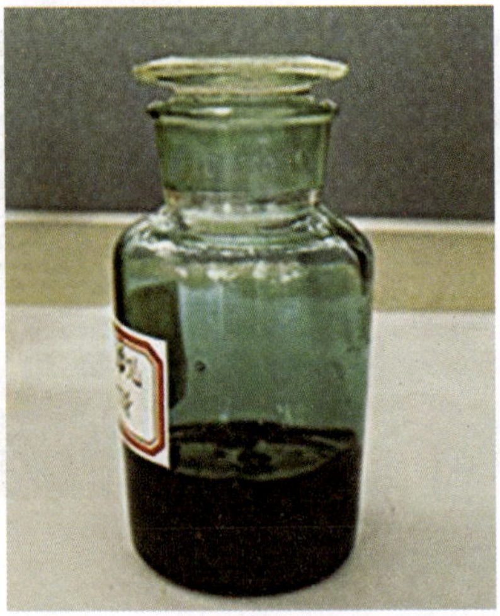

Fig. 9.84 Paraquat solution (with added dye)

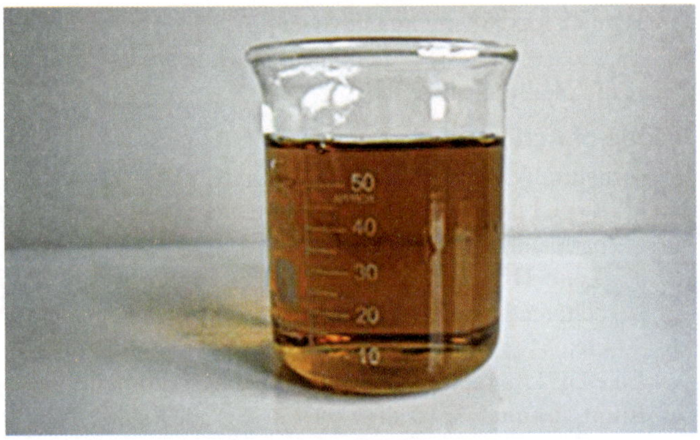

Fig. 9.85 Paraquat solution (without added dye)

Mode of Action

- Paraquat is a rapidly-acting herbicide. It kills the tissues of green plants by contact action with foliage and by some amount of translocation to the xylem. In the presence of light, paraquat generates **reactive oxygen radicals** including **hydrogen peroxide** that disrupt cell membrane integrity. The above-ground portion of the plant collapses rapidly ("burn down") although regrowth can occur from the roots of perennials. It is rapidly inactivated by adsorption to soil.
- When paraquat is ingested, it exerts maximum toxicity in the lungs leading to an **acute alveolitis**, followed by diffuse alveolar collapse, vascular congestion and adherence of activated platelets and polymorphonuclear leucocytes to the vascular endothelium. There is apoptosis of affected cells. The primary target of toxicity in the lung is the alveolar epithelium. Sloughing of the alveoli is associated with pulmonary oedema. This initial '***destructive***' phase is followed by a '***proliferative***' phase during which the alveolar space becomes filled with mononuclear profibroblasts which mature into fibroblasts over a period of days to weeks. The last stage is characterized by **lung fibrosis**.
- **Kidneys** exposed to paraquat demonstrate vacuolation in proximal convoluted tubules which leads to **necrosis**.

- Corneal injury and protracted opacification of the cornea may result following eye exposure to paraquat. Irritation of the skin and mucous membranes may be severe following paraquat exposure.
- After ingestion, sore throat and difficulty in swallowing can occur. Concentrated solutions of paraquat corrode the GI mucosa.
- *Mechanism of Action*:
  - Paraquat exerts most of its toxicity by a process of **redox-cycling**, with subsequent generation of **reactive oxygen species (ROS)**. Paraquat is metabolized by several enzyme systems, and its metabolism by these systems generates a paraquat mono-cation radical ($PQ^{\cdot+}$). Inside the cell, $PQ^{\cdot+}$ rapidly gets re-oxidized to PQ^{2+} and in the process it generates **superoxide ($O_2^{\cdot-}$)**. O_2 acts as an electron acceptor and NADP as an electron donor in this reaction. This further gives rise to formation of the **hydroxyl free radical (HO·)** in the presence of iron via the Fenton reaction. NO· combines with $O_2^{\cdot-}$ to generate **peroxinitrite ($ONOO^-$)** which is a very strong oxidant and a nitrating intermediate. Generation of these highly reactive oxygen and nitrite species results in toxicity in most organs, but the toxicity is most severe in the lungs as paraquat is taken up against a concentration gradient in to the lung.
  - Paraquat can also induce **lipid peroxidation**, which compromises cell membrane function and triggers apoptosis.

Usual Fatal Dose

- **Estimated lethal dose is 10–15 mL of the concentrate.**
- **Ingestion of 30–50 mg of paraquat ion per kg results in death in most cases.**

Clinical Features

1. **Typical Form** (*ingestion of 30–50 mg/kg of paraquat*):
   a. Initial Phase – Pain in the mouth, oesophagus and stomach due to corrosion, vomiting, diarrhoea, dysphagia, aphonia. Mucosal lesions of the mouth and the tongue ('**paraquat tongue**') **(Fig. 9.86)** begin to appear within the first few days and may become ulcerated with bleeding. There may be gastric perforation/gastrointestinal haemorrhage.
   b. Second Phase – begins after 2–5 days and is characterised by renal and hepatic toxicity, i.e., renal tubulopathy and centrilobular hepatic necrosis, respectively.
   c. Third Phase – begins after 5 days and is characterised by **pulmonary fibrosis** (**Fig. 9.87**) which leads to progressive respiratory failure.
2. **Hyperacute Form** (*ingestion of more than 50 mg/kg of paraquat*)
   a. There is rapid development of cardiogenic shock ending in death in 3–4 days.
   b. Renal and hepatic lesions are also common.
3. **Subacute Form** (*ingestion of <30 mg/kg of paraquat*):
   a. This is characterised only by gastrointestinal manifestations.

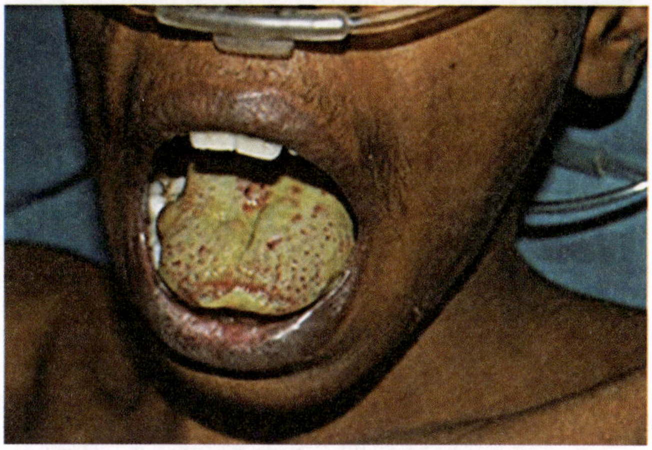

Fig. 9.86 Paraquat tongue (*Courtesy*: *Dr N Ganapathy*)

Mortality in paraquat poisoning can be high and is related to two factors – concentration and quantity. Ingestion of 20% solution is associated with high mortality. Swallowing more than a mouthful can cause death in 72 hrs, because it corresponds to ingestion of more than 50 mg/kg. If it is less than a mouthful, death may be delayed up to 70 days and is usually due to pulmonary fibrosis.

Adrenal cortical necrosis is often observed, particularly in severely poisoned patients with multiple organ failure. A polymorphonuclear leucocytosis is a frequent finding. Metabolic acidosis, probably secondary to cardiovascular collapse and hypoxia, is a common complication; an increase in the arterial lactate concentration is frequent in non-survivors. An increase in transaminase activity is common.

Survivors of severe paraquat poisoning often develop **progressive pulmonary fibrosis** within 5–10 days or longer after exposure. Continued survival is dependent on the extent of lung involvement.

Paraquat in concentrated formulations, has a strong irritant action on various types of epithelia. It will cause erythema, blistering, irritation and ulceration of the skin and eczematous

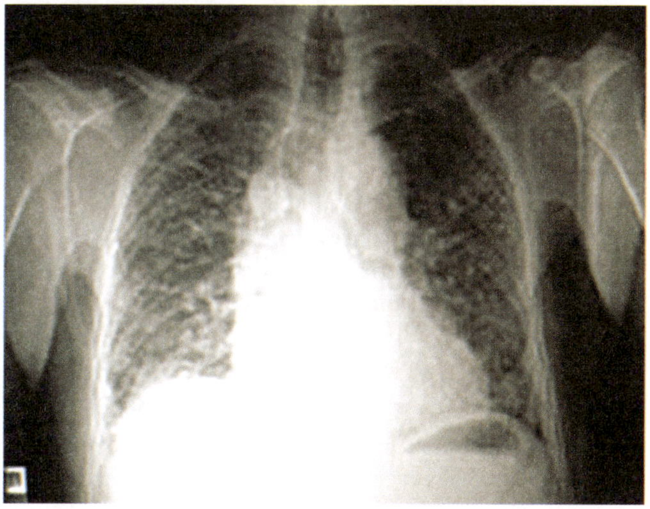

Fig. 9.87 Lung fibrosis – Paraquat exposure

dermatitis. Concentrated solutions of paraquat may also cause localised discolouration or a transverse band of white discoloration affecting the nail plate. Transverse ridging and furrowing of the nail progressing to gross irregular deformity of the nail plate and loss of nail may also occur. Normal nail growth resumes once exposure has ceased.

Diagnosis

1. **X-ray of the chest** may reveal patchy infiltration in the early stages, and opacification of one or both lung fields in later stages. However, if death is due to the hyperacute form of presentation, no abnormalities may be noted on the chest X-ray.
2. **Plasma paraquat level** can be assayed by spectroscopy, radioimmunoassay, or HPLC. Serum levels > 0.2 μg/mL at 24 hrs, and 0.1 μg/mL at 48 hrs are associated with high mortality.
3. **Sodium dithionite test**: Urine can be tested for paraquat by alkalizing 5 mL with a few mg of sodium bicarbonate, and adding a few mg of sodium dithionite. An intense blue (or green) colour is a positive test (**Fig. 9.88**).

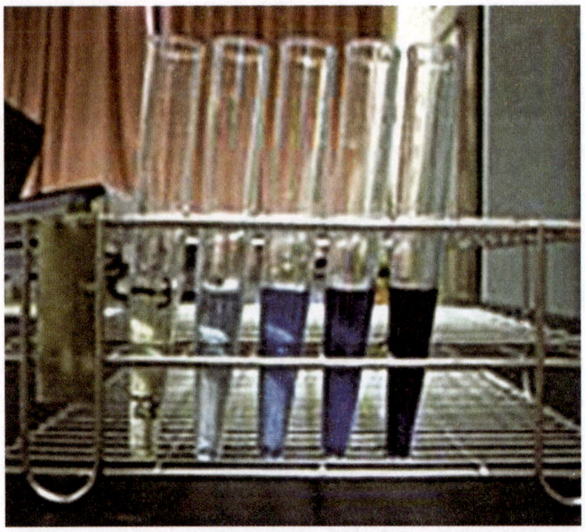

Fig. 9.88 Sodium dithionite test – Paraquat

4. **Urine paraquat level** can be assayed by spectrophotometry. Survival is usually associated with levels less than 1 μg/mL, while mortality is high when the level exceeds 10 μg/mL.
5. Monitor **renal and liver function tests** carefully. Obtain baseline urinalysis and monitor urine output.
6. Obtain **baseline pulmonary function tests, chest X-ray** and **ABGs** and monitor serially for several days.

   When submitting samples for chemical analysis, it must be ensured that only plastic containers are used, since paraquat binds to glass.

Treatment

All cases of paraquat ingestions should be considered as medical emergencies even if the patient is asymptomatic.

1. As paraquat is well adsorbed by **activated charcoal,** it must be administered in the usual dose to all patients who present within 1 hr of ingestion of paraquat. It can be given up to 2–3 hrs after ingestion, beyond which time it becomes practically useless.
   a. If activated charcoal is not available, **Fuller's earth** can be given, or even **garden clay** as an emergency measure. These adsorbents can sometimes make a difference of survival or death.
   b. Gastric lavage is contraindicated as paraquat ingestion causes caustic injury, and it is not likely to provide any added benefit.
   c. Perform upper gastrointestinal endoscopy to identify the extent and severity of corrosion.
2. Pain due to corrosion may be relieved by ice-cold fluids (e.g., ice cream), mouthwashes, local anaesthetic sprays and lozenges. Strong analgesics may be required for ulceration of the oropharynx. Opiates may be required in some cases.
3. In addition to the estimation of paraquat in body fluids as discussed under "**Diagnosis**", routine biochemistries (electrolytes and renal and liver function tests) and haematological investigations (full blood count) must be done at least daily.
4. A chest radiograph should be performed, if pneumomediastinum, pneumothorax or lung fibrosis is suspected. A CT scan of the chest may be useful in detecting early lung fibrosis or assessing long-term damage in survivors.
5. Patients should be monitored for the development of:
   a. *Acute renal failure*: Adequate fluid balance should be maintained to ensure a good urine output without overloading the patient.
   b. *Liver toxicity*: Examine for jaundice and right hypochondrial pain.
   c. *Respiratory failure*: Respiratory rate, auscultation of the lungs (for crepitations) and measurement of peripheral oxygen saturation should be performed at least every 12 hrs. However, **supplementary oxygen should not be given except as a palliative measure** in patients determined to be in terminal decline.
   d. *GI mucosal injury*: Oral ulcers usually prevent patients from taking adequate food or fluids. It is important that early insertion of a nasogastric tube is undertaken to ensure adequate nutrition. Pain relief with opiates is often required.
6. **Haemodialysis** and **haemoperfusion** are part of standard treatment in paraquat poisoning. However, the real benefits of these methods of enhanced elimination are doubtful, because the endogenous clearance of paraquat is high in the first 6–12 hrs and most of it is eliminated rapidly.
7. Supportive measures form the mainstay of treatment: Protection of airway, maintenance of circulation, treatment of secondary infection, prevention or treatment of renal failure and treatment of complications. **Oxygen must not be administered as far as possible since it enhances lung damage.** Allow additional oxygen only in victims considered beyond rescue to relieve air hunger and terminal disease.

8. '**Immunosuppression**' is widely practised as a treatment of paraquat self-poisoning. The theory is that as paraquat leads to an acute inflammatory response, interference with this may inhibit the processes that follow that then lead to lung fibrosis and death.
   a. The most widely studied regimen uses **cyclophosphamide, MESNA, methylprednisolone** & **dexamethasone**.
   b. However, there are no studies that have demonstrated real benefits of this 'immunosuppression' combination in experimental paraquat poisoning. Clinical evidence of benefit is also very limited.
9. Several **antioxidants** have been tested as potential antidotes for paraquat poisoning. As a general statement they have had impressive results *in vitro*, with mixed but modest results in animal studies. Human studies have either been absent or small and uncontrolled. The following are some therapeutic preparations of antioxidants for which there is reliable information: **Vitamin E, Vitamin C, N-acetylcysteine (NAC), Desferrioxamine (DFO), Salicylic acid**.
10. Pulmonary damage may be ameliorated by **radiotherapy**. However the current consensus is NOT to undertake radiotherapy because of lack of clinical evidence of efficacy.
11. **Lung transplantation** has not met with success in most cases where it was attempted.
12. **Eye exposure**: Remove contact lenses, if present and immediately irrigate the affected eye thoroughly with water or 0.9% saline for at least 10–15 min. Continue until the conjunctival sac pH is normal (7.5–8.0). Corneal damage may be detected by instillation of fluorescein.

Autopsy Features

- Ulceration around lips and mouth, reddened or desquamated oral and oesophageal mucosa, erosion and patchy haemorrhages in the stomach.
- Liver may show pallor or mottled fatty change; centrilobular necrosis.
- Lungs often appear stiffened. There may be evidence of proliferative pulmonary fibrosis, fibrinous pleurisy, or scanty blood-stained pleural effusion. Cut surface reveals oedema.
- Kidneys may reveal evidence of tubular damage.

Forensic Issues

- Paraquat is increasingly being reported in suicidal cases.
- Accidental poisoning can occur, if the solution is stored carelessly, e.g., in a soft drink bottle.
- Homicidal poisoning has been reported.

ALUMINIUM PHOSPHIDE

Physical Appearance

- Aluminium phosphide is marketed in India under various trade names (commonest being *Celphos*), and is generally available as greyish green tablets of 3 g each, mixed with urea and ammonium carbonate (**Fig. 9.89**).

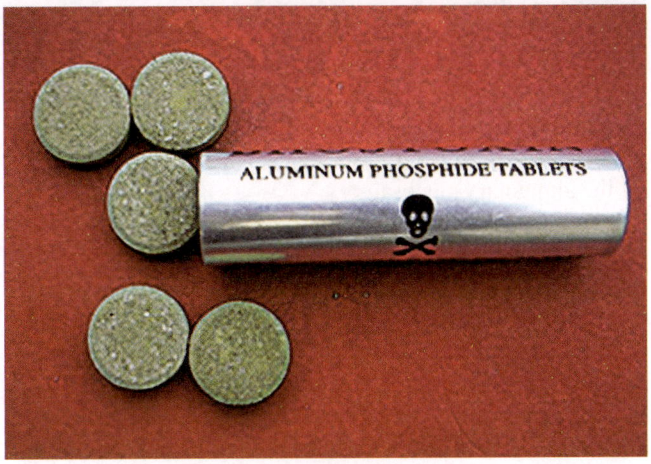

Fig. 9.89 Aluminium phosphide tablets

- Despite the addition of ammonium carbonate to reduce the potential for spontaneous ignition or explosions, both events may occasionally occur during the handling of aluminium phosphide. Spontaneous ignition has also been reported in individuals that have ingested aluminium phosphide.
- Each tablet liberates 1 g of phosphine.

Uses

- **Grain preservative**: Aluminium phosphide is said to be the most ideal grain preservative since it is relatively cheap while being very effective in repelling pests. The required number of tablets are removed from the airtight container and placed among the grain. On exposure to moisture, **phosphine** is released which percolates among the grain. When fumigated grains are subsequently well aerated, phosphine evaporates rapidly leaving behind virtually no residue.*
- Phosphine is oxidised to hypophosphite ($H_2PO_2^-$), phosphate (PO_4^{3-}) and phosphite (HPO_3^{2-}), none of which are toxic.
- Aluminium phosphide can also be used as an oral pesticide.
- As a rodenticide, aluminium phosphide pellets are provided as a mixture with food for consumption by the rodents. The acid in the digestive system of the rodent reacts with the phosphide to generate the toxic phosphine gas.

Usual Fatal Dose

- **One to three tablets.**
- Phosphide ingestions over **1 g** are potentially fatal.

Mode of Action

- When exposed to air and moisture, aluminium phosphide liberates **phosphine** which causes multi-organ damage.

$$AlP + 3H_2O \rightarrow Al(OH)_3 + PH_3$$

*__Note__: *Even if some residue remains, it is invariably less than the WHO/FRO recommended permissible level of 0.1 mg/kg of phosphine for raw cereals.*

Pillay – Textbook of Forensic Medicine & Toxicology

Clinical Features

- The short interval between ingestion of aluminium phosphide and the appearance of features of systemic phosphine toxicity indicates that aluminium phosphide is hydrolysed rapidly to **phosphine**, which is absorbed through the alimentary mucosa.
- Common presenting symptoms include metallic taste, vomiting, garlicky (or fishy) odour of breath, intense thirst, burning epigastric pain and diarrhoea.
- In severe cases, there are cardiovascular manifestations such as hypotension, tachy/bradycadia and ECG abnormalities (sinus tachycardia, sinus arrhythmia with ST segment depression, and AVF, ST elevation, atrial fibrillation, ventricular premature complexes followed by ventricular tachycardia, T wave inversion, sinus arrest, complete heart block).
- Patients often suffer shock after ingestion of aluminium phosphide tablets and develop adult respiratory distress syndrome within 6 hrs.
- Convulsions have been reported in some cases. Coma supervenes in later stages.
- Hepatic damage, renal failure and metabolic acidosis are possible.
- Respiratory distress is invariably present with cyanosis, and cold, clammy skin.

Diagnosis

1. **Garlicky odour** in the breath.
2. Urinalysis may reveal occult blood, bilirubin, glucose and albumin.
3. Liver function tests are often abnormal.
4. Blood urea and serum creatinine are usually higher than normal.
5. Hypo/Hypermagnesaemia; Hypo/hyperphosphataemia.
6. Hypo/Hyperglycaemia.
7. Hypokalaemia is common and is probably secondary to vomiting.
8. Metabolic acidosis is frequently seen.
9. ECG changes (mentioned under **Clinical Features**): Perform a 12-lead ECG in all patients who require assessment. Check cardiac rhythm, QRS duration and QT interval.
10. Qualitative tests for detecting phosphine in the breath and gastric aspirate:
    a. **Breath test**: A piece of filter paper impregnated with 0.1N silver nitrate solution is used in the form of a mask through which the patient is asked to breathe in and out for 5–10 min. Blackening of the paper is indicative of the presence of phosphine in the breath, since silver nitrate is reduced to silver on exposure to it. Similar reaction is also produced by hydrogen sulphide.
    b. **Biological sample test**: A small amount of gastric aspirate (5–10 mL) or minced tissue (5–10 g of liver)* is taken into a steam distillation flask to which an equal quantity of water is added and then acidified with dilute HCl or H_2SO_4, followed by heating up to 50°C for 15 min. The distillate is collected in an ice cold receiver containing 5 mL of 1% silver nitrate solution by dipping the adapter into it. If phosphine is present, the solution will turn black.

Treatment

- There is no specific treatment. Emesis is not to be induced.
- While there were initial reports eulogising the efficacy of magnesium sulphate, particularly in relieving cardiovascular manifestations, later studies could not sustain such a view.
- Presently, the suggested measures include the following:
  - Management of circulatory shock with IV fluids (4–6 L over 6 hrs), while monitoring the central venous pressure and/or pulmonary wedge pressure. Dopamine can be given IV at a dose of 4–6 µg/kg/min (maximum 10 µg/kg/min).
- Management of respiratory distress with 100% humidified oxygen, intubation and assisted ventilation.
- If metabolic acidosis persists despite correction of hypoxia and adequate fluid resuscitation consider correction with IV sodium bicarbonate. In adults, an initial dose of 50 mmol may be given and repeated as necessary, guided by arterial blood gas monitoring (aim for a pH of 7.44 [Hydrogen ion concentration 36]). In children, use 8.4% sodium bicarbonate diluted in an equal volume of 5% glucose and give a "calculated" dose: dose (in mmol) = desired change in base deficit (current-target) × 0.3 × weight of child up to a maximum of 50 mmol. Administer at a rate of 1 mmol/min.
- Control of convulsions with anticonvulsants (benzodaizepines, barbiturates, etc.).
- **Magnesium sulphate therapy**: Given IV as a 3-g bolus, followed by 6-g infusion over 24 hrs for 5–7 days. Alternatively, 1 g can be given IV to begin with, followed each hour by the same dose for 3 consecutive hours, and then 1 g every 6 hrs for 5 days. Magnesium sulphate is said to be beneficial in the management of cardiac arrhythmias. Conventional antiarrhythmic drugs such as digoxin and lidocaine are ineffective.
- Ranitidine 50 mg IV 8th hourly to counter the severe epigastric pain.
- Though there is often intense thirst, do not administer water since whatever aluminium phosphide is still remaining in the stomach will react with it, releasing phosphine. For the same reason, stomach wash is said to be contraindicated. While activated charcoal can be administered, it should be mixed with sorbitol (and not water), using 240 mL for every 30 g. However, today most authorities recommend the performance of gastric lavage as well as the administration of activated charcoal using aqueous solutions. Some investigators claim that **coconut oil** has a beneficial effect and can be used as an antidote in acute aluminium phosphide poisoning in humans.

**Note: Applicable only to autopsied cases!*

Autopsy Features

- There is widespread hypoxic organ damage with congestion and petechiae.
- There may be a garlicky odour around the mouth and in the vicinity of the body.
- The face is usually livid with distinct bluish discolouration and blood mixed froth from and around the nostrils.
- Internal examination often reveals froth in the trachea and oedematous lungs with haemorrhages in the interlobular areas and at the margins of the lungs.
- Contents of stomach are often haemorrhagic with mucosal shedding, and there is usually an intense **garlicky odour**. Stomach may reveal grayish brown fluid or pasty material. The mucous membrane of stomach is rendered corrugated, loosened or hardened and inflamed, along with inflamed intestines.
- Histopathological examination may reveal varying degree of congestion, oedema and leucocytic infiltration, suggesting cellular hypoxia in aluminium phosphide poisoning. The most dramatic effects are evident in the lungs, kidneys and adrenals.

Forensic Issues

- Prior to 1980, aluminium phosphide poisoning was virtually unreported in India. Today it is one of the leading causes of suicidal (and sometimes accidental) death in northern Indian states such as Punjab, Haryana, Uttar Pradesh, Madhya Pradesh and Rajasthan. Southern states have so far not been significantly affected since aluminium phosphide is yet to make inroads into the agricultural sector here. But, there are ominous indications of a gradual rise in the number of cases being reported.
- The onset of symptoms is usually very rapid and mortality is high.
- Homicidal poisoning with aluminium phosphide has been reported.

ZINC PHOSPHIDE

Physical Appearance

- Zinc phosphide is available as dark grey tetragonal crystals or grey-to-black cystalline powder (**Fig. 9.90**) marketed under various trade names (commonest being *Ratol*).
- It has a repulsive odour of **rotten fish**.

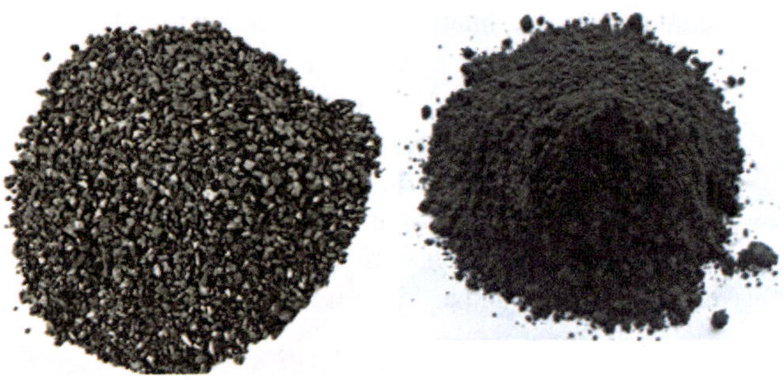

Fig. 9.90 Zinc phosphide crystals (L) and powder (R)

Uses

- Zinc phosphide is a widely used **rodenticide** in India. Rodenticide-grade zinc phosphide usually contains 75% of zinc phosphide and 25% of antimony potassium tartrate, an emetic to cause vomiting, if the material is accidentally ingested by humans or domestic animals. However, it is still effective against rats, mice, guinea pigs and rabbits, none of which have a vomiting reflex.

Usual Fatal Dose

2–4 g.

Mode of Action, Clinical Features, Diagnosis, Treatment and Autopsy Features

- Same as for aluminium phosphide.
  - Zinc phosphide is more hepatotoxic than aluminium phosphide; the latter is more cardiotoxic.
- In symptomatic patients monitor FBC, U&Es, LFTs, cardiac enzymes, phosphate, blood glucose, calcium, magnesium and blood gases.
- Perform a chest X-ray and monitor cardiac rhythm.
- Treat renal failure conventionally with haemodialysis, haemodialfiltration or haemofiltration.
- Hepatic damage can be ameliorated to some extent with N-acetylcysteine.

Forensic Issues

- Accidental and suicidal poisonings have been reported involving the consumption of rat powder/pastes containing zinc phosphide. Some of these brands are marketed in tubes that look very similar to toothpaste tubes leading to accidental use (**Fig. 9.91**).

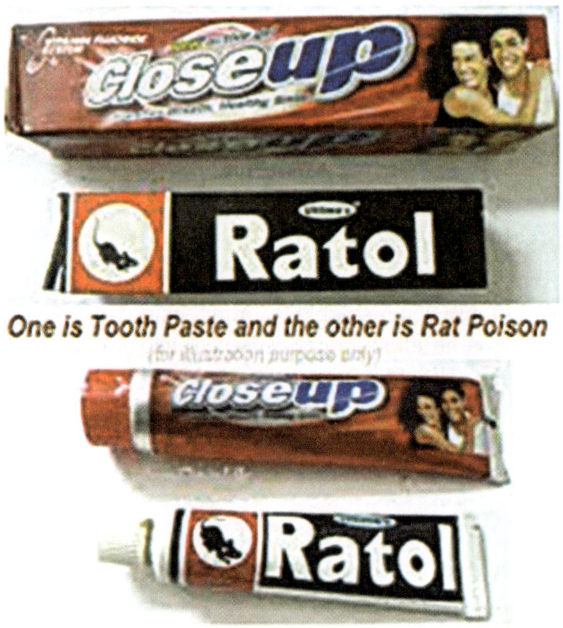

Fig. 9.91 Tooth paste and Rat paste tubes

> **FM 9.6: Core – Written/Viva Voce/ Objective Structured Clinical Examination (OSCE)**
> - Describe general principles and basic methodologies in treatment of poisoning: decontamination, supportive therapy, antidote therapy, procedures of enhanced elimination with regard to:
>   - Ammonia
>   - Carbon monoxide
>   - Hydrogen cyanide & derivatives
>   - Methyl isocyanate
>   - Tear (riot control) gases

All the above are asphyxiant gases (toxic inhalants).

CLASSIFICATION OF ASPHYXIANTS

1. **Simple Asphyxiants** – These gases displace oxygen from the ambient air and reduce the partial pressure of available oxygen.
   a. Examples include **carbon dioxide, nitrogen, aliphatic hydrocarbon gases** (butane, ethane, methane and propane)
   b. Noble gases (argon, helium, neon, radon and xenon).
2. **Respiratory Irritants** – These gases damage the respiratory tract by destroying the integrity of the mucosal barrier.
   a. Examples include acrolein, **ammonia**, chloramine, **chlorine**, formaldehyde, **hydrogen sulphide**, methyl bromide, **methyl isocyanate**, oxides of nitrogen, osmium tetroxide, ozone, phosgene and sulphur dioxide.
   b. Heavy metal-related gases also come under this category (cadmium fumes, copper fumes, mercury vapour, zinc chloride and zinc oxide).
3. **Systemic Asphyxiants** – These gases produce significant systemic toxicity by specialised mechanisms.
   a. Examples include **carbon monoxide, cyanide** and smoke.

The **asphyxiant gases** listed in the new curriculum will now be discussed. There will be no discussion with regard to other toxic gases, though some of these are actually as important, if not more important than the ones mentioned in the curriculum.

AMMONIA

Physical Appearance

- Extremely irritant gas with a penetrating odour.
- It is highly water soluble (forming ammonium hydroxide which is an alkaline corrosive). Aqueous ammonia is a colourless liquid with a strong alkaline reaction (pH 11.6) and a penetrating pungent (urine-like) odour.

Molecular Formula

NH_3

Uses

- Agriculture (fertilizer)
- Mining
- Manufacture of plastics and explosives
- Refrigerant
- Cleaning and bleaching agent
- Treatment of syncope in the form of **smelling salts**: preparation of ammonium carbonate and perfume, sniffed as a restorative or stimulant. Traditionally, they were sniffed as a stimulant to relieve faintness or swooning.

Mode of Action

- Anhydrous ammonia (liquid or gas) reacts with tissue water to form the strongly alkaline solution ammonium hydroxide. This reaction is exothermic and capable of causing significant thermal injury.
- Tissue damage from alkali is caused by liquefaction necrosis and tissue penetration may be deeper than that caused by an equipotent acid.

Usual Fatal Dose

- **5–10 mL of liquid ammonia.**
- Inhalation of the gas at concentrations above 5000 ppm can be rapidly fatal.

Clinical Features

- Inhalation produces such severe upper airway irritation that the victim seldom remains exposed for more than an instant, unless he is trapped.
- Symptoms include lacrimation, cough, dyspnoea, convulsions, coma and death.
- There is glottic and laryngeal oedema, sloughing of bronchial mucosa and chemical pneumonitis with pulmonary oedema.
- If recovery from the acute event is incomplete, a chronic condition may set in called **reactive airways dysfunction syndrome** or **RADS**. This is a persistent, asthma-like syndrome and is also referred to as **irritant induced asthma**. It is different from **occupational asthma**, since there is no evidence of atopy in individuals suffering from RADS, and the agents involved are generally not considered to be immunologically sensitizing.
- Ingestion of ammonia solution produces corrosion of the alimentary tract and aspiration pneumonia. Nausea and vomiting occur frequently following ingestion. Swelling of the lips, mouth and larynx, and oral or oesophageal burns may occur, if concentrated ammonia solutions are ingested.
- Dermal contact can result in deep, penetrating burns. Exposure to anhydrous ammonia stored at minus 28°F may produce frostbite injury with thrombosis of surface vessels and subsequent ischaemia and necrosis.
- Ocular exposure can result in immediate and serious chemical burn with rapid penetration into the interior of the eye. Conjunctivitis, lacrimation, corneal irritation and temporary or permanent blindness can result.
- Chronic exposure in workers may lead to initial complaints of chronic cough, dyspnoea on effort, bilateral infiltrates on chest X-ray and lung function indices reflecting ventilatory and diffusion abnormalities. Asthma & laryngitis have been reported in workers chronically exposed to ammonia. Workplace exposure has led to interstitial lung fibrosis.

Diagnosis

1. Chest X-ray in dyspnoeic patients.
2. Early endoscopy to determine the extent of injury.

3. Barium swallow after 1–2 weeks to rule out oesophageal strictures.
4. Presence of ammonia in an unknown solution, stomach contents or vomitus can be confirmed by placing an open bottle of conc HCl in the vicinity. This will produce copious white fumes of ammonium chloride.

Treatment

1. Ocular exposure should be treated with prolonged irrigation with water (30 min or more) until the eye reaches neutral pH as tested with a litmus paper in the conjunctival sac.
2. Dermal exposure requires washing with soap and water, followed by copious irrigation with water alone. Frostbite should be treated in the standard manner.
3. Inhalation should be treated with oxygen, PEEP (positive end expiratory pressure), intubation and bronchodilators. Intubation or tracheostomy may be life-saving following severe exposure if stridor, indicating laryngeal oedema, is present.
4. If bronchospasm and wheezing occur, consider treatment with inhaled sympathomimetic agents.
5. In the case of ingestion, a small quantity of water or milk can be administered as a first-aid measure to dilute the chemical. Neutralisation with vinegar or weak acids is not recommended. Demulcents can be given.
6. Activated charcoal is of no benefit, and may induce vomiting and obscure endoscopy findings.
7. Stomach wash and emetics are contraindicated.
8. Obtain consultation concerning endoscopy as soon as possible, and perform endoscopy within the first 24 hrs when indicated.
9. Antibiotics are indicated only when there is evidence of infection.
10. The use of corticosteroids for the treatment of caustic ingestion is controversial.

Forensic Issues

- While poisoning with ammonia is not very common, most of the cases reported are suicidal in nature.
- Since the solution or gas even when weak has a distinct irritant smell, accidental poisoning is unlikely.
- Obviously, its properties preclude its choice for murder.
- However, of late ammonia is being used as a spray to incapacitate victims of robbery. Serious eye injuries can result.

CARBON MONOXIDE

Synonyms

Carbon oxide, Exhaust gas, Flue gas

Physical Appearance

- Pure carbon monoxide is an odourless, colourless, non-irritating gas, which is lighter than air.

Sources

- Incomplete combustion of almost any form of fuel (wood, charcoal, gas, kerosene).
- Automobile exhaust.
- Fires.
- Paint remover (especially methylene chloride).
- Tobacco smoke.

Endogenous CO resulting from haem degradation can never reach toxic levels on its own. Normal CO level in plasma is in the range of 1–5% and may rise up to 7–8% in smokers.

It is important to note that **domestic gas** does not contain CO. It is a mixture of methane 90–95%, ethane 3% and nitrogen 1–2.5%, with small amounts of propane, butane, higher hydrocarbons and carbon dioxide (up to 5%).

Usual Fatal Dose

- This is usually expressed in terms of plasma concentration of the gas (carboxyhaemoglobin or COHb).
  - **COHb level exceeding 50–60% is potentially lethal.**
- A carbon monoxide concentration of 5000 ppm in air is lethal to humans after 5 min of exposure.

Toxicokinetics

- The lungs avidly absorb CO which combines with haemoglobin (85%) and myoglobin (15%).
- Elimination occurs exclusively through the lungs.

Mode of Action

- **Carbon monoxide has an affinity for haemoglobin which is 230–270 times greater than that of oxygen**. Therefore, in spite of adequate partial pressure of oxygen (pO_2) in blood, there is reduced arterial oxygen content. Further, CO causes a leftward shift of the oxyhaemoglobin dissociation curve, thus affecting the offloading of oxygen from haemoglobin to the tissues. The net result of all this is the decreased ability of oxygen to be carried by the blood and released to tissues.
- Apart from the COHb-mediated hypoxia described, it is postulated that CO may also interfere with cellular respiration by inactivating mitochondrial cytochrome oxidase.

Clinical Features

I. **Acute Poisoning**:
   a. Mentioned in relation to severity of exposure in **Table 9.20**.
   b. The earliest manifestations are often non-specific and may be confused with other conditions. **Table 9.21** outlines the important conditions in the differential diagnosis.
   c. Two of the "classical" features of CO poisoning mentioned in several textbooks on toxicology are actually quite rarely encountered in clinical practice:
      i. **Cherry red colour of blood and tissues** (including skin) is seen only in 2–3% of cases (**Fig. 9.92**). It is important that every doctor understands what is meant by "cherry red" or "cherry pink" colour (**Fig. 9.93**).
      ii. Development of **cutaneous bullae (blisters)** is another uncommon finding in clinical practice.
   d. It has been suggested that a more thorough examination of the eye (i.e., electrodiagnostic tests) would

Table 9.20 Acute Carbon Monoxide Poisoning

Severity	Symptoms and Signs
Mild (COHb < 30%)	Headache, nausea, vomiting, dizziness, exertional dyspnoea.
Moderate (COHb 30–40%)	Chest pain, blurred vision, confusion, weakness, increasing dyspnoea, tachycardia, tachypnoea, ataxia, severe headache, syncope, cyanosis, perspiration, impaired sensorimotor task performance, prolonged reaction time, impaired judgement, loss of muscular control, tinnitus, drowsiness, hallucinations and cardiovascular toxicity.
Severe (COHb > 40%)	Trismus, muscle spasms, convulsions, palpitations, disorientation, ventricular dysrhythmias, hypotension, myocardial ischaemia, skin blisters, pulmonary oedema, respiratory failure, coma, collapse and death.

Table 9.21 Differential Diagnosis of Carbon Monoxide Poisoning

- Alcoholic intoxication
- Cerebrovascular accident
- Epilepsy
- Food poisoning
- Hyperventilation syndrome
- Meningitis, encephalitis
- Myocardial infarction
- Pneumonia

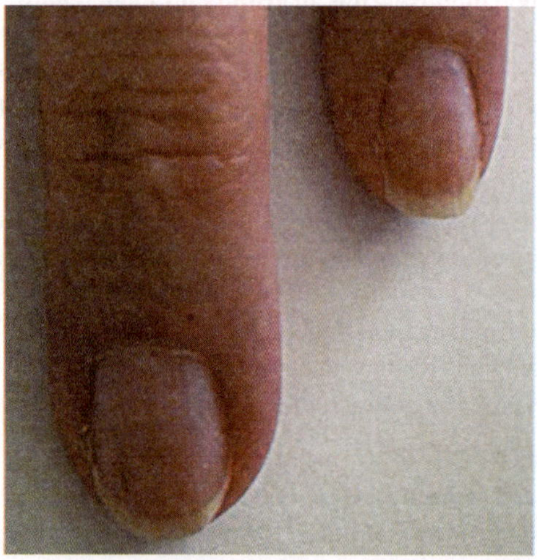

Fig. 9.92 Cherry red colour of fingertips – Carbon monoxide poisoning

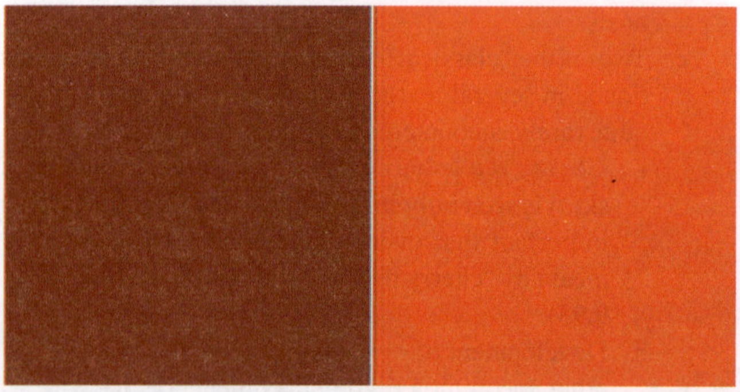

Fig. 9.93 Cherry red (L) and Bright red (R)

reveal that retinal haemorrhage may occur frequently, and that it can occur superficially or deeper in the nerve fibre layer (flame haemorrhage), and is often peripapillary. These changes reflect the hypoxic injury to the retina due to CO poisoning. Paracentral scotomata, homonymous hemianopia, tunnel vision and temporary/permanent blindness are known sequelae.

e. Myocardial ischaemia may be precipitated or aggravated by CO; reported even with low CO levels in patients with preexisting coronary artery disease. ECG changes of CO poisoning include S-T segment depression or elevation, T wave abnormalities, atrial fibrillation and intraventricular conduction block.
f. Muscle necrosis, rhabdomyolysis, compartment syndrome and elevated CPK have been reported following toxic exposures.
g. Haematuria, albuminuria, renal failure, myoglobinuria and acute tubular necrosis have developed with severe poisoning.
h. Lactic acidosis may occur.
i. Bullous lesions associated with carbon monoxide poisoning generally appear within 24 hrs of exposure and are usually located on the palms and soles. They are not a common occurrence.
j. High susceptibility groups to CO poisoning include infants (high respiratory and metabolic rates), pregnant women, the elderly, individuals with anaemia, haematologic disorders and patients with a history of ischaemic heart disease or chronic obstructive lung disease.
k. A **"post-CO syndrome,"** including headache, nausea, and weakness may persist for 2–3 weeks following exposure to carbon monoxide.
l. Recovery from the acute episode may be followed by permanent neurological sequelae such as dementia, amnesia, psychosis, parkinsonism, paralysis, chorea, blindness, etc. Personality changes may also occur, with increased irritability, verbal aggression, violence, impulsivity and moodiness.

m. CO exposure during pregnancy is teratogenic. Exposure to the foetus can result in permanent brain damage, including mental retardation, limb malformation, hypotonia, basal ganglia damage, microcephalus, low infant birth weight, seizures and stillbirth.

II. **Chronic Poisoning**:
   a. Headache, dizziness, confusion.
   b. Weakness, nausea, vomiting, abdominal pain.
   c. Paraesthesias.
   d. Visual disturbances: homonymous hemianopia, papilloedema, scotomata, retinal haemorrhages.
   e. Hypertension, hyperthermia.
   f. Cherry red skin.
   g. Palpitations, aggravation of angina, intermittent claudication.
   h. Elevated RBC and WBC count.
   i. Albuminuria, glycosuria.
   j. Permanent neurological sequelae: amnesia, agnosia, rigidity, personality changes, psychosis, blindness and hearing impairment.

Diagnosis

Summary – Determine COHb level when the patient is first seen and repeat every 2–4 hrs until patient is asymptomatic, or level is within the normal range. Monitor ECG, electrolytes, CPK, urinalysis, arterial blood gases, if symptomatic, or if the COHb level is greater than 20%. Pulse oximetry may not provide a reliable estimate of oxyhaemoglobin saturation. Monitor cardiac function. CT scan or MRI should be considered, if neurologic symptoms persist.

1. *Estimation of carboxyhaemoglobin level (COHb)*: Normal levels range from 0 to 5%, but in heavy smokers it may be as high as 10%. The usual method of estimation is a **co-oximeter**, which spectrophotometrically reads the percentage of total haemoglobin saturated with CO. Either arterial blood or venous blood can be used. It must be borne in mind that COHb levels do not always correlate with clinical manifestations or the final outcome.
2. *Pulse oximetry*: It is a non-invasive method of measuring oxygen saturation and is relatively easy to perform, painless, rapid and accurate. But in CO poisoning, pulse oximetry gives higher readings than the true HbO_2 (oxyhaemoglobin) levels and may fail to alert the physician to potentially lethal hypoxia. COHb absorbs light almost identically to HbO_2 at 660 nm. The oximeter responds to COHb as if it were HbO_2.
3. *Arterial blood gases*: Partial pressure of oxygen is usually normal, but the oxygen saturation expressed as a percentage is decreased. A gap between the measured percentage HbO_2 and the calculated percentage HbO_2 indicates the necessity for measuring COHb. PCO_2 may be normal or slightly decreased. Metabolic acidosis is invariably present.
4. *ECG*: This may reveal myocardial damage in the form of ST depression or elevation, T-wave flattening or inversion and dysrhythmias.
5. *Chest X-ray*: This may reveal ground-glass appearance, perihilar haze, peribronchial cuffing and intra-alveolar oedema.
6. *CAT Scan*: This may reveal low-density globus pallidus lesions which are predictive of neurological sequelae. Lucencies of the basal ganglia, particularly the globus pallidus is characteristic of severe carbon monoxide poisoning.
7. *MRI*: Cytotoxic oedema and demyelination, as well as damage to white matter and basal ganglia are often detected accurately by MRI.
8. *Ancillary Investigations*:
   a. Routine laboratory investigations often reveal elevated serum creatine kinase and lactate dehydrogenase levels, as well as creatinine. Hypokalaemia and hyperglycaemia are also usually present.
   b. Retinal haemorrhage is a common finding in CO poisoning. It has been suggested that careful eye exam may provide useful diagnostic information. Findings include superficial or deep retinal haemorrhage, venous changes (i.e., engorgement and tortuosity) and oedema of the optic disc.
9. *Bedside Tests*:
   a. Take 1 drop of blood and dilute with 10–15 mL of water. Compare with normal blood diluted in the same manner. Blood containing carbon monoxide is pink.
   b. Add 0.1 mL of blood to 2 mL of ammonium hydroxide solution (0.01 mol/L), and vortex-mix for 5 sec. A pink tint in comparison with the colour obtained from a normal blood specimen suggests the presence of COHb.*
   c. Dilute 1 mL of the patient's blood with 10 mL of water in a test tube and add to it 1 mL of a 5% solution of sodium hydroxide. If COHb is present, the solution will turn straw yellow (20% COHb) or pink (>20% COHb). In the case of normal blood (HbO_2) the solution turns brown in colour.

   All the bedside tests are only screening tests and the results must be confirmed by other methods mentioned earlier, especially spectrophotometric estimation of COHb level.

Treatment

1. Immediate removal from the contaminated environment.
2. Oxygen (100%) through a tight-fitting mask or endotracheal tube, until COHb falls to 15–20%.
3. Monitor cardiac and respiratory status.
4. Patients who only develop minor symptoms such as headache, nausea and transient vomiting, who have normal mental status examinations, and who are not pregnant may be treated with 100% oxygen, and discharged when asymptomatic.
5. Watch for the development of cerebral oedema with serial neurologic exams, CAT scans and fundoscopic examination. Hyperventilation (PCO_2 25–30 mm Hg), head eleva-

Note: *Cyanide also gives a similar tint and hence must be ruled out.*

tion (35°) and mannitol (0.25–1 g/kg of 20% solution over 30 min) are recommended as initial management of raised intracranial pressure.

6. If metabolic acidosis persists despite correction of hypoxia and adequate fluid resuscitation consider correction with IV sodium bicarbonate.
7. Administer supplemental glucose to prevent hypoglycaemia.
8. Convulsions can be controlled with IV diazepam or phenytoin in the usual manner.
9. Correct hypotension by adequate fluid resuscitation with a crystalloid. Treat brady and tachyarrhythmias appropriately. Vasopressors and inotropes can be initiated in an emergency through peripheral venous access.
10. Physical activity should be restricted for at least 1 month after the exposure to minimise the incidence of cerebral demyelination.
11. **Antidote**: Several authorities consider administration of **hyperbaric oxygen (HBO)** to be antidotal in its effects in carbon monoxide poisoning (**Fig. 9.94**). It involves inhalation of oxygen at a pressure greater than 1 atmosphere absolute (ATA). 100% oxygen at ambient pressure reduces the half-life of COHb to 40 min, while at 2.5 atmospheres absolute it is reduced to just 20 min. Hyperbaric oxygen should be instituted with 30 min of 100% oxygen at 3 ATA, followed by 2 ATA for 60 min or until a COHb level less than 10% is achieved.
    a. It must be borne in mind, however that HBO therapy is associated with serious risks such as cerebral gas embolism, rupture of tympanic membranes, visual deficits, reversible myopia, sweating, palpitations, syncope, claustrophobia and oxygen toxicity (convulsions and pulmonary oedema). So, the routine administration of HBO is not recommended in every case of CO poisoning.
    b. Hyperbaric oxygen is also used in the treatment of poisoning due to cyanide, hydrogen sulphide, smoke, methylene chloride and carbon tetrachloride.

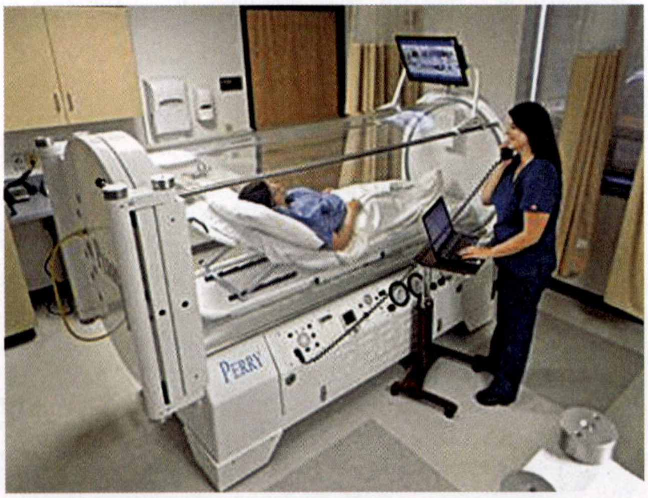

Fig. 9.94 Hyperbaric chamber with reclining facility

Autopsy Features

- Cherry red (pink) colour of skin, especially noticeable in the areas of postmortem lividity. In dark complexioned individuals, the colour can be made out more easily in the inner aspects of lips, nail beds, tongue and palms and soles.
- Cutaneous bullae (skin blisters) are sometimes seen in the regions of the calves, buttocks, wrists and knees.
- Cherry pink colour of blood and tissues. If blood is diluted with water in a test tube and held against light or a white background, the pink colour will be more easily made out.
- Pulmonary oedema.
- The white matter of the brain is said to be firmer than usual in CO poisoning, and the brain as a whole retains its shape better after removal from the skull cavity.
- In delayed deaths, necrosis and cavitation of basal ganglia, especially globus pallidus and putamen are commonly described features. Petechiae and ring shaped haemorrhages may be seen in the white matter. Heart may show focal areas of necrosis.
- It is mandatory to collect blood for chemical analysis preferably from a peripheral vein. But unlike in other cases of poisoning, if blood is difficult to obtain from a vein, heart blood or blood from body cavities or even bone marrow can be used for analysis. Sodium fluoride may be added as a preservative.

Forensic Issues

- Next to carbon dioxide, carbon monoxide is the most abundant atmospheric pollutant and is progressively increasing in concentration. Apart from its role as an environmental contaminant, CO is responsible for a significant number of deaths encountered in forensic practice. Once upon a time, when domestic gas consisted of **coal gas** (which contained upto 7% CO), suicides accomplished with it at home were very common in Western countries. "Putting the head in the gas oven" was the most common form of self-destruction in countries such as the UK. Now that coal gas has been replaced by **natural gas** (which contains little or no CO), a major means of domestic suicide has been removed. But, incomplete combustion of natural gas can release CO which can cause accidental poisoning in ill-ventilated areas.
- Today, the suicidal use of CO is utilised in a different way. The victim utilises the exhaust fumes of a motor car either by merely sitting in a closed garage with a window of the car open while the fumes build up in the enclosed area, or a device is fitted (e.g., a hose) to pipe the gas into the interior of the car with all windows rolled up (**Fig. 9.95**). Such cases are however less common in India and other Asian countries while they are quite frequently reported in Western countries. The use of catalytic converters in automobiles has lessened the likelihood of death resulting from a suicide attempt via inhalation of exhaust fumes.
- Accidental CO poisoning can occur in several other situations apart from domestic exposure. Internal combustion engine exhaust fumes, malfunctioning home heating systems, gas hot water heaters, gas clothes dryers, charcoal

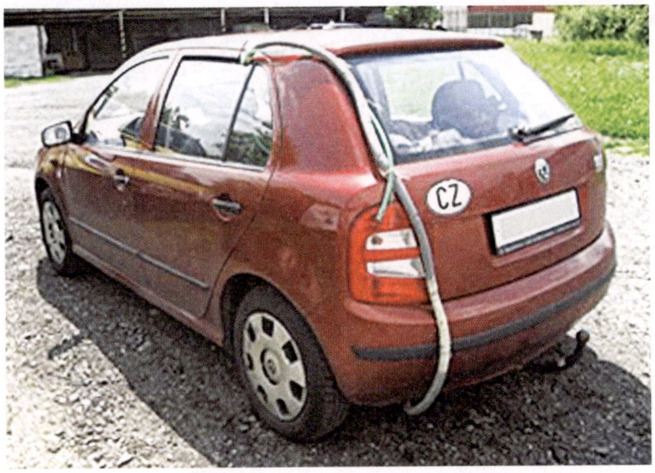

Fig. 9.95 Car with exhaust pipe connection into interior for suicide

and poorly vented wood/coal stoves, space heaters, gas and kerosene lanterns, and fires in buildings are common sources of carbon monoxide poisoning. Defective exhaust system of an automobile can allow gas to percolate through the floor or engine bulkhead into the interior. Sometimes, the driver may become so affected that he loses control of the vehicle resulting in a crash.

- **Tobacco smoke** is an important source of carbon monoxide contamination of environment. Mainstream cigarette smoke, which is inhaled into the smoker's lungs can contain as much as 5% carbon monoxide by volume. Sidestream smoke, the source of environmental exposures, contains between 70% and 90% of the total CO per cigarette.
- A common cause of accidental CO poisoning resulting in mass deaths is a **conflagration**, wherein a large building (hotel, theatre, block of flats, etc.) goes up in flames. The majority of deaths in such cases are caused by inhalation of smoke (containing CO) rather than by burns.
- Homicidal poisoning with CO is rare, but cases have been reported (and continue to be reported) from time to time.

CYANIDE

Physical Appearance

- **Cyanide** occurs as a gas or liquid or solid.
  - In its gaseous state, it is referred to as **hydrogen cyanide (HCN)**.
  - The liquid form is referred to as **hydrocyanic acid** or **Prussic acid**.
  - Salts of cyanide occur as solids (white, crystalline powder): **Sodium cyanide, Potassium cyanide**, etc.
- The **odour** of cyanide, especially the gas, is described as "**bitter almond**" in nature. However, it cannot be perceived by everybody. 20–40% of the human population (mostly males) do not possess this capacity which is inherited as a sex-linked recessive trait. Some sources put this at 40–60%.
- **Hydrogen cyanide** is a colourless flammable gas with a faint bitter almond odour. It exists as a yellow/brown liquid below 26°C.
- **Hydrocyanic acid** is a bluish-white liquid with a faint, bitter almond odour.
- **Cyanogen** is a colourless, flammable gas with a pungent, almond-like odour. Salts include cyanogen bromide, cyanogen chloride and cyanogen azide.
- **Potassium, sodium and calcium cyanides** are white, deliquescent, noncombustible solids with a faint bitter almond odour.
- The taste of cyanide has been described as bitter and burning in nature.

Uses

1. *Industrial*: Electroplating, metal processing, production of synthetic rubber, and manufacture of plastics.
2. *Agriculture*: Insecticide and rodenticide; hydrogen cyanide is used as a fumigant pesticide.
3. *Medicinal*:
   a. **Laetrile** (synthetic amygdalin) is sometimes used as a chemotherapeutic agent for cancer, though studies have shown it is not efficacious, and in fact can be hazardous.
   b. **Sodium nitroprusside** is an effective antihypertensive and is especially useful in treating hypertensive crisis as an intravenous infusion. But, it is metabolised in the body to cyanide and infusions exceeding the recommended dose can lead to cyanide toxicity.
4. *Laboratory*: Cyanide is used in various laboratory processes.
5. *Household*: Household uses of cyanide include silver-polishing, and as fertilizers, rodenticides, and insecticides.

Sources

1. *Plants*: Cyanide is present in the form of **cyanogenic glycosides** in a wide variety of plants and plant parts (**Table 9.22**). Hydrolysis of these glycosides by digestive enzymes can release cyanide in the GI tract. The **seeds** (often called kernels) of many species of plants belonging to family Rosaceae, especially prunus and malus species, lie within the fruit stone (**endocarp**; also called pits). The fruit stones and surrounding fruit are generally not toxic; however, seeds within the fruit stones could contain cyanogenic glycosides.
2. *Combustion*:
   a. Burning of plastic furniture (polyurethane or polyacrylonitrile).
   b. Burning of silk or wool.
   c. Cigarette smoking – each cigarette liberates 150–200 mcg of HCN.
3. Cyanide can be released by hepatic metabolism from various nitrile compounds, such as malononitrile, succinonitrile, acetonitrile, etc., following absorption into the body.

Usual Fatal Dose

- **Hydrogen cyanide**:
  - Inhalation of 1 part in 2000 can kill instantaneously, 1 part in 10,000 within a few minutes, 1 part in 50,000 within a few hours.
- **Hydrocyanic acid: 50–100 mg**.

Table 9.22 Cyanogenic Plants

Plant	Toxic Part	Cyanogenic Glycoside
Prunus species: cherry laurel, chokeberry, bitter almond, peach, apricot, plum	Leaf, bark, seed	Prunasin or Amygdalin
Sorghum species: sorghum, sudan grass, arrow grass	Grain, shoot	Dhurrin
Malus species: apple, pear	Seed	Amygdalin
Cassava, lima beans	Bean, root	Linamarin
Miscellany: christmas berry, elderberry, bamboo, cycad nut	Seed, leaf, shoot	Unclear

- **Cyanide salts (sodium, potassium or calcium): 100–200 mg**. Specifically for potassium or sodium cyanide, the minimum lethal dose has been estimated to be about 3 mg/kg.
- **Bitter almonds** (derived from *Prunus amygdalus var. amara*, a plant which grows in Kashmir) (**Fig. 9.96**): 50–80 in number.

Toxicokinetics

- Absorption is rapid across mucous membranes. Cyanogen is readily absorbed through intact skin resulting in systemic toxicity.
- Ingestion of cyanide salts results in the release of HCN through the action of hydrochloric acid in the stomach, and is subsequently absorbed as the cyanide ion (CN^-).
- Cyanide is distributed to all organs and tissues via the blood, where its concentration in red cells is greater than that in plasma by a factor of 2 or 3.
- Metabolism occurs mainly in the form of conversion to thiocyanate by the enzyme ***rhodanese*** (present in the mitochondria of liver and kidneys), which needs sodium thiosulphate for effective functioning.
- Once the relatively nontoxic metabolite thiocyanate is formed, it is excreted mainly in the urine. Small amounts of cyanide are excreted in the breath and sweat producing the characteristic bitter almond odour.
- About 80% of cyanide detoxification occurs by the route described above. Other endogenous methods of cyanide detoxification include binding to methaemoglobin, reaction with cysteine and incorporation into choline and methionine.
  - Some of the cyanide is converted to cyanacobalamin (vitamin B_{12}) in the presence of hydroxocobalamin (vitamin B_{12a}).

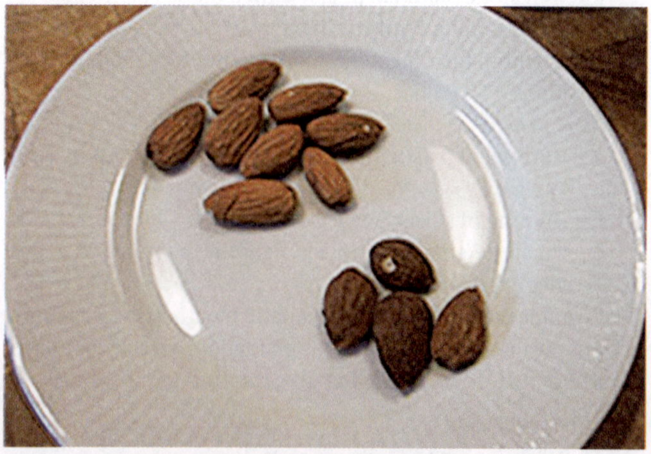

Fig. 9.96 Normal almonds and Bitter almonds

Mode of Action

- The toxic effect of cyanide is mainly attributed to its production of a **histotoxic anoxia by inhibition of cytochrome oxidase**. This is a metalloenzyme essential for oxidative phosphorylation which is responsible for aerobic energy production. Cyanide inhibits cytochrome oxidase at the cytochrome aa_3 portion of the enzyme. As a result of the consequent reduced ATP production, tissues resort to anaerobic energy production which is a less efficient alternative pathway for formation of ATP. Pyruvic acid no longer enters the Krebs cycle, but is converted to lactic acid which accumulates and results in metabolic (lactic) acidosis. The degree of lactic acidosis correlates with the severity of poisoning.
- Aside from cytochrome oxidase, cyanide also inhibits succinic dehydrogenase, superoxide dismutase, carbonic anhydrase and several other enzymes.

Clinical Features

I. **Acute Poisoning**:

1. Inhalation produces the most rapid and serious exposures resulting in almost immediate coma, while ingestion causes less rapid onset because of slower entry into the circulation, and passage of cyanide through the portal system where the liver metabolises some of it by the first-pass effect.*
2. *CNS*: Headache, anxiety, agitation, confusion, convulsions and coma. Pupils are often dilated.

**Note*: *Rapid onset of coma in suspected poisoning usually indicates one of the following: cyanide, carbon monoxide, hydrogen sulphide, nicotine or powerful opiate/barbiturate.*

3. *CVS*: Initial tachycardia and hypertension, followed by bradycardia and hypotension and ventricular dysrhythmias.
4. *RS*: Tachypnoea followed by bradypnoea, and cardiogenic or non-cardiogenic pulmonary oedema. Cyanosis is generally a late finding.
5. *GIT*: Ingestion of cyanide salts results in nausea, vomiting and abdominal pain. Some salts cause corrosion.
6. *Skin*:
   i. **Bright (brick) red colour** of skin and mucous membranes is said to be characteristic. It is due to increased haemoglobin oxygen saturation in venous blood because of decreased utilisation of oxygen by tissues. It can be made out better in retinal vessels on fundoscopic examination.
   ii. The skin feels cold and clammy to the touch.
7. *Acid–base*: Anion gap metabolic acidosis and lactic acidosis are common.

II. **Chronic Poisoning**:
1. Survivors of serious poisoning may develop delayed neurologic sequelae, especially in the form of Parkinsonian symptoms – akinesia, rigidity (*cog wheel type*), dystonia, dysarthria and tremor. CAT scan or MRI often reveals basal ganglia damage. Cases of patients developing sequelae such as personality changes, paranoid psychosis and memory deficits have also been reported.
2. Chronic exposure is associated with headache, vertigo, tremors, weakness, fatigue, dizziness, confusion, motor aphasia, optic neuropathy, seizures, paresis/hemiparesis, myelopathy and permanent mental impairment.
3. Chronic, low-level exposure may result in any of the following:
   i. ***Tobacco amblyopia***: Progressive loss of visual function seen in heavy smokers. Cessation of smoking and administration of hydroxocobalamin may reverse the visual impairment.
   ii. ***Leber's hereditary optic atrophy***: Congenital deficiency of rhodanese is suspected in this condition which exclusively affects males and results in acute visual failure due to the sensitivity of optic nerve to cyanide. Hydroxocobalamin may be beneficial.
   iii. ***Tropical ataxic neuropathy (Nigerian nutritional ataxic neuropathy)***: It is prevalent among populations consuming large quantities of **cassava** or **tapioca (*manihot*)** (**Fig. 9.97**). This tuber contains two cyanogens – linamarin and lotaustralin which can be removed only by proper fermentation techniques. Symptoms include peripheral sensory neuropathy, optic atrophy (tropical amblyopia), ataxia, deafness, glossitis, stomatitis and scrotal dermatitis.
   iv. A related condition resulting from chronic consumption of improperly processed bitter cassava is ***Konzo*** which produces spastic paraparesis.

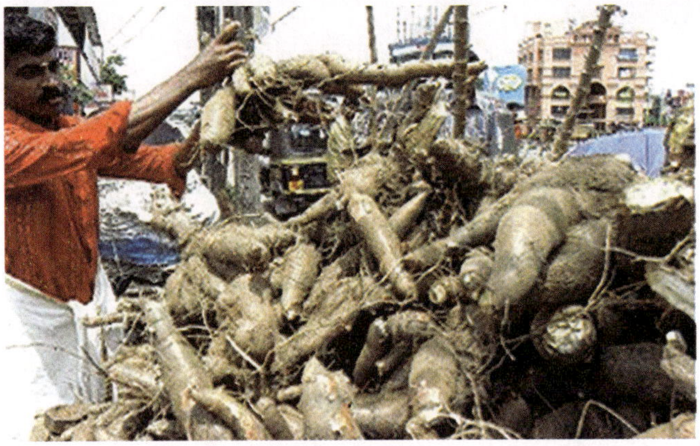

Fig. 9.97 Cassava (Tapioca) roots

   v. Workers, such as electroplaters and picklers, who are exposed daily to cyanide solutions may develop a "**cyanide rash**", characterized by itching, and by macular, papular and vesicular eruptions.
   vi. Abnormal thyroid function tests have been reported following chronic cyanide exposure in the occupational setting.

Diagnosis

- Characteristic **bitter almond odour** in the vicinity of the patient.
- ***Lee-Jones test***:
  - Add a few crystals of ferrous sulphate to 5 mL of gastric aspirate.
  - Add 5 drops of 2% sodium hydroxide
  - Boil and cool.
  - Add 10 drops of 10% hydrochloric acid.
  - Interpret: Greenish-blue colour indicates cyanide, while purplish colour indicates salicylates.
- *Serum cyanide level*: This is confirmatory, but difficult to accomplish in practice. Normal serum level is less than 0.004 μg/ml for non-smokers and 0.006 μg/mL for smokers. Whole-blood levels are higher than serum levels – 0.016 μg/mL for non-smokers and 0.041 μg/ml for smokers.
  - Blood cyanide levels greater than 3 μg/mL (SI = 115 μmol/L) are generaly fatal.
- *Laboratory findings*:
  - Serum lactate level more than 7–10 mmol/L. The degree of lactic acidosis correlates well with the severity of poisoning.
  - Elevated serum anion gap.
  - Elevated venous oxygen saturation.
- *ECG*: Erratic atrial and ventricular cardiac rhythms with varying degrees of AV block, followed by asystole may be seen in severe cyanide poisoning. ST-T segment elevation or depression may occur.
- *Fundoscopic examination*: Retinal arteries and veins that appear equally red on fundoscopic examination is suggestive of cyanide poisoning.

Treatment

Time is of The Essence! Do Not Delay!

1. *Stabilisation*: Assisted ventilation, 100% oxygen, cardiac monitoring, IV access, treatment of metabolic acidosis, vasopressors for hypotension.
2. *Decontamination*:
   a. Cutaneous exposure – Remove clothing and wash skin with soap and water.
   b. Ingestion – Stomach wash (preferably with 5% sodium thiosulphate solution), activated charcoal and cathartics, after antidotal therapy has been instituted.
   c. Haemodialysis and haemoperfusion are NOT effective.
3. *Antidotal therapy*:
   a. ***The 3-step Eli Lilly cyanide kit approach***
      i. **First step**:
         - **Amyl nitrite** (one perle of 0.2 mL is crushed and inhaled for 30 sec) every min until the 2nd step is begun.
         - *Alternative administration methods*:
           - Administer amyl nitrite via a nebulizer or
           - Give amyl nitrite via an inhaler device; may be particularly useful, if there are many victims
      ii. **Second step**:
         - **Sodium nitrite** (3% soln) slow IV, i.e., over 5–10 min.
         - Adult dose – 10 mL (300 mg).
         - Paediatric dose – 0.33 mL/kg, up to a maximum of 10 mL.
         - Exceeding the recommended dose can result in fatality.
         - Methaemoglobinaemia.
      iii. **Third step**
         - **Sodium thiosulphate** (25% soln), 3–5 mL/min, IV Adult dose – 50 mL (12.5 g).
         - Paediatric dose – 1.65 ml/kg (412.5 mg/kg), up to a maximum of 50 mL.
         - Both sodium nitrite and sodium thiosulphate can be repeated at half the initial dose at the end of 1 hr, if symptoms persist or reappear.
         - *Mechanism of action of nitrites:* Nitrites induce methaemoglobinaemia which causes the detachment of cyanide from the haem group of cytochrome oxidase. Amyl nitrite perles are meant to be a temporizing measure until sodium nitrite can be administered intravenously. If vascular access is easy, and the patient is severely poisoned, amyl nitrite may be omitted and IV sodium nitrite and sodium thiosulphate should be administered.
         - *Mechanism of action of sodium thiosulphate:* It enables the enzyme rhodanese to catabolise cyanide to non-toxic thiocyanate which is excreted in the urine.
   b. ***Other Antidotes***:
      i. **4-Dimethylaminophenol (4-DMAP)**: It is the agent of choice to induce methaemoglobinaemia in Europe (as opposed to the USA where nitrites are more popular). 4-DMAP can sometimes produce unexpectedly high levels of methaemoglobin which can be life-threatening. Dose: 3 mg/kg, IV
      ii. **Dicobalt edetate (Cobalt-EDTA)**: It acts by chelating cyanide without inducing methaemoglobinaemia. Cobalt-EDTA is used in Britain and France under the brand name ***Kelocyanor***. The edetate (ethylene diamine tetra acetate) part of the antidote is included only to minimise the toxicity of cobalt.
      Dose: 20 mL of 1.5% soln (300 mg) IV over 1 min followed by 50 mL of 50% dextrose.
      iii. **Hydroxocobalamin** (Vitamin B_{12} precursor): It combines with cyanide to form cyanacobalamin (vitamin B_{12}), which is excreted in the urine.
      Dose: 200 mL of 25 mg/mL (5 g) IV over 15 min. A second dose of 5 g can be given over 15 min to 2 hrs depending on the severity of the poisoning.
      iv. **Alpha-ketoglutaric acid**: It is presently only in the experimental stage, but shows a great deal of promise since it binds with cyanide to render it non-toxic without inducing methaemoglobinaemia.
      v. **Pyruvate, mercaptopyruvate, sulphur sulphanes, and stroma-free methaemoglobin solutions** have been tried in animal studies, but are not yet recommended for human use.
      vi. **Hyperbaric oxygen**: The Undersea Medical Society has classified cyanide poisoning as a disorder for which hyperbaric oxygen therapy is useful. However, existing medical literature indicates that the role of hyperbaric oxygen is of doubtful value.
      vii. **Methylene blue is NOT an antidote for cyanide** and must NOT be used. However, if significant methaemoglobinaemia occurs due to use of amyl/sodium nitrite, methylene blue may have to be administered.
4. *Other measures*:
   a. If metabolic acidosis persists despite correction of hypoxia and adequate fluid resuscitation consider correction with IV sodium bicarbonate. In adults, an initial dose of 50 mmol may be given and repeated as necessary, guided by arterial blood gas monitoring (aim for a pH of 7.44 [Hydrogen ion concentration 36]). In children, use 8.4% sodium bicarbonate diluted in an equal volume of 5% glucose and give a "calculated" dose: dose (in mmol) = desired change in base deficit (current-target) × 0.3 × weight of child up to a maximum of 50 mmol. Administer at a rate of 1 mmol/minute.
   b. Control convulsions that are frequent or prolonged with IV diazepam (10–20 mg in adults; 0.1-0.3 mg/kg in children), lorazepam (4 mg in adults and 0.1 mg/kg in children), or midazolam (5–10 mg in adults; 0.05–0.15 mg/kg in children). If convulsions are unresponsive to initial treatment, second-line therapy is phenobarbitone sodium (10 mg/kg at maximum rate of 100 mg/min; maxi-

mum dose 1 g). An alternative is phenytoin (loading dose 18 mg/kg IV infusion in adults and children, given via slow IV [maximum rate 50 mg/min] over 20–30 min with BP and ECG monitoring). Thiopentone sodium is the preferred antiepileptic for status epilepticus not responding to the above measures.

c. Correct hypotension by adequate fluid resuscitation with a crystalloid. Treat brady and tachyarrhythmias appropriately. Poisoned patients with fluid-resistant hypotension can deteriorate extremely rapidly and should be managed by experienced physicians. Vasopressors and inotropes can be initiated in an emergency through peripheral venous access.

d. For acute lung injury: Maintain adequate ventilation and oxygenation with frequent monitoring of arterial blood gases and/or pulse oximetry. If a high FIO_2 is required to maintain adequate oxygenation, mechanical ventilation and positive-end-expiratory pressure (PEEP) may be required.

Autopsy Features

I. **External**:
1. Odour of bitter almonds.
2. Bright (brick) red colour of skin (**Fig. 9.98**) and mucous membranes. It is especially evident in areas of postmortem lividity.
3. Cyanosis of extremities.
4. Froth at mouth and nostrils (may be blood-stained).

II. **Internal**:
1. Haemorrhagic gastritis (ingestion death). Stomach wall may appear hardened.
2. Pulmonary and cerebral oedema.
3. Disseminated petechiae in brain, meninges, pleura, lungs and pericardium.

The most appropriate fluids and tissues to remove for chemical analysis are blood, stomach contents, lung, liver, kidney, brain, heart and spleen. Lung should be sent intact, sealed in a nylon bag (**not** a plastic or polyvinylchloride bag). **Spleen** is said to be the best specimen for cyanide analysis, since it generally has the highest concentration of the poison owing to a strong presence of RBC.

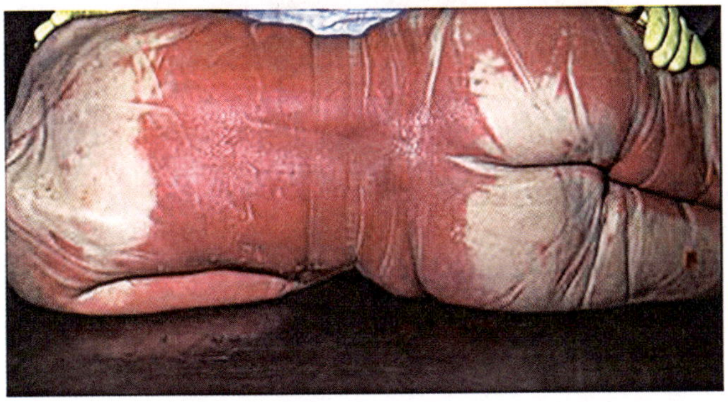

Fig. 9.98 Bright (brick) red colour of postmortem lividity – Cyanide poisoning

Forensic Issues

1. **Homicide**:

The very mention of cyanide to a lay person would make him think of murder. Like arsenic and strychnine, cyanide has a reputation (quite unfounded) of being a homicidal poisoner's favourite, probably because of the perpetuation of such a notion in popular detective fiction. But, the reality is that except for certain exceptional situations, its employment in murder has been quite rare.

There are at least two features that go against the concept of cyanide being an ideal homicidal poison – its possible detection by smell, and the suspicion likely to be aroused by the dramatic nature of death. However, a few notorious killers in India (especially serial killers) have used cyanide quite successfully without arousing suspicion (**Box 9.5**).

Elsewhere in the world, cyanide has been more commonly employed in the commission of **mass murder**, for e.g., the **genocide of Jews** perpetrated by the **Nazis** during the second world war. Initially, the Nazis used carbon monoxide, but later in order to expedite their gory task, they began employing hydrogen cyanide (***zyklon B***) (**Fig. 9.99**). Up to 10,000 innocent people per day were butchered by this "efficient" gas and the final tally ran into millions. Earlier during the first world war, HCN was used as a war gas but was quickly replaced by other more effective war gases such as nitrogen mustard.

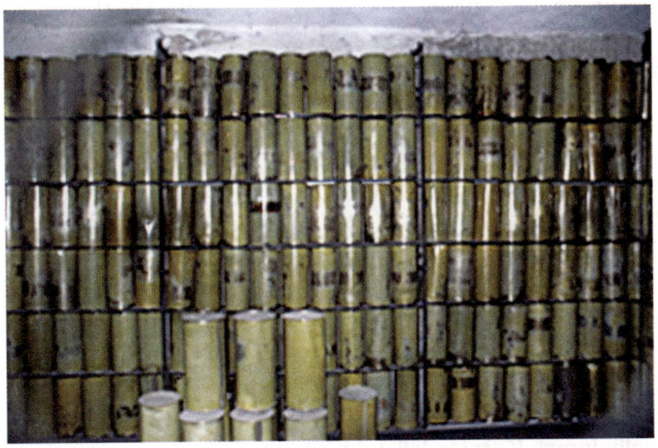

Fig. 9.99 Empty canisters of Zyklon B recovered from a Nazi concentration camp

Box 9.5—India's Serial Cyanide Killers

KD Kempamma (Cyanide Mallika), is India's first convicted female serial killer. Commencing with her first murder in 1999, Kempamma killed 6 women over the next 8 years. She befriended victims from female temple devotees and portrayed herself as a deeply pious woman. After gaining their confidence, she would call them to another temple, ask them to dress in their best clothing and jewellery, and give them 'holy water' with cyanide to drink. She was caught

contd.

by police trying to dispose of some of the jewellery, and confessed under interrogation. She was the first woman to be sentenced to death in Karnataka (now commuted to life in prison).

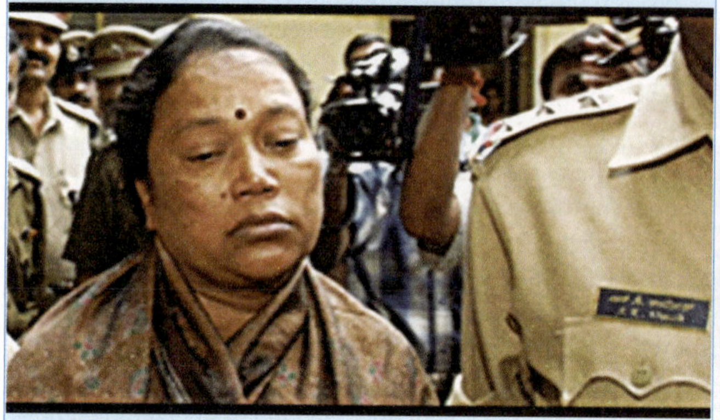

KD Kempamma

Mohan Kumar Vivekanand (Cyanide Mohan), is a serial killer who preyed on women looking for marriage. He was a primary school physical education teacher before embarking on a life of crime. A Mangalore fast track court tried and convicted him for the murder of 20 women. He was accused of luring women who were unable to pay dowry, or were unable to find suitable husbands. He would kill them by giving them cyanide pills, claiming they were contraceptives, and rob them of their jewellery. Mohan Kumar was charged with 20 murders and unsuccessfully defended himself in court. He was sentenced to death in December 2013.

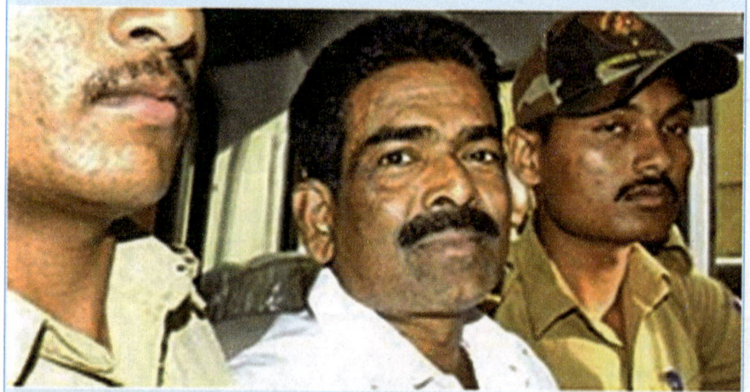

Mohan Kumar

Jolly Joseph (Cyanide Jolly) is the prime suspect in the murder of six members of the family she married into, in the Kozhikode district of Kerala. Jolly is originally from Idukki district, and a first year college dropout. She married her first husband Roy Thomas in 1997. Jolly and Roy had two sons. Jolly lied to neighbours about being an MCom graduate and having a job at the prestigious National Institute of Technology, Calicut. However, her true where abouts during her daily outings to fake her "job" remains uncertain. In 2011, her husband Roy Thomas died under mysterious circumstances, followed by 5 more unnatural deaths in her family over a period of 14 years. Following the murder of Shaju Zachariah's wife (a relative) in 2016, Jolly married him. It was Rojo Thomas, Roy Thomas' brother, who complained to the police about the six unnatural deaths in the family, the investigation of which led to Jolly Joseph. Following her arrest in October 2019, Jolly confessed to using cyanide to kill the six aforementioned people. She allegedly obtained the cyanide with the help of another relative who was friends with a goldsmith having access to cyanide. **Jolly is awaiting trial and has not been convicted yet**.

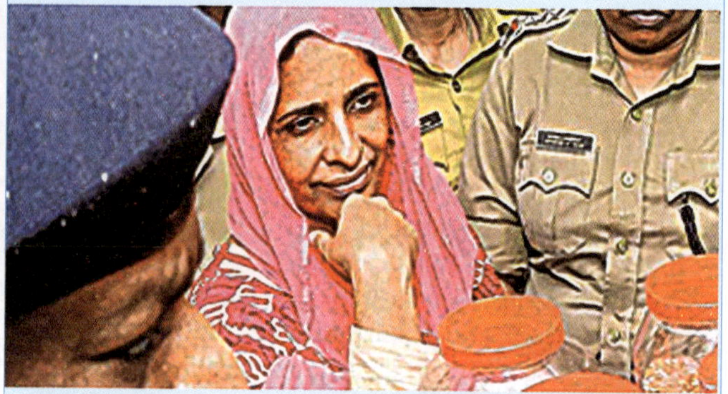

Jolly Joseph

Velanki Simhadri (Cyanide Siva) was arrested by the Andhra Pradesh Police for 10 murders in 2019. He used cyanide to eliminate his victims. Those murdered included Siva's grandmother and his sister-in-law. He gave cyanide to his victims as "prasad" to help them get rid of their problems. Once the victim died, he would steal his/her gold and cash. Relatives of one of the victims got suspicious about the cause of death that took place on Oct 16. At the time of his death, the victim (Nagaraju) was carrying with him Rs 2 lakhs and five gold sovereigns. But when the body was found, gold and cash were missing. Police sources said, "After a formal police complaint was filed, CCTV footage retracing Nagaraju's movements was scanned and it was seen that Nagaraju was talking to the accused. Initially, he admitted to Nagaraju's murder only, but on examining his call record, we found he was linked to several other deaths. He later admitted to have killed nine others". Siva had suffered major losses in property business. To make good those losses, he murdered his victims by administering them cyanide, and gathered around Rs 24 lakhs in cash and gold worth 35 sovereigns. **He is awaiting trial and has not been convicted yet**.

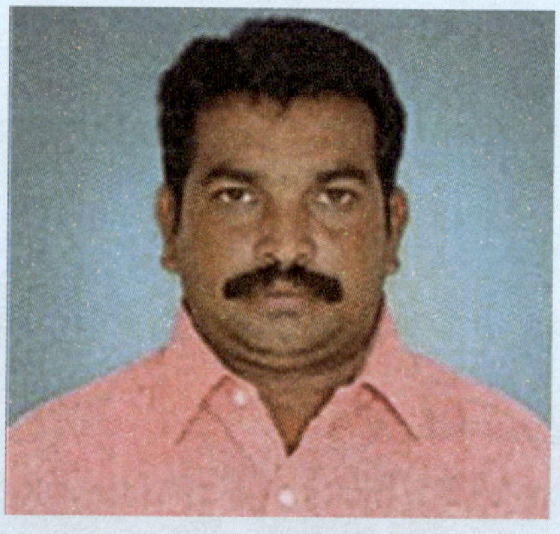

Velanki Simhadri

More recently, mass homicide (albeit on a much smaller scale) was accomplished with the help of cyanide by **Jim Jones** (**Fig. 9.100**), a self-styled preacher who founded a cult called the **People's Temple** in 1974, in California, USA. This "religious" sect comprising mainly mentally afflicted individuals, cripples, drug addicts and ex-convicts, soon moved to Guyana due to local public disapproval. In November 1978, most of them (numbering around 900) died after drinking a cyanide solution prepared by Dr Schat, a medical officer of the cult on instructions issued by Jones. The latter shot himself to death. The reason for such an abrupt and bizarre end to this cult is unclear, though it may have been triggered off by rumours of imminent investigations into the sect's activities by a group of relatives of some cult members.

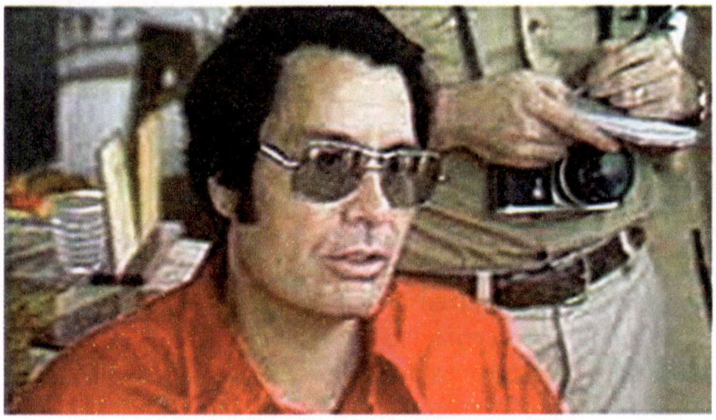

Fig. 9.100 Jim Jones

A different type of mass poisoning resulted in 1982 in Chicago, USA, when paracetamol capsules (*Tylenol*) were deliberately tampered and laced with hydrogen cyanide. Seven innocent victims died. In 1986, capsules of another brand of analgesic (*Excedrin*) were tampered and laced with cyanide by a woman, Stella Nichols whose intended victim was her own husband, Bruce Nichols. She succeeded, but also inadvertently killed another victim in the process (Susan Snow). Stella was convicted and sentenced to life imprisonment on May 9, 1988.

Cyanide has been used to kill convicted criminals in some of the states of the USA, gassing with it being the **official mode of execution** in these states. However, most of these states have of late either switched over to lethal injection, or offer the latter as an option to gassing. Only 6 states (Arizona, California, Maryland, Mississippi, Missouri, Wyoming) authorize lethal gas, and that too only if lethal injection is not possible, or the condemned person chooses to die in the gas chamber.

While cyanide has always been touted as a rapidly acting, sure-fire killer, there have been some notable instances where it failed to live up to its reputation. One such celebrated case involved the murder of the Russian monk **Grigori Rasputin** (**Fig. 9.101**) by Prince Yussoupov, who resented the former's increasing power and influence. The Prince invited Rasputin one day to his mansion for dinner

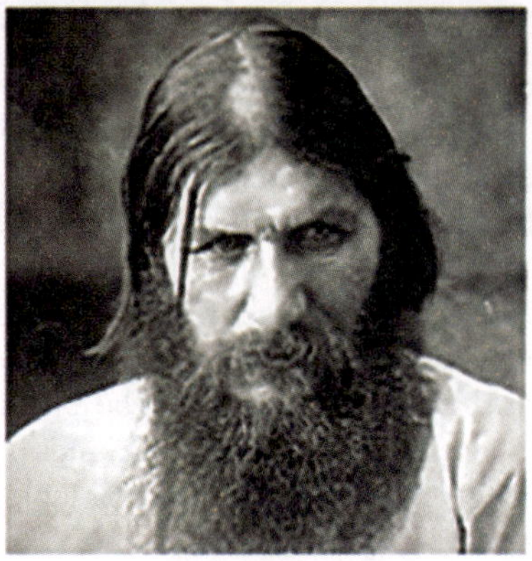

Fig. 9.101 Grigori Rasputin

and plied him with cyanide-laced cakes. The monk ate two of the cakes with great relish which should have been sufficient in the normal course to have killed several men, and yet he suffered no ill effects.

Subsequently, Prince Yussoupov and his fellow conspirators had to shoot him, club him and drown him in ice cold water of a nearby river before Rasputin finally succumbed.

2. **Suicide**:
The use of cyanide for suicide is relatively uncommon in the general population, but in certain occupational groups having ready access to cyanide it may be employed more frequently, e.g., pharmacists, chemists and medical or paramedical personnel.

It is perhaps poetic justice that at the conclusion of the Second World War, several Nazi officers (responsible for the gassing to death of thousands of Jews with cyanide gas) themselves committed suicide with this chemical. Hermann Goering the Field Marshall was one of them.

One of the myths associated with cyanide is that it kills with lightning speed, and while this may be true to a certain extent in some cases of inhalation of the poison in its gaseous form, there is ample evidence to show that in many instances death is delayed for several minutes or even hours.

3. **Accident**:
Accidental exposure to cyanide can occur in a number of ways. Since hydrogen cyanide is occasionally used for fumigation (ships, greenhouses), deaths can occur from negligence. Industrial and laboratory mishaps involving this chemical are also not infrequent.

The significant presence of cyanide in smoke emitted by the combustion of polyurethane articles, silk and woollen clothing, as well as celluloid film is now a well-established fact. This undoubtedly contributes to the mortality in conflagrations.

A comparitively lesser known danger is that associated with the seeds and kernels of **cyanogenic fruits**. Serious poisoning and even deaths have been reported (especially in children) from the ingestion of apricot kernels which is considered a delicacy in some countries of the Middle

East. Apricot kernels are sometimes also ingested as a cure for cancer. Therefore, case reports often relate to patients who have (intentionally) ingested large numbers of apricot kernels as an alternative remedy. The most toxic of all cyanogenic fruits is bitter almond (**Fig. 9.96**), the oil of which is sometimes used as a flavouring agent and can occasionally cause serious poisoning. Sweet almonds are non-toxic. Bitter almonds are reported to be poisonous in small quantities, with 10 bitter almonds said to be a fatal dose in children. Chronic consumption of certain kinds of foods rich in cyanogenic glycosides (e.g., cassava or tapioca) can cause debilitating neurological ailments.

METHYL ISOCYANATE

Synonyms

Isocyanatomethane, Isocyanic acid, Methyl ester, MIC

Physical Appearance

- Colourless liquid with a sharp odour, which becomes gaseous at 39°C.
- It is an extremely reactive chemical and needs to be stored carefully. Contact with water results in an exothermic reaction.

Uses

- Manufacture of carbaryl (a carbamate pesticide).
- Manufacture of polyurethane articles (plastics, urethane foam, adhesives, etc.).

Mode of Action

- Isocyanate compounds (including MIC) cause toxic effects by two mechanisms: they cause irritation to the mucous membranes, eyes and respiratory tract; and they also cause sensitisation, and by this means can induce an immunological response, particularly bronchospasm.
- The exact immunological mechanism remains uncertain, but acute exposure has been associated with a type I hypersensitivity response that causes an early asthmatic response. High concentrations or repeated exposure may also cause delayed IgG mediated hypersensitivity associated with airway inflammation that persists for months or years after initial exposure.

Usual Fatal Dose

- At 2 ppm, no odour is generally discernible, but irritation and lacrimation may be noted. Symptoms become more marked at 4 ppm and unbearable at 21 ppm.

Clinical Features

- Inhalation of MIC gas produces immediate lacrimation, photophobia, lid swelling, and corneal ulceration; cough, choking sensation, dyspnoea, chest pain, haemoptysis, pink frothy discharge from nose and pulmonary oedema; less commonly vomiting, convulsions and coma. Metabolic acidosis has been reported.
- A single exposure can result in sensitisation with subsequent re-exposure causing a delayed severe asthma-like attack. Airway responses can be immediate (onset of symptoms within 30 min), late (after 1 hr or more) or dual, with both immediate and late onset of symptoms.
- Dermal exposure results in erythema and vesiculation.
- Ocular exposure can cause permanent damage. Eyelids are often affected with trachoma formation ("***Bhopal eye syndrome***"). There can also be cataract formation.
- Long-term effects after survival include ***RADS*** (***Reactive Airways Dysfunction Syndrome***), and pregnancy-related problems: high incidence of abortions, and increased perinatal mortality.

Treatment

1. Decontamination of skin and eyes with saline. Remove contact lenses and irrigate exposed eyes with copious amounts of room temperature 0.9% saline or water for at least 15 min. If irritation, pain, swelling, lacrimation or photophobia persist after 15 min of irrigation, an ophthalmologic examination should be performed. Topical antibiotics may be useful in secondary infection. Severe iritis may be treated with topical atropine or homatropine.
2. *Ingestion*: Activated charcoal may be beneficial. Stomach wash is contraindicated. A glass of milk or water to drink may provide symptomatic improvement provided the airway can be protected.
3. *Inhalation*: Covering the face with a wet cloth immediately during exposure may minimize toxicity. Move patient from the toxic environment to fresh air. Monitor for respiratory distress. Observation for 72 hrs is advisable to detect delayed onset of acute lung injury. If cough or difficulty in breathing develops, evaluate for hypoxia, respiratory tract irritation, bronchitis or pneumonitis.
   a. Oxygen, endotracheal intubation, assisted ventilation as required.
   b. Bronchodilators and corticosteroids may be beneficial. Administer $beta_2$ adrenergic agonists, inhaled ipratropium and systemic corticosteroids (e.g., prednisone 1–2 mg/kg/day).
   c. Treat pulmonary oedema and/or acute lung injury with continuous positive airway pressure (CPAP) or in severe cases with IPPV and PEEP.
   d. Antibiotics are indicated only when there is evidence of infection.
4. Supportive measures.

Isocyanates are **not** the same as cyanides and antidotes for the latter such as nitrites and sodium thiosulphate must **not** be used for the former.

Autopsy Features

- Haemorrhages and cerebral oedema, cherry red colour of blood, fatty infiltration of the liver and renal tubular necrosis were the principal autopsy findings of Bhopal victims.
- Signs of asphyxia.
- Pulmonary and cerebral oedema.
- Generalised visceral congestion.

Forensic Issues

- MIC was involved in one of the most devastating gas disasters, which occurred in Bhopal, Madhya Pradesh in 1984, which is by far the most devastating industrial gas accident to ever occur, leaving more than 2000 people dead (unofficial estimates put the figure at more than 10,000), and more than 200,000 injured. It is commonly referred to as the "**Bhopal Gas Tragedy**".
  - The incident occurred in a small pesticides division of Union Carbide Company manufacturing carbaryl (a carbamate) (**Fig. 9.102**), for which methyl isocyanate is required. This deadly chemical was stored in huge, double-walled stainless steel tanks, one of which burst on the night of Dec 02, 1984. More than 24,000 kg of MIC gas escaped over the next several hours into the atmosphere forming an ominous white cloud that drifted rapidly over the surrounding heavily populated neighbourhood killing thousands in their sleep and incapacitating several thousands more (**Fig. 9.103**). Civil and criminal cases were filed in the District Court of Bhopal, India, involving UCC and Warren Anderson, UCC CEO at the time of the disaster.
  - In 2007, more than 10 lakh cases were registered. Number of awarded cases comprised more than 500,000. Total compensation awarded was US$250 million. On 24th June 2010, the Union Cabinet of the Govt of India approved a US$200 million aid package which would be funded by Indian taxpayers through the government.
  - In June 2010, seven ex-employees, including the former UCIL chairman, were convicted in Bhopal of causing death by negligence and sentenced to 2 years imprisonment and a fine of Rs. 1 lakh each. An eighth former employee was also convicted, but died before the judgement was passed.
  - Today, however there is some controversy as to whether MIC was entirely responsible for the disaster. Evidence that hydrogen cyanide gas was the toxic component:
    - Reported cherry-red colour of victims' viscera and blood.
    - Increased thiocyanate levels in the urine of some survivors.
    - Reports of symptomatic relief after administration of sodium thiosulphate.
  - Evidence that hydrogen cyanide gas was **not** the toxic component:
    - No HCN residue was detected in or around the plant or in the most severely affected neighbourhoods surrounding it.
    - No cyanide was reported in tissue samples of victims.
    - The temporal pattern of mortality was not consistent with death due to hydrogen cyanide poisoning.

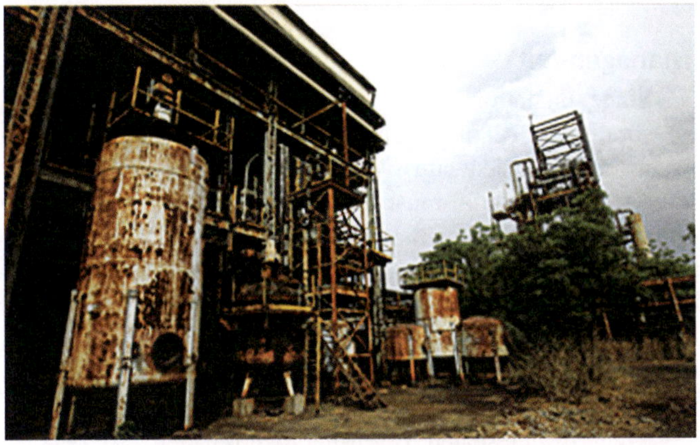

Fig. 9.102 Remains of the Union Carbide Company at Bhopal

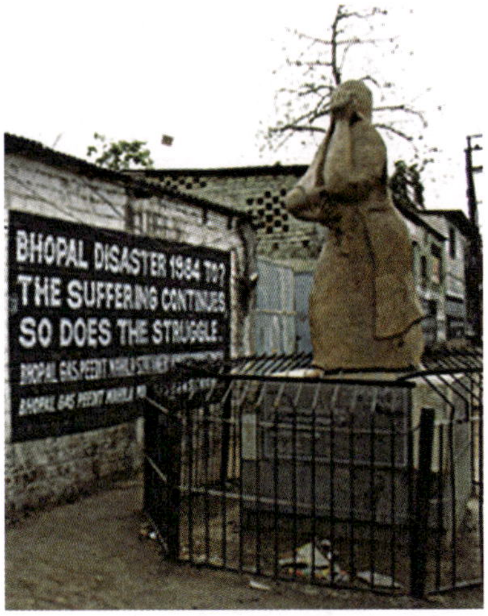
BHOPAL DISASTER 1984
THE SUFFERING CONTINUES
SO DOES THE STRUGGLE

Fig. 9.103 Bhopal memorial for those killed and disabled by the 1984 MIC release

RIOT CONTROL AGENTS

(TEAR GASES; NON-LETHAL LACRIMATORS)

Definition

- A **riot control agent** (formerly referred to as "**tear gas**") is a chemical compound that temporarily incapacitates a person, and makes him/her unable to function by causing irritation to the eyes, mouth, throat, lungs and skin.

Examples

- Chloroacetophenone (CN)
- Chlorobenzylidenemalononitrile (CS)
- Chloropicrin (PS)
- Bromobenzylcyanide (CA)
- Dibenzoxazepine (CR)

Uses

- Riot control agents are used by law enforcement officials for **crowd control**.
- Individuals and the general public can use them for **personal protection**.
  - For this purpose, the commonest agent used is ***capsaicin***, an alkaloid present in Capsicum, which is dispensed

in the form of a spray from a hand-held canister (**pepper spray**) (**Fig. 9.104**).

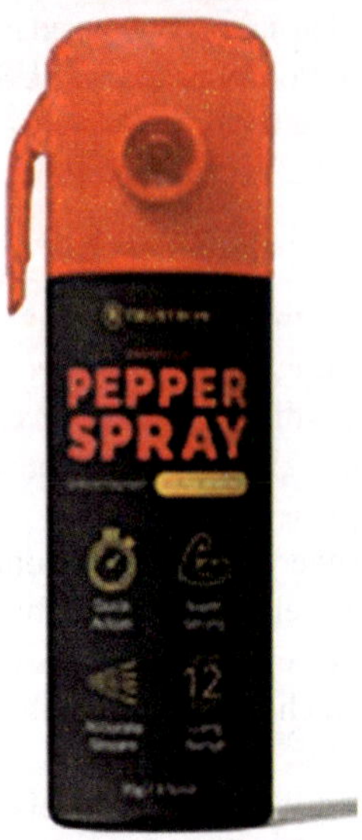

Fig. 9.104 Pepper spray canister

Effects

- Because these agents are either liquids or very fine powder, they are released into the air in the form of grenades which are cast into a rioting crowd, or fired from specialized equipment.
- The crowd gets exposed to these agents through skin contact, eye contact or respiratory system via nose and mouth.
- The effects will depend on the amount of riot control agent to which a person was exposed, the location of exposure (indoors versus outdoors), how the person was exposed and the length of time of the exposure.
- Riot control agents work by causing irritation to the area of contact (e.g., eyes, skin, nose) within seconds of exposure.
- The effects of exposure are usually short-lived (15–30 min) after the person has been removed from the source, and decontaminated (cleaned off).
- People exposed to riot control agents may experience some or all of the following symptoms immediately after exposure:
  - *Eyes*: Excessive tearing, burning, blurred vision, redness.
  - *Nose*: Runny nose, burning, swelling.
  - *Mouth*: Burning, irritation, difficulty swallowing, drooling.
  - *Lungs*: Chest tightness, coughing, choking sensation, wheezing, breathlessness.
  - *Skin*: Burns, rash.
  - *Other*: Nausea and vomiting.
- Long-lasting exposure or exposure to a large dose of riot control agent, especially in a closed setting, may cause severe effects such as the following:
  - Blindness
  - Glaucoma
  - Immediate death due to severe chemical burns to the throat and lungs
  - Respiratory failure possibly resulting in death
- Long-term health effects of exposure to riot control agents:
  - Prolonged exposure, especially in an enclosed area, may lead to long-term effects such as eye problems (scarring, glaucoma, cataracts), breathing problems (asthma), etc.

Management

- Since inhalation is likely to be the primary route of exposure, the affected person must be **evacuated** immediately from the incident site to a location where there is fresh air.
- Affected clothing must be removed and the entire **body should be washed with soap and water**.
- If the eyes are burning or the vision is blurred, **rinsing the eyes** gently with **plain water** is essential (for at least 10–15 min). If the patient is wearing contact lenses, they must be removed and discarded.
- Discarded clothing must be placed inside a plastic bag, which is then sealed for further disposal.
- Hospital admission and **oxygen administration** may be required, if the respiratory tract has been affected. **Bronchodilators** and **steroids** may be needed.
- Burn injuries to the skin are treated with standard **burn management techniques**, including use of medicated bandages.

Topic 10

PHARMACEUTICAL TOXICOLOGY

(Number of Competencies – 1: FM 10.1)

Teachers and students, please note:

- Topics 9–13 deal with specific categories of poisons with regard to clinical features, diagnosis and management, upon exposure to them. It is to be noted that except for Topic 13, the ***new curriculum does not mention medicolegal aspects at all***! So, it is a moot point whether students can be assessed on these aspects.
- However, as the editor feels it is important, this book lists medicolegal aspects too (under 'Forensic Issues') for all the poisons.
- Also, there is always a possibility of a revised (corrected) curriculum being released incorporating medicolegal aspects, anytime in the future. So, it is better to be prepared!

FM 10.1: Core – Written/Viva Voce/ Objective Structured Clinical Examination (OSCE)

- Describe general principles and basic methodologies in treatment of poisoning: decontamination, supportive therapy, antidote therapy, procedures of enhanced elimination with regard to:
  - Antipyretics
    - Paracetamol, Salicylates
  - Anti-infectives
    - Common Antibiotics – An overview
  - Neuropsychotoxicology
    - Barbiturates
    - Benzodiazepines
    - Phenytoin
    - Lithium
    - Haloperidol
    - Neuroleptics
    - Tricyclics
  - Narcotic Analgesics, Anaesthetics, Muscle Relaxants
  - Cardiovascular Toxicology
    - Cardiotoxic Plants – Oleander, Odollam, Aconite, Digitalis
  - Gastrointestinal and Endocrinal Drugs – Insulin

ANTIPYRETICS

Salicylates

- These compounds are derivatives of **salicylic acid** and include **acetyl salicylic acid**, **sodium salicylate** and **methyl salicylate**.
- **Salicin**, a naturally occurring salicylate is a constituent of several plants but is present in highest concentration in the **Willow tree** (*Salix alba*) (**Fig. 10.1**), which grows near lakes and rivers in temperate climates and whose branches are used to make cricket bats and baskets.
- **Hoffman**, a chemist at Bayer Company first synthesised acetyl salicylic acid in the laboratory in **1897**.
- The name "**aspirin**" was coined in **1899**, and since then the drug has marched through time displaying a rare and astonishing staying power.

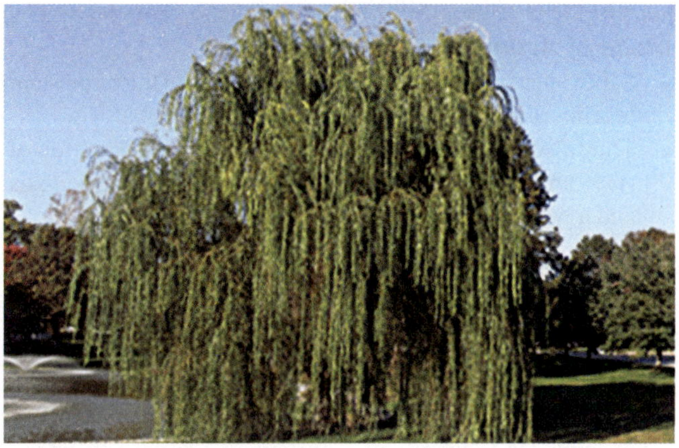

Fig. 10.1 Willow tree

Examples

Aspirin, Methyl salicylate, Salicylic acid, Sodium salicylate

Physical Appearance

- **Acetyl salicylic acid** (Aspirin): Odourless, white, crystalline powder with an unpleasant saline taste.
- **Sodium salicylate**: Odourless, white scaly crystals with the same unpleasant saline taste.
- **Methyl salicylate** is a colourless liquid with aromatic odour and sweetish taste.

Uses

- **Sodium salicylate & Acetyl salicylic acid**:
  - Antipyretic
  - Analgesic
  - Treatment of rheumatoid arthritis.
  - **Low-dose aspirin** is used in the prophylaxis of cerebrovascular ischaemic events and angina pectoris.
- **Methyl salicylate** (***oil of wintergreen***, ***sweet birch oil***, ***gautheria oil***) is used for the local treatment of musculoskeletal pain and inflammation.

Usual Fatal Dose

- **Sodium salicylate, aspirin: 15–20 g**.
- **Methyl salicylate: 5–15 mL**.

Toxicokinetics

- Salicylates are rapidly absorbed from the stomach, and to a slightly lesser extent from the small intestine. Delayed ab sorption is seen in the following situations: enteric coated preparations, pylorospasm, pyloric stenosis and bezoar formation.

- Methyl salicylate is readily absorbed through intact skin.
- Metabolism occurs chiefly in the liver, where salicylates are broken down into salicyluric acid, ether glucuronide, ester glucuronide and gentisic acid.
- Excretion is mainly through urine. Up to 10% excretion may be in the form of free salicylic acid, and this is greatly enhanced in alkaline urine.
- Sustained release preparations of aspirin contain aspirin released over a 12-hr or longer period of time. Prolonged absorption and persistently elevated salicylate levels may occur following overdose.

Mode of Action

- Salicylates stimulate the respiratory centre in the brain stem leading to hyperventilation and respiratory alkalosis.
- They also interfere with Krebs cycle, inhibit production of ATP, and increase lactate production, leading to ketosis and a wide anion-gap metabolic acidosis.
- The mechanism for ototoxicity is thought to be multifactoral: vasoconstriction causes reduced cochlear blood flow; membrane permeability changes cause loss of outer hair cell turgor in the organ of Corti.
- Respiratory acidosis in salicylate overdose indicates grave prognosis and is seen in salicylate-induced pulmonary oedema, CNS depression from mixed overdose or severe fatigue due to prolonged hyperventilation.
- Salicylates are extremely irritating to the GI mucosa, and overdose often results in haemorrhagic gastritis.
- Aspirin is commonly involved in allergic reactions, ranging in severity from urticaria or angioedema to acute anaphylaxis.

Clinical Features

I. **Acute Poisoning**
   1. *Mild* (peak salicylate concentration of less than 300 mg/L) – Nausea, vomiting, deafness, tinnitus (ringing or hissing), vertigo and lethargy.
   2. *Moderate* (peak salicylate concentration 300–700 mg/L) – Dehydration, restlessness, sweating, warm extremities with bounding pulse, tachypnoea and hyperventilation. Respiratory alkalosis is often present at lower concentrations; metabolic acidosis may co-exist.
   3. *Severe* (peak salicylate concentration >700 mg/L) – Cardiac arrhythmias, acute non-cardiogenic pulmonary oedema, cerebral oedema, convulsions, confusion, coma, hyperpyrexia, heart failure, renal failure and worsening metabolic acidosis.
      i. A **mixed respiratory alkalosis and metabolic acidosis** with normal or high arterial pH is often seen.
      ii. **Anion gap is increased** in severe cases.
   4. Salicylates must **not** be therapeutically administered to children under 15 years of age, especially if they are suffering from chicken pox or influenza. There is a serious (though rare) risk of precipitating **Reye's syndrome** which can be fatal (**Table 10.1**).
      i. The main features are acute onset of hepatic failure and encephalopathy.
      ii. It probably results from damage to mitochondria in liver cells.
      iii. Recovery is associated usually with permanent neurological sequelae.

II. **Chronic Poisoning** (Salicylism)
   1. Slow onset of confusion, agitation, lethargy, disorientation, slurred speech, hallucinations, convulsions and coma. There may also be tinnitus, hearing loss, nausea, dyspnoea, tachycardia and fever.
   2. Sometimes Salicylism presents as ***psuedosepsis syndrome*** characterised by fever, leukocytosis, hypotension and multi-organ system failure.

Diagnosis

I. **Laboratory Findings**:
   1. Anion-gap acidosis.
   2. Hypokalaemia (acidosis may mask it).
   3. Hypocalcaemia.
   4. Hypoglycaemia.

II. **Bed-side Tests**:
   1. ***Ferric chloride test*** – Add a few drops of 10% ferric chloride solution to 1 mL of urine. A purple colour indicates the presence of salicylates.

Table 10.1 Reye's Syndrome

Stage	Manifestations
I	Lethargic
II	Stuporous, sluggish pupillary reaction, conjugate deviation of eyes (oculocephalic reflex)
III	Comatose, decorticate posture, sluggish pupillary reaction, conjugate deviation of eyes (oculocephalic reflex)
IV	Comatose, decerebrate posture, sluggish pupillary reaction, inconsistent response (oculocephalic reflex)
V	Comatose, flaccid posture, no pupillary reaction, no response to painful stimuli, no response to oculocephalic reflex

2. ***Trinder's test*** – The test can be done on urine, stomach contents or scene residue. Add 0.1 mL of Trinder's reagent to 2 mL of sample and mix for 5 sec. A strong violet colour indicates the presence of salicylates.

III. **Confirmatory Test**: The only confirmatory test is to estimate the **serum salicylate level**. Unfortunately, the seriousness of poisoning correlates poorly with serum levels. Previously, the ***Done nomogram*** (first published in **1960**) was highly recommended to correlate serum salicylate level with the degree of intoxication at varying intervals after acute ingestion of aspirin. But, there are severe limitations to its use and is now **not considered to be reliable**.

Treatment

1. **Stomach wash** is said to be beneficial up to 12 hrs after ingestion, since toxic doses of salicylates can cause pylorospasm and delayed gastric emptying.
2. **Whole bowel irrigation** might be useful in patients with bezoars, or patients who have ingested enteric coated or sustained release products.
3. **Activated charcoal (AC)**: Very efficacious in the treatment of salicylate poisoning, since each gram of AC can adsorb 550 mg of the drug. A 10:1 ratio of AC to salicylate results in maximum efficiency.
4. **Urinary alkalinisation**: This should not be confused with *forced diuresis* which was recommended in the past, where the accent was on increasing urinary flow rate in order to increase salicylate clearance. It carries with it, the risk of fluid overload with attendant complications.
   a. Alkalinisation of both blood and urine can be achieved with intravenous sodium bicarbonate. 1 mEq/kg of $NaHCO_3$ is added to the first bottle of 5% dextrose.
   b. If alkalinisation (urinary pH 7.5–8.5) is not achieved in a few hrs, it can be repeated.
   c. Alkalinisation should be stopped when serum salicylate level falls below 35 mg/100 mL.
5. **Haemodialysis or haemodiafiltration**:
   a. They are very effective in salicylate poisoning and must always be considered in the presence of cardiac or renal failure, intractable acidosis, convulsions, severe fluid imbalance, or a serum salicylate concentration of greater than 700 mg/L with metabolic acidosis.
6. **Supportive measures**:
   a. Avoid intubation unless the patient actually has respiratory failure (worsening respiratory acidosis, hypoxaemia). Loss of hyperventilatory drive can result in sudden decompensation and death.
   b. Correction of fluid and electrolyte imbalance.
   c. Hypoprothrombinaemia can be corrected by 2.5–5 mg of vitamin K IV every day.
   d. Hyperpyrexia must be tackled by cooling measures (e.g., ice in the axilla and groin). When body temperature exceeds 39°C, urgent cooling measures such as ice-baths and internal cooling devices should be used. If hyperthermia is persistent, dantrolene may be considered (1 mg/kg IV to a maximum of 10 mg/kg).
   e. Correction of hypocalcaemia with calcium gluconate IV (5–10 mL in adults).
   f. Correct hypokalaemia as needed.
   g. Correction of hypoglycaemia with glucose IV (50 mL of 5% dextrose or 1 mL/kg).
   h. Correct metabolic acidosis with IV sodium bicarbonate 50–100 mmol given over 30 min.
   i. Treatment of convulsions with benzodiazepines.
7. **Treatment of Reye's syndrome**:
   a. Admit the patient to an intensive care unit.
   b. Raise the head-end of bed (40°).
   c. Mannitol IV (0.2–1.0 g/kg.).
   d. Acute hyperventilation may be helpful.
   e. Short acting barbiturates in resistant cases.

Autopsy Features

- Petechiae in the skin (occasionally).
- Erosions of gastric mucosa. Black, altered blood may lie in the stomach. Sometimes massed concretions of tablets are present.
- Petechiae in various organs and serous membranes (parietal pleura, pericardium).
- Pulmonary and cerebral oedema.

Forensic Issues

- Most of the cases of overdose are suicidal in nature; a few may be accidental.
- In some individuals, a small dose of aspirin can provoke a fatal hypersensitivity reaction. The patient is usually (curiously) a middle-aged female, and often has nasal polyps. Within minutes of ingestion there is an acute vasomotor rhinitis, angioneurotic oedema and urticaria. Death results from laryngeal oedema, hypotension or shock.
- Salicylate poisoning can also result from extensive application of salicylate-containing ointments, keratolytic agents or other agents containing methyl salicylate.

PARACETAMOL

Synonyms

Acetaminophen

The word "acetaminophen" is a shortened form of N-**acet**yl **aminophen**ol, and is the preferred term in the US, while the word "paracetamol" is a shortened form of **para**-**acet**yl-**am**ino-phen**ol**, and is the preferred term in the UK.

Uses

1. **Antipyretic**:
   a. **Phenacetin** was synthesized and introduced in **1887** as an effective antipyretic. This was extensively used until its role in ***analgesic nephropathy**** became clear and led to its withdrawal.
   b. In **1893**, **von Mering** introduced **paracetamol**, and a

*__Note__: *Prolonged duration of phenacetin therapy causes chronic interstitial nephritis and renal failure.*

hundred years later, it is still going strong. In fact, paracetamol is the active metabolite of phenacetin.

2. **Analgesic.**

Usual Fatal Dose

- **20–25 g.**
- However, ingestion of even 150 mg/kg or 7.5 g has caused serious liver injury.

Toxicokinetics and Mode of Action

- Paracetamol is rapidly and completely absorbed from the GI tract. Peak plasma levels are reached in ½ to 1 hr, while the plasma half-life is about 2 hrs.
- Normally about 90% of the drug undergoes hepatic conjugation with glucuronide and sulphuric acid to form harmless metabolites, while 10% is oxidised (through P450 mediation) to **N-acetyl-p-benzoquinoneimine (NAPQI)** which is a highly reactive intermediate.
  - NAPQI is capable of covalent binding and arylating critical cell proteins inducing a series of events that result in cell death.
  - In the normal course, glutathione rapidly detoxifies this intermediate to cysteine and mercapturate conjugates.
  - In the overdose situation, glutathione stores become depleted and the toxic NAPQI binds covalently with hepatocytes of the liver causing **centrilobular hepatic necrosis**.

Clinical Features

I. **Acute Poisoning**

1. *Stage I* (½ to 24 hrs): Anorexia, vomiting, sweating, malaise.
2. *Stage II* (24–72 hrs): Relatively symptom-free. There may be right upper quadrant pain. Liver function tests may be abnormal.
3. *Stage III* (72–96 hrs): Hepatic necrosis sets in with coagulation defects, jaundice and encephalopathy. Nausea and vomiting reappear. Renal failure and myocardial damage are frequently present. Death is usually due to hepatic failure and is preceded by coma.
4. *Stage IV* (4 days to 2 weeks): If the patient survives the IIIrd stage, complete resolution of hepatic damage is the rule rather than the exception. There are no reported cases of chronic hepatic dysfunction from paracetamol.

Elevated blood levels of liver enzymes (SGOT/ALT, SGPT/AST) may begin to develop within 24 hrs after overdose, and peak 2–3 days post-ingestion.

Nephrotoxic effects include acute tubular necrosis, flank pain, haematuria and proteinuria.

Metabolic acidosis and high blood lactate levels may be seen early (12 hrs), especially in severe overdoses.

Hyperphosphataemia (>1.2 mmol/L) appears to be an early predictor of non-survival in severe paracetamol-induced hepatotoxicity at 48–96 hrs post-ingestion.

II. **Chronic Poisoning**

1. This is uncommon, but cases have been reported wherein an individual has consumed large doses of paracetamol over a period of time for relief of chronic pain which resulted in toxic hepatitis.
2. This is more common in alcoholics, AIDS patients (in whom there is depletion of glutathione) and patients receiving other medications which are cytochrome P450 inducers, e.g., isoniazid, rifampicin, phenytoin, carbamazepine and barbiturates.
3. Chronic overdose among children is more common than in adults mainly because of dose miscalculation by parents. Features include anorexia, vomiting, lethargy, low body temperature, hepatomegaly and oliguria.

Diagnosis

1. *Evidence of hypoglycaemia, metabolic acidosis.*
2. *Evidence of hepatocellular injury*:
   a. Elevated aspartate aminotransferase (AST), alanine aminotransferase (ALT), bilirubin and prothrombin time.
   b. Hypophosphataemia is often present. Hyperphosphataemia (>1.2 mmol/L), occurring 48–96 hrs after the overdose, and in the presence of both renal and hepatic dysfunction, is a poor prognostic indicator.
   c. Decreased serum interleukin-6 (IL-6) or C-reactive protein (a surrogate for IL-6) levels following acute paracetamol overdose have been found to be statistically associated with hepatic injury and may serve as prognostic factors for predicting impending hepatic injury.
3. *Evidence of renal damage*: Proteinuria, phosphaturia.
4. *Evidence of myocardial damage*: ECG changes indicative of arrhythmias.
5. ***Serum paracetamol level***: The lowest acute dose of paracetamol capable of toxicity is generally regarded as 7.5 g in an adult and 150 mg/kg in a child.
   a. Interpretation of serum paracetamol levels is usually done on the basis of the **Rumack-Matthew nomogram** which has undergone some modification and is depicted in **Fig. 10.2**. The original nomogram was based on the fact that patients in whom the AST or ALT values would rise (more than 1000 IU/L) could be separated from those in whom this would not happen on the basis of initial paracetamol level (PL). The nomogram line was constructed on a plot of PL versus time since ingestion. The line chosen started at a PL of 200 µg/mL, 4 hrs post-ingestion; declined with a 4-hr half-life through 50 µg/mL, 12 hrs post-ingestion; and ended at 6.25 µg/mL, 24 hrs post-ingestion. The line is based solely on ALT elevation rather than hepatic failure and is very sensitive though not very specific.
   b. While the original line is still widely in use, the line used more commonly today has been lowered by 25% in order to enhance sensitivity. This is depicted in **Fig. 10.2** as a second, lower line (beginning at 150 µg/mL instead of 200 µg/mL). By using this modified nomogram it is said that nomogram failures are virtually non-existent.
   c. The purpose of the Rumack-Matthew nomogram is to predict the risk of hepatic injury at the outset and begin

antidotal therapy well in time. Levels obtained before 4 hrs or after 24 hrs cannot be interpreted, nor can levels obtained after chronic overdose. In those cases where the time of ingestion is unknown and cannot be determined, it is advisable to determine both PL and AST. If the AST is elevated regardless of PL, begin antidotal therapy. If the PL is less than 10 μg/mL and AST level is normal, the antidote (N-acetylcysteine) can be withheld.

d. If it is not possible for any reason to estimate the paracetamol level at all, then the risk of hepatic injury should be predicted on the basis of the history. Do not delay antidotal therapy for lack of a paracetamol level. Administer loading dose, then discontinue if level comes back below the nomogram treatment line.

e. The nomogram is unreliable if the timing of ingestion is uncertain. If there is any uncertainty about whether the patient's paracetamol concentration is above or below the nomogram line, the patient should be treated with acetylcysteine. The nomogram is also unreliable if the overdose is staggered (taken over longer than 1 hr).

Treatment

1. **Stomach wash**: useful only in cases of very early presentation (<1 hr), or in concomitant ingestion of other drugs which delay GI absorption.
2. **Activated charcoal** can adsorb paracetamol, but it can also adsorb the antidote (N-acetylcysteine) and hence must be administered earlier to 4 hrs post-ingestion. It is most effective, if given within 1 hr of ingestion.
3. **Anti-emetic**, if the patient is vomiting repeatedly.*

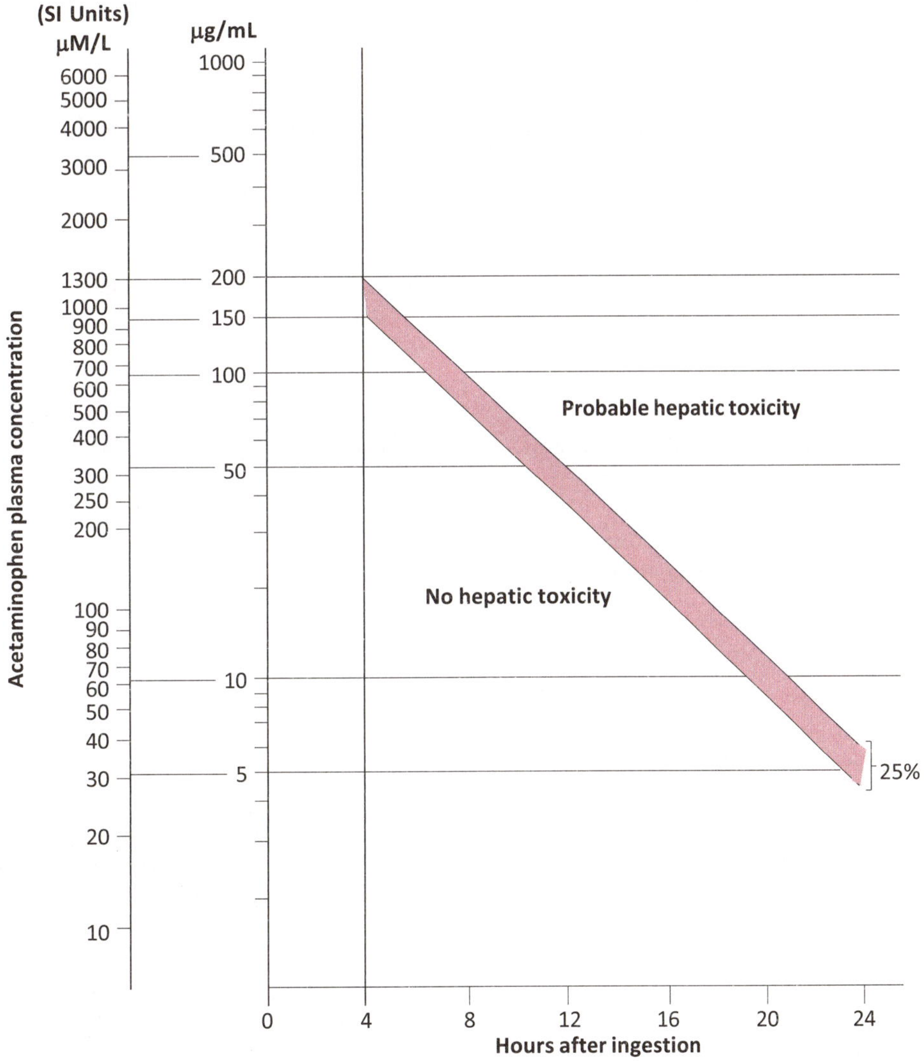

The upper line characterizes serum paracetamol levels associated with hepatotoxicity.
The lower line is a 25% allowance for possible errors in history and laboratory analysis.

Fig. 10.2 Rumack Matthew Nomogram

Note: *Since the antidote (N-acetylcysteine) can be orally administered, if vomiting is not controlled it will be difficult to administer the same.*

4. **Supportive measures**:
   a. 10–20% dextrose for hypoglycaemia.
   b. Vitamin K_1, if PT is elevated.
   c. Fresh-frozen plasma, if there is overt bleeding.
   d. Mannitol (0.5 g/kg given over 10 min) for cerebral oedema.
   e. Broad spectrum antibiotics IV (ceftazidime or fluoxacillin), if necessary.
   f. H_2 antagonists to prevent upper GI haemorrhage.
   g. Do **not** give sedatives, benzodiazepines or NSAIDs.
5. **Antidotal therapy**:
   a. **Methionine** – This is an oral antidote that is popular in the UK and some other countries, but is presently not available in India.
   b. **N-Acetylcysteine (NAC)** – It is a derivative of L-cysteine, a naturally occurring amino acid.
      - **Indications**: NAC is indicated in paracetamol overdose if
        - PL estimated between 4 and 12 hrs post-ingestion lies above the nomogram line (**Fig. 10.2**).
        - Paracetamol ingested is more than 100 mg/kg.
        - Likelihood exists of paracetamol-induced hepatic failure.
      - **NAC is the antidote of choice for paracetamol poisoning in India.** It gives maximum protection against hepatotoxicity when administered within 10 hrs of paracetamol overdose, but can be given with (lesser) benefit up to 36 hrs.
        - **Dose**:
          Oral: 5% solution given as loading dose of 140 mg/kg. This is followed by 17 more doses at 70 mg/kg, 4th hourly, total making up to 1330 mg/kg over 72 hrs. The calculated dose can be administered mixed with water, or flavoured or carbonated drink.
          Intravenous:
          21-hr regimen →
          First infusion: 150 mg/kg in 200 mL of 5% dextrose given IV over 1 hr.
          Second infusion: 50 mg/kg in 500 mL of 5% dextrose over 4 hrs.
          Third infusion: 100 mg/kg in 1 L of 5% dextrose over 16 hrs.
          The total dose usually works out to 300 mg/kg given over 21 hrs.
          48-hr regimen → Useful in delayed admissions and massive ingestion.
          A loading dose of 140 mg IV is given over 1 hr, followed 4 hrs later by the first of 12 maintenance doses of 70 mg/kg, each administered over 1 hr. The total dose of NAC works out to 980 mg/kg in just over 48 hrs.
          Oral acetylcysteine therapy – If oral therapy is required (e.g., complete absence of venous access in an intravenous drug abuser), oral therapy using the IV preparation may be used. The taste of NAC is unpleasant and can be masked using fruit juice or cola.
          Loading dose: 140 mg/kg given as a 5% solution.
          Maintenance doses: 17 doses of 70 mg/kg as a 5% solution every 4 hrs to a total of 1330 mg/kg over 72 hrs.
      - **Adverse effects**:
        - *Oral* – Drinking NAC through a straw minimises its unpleasant odour. The main problem with oral NAC is induction of vomiting. Metoclopramide or ondansetron may have to be administered.
        - *Intravenous* – Anaphylactoid reaction. If it occurs, it should be managed in the usual way with antihistamines, epinephrine, etc.
        - Isolated effects include pruritus, angioedema, nausea and vomiting, bronchospasm, tachycardia, hypotension and hypertension. Facial or chest flushing is common.
   c. **Cysteamine** – It was formerly popular, but efficacy is greatly diminished if administered more than 10 hrs post-ingestion. Cysteamine also suffers from serious adverse effects. **It is no more recommended today**.
6. **Liver transplantation**: When fulminant liver failure develops after a massive paracetamol overdose, virtually the only treatment modality available is liver transplantation.
   Indications:
   - pH < 7.3.
   - PT > 100 sec, and serum creatinine > 3.4 mg/100 mL in patients with grade III or IV encephalopathy.
7. Renal failure may occur as part of acute hepatic injury (hepatorenal syndrome) or, rarely, in the absence of hepatic injury. Treat renal failure conventionally. Recovery is the norm.
8. Forced diuresis, haemodialysis and charcoal haemoperfusion are of little value in preventing paracetamol induced hepatotoxicity.

Autopsy Features

- Liver may be enlarged and yellowish in colour. Microscopy reveals **centrilobular necrosis** (**Fig. 10.3**).

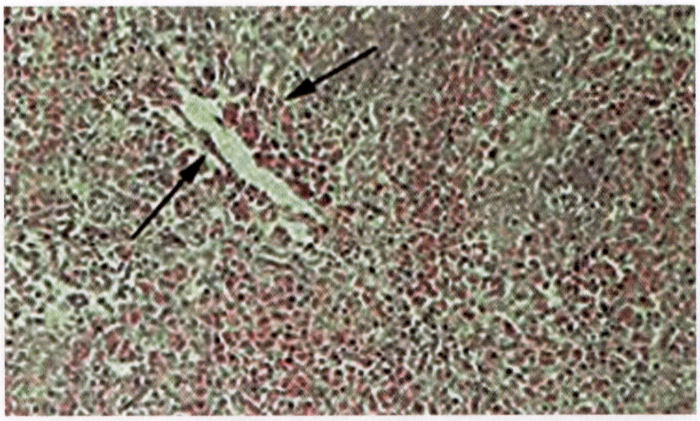

Fig. 10.3 Centrilobular necrosis of liver – Paracetamol overdose

- Histological evidence of renal damage.
- Cerebral oedema.
- Cardiac findings in fatal overdoses have included subendocardial haemorrhages, fatty degeneration and focal necrosis.

Forensic Issues

- Attempted suicide with paracetamol accounts for a staggering 15–30% of cases of poisoning in the UK; a similar scenario exists in the USA, where paracetamol overdose accounts for more hospitalisations than any other pharmaceutical agent. While the situation at present is not as bad in India, there are alarming indications of rising incidence.
- Accidental poisoning most often results from inadvertent therapeutic overdose either as an acute or as a chronic phenomenon. A few cases result from hypersensitivity reactions which (though rare) may sometimes produce serious manifestations ranging from dermal to respiratory to anaphylactoid reactions.
- The FDA (USA) requires an **alcohol warning** on all over-the-counter pain relievers, which includes paracetamol, aspirin, other salicylates, ibuprofen, ketoprofen and naproxen sodium due to a potential drug interaction resulting in upper GI bleeding or liver damage.

ANTI-INFECTIVES

Anti-infective drugs are those which fight infections caused by bacteria, viruses, fungi and protozoa, as well as infestations resulting from parasites such as helminths.

I. **Antimicrobial Agents**:
   A. ***Antibacterial Drugs***
      1. Sulphonamides
      2. Quinolones & Fluoroquinolones
      3. Penicillins
      4. Cephalosporines
      5. Aminoglycosides
      6. Tetracyclines
      7. Chloramphenicol
      8. Macrolides & Ketolides
      9. Antitubercular Drugs
      10. Antileprotic Drugs
      11. Other Antibacterial Drugs
   B. ***Antiviral Drugs***
      1. Antiherpesvirus Drugs
      2. Antiretrovirus Drugs
      3. Other Antiviral Drugs
   C. ***Antifungal Drugs***
II. **Antiprotozoal Agents**:
   A. ***Antimalarial Drugs***
   B. ***Antiamoebic Drugs***
   C. ***Other Antiprotozoal Drugs***
III. **Antihelminthic Agents**

ANTIBIOTICS (*An Overview*)

Note: As the new curriculum specifies only "Antibiotics" under Competency **FM 10.1**, the discussion on "Anti-infectives" will be limited only to antibiotics.

Definition

- Sometimes, the term **antibiotic** (which literally means "opposing life", from the Greek roots *anti*, "against" and *bios*, "life") is broadly used to refer to any substance used against microbes, but in the usual medical usage, antibiotics (such as penicillin) are those produced naturally (by one microorganism fighting another), whereas non-antibiotic **antibacterials** (such as sulphonamides and antiseptics) are fully synthetic.
  - However, both classes have the same goal of killing or preventing the growth of microorganisms, and both are included in **antimicrobial chemotherapy**.
  - "**Antibacterials**" include antiseptic drugs, antibacterial soaps and chemical disinfectants, whereas **antibiotics** are an important class of antibacterials used more specifically in medicine.

COMMON ANTIBIOTICS

Penicillins

Examples

1. **Aminopenicillins**
   a. Amoxycillin
   b. Ampicillin
2. **Extended Spectrum**
   a. Carbenicillin
   b. Piperacillin
   c. Ticarcillin
3. **Natural Penicillins**
   a. Penicillin G
   b. Penicillin V
4. **Penicillinase-resistant**
   a. Cloxacillin
   b. Methicillin

Adverse Effects

1. **Hypersensitivity Reactions**: Penicillins are the most common agents implicated in drug allergy. In decreasing order of frequency, allergic reactions to penicillins include maculopapular rash, urticarial rash, fever, bronchospasm, vasculitis, serum sickness, exfoliative dermatitis, Stevens-Johnson syndrome and **anaphylaxis**.
   a. **Anaphylaxis** –
      Grades of anaphylaxis:
      I – Local cutaneous reaction (> 15 cm)
      II – Generalised urticaria
      III – Asthma, angioedema
      IV –
         a) Airway type – asthma, swelling of tongue, dysphagia, laryngeal oedema.
         b) Cardiovascular type – hypotension, cardiovascular collapse.

      Treatment (for Grade II, III or IV):
      - Adrenaline – 0.01 mL/kg (0.5 mL) of 1:1000 solution, subcutaneously, every 15 min.
      - Oxygen – 40–100%.

- β_2-Adrenergic stimulants – preferably by nebulisation.
- Corticosteroids – preferably methylprednisolone.
- Antihistamines – preferably diphenhydramine.
- Aminophylline – IV infusion.
- IV fluids – 10–30 mL/kg (titrated to effect).
- Activated charcoal – 1 g/kg (if reaction has occurred to oral penicillin)

2. Orally administered penicillins can alter the composition of microflora by eliminating sensitive microorganisms, which can result in superinfection by resistant microbes. Occasionally, **pseudomembranous colitis** may develop due to overgrowth and production of toxin by *Clostridium difficile*. There is formation of a pseudomembrane on the mucosa of the colon (**Fig. 10.4**) with diarrhoea (mixed with blood and mucus), abdominal cramps, fever and leukocytosis. Treatment involves immediate cessation of penicillin and administration of vancomycin or metronidazole.

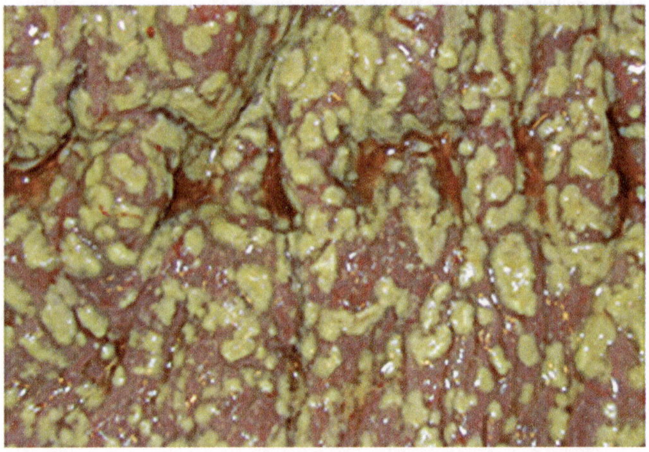

Fig. 10.4 Pseudomembranous colitis

Toxic Effects

- Overdose with penicillins is rare and almost never life-threatening. Manifestations include nausea, vomiting, diarrhoea and occasionally electrolyte abnormalities.
- Large intravenous doses of penicillins can produce convulsions.
- Accidental injection of penicillin into sciatic nerve during deep intamuscular administration of the drug in the region of the buttock can cause severe pain and nerve dysfunction which can persist for weeks.

Treatment

1. The minimum oral amount reported in the literature to produce systemic effects is 11 times the maximum daily therapeutic dose (574 mg/kg). Toxicity is unlikely with doses of 250 mg/kg or less.
2. Patients without a history of penicillin allergy and with ingestion of small to moderate doses of penicillin can almost always be managed at home.
3. Patients ingesting large doses of penicillin (e.g., over 11 times the usual single therapeutic dose or over 250 mg/kg) should receive gastric decontamination and should be evaluated in a health care facility.
4. Control convulsions that are frequent or prolonged with IV diazepam, lorazepam or midazolam. If convulsions are unresponsive, second-line therapy is phenobarbitone sodium.
5. Cardiac arrhythmias should be treated with standard antiarrhythmic drugs, if necessary.
6. In severe overdosage, dialysis may be considered for correction of acidosis and electrolytes, rather than for removal of penicillins.

Quinolones & Fluoroquinolones

Among the very few members of the classic **quinolones** used today is nalidixic acid, while there are several **fluorinated 4-quinolones** (**fluoroquinolones**) which are very popular as broad spectrum antibacterials. Examples include ciprofloxacin, gatifloxacin, levofloxacin, norfloxacin, ofloxacin, pefloxacin, etc.

Adverse Effects

- While the quinolones and fluoroquinolones are generally well tolerated, the following adverse effects have been reported: skin rash, nausea, abdominal discomfort, headache, vertigo and rarely, delirium with hallucinations.
- Crystalluria and nephrolithiasis have been reported with therapeutic use.
- Arthralgias, myalgias and polyarthritis have also been reported.
- **Fluoroquinolones** are not recommended for children (under 15 years) because of the risk of inducing arthralgia and joint swelling. Rare adverse effects include rhabdomyolysis, tendonitis, tendon rupture, delirium, altered mental status, QT prolongation and ventricular arrhythmias.
  - Tendinopathy (a rare effect) appears to be a class-related adverse effect of fluoroquinolones and includes first and second generation drugs. In one study, drug monitoring indicated that levofloxacin had the highest rate of tendinopathies.
  - Due to the theoretical risk of arthropathy, the use of quinolones and fluroquinolones in pregnancy is not generally recommended, except for the treatment of serious or life-threatening conditions unresponsive to standard antibiotic therapy.

Toxic Effects

- Every case of alleged overdose must be observed for at least 4 hrs after ingestion.
- Acute toxicity with nalidixic acid is relatively common, resulting in vomiting, convulsions, hyperglycaemia, benign intracranial hypertension, behaviour disorders, lethargy, toxic psychosis and metabolic acidosis. Visual disturbances (hazy vision, halos, colour perception changes, diplopia, photophobia) have also been reported.
- Overdose with fluoroquinolones has caused dizziness, drowsiness, disorientation, slurred speech, nausea, vomiting and tremors.
- Hepatic injury including hepatitis, acute liver failure and subfulminant hepatic failure have been reported with the use of fluoroquinolones in both short and long term use.

- At therapeutic doses, haematuria, crystalluria and interstitial nephritis have been associated with ciprofloxacin therapy.

Treatment

1. Stomach wash (within 2 hrs of ingestion).
2. Activated charcoal may be helpful.
3. Control convulsions that are frequent or prolonged with IV diazepam, lorazepam or midazolam. If convulsions are unresponsive, second-line therapy is phenobarbitone sodium
4. Periodic evaluation of renal function: urinalysis for crystalluria, serum creatinine, blood urea nitrogen.
5. Adequate hydration (to prevent crystalluria).
6. If metabolic acidosis persists despite correction of hypoxia and adequate fluid resuscitation consider correction with IV sodium bicarbonate.
7. Supportive care including replacement of fluid and electrolytes lost during prolonged vomiting remains the cornerstone of treatment.
8. Steroids may help in ameliorating arthralgias and interstitial nephritis, if present.

Cephalosporines

1. **First generation cephalosporines** – Cefadroxil, cefalexin, cefalothin, etc.
2. **Second generation cephalosporines** – Cefaclor, efuroxime.
3. **Third generation cephalosporines** – Cefixime, cefotaxime, cefpodoxime, ceftriaxone, etc.
4. **Fourth generation cephalosporines** – Cefclidine, cefepime, cefpirome, etc.
5. **Fifth generation cephalosporines** – Ceftobiprole, ceftaroline

Adverse Effects

- The most important adverse effects arise out of **hypersensitivity** in the same manner as penicillins. Manifestations of allergy include skin rashes, bronchospasm, fever and anaphylaxis.
- Seizures have been reported following therapeutic administration.
- Vomiting, diarrhoea and pancreatitis may occur.
- A **disulfiram-like reaction** can develop following the use of some cephalosporines with ethanol ingestion.

Toxic Effects

- Acute overdose produces manifestations similar to those seen with penicillin, including the possibility of convulsions. Treatment is supportive.
- Chronic effects of cephalosporine therapy include serum sickness, interstitial nephritis, hepatitis.

Treatment

1. Urinalysis should be monitored following very large doses of cephalosporines.
2. Activated charcoal is indicated following a large overdose (more than 15 times the therapeutic dose).
3. Treatment of allergic reactions in the usual manner.
4. Supportive measures.
5. In severe overdosage where increased absorption may have occurred and there exists severe renal impairment, dialysis may be considered.

Aminoglycosides

Examples

Amikacin, gentamicin, kanamycin, neomycin, streptomycin, tobramycin.

Adverse Effects

1. **Ototoxicity**:
   a. Any of the aminoglycosides can cause both vestibular and auditory dysfunction which may be irreversible, owing to destruction of vestibular and cochlear sensory cells.
      i. Symptoms include tinnitus, deafness and dysequilibrium characterised by ataxic gait, stumbling and loss of balance on turning. Onset may be sudden and is usually progressive over 6–10 months.
      ii. Ototoxicity after acute single overdose is not well documented.
2. **Nephrotoxicity**:
   a. Typically, acute tubular necrosis sets in after 7–10 days of therapy.
   b. Most cases are reversible.
3. **Neuromuscular blockade**:
   a. All aminoglycosides are capable (rarely) of causing neuromuscular blockade with consequent paralysis.
4. **Other effects**:
   a. Optic nerve toxicity has been reported with streptomycin, as also peripheral neuritis and paraesthesia. Intramuscular injections involving this drug are extremely painful.
   b. Aminoglycosides are in **pregnancy category D**, that is, there is positive evidence of human foetal risk based on adverse reaction data, but potential benefits may warrant use of the drug in pregnant women despite these risks.

Treatment

- Acute overdoses of aminoglycoside antibiotics are almost invariably the result of dosage errors (especially in infants). Fortunately these overdoses are rarely life threatening, and most patients can be successfully managed with supportive measures.
- Charcoal administration can be considered if the patient is seen within a short time following ingestion.
- Maintain good urine output (3–6 mL/kg/hr) with intravenous fluids.
- Peritoneal or haemodialysis is effective, the latter being preferable.

Tetracyclines

Examples

Chlortetracycline, oxytetracycline demeclocycline, tetracycline, doxycycline, minocycline.

Adverse & Toxic Effects

- Acute overdose of tetracyclines is generally not attended with serious toxicity.
- Gastro-intestinal distress is common, manifested by nausea, vomiting, epigastric pain and occasionally diarrhoea. Rarely, there is development of oesophagitis, oesophageal ulcers, and even pancreatitis.
- Hepatic damage results from large doses, and is characterised by jaundice, azotaemia, acidosis and shock.
- Renal toxicity has also been reported.
    - Ingestion of outdated or degraded tetracycline can result in the development of a variant of **Fanconi syndrome** characterised by vomiting, polydipsia, polyuria, proteinuria, acidosis, glycosuria and aminoaciduria.
- Patients administered tetracyclines (especially doxycycline and demeclocycline) should avoid exposure to sunlight, or else **photosensitivity reactions** may occur in the skin, as also onycholysis and pigmentation of nails. Skin hyperpigmentation consisting of dark-grey discolouration of sun-exposed areas has been reported.
- **Tetracyclines should not be administered to pregnant women, and also to children under the age of 8 years.**
    - Hepatotoxicity, pancreatitis and renal failure may occur in pregnant women following ingestion of tetracyclines during pregnancy.
    - Maternal ingestion of tetracyclines during pregnancy, particularly during the first trimester, may cause various congenital defects, including cardiovascular defects, oral clefts, polydactyly, hypospadias, limb hypoplasias and inguinal hernias.
    - Use in the second or third trimester can cause **discolouration of teeth and bones**.
    - Children administered tetracycline develop **brown discolouration of teeth** (**Fig. 10.5**) due to the formation of a tetracycline–calcium–orthophosphate complex. The same applies to children of mothers who had received the drug during pregnancy. Permanent teeth are not affected by prenatal exposure to tetracycline as calcification does not begin until after birth. Tetracyclines also get deposited in the skeleton during gestation and childhood resulting in depression of bone growth.
- Intravenous administration of tetracyclines can result in severe thrombophlebitis.
- Long-term therapy with tetracyclines is associated with leukocytosis, atypical lymphocytes, toxic granulation of granulocytes and thrombocytopenic purpura.

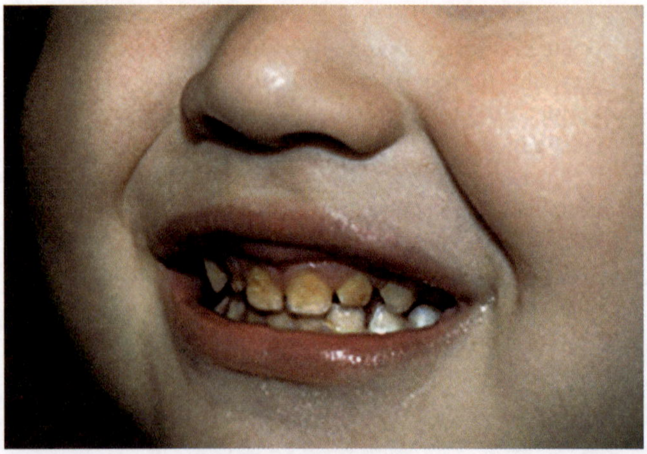

Fig. 10.5 Tetracycline stained teeth

Treatment

- Withdrawal of the drug and institution of supportive measures.
- Renal and hepatic monitoring steps should be instituted when prolonged use of large doses of tetracyclines has occurred.
- Severe toxicity is unlikely after ingestion.
- Gastrointestinal decontamination is generally not required.
- Antacids may be useful in treating gastric irritation.

Chloramphenicol (Chloromycetin)

Though chloramphenicol is one of the "**broad spectrum**" antibiotics, its serious adverse effects restricts its use only for certain cases of **meningitis**, **typhus** and **typhoid fever**, as well as **Rocky Mountain spotted fever**.

Adverse Effects

- Skin rashes, fever and angioedema are uncommonly reported hypersensitivity reactions to chloramphenicol.
- Serious adverse reactions to chloramphenicol include anaemia, leukopenia and thrombocytopenia.
    - **Aplastic anaemia** is not dose-related, but is instead an idiosyncratic reaction. The risk while being low, is potentially fatal if it does materialise. Even if recovery occurs, there is a subsequent increased predisposition to acute leukaemia.

Toxic Effects

1. Oral administration of large doses causes nausea, vomiting, unpleasant taste and diarrhoea. Glossitis, stomatitis or enterocolitis may occur.
2. Blurring of vision, optic neuritis and digital paraesthesias.
3. Metabolic acidosis (an early sign, more common with chronic toxicity).
4. Hypotension, hypothermia, sudden cardiovascular collapse.
5. **Chronic toxicity**: Anaemia and leukopenia (reversible after discontinuation), metabolic acidosis, optic neuritis and peripheral neuritis
6. **Overdose in neonates** can result in **Gray baby syndrome**,* characterised by vomiting, refusal to feed, tachypnoea, abdominal distension, cyanosis (**Fig. 10.6**) and loose, greenish stools. Within 24 hrs the baby becomes flaccid, hypothermic, and turns ashen-gray in colour. Mortality is around 40%.

Note*: ***Gray syndrome* *with similar manifestations can occur rarely in adults.*

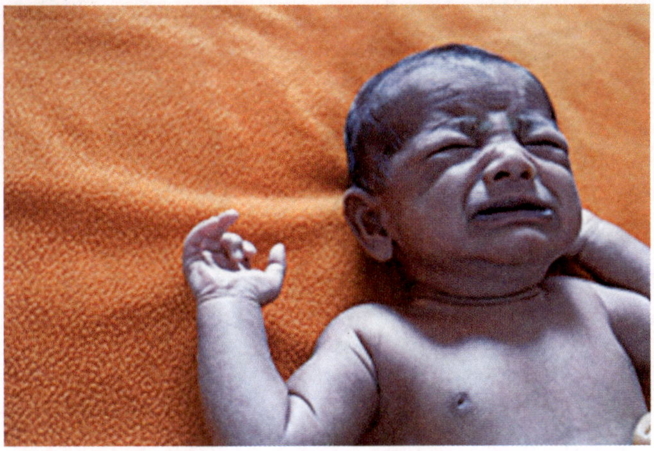

Fig. 10.6 Gray baby syndrome

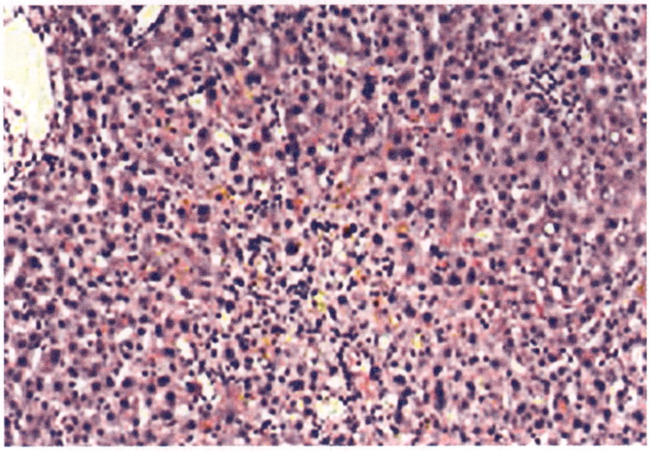

Fig. 10.7 Erythromycin-induced cholestatic hepatitis

7. **Idiosyncratic reaction**: **Aplastic anaemia**, which does not appear to be dose-related, may occur weeks or months after therapy has been discontinued; it has occurred after IV, oral and ocular routes. It carries high mortality (>50% mortality).

Treatment

1. Gastric lavage may be helpful for recent ingestions.
2. Activated charcoal can be administered subsequently (1 g/kg).
3. For optic neuritis, with or without peripheral neuritis: administration of vitamins B_6 and B_{12} has been recommended.
4. Chloramphenicol is not well dialysed. However, in patients with impaired renal function, clearance is moderately increased by haemodialysis.
5. Charcoal haemoperfusion is said to be beneficial.

Macrolides

Examples

Azithromycin, clarithromycin, erythromycin, roxithromycin.

Adverse & Toxic Effects

- In general, macrolide antibiotics are considered to have fewer, less severe toxic effects than most other antimicrobial agents.
- Allergic reactions are uncommon (fever, eosinophilia and skin eruptions).
- The most striking side-effect, especially associated with erythromycin estolate is **cholestatic hepatitis (Fig. 10.7)**, which is probably immune-mediated. Cholestasis is characterized by elevated liver enzymes, fever, abdominal pain and jaundice. Discontinuation of the drug usually results in resolution of hepatotoxic effects.
- Large doses of macrolides are also associated with reversible high-frequency **sensorineural hearing loss**.
- Acute oral overdoses of macrolide antibiotics are usually not life-threatening, and comprise mainly gastrointestinal manifestations. Seizures may occur. Treatment is the same as for penicillin overdose.

Treatment

1. Observe asymptomatic patients for at least 6 hrs after ingestion of more than a toxic dose. Further observation may be required in symptomatic patients.
2. Severe toxicity is unusual after ingestion; prehospital decontamination is generally not necessary. Discontinuation of the drug usually results in the resolution of the toxic effects.
3. Food, milk or an antacid may be administered for treatment of gastrointestinal distress.
4. Liver enzyme levels may aid in diagnosing or following a patient with evidence of cholestasis or hepatitis.

NEUROPSYCHOTOXICOLOGY

Barbiturates

Barbiturates are derivatives of **barbituric acid** and were extensively used as sedative-hypnotics till the 1960s when the benzodiazepines arrived and quickly displaced them.

Examples

1. **Long acting** (duration of action 6–12 hrs)
   a. Barbitone
   b. Mephobarbitone
   c. Phenobarbitone
2. **Intermediate acting** (duration of action 3–6 hrs)
   a. Amobarbitone (Sodium amytal)
   b. Aprobarbitone
   c. Butobarbitone
3. **Short acting** (duration of action <3 hrs)
   a. Hexobarbitone
   b. Pentobarbitone
   c. Secobarbitone (Quinalbarbitone)
4. **Ultra-short acting** (duration of action <15–20 min)
   a. Thiopentone
   b. Methohexitone

Uses

1. Sedative-hypnotic.
2. Pre-operative sedation.
3. Treatment of seizure disorders.

Usual Fatal Dose

- **Phenobarbitone: 6–10 g.**
- **Amobarbitone, pentobarbitone, secobarbitone: 2–3 g.**
- Lethal blood level
  - Short- and intermediate-acting barbiturates: 3–4 mg/100 mL
  - Phenobarbitone: 8–15 mg/100 mL.
- Ingestion of any amount of thiopentone should always be considered a toxic amount.

Toxicokinetics

- Most barbiturates are administered orally. Intravenous route is usually reserved for management of status epilepticus or induction/maintenance of general anaesthesia.
- Following absorption, barbiturates are distributed widely. The long acting barbiturates have a plasma half-life of about 80 hrs.
- Metabolism occurs by oxidation in the liver resulting in the formation of alcohols, ketones, phenols or carboxylic acids which are excreted in the urine as such, or in the form of glucuronic acid conjugates.

Adverse Effects

- Paradoxical excitement (especially in the elderly).
- Hypersensitivity reaction – swelling of eyelid, cheek or lip; dermatitis.
- Synergistic action with ethanol and antihistamines.

Clinical (Toxic) Features

1. Slurred speech (dysarthria), ataxia, lethargy, confusion, headache, nystagmus.
2. CNS depression, coma, shock. Barbiturates decrease gut motility, which may lead to a slow onset and worsening of symptoms, or cyclical improvement and worsening of symptoms.
3. Pupils are at first constricted, but later dilate because of hypoxia.
4. Hypothermia, hypotonia, hyporeflexia, hypotension.
5. Cutaneous bullae (“***barb burns***”, ***barbiturate blisters***): These are clear, erythematous or haemorrhagic blisters, and occur in various areas of the body, most typically on the hands (**Fig. 10.8**), buttocks, and between the ankles and knees, usually over pressure points.
6. Death may occur from respiratory arrest or cardiovascular collapse.
7. Chronic barbiturate (ab)use is associated with the development of tolerance which is responsible for decreasing the therapeutic to toxic index. An addict may obtain therapeutic benefit only with 5–6 times the normal dose!
   a. Abrupt withdrawal results in anorexia, tremor, insomnia, cramps, seizures, delirium and orthostatic hypotension.

Diagnosis

- Thin layer chromatography (for urine, stomach contents or scene residue).

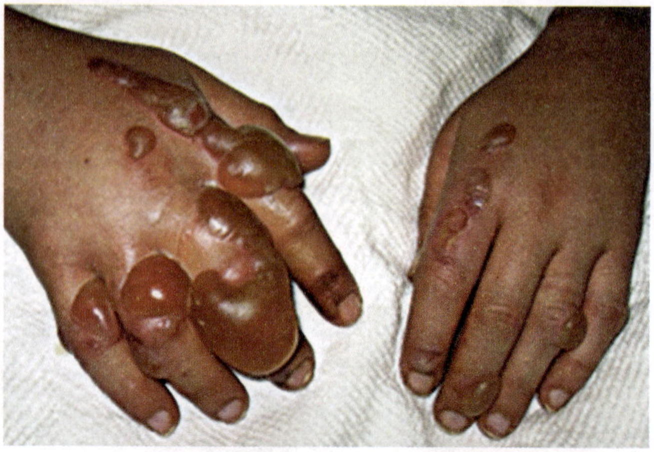

Fig. 10.8 Barbiturate blisters

- Gas chromatography or high pressure liquid chromatography.
- Serial plasma levels may be useful in the management of phenobarbitone overdose. Plasma levels exceeding 8 mg/100 mL are generally associated with coma.
- EEG : Alpha coma* indicates poor prognosis.

Treatment

1. Gastric lavage can be done with benefit up to 12–24 hrs post-ingestion.
2. Activated charcoal in the usual dose.
3. **Alkaline diuresis** is said to be particularly useful in phenobarbitone poisoning. The following procedure may be followed:
   - 1 mEq/kg of sodium bicarbonate by IV bolus with 20–40 mEq/L potassium chloride in 5% dextrose in water, at a rate sufficient to produce a urine pH of at least 7.5.
4. **Haemodialysis** or **haemoperfusion**: In patients who are severely intoxicated with any barbiturate (i.e., coma or needing respiratory or circulatory support), charcoal haemoperfusion or haemodialysis should be considered to increase elimination of barbiturates.
5. Exchange transfusion has been successful in decreasing plasma phenobarbitone levels in a few cases.
6. For hypotension: First administer 10–20 mL/kg of isotonic intravenous fluids and place in Trendelenburg position. If the patient is unresponsive to isotonic fluid therapy administer a vasopressor. Dopamine or noradrenaline should be titrated to desired response.
7. Monitor core temperature with rectal or bladder probe. Initiate external rewarming with warm blankets, IV fluids and warm humidified oxygen until temperature is greater than 32.2°C. For severe hypothermia, provide gastric or peritoneal lavage with warm fluids.
8. Supportive measures: Supplemental oxygen, intubation, assisted ventilation, IV fluids.
9. Treat skin blisters as burns.

Note: Normally, alpha activity in the EEG is associated with wakefulness. When it occurs in coma, it is referred to as **alpha coma.*

10. Withdrawal may be treated by reinstitution of the phenobarbitone, and a program of gradual reduction over three weeks. A tapering schedule of 10% every 3 days has been used successfully.

Autopsy Features

- Peripheral cyanosis.
- Froth at the mouth and nose.
- ***Barbiturate blisters*** on the dependent parts of skin surface*: buttocks, inner aspects or back of thighs, calves and forearms.
- Intensely congested lungs.
- Congestion or even erosion of the stomach.

Forensic Issues

- The incidence of poisoning with barbiturates has declined dramatically in recent years as a direct result of decline in their use as sedative-hypnotics. However, cases do get reported even today, mostly the result of deliberate self-ingestion. This type of (suicidal) poisoning was rampant in the 1960s, when these drugs were widely prescribed and consequently abused. One of the most famous cases during this period concerned immortal Hollywood actress **Marilyn Monroe** (**Fig. 10.9**) who at the end of her short, tempestuous career became hopelessly addicted to alcohol and barbiturates. In 1962, at the age of 36, Marilyn Monroe was found dead at home following an overdose of barbiturates.

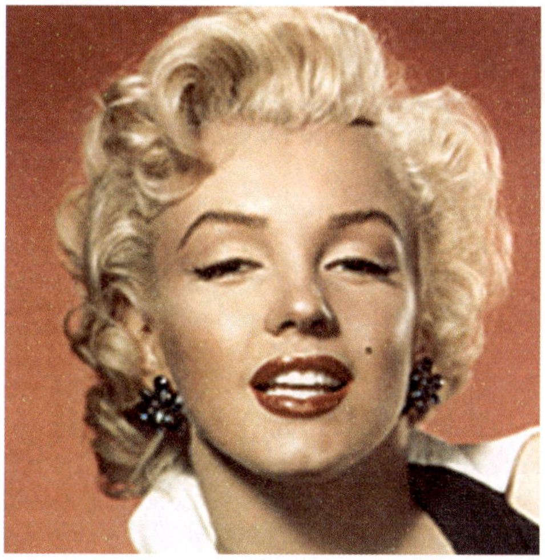

Fig. 10.9 Marilyn Monroe

- In most parts of the world today, the few barbiturates still used in therapeutics comprise phenobarbitone and thiopentone. The latter being available only as an injectable preparation has never been popular for committing suicide. Nevertheless there have been reported cases.
  - A recent trend involves the use of barbiturates in **euthanasia** which is permissible in some Western countries within certain specified guidelines. For example, in Switzerland, the Exit Association which is an organisation providing conditional assistance to individuals wishing to end their own lives, utilises oral pentobarbitone for the purpose.
- Accidental barbiturate poisoning due to inadvertent overdose is not uncommon among addicts because of their phenomenon of tolerance. But, earlier hypotheses that a patient could overdose himself to death by so-called **automatic behaviour** brought on by sleepy confusion have not withstood scientific analysis (*Barbiturate Automatism*).
- Intravenous thiopentone has been used as **truth serum** to extract confessions during interrogation by inducing a state of drowsy disorientation in the course of which the person may reveal the truth. This controversial practice is closely related to the legitimate psychiatric practice of **narcoanalysis** used to diagnose certain mental ailments by placing the patient in a reclining position and administering amylobarbitone or some other short-acting barbiturate intravenously until lateral nystagmus is induced or drowsiness is noted, when the interview is begun and sustained in a gentle fashion with periodic maintenance doses of the drug. This is sometimes referred to as the "**Amytal interview**", amytal being a synonym for amobarbitone in some Western countries.

Benzodiazepines

Examples

Alprazolam, chlordiazepoxide, clonazepam, diazepam, flurazepam, lorazepam, midazolam, nitrazepam, oxazepam, temazepam, triazolam.

Slang Terms

- **Benzodiazepines**: Roches, pumpkin seeds
- **Clonazepam**: Pins
- **Diazepam**: Blue bombers, blue boys, blue thunder, valleys (*esp. Valium*)
- **Flunitrazepam**: Circles, date rape drug, forget me pill, Mexican valium, roofies
- **Chlordiazepoxide**: Green & blacks, green apples
- **Temazepam**: Jelly babies, yellow eggs

Uses

Management of:

- Anxiety disorders
- Seizure disorders
- Insomnia

Usual Fatal Dose

Uncertain for most benzodiazepines. Even ingestion of up to 2000 mg diazepam has not resulted in death, or for that matter, even serious morbidity. However, several cases of fatality due to triazolam and flunitrazepam overdose have been described.

Mode of Action

- Benzodiazepines act by stimulating a subset of the GABA (gamma-aminobutyric acid) receptors, thereby opening up the chloride ion channel in the receptor complex, resulting

**Note*: *Similar blisters may be seen in poisoning due to tricyclics, carbon monoxide, meprobamate and methaqualone.*

in the increased conductance of chloride ion across the nerve cell membrane.

- The subset of $GABA_A$ receptors that bind benzodiazepines are referred to as benzodiazepine receptors (BzR). Once bound to the benzodiazepine receptor, the benzodiazepine ligand locks the benzodiazepine receptor into a conformation in which it has a greater affinity for the GABA neurotransmitter. This increases the frequency of the opening of the associated chloride ion channel and hyperpolarizes the membrane of the associated neuron. The inhibitory effect of the available GABA is potentiated, leading to sedatory and anxiolytic effects.

Toxicokinetics

- Most benzodiazepines are administered orally or by IV injection. Lorazepam and midazolam can also be given IM.
- Following absorption, all benzodiazepines are bound to plasma proteins to the extent of 70–99%, and are metabolised by microsomal enzyme systems in the liver.

Adverse Effects

- Weakness, headache, amnesia, vertigo, diplopia, nausea.
- Paradoxical effects (***disinhibition*** or ***dyscontrol reaction***) may sometimes occur characterised by restlessness, agitation and hallucinations.

Clinical (Toxic) Features

- Benzodiazepines are remarkably safe drugs and rarely produce serious toxic effects even with substantial ingestion. Death is uncommon unless other synergistic drugs have also been ingested. However, newer benzodiazepines such as alprazolam, triazolam and temazepam are associated with fatalities.
- **Acute Poisoning**:
  - *Mild*: Drowsiness, ataxia, weakness.
  - *Moderate* to *Severe*:
    - Vertigo, slurred speech, nystagmus, partial ptosis, lethargy, coma. Hypotension and respiratory depression supervene in potentially lethal ingestions. Both miosis and mydriasis have been reported. Nystagmus occurs occasionally.
    - Respiratory depression is the primary clinical concern in benzodiazepine overdose. Respiratory arrest has occurred following rapid IV administration.
    - Administration of benzodiazepines to a pregnant woman prior to delivery may produce signs of poisoning in the neonate. A condition called "***floppy infant syndrome***", characterized by hypotonia that may last several days, may occur following maternal diazepam use.
- **Chronic Poisoning**:
  - Long-term use of benzodiazepines is associated with the development of tolerance. Abrupt cessation provokes a withdrawal reaction (**Table 10.2**).

Table 10.2 Benzodiazepine Withdrawal Syndrome

▪ Anxiety
▪ Irritability
▪ Insomnia
▪ Fatigue
▪ Headache
▪ Muscle ache, twitching
▪ Tremor
▪ Sweating
▪ Vertigo
▪ Nausea, loss of appetite
▪ Depression
▪ Difficulty in concentration
▪ Abnormal perception

Diagnosis

- Estimation of plasma levels of benzodiazepines is usually not necessary. Qualitative testing for presence of benzodiazepine is helpful to confirm presence, especially when overdose history is sketchy. Quantitative levels are not usually clinically useful.
- Blisters of skin (bullae) can occur following overdose with nitrazepam, oxazepam and temazepam.

Treatment

- **Acute Poisoning**:
  - ***Decontamination***: Stomach wash may be helpful, if the patient is seen within 6–12 hrs after the ingestion. Cuffed endotracheal intubation is a prerequisite in comatose patients. Activated charcoal adsorbs benzodiazepines and can be administered in the usual manner.
  - Establish clear airway. Oxygen and assisted ventilation are often necessary.
  - Monitor level of consciousness, respiratory rate, pulse oximetry and blood pressure in symptomatic patients. Consider arterial blood gas analysis in patients who have a reduced level of consciousness, or have reduced oxygen saturations on pulse oximetry.
  - IV fluids (Ringer's lactate at a rate of 150 mL/hr for adults).
  - Correction of hypotension: Begin by infusing 10–20 mL/kg of isotonic fluid, and place patient in Trendelenburg position. If hypotension persists, administer dopamine or noradrenaline.
  - ***Antidote***:
    - **Flumazenil** is effective in reversing the coma induced by benzodiazepines. The effect is however usually short-lived, and flumazenil also has the tendency to induce a withdrawal reaction in benzodiazepine-dependent patients.
    - The mode of action is competitive antagonism.
    - Recommended initial IV dose is 0.2 mg (2 mL), administered over 15 sec. If adequate consciousness is not obtained within 45 sec, a further dose of 0.2 mg (2 mL) may be repeated at 60-sec intervals to a maximum total dose of 1 mg (10 mL). Most patients will respond to 0.6–1 mg; titrate each case as needed.

- However, re-sedation occurs within ½-hr to 2 hrs, and therefore patients must be carefully monitored and subsequent doses of flumazenil should be administered as needed.
- It is not necessary or appropriate in cases of poisoning to fully reverse the benzodiazepine effect. Since flumazenil has a short half-life, an infusion may be required. The use of continuous flumazenil maintenance infusion over 5 –24 hrs seems of therapeutic value in the event of re-sedation after initial response.
- Flumazenil has also been reported to reverse cardiovascular depression secondary to benzodiazepine use.
- Flumazenil is contraindicated in mixed ingestions involving tricyclic antidepressants and drugs which induce seizures, e.g., theophylline, carbamazepine, chloroquine, etc.
- ***Adverse effects***:
  - Fatigue, vertigo, nausea, vomiting, hypertension, tachycardia, anxiety, confusion, restlessness, aggression, paraesthesia, and rarely convulsions and cardiac arrhythmias.

- **Chronic Poisoning**:
  - Phenobarbitone-substitution technique is recommended for benzodiazepine withdrawal which employs propranolol for acute somatic symptoms, while phenobarbitone is used for detoxification.
  - However the most frequently used method among clinicians is the replacement of a short half-life benzodiazepine (such as alprazolam) with a long half-life benzodiazepine (such as clonazepam), before initiating a taper and final discontinuation.

Forensic Issues

- Ever since the introduction of benzodiazepines in the 1960s, they have become progressively more popular as anxiolytic agents and sedatives, displacing the barbiturates from their previously held top spot. In spite of extensive use worldwide, there have been only a few cases reported involving fatalities, demonstrating the wide margin of safety of benzodiazepines. But complacency must be avoided and the safety profile of these drugs should not be taken for granted, as deaths have been reported in some recent cases even from unexpectedly low doses of certain benzodiazepines. There are also indications that some of the newer benzodiazepines have a slightly smaller margin of safety.
- An area of concern with long-term benzodiazepine use is the possibility of ***behavioural disinhibition*** which may induce a person to hostile acts, aggressive behaviour and verbal indecency.
- Yet another important issue is with reference to the use of benzodiazepines to deliberately induce amnesia in certain individuals in order to accomplish an immoral act (e.g., **date rape**). Many of these drugs, particularly flunitrazepam, are capable of causing retrograde amnesia. Flunitrazepam (Rohypnol®; "Roofies") (**Fig. 10.10**) has become popular as a drug of abuse, often combined with alcohol, marijuana or cocaine to produce an intense "high". It has been used as a "date rape" drug, both for its properties of lowering inhibitions and because it can cause retrograde amnesia.
- While addiction to benzodiazepines is an undeniable possibility among patients on long term therapy, the abuse potential is much less when compared to most other sedative-hypnotics such as the barbiturates. Withdrawal reactions are also generally less severe and more easily managed.

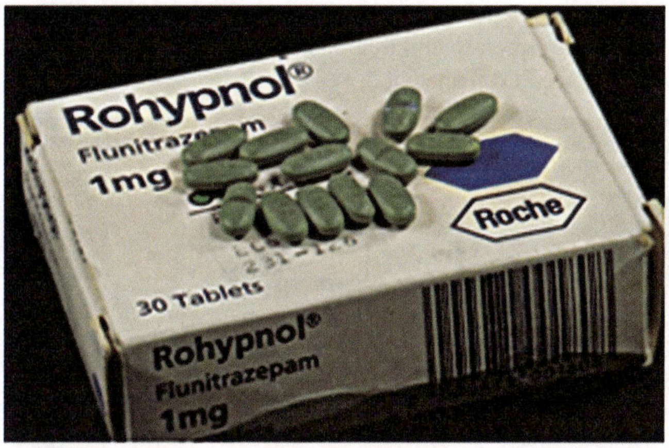

Fig. 10.10 Rohypnol tablets ("Roofies")

Phenytoin

Phenytoin (Diphenylhydantoin) was first synthesized in 1908, but its anticonvulsant property was discovered only in 1938. It is effective against all types of partial and tonic-clonic seizures, but not absence seizures.* Phenytoin is also used in the treatment of ventricular arrhythmias (especially digitalis-induced).

Fosphenytoin is another hydantoin anticonvulsant which is chemically related to phenytoin.

Toxicokinetics

- Phenytoin is reasonably well absorbed on oral administration. It is given intravenously in status epilepticus. Intravenous phenytoin should be administered only with saline and not with glucose as it precipitates in the latter. Intramuscular injection is not advisable since the drug gets precipitated at the site, and absorption is slow as well as erratic.
- In acute overdose, peak levels are frequently delayed for 24–48 hrs, and occasionally as long as 7 days. Toxicity may persist for 7–10 days.

Mode of Action

- Phenytoin acts on the motor cortex preventing the spread of seizure activity. It stabilises the threshold for hyperexcitability and reduces post-tetanic potentiation at synapses.

****Note***: *An "absence seizure" is characterised by abrupt onset of impaired consciousness associated with staring and cessation of activities, typically lasting less than 30 sec. There is no muscular activity or contraction.*

- Further, phenytoin reduces brainstem activity which is responsible for the tonic phase of tonic-clonic convulsion.

Adverse Effects

- Therapeutic doses (especially when administered over a prolonged period of time) can result in dyskinesia, peripheral neuropathy, hirsutism, hypokalaemia, macrocytic anaemia, hepatitis, thyroiditis, skin rashes, vertigo, mild sedation and CNS depression, ataxia, dysarthria, nystagmus and diplopia. Chronic high blood levels may cause a "**phenytoin encephalopathy**" with increase in seizure frequency and the development of more tonic or opisthotonic components.
- **Gingival hypertrophy** (**Fig. 10.11**) occurs in about 20% of patients (mostly children or adolescents), and is due to altered collagen metabolism.

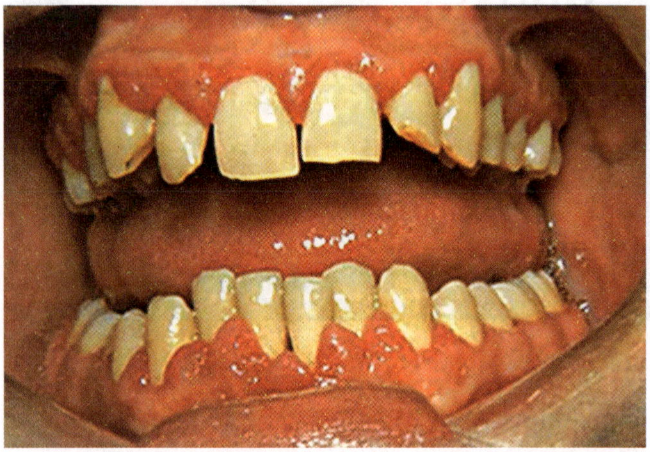

Fig. 10.11 Gingival hypertrophy due to phenytoin

- Hypersensitivity reactions are known to occur with phenytoin and usually manifest as fever, rash, lymphadenopathy and hepatosplenomegaly, 3 weeks to 3 months after initiation of therapy. Such a reaction (**phenytoin hypersensitivity syndrome**) can be potentially fatal.
- **Purple glove syndrome** has been reported following intravenous phenytoin. It is a progressive development of limb oedema, discolouration and pain after phenytoin administration, with some patients developing skin ulceration.
- Phenytoin is a known teratogen and can cause a number of defects in the newborn, together referred to as **foetal hydantoin syndrome** (**Table 10.3**) (**Fig. 10.12**). This is especially likely, if phenytoin is used during the first trimester of pregnancy. Increased risk of neural-tube defects, cardiovascular defects, oral clefts and urinary tract defects have been reported.

Toxic Effects

- Overdose with phenytoin causes at first lateral gaze nystagmus, ataxia and drowsiness, followed by vertical or horizontal nystagms, oscillopsia (a very fine vertical or horizontal periodic dancing of the eyes), slurred speech, lurching gait, coarse tremor of the extremities, mental confusion and disorientation.
- True coma is uncommon. Severe poisonings may rarely result in respiratory depression.
- Sometimes, paradoxical intoxication occurs characterised by increased seizure activity.
- Hypotension appears to be common following intravenous phenytoin, and is concentration- and dose-related.
- Death is rare, and if it does occur, it is invariably due to cardiac arrest or ventricular fibrillation.

Usual Fatal Dose

- An upper limit for therapeutic phenytoin serum concentration is generally considered as 20 μg/mL.
- Toxic effects are usually seen at levels >30 μg/mL.

Treatment

1. *Decontamination*: Stomach wash and activated charcoal are beneficial.
2. *Stabilisation*:
   a. Cardiac monitoring is advisable following parenteral overdose or rapid infusions.
   b. Treat hypotension by Trendelenberg position, fluid infusion and pressor amines (dopamine or noradrenaline).
   c. Treat heart block with atropine or pacemaker.

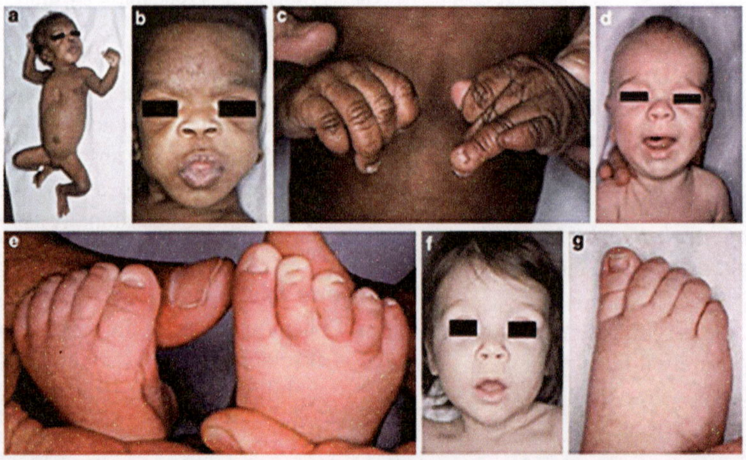

Fig. 10.12 Infants afflicted with foetal hydantoin syndrome

Table 10.3 Foetal Hydantoin Syndrome

Chest Anomalies	Cranio-facial Anomalies	Limb Anomalies	Other Anomalies
▪ Widespread nipples ▪ Chest wall deformities	▪ Mental retardation ▪ Broad nasal bridge ▪ Low-set hairline ▪ Short neck ▪ Ocular hypertelorism ▪ Microcephaly ▪ Cleft lip/palate ▪ Low-set ears ▪ Epicanthic folds ▪ Ptosis	▪ Small nails ▪ Digital thumb ▪ Dislocated hip	▪ Pilonidal sinus ▪ Hernia ▪ Abnormal genitals ▪ Neuroblastoma ▪ Acne vulgaris ▪ Hirsutism

d. For seizures (paradoxical intoxication), use diazepam. If seizures persist or recur, administer phenobarbitone.
e. *Supportive measures*: Hypersensitivity reactions may respond to corticosteroids.
f. Forced diuresis, peritoneal dialysis and haemodialysis are generally ineffective.

Lithium

Lithium, the lightest of all metals is the drug of choice even today (more than 50 years after its introduction) for the treatment of manic-depressive psychosis, i.e., bipolar affective disorder. It is also useful as adjunctive therapy for depression, mania in children and young adults, alcoholism and as a prophylaxis for cluster headaches.

Toxicokinetics

- Lithium is rapidly absorbed on oral administration and peak levels are achieved in 2–4 hrs. It is evenly distributed among the tissue compartments.
- The therapeutic elimination half-life is about 20–24 hrs, and 95% of the drug is excreted by the kidney of which 80% is reabsorbed, while the remaining 20% appears in the urine unchanged.

Mode of Action

- The exact mechanism of action is so unclear that there have been innumerable theories propounded to explain the therapeutic efficacy of lithium in bipolar disorders none of which have been conclusively demonstrated to be correct.
- The main premise is as follows: since lithium crosses cell membranes by various methods including the sodium pump, the sodium leak canal, a lithium–bicarbonate exchange and the sodium–lithium counter-exchange system, it is believed that the chemical exerts its therapeutic effect by substituting for sodium in these transmembranal ion exchanges.

Adverse Effects

- Thirst, polyuria, tremor, acne, hypothyroidism, impaired concentration, ataxia and dysarthria.
- Less commonly there may be alopecia, psoriasis of fingernails and restless legs syndrome.

Toxic Effects

There are three types of lithium poisoning:

1. Acute poisoning in patients ***not*** under lithium treatment – mild or moderately severe manifestations.
2. Acute poisoning in patients under lithium treatment – severe manifestations.
3. Chronic poisoning in patients under lithium treatment.

Table 10.4 lists the manifestations of lithium toxicity.

There are indications that lithium intake during pregnancy may be associated with cardiovascular and other congenital malformations. Congenital malformations, including cardiac defects have been reported in infants of mothers receiving lithium therapy in the first trimester. Lithium toxicity may be one of the causes of **Floppy baby syndrome**, which manifests as cyanosis with hypotonia.

Diagnosis

1. Blood lithium level (BLL):
   a. Therapeutic levels generally range from 0.6 to 1.2 mEq/L.
   b. Toxicity is associated with levels over 2 mEq/L.
   c. Death is likely, if the BLL crosses 5 mEq/L.
2. Toxicity is unlikely in patients who ingest <50 mg/kg lithium carbonate.
3. Lithium can be measured by atomic spectrophotometry, ion-selective electrode or emission photometery.
4. Evidence of hypernatraemia, hypocalcaemia and hypoparathyroidism.

Treatment

1. **Stabilisation**: Maintenance of airway, breathing and circulation. Cardiac monitoring is desirable.
2. In the case of hypotension, infuse 10–20 mL/kg of isotonic fluid and place in Trendelenburg position. If hypotension persists, administer dopamine or noradrenaline.
3. **Decontamination**: Activated charcoal is ineffective. Stomach wash may help if the patient is seen early. Whole-bowel irrigation with polyethylene-electrolyte solution (PEG-ELS) is said to be quite beneficial. The recommended rates of administration are 2 L/hr (adult) and 500 mL/hr (child).
4. **Elimination enhancement**: Haemodialysis is indicated in the following situations:

a. Severe intoxication with coma, convulsions or respiratory failure.
b. > Grade 3 coma.
c. Progressive deterioration.
d. Rising serum concentration.
e. >4 mEq/L of serum concentration.

5. **Supportive measures**.

Neuroleptics

These drugs are also referred to as **major tranquillisers** or **antipsychotics**. Many of these drugs act as dopamine receptor antagonists, though a few of them do not (e.g., clozapine).

I. ***Typical or First Generation Antipsychotics***:
   1. **Phenothiazines**: Chlorpromazine, triflupromazine. trifluoperazine, prochlorperazine, fluphenazine, thioridazine.
   2. **Thioxanthenes**: Chlorprothixene, clopenthixol, flupenthixol,
   3. **Butyrophenones**: Droperidol, haloperidol, benperidol

II. ***Atypical or Second Generation Antipsychotics***:
   1. **Dibenzodiazepines**: Clozapine, olanzapine
   2. **Benzisoxazoles**: Risperidone
   3. **Dibenzothiazepine**: Quetiapine

III. ***Third Generation Antipsychotics***:
   1. Aripiprazole

Mode of Action

- Neuroleptics inhibit the activity of a variety of receptors – dopaminergic, cholinergic, $alpha_1$ & $alpha_2$ adrenergic, histaminic and serotonergic ($5HT_2$).
- Neuroleptic activity is thought to be related to the dopamine-receptor blocking activity in the limbic system. Most neuroleptics have a high affinity for D_2 and D_3 receptors.

Uses

- Neuroleptics are used in the treatment of schizophrenia, manic phase of manic-depressive illness, severe depression associated with psychosis and organic psychotic states.
- Haloperidol is frequently used for agitation or aggressive behaviour, especially in elderly patients.

Toxicokinetics

- All dopamine receptor antagonists are generally well absorbed on oral or parenteral administration. Haloperidol is readily absorbed (60–70%) from the gastrointestinal tract.
- Plasma concentrations usually peak 1–4 hrs after ingestion and ½ to 1 hr after intramuscular injection.
- Most antipsychotics are highly lipophilic and accumulate in fat, lungs and brain. They are generally highly protein-bound.
- Metabolism is largely hepatic and occurs through conjugation with glucuronic acid, hydroxylation, oxidation, demethylation and sulphoxide formation.

Adverse & Toxic Effects

1. **Neurological**:
   a. **Neuroleptic malignant syndrome (NMS)**:
      i. This is a rare complication occurring in about 0.02–2.4% of patients taking antipsychotic medication.
      ii. NMS can be caused by other drugs also.
      iii. Among the neuroleptics, NMS is most frequently associated with phenothiazines, butyrophenones and thioxanthines.
      iv. NMS is believed to be an idiosyncratic reaction and carries with it a high mortality (20–40%). The syndrome is twice as common in males as in females, and is more likely to occur in younger patients.
      v. The pathophysiology is thought to be central dopamine blockade, and symptoms usually begin 3–9 days after neuroleptic treatment, lasting for about 5–10 days even after discontinuing the drug.

Table 10.4 Lithium Poisoning

System	Acute	Chronic
GIT	Nausea, vomiting	Nausea
CNS	Weakness, vertigo, tremor, twitching, hyperreflexia, muscle rigidity, ataxia, agitation, tinnitus, drowsiness, slurred speech, confusion, convulsions, extrapyramidal symptoms, CNS depression, coma	Parkinsonism, psychosis, photophobia, blurred vision
CVS	Prolonged QT interval, ST and T wave anomalies, hypotension	Myocarditis, T wave changes, bundle branch blocks, bradycardia, hypotension
Blood	Leukocytosis	Aplastic anaemia
Renal	Polyuria	Nephrogenic diabetes insipidus, interstitial nephritis, renal failure
Endocrine	–	Hypothyroidism
Skin	–	Dermatitis, ulcers

In essence, NMS is a severe form of extrapyramidal reaction and is manifested by hyperthermia (39–42°C), muscular hypertonicity (generalised "lead pipe" rigidity, akinesia, tremor, choreoathetosis), fluctuating mental status (confusion, agitation, stupor) and autonomic irregularities (tachycardia, labile blood pressure, tachypnoea, urinary incontinence, respiratory stridor, sweating, cardiac arrest).

- **Complications** include rhabdomyolysis, aspiration pneumonia, pulmonary embolism, pulmonary oedema, ARDS, DIC, seizures, myocardial infarction, peripheral neuropathy and death.

vi. **Laboratory investigations** indicate the presence of metabolic acidosis, liver enzyme abnormalities, leukocytosis and elevation of creatinine as well as creatine phosphokinase.

b. **Acute extrapyramidal syndromes**: These syndromes result from decreased dopamine activity in the basal ganglia and have their onset soon after initiation of antipsychotic drug therapy, but disappear once the drug use is discontinued.

i. **Akathisia** – It is the most common and most distressing of the acute extrapyramidal syndromes resulting from antipsychotic therapy and is characterised by a sensation of restlessness manifesting as agitation, fidgeting, restless legs, hostility and belligerence.

ii. **Acute dystonia** – This is characterised by oculogyric crisis (upward gaze paralysis), spasms of jaw and throat, tongue protrusion, torticollis (neck twisting), retrocollis (spasm of back of neck), opisthotonus, facial grimacing, tortipelvis (abdominal wall spasm) and laryngeal dystonia which can be life threatening.

iii. **Parkinsonism** – This is more common in elderly patients and manifests classically as akinesia, rigidity, shuffling gait, mask-like facies and tremor. Examination often reveals a positive glabella tap.

c. **Chronic extrapyramidal syndromes**:

i. **Tardive dyskinesia** – This is the most serious side effect of long-term phenothiazine and haloperidol treatment. Manifestations are quite disabling and comprise facial gimacing, eye blinking, furrowing of eyebrows, lip smacking, tongue protrusion, jaw deviation and choreoathetoid-like movements of the limbs. These features are completely absent in sleep. Once established, tardive dyskinesia may take a long time to disappear, and sometimes becomes permanent.

ii. **Rabbit syndrome** – This is characterised by rhythmic involuntary movements of the oral and masticatory musculature mimicking the chewing movements of a rabbit. It may be irreversible.

2. **Cardiovascular**: Common cardiovascular adverse effects include orthostatic (or postural) hypotension, cardiac arrhythmias and ECG anomalies (prolongation of PR, QRS, & QTc intervals, blunt T waves and depressed ST segments).
3. **Gastrointestinal**: Gastrointestinal toxic effects manifest as dry mouth and constipation; less commonly there may be vomiting or diarrhoea.
4. **Other systems**:
   a. Urinary retention may result from the anticholinergic effect of many of these drugs.
   b. Leukopenia, thrombocytopenia, agranulocytosis and pancytopenia are rare complications.
   c. Skin rash occasionally occurs. Photosensitivity reactions are not uncommon, and therefore patients should be instructed to avoid direct sunlight.
   d. Female patients may experience galactorrhoea, breast enlargement and irregular menses while on antipsychotic medication owing to increased circulating prolactin concentrations. In males, there may be decreased libido, erectile disturbances and ejaculatory problems.
   e. Hepatic disease has been associated with almost all of the phenothiazines. Cholestatic jaundice or mixed cholestatic and hepatocellular jaundice are the most common hepatic problems associated with therapeutic use and overdose.
5. **Acute overdose**:
   a. Result in the exaggeration of the usual adverse effects already described, and summarised in **Table 10.5**.

Laboratory Investigations

- Monitor acid–base status, fluid and electrolyte balance, hepatic enzyme levels (serum ALP, SGOT and SGPT), renal function and urine output.
- Patients with clinical signs of neuroleptic malignant syndrome should be monitored for rising serum CPK levels and leukocyte count. Institute continuous cardiac monitoring and follow serial ECGs.
- Unabsorbed phenothiazines are radiopaque in the gastrointestinal tract, and the diagnosis of phenothiazine ingestion can be made radiographically. Absence of radiopacity does not rule out phenothiazine overdose.
- Phenothiazines have been reported to impart a pink or red colour to the urine.

Treatment

1. **Neuroleptic malignant syndrome**:
   a. Discontinue neuroleptic therapy.

Table 10.5 Neuroleptic Drug Overdose

- Severe rigidity, dystonia
- Sedation, delirium, restlessness
- Convulsions
- Fever
- Hypotension, ECG changes, cardiac arrhythmias
- Mydriasis
- Anticholinergic effects: Dry mouth, ileus, urinary retention
- Coma, respiratory depression

b. Diazepam 10–20 mg or lorazepam 1–2 mg every 4–6 hrs, is recommended in mild to moderate NMS.
c. Management of hyperthermia by rapid external cooling with ice.
d. Dantrolene sodium: 1–2.5 mg/kg, IV every 6 hrs for 48 hrs.
e. Bromocriptine: Initially 2.5 mg 8 hourly, orally or by nasogastric tube. Can be increased to a maximum of 45 mg/day.
f. Amanditine: 100 mg 8–12 hourly orally or by nasogastric tube can be given in place of bromocriptine.
g. Perform a 12-lead ECG and measure the QRS duration and QT interval.
h. Supportive measures: Correction of fluid and electrolyte imbalance, management of hypo/hypertension, maintaining pulmonary, cardiovascular & renal functions and sedation.

2. **Acute extrapyramidal syndromes**:
   a. **Akathisia**:
      i. Reduce dose of neuroleptic drug.
      ii. Administer antiparkinsonian drugs or benzodiazepines, or both.
   b. **Acute dystonia**:
      i. Diphenhydramine, 1–2 mg/kg, IV (maximum 100 mg), **or** benztropine mesylate, 1–2 mg, IV
   c. **Parkinsonism**: Administration of antiparkinsonian drugs.
3. **Chronic extrapyramidal syndromes**:
   a. **Tardive dyskinesia**:
      i. Treatment of tardive dyskinesia has been attempted with a wide variety of drugs with little or no success. They include the following: serotonergic drugs (tryptophan, cyproheptadine), noradrenergic drugs (lithium), beta-adrenergic receptor antagonists (propranolol) and alpha-adrenergic agonists (clonidine). Benzodiazepines may give temporary relief, but sometimes there is exacerbation.
   b. **Rabbit syndrome**:
      i. Discontinue neuroleptic therapy.
      ii. Administer antiparkinsonian drugs.
4. **Cardiovascular toxicity**:
   a. Arrhythmias can be managed effectively by temporary cardiac pacing which should preferably last for 10 days, especially in patients who have presented with ventricular tachycardia associated with AV block I or II. Cardioversion is often required for ventricular tachycardia, and is the initial treatment for ventricular fibrillation, but the arrhythmias are often resistant.
   b. Hypotension usually responds to Trendelenberg position and Ringer's lactate. If vasopressors are considered necessary, alpha-adrenergic agonists such as noradrenaline are the drugs of choice.
5. **Gastrointestinal symptoms**: Patients who experience a severely dry mouth should be advised to rinse their mouth frequently, and to chew gum (preferably sugar-less) or candy.
6. **Acute neuroleptic overdose**:
   a. Stabilisation: Intubation, assisted ventilation, IV line, cardiac monitoring.
   b. Decontamination: Gastric lavage, activated charcoal.
   c. Elimination enhancement: Haemodialysis, haemoperfusion, etc., do not appear to be beneficial.
   d. Management of convulsions with diazepam or phenytoin. If seizures recur, administer phenobarbitone.
   e. Management of hypotension: Fluid challenge is sufficient for correction of hypotension in most patients.
   f. Cardiac monitoring: Since the phenothiazines produce "quinidine-like" effects on the myocardium, quinidine, procainamide and disopyramide should be avoided. Lignocaine is usually effective for ventricular arrhythmias. Cardioversion is often required for ventricular tachycardia, and is the initial treatment for ventricular fibrillation, but the dysrhythmias are often resistant. A pacing wire may be the only effective treatment, especially if atrioventricular block is present.
   g. Management of rhabdomyolysis.

Antidepressants

Major depression is one of the affective disorders, and is perhaps the commonest mental illness worldwide. It is characterised by feelings of intense sadness and despair, slowing of thought process, impaired concentration, constant worry, agitation and self-deprecation.

1. **Cyclic antidepressants**:
   a. **Tricyclic antidepressants (TCAs)**: Amitriptyline, clomipramine, desipramine, doxepin, imipramine, nortriptyline.
   b. **Tetracyclic antidepressants (TeCAs)**: Amoxapine, maprotiline, mirtazapine.
2. **Selective serotonin reuptake inhibitors (SSRIs)**: Citalopram, escitalopram, fluoxetine, fluvoxamine, paroxetine, sertraline.
3. **Monoamine oxidase inhibitors (MAOIs)**: Isocarboxacid, phenelzine, tranylcypromine, selegiline, moclobemide.
4. **Norepinephrine (noradrenaline) reuptake inhibitors (NRIs)**: Reboxetine, viloxazine.
5. **Serotonin-norepinephrine (serotonin-noradrenaline) reuptake inhibitors (SNRIs)**: Desvenlafaxine, duloxetine, venlafaxine.
6. **Serotonin antagonists and reuptake inhibitors (SARIs)**: Nefazodone, trazodone.
7. **Atypical antidepressants**: Bupropion.

The toxicity of only **tricyclic antidepressants** among these groups will be discussed here, since the other drugs are not mentioned in the new curriculum.

Cyclic Antidepressants

The foundation for the **norepinephrine hypothesis of depression** was laid by the discovery in **1957** of the antidepressant property of imipramine. During the next two decades several more compounds were developed which also had similar antidepressant properties and came to be called the "**tricyclics**" or "**cyclic antidepressants.**"

- **Tricyclic antidepressants (TCAs)**: Amitriptyline, clomipramine, desipramine, doxepin, imipramine, nortriptyline.
- **Tetracyclic antidepressants (TeCAs)**: Amoxapine, maprotiline, mirtazapine.

Toxicokinetics

- All cyclic antidepressants are rapidly absorbed from the GI tract and have large volumes of distribution.
- They are all highly lipophilic, sparingly water soluble and substantially metabolised by first-pass in the liver.

Mode of Action

- Tricyclics are structurally similar to the phenothiazines with similar anticholinergic, adrenergic and alpha-blocking properties of the phenothiazines.
- They act by inhibiting voltage-gated sodium channels in myocardial cells, blocking of H_1, H_2 and D_2 receptors, as well as muscarinic receptors, inhibiting alpha-adrenergic receptors, interacting with GABA receptors, and inhibiting the transport and reuptake of biogenic amines at nerve terminals.

Adverse Effects

- Postural hypotension, cardiac arrhythmias, vertigo, weakness, tremor, confusion, weight gain, agranulocytosis and thrombocytopenia.
- Anticholinergic effects are common: Tachycardia, hypertension, mydriasis, dry and flushed skin, visual blurring, decreased GI motility, urinary retention, and delirium with hallucinations and convulsions.

Toxic Effects

- Overdose results in seizures, tachycardia, hypotension, agitation, hallucinations, confusion, delirium, hyperthermia, ataxia, urinary retention and coma.
- Neuroleptic malignant syndrome (NMS) has been reported.
- Cardiovascular toxicity results in myocardial depression, ventricular tachycardia and fibrillation. A variety of ECG findings have been described: prolongation of the PR, QRS and QT intervals, non-specific ST segment and T wave changes and atrioventricular block.

Usual Fatal Dose

- Serum drug level of more than 1000 ng/mL (10–20 mg/kg). The therapeutic range for most tricyclic antidepressants is 100–260 ng/mL.
- About 10 times the therapeutic daily dose of a cyclic antidepressant is potentially fatal.

Diagnosis

1. ECG changes (*vide supra*). Monitor serial ECGs and institute continuous cardiac monitoring in all patients with suspected tricyclic overdose.
2. Elevation of creatine kinase and lactic acid dehydrogenase levels.
3. Chest X-ray to detect pulmonary oedema.

Treatment

1. *Supportive measures*:
   a. Maintain airway; intubate, if indicated.
   b. Monitor arterial blood gases.
   c. Administer oxygen, if necessary.
   d. Treat hypotension with IV crystalloids, inotropes (dopamine), vasopressors (noradrenaline), etc., as necessary.
2. *Reduce drug absorption*:
   a. Stomach wash (within the first 6 hrs).
   b. Consider activated charcoal (dose: 50 g for adults, 1 g/kg body weight for children) by mouth or naso-gastric tube, if the patient presents within 1 hr of ingesting a toxic dose.
3. *Enhance drug elimination*:
   a. Multiple-dose activated charcoal.
   b. Forced diuresis, haemodialysis and haemoperfusion are of no value due to the large volume of distribution of tricyclic antidepressants.
4. *Treat convulsions*:
   a. Control convulsions that are frequent or prolonged with IV diazepam (10–20 mg in adults; 0.1–0.3 mg/kg in children), lorazepam (4 mg in adults; 0.1 mg/kg in children), or midazolam (5–10 mg in adults; 0.05–0.15 mg/kg in children).
   b. Phenytoin 15 mg/kg IV infusion.
5. *Treat arrhythmias*:
   a. Perform a 12-lead ECG and measure the QRS duration and QT interval. A repeat 12-lead ECG is recommended, especially in symptomatic patients or in those who have ingested slow release preparations.
   b. QT prolongation occurs due to potassium channel blockade and may provoke torsade de pointes ventricular tachycardia. Magnesium sulphate should be administered urgently to patients with torsade de pointes.
   c. Serum alkalinization to a pH of 7.45–7.55 using intravenous boluses of sodium bicarbonate is recommended for patients with arrhythmias or QRS widening.
   d. If cardiotoxicity is unresponsive, consider the use of a lipid emulsion.
6. *Other measures:*
   a. If metabolic acidosis persists despite correction of hypoxia and adequate fluid resuscitation consider correction with IV sodium bicarbonate.
   b. Agitated adults can be sedated with an initial dose of oral or IV diazepam (0.1–0.3 mg/kg). Consider oral (5–10 mg) or parenteral (2–10 mg) haloperidol in the elderly. In children, it is better to manage agitation without sedation, and exclude other causes (e.g., hypoxia, infection, hypoglycaemia and raised ICP).
   c. Mild hyperthermia should be treated with conventional cooling measures. In patients with pyrexia, monitor renal function and creatine kinase activity. Ensure adequate hydration and monitor urine output carefully. When body temperature exceeds 39°C, urgent cooling measures such as ice-baths, internal cooling devices

and sedation should be used, depending on availability. Dantrolene may be considered (1 mg/kg by IV injection to a maximum of 10 mg/kg).

NARCOTIC ANALGESICS

Though the new curriculum mentions these as **Narcotic Analgesics**, the correct term is just **Narcotics** or **Narcotic Drugs**, as some of these are not analgesics at all.

NARCOTICS (SOMNIFEROUS DRUGS)

Opium

Opium refers to the dried extract of the **poppy plant** (*Papaver somniferum*) which belongs to the family Papaveraceae and is a herb growing up to 1 m in height. The leaves are oblong, irregularly toothed and slightly lobed. Flowers are large and may be pink, purple or white in colour (**Fig. 10.13**). Each plant bears 5–8 capsules which are incised in their unripe state to extract a milky fluid that on drying yields opium (**Fig. 10.14**). *Papaver somniferum* grows well in India, but its **cultivation is banned** except on license obtained from the central government, for growing the plant strictly for the pharmaceutical industry. Such a **license** is issued only for the states of **Rajasthan**, **Uttar Pradesh** and **Madhya Pradesh**.* India produces 70–80% of opium that is used worldwide by pharmaceutical companies to manufacture several vital drugs including morphine, codeine and pethidine. Unfortunately, a significant quantity of opium is funnelled clandestinely into a global smuggling racket which feeds the illicit drug trade flourishing in Western countries.

While "narcosis" is virtually synonymous with "hypnosis" in the sense that both words refer to *induction of sleep*, the former has come to be associated almost exclusively with the state of mind induced by opium and its derivatives, many of which produce analgesia in addition to somnolence. Hence, all **opiates** and **opioids** are referred to as **narcotic drugs** (or just **narcotics**).

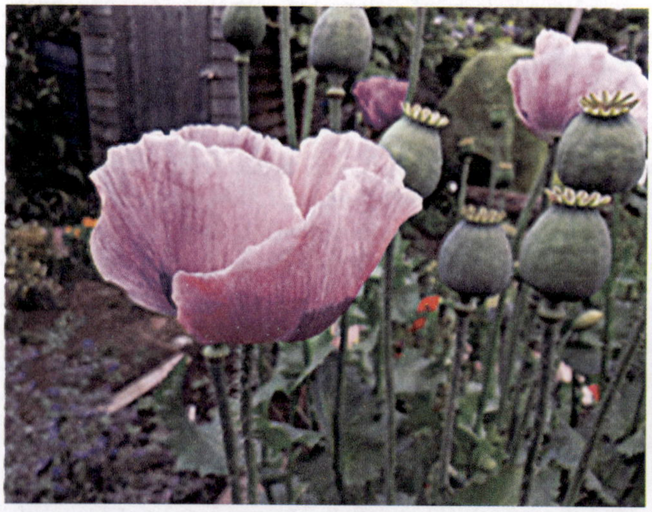

Fig. 10.13 Papaver somniferum

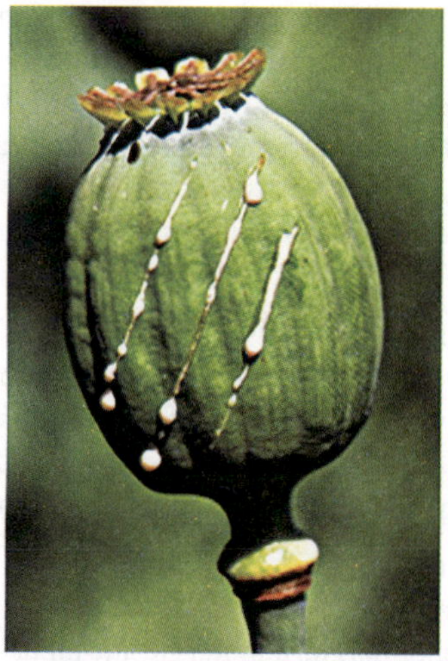

Fig. 10.14 Incised poppy capsule with exudation of juice

Physical Appearance

- Crude opium is a dark brown or grey irregular mass (**Fig. 10.15**) with a characteristic odour and bitter taste, obtained from unripe poppy fruit capsule or poppy straw.
- Raw opium typically contains approximately 10% morphine.
- Poppy seeds (**Fig. 10.16**) contain very low levels of opiates, and the oil extracted from them contains even less.

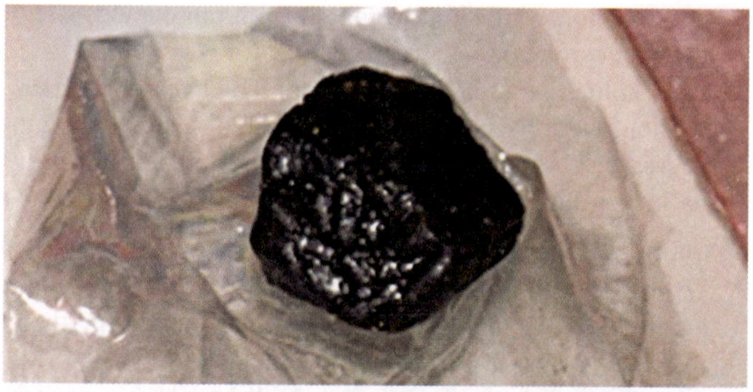

Fig. 10.15 Crude (black tar) opium

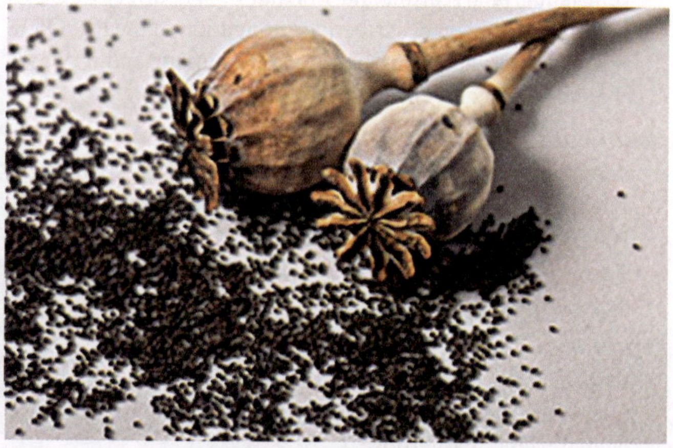

Fig. 10.16 Poppy capsules with seeds spilling out

**Note: Easy to remember: RUM!*

They are commonly used in cuisine from many different cultures. Poppy seeds are a common and flavoursome topping for breads and cakes. One gram of poppy seeds contains up to 33 μg of morphine and 14 μg of codeine.

Toxic Part

- **Fruit capsule (unripe)**

Toxic Principles

- Opium contains a number of alkaloids which fall into two groups:
  1. *Phenanthrene group*: Morphine, codeine and thebaine.
  2. *Benzylisoquinoline group*: Papaverine and noscapine (narcotine).
- Apart from these natural derivatives there are several other drugs used in pharmacotherapeutics which are either semisynthetic or synthetic analogues (**Table 10.6**).
  - When referring to these derivatives, there has always been confusion in terminology. While strictly speaking, the term "**opiate**" refers to natural and semisynthetic derivatives, and the term "**opioid**" is a more inclusive term applying to all agonists and antagonists with morphine-like activity, for the sake of convenience (and to avoid confusion), the former term will be used in this book as an umbrella-expression to cover all derivatives of opium – natural, semisynthetic and synthetic.

Uses

Opiates have tremendous pharmacological importance, and are used for various therapeutic purposes (**Table 10.6**).

Usual Fatal Dose

The usual fatal doses (as well as usual therapeutic doses) of common opiates are listed in **Table 10.7**.

Mode of Action

Today, it is believed that there are three major classes of opiate receptors to which different opiates bind with differing affinity:

Table 10.6 Pharmacological Uses of Opiates

Derivative	Nature	Use
Buprenorphine	Semisynthetic	Analgesic, pre-anaesthetic medication
Butorphanol	Semisynthetic	Analgesic
Codeine	Natural	Antitussive
Dextromethorphan	Semisynthetic	Antitussive
Diphenoxylate	Synthetic	Antidiarrhoeal
Fentanyl	Synthetic	Adjunct to anaesthesia
Heroin	Semisynthetic	–
Loperamide	Synthetic	Antidiarrhoeal
Methadone	Synthetic	Analgesic, treatment of opiate abstinence syndrome
Morphine	Natural	Analgesic
Nalbuphine	Semisynthetic	Analgesic
Nalmefene	Semisynthetic	Treatment of acute opiate poisoning
Naloxone	Semisynthetic	Treatment of acute opiate poisoning
Naltrexone	Semisynthetic	Treatment of opiate addiction
Oxycodone	Semisynthetic	Analgesic
Pentazocine	Semisynthetic	Analgesic
Pethidine (Meperidine)	Synthetic	Analgesic
Propoxyphene	Synthetic	Analgesic
Tramadol	Synthetic	Analgesic

Table 10.7 Usual Fatal Dose & Usual Therapeutic Dose for Common Opiates

Opiate	Usual Fatal Dose	Usual Therapeutic Dose
Morphine	200 mg	10–15 mg
Codeine	800 mg (7–14 mg/kg)	10–60 mg
Heroin	50 mg	–
Crude Opium	500 mg	–
Pethidine	1 g	50–150 mg

- The μ **(mu) receptor** is also known as $\mathbf{OP_3}$ and consists of 2 sub-types: $\mu_1$and μ_2 (OP_{3A} and OP_{3B}). Most of the clinically used opiates are relatively selective for μ receptors reflecting their similarity to morphine.
- The **κ (kappa)** receptor is also known as $\mathbf{OP_2}$ and consists of 3 subtypes: κ_1, κ_2 and κ_3 (OP_{2A}, OP_{2B} and OP_{2C}).
- The **δ (delta)** receptor is also known as $\mathbf{OP_1}$.

Toxicokinetics

- In general, most opiates are readily absorbed from the GI tract, and also can be administered by subcutaneous, intramuscular or intravenous injection. However, the effect of an oral dose is usually much less than that obtained on parenteral administration due to significant first-pass metabolism in the liver.
- The major metabolic pathway of morphine is conjugation with glucuronic acid to produce morphine-6-glucuronide which is also pharmacologically active. Excretion occurs in the urine as morphine-3-glucuronide.
- Duration of action of opiates varies from 2 hrs (pentazocine, pethidine) to 4 hrs (morphine, codeine, heroin), to 8 hrs (methadone, buprenorphine). Fentanyl, alfentanil, and surfentanil are ultra-short acting (few minutes to 1 hr).

Adverse Effects

- Respiratory depression, vomiting, vertigo, dysphoria, miosis, constipation, hypotension, urinary retention and pruritis are commonly encountered.

Clinical (Toxic) Features

1. **Acute Poisoning**:
   a. The triad of ***coma, pinpoint pupils*** and ***respiratory depression*** is said to be almost pathognomonic for opiate poisoning.
   b. The important clinical manifestations are summarised in **Table 10.8**. Pupils are usually pinpoint (**Fig. 10.17**) but may be dilated in the presence of severe acidosis, hypoxia or respiratory depression. Pethidine often causes mydriasis.
   c. Some opiates cause cardiotoxicity, e.g., methadone, causing prolonged QT and dextropropoxyphene, causing sodium channel blockade and QRS prolongation. Bradycardia is said to be common.
   d. Bradypnoea is also common in opiate poisoning.
   e. Non-cardiogenic pulmonary oedema ("**heroin-lung**") is an infrequent, but severe, complication of heroin overdose and is generally abrupt in onset (immediate to 2 hrs) following intravenous heroin overdose. Manifestations include rales, pink frothy sputum, significant hypoxia and bilateral fluffy infiltrates on chest X-ray.

Table 10.8 Acute Opiate Poisoning

- Pinpoint pupils (may be dilated, if hypoxia is severe)
- Bradypnoea
- Cyanosis
- Non-cardiogenic pulmonary oedema
- Bradycardia
- Hypotension
- Hypothermia
- Cold, clammy skin
- Urinary retention
- Convulsions
- Coma

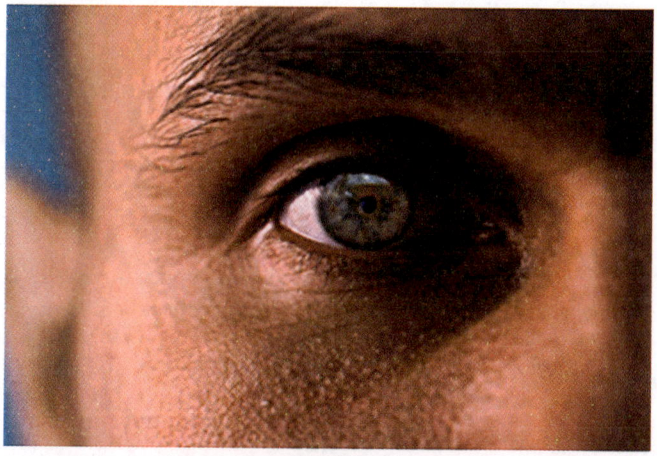

Fig. 10.17 Pinpoint pupil

   f. Bronchospasm and wheezing have been reported in both intravenous and inhalational abusers of heroin. Respiratory distress can occur with any opiate.
   g. Cramping and constipation as well as sphincter of Oddi spasm may occur.
   h. Hyperkalaemia may occur following an overdose, especially in the presence of rhabdomyolysis and acute renal failure.
   i. Most opiates cross the human placenta. They have been shown to appear in the foetal circulation within 5 min following maternal IV injection.
   j. Increased risk of congenital malformation has been reported following *in utero* exposure to opiates as a group, and for certain individual opiates.
2. **Chronic Poisoning (Addiction)**:
   a. The following are some useful pointers which indicate opiate addiction:
      i. Unusual mood swings, periods of depression alternating with euphoria.

ii. Withdrawal from family, friends and social activities.
iii. Frequent domestic strife.
iv. Long hours of unexplained absence from home.
v. Unexplained overspending.
vi. Frequent conflicts with law (e.g., driving offences).
vii. Dwindling sexual drive.
viii. Pills, syringes, etc., lying around the house.
ix. Bloody swabs or tissues lying around the home or in the working place.
x. Periodic disappearances into a locked room (bathroom, bedroom, etc.).
xi. Pinpoint pupils.
xii. Weight loss, pallor.
xiii. Chronic constipation.
xiv. Periodic withdrawal manifestations: Sweating, tremors.

b. In addition, an addict may have dermal scars (from intravenous abuse) (**Fig. 10.18**), and suffer from amnesia, confusion and occasional hallucinations.

3. **Withdrawal Syndrome**:
Abrupt cessation of opiate intake can cause a withdrawal reaction (***cold turkey***).* Common manifestations are mentioned in **Table 10.9**. Symptoms of opiate withdrawal may occur within 6–12 hrs of cessation of short-acting opiates such as heroin, or 24–36 hrs of long-acting opiates such as methadone or buprenorphine. Neonatal withdrawal may be seen in the infants of addicted mothers 12–72 hrs after birth.

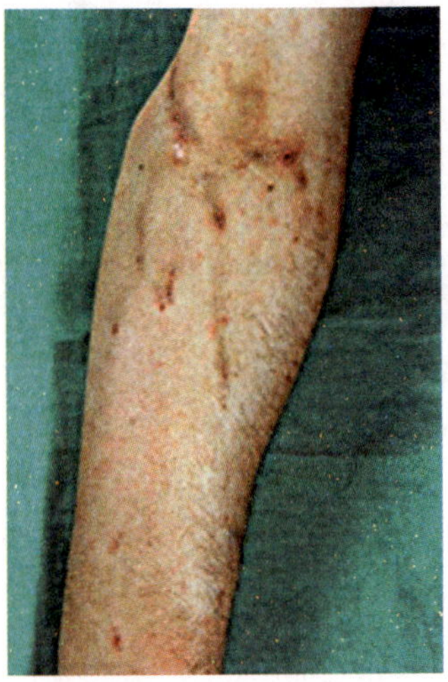

Fig. 10.18 Dermal scars from IV drug abuse

Diagnosis

1. Needle marks, dermal scars (suggestive of addiction).
2. Evidence of hypoglycaemia, hypoxia and hypothermia.
3. Most opiates can be detected in urine or blood by RIA, GC–MS or HPLC.
4. Empirical administration of naloxone (*can precipitate reaction in addicts*).
5. Past opiate usage can be detected by means of hair analysis.

Treatment

I. **Acute Poisoning**:

a. **Supportive measures**:
   i. Maintenance of patent airway.
   ii. Endotracheal intubation, assisted ventilation. Maintain adequate ventilation and oxygenation with frequent monitoring of arterial blood gases and/or pulse oximetry.

b. Consider prehospital administration of **activated charcoal** as an aqueous slurry in patients with a potentially toxic ingestion who are awake and able to protect their airway. Activated charcoal is most effective when administered within one hour of ingestion.

c. **Naloxone** is the **antidote of choice** for opiate poisoning (**Box 10.1**). The use of **physostigmine salicylate** (0.04 mg/kg IV) has been suggested for reversing respiratory depression, if the regular opiate antidotes are not available, since it increases the acetylcholine content of the reticular formation of the brainstem which is suppressed by opiates. However, there is controversy regarding such a measure since physostigmine (unlike regular opiate antagonists) is a dangerous antidote with serious adverse effects.

d. The use of drugs such as levorphanol and amiphenazole is no more recommended today.

Table 10.9 Opiate Withdrawal*

Anticipatory (*3–4 hrs*)	**Early** (*8–10 hrs*)	**Fully Developed** (*1–3 days*)	**Protracted Abstinence** (*up to 6 months*)
Anxiety, craving, drug-seeking behaviour	Restlessness, yawning, nausea, sweating, rhinorrhoea, lacrimation, mydriasis, stomach cramps, drug-seeking behaviour	Tremor, piloerection, vomiting, diarrhoea, muscle spasm, hypertension, tachycardia, fever, chills, impulse-driven drug-seeking behaviour	Hypotension, bradycardia, insomnia, anorexia, stimulus-driven opiate craving

Timings mentioned in the table refer to* ***heroin*.

**Note*: *This expression is derived from the nodular appearance of skin of an addict withdrawing from opiate addiction, which is due to goose-fleshing and hypothermia.*

e. **Convulsions** may be treated with benzodiazepines in the usual manner (5–10 mg initially, repeat every 5–10 minutes as needed), though this is frequently not necessary, if naloxone is available.

f. **For hypotension**: Infuse 10–20 mL/kg of isotonic fluid and place in Trendelenburg position. If hypotension persists, administer dopamine (5 μg/kg/min, progressing in 5 μg/kg/min increments as needed) or noradrenaline (0.5–1 μg/min, and titrate to maintain adequate blood pressure).

g. **Magnesium sulphate** should be administered urgently to patients with torsade de pointes.

h. **Prevention of rhabdomyolysis**: Early aggressive fluid replacement is the mainstay of therapy and may help prevent renal insufficiency. Diuretics such as mannitol or furosemide may be needed to maintain urine output. Urinary alkalinization is not routinely recommended.

II. **Chronic Poisoning**:

a. Gradual withdrawal of the opiate.

b. **Substitution therapy** (*methadone*: 30–40 mg/day & gradually tapered off).

c. A beta adrenergic blocker like propranolol (80 mg) is said to be effective in relieving the anxiety and craving associated with opiate addiction, but has no effect on physical symptoms. Alternatively, drugs such as clonidine can be used. Buprenorphine or naltrexone can also be used.

d. Antispamodics for abdominal cramps associated with vomiting and diarrhoea.

e. Tranquillisers or bed time sedation, if necessary.

f. Psychiatric counselling.

g. Withdrawal syndrome must be managed in an ICU by supportive and symptomatic measures.

Autopsy Features

- Injection marks, dermal abscesses, scarring. Look for injection marks in the antecubital fossae, forearms, back of the hands, neck, groin and ankles.
- Tattooing (a common feature of the drug subculture) (**Fig. 10.19**).

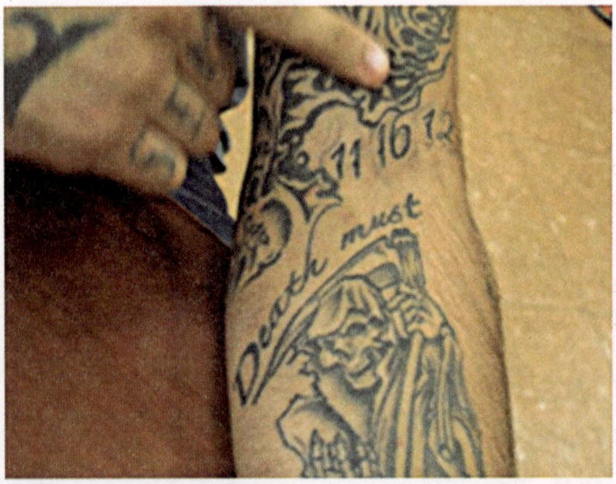

Fig. 10.19 Tattooing to conceal IV drug abuse

- Emaciation, unkempt appearance.
- Gross pulmonary oedema with froth exuding out of mouth and nostrils, especially in sudden heroin-related death. Another frequent autopsy finding in heroin fatalities is undiagnosed pneumonia.
- Autopsy findings of heroin-induced spongiform leukoencephalopathy include spongiform degeneration of white matter, vacuolization and fluid accumulation in myelin sheaths.
- Cerebral oedema.
- Congestion of liver with enlargement of hepatic lymph nodes. Chemical analysis of lymph nodes may reveal presence of morphine.
  - Even if heroin was being abused by the victim, it is metabolised into morphine in the body.

Box 10.1—Antidotes for Opiates

The first opiate antagonist to be introduced into practice was N-Allylnorcodeine in 1915. Nalorphine was developed in 1954, Naloxone in 1960 and Naltrexone in 1963. The most recent entrant is Nalmefene.

Nalorphine and Levallorphan (a related antagonist) are no more used today, since both are weak competitive antagonists with undesirable properties.

Naloxone, naltrexone and nalmefene are pure competitive antagonists at μ, κ and δ receptors. They are recommended today as approved antidotes.

Naloxone:

It is effective against all opiates except buprenorphine. It can be given IV, IM, SC or intranasally.

***Dose*:**

- *For adults*:
  - Give an initial dose of 400 μg (0.4 mg) IV.
  - If there is no response after 60 sec, give a further 800 μg (0.8 mg).
  - If there is still no response after another 60 sec, give another 800 μg (0.8 mg).
  - If still no response (after a total of 2 mg), give a further 2 mg dose. Large doses (4 mg) may be required in a seriously poisoned patient.
  - Aim for reversal of respiratory depression, not full reversal of consciousness.
  - Once an adequate response has occurred, monitor blood gases, oxygen saturation and respiratory rate.
- *For children (under 12 years of age)*:
  - Give an initial dose of 100 μg/kg (0.1 mg/kg) up to a maximum of 2 mg.
  - If there is no response after 60 sec give another 100 μg/kg (0.1 mg/kg) and repeat until a satisfactory response has been obtained or a maximum of 2 mg has been given.

Naltrexone:

Naltrexone is a long-acting opiate antagonist which can be administered orally. It is usually used for treating opiate addiction. However, it must not be given to an opiate-dependent patient who has not been detoxified.

contd.

Naltrexone is also beneficial in the management of alcohol addiction, infantile autism and Tourette's syndrome.
Dose: 50 mg/day orally, which may have to be continued for several weeks or months.

Nalmefene:
Nalmefene is a naltrexone derivative with pure opiate antagonistic effects, and has a longer duration of effect than naloxone in acute opiate poisoning.

It is usually given intravenously beginning with 0.1 mg, and if withdrawal reaction does not occur, 0.5 mg is administered, followed by 1 mg in 2–5 min (if necessary). Nalmefene can also be given intramuscularly or subcutaneously.

Samples of blood, urine, brain, liver, bile must be preserved for chemical analysis.

Human hair analysis has been explored as a way to test the drug history of an individual from sampling time to several months previous.

It is important to remember that infections such as serum hepatitis and AIDS are common among intravenous drug abusers, and hence autopsies conducted in drug-related deaths must be done cautiously with necessary precautions.

Forensic Issues

- Opiates are among the commonest of the drugs abused today in India. Heroin (**brown sugar**) is popular among all classes of addicts in metropolitan cities such as Mumbai, Delhi, Bangalore, etc. Opiates used for therapeutic purposes, e.g., morphine, pethidine and pentazocine are more commonly abused by medical and paramedical personnel. Codeine which is easily available over the counter in the form of antitussive preparations is being increasingly abused especially by college-going youth.
- Accidental deaths are not infrequent from overdose, particularly among intravenous abusers of heroin ("***death on the needle***").
- "**Cotton fever**" is common among IV abusers, which is a febrile reaction that develops because these drugs are often filtered through cotton balls prior to being injected.
- Chronic parenteral opiate abuse can result in abscesses, acute transverse myelitis, anaphylaxis, AIDS, arrhythmias, wound botulism, cellulitis, endocarditis, glomerulonephritis, osteomyelitis, tetanus, thrombophlebitis, nephropathy, hepatitis, mycotic aneurysms or leukoencephalopathy.
- Suicidal deaths are also reported from time to time, since opiates are reputed to cause a painless death. Homicides are rare, but a few cases have been documented in medical literature.
- **Body Packer Syndrome**:
  - Although this is more commonly associated with smuggling of cocaine, it has also been reported in the case of other drugs such as heroin, amphetamines and cannabis.
  - A "**bodypacker**" or "**mule**" is an individual who attempts to transport illicit drugs from one country to another by ingesting wrapped packages, or condoms, or balloons containing concentrated drug, especially cocaine or heroin.*
  - "**Body-stuffers**" (also known as "**Contact Precipitated Concealers**") constitute a different entity, and refer to those individuals who rapidly ingest illegal drugs to avoid detection or arrest, often using flimsy wrapping (e.g. 'cling film-type' or a single-layer cellophane bag).
  - The term "**Parachuting**" is used when the intent is to purposefully delay absorption. There is often early leakage of drugs from the package, generally within 8 hrs of ingestion.
  - After arrival at the destination, cathartics are self-administered and the packets are defaecated out (**Fig. 10.20**). Sometimes rectal suppositories or disposable enemas are used.
  - Although generally asymptomatic, in a few cases serious toxicity may result due to rupture of packets. Death due to intestinal obstruction and perforation has been reported in body packers.
  - Diagnosis of an asymptomatic body packer can be accomplished with the help of an abdominal X-ray (**Fig. 10.21**), ultrasound or CT scan. The last two methods should be resorted to only if X-ray is unclear. In some cases, faecal examination over a period of a few days may be necessary.

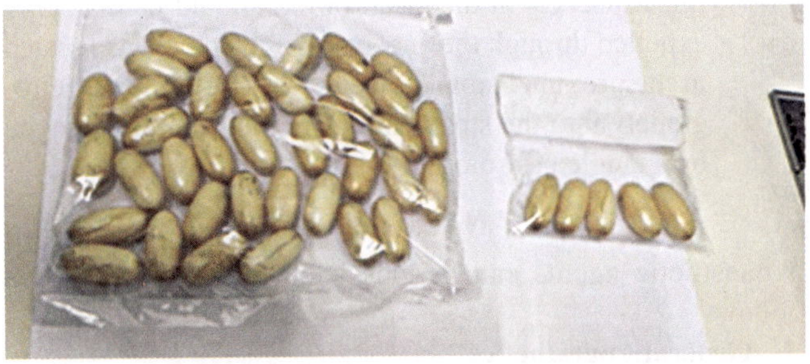

Fig. 10.20 Drug filled packets recovered from a 'mule'

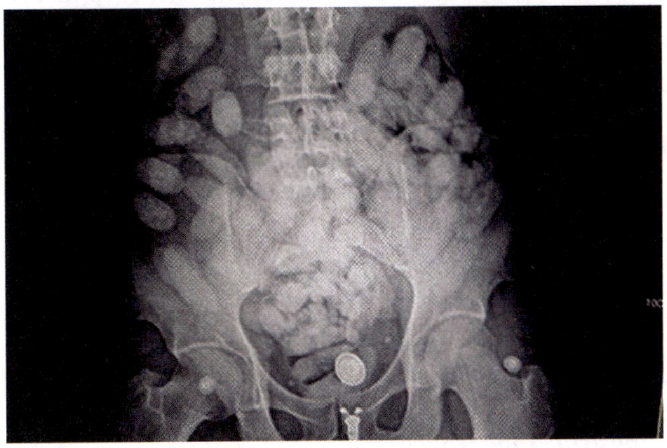

Fig. 10.21 Abdominal X-ray of a 'bodypacker' revealing numerous packets in the intestinal tract

Note: *Bodypacking can also refer to inserting drugs/drug packets into the rectum or vagina.*

- Asymptomatic patients should be treated by whole bowel irrigation with polyethylene glycol solution. However, some investigators do not approve of this method since the polyethylene glycol can dissolve the heroin from a package, rupturing it and increasing absorption of heroin. Instead, a period of waiting is recommended so that all packages pass into the colon from the stomach, and then low-volume phosphosoda enemas or high-volume saline enemas are administered. Food ingestion must not be permitted until all packages have moved into the colon.
- Surgical intervention for bowel obstruction is said to be necessary in 3–5% of body-packers.
- Body packers remain at risk of severe intoxication until complete evacuation of **all** packages, usually indicated by the passage of two consecutive package-free stools. Repeat radiology (CT) may be necessary for confirmation of evacuation in some cases, e.g., when patients exhibit intoxication even after stools remain package-free.
- Symptomatic patients must be managed with continuous-infusion naloxone, activated charcoal and whole bowel irrigation. Intestinal perforation or obstruction by packets requires surgical intervention. Whenever possible a CT scan (without oral contrast) should be performed prior to operative intervention, but this should not be allowed to delay surgical intervention. Intact packets in the distal bowel should be manually expelled through the anal canal. Intact packets located in the proximal small bowel should be 'milked' retrogradely into the stomach, where they can be removed by a single gastrotomy.

ANAESTHETICS

Anaesthetic agents can be classified into two groups as follows:

1. **General Anaesthetics**:
   a. *Inhalational Agents*: Nitrous oxide, halothane, isoflurane, enflurane, methoxyflurane, sevoflurane, desflurane.
   b. *Intravenous Agents**: Thiopentone, amobarbitone (Amytal), methohexitone, ketamine, fentanyl & its derivatives and propofol.
2. **Local Anaesthetics**: Cocaine, lignocaine, bupivacaine, mepivacaine, prilocaine, procaine, ropivacaine, tetracaine, benzocaine and many more.

INHALATIONAL ANAESTHETICS

Nitrous Oxide

Synonyms

Dinitrogen monoxide; Laughing gas

Physical Appearance

- Nitrous oxide is a colourless gas with a slightly sweetish odour and taste.

Uses

- As a sole agent, nitrous oxide is used intermittently to provide analgesia for dental and obstetric procedures.
- In combination with other agents, nitrous oxide is used as a general anaesthetic.

Adverse Effects

- Nitrous oxide is 35 times more soluble in blood than nitrogen. When it is inhaled, compliant air-containing spaces such as the bowel will increase in size, while non-compliant spaces such as eustachian tubes will increase in pressure. This can lead to bowel distension, tympanic membrane rupture, etc.

Toxic Effects

- Respiratory depression, increased muscle tone, hypertension, mydriasis, cardiovascular failure.
- "**Nagging**" or "**nanging**" are terms used to describe the recreational use of nitrous oxide, derived from the repetitive sound distortions experienced by nitrous oxide users. Nitrous oxide is readily available from most supermarkets and online, as it is used as the aerator and propellant for **whipped-cream dispensers**. The average bulb used for aerating whipped cream contains 8 g of nitrous oxide.
- Chronic use (or abuse) can lead to bone marrow depression, polyneuropathy, megaloblastic changes and death. Chronic abuse can also cause myeloneuropathy.

Usual Fatal Dose

- Inhalation of 40% nitrous oxide in air can cause confusion and sedation, while an 80% level causes unconsciousness in most individuals.

Treatment

1. Removal from source of exposure.
2. Cerebral oedema and elevated intracranial pressure (ICP) may occur. Emergent management includes head elevation and administration of mannitol.
3. Vitamin B_{12}: Case reports suggest that administration of folate and vitamin B_{12} supplements may help reverse myeloneuropathy associated with chronic nitrous oxide abuse.
4. Folinic acid, 30 mg, IV, for bone marrow abnormalities.
5. Supportive measures:
   a. Treatment of hypoxia.
   b. Control of seizures.
   c. Treatment of pulmonary oedema.
   d. Continuous cardiac monitoring.

Halothane

Physical Appearance

- Halothane is a non-flammable, volatile liquid.
- It is colourless and has a sweetish odour.
- It is light-sensitive.

****Note***: *Also referred to as Induction agents.*

Uses

- Halothane can be used in combination with oxygen, or other gas mixtures such as nitrous oxide and oxygen for general anaesthesia.

Adverse Effects

- Hypotension, cardiac rhythm disturbances, **malignant hyperthermia** (which has been reported in patients given halothane with and without suxamethonium, i.e., succinylcholine).

Toxic Effects

- The most important toxic effect is **hepatitis**. Two types of hepatitis have been observed. The first is a mild dysfunction which develops in about 20% of exposed patients, is characterised by moderate elevation of serum aminotransferase level, and is associated with complete recovery. The second is a life-threatening hepatitis occurring in about 1 in 10,000 exposed patients which can terminate in massive hepatic necrosis.
- Halothane is known for its abuse potential among hospital personnel, since inhalation of small amounts produces pleasurable effects. A popular method of halothane abuse is to drip the liquid onto a pad held over the face.

Treatment

- Full recovery is usual with supportive care.
- N-Acetylcysteine has been an effective pre-treatment in protecting against halothane-induced hepatotoxicity.

INTRAVENOUS ANAESTHETICS

Ketamine

- Ketamine is a phencyclidine derivative.
- It is a general anaesthetic that is rapid acting, producing profound analgesia with normal laryngeal-pharyngeal reflexes, skeletal muscle tone, and cardiovascular and respiratory stimulation. When given intravenously, it induces sedation associated with immobility, amnesia and analgesia (***dissociative anaesthesia***).
- Ketamine is popular as an anaesthetic in cases of trauma and emergency surgical procedures. It is also frequently used for short-term sedation during clinical procedures; most frequently in the paediatric population.
- During the period of unconsciousness, patients are usually non-communicative, though the eyes may be open and they appear to be awake. Skeletal muscle spasm is often present.
- Following usual anaesthetic doses, side effects include significant transient increases in blood pressure and heart rate, respiratory depression, airway obstruction, apnoea, muscular hypertonus, psychomotor, psychomimetic and acute dystonic reactions. Ketamine elevates intracranial and intraocular pressure. Mydriasis and nystagmus may occur.
- Emergence phenomena are also commonly reported characterised by vivid dreams, nightmares, hallucinations, screaming, crying, disorientation and delirium.
- Overdose is associated with convulsions, hypertension, tachycardia and respiratory depression.
- Ketamine is increasingly gaining popularity as a recreational drug and is employed in "**rave parties**" for its dissociative hallucinatory effects. It is usually taken intranasally or by inhalation, but may also be injected (IM or IV). Users describe the effects of ketamine as an "out of body" experience or "near death", characterised by exhilarating sensations of immobility and a disregard for death.

Treatment of the adverse and toxic effects of ketamine involves mainly symptomatic and supportive measures. Plasma ketamine levels are not clinically useful. Airway control and ventilatory support are essential.

Propofol

- Propofol is a synthetic intravenous anaesthetic which is an oil at room temperature and is supplied as a 1% emulsion (in 10% soyabean oil, 2.25% glycerol and 1.2% purified egg phosphatide).
- It is useful in the induction and maintenance of general anaesthesia as part of inpatient or outpatient surgery.
- Propofol is known to cause hypotension, bradycardia and even cardiac arrest. In children, it may induce choreiform movements, rigidity and ataxia, if the usual dose is exceeded.
- Several paediatric (and adult) case reports of "**propofol infusion syndrome**" following prolonged propofol use for intensive care sedation have been described. The syndrome, which may be fatal, is characterized by fever, metabolic acidosis, bradyarrhythmias, rhabdomyolysis, hyperkalaemia, hyperlipidaemia, ketonuria, myoglobinuria, elevated creatine kinase, acute renal failure, elevated liver enzymes, fatty liver and myocardial failure.
- Anaphylactic reactions have occurred during propofol administration.
- Discoloured urine (olive green, rusty brown, tea-coloured) has been reported in several paediatric exposures to prolonged propofol infusions used for intensive care sedation (**Fig. 10.22**).
- Adverse events are as follows: Pain on injection, nausea or vomiting, excitement, hypotension, bradycardia, confusion, arrhythmias, cardiac arrest, pulmonary oedema, bronchospasm, chest pain.

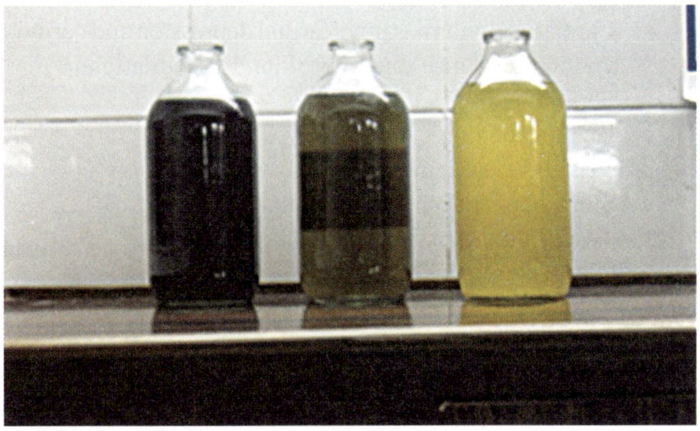

Fig. 10.22 Propofol – Urine discolouration (toxicity to recovery) (*Courtesy: S Senthil kumaran*)

- It appears that propofol has both anti-convulsant and pro-convulsant activity. There have been several reports of seizure activity following the use of propofol in the literature.
- Propofol is susceptible to contamination with microorganisms (*S. aureus*, *E. coli*, *P. aeruginosa*, *C. albicans*, etc.), and cases have been recorded, where bacteraemia has resulted from its use in patients. It is recommended that propofol ampoules should be wiped with alcohol before use, and strict aseptic techniques should be followed when preparing infusions.

LOCAL ANAESTHETICS

Procaine, introduced in 1905, was the first synthetic local anaesthetic and is an amino ester. The other amino esters include **amylocaine**, **benzocaine**, **butacaine**, **tetracaine (amethocaine)** and of course **cocaine**.

A second group of local anaesthetics comprise the amino amides – **bupivacaine, lignocaine (lidocaine), mepivacaine, prilocaine** and **ropivacaine**.*

The most commonly used local anaesthetics are **lignocaine** and **bupivacaine**.

Toxic Effects

1. **Allergic Reactions**: Generally rare and usually associated with ester compounds.
   a. Idiosyncrasy – Vasovagal attack or hysterical reactions. Anxiety, panic attacks, hallucinations and psychotic reactions have occurred.
   b. Local Effects – Accidental subarachnoid injection of chloroprocaine may cause adhesive arachnoiditis or cauda equina syndrome. Intravenous use is associated with venous thrombosis.
   c. Systemic Effects – Usually result from inadvertent intravascular injection of local anaesthetics. The following manifestations occur: perioral numbness, tingling, auditory and visual disturbances, twitching, convulsions, cardiac arrhythmias, coma and death.
2. **Systemic Toxicity**: Toxicity may occur after ingestion, topical use or parenteral administration. It may result from an excessive dose, mistaken drug identity, enhanced drug absorption, inadvertent intravascular injection, altered protein binding, slowed redistribution and/or elimination.
   a. Cardiac arrhythmias, myocardial depression and cardiovascular collapse due to profound vasodilation.
   b. Perioral numbness.
   c. Lightheadedness, tinnitus.
   d. Visual disturbances, miosis.
   e. Slurring of speech, irrational talk.
   f. Twitching, convulsions.
   g. Coma, apnoea.

Usual Fatal Dose

The minimum IV toxic doses of some local anaesthetics are listed in **Table 10.10**.

Diagnosis

Therapeutic blood levels of lignocaine vary between 1 and 5 µg/mL. Serious poisoning may occur at levels above 5 µg/mL for lignocaine, mepivacaine or procaine. For bupivacaine, therapeutic plasma concentrations are less than 3 µg/mL.

Bupivacaine is more toxic than lignocaine when given intravenously.

Table 10.10 Minimum IV Toxic Doses of Local Anaesthetics

Drug	Toxic Dose (mg/kg)
Bupivacaine	1.6
Lignocaine	6.4
Mepivacaine	9.8
Procaine	19.2

*Treatment***

1. Maintain airway; ventilate with 100% oxygen.
2. Treat acidosis (presence of acidosis increases toxicity). Consider sodium bicarbonate in patients with severe metabolic acidosis.
3. Treat convulsions with thiopentone IV (50–100 mg), diazepam (10 mg) or midazolam (2 mg). If seizures persist or recur administer barbiturates.
4. Treat hypotension with IV fluids, pressors (e.g., dopamine), Trendelenberg position.
5. Treat bradycardia with atropine, tachycardia or ventricular fibrillation with electrical cardioversion, or bretylium (5 mg/kg IV).
6. Acute lignocaine toxicity can usually be managed with supportive measures. Massive overdose may necessitate atrioventricular cardiac pacing, or extracorporeal pump assistance.
7. Methaemoglobinaemia resulting from lignocaine and prilocaine can be treated with methylene blue (1–2 mg/kg/dose or 0.1– 0.2 mL/kg/dose IV over 5 min as needed every 4 hrs).

Forensic Issues (Anaesthetics)

- In contrast to earlier years, anaesthesia is associated with low mortality today and is estimated to be just 1 in 10,000 with proper care in administration. Low blood volume, underventilation, aspiration and vomiting, and collapse following intravenous block are the main factors in the few deaths reported.
- Increased susceptibility to mortality is associated with heart disease, advanced age and high-risk surgery (cardiovascular, thoracic, abdominal or neurologic).

Table 10.11 mentions important causes of death during anaesthesia.

*Note: *If a local anaesthetic has the letter "i" within the first four letters of its name, it is an amide. If not, it is an ester.*

Note: *A useful mnemonic to remember the principal points in treatment of local anaesthetic toxicity is **SAVED, where S—**Stop** injection; A—**Airway maintenance**; V—**Ventilation**; E—**Evaluation of circulation**; D—**Drugs**.*

Table 10.11 Common Causes of Anaesthetic Deaths

- Aspiration of gastric contents
- Overdose of anaesthetic agents
- Hypoxia
- Airway problems
- Polypharmacy
- Errors in choice of anaesthetic or technique
- Errors in evaluation or preparation of patient
- Inadequate monitoring of patient's status during anaesthesia
- Inadequate ventilation

- There is evidence to suggest that operating room workers may suffer from the results of occupational exposure to general (inhalational) anaesthetics, if precautions are not taken – proper connection of scavenging equipment, turning the gas off when breathing system is disconnected from patient, and use of properly fitting masks on patients.
- Anaesthetic drug abuse is a significant problem among anaesthesia personnel in the Western countries, while similar data are not available in the Indian context. Common agents abused include alcohol, narcotic drugs, barbiturates, tranquillisers and nitrous oxide. Halothane and ketamine are also being increasingly abused.
- Nitrous oxide is used as a propellant gas in food aerosols (i.e., foaming agent for whipped cream). "**Whippet**" or "**Whip-it**" is a slang term or brand name for a cylinder or cartridge designed to charge whipped cream dispensers (**Fig. 10.23**). The term "***nanging***" has been used to describe the recreational use of this agent via cartridges of nitrous oxide. Widespread abuse of this agent has been reported in the United States. These cartridges may be commercially available in supermarkets, adult bookstores, bar supply shops and by mail order.
- Propofol is increasingly being used as an intravenous drug of abuse.
  - The case of the famous pop singer **Michael Jackson** (**Fig. 10.24**) who is alleged to have died as a result of overdose with propofol is well known. Michael Jackson was an American singer, songwriter and dancer. Called the King of Pop, his contributions to music and dance, along with his publicized personal life, made him a global figure in popular culture for over four decades. Through stage and video performances, Jackson popularized a number of complicated dance techniques, such as the robot and the moonwalk, to which he gave the name. His distinctive sound and style has influenced numerous hip hop, post-disco, contemporary R&B, pop and rock artists.

    While preparing for his comeback concert series titled "This Is It", Jackson died of acute propofol and benzodiazepine intoxication on June 25, 2009, after suffering from cardiac arrest. The Los Angeles County Coroner ruled his death a homicide, and his personal physician Conrad Murray was convicted of involuntary manslaughter.

    The County Coroner stated that Jackson died from a combination of drugs in his body, with the most significant drugs being the anaesthetic propofol (**Fig. 10.25**) and the anxiolytic lorazepam. Less significant drugs found in Jackson's body were midazolam, diazepam, lidocaine and ephedrine.
- Procaine may produce a stimulant effect, similar to cocaine, when inhaled and is sometimes called "**synthetic cocaine**."

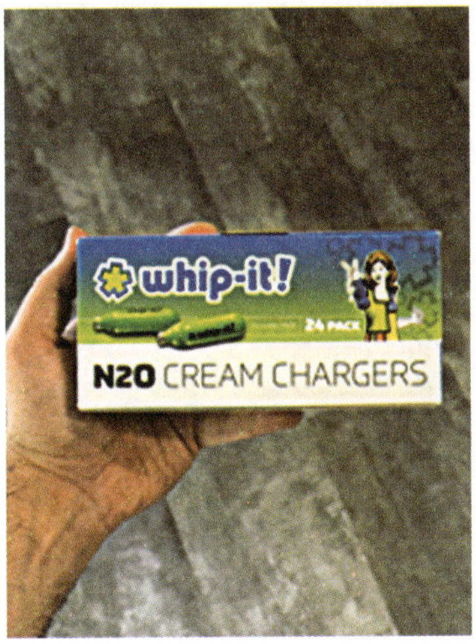

Fig. 10.23 Whip-it cream charger

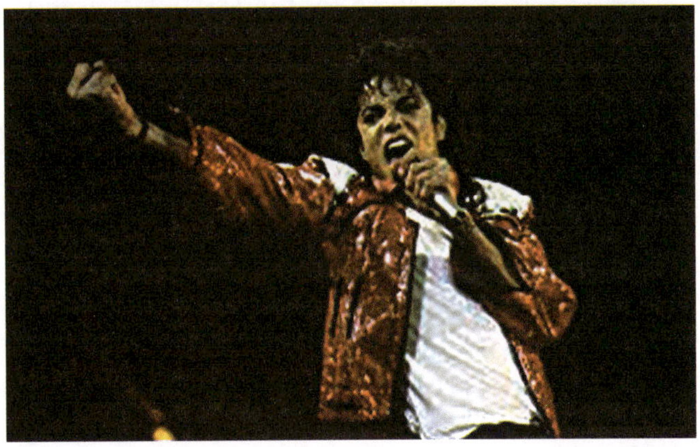

Fig. 10.24 Michael Jackson

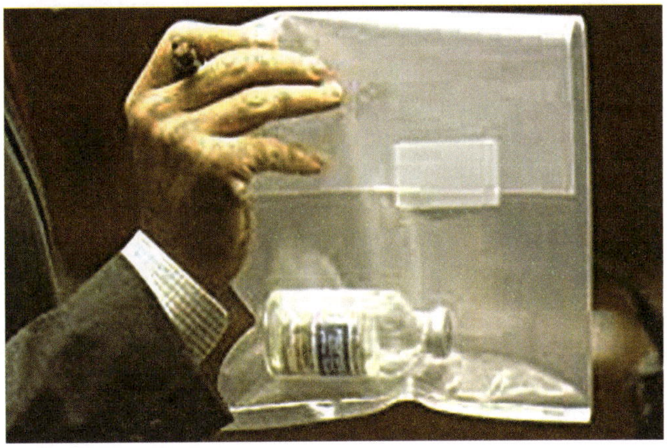

Fig. 10.25 Propofol vial recovered from the scene

Powdered procaine is commonly used to "cut" cocaine and has been sold as cocaine when mixed with mannitol or lactose.

- Anaesthetic agents are not uncommonly employed for suicide. Homicides are rare.

MUSCLE RELAXANTS

1. **Central Skeletal Muscle Relaxants**: Baclofen, carisoprodol, chlormezanone, chlorzoxazone, methocarbamol.
2. **Neuromuscular Blocking Agents**:
   a. Depolarisers: Succinylcholine, decamethonium.
   b. Non-depolarisers:
      i. Benzylisoquinolines – Atracurium, doxacurium, mivacurium, tubocurarine.
      ii. Ammoniosteroids – Pancuronium, rocuronium, vecuronium.
3. **Miscellaneous Drugs** – Orphenadrine, dantrolene, cyclobenzaprine.

CENTRAL SKELETAL MUSCLE RELAXANTS

Baclofen

- Baclofen is a derivative of the inhibitory neurotransmitter GABA (*gamma amino butyric acid*). It inhibits both monosynaptic and polysynaptic reflexes at spinal level and also has CNS depressant effects.
- At therapeutic doses (40–80 mg/day), baclofen is relatively free of adverse effects, and toxicity usually manifests only at daily doses exceeding 150–200 mg/day.
- **Overdose** is characterised by agitation, involuntary movements, twitching, convulsions, delirium, flaccidity, coma and respiratory depression. Nausea and vomiting are common.
- Long-term administration of therapeutic doses of baclofen may cause fatigue, vertigo, nausea, confusion, depression, headache and muscle weakness.
- **Treatment**:
  - Admission to an intensive care facility, with gastric lavage and activated charcoal, has been recommended for adults ingesting over 100 mg and children ingesting over 5 mg/kg of baclofen.
  - Treatment of overdose involves oxygen administration, assisted ventilation, gastric lavage, activated charcoal, IV diazepam for convulsions, and Trendeleberg position, IV fluids and pressor amines (dopamine or noradrenaline) for hypotension.
  - Physostigmine is said to be effective in reversing respiratory depression, arreflexia and coma. The usual dose is 1–2 mg by slow IV infusion, repeated cautiously if required, all the while watching out for adverse effects.
  - Forced diuresis may be helpful in enhancing the elimination of baclofen.

NEUROMUSCULAR BLOCKING AGENTS

- Neuromuscular blocking agents or neuromuscular blockers (NMBs) are widely employed to achieve muscle relaxation during anaesthesia.
- The essential mechanism of action of all NMBs is inhibition of the effects of acetylcholine (ACH) on nicotinic receptors at the neuromuscular junction (NMJ).
  - The depolarising NMBs (or DNMBs) such as succinylcholine (suxamethonium) produce muscle depolarisation in the same way as ACH.
  - The nondepolarising NMBs (or NDNMBs) act by competitive inhibition of ACH at nicotinic receptors, and their action is in general of shorter duration.

Uses

1. Adjuvant in surgical anaesthesia to obtain skeletal muscle relaxation.
2. Fascilitation of orthopaedic procedures such as correction of dislocations and alignment of fractures.
3. Fascilitation of endotracheal intubation, laryngoscopy, bronchoscopy, oesophagoscopy, etc.
4. Prevention of trauma during electroconvulsive therapy.

Adverse Effects

- Prolonged apnoea and respiratory paralysis.
- Cardiovascular collapse preceded by tachy- or bradycardia and hypo- or hypertension.
- Histamine-release effects: Bronchospasm, hypotension, excessive airway secretions.
- Hyperkalaemia (with succinylcholine).
- ***Malignant hyperthermia*** (with succinylcholine). **Box 10.2** outlines the details of this rare, but serious complication. Succinylcholine-induced rhabdomyolysis from prolonged fasciculations or malignant hyperthermia can lead to renal failure.
- Persistent weakness (especially in critically ill patients subjected to prolonged ventilation) referred to as ***ICU neuromuscular syndrome***. Recovery may take up to 6 months.

Box 10.2—Malignant Hyperthermia

Malignant hyperthermia (MH) is a rare, genetically influenced, potentially lethal complication associated with the use of inhalational anaesthetics, amino-amide local anaesthetics and some muscle relaxants (succinylcholine, decamethonium, d-tubocurarine and gallamine).

Manifestations:
- Tachycardia (unexplained).
- Tachypnoea, cyanosis (unexplained).
- Rigidity (masseters fail to relax for intubation).
- Marked hyperthermia (late sign).
- Hypotension, arrhythmias.
- Metabolic acidosis.
- Hyperkalaemia, hypercalcaemia.
- Electrolyte disturbances.
- Rhabdomyolysis, disseminated intravascular coagulation (DIC), renal failure.
- Pulmonary oedema.

Treatment:
- Hyperventilate with 100% oxygen (10 L/min).
- Give dantrolene sodium 2–3 mg/kg IV bolus, followed by increments up to a maximum of 10 mg/kg.

contd.

- Give sodium bicarbonate to correct metabolic acidosis (1–2 mEq/kg).
- Treat hyperthermia with:
  - IV iced saline, 15 mL/kg, q15 min × 3.
  - Lavage of stomach, bladder and rectum with iced saline.
  - Skin surface cooling with ice.
- Treat persistent arrhythmias with standard anti-arrhythmic drugs.
- Treat hyperkalaemia with hyperventilation, sodium bicarbonate, IV glucose and insulin.
- Ensure adequate urine output (more than 2 mL/kg/hr).

Toxic Effects

- Succinylcholine (suxamethonium) is a bis-quaternary ammonium ion composed of two acetylcholine molecules connected by their acetate groups.
- The dose necessary to produce neuromuscular blockade and respiratory paralysis in adults ranges from 0.3 to 1.1 mg/kg in adults (mean 0.6 mg/kg). Prolonged respiratory paralysis may occur following therapeutic doses in individuals with a deficiency of pseudocholinesterase.
- Succinylcholine use is sometimes associated with prolonged apnoea which may be due to genetically determined atypical pseudocholinesterase (incidence 1:2500), or due to exposure to cholinesterase inhibitors such as organophosphates.
- Adverse effects of succinylcholine include cardiac arrhythmias, hyperkalaemia, increased intracranial pressure, increased intraocular pressure, increased intragastric pressure, myalgia, muscle fasciculations, muscle rigidity (especially masseters), malignant hyperthermia, rhabdomyolysis and myoglobinuria.
- Succinylcholine is also well known for causing anaphylaxis in susceptible individuals (mostly women) which manifests as rapid circulatory collapse without other conventional signs such as skin rash or wheezing.
- **Overdose** of tubocurarine and all other curariform blocking agents produce complete skeletal muscle paralysis without affecting consciousness. Initially, the small muscles of the eyes, ears, fingers and toes are paralysed, followed by face and neck, upper and lower limbs, and finally the diaphragm and intercostal muscles, leading to respiratory failure.
- Pancuronium is a synthetic bis-quaternary aminosteroid which has a selective cardiac antimuscarinic (atropine-like) action resulting in increased heart rate and blood pressure.

Treatment

1. Reversal of NDNMB block can be achieved by anticholinesterases such as neostigmine, pyridostigmine or edrophonium in combination with antimuscarinic agents such as glycopyrrolate or atropine.
2. Overdose with depolarising agents such as succinylcholine cannot be reversed pharmacologically, and must be managed with prolonged assisted ventilation. Physostigmine, neostigmine and other anticholinesterase drugs, including edrophonium, are contraindicated as antidotes to succinylcholine because they actually prolong its action by interfering with metabolism by cholinesterase.
3. Maintain patent airway and supply 100% oxygen. Assisted ventilation is usually required.
4. Malignant hyperthermia is treated on the lines mentioned earlier (*vide supra*).
5. Treat cardiovascular failure in the usual way.
6. Treat severe hyperkalaemia (associated arrhythmias, QRS widening) aggressively. Monitor ECG continuously during and after therapy.

Dantrolene

- Dantrolene is a hydantoin derivative which is structurally similar to both anticonvulsants and local anaesthetics, but does not possess their properties.
- The most important use of dantrolene is to treat malignant hyperthemia. It is also sometimes employed in the control of fever in thyrotoxicosis.
- **Overdose** results in muscle weakness, visual disturbances, lethargy, nausea, vertigo, pulmonary oedema, convulsions, hepatic toxicity (hepatitis), aplastic anaemia and leukopenia.
- **Treatment** involves symptomatic and supportive measures.

Forensic Issues (Muscle Relaxants)

- Accidental overdose involving these drugs is not uncommon. Morbidity and mortality associated with pure skeletal muscle relaxant ingestion are low.
- Suicides have been reported with many of these drugs, and most of them have involved medical or paramedical personnel.
- Homicides are increasingly being reported, especially with regard to neuromuscular blocking agents.
- Some of these drugs are subject to being abused, e.g., orphenadrine, baclofen.

CARDIOVASCULAR TOXICOLOGY

Cardiovascular Toxicology deals with toxicity resulting from **Cardiac Drugs** (drugs used in heart failure, anti-anginal drugs, lipoprotein lowering drugs), **Antihypertensives**, **Anticoagulants**, etc., but the new curriculum specifies only **Cardiotoxic Plants**.

Cardiotoxic Plants: **Aconite**, Azalea, Death camas, False hellebore, **Foxglove (Digitalis)**, Lily of the valley, Meadow saffron, Mountain laurel, **Oleander**, Rhododendron, **Suicide tree (Odollam)**, Yew.

Most of these plants contain various cardiac glycosides which act in similar fashion. Some of these glycosides are useful in pharmacotherapeutics (e.g., digitalis derived from foxglove). Only the cardiotoxic plants mentioned in the curriculum will be discussed here (highlighted in red colour in the examples listed above).

CARDIOTOXIC PLANTS

Digitalis

Botanical Name

Digitalis purpurea

Common Names

Foxglove; Dead men's bells

Physical Appearance

- The plant grows well in the hilly regions of Darjeeling, Nilgiris and Kashmir, and is a biennial or perennial herb growing up to 1–1.5 m in height.
- Leaves are ovate, toothed and grey-green in colour, while the flowers are tubular and pink or white in colour (**Fig. 10.26**).
- There is a related species, ***Digitalis lanata*** (**Fig. 10.27**), which is also rich in cardiac glycosides. Leaves constitute the main source of glycosides in both plants.
- The following discussion will be mainly with reference to the digitalis glycosides **digoxin** and **digitoxin**, which are the most widely used cardiac glycosides. Other less commonly used glycosides include **gitoxin**, **gitalin**, **digitonin**, **digitin** (all from ***D. purpurea***), **lanatoside C** and **deslanoside** (both from ***D. lanata***).*

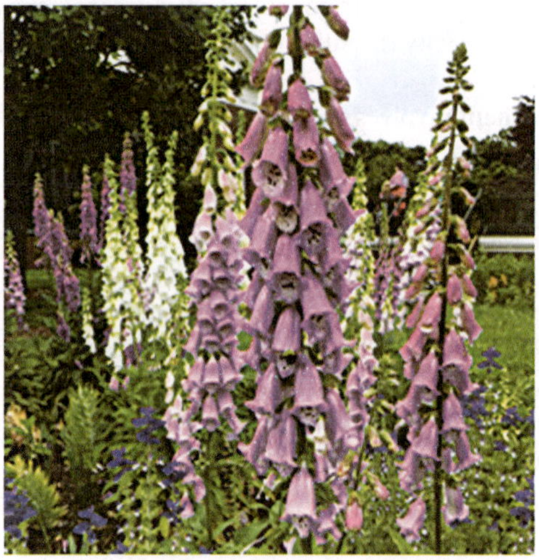

Fig. 10.26 *Digitalis purpurea*

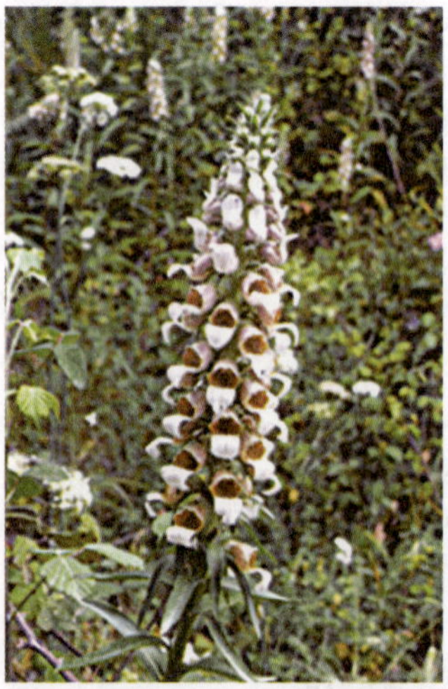

Fig. 10.27 *Digitalis lanata*

Uses

- Digoxin, once considered first line therapy for heart failure, is today used only if the condition cannot be controlled by other medications, and occasionally for the treatment of atrial fibrillation and atrial flutter.

Toxicokinetics

- Both digoxin and digitoxin are well absorbed orally, but while the former is only moderately protein bound (25%), and has a large apparent volume of distribution, digitoxin is highly protein bound (97%) and has a low apparent volume of distribution.
- Peak serum concentrations of digoxin occur within 1.5–6 hrs after an oral dose.
- After a single dose, digoxin is the major serum and urine metabolite of digitoxin.

Mode of Action

- Digitalis glycosides inhibit active transport of Na^+ and K^+ across cell membranes by binding onto a specific site on the extracytoplasmic face of the a subunit of Na^+-K^+-ATPase.
- The force of contraction of the heart (positive inotropic effect) is increased due to increase in cytosolic Ca^{2+} during systole.
- Both Na^+ and Ca^{2+} enter the myocardial cells during each cycle of depolarisation, contraction and repolarisation. During repolarisation and relaxation, Ca^{2+} is pumped back into the sarcoplasmic reticulum.
- In acute overdose, the sodium–potassium pump is poisoned, producing a fall in intracellular potassium and a rise in extracellular potassium, which may be marked. The normal membrane resting potential is reduced, and electrical conduction is slowed, with eventual complete loss of myocardial electrical function. Clinically, this results in high grade heart block, and eventually in asystole, which may not respond to electrical pacing.

Adverse Effects

1. *CVS*: Arrhythmias are induced, the more common types comprising non-paroxysmal atrial tachycardia, premature ventricular extrasystoles, premature atrial and junctional extrasystoles, and all grades of A-V block. **The most serious arrhythmias are ventricular tachycardia and ventricular fibrillation**.
2. *GIT*: Anorexia, nausea, vomiting, weakness.
3. *CNS*: Confusion, disorientation, headache and hallucinations (***digitalis delirium***).
4. *Eye*: Transient amblyopia, blurred vision, scotomata, photophobia and chromatopsia.**

****Note***: *Cardiac glycosides are also present in Oleander (Nerium oleander and Cerbera thevetia), Lily of the valley (Convollaria majalis) and Red squill (Urginea maritima). But, they are not used in pharmacotherapeutics.*

*****Note***: *Refers to aberrations of colour vision such as yellow halos around light (xanthopsia).*

5. *Miscellaneous*: Gynaecomastia, restlessness, diarrhoea in elderly.

Toxic Effects

- All parts of the plant are toxic to varying extent.
- Poisoning may be **acute** or **chronic**. In an **acute ingestion**, nausea and vomiting are prominent as well as evidence of cardiotoxicity. In **chronic poisoning**, nonspecific symptoms, such as malaise and weakness predominate, as well as the classic, but rare, visual disturbances.
- Lethargy, drowsiness, weakness, paraesthesias and headache may occur with digoxin toxicity.
- Signs of toxic psychosis, including hallucinations, paranoia, agitation, confusion and delirium, may also occur. Often, CNS signs will be the only presentation of digitalis toxicity, before cardiac or gastrointestinal symptoms.
- In many patients, though, the sole evidence for **digitalis toxicity** is the appearance of a **cardiac arrhythmia**. Every known type of arrhythmia has been associated with digitalis intoxication, but commonly appearing aberrations include **frequent premature ventricular beats, bradyarrhythmias, paroxysmal atrial tachycardia with block, junctional tachycardia** and **bidirectional ventricular tachycardia**.
- Nausea, vomiting and abdominal pain are early manifestations of acute and chronic toxicity. The most common presenting symptoms in a **paediatric patient** are **gastrointestinal complaints, sinus bradycardia** or **first-degree AV block**.
- Hypotension and cardiac arrest may occur.
- **Hyperkalaemia** is common in severe poisoning as a result of blockade of the Na-K-ATPase pump causing potassium shift from the intracellular to the extracellular space. It is a useful marker of toxicity in acute overdose.
- Photophobia, amblyopia, miosis and **aberrations of colour** (predominance of yellow-green), are associated primarily with **chronic toxicity**.

Usual Fatal Dose

- **Digitoxin: 3 mg**
- **Digoxin: 10 mg**
- **Digitalis leaf: 2 g (2–3 leaves)**
- Therapeutic plasma concentration of digoxin should not exceed 2 ng/mL (range – 0.5–2 ng/mL). Concentrations exceeding **15 ng/mL** are potentially **fatal**.

Treatment

1. **Initial Treatment**:
   a. *Decontamination*: Lavage, activated charcoal,* cathartic (as applicable). Stomach wash may enhance vagal stimulation and exacerbate bradycardia or heart block. While digoxin immune Fab fragments are the preferred treatment for severe or life-threatening cardiac glycoside intoxication, multiple dose activated charcoal may be useful in situations in which Fab fragments are not available. Whole bowel irrigation may be useful after large ingestions.
   b. Forced diuresis, haemodialysis and haemoperfusion are generally ineffective.
   c. Monitor serum glycoside and potassium levels frequently. Hyper- or hypokalaemia may occur.
   d. All patients with a history of cardiac glycoside® ingestion should have a baseline electrocardiogram, and serial serum levels and electrolytes.
2. **Advanced Treatment**:
   a. **Antidote: Digoxin-specific antibody fragments (Fab)**
      i. Fab therapy is of proven efficacy in not only digitalis overdose, but also in red squill and oleander poisoning.
      ii. Fab fragments are administered intravenously. They bind intravascular free digoxin and then diffuse into the interstitial space and bind free digoxin there.
      iii. *Indications for antidotal treatment include*:
         - Ingestion of greater than 10 mg digoxin by an adult (4 mg by a child).
         - Potassium concentration exceeding 5 mEq/L.
         - Serum digoxin level of more than 15 ng/mL.
         - Progressive bradyarrhythmias or severe ventricular arrhythmias.
         - Rapidly progressing clinical symptomatology.
      iv. *Dose*:
         - Use an empiric dose based on average requirements for an acute or chronic overdose in an adult, as mentioned below:
           Adult = 10–20 vials (*acute poisoning*), 3–6 vials (*chronic poisoning*).
      v. *Mode of Administration*: Intravenous, over 30 min. Reconstitute each vial with 4 mL of sterile water and use immediately (or within 4 hrs, if refrigerated).
      vi. *Adverse effects*: Allergic reactions (rare).
      vii. *Disadvantages*: Not easily available in India. Can be procured from abroad, but is extremely expensive. A full course of antidotal therapy with Fab fragments can cost several thousand dollars! The FDA (USA) has approved for licensing, **DigiFab**®, which is available as a lyophilized powder in a vial containing 40 mg digoxin immune Fab.
   b. In the absence of Fab fragments, ventricular irritability can be treated with phenytoin or lidocaine. Antiarrhythmics that may be useful include atropine, phenytoin and lidocaine.
   c. Atropine is useful in the management of bradycardia, and varying degrees of heart block. In patients with severe supraventricular bradyarrhythmias, or high degrees of AV block, 0.5 mg of atropine is given IV in an adult. This dose can be repeated every 5 min as necessary.

**Note: In place of activated charcoal, steroid-binding resins such as cholestyramine (12–16 g/day orally), or colestipol may be used to equally good effect.*

d. Magnesium (20 mL of 20% solution over 20 min by slow infusion) has been reported to reverse digoxin-induced arrhythmias.
e. External or transvenous pacemaker: Pacemaker use should be considered in severe bradycardia and/or slow ventricular rate due to second or high-degree AV block that fails to respond to atropine and/or phenytoin when digoxin Fab are not available.
f. Percutaneous cardiopulmonary bypass has been used for therapy resistant cardiac arrest due to digoxin overdose.
g. Haemodialysis is ineffective in removing cardiac glycosides, but may assist in restoring serum potassium to normal levels.
h. Treatment of hypo-/hyperkalaemia as follows: *Hypokalaemia*: IV potassium chloride in 0.9% or 0.45% sodium chloride, at a rate of 0.5–1.0 mEq/min (1 mEq/kg/hr in a child).
Hyperkalaemia: IV insulin, dextrose, sodium bicarbonate and oral ion-exchange resins (sodium polystyrene sulfonate). Digoxin immune Fab is first-line treatment.

Forensic Issues

- Digitalis poisoning (acute and chronic) is an important pharmacotoxicological problem. Acute toxicity may result from accidental ingestions (children), deliberate overdose (adults) or inadvertent dosing errors (elderly). Chronic toxicity is usually iatrogenic.
- Accidental ingestion has occurred following confusion of foxglove with **Comfrey*** (**Fig. 10.28**), while preparing herbal tea.

Aconite

Other Common Names

Monkshood, Wolfsbane, Helmet flower, Soldier's cap, Old wife's hood, Friar's cap

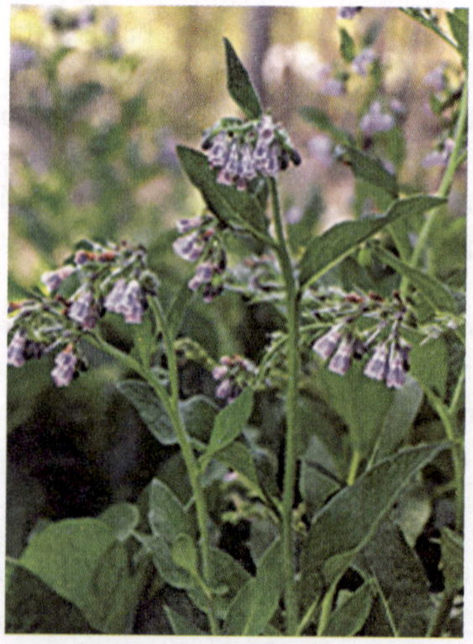

Fig. 10.28 Comfrey

Botanical Name

Aconitum species, of which there are 350 worldwide.

Aconitum napellus is the European variety, while Indian species include *A. ferox* (**Fig. 10.29**), *A. chasmanthum*, *A. cordatum* and *A. balfouri*.

Physical Appearance

- This plant grows well in the hilly regions of Northern and Eastern parts of India, extending from Assam to Kashmir.
- It is a perennial herb with distinctive helmet shaped flowers (**Fig. 10.30**), which may be blue, purple or pinkish white in colour.
- The root is stout and dark, and has a superficial resemblance to **horseradish**.
- Fruits form in groups, green to brown in colour and have many seeds which are white to brown, and are angled/winged.

Uses

- The tuber is very popular in Chinese medicine for the treatment of various ailments. The root is usually processed by

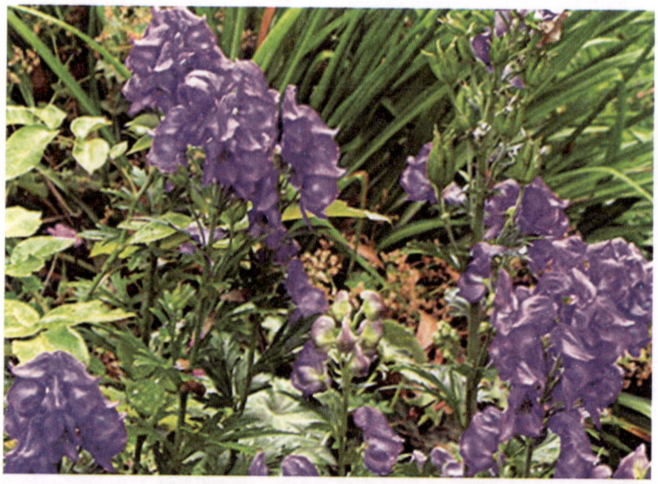

Fig. 10.29 *Aconitum ferox*

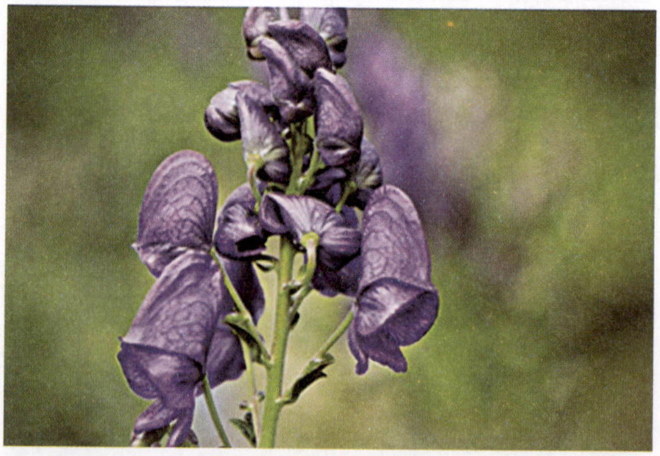

Fig. 10.30 Aconite flowers

****Note***: *Comfrey is a plant that has been used in herbal medicine, and is claimed to be effective in a wide variety of ailments ranging from bronchial problems, broken bones, sprains, arthritis, gastric and varicose ulcers, severe burns and acne.*

drying, soaking or boiling, which significantly reduces its toxicity. Raw aconite roots are highly toxic. Herbal decoctions of aconite are generally prepared by soaking the roots in water or saturated lime water and then boiling. This causes hydrolysis of aconite alkaloids to less toxic benzylaconine and aconine derivatives.

- Aconite is also used in Indian folk remedies. It is also used as an antipyretic in Ayurvedic medicine, after "detoxification."
- Formerly, aconite found mention in the British Pharmacopoeia (until 1953), but today it is only used in allopathic medicine as a proarrhythmic agent in animal studies to test the efficacy of antiarrhythmic agents. It is however quite popular in homoeopathy, though in trace concentrations, which are not likely to cause toxicity.
- Aconite is sometimes used as an abortifacient.

Toxic Part

All parts, but the **root** (**Fig. 10.31**) is most toxic. It is said to have a bitter-sweet taste.*

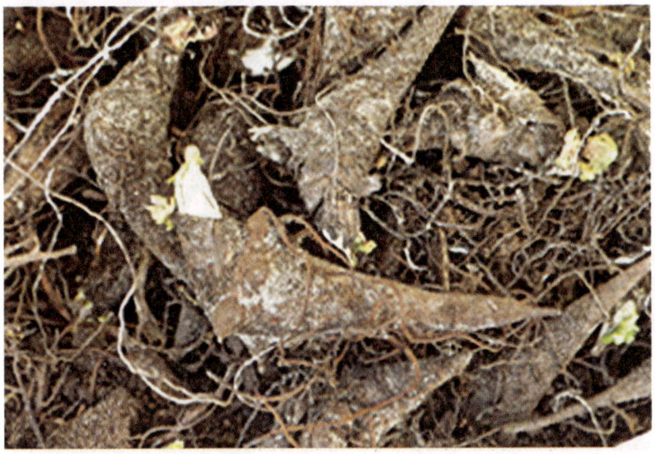

Fig. 10.31 Aconite roots

Toxic Principles

- European and American species contain **aconitine**, mesaconitine and jesaconitine.
- Indian species contain **hypoaconitine** and **mesoaconitine** which are less potent.

Mode of Action

- Aconitine acts on nerve axons by opening sodium channels, as well as by inhibiting complete repolarisation of the membrane of myocardial tissue, causing repetitive firing.
- Aconitine also stimulates the vagal medullary centre.

Toxic Effects

1. *GIT*: Nausea, hypersalivation, vomiting, diarrhoea. Chewing on a root may cause swelling of the lips, tongue and mouth, making speech difficult.
2. *CVS*: Palpitations, hypotension, ventricular ectopics, arrhythmias, A-V block.
   - Vagal slowing is seen in 10–20% of fatal intoxications. In severe cases, supraventricular tachycardia, ventricular tachycardia, torsades de pointes and other conduction disturbances are seen. Ventricular fibrillation is often the cause of death.
3. *CNS*: Tingling and numbness of mouth and lips which may extend to the limbs, followed by convulsions. Initial feelings of numbness may progress to paralysis of the skeletal muscles. Vertigo is often present.
4. *RS*: A few patients have reported breathing difficulty after ingesting aconite-containing herbals. Pulmonary oedema often occurs in the terminal stages.
5. *Eye*: Visual blurring, fluctuant or alternately contracting and dilating pupils (**pupillary hippus**; **pupillary athetosis**), mydriasis. Miosis may be seen until the patient develops hypoxia. Xanthopsia (yellow halos around objects) has been reported.
6. Death usually occurs from ventricular arrhythmias or respiratory paralysis, and this may happen in just a few minutes, or take several days.

Usual Fatal Dose

- **9–18 g of root.**
- **3–5 mg of aconitine.**
- **10–15 mL of tincture.**

Drying and storing these plants could result in changes in the composition and even transformation of the alkaloidal content, thus altering toxicity of individual exposures. Thus, the specimen of aconite placed in the museum of the forensic medicine department of an average medical college in India may actually be completely non-toxic!

Treatment

1. Gastric decontamination (lavage, charcoal).
2. Perform an arterial blood gas, serum electrolytes, creatine phosphokinase (fractionated) and an ECG.
3. Provide airway support, and establish vascular access.
4. Extensive vomiting and diarrhoea often necessitate fluid and electrolytes to be given in substantial doses.
5. There is no specific antidote. Treatment is symptomatic and supportive after decontamination.
6. Treat convulsions with benzodiazepines, followed by phenytoin, if required.
7. Treat metabolic acidosis and hypokalaemia.
8. Bradyarrhythmia and hypersalivation respond to atropine.
9. Perform a 12-lead ECG and measure the QRS duration and QT interval. Repeat 12-lead ECGs are recommended, especially in symptomatic patients. QT prolongation occurs due to potassium channel blockade and may provoke torsade de pointes ventricular tachycardia. Magnesium sulphate should be administered urgently to patients with torsade de pointes.
10. Arrhythmias are unfortunately often refractory to drug management.

*__Note__: *That is why aconite is referred to as "mitha zahar" in Hindi, which means "sweet poison."*

a. No single antiarrhythmic agent has been found to be uniformly effective for controlling tachyarrhythmias. DC cardioversion is not effective.
b. For symptomatic bradycardia, give atropine intravenously, 0.5–1.2 mg for an adult or 0.02 mg/kg for a child. Repeat doses may be necessary. Temporary pacemaker insertion may be required, alternatively external pacing may be used.
c. Calcium gluconate or chloride may help reverse arrhythmias in some cases. They must be followed up with magnesium sulphate.
d. If cardiotoxicity is unresponsive to the above consider the use of a lipid emulsion.
e. In patients with life-threatening haemodynamic instability, veno-arterial extracorporeal membrane oxygenation (VA-ECMO) has been used as a bridge to recovery in a few reported cases.

Forensic Issues

- Poisoning with aconite has never been common. Most reported cases are accidental in nature, resulting from therapeutic misadventures. Aconite is used in herbal medicines (cold preparation, antipyretic, digestive and general tonic, etc.), or to increase the intoxicating effect of alcoholic beverages. Fatalities have been reported with the use of tincture aconite added to liquor.
- A few cases result from mistaken identity with horseradish (**Fig. 10.32**).* Rarely, suicides and homicides have been reported.

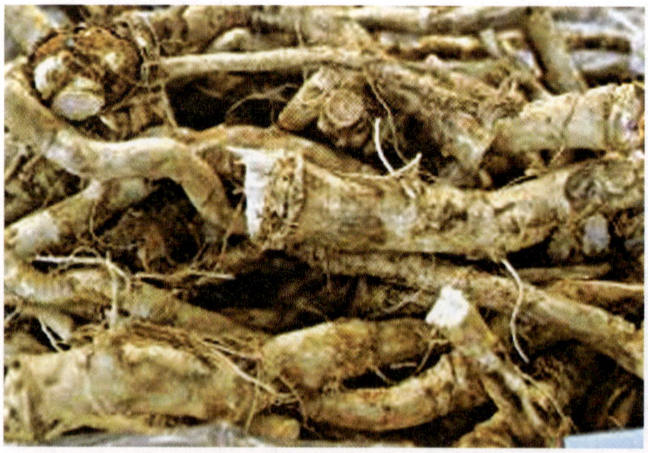

Fig. 10.32 Horseradish

Oleander – Common Oleander

Other Common Names

White oleander, Pink oleander, Rose laurel, Rosa francesca, Laurier rose

Botanical Name

Nerium oleander

Physical Characteristics

- This plant is a large evergreen ornamental shrub (**Fig. 10.33**) with long, lanceolate, leathery leaves and clusters of pink or white flowers (**Fig. 10.34**).
- The leaves produce a clear, thick sap.

Uses

- Decoction of the leaves and root are used in Indian traditional medicine as local applications for various skin ailments.
- Root is used by rural folk as abortifacient.
- Common oleander is a popular ornamental garden plant.

Toxic Part

All parts, especially the **root**.

Toxic Principles

- The seeds, stem and root are rich in the following **cardiac glycosides**: Oleandrin, neriin, folinerin, rosagenin and digitoxigenin.
- Leaves contain oxalate crystals.

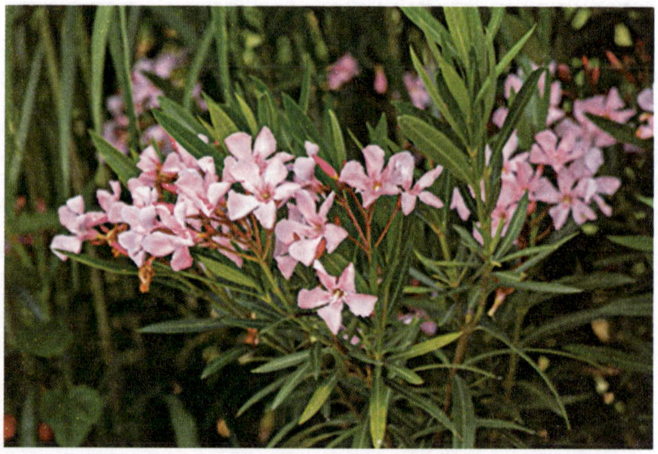

Fig. 10.33 *Nerium oleander* plant

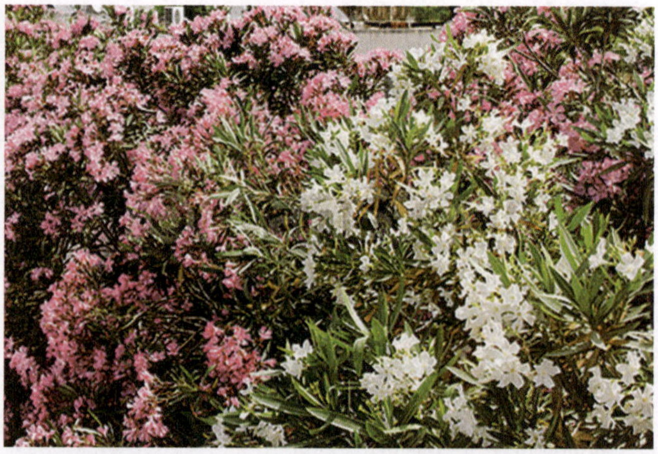

Fig. 10.34 *Nerium oleander* – Pink and white flowers

****Note***: *One way of distinguishing the two is to cut the root. Aconite will turn pinkish on exposure to air. Horseradish will show no change.*

Mode of Action

- All the glycosides have digoxin-like effects; they inhibit sodium-potassium ATPase.

Toxic Effects

1. *GIT*: Nausea, vomiting, diarrhoea.
2. *CVS*:
    a. Marked bradycardia with PR and QRS prolongation.
    b. Sinus arrest, varying degrees of AV block with dissociation or escape rhythms may occur, including paroxysmal atrial tachycardia with AV block, junctional tachycardia, frequent ventricular ectopics and bigeminy.
    c. Hypotension may occur.
    d. Ventricular fibrillation is potentially lethal.
3. *CNS*:
    a. Delirium, lethargy, dizziness, drowsiness, headache.
    b. Occasionally, there may be seizures and coma.
    c. Rarely, blurred vision or alteration in colour perception (classically xanthopsia) may also occur.
4. Hyperkalaemia is common in severe poisoning as a result of blockade of the Na-K-ATPase pump causing potassium shift from the intracellular to the extracellular space.
5. Metabolic acidosis may occur.
6. Skin contact, particularly with the sap, may produce dermatitis.

Usual Fatal Dose

- **5–15 leaves.**
- **15 g of root.**

Diagnosis

- Because oleander-derived cardiac glycosides are cross-reactive with the frequently used radio-immunoassays for digoxin, an elevated level may help confirm suspicion of oleander poisoning
- Thin-layer chromatography and fluorescence spectrophotometry can also be used to identify oleander glycosides.
- HPLC and LC/MS are confirmatory.

Treatment

1. Gastric lavage, activated charcoal:
    a. Gastric lavage is of limited benefit in patients ingesting plant parts, particularly children, because of the size of the plant parts relative to the lavage tube. Also, the procedure may worsen bradycardia secondary to vagal stimulation.
    b. Whole gut lavage may be more useful in such situations.
    c. Consider activated charcoal (50 g for adults; 1 g/kg for children), if the patient is symptomatic or presents within 4 hrs of ingestion.
2. Measure urea, electrolytes, magnesium and creatinine in all patients. Serum potassium correlates with cardiotoxicity, and careful measurement is one of the most important laboratory tests to be done, since hyperkalaemia is quite common.
3. The emergency management of life-threatening hyperkalaemia (potassium levels > 6.5 mEq/L) includes IV bicarbonate, glucose and insulin (administer 0.2 unit/kg of regular insulin with 200–400 mg/kg glucose). Concurrent administration of IV sodium bicarbonate (about 1 mEq/kg) is of additive value in rapidly lowering serum potassium levels.
4. Severe hyperkalaemia is normally an indication for digoxin-specific antibody therapy.
5. Perform a 12-lead ECG in all patients who require assessment. Repeat 12-lead ECGs are recommended, especially in symptomatic patients. Check cardiac rhythm, QRS duration and QT interval.
6. Atropine for sinus bradycardia and A-V block: 1 mg IV; repeat in 3–5 min, if asystolic cardiac arrest persists.
7. Antiarrhythmics (e.g., lignocaine): Lignocaine is useful in the management of ventricular tachy-arrhythmias, PVCs and bigeminy.
8. **Digoxin-specific antibodies** are the treatment of choice for severe **bradyarrhythmias with hypotension** unresponsive to atropine and life-threatening **ventricular arrhythmias**. An antidote effect is usually seen within 15–30 min of administration. Digoxin-specific antibodies are also the treatment of choice in managing severe **hyperkalaemia**.
9. Correct hypotension by adequate fluid resuscitation with a crystalloid. Treat brady and tachyarrhythmias appropriately. Vasopressors and inotropes can be initiated in an emergency through peripheral venous access.
10. If metabolic acidosis persists despite correction of hypoxia and adequate fluid resuscitation consider correction with IV sodium bicarbonate.
11. Haemodialysis or haemoperfusion are unlikely to enhance the elimination of cardiac glycosides, as they have a large volume of distribution and are highly protein bound.

Forensic Issues

- Accidental poisoning from its use in traditional medicine or 'herbal tea'.
- **Comfrey** (***Symphytum officinale***) leaves resemble those of **Foxglove** (***Digitalis purpurea***), when the plant is not in bloom and, therefore, cardiac glycoside poisoning may occur when people confuse foxglove with comfrey (**Fig. 10.35**).

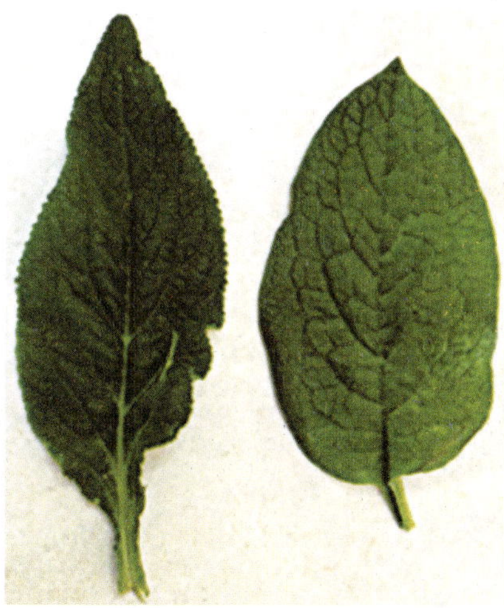

Fig. 10.35 Digitalis leaf (*left: serrated margins*) and Comfrey leaf (*right: smooth margins*)

- Suicidal ingestion of decoction prepared from leaves or root is fairly common in rural areas.
- Homicidal cases are rare, but have been reported.

Yellow Oleander

Other Common Names

Bastard oleander, Exile oleander, Be-still tree, Lucky nut, Tiger apple

Botanical Names

Cerbera thevetia, Thevetia peruviana, T. neriifolia

Physical Characteristics

- It is an ornamental shrub (that grows to about 30 feet height) (**Fig. 10.36**), with longish (about15 cm long) leaves yielding a milky sap and yellowish funnel-shaped flowers (**Fig. 10.37**).
- The leaves are pointed, with dark green upper surface and lighter green undersides.
- Fruit is diamond shaped or clam shaped (**Fig. 10.38**), and has 2–4 seeds in its stony inner section. It is about ½ inch in size, greenish at first and turning yellow when ripe, and may even appear blackish in the later stages. The kernel (seed) is very toxic.
- All parts of the plant contain a milky juice or sap.

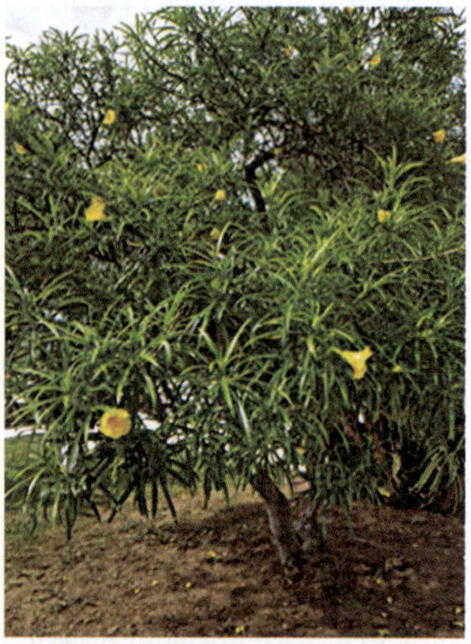

Fig. 10.36 Yellow oleander plant

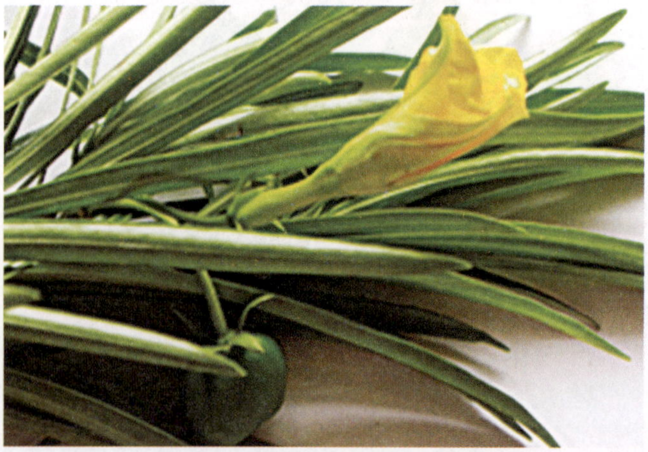

Fig. 10.37 Yellow oleander – flower (*Courtesy*: *Dr Shashidhar C Mestri*)

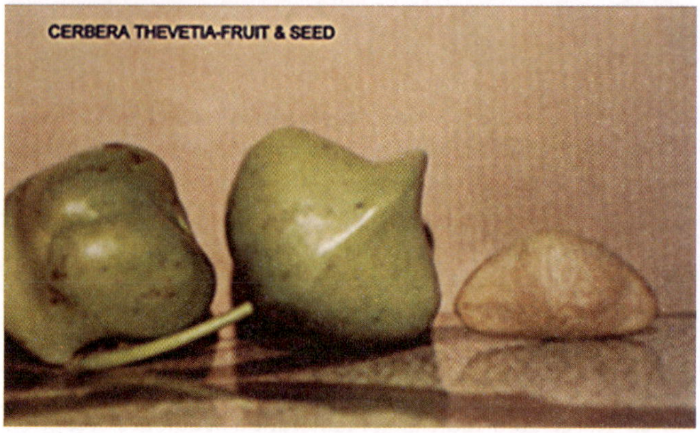

Fig. 10.38 Yellow oleander – Fruit and seed (*Courtesy*: *Dr Shashidhar C Mestri*)

Uses

- Like common oleander, yellow oleander is also used in traditional Indian medicine for the treatment of various ailments.

Toxic Part

- All parts, particularly **seeds** and **root**.
- Yellow oleander plant parts are generally more toxic than *Nerium oleander*.

Toxic Principles

- Cerberin
- Nerifolin
- Peruvoside
- Ruvoside
- Thevetin A & B

Usual Fatal Dose

- **8–10 seeds**
- **15–20 g of root**

Toxic Effects

- The commonest manifestations associated with yellow oleander poisoning include bradycardia with AV block, hypotension, lethargy, dizziness and GI distress.
- Convulsions, electrolyte disturbances, hypertension and coma have also been reported.
- Mydriasis may occur.
- Numbness and burning sensation of the mouth may develop after chewing a single seed.
- The sap of yellow oleander tree may cause blistering or dermatitis on contact.

Diagnosis

- Cardiac glycosides of this plant are best identified by radioimmunoassay.

Treatment

- As far as specific treatment is concerned, it has been shown that anti-digoxin Fab fragments are effective in the management of yellow oleander-induced arrhythmias. They rapidly restore sinus rhythm, and revert bradycardia and hyperkalaemia back to normalcy.
- **Digoxin Fab fragments** are indicated, if the potassium concentration exceeds the upper limit of the normal range (5 mEq/L), in association with other severe symptoms. Even if the exact cause is uncertain as to whether yellow oleander is the culprit in a given case, some investigators recommend the empiric administration of 10 vials of digoxin-specific Fab. However, serum potassium can drop steeply, and must be monitored frequently for several hours post administration.
- Combination therapy (glucose, insulin and bicarbonate) must be tried, if Fab fragments are not available.
- Atropine is useful in the management of bradycardia, and varying degrees of heart block.
- Lignocaine is useful in the management of ventricular tachyarrhythmias, PVCs and bigeminy.

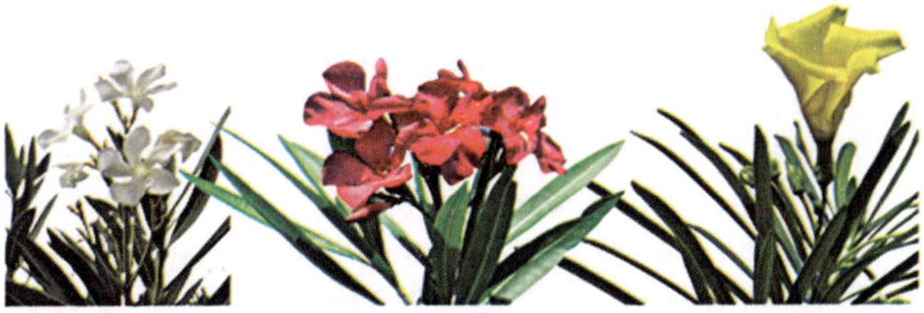

Nerium oleander WHITE FLOWER — *Nerium oleander* PINK FLOWER — *Thevetia neriifolia* YELLOW FLOWER

Suicide Tree (Odollam)

Other Common Names

Ordeal tree, Tangena nut, Pong-pong

Botanical Name

Cerbera odollam

Physical Characteristics

- It is a small tree (**Fig. 10.39**) that grows well in South India, especially Kerala.
- It bears fruits which resemble unripe (green) mangoes (**Fig. 10.40**). The fruit contains generally two hemispherical seeds with a tough, horny, granular envelope (kernel) (**Fig. 10.41**).
- The seeds are employed in folk medicine as an emeto-cathartic, while the bark, the latex and the leaves are used as purgatives, but all are dangerous.

Toxic Part

Kernel of fruit

Toxic Principle

- **Cerberin**: The seeds contain a colourless, crystallizable glycoside *Cerberin*, which is very toxic, especially on the heart. It blocks the calcium ion channels in heart muscle, causing disruption of the heartbeat.

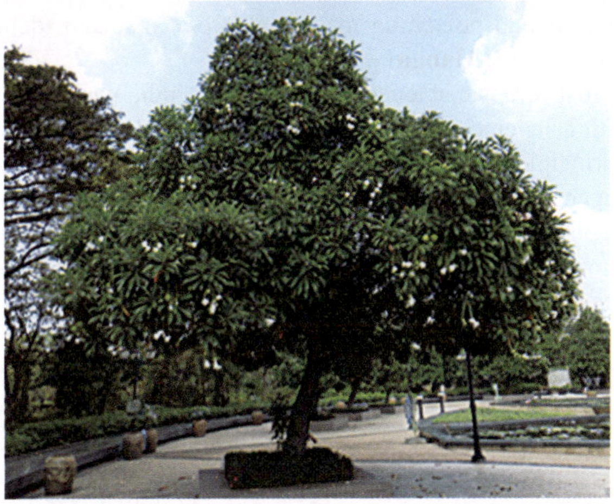

Fig. 10.39 *Cerbera odallum*

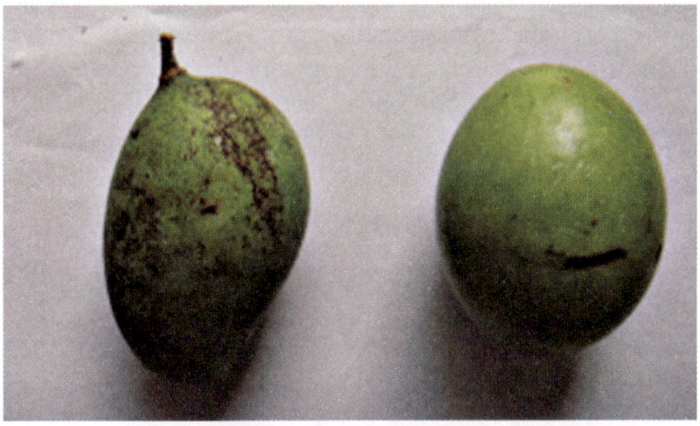

Fig. 10.40 Unripe mango and *Cerbera odallum* (*Courtesy: Dr S Sivasuthan*)

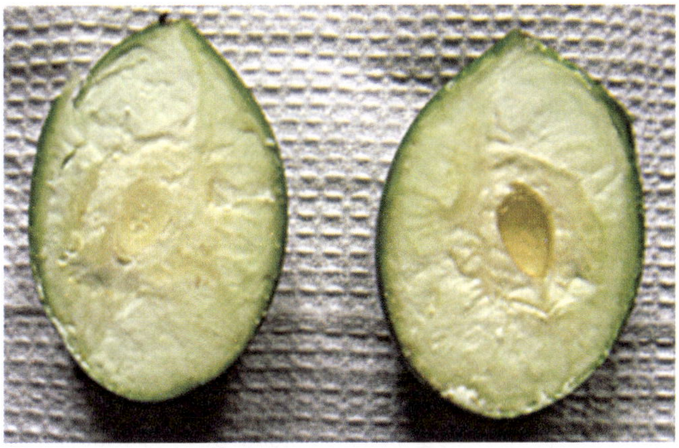

Fig. 10.41 *Cerbera odallum* – cut open (*Courtesy: Dr S Sivasuthan*)

Toxic Effects and Treatment

Manifestations of poisoning as well as treatment are the same as that for oleander.

Forensic Issues

- Cerberin is difficult to detect in autopsies and its taste can be masked with strong spices. Therefore, it is a common method in both homicide and suicide in India.

- Accidental poisoning may result from mistaken identity (with unripe **Mango**).
- Most forensic science laboratories in India perform TLC (thin layer chromatography) assays for detecting active principles of *Cerbera odollam*, which is a common suicidal agent in states like Kerala. There have been instances where a positive report for *Cerbera odollam* was furnished, where no such history of ingestion was available. In some of these cases, there was history of ingestion of **Cassava** (***Manihot esculenta***), which is a staple food in some communities. The suspicion naturally arose as to whether the active principles of these two plants (one edible, the other poisonous) exhibit similar TLC profiles leading to the confusion. The TLC patterns of the glycosides present in *Cerbera odollam* and *Manihot esculenta* were studied in the analytical toxicology laboratory of Amrita Institute of Medical Sciences, Cochin, which revealed that this was indeed the case. This makes it imperative that alternative methods must be used in suspected poisoning with *Cerbera odollam*, in order to avoid confusion in medicolegal cases. It is clear that the glycosides present in both odollam and cassava cross-react with each other giving similar TLC results.

GASTROINTESTINAL AND ENDOCRINAL DRUGS

A. Gastrointestinal Drugs
   a. Antacids and Anti-ulcer Agents
   b. Laxatives
   c. Anti-diarrhoeals
   d. Antiemetics and Prokinetic Drugs
   e. Bile Acids and Pancreatic Enzymes

B. Endocrinal Drugs
   a. Anterior Pituitary Hormones
   b. Thyroid and Anti-thyroid Drugs
   c. Oestrogens, Progestins and Antagonists
   d. Adrenocorticotropic Hormone and Corticosteroids
   e. Insulin and Oral Hypoglycaemics

Of the innumerable categories and examples of gastrointestinal and endocrinal drugs used in medical practice (listed above), fortunately, even if strangely, the new curriculum specifies only one: **Insulin**. Even other anti-diabetic drugs (oral hypoglycaemics) are not included. Hence in this book, discussion will be confined only to insulin.

Insulin

Insulin is a hormone that facilitates the penetration of glucose and amino acids through cell membranes of skeletal and heart muscle.

Preparations

1. **Short-acting insulins**: Insulin (neutral insulin, soluble insulin), insulin aspart, insulin glulisine.
2. **Intermediate and long-acting insulins**: Insulin glargine, insulin zinc suspension, isophane insulin, protamine zinc insulin.
3. **Biphasic insulins**: Biphasic insulin aspart, biphasic insulin lispro, biphasic isophane infusion.

Uses

1. Subcutaneous administration of insulin is the primary treatment for all patients with IDDM (*insulin-dependent diabetes mellitus* or *Type I DM*), and for patients with NIDDM (*non-insulin-dependent diabetes mellitus* or *Type II DM*), that is not adequately controlled by diet or oral hypoglycaemics.
2. Management of diabetic ketoacidosis.

Toxicokinetics

- Insulin is usually administered by subcutaneous injection. Commercial preparations are available for either subcutaneous or intravenous injection which differ in respect to onset and duration of action.
- Insulin is not absorbed from the GI tract.
- Metabolism to the extent of 50% of the administered dose occurs in the liver. Insulin is 5% protein bound.
- Insulin is reabsorbed in the proximal renal tubule (up to 98%), and 60% is returned to the venous blood. Less than 2% is excreted unchanged.

Adverse Effects

1. **Hypoglycaemia**: This remains one of the potential hazards of insulin therapy, and is invariably the result of inadvertent overdose. Symptoms will depend on the extent of overdose and the time elapsed since administration (**Table 10.12**).

   It is important to remember the differential diagnosis of hypoglycaemia since the condition can result from a number of causes (**Table 10.13**).

   Prolonged hypoglycaemia can produce behaviour disturbances, convulsions, coma and death. Irreversible neurologic sequelae are likely to occur when the duration of untreated hypoglycaemia approaches 7 hrs following over-dose. Sequelae may include amnesia, dementia and confusion.
2. **Sensitivity reactions**: These are more common with bovine preparations than with porcine insulin, while human insulin is associated with negligible incidence of allergic reactions. Cutaneous manifestations are most common, while in some cases there may be systemic effects.
3. **Lipoatrophy and lipohypertrophy**: The former is said to be a variant of an immune response to insulin, while the latter is because of lipogenic action of high local concentrations of insulin. Both are rare with purified insulin preparations. It is advisable to rotate the site of injection frequently to avoid these effects.
4. **Insulin oedema**: Sodium retention consequent to insulin administration can result in oedema, abdominal bloating, weight gain and blurred vision.

Toxic Effects

1. **Acute Poisoning**
   a. *General*:
      i. Patients with intermediate or extended insulin overdose may not develop symptoms for 18–36 hrs except for vomiting and lethargy. With long acting insulin, there is a compensatory mechanism in the first

Table 10.12 Hypoglycaemia Due To Insulin

Time after insulin administration	Symptoms
30 min	Sweating, salivation, drowsiness, restlessness, tachycardia (when stimulated), bradycardia (when somnolent).
2–4 hrs	Loss of contact with environment, myoclonus, primitive reflexes (grasping, sucking), mydriasis.
4–5 hrs	Comatose, roving eye movements, tonic and torsion muscular spasms, extensor plantar response.
5–6 hrs	Decerebrate rigidity.
6–7 hrs	Miosis, bradycardia, flaccid tone, depressed reflexes.

Table 10.13 Causes of Hypoglycaemia

Endocrine Disorders	Addison's disease, Glucagon deficiency, Panhypopituitarism (*Sheehan syndrome*).
Hepatic Disease	Alcoholism, Cirrhosis, Galactose or Fructose intolerance, Glycogen storage disease
Renal Disease	Chronic renal insufficiency.
Drug-Induced	Salicylates, beta blockers, β_2 agonists, quinine and quinidine, ACE inhibitors, MAOIs, paracetamol, tricyclics, tetracycline, mebendazole, fluoxetine, ethanol, lithium, cocaine
Miscellaneous	AIDS, Autoimmune disorders, Burns, Shock, Septicaemia, Pregnancy

24 hrs which helps to maintain normoglycaemia. Later this is exhausted, leading to irreversible brain and myocardial damage due to severe hypoglycaemia.

ii. After an insulin overdose, up to 12 days of treatment may be required before insulin needs return to normal. Nondiabetic patients are found to be more likely to present with hypoglycaemia, and develop recurrent hypoglycaemia despite oral intake and IV glucose infusion following intentional misuse.

iii. Hypoglycaemia can occur with therapeutic doses of insulin in diabetics on an uncontrolled diet, with too much exercise, or in patients with brittle diabetes. It is difficult to predict the minimum toxic or lethal dose of insulin and severity of intoxication must be based on clinical findings.

iv. Although insulin is not expected to cause toxicity when ingested due to enzymatic degradation in the gut, massive ingestion has been associated with hypoglycaemia in a few cases.

b. *Specific*:

i. Eyes: Mydriasis, sluggish external ocular movements.

ii. CNS: Drowsiness, confusion, headache, restlessness, extensor plantar reflexes, absent gag reflex. Generalized seizures may accompany severe hypoglycaemia following overdose. Aphasia, maniacal behaviour and other personality changes secondary to hypoglycaemia can also occur.

iii. Skin: Cold, clammy, pale, with profuse sweating.

iv. Respiratory system: Breathing is deep and heavy, with periods of apnoea. Pulmonary oedema may occur.

v. CVS: Tachycardia.

vi. Extremities: Pain, cramps, twitching.

vii. Hypokalaemia may occur along with other electrolyte abnormalities.

2. **Chronic Poisoning**: This is usually the result of chronic overtreatment with insulin.

Wilson's clues – Recurrent, episodic hypoglycaemia characterised by:

i. Pallor, restlessness, stertorous respiration, depression, inattentiveness.

ii. Sweating.

iii. Nightmares, night sweats, difficulty in awakening.

iv. Glycogen-laden hepatomegaly.

v. Morning hypothermia.

Diagnosis

Monitor blood sugar levels regularly. Plasma glucose levels of 30 mg/dL or lower are common following large overdosage.

1. Plasma insulin levels do not correlate well with severity of hypoglycaemia.
2. Leukocytosis is commonly observed.
3. Potassium levels may be depressed.

4. *ECG*: Sinus tachycardia, occasional premature ventricular beats, elevated ST segments.
5. *EEG*: Slow diffuse waves without lateralising discharges.
6. *Urinalysis*: Albuminuria, hyaline casts.
7. Chronic insulin-induced hypoglycaemia is often associated with the presence of insulin-binding antibodies and low C-peptide levels.

Treatment

1. *Stabilisation*: Airway, breathing and circulation must be established and maintained. Endotracheal intubation and assisted ventilation may be necessary. Asymptomatic patients should be observed in hospital for a minimum of 12–24 hrs.
2. *Antidote*:
   a. **Glucose is the specific antidote and must be administered without delay.** Correct hypoglycaemia as quickly as possible. If the patient is awake give oral glucose followed by a carbohydrate meal.
      i. Adults: If the patient is drowsy or unconscious give up to 250 mL 10% or 125 mL 20% glucose IV rapidly (titrated to patient responsiveness). If hypoglycaemia persists 50 mL 50% glucose IV may be given but is irritant to veins and can cause skin necrosis in cases of extravasation.
      ii. Children: Give 2 mL/kg bolus of 10% glucose followed by an IV infusion containing glucose (0.45% NaCl/10% glucose) at an appropriate rate to maintain adequate blood sugar. Persistent hypoglycaemia should be treated with repeated boluses of 10% glucose initially, though continuous infusions of higher concentrations of glucose may be required in severe cases.
   b. **Glucagon** 1–2 mg IM (1 mg in children over 25 kg body weight; and 0.5 mg in children under 25 kg) may also be used, if IV access is difficult or the patient is combative but its effects are dependent on available glycogen stores.
3. Adrenaline (1:1000), 1 mg, subcutaneously, can be beneficial in some cases.
4. Cerebral oedema is treated with mannitol and dexamethasone.
5. Hypokalaemia is managed by potassium supplements. Administer intravenous potassium chloride (20–60 mEq/L of fluid).
6. Administer 300 g daily or more of carbohydrates when the patient awakens, to supplement intravenous glucose and prevent secondary hypoglycaemia.

Forensic Issues

- Most cases of toxicity are iatrogenic due to inadvertent overdoses. However, there have been several cases of intentional insulin overdose among depressed patients intent on committing suicide. A few of these cases may represent factitious administration. Surreptitious insulin administration may be a symptom of serious underlying psychiatric disorder (especially in adolescents with insulin-dependent diabetes mellitus).
- Insulin has been used as a performance-enhancing drug by body builders. It can often be obtained on the "black market" by users identified as anabolic androgenic steroid injectors to promote anabolic processes and inhibit catabolism.
- Insulin injections have been used in cases of deliberate poisoning in both children and adults (Munchausen syndrome and Munchausen by proxy) and should be considered as a cause of unexplained hypoglycaemia.
- While homicidal poisoning with insulin and oral hypoglycaemics is quite rare, a few cases have been reported, and doctors must always be alert to this macabre possibility (**Box 10.3**).

Box 10.3—Homicides with Insulin

- The first published case involved a healthcare worker named **Kenneth Barlow**, a registered nurse, in Yorkshire, England in 1957. He murdered his pregnant 32-year-old wife, at home in the bath, trying to make out that she had unfortunately drowned by accident. His account of events was suspicious and a second examination of her body revealed two injection sites in each buttock. This was over 60 years ago when limited assays available to measure insulin relied on finding the dose of insulin which caused hypoglycaemic convulsions in mice. Extracts of tissues from the victim's buttocks were injected into mice, producing measurable quantities of insulin. He was sentenced to life imprisonment and released 26 years later, in 1984, still maintaining his innocence.

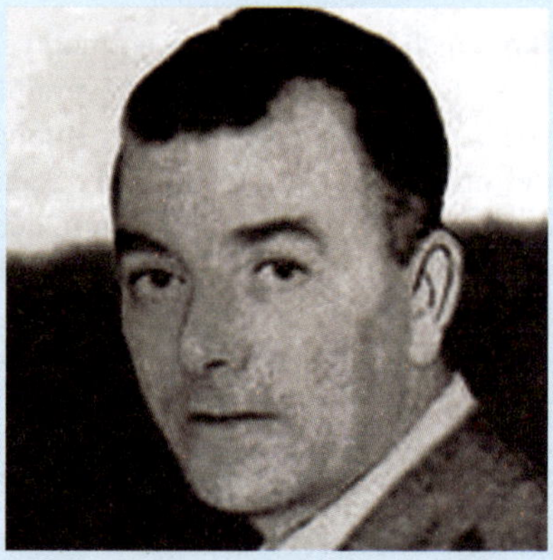

Kenneth Barlow

- In 1991, several unexpected infant deaths and unexplained illness occurred on the children's ward of Grantham Hospital, England. Suspicion fell on **Beverley Allitt**, a State Enrolled Nurse who worked in the same ward. Painstaking investigations provided convincing evidence of insulin as the murder weapon, in at least two of the cases. Toxicological assays revealed very high levels of immune-reactive insulin, accompanied by very low C peptide. These findings, along with Allitt's attendance during these attacks, finally led to her arrest. She was convicted of murdering four children, attempting to murder three other children, and causing grievous bodily harm to a further six. Sentenced to life

contd.

imprisonment in 1993, she is currently detained in a psychiatric facility. Perhaps the most notorious British serial child killer, Allitt was the subject of a book and a BBC dramatisation of the case, Angel of Death (2005).

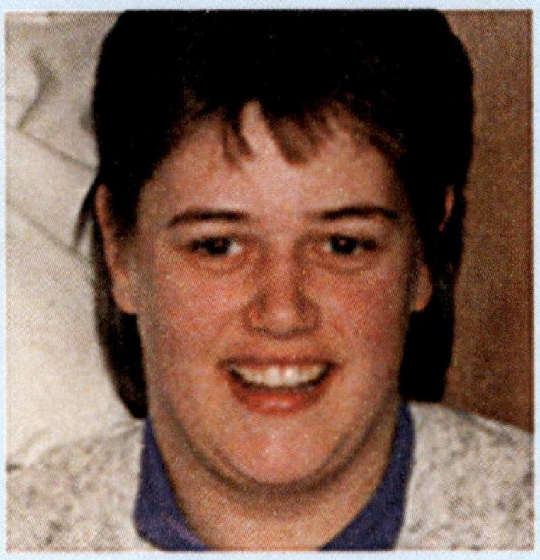

Beverley Allitt

- The "**Stockport Murders**" reflected a different kind of healthcare worker serial killer, whereby the victims were seemingly chosen at random. **Victorino Chua**, a hospital nurse, injected insulin into saline bags and ampoules while working on two acute wards at Stepping Hill Hospital, Stockport, England in 2011. He left these contaminated products in the treatment rooms, not knowing who would fall victim to his actions. These were then unwittingly used by other nurses on the ward, leading to a series of insulin overdoses. In 2015, he was convicted by a jury at Manchester Crown Court of murdering two patients and 22 counts of attempted grievous bodily harm alongside other charges. During the 3-month trial, no motive ever really emerged for why Chua decided to kill his patients. He was jailed for life.

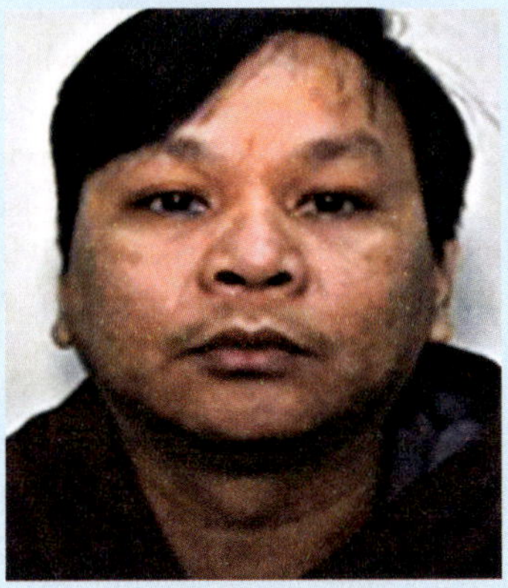

Victorino Chua

- In 2018, in India, **Dr Govind Prakash**, a diabetologist, allegedly killed his mother and sister by injecting them with an overdose of insulin and tried, unsuccessfully, to end his own life by the same method. It appeared to be a suicide pact as a suicide note written by Dr Govind states that all three decided to end their lives as they were suffering from migraines and disk prolapse. The letter also states that no one else is responsible for their death.

Topic 11

BIOTOXICOLOGY

(Number of Competencies – 1: FM 11.1)

Teachers and students, please note:

- Topics 9–13 deal with specific categories of poisons with regard to clinical features, diagnosis and management, upon exposure to them. It is to be noted that except for Topic 13, the new curriculum does not mention medicolegal aspects at all! So, it is a moot point whether students can be assessed on these aspects.
- However, as the editor feels it is important, this book lists medicolegal aspects too (under 'Forensic Issues') for all the poisons.
- Also, there is always a possibility of a revised (corrected) curriculum being released incorporating medicolegal aspects, anytime in the future. So, it is better to be prepared!

FM 11.1: Core – Written/Viva Voce
- Describe features and management of:
  - Snake bite
  - Scorpion sting
  - Bee and Wasp sting
  - Spider bite

There are hundreds of **venomous creatures** that exist around the world. These creatures are capable of delivering toxic venom into tissues by way of injection either by biting or stinging. They need to be differentiated from **poisonous creatures** that cause toxicity usually upon consumption or some other form of exposure, but do not possess venom, or even biting or stinging apparatus. While some of these creatures may be able to deliver a bite, e.g., non-venomous snakes, no venom is injected.

SNAKES

- **Snakes** (or '**serpents**') are elongated, legless, carnivorous reptiles that can be distinguished from legless lizards by their lack of eyelids and external ears.
- The body is divided into head, trunk and tail. The head may be oval, triangular or the same width as the trunk, ending as a blunt snout. The head bears two eyes, two nostrils and a mouth. External ears are absent since snakes do not possess auditory apparatus. However, though a snake cannot perceive sounds, it senses vibrations on the ground, which enables it to hunt prey and keep clear of predators. The eyes of a snake lack eyelids, each being covered by a transparent scale. This is the reason for the steady unwinking stare that snakes are well known for. Pupils may be round or elliptical.
- Living snakes are found on every continent except **Antarctica**; as also **Ireland**, **Iceland**, **Greenland**, **Hawaii** and **New Zealand**.
- More than 20 families are currently recognized, comprising about 520 genera and about 3600 species.
- Snakes are essentially carnivorous and feed mostly on mice, rats, lizards, or frogs. Water snakes feed on fish. Some are cannibals and feed on other snakes, e.g., Krait, King cobra, etc.
- Most snakes have four rows of teeth in the upper jaw, and two rows of teeth in the lower jaw.
- Venomous snakes have modified teeth called **fangs** in addition to ordinary teeth. Fangs are usually two in number, invariably located one on each side of the upper jaw. They may be grooved or canalized, and are connected to the venom glands which are a pair of modified parotid salivary glands located one on each side, just below and behind the eye.
  - The most primitive type of biting apparatus is seen in colubrid snakes, which were previously considered "non-venomous." These snakes have short, immobile fangs or enlarged solid teeth at the rear end of the maxilla. Significant human envenomation is extremely rare, and is possible only if the snake seizes and chews at a finger of the victim.
  - The elapids and hydrophids have grooved fangs situated anteriorly, which are immobile, while the vipers have highly developed long, curved, hinged front fangs which have a closed venom channel, giving them a structure like a hypodermic needle. Because of this seemingly superior injection mechanism, it has always been believed that viper bites are invariably associated with effective instillation of substantial quantities of venom deep under the skin. However, the discharge orifice of a viper fang is usually well above its tip, so the point of the fang can penetrate deeply, and yet part or most of the venom may be ejected superficially or externally without really entering the wound. Even a thin layer of clothing may afford great protection. Because of the superficial injection of venom not only by the vipers, but also by elapids and hydrophids, as many as 1/5th of patients bitten by venomous snakes show no evidence of envenomation even though the fangs have penetrated the skin. It is also true that "**dry bites**" may occur in up to 20–30% of strikes, where no venom at all has been ejected! This suggests that snakes might be capable of biting defensively without injecting venom, and is particularly true of some species, e.g., pit vipers.

- The snake's venom apparatus (**Fig. 11.1**) has been evolved to deliver a mechanically effective bite with injection of a lethal dose of venom into the snake's natural prey, comprising usually small creatures such as rodents, frogs and lizards. When the snake strikes at a human foot or ankle (the most common bitesite), it is far less likely, for purely anatomical reasons, that an adequate injection of venom will be achieved.

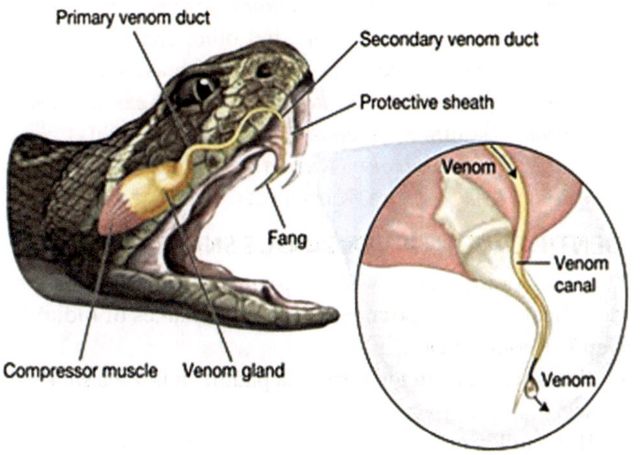

Fig. 11.1 Snake – Venom delivery

- Symptomless envenomation is said to be most common in sea snakebites, where up to 80% of cases show no manifestations at all. Since most venomous snakes have either a single or a pair of fangs, examination of the bitten area in a victim will show usually one or two puncture wounds. Non-venomous snakes leave behind multiple teeth impressions, which are not deep. However, such an appearance does not necessarily exclude the bite of a venomous snake. While it is true that fang marks are not seen with non-venomous snakebites, venomous snakes do have other teeth in addition to fangs, and multiple teeth impressions may be seen in conjunction with a venomous bite. It is also to be noted that the exact number of actual fang marks may vary because of glancing blows, multiple fangs, multiple strikes, or from protection of clothing or shoes.
- Sometimes the offending snake may have been killed by bystanders, and produced for inspection. The mouth can then be examined for the presence of fangs, but these may sometimes be difficult to identify, either because they are too small (colubrids, elapids and hydrophids), or because they are folded back inside a sheath (vipers). While examining an apparently dead snake, it must be remembered that sometimes reflex action occurs on handling, resulting in a bite. This is possible up to 1 hr after death.

▪ The tongue of a snake is forked and can be flicked in and out of the mouth rapidly. It is not adapted for licking or sucking, but is actually a device to pick up scent particles from the exterior and transfer them to the Jacobson's organ in the roof of the mouth. Thus, the snake is able to track its prey, locate suitable mates and smell out predators such as mongoose or humans.

▪ The nostrils enable a snake to inhale air into its lungs. Hissing is accomplished by the forcible expulsion of air through the nostrils, and is an act of aggression or defence. Russell's viper and puff adder are noted for their very loud hiss. In some (Crotalid) snakes, there is a pit between the eye and nostrils, which is a heat sensitive organ that helps in detecting warm-blooded prey.

▪ Snakes are encountered in all kinds of geographical locations, such as on land, in marshes and in water (fresh water and the sea). Most snakes can climb trees, and a few can burrow into the ground. Land snakes can swim in water, but sea snakes cannot survive on land.

▪ Snakes regularly moult, i.e., they shed their skin periodically (usually every 2 months). The skin which is cast off, is turned inside out, in the manner of a glove being removed from the hand. Moulting enables a snake to become more alert and active.

▪ Sexes are distinct in snakes. Each species breeds true, and hybrids are virtually unknown. Most snakes lay eggs (oviparous) while a few species bring forth their young alive (viviparous). Snakes usually survive for many years, a few species living up to 20 years or more.

CLASSIFICATION OF SNAKES

▪ Snakes are classified on the basis of morphological characteristics such as arrangement of scales (***lepidosis***), dentition, osteology, myology, sensory organs and the form of the hemipenes, as well as on the basis of immunological analysis of venom and serum proteins, and sequence analysis of DNA that encodes mitochondrial and other enzymes.

▪ There are about 3600 known species of snakes in the world, of which less than 350 species are venomous. Only about 200 species have caused death or permanent disability by biting humans.

▪ Among non-venomous snakes, only the **giant constrictors** belonging to family Boidae are dangerous to man.
  - Examples include **rock python** (*Python sebae*) of Africa, **reticulated python** (*Python reticulatus*) of South East Asia, especially Indonesia and **anaconda** (*Eunectes murinus*) of South America.
  - The **Indian rock python** (*Python molurus*) (**Fig. 11.2**) is seen all over India, and grows up to 3 m, but not a single case of human fatality has been reported that can be definitely attributed to this snake.
  - The **regal python** of Nepal grows up to 10 m in length, and is said to be the **largest snake in the world**.
  - The giant constrictors act by coiling around the victim and crushing him to death.

▪ **Venomous snakes** belong to **5 families**:
  - **Colubridae**: These have short immobile fangs, or enlarged solid teeth at the posterior end of the maxilla. They are mostly arboreal snakes, e.g., **African boomslang** and **twig snakes**.

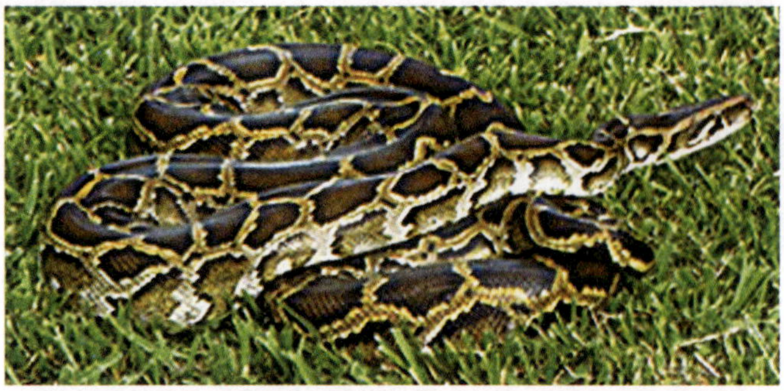

Fig. 11.2 Indian rock python (*Python molurus*)

- **Atractaspididae**: Comprises of African and Middle Eastern **burrowing asps** or **stilleto snakes**, which have long front fangs used for immobilizing their prey by a side-swiping motion. These fangs often protrude from the corner of the partially closed mouth.
- **Elapidae**: These snakes have relatively short, fixed front fangs. Examples include:
  - **Cobras** (*Naja*)
  - **Kraits** (*Bungarus*)
  - **Coral snakes** (*Calliophis, Maticora, Micrurus*)
  - **Mambas** (*Dendroaspis*)
- **Viperidae**: These snakes have highly developed long curved, hinged, front fangs, which are channelised in the form of a hypodermic needle. There are two subfamilies:
  - **Viperinae** or **true vipers**: Vipers and adders
  - **Crotalinae** or **pit vipers**: **Rattle snakes** (*Crotalus, Sistrurus*), **moccasins** (*Agkistrodon*) and **Asian pit vipers** (*Agkistrodon, Deinagkistrodon, Calloselasma, Trimeresurus, Hypnale*).
- **Hydrophidae**: This family comprises **sea snakes**, which have short fixed fangs as in the case of the elapids.

- Approximately, 330 species of snakes exist in India, of which about 70 species are venomous (40 land snakes and 30 sea snakes).
  - The commonest Indian venomous snakes are:
    - **Common krait** (*Bungarus caeruleus*)
    - **Common cobra** (*Naja naja*)
    - **Saw-scaled viper** (*Echis carinatus*)
    - **Russell's viper** (*Daboia russelli*).*
  - Of the remaining, the following are important: **King cobra** (*Ophiophagus hannah*) and **Common Indian coral snake** (*Hemibungarus nigrescens*).
  - The commonest sea snake encountered in Indian seas is the **Hook-nosed sea snake** (*Enhydrina schistosa*).
- The most venomous snakes of the world in order of lethal potency are listed in **Table 11.1**.
- In terms of mortality from snakebite, India suffers the highest level in terms of absolute numbers.
- The Registrar-General of India's "**Million Death Study**", 2001–2003, provides reliable evidence of substantial mortality (**exceeding 50,000 per year**) as it is based on Representative, Re-sampled, Routine Household Interview of Mortality with Medical Evaluation ("RHIME"), covering all age groups across the entire country with geographical, seasonal and occupational data.
- "**The Big Four**" medically important species had been considered to be *Naja naja, Bungarus caeruleus, Daboia russelii* and *Echis carinatus*, but other species have now been proved important in particular areas, such as *Naja oxiana* (north-west), *N. kaouthia* (north-east), *Hypnale hypnale* (south-west coast and Western Ghats), *Echis carinatus sochureki* (Rajasthan) and *Trimeresurus malabaricus* (Mysore, Karnataka).

IDENTIFICATION OF VENOMOUS SNAKES

The following step-wise approach helps in the easy identification of the common venomous snakes of India**:

Step 1: Look at the **tail**.

- If it is flattened in the form of a paddle, it is a sea snake. All sea snakes are venomous.
- If the tail is cylindrical and tapers very gradually to a fine point, it is a land snake (most probably arboreal or tree-snake), which is non-venomous or mildly venomous.
- However, if the tail is cylindrical and tapers abruptly, it could be venomous.

Step 2: Look at the ventral part (**belly** or undersurface) of the snake.

- If the belly scales are small like those on the back or dorsal surface, or they are broad but do not extend across the entire width, the snake is non-venomous.
- If the scales are broad enough to extend across the entire width of the belly, the snake could be either venomous or non-venomous, and it is necessary to proceed to the next step of the identification process.

Step 3: Look at the **head** scales.

- If these are small, or if there is a pit between the eye and the nostril, it is a venomous snake (true viper and pit viper, respectively).
- Vipers usually have a triangular head which is an additional point of importance.
- If the head scales are large and the belly scales are broad, proceed to the fourth step.

Step 4: If the head has large scales (or shields), look for a **hood** in the region of the neck.

- If a hood is discernible, it is a cobra.
- The common cobra has in addition a spectacle (binocellate) mark on the neck.
- A cobra can also be identified by the presence of 2 or 3 series of dark plates on the undersurface of the neck.

Step 5: Look closely at the **scales** on the head.

**Note*: *Referred to as the "Big Four".*

***Note*: *Must be attempted only in a killed snake! It should be noted that reflex bites can occur up to 1 hr after death even in the case of a killed snake which is being handled. Extreme caution is therefore advised at all times.*

Table 11.1 Top Venomous Snakes
(in descending order of lethal potency of venom)

Snake	Region
Inland taipan	Australia
Forest cobra	Coral Sea, Arafura Sea, Timor Sea and Indian Ocean
Eastern brown snake	Australia, Papua New Guinea, Indonesia
Yellow bellied sea snake	Tropical oceanic waters
Peron's sea snake	Gulf of Siam, Strait of Taiwan, Coral sea islands and other places
Coastal Taipan	Australia
Many-banded krait	Mainland China, Taiwan, Vietnam, Laos, Burma
Black-banded sea krait	Eastern coast of the Malay Peninsula and Brunei, and in Halmahera, Indonesia
Black Tiger snake	Australia
Western Australian Tiger snake	Australia
Beaked sea snake	Tropical Indo-Pacific

***Source**: Australian Venom Research Unit (2014). Facts and Figures: World's Most Venomous Snakes. University of Melbourne.*

- If the 3rd upper lip shield touches the shield of the nose and the eye, it could be a cobra or a coral snake.
- A common cobra would have in addition, a small wedge shaped shield between the 4th and 5th lower lip shields, called the "cuneate."
- King cobra has two large occipital shields behind the parietals on the head.
- Coral snakes have "coral spots" on their belly. Also they usually have red, yellow and black bands on the back.

Step 6: If none of the features characteristic of a cobra or coral snake is evident as mentioned in the previous two steps, it becomes important to determine whether the snake is a krait. This can be done by looking at the **back** (dorsal surface) of the body.

- The scales in the middle of the back are enlarged and hexagonal in a krait.
- In addition, the common krait is usually dark grey or brownish in colour, with paired white bands or half-rings over the entire back.
- Also, the 4th infralabial (lower lip) scale is the largest of all the infralabials.
- A banded krait has an unmistakable series of glistening black and yellow broad bands on the back.
- Scales on the undersurface of the tail (subcaudals) of a krait are usually undivided.

General features of venomous snakes are listed in **Table 11.2**.

COMMON INDIAN VENOMOUS SNAKES

THE BIG FOUR

Common Cobra

This snake is revered in Indian mythology and culture, and is often seen with snake charmers. It is now protected in India under the *Indian Wildlife Protection Act* (1972).

Scientific Name

Naja naja

Other Common Names

Indian Cobra, Spectacled Cobra, Binocellate Cobra

Geographical Distribution

All over India (except the North East, where it is rarely encountered).

Table 11.2 Features Indicative of Venomous Snake

Usually dull coloured: brown, black, grey, dull green, etc.
Stout body with abruptly tapering tail.
Compressed tail.
Broad belly scales extending across entire width of belly.
Small scales on triangular head.
Pit between eye and nostril.
Presence of hood with or without markings.
Presence of fangs.
Presence of rattle at the end of tail.

Physical Appearance

- The common cobra is usually brown or black in colour.
- It is a distinctive snake growing up to 5–6 feet in length, with a distensible neck that can be expanded into a hood (**Fig. 11.3**). On the dorsal side of the hood, there may be a monocellate (monocle) or binocellate (spectacle) mark (**Fig. 11.4**).
- On the ventral surface of the hood are faint, broad, black stripes above which are two dark spots that extend over 3–4 scales.
- The head is small, and pupils are round.
- The most important distinguishing feature of this snake is the fact that the 3rd supralabial shield touches the eye and nose shield. Also, a small wedge-shaped scale ("cuneate") is present between the 4th and 5th infralabials.
- The **Indian rat snake** (*Ptyas mucosa*) (**Fig. 11.5**) is often mistaken for the cobra; however, this snake is much longer and can easily be distinguished by the more prominent ridged appearance of its body.

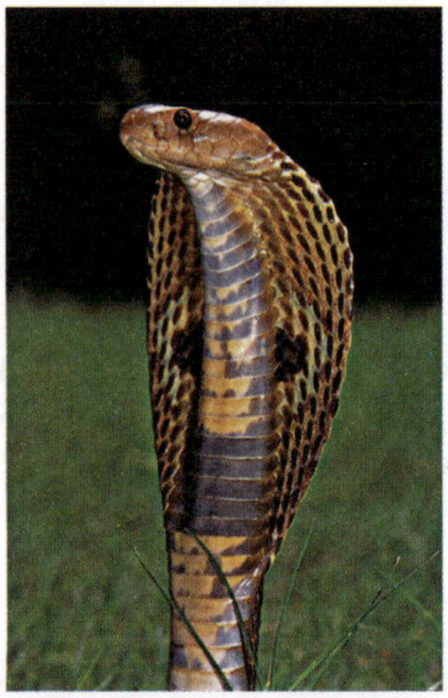

Fig. 11.3 Common cobra (*Naja naja*) – Hood expanded (*Courtesy: Ashok Captain*)

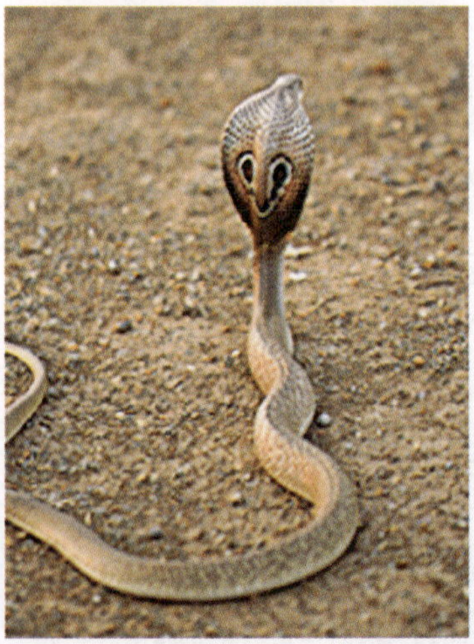

Fig. 11.4 Common cobra – Binocellate mark on hood

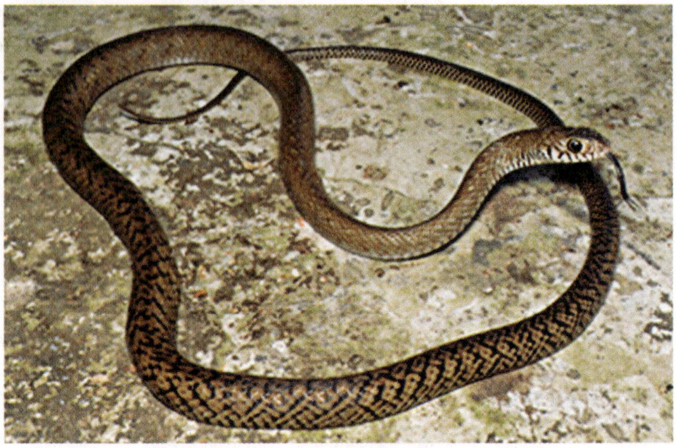

Fig. 11.5 Indian rat snake (*Ptyas mucosa*)

Habitat

- The **Indian Cobra** inhabits a wide range of habitats throughout its geographical range. It can be found in dense or open forests, plains, agricultural lands (rice paddy fields, wheat crops), rocky terrain, wetlands and it can even be found in heavily populated urban areas such as villages and city outskirts.

Nature of Venom

Predominantly **neurotoxic**.

Common Krait

Scientific Name

Bungarus caeruleus

Other Common Names

Indian krait, Blue krait

Geographical Distribution

All over India

Physical Appearance

- The common krait is a steel-blue snake growing up to 3–4 feet in length, with whitish bands or half-rings throughout its back (**Fig. 11.6**).
- The most distinctive features comprise the following:
  - A chain of hexagonal large scales throughout the mid-dorsal aspect of the body.

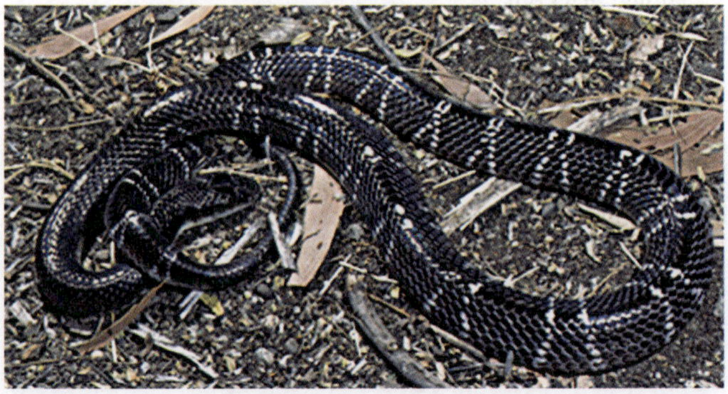

Fig. 11.6 Indian krait (*Bungarus caeruleus*)

- The subcaudals (ventral scales distal to the vent) are undivided, unlike other elapids.
- The 4th infralabial scale is the largest of the infralabials.

- The **common wolf snake** (*Lycodon aulicus*) (**Fig. 11.7**) looks very similar to the krait. One of the most important features differentiating it from the latter is that it has bands on its body that are equidistant from each other, while the bands in the Indian krait are paired (**Fig. 11.8**).

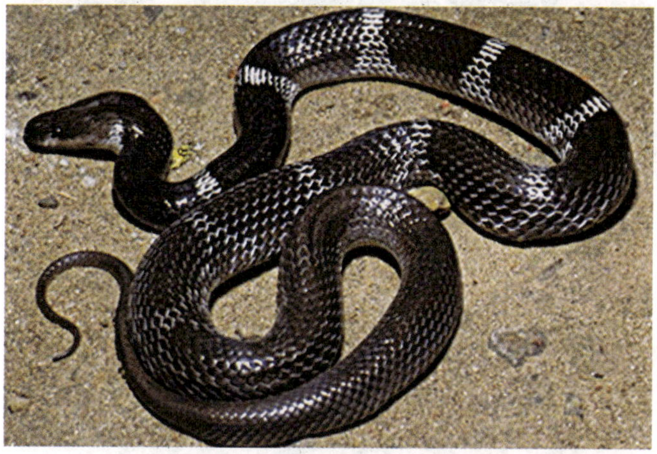

Fig. 11.7 Common wolf snake (*Lycodon aulicus*)

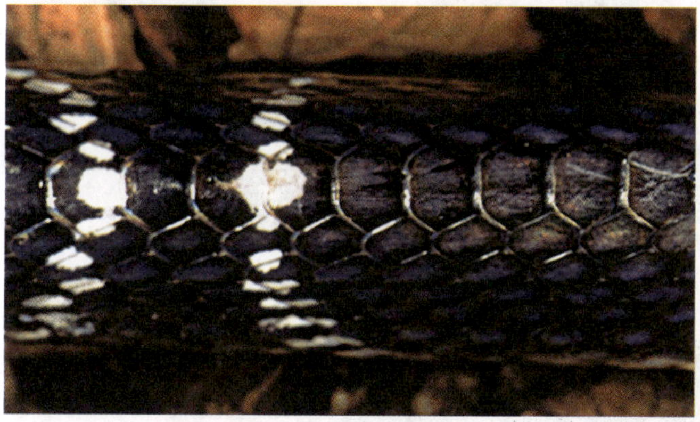

Fig. 11.8 Indian Krait – paired bands on the back (*Courtesy: Ashok Captain*)

Habitat

- The Indian krait is found in fields and low scrub jungle, as well as inhabited areas.
- This is a reclusive snake which prefers to reside in crevices of rocks or logs of wood, and being nocturnal, emerges only during the night to hunt for prey. It may enter human habitations and hide in dark corners, cupboards, bookshelves, etc.

Nature of Venom

Predominantly **neurotoxic.**

It is the most venomous snake of India.

Saw-scaled Viper

Scientific Name

Echis carinatus

Other Common Names

Carpet viper, Little Indian viper

Geographical Distribution

All over India (especially plains and deserts).

Physical Appearance

- The saw-scaled viper is a small snake, about 1½ to 2 feet long, and is usually brown in colour (**Fig. 11.9**). There is a wavy white line along the entire length of each flank, while diamond-shaped markings extend over the back, numbering usually 25–30.
- The head is triangular with small scales. A characteristic whitish, arrow-shaped or crow's foot mark is often present on the head. The pupils are vertical.
- The saw-scaled viper is named as such because its **scales are serrated**. When agitated, it throws itself into a double coil (in the manner of a "figure of eight"), and rubs the coils together vigorously, producing a harsh, rasping sound, akin to the sound of a sandpaper being scraped over a rough surface. At the same time, it also hisses loudly by exhaling forcefully through the nostrils.
- Like other vipers, the saw-scaled viper is viviparous.
- The echis is an aggressive snake and may bite on the slightest provocation.

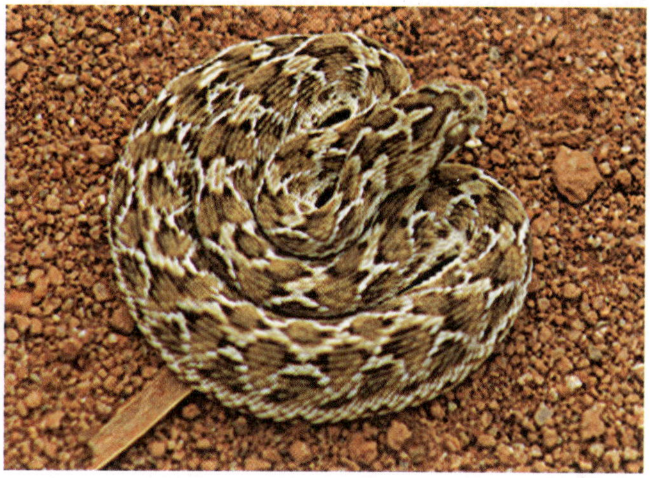

Fig. 11.9 Saw-scaled viper (*Echis carinatus*)

Habitat

E. carinatus prefers desert regions, and is often found basking in the sun during the daytime, among rocks or in sandy soil. It may enter human habitations especially tents, in search of prey.

Nature of Venom

Vasculo- and haemotoxic.

Russell's Viper

Scientific Name

Vipera russelii, Daboia russelii

Other Common Names

Chain viper, Seven pacer, Scissors snake

Geographical Distribution

All over India. It is abundant in Punjab, very common along the West Coast and its hills, in Southern India, and parts of Bengal. It is uncommon to rare in the Ganges valley, northern Bengal and Assam.

Physical Appearance

- *D. russelii* averages about 4 feet in length.
- Like all vipers, it is a nocturnal snake, but unfortunately for humans, during the daytime hours it rests up under bushes, at the base of trees and in leaf litter. It is therefore frequently encountered by rural workers as they carry out general agricultural activities.
- The Russell's viper is known to hiss loudly when agitated.
- Dorsally, the colour pattern consists of a deep yellow, tan or brown ground colour, with three series of dark brown spots that run the length of the body (**Fig. 11.10**). The head has a pair of distinct dark patches, one on each temple, together with a pinkish or brownish V marking that forms an apex towards the snout.
- Superficially, the **rough-scaled sand boa** (*Gongylophis conicus*) (**Fig. 11.11**) has a colour pattern that looks like that of *D. russelii*, though it is completely harmless.

Habitat

- *D. russelii* is mostly found in open, grassy or bushy areas.
- *D. russelii* does not associate as closely with human habitation as *Naja* and *Bungarus* species (cobras and kraits).
- When threatened, these snakes form a series of S-loops, raise the first third of the body, and produce a hiss that is supposedly louder than that of any other snake. When striking from this position, they can exert a great deal of force. As the fangs are relatively long (**Fig. 11.12**), the injection mechanism is quite effective as compared to many other venomous snakes.

Nature of Venom

Predominantly **vasculo- and haemotoxic**, but is able to produce **neurotoxic** effects also.

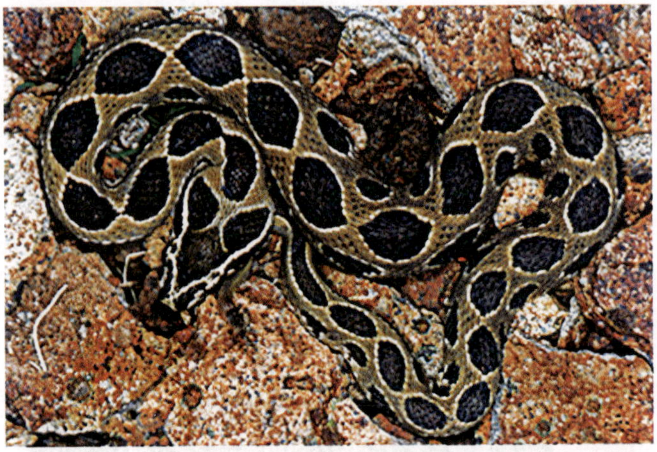

Fig. 11.10 Russell's viper (*Daboia ruselii*) (*Courtesy*: *Ashok Captain*)

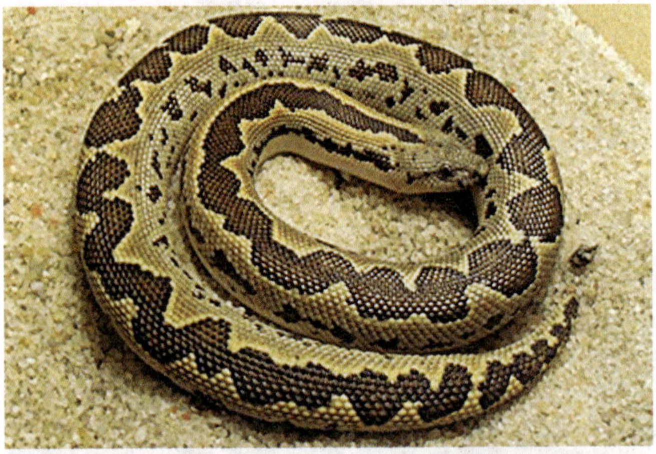

Fig. 11.11 Rough scaled sand boa (*Gongylophis conicus*)

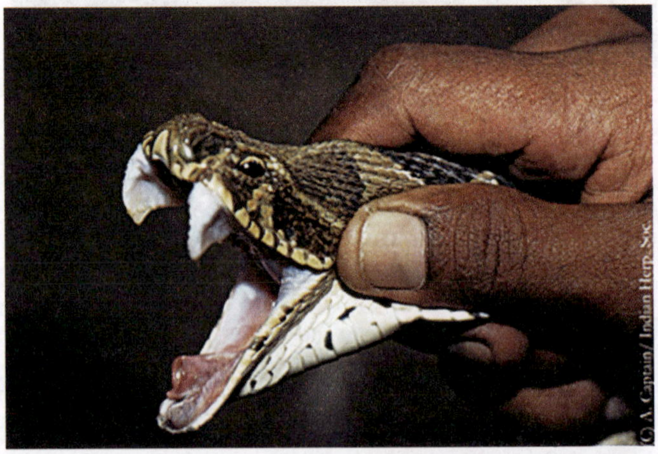

Fig. 11.12 Russell's viper fangs (*Courtesy*: *Ashok Captain*)

OTHER SNAKES

King Cobra

Scientific Name

Ophiophagus hannah

Other Common Names

Hamadryad

Geographical Distribution

- Himalayan region, Bengal, Assam, and hills and forests of South India. It lives in dense highland forests, preferring areas dotted with lakes and streams.
- King cobras are placed under Schedule II of Wildlife Protection Act, 1972 (as amended), and a person guilty of killing the snake can be imprisoned for up to 6 years.

Physical Appearance

- The king cobra is the **largest venomous snake in the world**, and grows up to 8–12 feet or more in length (maximum length 18.8 feet).
- The skin of this snake is either brown or black, and it has faint, pale yellow cross bands down the length of the body.
- Like the common cobra, it has a hood (**Fig. 11.13**), but lacks the monocellate or binocellate marking.

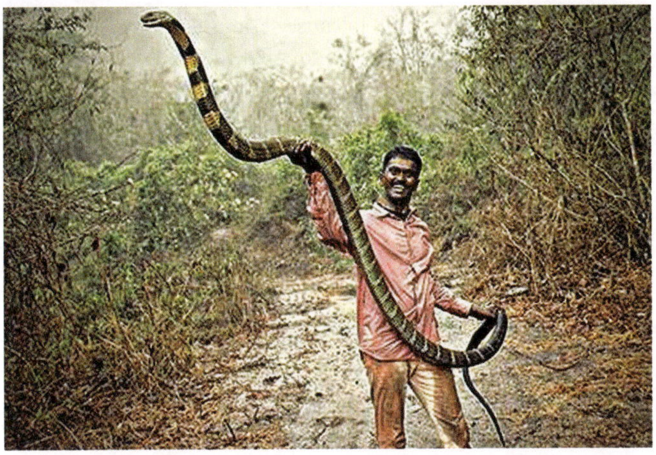

Fig. 11.13 King cobra (*Ophiophagus hannah*) (*In the pic*: *Vava Suresh, Snake Conservationist, Kerala*)

Nature of Venom

Predominantly **neurotoxic**.

Banded Krait

Scientific Name

Bungarus fasciatus

Geographical Distribution

In India, the banded krait is most commonly encountered in Northeast India, Odisha, Assam and West Bengal.

Habitat

- Banded kraits are seen in a variety of habitats, ranging from forests to agricultural lands.
- They prefer open plains of the countryside.

Physical Appearance

- The most distinctive feature of this snake is the presence of glistening, broad bands of yellow, alternating with black (**Fig. 11.14**). These alternating bands encircle the body and are almost equal in width.

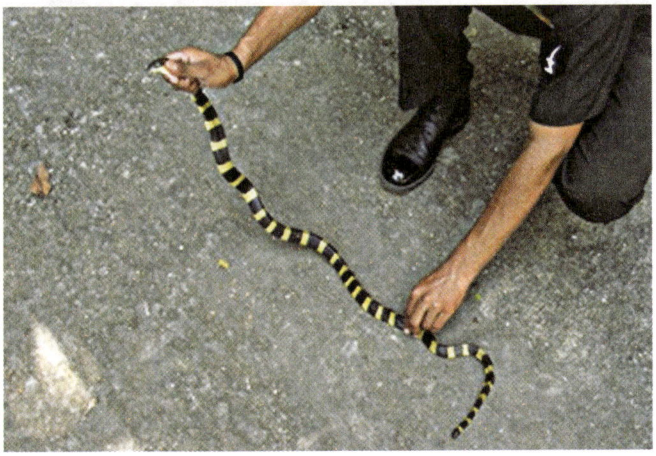

Fig. 11.14 Banded krait (*Bungarus fasciatus*) captured in Binnaguri, North Bengal, India (*Courtesy*: AshLin)

- It is a large snake averaging 5 ft in length. It has a triangular body cross-section due to the marked vertebral ridge consisting of enlarged vertebral shields along its body.

Nature of Venom

Predominantly **neurotoxic**.

Pit Vipers

The Crotalinae, commonly known as **pit vipers**, **crotaline snakes** or **pit adders**, are a subfamily of venomous vipers found in Eurasia and America. They are distinguished by the presence of a heat-sensing pit organ located between the eye and the nostril on either side of the head.

There are two kinds of Indian pit vipers:

1. **Pit Vipers with small head scales**:
   a. **Common Green Pit Viper**: It is also referred to as the **bamboo pit viper** or **Indian green pit viper**, and its scientific name is *Trimeresurus gramineus*. It is the commonest of the pit vipers, and is found in most of the hilly regions of Southern India. It is vivid green or yellow in colour (**Fig. 11.15**) with a whitish or yellowish line on each flank. Length varies from 2 to 3 feet or more. As the name suggests, it prefers to reside among bamboo trees.

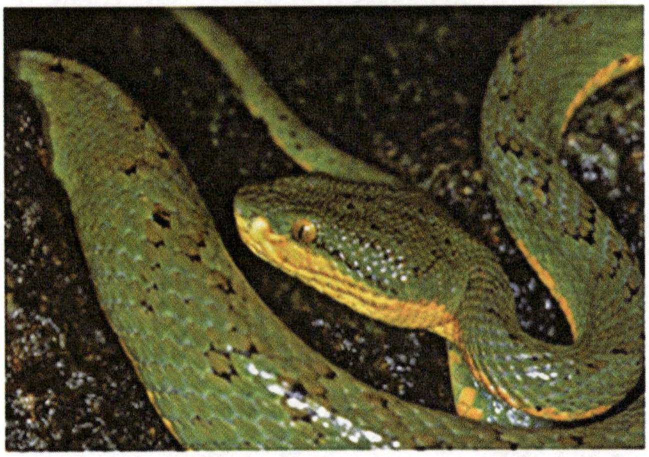

Fig. 11.15 Common green pit viper (*Trimeresurus gramineus*) (*Courtesy*: Thomas Brown)

   b. **Mountain Pit Viper**: The scientific name of this snake is *Ovophis monticola*. It is encountered in Assam, Sikkim, Mizoram and Nagaland, and is brownish in colour, growing up to 3 feet in length (**Fig. 11.16**).
   c. **South Indian Pit Vipers**: The **horse-shoe viper** (*Trimeresurus strigatus*) is encountered in the Western Ghats and the Nilgiris, while the **Malabar pit viper** (*Trimeresurus malabaricus*) (**Fig. 11.17**) is found in southern and western India, including the Western Ghats.
2. **Pit Vipers with shields on the head**:
   a. **Himalayan Pit Viper** (*Gloydius himalayanus*): This is the commonest pit viper in the Himalayan region and Kashmir (**Fig. 11.18**). Bites from this species result in intense local pain and swelling, which usually subsides within 2–3 days, even without treatment.

Pillay – Textbook of Forensic Medicine & Toxicology

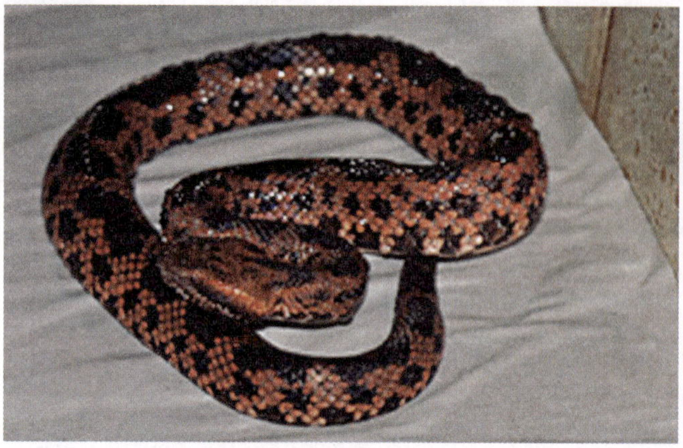

Fig. 11.16 Mountain pit viper (*Ovophis monticola*) (*Courtesy*: *Zhimin Wang*)

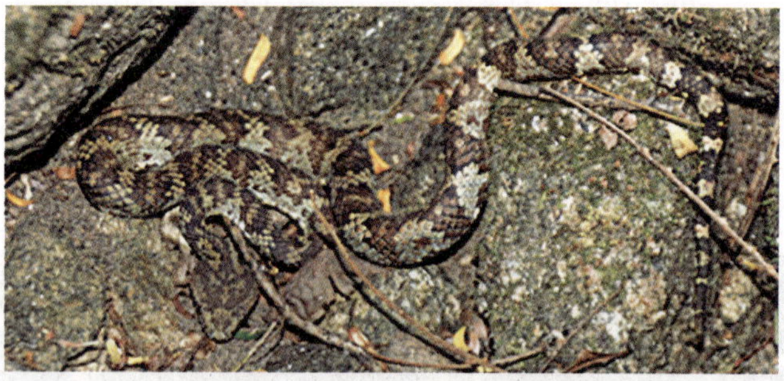

Fig. 11.17 Malabar pit viper (*Trimeresurus malabaricus*) (*Courtesy*: *K Shaji Kumar/Dr Jaideep C Menon*)

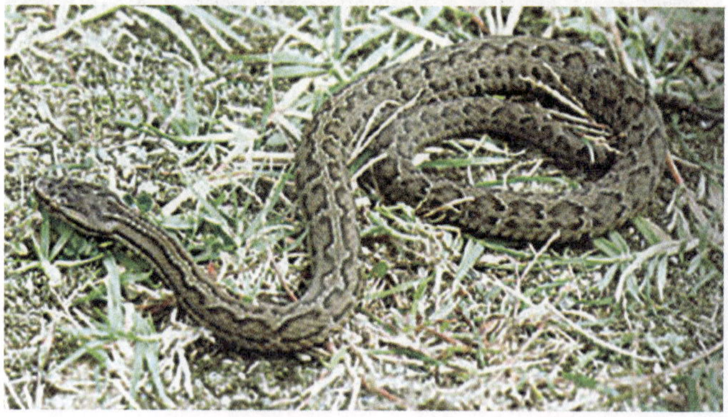

Fig. 11.18 Himalayan pit viper (*Gloydius himalayanus*) (*Courtesy*: *Steven Gilbert*)

b. **Hump-nosed Pit Viper** (*Hypnale hypnale*): This snake is also referred to as **Merrem's hump-nosed viper**. It is called 'Churutta' in Malayalam and is quite common in Kerala, aside from other hilly regions of South India. *H. hypnale* is found in dense jungle and coffee plantations in hilly areas. It grows to an average of 30–45 cm length. The snout is pointed and turned upwards, ending in a hump (hence the name) (**Fig. 11.19**). The colour pattern is greyish with heavy brown mottling, overlaid with a double row of large dark spots. Bites from *H. hypnale*, although previously thought to be innocuous, are now known to cause serious complications such as coagulopathy and acute renal failure (ARF).

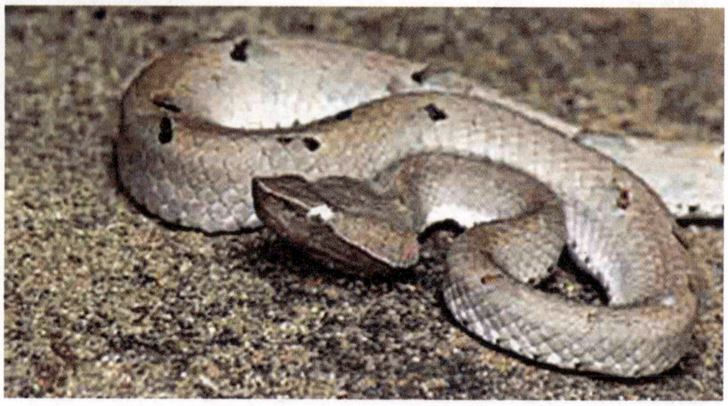

Fig. 11.19 Hump nosed pit viper (*Hypnale hypnale*), Agastyavanam Biosphere Reserve, Thiruvananthapuram, Kerala

The venom of pit vipers is predominantly **vasculo- and haemotoxic**, though **neurotoxic features** are also quite common.

Sea Snakes

Sea snakes comprise more than 60 species of highly venomous marine snakes of family Elapidae. There are two independently evolved groups: the **true sea snakes** (subfamily: Hydrophiinae), which are related to Australian terrestrial elapids, and the **sea kraits** (subfamily: Laticaudinae) (**Fig. 11.20**), which are related to the Asian cobras. Although their venom is the **most potent of all snakes**, human fatalities are rare because sea snakes are not aggressive, their venom output is small, and their fangs are very short.

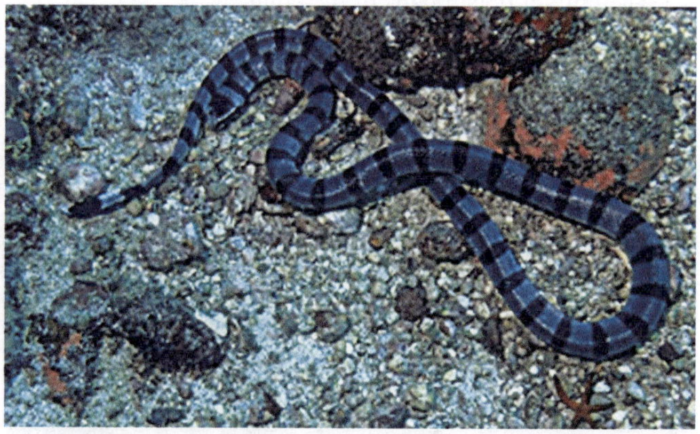

Fig. 11.20 Sea krait

All the Indian seas (Indian Ocean, Bay of Bengal and Arabian Sea) abound in venomous sea snakes which are characterized by their **flattened, paddle shaped tails** (**Fig. 11.21**). Apart from the paddle shaped tail, these snakes can be distinguished by the nostrils which (unlike in land snakes) are situated on the top of the snout. This enables them to breathe while in water. The venom of sea snakes is predominantly **myotoxic**.

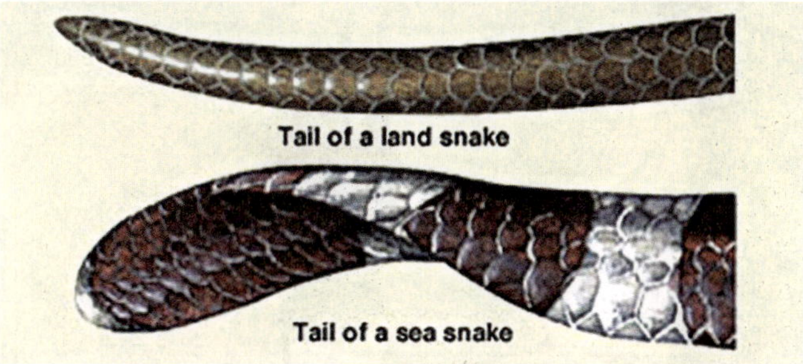

Fig. 11.21 Comparison between the tail of land snake with sea snake

SNAKE VENOM

- Snake venom is the **toxic saliva** secreted by modified parotid glands, and is a clear, amber-coloured fluid when fresh.
- It is a complex poison, containing more than 20 components. Most of the dry weight of venom is constituted by protein, comprising a variety of enzymes and polypeptides. Non-protein ingredients of venom include carbohydrates and metals (in the form of glycoprotein metalloprotein enzymes), lipids and amino acids.
- The lethal fractions of snake venom are peptides and proteins of relatively low-molecular weight (6000–30,000). About 90% of viperid and 25–65% of elapid venom consists of enzymes such as hydrolases and elements which generate or inhibit a physiological process. In addition, most venom contains phospholipase A_2, L-amino acid oxidase and peptidases. Viper venoms also contain enzymes which activate prothrombin and Factor X. Polypeptide toxins (neurotoxins) are found mainly in elapid and hydrophid venoms.
- Snake toxins vary greatly in their functions. Two broad classes of toxins found in snake venoms are **neurotoxins** (mostly found in **elapids**) and **haemotoxins** (mostly found in **viperids**).
- Hyaluronidase may serve to promote the spread of venom through tissues. Proteolytic enzymes (hydrolases) may be responsible for local changes in vascular permeability leading to oedema, blistering, and bruising, and to necrosis. Biological amines such as histamine and 5-hydroxytryptamine may contribute to local pain and permeability changes at the site of a snakebite.
- Since snake venom is mostly comprised of protein, it is not surprising that anaphylactic shock can be induced, if a person is bitten by the same species of snake a second time, after a variable interval following upon the first bite. Some data connected with venoms of common Indian snakes are mentioned in **Table 11.3**.

SNAKEBITE

Epidemiology

- Estimates put the number of snakebites at 1.2–5.5 million snakebites globally, around 1.8 million envenomings, and 70,000–94,000 deaths.
- Most snake envenomings and fatalities occur in Asia and Africa, with India reporting the most snakebite deaths of any country (around 25,000–50,000 annually).
- On the Indian subcontinent, almost all snakebite deaths have traditionally been attributed to the **Big Four**, consisting of the Russell's viper, Indian cobra, saw-scaled viper, and the common krait. However, studies have shown that the hump-nosed viper, and other pit vipers, as well as banded krait are other species involved in a significant number of venomous bites.

Clinical Features

Non-Venomous Snakebite

- A significant proportion of snakebites is said to be due to non-venomous snakes. Since the question of envenomation does not arise in such cases, systemic manifestations are non-existent, except those due to psychological shock.
- As a result of the fear and apprehension associated with snakes, every bite (venomous or otherwise) is attended by some degree of shock characterized by giddiness, syncope, sweating, palpitation, tachycardia and hypotension.
- Consequent upon reassurance especially by a doctor, about the non-venomous nature of the bite, these symptoms usually resolve rapidly.

Venomous Snakebite

1. ***Without Envenomation***:
   a. It is well known that even when a highly venomous snake bites a human, serious envenomation may not occur. In fact, it has been suggested that 20–50% of venomous bites are not attended with serious toxicity.
   b. Reasons for lack of envenomation in venomous bites include the following:
      - **Dry bite**: A snake does not always inject venom at the time of biting.
      - **Protective gear**: Envenomation may not occur in the case of bites inflicted on shod feet or heavily clothed parts.

Table 11.3 Toxicity of common Indian snake venoms

Species	Approximate yield of dry venom (*mg*)	Intravenous LD 50 (*mg/kg*)
Common cobra	170–325	0.4
Common krait	8–20	0.09
Russell's viper	130–250	0.08
Saw-scaled viper	20–35	2.3
Pit viper	40–60	6.2

- **Leakage of venom**: Head-on bites often result in efficient injection of venom, while sideswipes may cause some (or all) of the venom to escape outside the bitesite.
- **Superficial bite**: Since humans do not constitute normal prey for most venomous snakes, they bite only to defend themselves before making a quick get-away. In such instances, the snake often deliberately does not bite deeply, but instead only strikes superficially, thereby conserving precious venom for its genuine prey.

2. ***With Envenomation***:
   a. **Colubrid bite**:
      - Clinical effects of colubrid snakebite are generally localized, and comprise pain, oedema, erythema, ecchymosis and numbness, which resolve over 1–2 weeks.
      - Occasionally, there may be systemic effects involving other organ systems.

   b. **Elapid bite**:
      - *Local Effects*: In general, elapid bites are associated with minimal local manifestations (**Fig. 11.22**). Pain and swelling are relatively less intense, and often there is only a serosanguinous ooze from the bitesite with mild pain, tenderness and blistering. However, cobras can occasionally cause significant local swelling, blistering and regional lymphadenopathy. The lesion may emit a putrid smell, and break down with loss of skin and subcutaneous tissue (**Fig. 11.23**). Elapid bites sometimes cause early onset of gangrene (of the wet type), while viperid bites progress more slowly, and the gangrene is usually of dry type. Secondary infections, e.g., tetanus, gas gangrene, etc., are relatively less common.
      - *Systemic Effects*: Neurotoxicity is the dominant clinical feature of elapid bites. Symptoms usually occur earlier (within 15 min to ½ hr) in cobra bite, while they are often delayed (up to several hours) in krait bite.

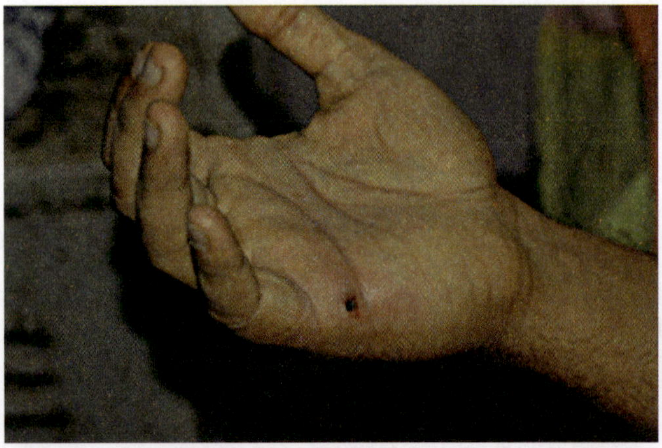

Fig. 11.22 Cobra bite – Minimal local effects (*Courtesy*: *Dr HS Bawaskar*)

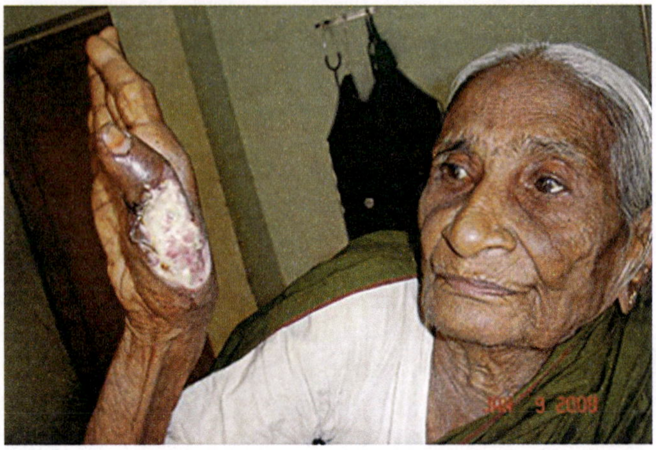

Fig. 11.23 Cobra bite – Local necrosis (*Courtesy*: *Dr DRK Prasad*)

i. Preparalytic Stage:
   - Vomiting
   - Ptosis (preceded by contraction of frontalis muscle) (**Fig. 11.24**)
   - Blurred vision, external ophthalmoplegia
   - Paraesthesiae around the mouth
   - Hyperacusis
   - Headache, myalgia
   - Vertigo
   - Hypersalivation (due to autonomic stimulation).

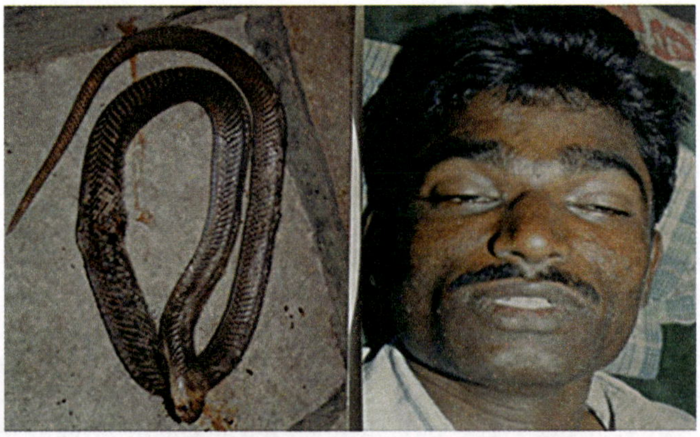

Fig. 11.24 Cobra bite – Ptosis (killed snake on the left) (*Courtesy*: *Dr HS Bawaskar*)

ii. Paralytic Stage:
   - The facial muscles, palate, jaws, tongue, vocal cords, neck muscles and muscles of deglutition all become progressively flaccidly paralysed. Many patients find it difficult to open their mouths and speak.
   - Respiratory arrest may occur due to obstruction of upper airway by the paralysed tongue or inhaled vomitus, or due to paralysis of intercostal muscles and diaphragm. Paradoxi-

cal respiration, as a result of the intercostal muscles becoming paralysed is said to be a frequent sign.

- Although a patient appears unconscious, most are able to follow simple commands as noted by purposeful movement of the fingers or toes. Loss of consciousness and convulsions are terminal phenomena resulting from hypoxaemia.
- Local pain and swelling develops within 2–3 hrs and becomes maximal in 24–48 hrs. Blisters and skin discolouration may develop, and may be followed by necrosis of subcutaneous tissue with sloughing.
- Renal complications are rare in elapid bites.

c. **Viperid bite**:

- *Local Effects:*
  i. Vipers cause marked local manifestations which develop rapidly, usually within ½ hr, but may occasionally be delayed for several hours.
  ii. Swelling first appears around the bitesite, and then spreads quickly to involve the whole limb (**Fig. 11.25**) and adjacent trunk. There is associated pain, tenderness and regional lymphadenopathy. Bruising is commonly seen over the path of superficial lymphatics and over regional lymph nodes. Persistent bleeding from bitesite is a constant feature.
  iii. Blisters begin to appear in about 12 hrs in and around the bitesite, progressing subsequently to involve the entire limb. They may contain either clear or bloodstained fluid. Extensive necrosis of skin, subcutaneous tissues and muscles may occur.
  iv. Raised intracompartmental pressure adds to the problem in regions with tight fascial compartments such as anterior tibial compartment. This is characterized by severe pain, tense swelling, subcutaneous anaesthesia and increased pain on stretching intracompartmental muscles.

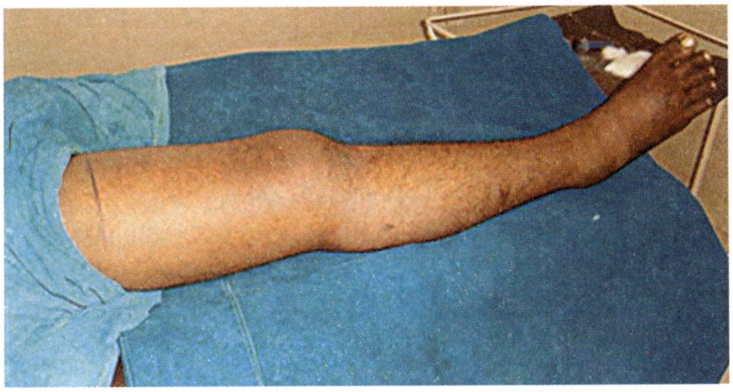

Fig. 11.25 Viper bite – Extensive swelling of lower limb (*Courtesy: Dr DRK Prasad*)

- *Systemic Effects:*
  i. Haemostatic abnormalities are very characteristic of viperid bites. The first evidence of this is persistent bleeding from the bitesite. Haematuria may be seen within a few hours of the bite (**Fig. 11.26**). Later gingival bleeding occurs (**Fig. 11.27**), followed by epistaxis, haemoptysis (relatively rare), haematemesis (**Fig. 11.28**), ecchymoses, intracranial and sub-conjuctival haemorrhages, and bleeding into the floor of the mouth, tympanic membrane, gastrointestinal tract and genitourinary tract. Bleeding into anterior pituitary (causing a Sheehan-like syndrome) has been reported. Subarachnoid haemorrhage manifests as severe headache and meningism, while intracerebral haemorrhage may cause hemiplegia, loss of consciousness and convulsions. Retroperitoneal and intraperitoneal haemorrhages cause abdomi-

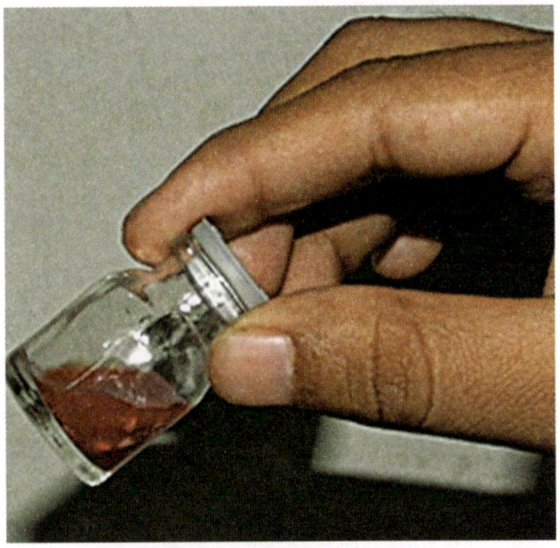

Fig. 11.26 Viper bite – Haematuria (*Courtesy: Dr HS Bawaskar*)

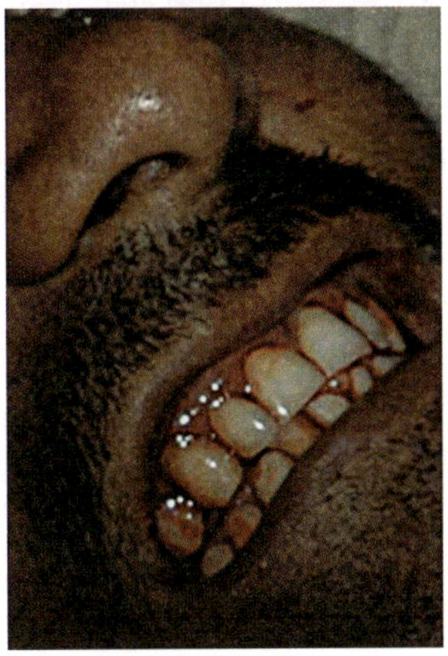

Fig. 11.27 Viper bite – Gingival bleeding (*Courtesy: Dr HS Bawaskar*)

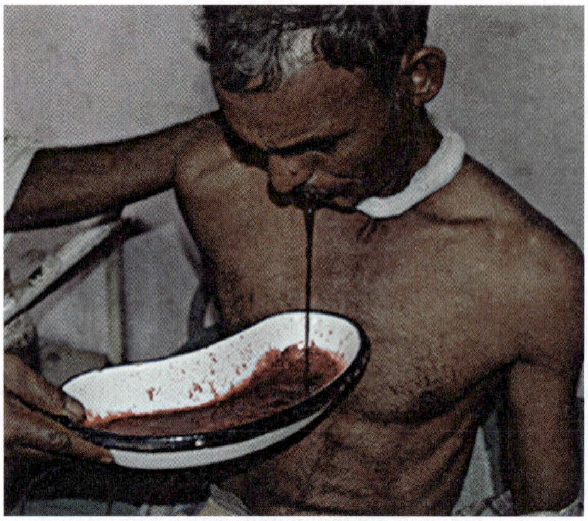

Fig. 11.28 Viper bite – Haematemesis (*Courtesy*: *Dr HS Bawaskar*)

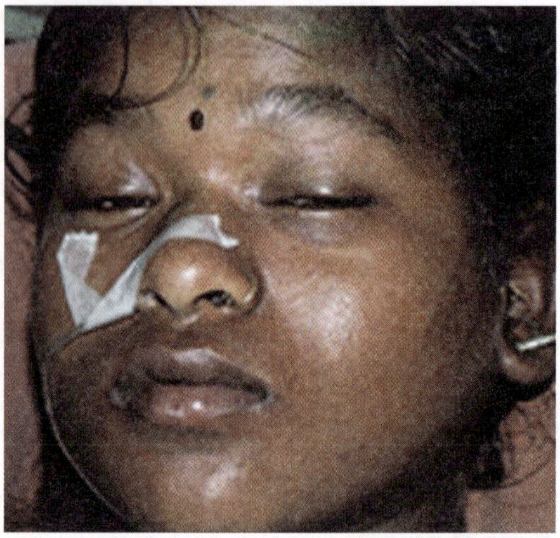

Fig. 11.29 Ptosis in Russell's viper bite (*Courtesy*: *Dr HS Bawaskar*)

nal distension, tenderness and peritonism, with signs of haemorrhagic shock.

ii. Viperid envenomation is almost synonymous with incoagulable blood, which results from defibrination. Intravascular haemolysis causing haemoglobinuria and renal failure is a frequent occurrence, especially in bites by Russell's viper. Acute renal failure is often associated with the presence of DIC which results in severe renal tubular and cortical necrosis with widespread microvascular fibrin deposition (microthrombi). The hump-nosed pit viper can also cause renal failure, but the saw-scaled viper usually does not.

iii. Hypotension is an important manifestation in all viper bites and is usually accompanied by tachycardia, unless the venom has affected the heart directly or reflexly, in which case the pulse may be slow or irregular.

iv. Cardiotoxicity (which may be seen in elapid bite also) produces a wide variety of ECG changes, including bradycardia with ST segment elevation or depression, T wave inversion, QT prolongation and changes due to hyperkalaemia, etc. Myocardial infarction has been reported.

v. It is important to note that ptosis and neurological symptoms may occur in the case of Russell's viper bite, and every clinician must be alert to this possibility. They can include drowsiness, paraesthesiae, abnormalities of taste and smell, ptosis (**Fig. 11.29**), external ophthalmoplegia, paralysis of facial muscles and other muscles innervated by the cranial nerves, etc. Conversely however, kraits and cobras **do not** cause coagulation abnormalities.

b. **Hydrophid bite**:

- *Local Effects*:
  i. Sea snakebites are well known to produce minimal local effects. The bite itself is often painless and the victim may not even realize he has been bitten. However, teeth are often left behind in the wound.
  ii. Local swelling is negligible, and regional lymphadenitis usually does not occur.
  iii. Fang marks may appear as one, two or more small circular dots, as though made by a pin or hypodermic needle.
- *Systemic Effects*:
  i. The dominant clinical feature is myalgia with stiffness and tenderness of muscles, which become apparent in ½ hr to 2 hrs. This is due to rhabdomyolysis, since hydrophid venom is predominantly myotoxic. Myoglobinaemia and myoglobinuria occur, resulting in acute tubular necrosis and renal failure.
  ii. Trismus is an early feature. Passive stretching of muscles is painful. Later, flaccid paralysis develops, beginning with ptosis (as in elapid bite).
  iii. Hyperkalaemia may be present due to release of potassium from damaged muscles. This may be severe enough to cause cardiac arrest. Tall, peaked T-waves and QRS prolongation suggest severe hyperkalaemia.
  iv. Neurotoxicity may include ptosis, ophthalmoplegia, dysarthria, blurred or double vision, mydriasis, inability to sit unassisted, depressed muscle stretch reflexes and flaccid paralysis.

Syndromic Approach to Snakebite

There are **5 syndromes** with regard to snakebite in the South East Asian Region (which includes India):

Syndrome 1:

- Local envenoming (swelling, etc.) with bleeding/clotting disturbances = All vipers.

Syndrome 2:

- Local envenoming (swelling, etc.)
  - With bleeding/clotting disturbances, shock or acute kidney injury = Russell's viper (hump-nosed pit viper in South India).
  - With ptosis, external ophthalmoplegia, facial paralysis etc., and dark brown urine = Russell's viper.

Syndrome 3:

- Local envenoming (swelling, etc.) with paralysis = Cobra or King cobra.

Syndrome 4:

- Paralysis with minimal or no local envenoming:
  - Bitten on land while sleeping on the ground = Krait.
  - Bitten in the sea = Sea snake.

Syndrome 5:

- Paralysis with dark brown urine and acute kidney injury:
  - Bitten on land (with bleeding/clotting disturbance) = Russell's viper.
  - Bitten on land while sleeping indoors = Krait.
  - Bitten in sea (no bleeding/clotting disturbances) = Sea snake.

Diagnosis of Snakebite

1. ***Fang Marks***: Classically, there should be two puncture wounds which are separated from each other by a distance varying from 8 mm to 4 cm, depending on the species involved (**Fig. 11.30**). However, a sideswipe may produce only a single puncture, while multiple bites could result in numerous fang marks.
2. ***Identification of Snake***: The method of identifying a venomous snake has been detailed in earlier sections (*page no. 560*). This can be attempted in those cases where the victim or his attendants bring with them the culprit (dead) snake. Extreme caution is imperative in this context: there are instances on record of killed snakes inflicting reflex bites on being handled! Even a completely severed head is not always innocuous in this regard.

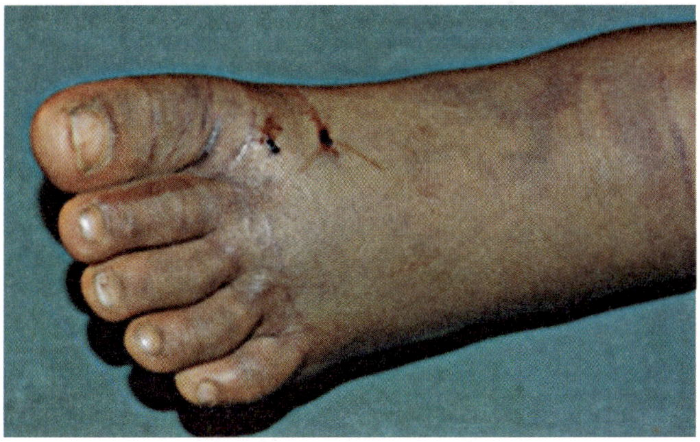

Fig. 11.30 Fang marks in viper bite (*Courtesy*: *Dr HS Bawaskar*)

3. ***Laboratory Investigations***:
   a. *Haematological* (mostly in vipers):
      i. WBC count: An early neutrophil leucocytosis is evidence of systemic envenoming from any species.
      ii. Thrombocytopenia in vipers.
      iii. Haematocrit: A transient increase indicates haemoconcentration resulting from a generalized increase in capillary permeability (e.g., in Russell's viper bite). More often, there is a decrease, reflecting blood loss or, in the case of Russell's viper bite, intravascular haemolysis.
      iv. Evidence of haemolysis: Fragmented RBC (schistocytes or helmet cells)
      v. Prolonged clotting time and prothrombin time
      vi. Prolonged partial thromboplastin time
      vii. Depressed fibrinogen levels
      viii. Elevated FDP (Fibrin degradation products)
      ix. **20-min whole blood clotting test (20WBCT)**: This very useful and informative bedside test requires very little skill and only one piece of apparatus – a new, clean, dry, glass vessel (tube or bottle).
         - Place 2 mL of freshly sampled venous blood in a small, new or heat cleaned, dry, glass vessel.
         - Leave undisturbed for 20 min at ambient temperature.
         - Tip the vessel once.
         - If the blood is still liquid (unclotted) and runs out, the patient has hypofibrinogenaemia ("incoagulable blood") as a result of venom-induced consumption coagulopathy.
         - In the South-East Asia region (including India), incoagulable blood is diagnostic of a viper bite and rules out an elapid bite.
         - If the vessel used for the test is not made of ordinary glass, or if it has been cleaned with detergent, its wall may not stimulate clotting of the blood sample (surface activation of factor XI – Hageman factor), and the test will be invalid.
         - If there is any doubt, repeat the test in duplicate, including a "control" (blood from a healthy person such as a relative).

   b. *ECG:* Common ECG changes include bradycardia with ST segment elevation or depression, T wave inversion, QT prolongation and changes due to hyperkalaemia.
   c. *Aminotransferases and muscle enzymes (creatine kinase, aldolase, etc.)* will be elevated, if there is severe local muscle damage or, particularly, if there is generalized muscle damage (sea snake, krait, Russell's viper bites). Potassium, creatinine, urea or blood urea nitrogen levels are raised in the renal failure of Russell's viper, hump-nosed viper bites and sea snakebites. Early hyperkalaemia may be seen following extensive rhabdomyolysis in sea snake-bites.

d. *Arterial blood gases* and *pH* may show evidence of respiratory failure (neurotoxic envenoming) and acidaemia (respiratory or metabolic acidosis).*

e. *Metabolic*:
   i. Hyperkalaemia
   ii. Hypoxaemia with respiratory acidosis
   iii. Metabolic acidosis or lactic acidosis (increased anion gap)

f. *Urine*: The colour of the urine (pink, red, brown, black) should be noted and the urine should be tested by dipsticks for blood or haemoglobin or myoglobin. Microscopy will confirm whether there are erythrocytes in the urine. Red cell casts indicate glomerular bleeding. Massive proteinuria is an early sign of the generalized increase in capillary permeability in Russell's viper envenoming and an early indicator of acute kidney injury.

g. *Renal*: In acute renal failure, all features of azotaemia will be present.

h. *Chest X-ray*:
   i. Pulmonary oedema
   ii. Intrapulmonary haemorrhages
   iii. Pleural effusion

i. *Immunodiagnosis*: Immunological detection of venom antigens in body fluids can be accomplished by ELISA. This is highly sensitive, but specificity may be inadequate to distinguish between different species of snakes.

Treatment of Snakebite

I. *First-Aid Measures*

1. ***Verbal reassurance***: Since most snakebites are either non-venomous or non-lethal, it is imperative to allay the anxiety that is inevitably experienced by a bitten victim, which can prove fatal (neurogenic shock).
2. ***Immobilization***: Since exertion can enhance systemic absorption of venom, there is universal consensus that the patient should be put at rest, and the bitten extremity immobilized by using a splint or sling. If available, firm binding of the splint with a crepe bandage is an effective form of immobilization (***Sutherland wrap***) (**Fig. 11.31**). However, while this may be true, in practice, it is difficult to judge how tightly to apply the crepe bandage, difficult for the patient to apply it by himself, and apprehensions have been raised about accentuation of locally necrotic effects of some snake venoms.
3. ***Immediate transportation to hospital***: A stretcher, bicycle, motorbike, cart, horse, motor vehicle, train or boat should be used, or the patient can be carried (e.g., using the "fireman's lift" method). If possible, patients should be placed in the recovery position, in case they vomit.

Snake-bite First Aid: Pressure Immobilization Method for Bites on the leg

Note: Do not attempt to remove pants as the movement will assist the venom to travel and enter the blood stream. If the pants are too tight to be rolled up, apply bandage over the pants. Keep the person as calm as possible.

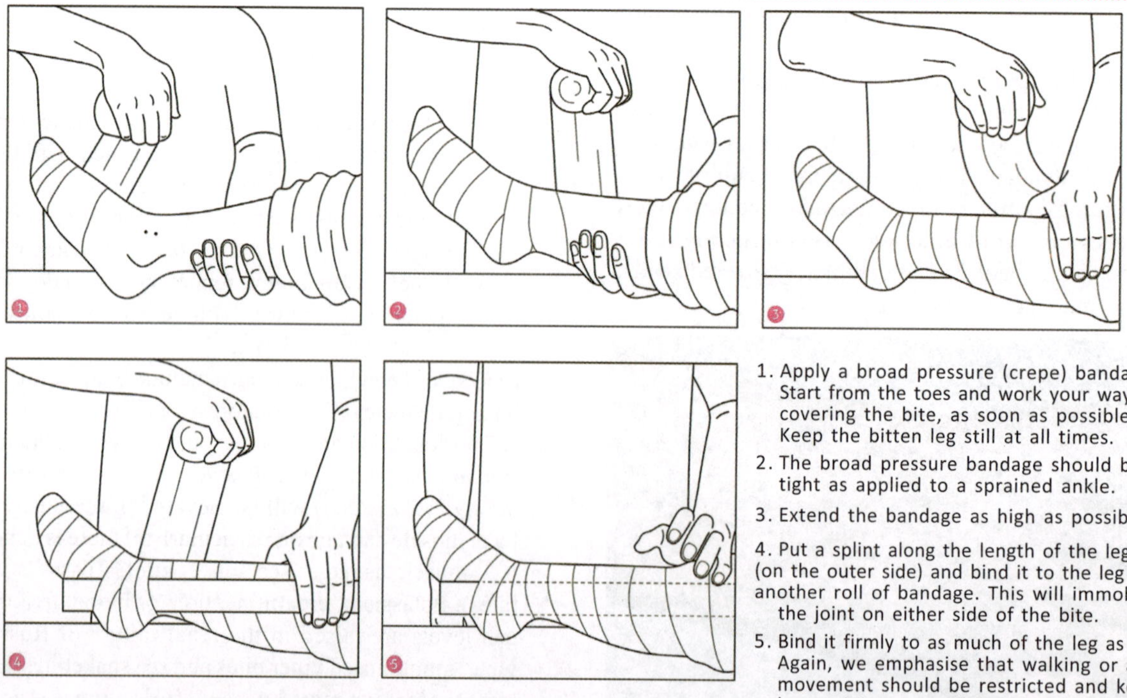

1. Apply a broad pressure (crepe) bandage. Start from the toes and work your way up covering the bite, as soon as possible. Keep the bitten leg still at all times.
2. The broad pressure bandage should be as tight as applied to a sprained ankle.
3. Extend the bandage as high as possible.
4. Put a splint along the length of the leg (on the outer side) and bind it to the leg using another roll of bandage. This will immobilse the joint on either side of the bite.
5. Bind it firmly to as much of the leg as possible. Again, we emphasise that walking or any movement should be restricted and kept to a bare minimum at all times.

Fig. 11.31 Method of application of Sutherland wrap

**Note*: *Arterial puncture is contraindicated in patients with haemostatic abnormalities (Viperidae).*

4. ***Beverages***: Use of "stimulating" beverages such as coffee is **inadvisable and ineffective**. In some cases, it can provoke vomiting, the tendency for which is usually present in the early hours following a bite. Alcohol must never be administered, since it increases the absorption of venom.
5. ***Tourniquet***: It is well known that systemic absorption of venom occurs mainly through superficial lymphatics, and therefore application of a tourniquet proximal to the bitesite of a bitten limb in order to prevent the spread has often been advocated. But, there are serious risks associated with tourniquets and other similar occlusive methods, which include ischaemia and gangrene (**Fig. 11.32**), damage to peripheral nerves (especially lateral popliteal nerve), increased fibrinolytic activity, congestion, swelling, increased bleeding and increased local effect of venom. It has also been claimed that subsequent release of a tourniquet which has been retained for some time, leads to a flooding of accumulated venom from the bitesite into the systemic circulation with life threatening consequences. Because of the dangers associated with it, the **general consensus is against application of a tourniquet**. If it is decided to be done, a wide constricting band loosely applied to limit lymphatic, but not venous flow may be placed a few inches proximal to the bite. It should be possible to insert a finger easily between the band and the skin. Before removing, it is better to start antivenom therapy.
6. **Incision and suction**: While there have been staunch advocates especially in the past, **the current view is generally against such a practice**. Most investigators are of the opinion that such a procedure can remove only about 20% of injected venom at the most. This is compounded by the serious risks associated with it, including uncontrolled bleeding in patients with incoagulable blood (viper bite), damage to nerves, blood vessels and tendons, and introduction of infection.

   Today, most authorities strongly condemn incision and suction as useless and hazardous.
7. **Cyrotherapy**: Local cooling (application of ice) in the region of the bitesite was previously recommended for minimizing the absorption of venom. Today, this is universally **condemned** because of serious risk of necrosis leading to gangrene, which may even necessitate amputation.
8. **Electric shock**: It has been suggested that if snake antivenom is not available to treat a venomous bite, local electric treatment may be done which is claimed to be life saving. The electric shock (25 kV, 1 mA) is to be applied direct to the bite by means of an insulated probe for a couple of seconds, and repeated 4–5 times at 5–10-sec intervals, taking care to ground the area as closely to the site of the bite as possible. However, the actual efficacy of this method has never been proved and it is **not recommended** any more.
9. **Drugs**:
   a. For mild to moderate pain, paracetamol can be given.

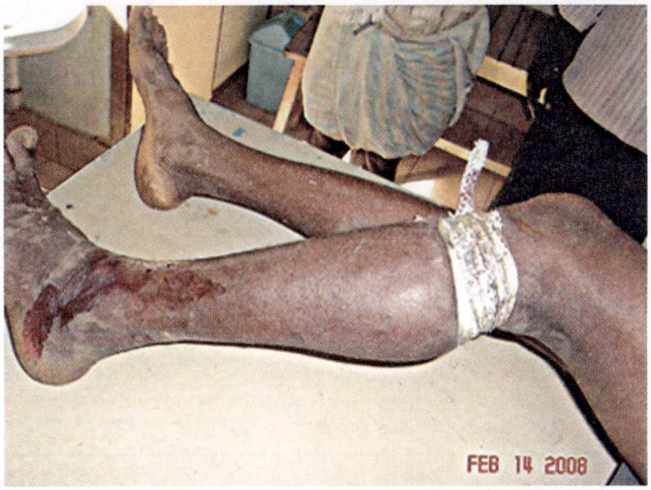

Fig. 11.32 Tight tourniquet leading to swelling & ischaemia of lower limb (*Courtesy*: *Dr DRK Prasad*)

   b. If pain is severe, several authorities recommend judicious use of narcotic analgesics such as pentazocine or pethidine, even though in some cases this can be hazardous, e.g., elapid bites, where there may be CNS depression.
   c. **Aspirin and non-steriodal anti-inflammatory drugs must not be used**, since they commonly cause gastric erosions, and could lead to persistent gastric bleeding in patients with incoagulable blood, as in the case of viper bites.
   d. Use of corticosteriods which were formerly administered routinely, is no longer advocated except in allergic reactions to antivenom. The same applies to antihistamines.
   e. Since vomiting is a common early symptom of systemic envenoming, patients should be made to lie on their side with the head down to avoid aspiration. Persistent vomiting can be treated with intravenous chlorpromazine. Intramuscular and subcutaneous injections should be avoided, especially in patients with incoagulable blood, since they can lead to haematoma formation. Pressure dressings should be applied to venepuncture sites to prevent oozing.
   f. While some authorities recommend prophylactic antibiotics to prevent infection, others denounce this as unnecessary. It is however a fact that the mouths of most snakes harbour various aerobic and anaerobic bacteria. Though *Clostridium tetani* has not been isolated, its ubiquitous nature prompts most authorities to emphasise the importance of **tetanus prophylaxis** in the form of tetanus toxoid. If the patient has not been previously immunized, tetanus antiserum or tetanus human globulin must be given.

Table 11.4 lists the so-called "first-aid measures" which are harmful, and must never be undertaken.

II. *Hospital Measures*

1. **Observe every case of alleged snakebite for a minimum period of 24 hrs**.

Table 11.4 How Not to Treat Snakebite

The following measures are potentially harmful, and must NOT be undertaken:
▪ Application of a tight tourniquet which occludes arterial supply.
▪ Cauterisation of bitesite.
▪ Multiple, deep incisions through bitesite.
▪ Making pricks/punctures ("tattooing").
▪ Suction by mouth, vacuum pump or syringe.
▪ Application of injurious substances such as potassium permanganate, phenol, etc.
▪ Application of electric shock.
▪ Application of ice (cryotherapy).
▪ Use of herbal, folk or Ayurvedic medicines or remedies.
▪ Use of (black) snake stones.

2. **Check for/monitor the following**:
   a. Pulse rate, respiratory rate, blood pressure and WBC count every hour.
   b. Blood urea, creatinine.
   c. Urine output.
   d. Vomiting, diarrhoea.
   e. Abnormal bleeds: Examine the skin and mucous membranes for evidence of petechiae, purpura, ecchymoses and, in the conjunctivae, for haemorrhages and chemosis. Thoroughly examine the gingival sulci, using a torch and tongue depressor, as these may show the earliest evidence of spontaneous systemic bleeding. Examine the nose for epistaxis. Abdominal tenderness may suggest gastrointestinal or retroperitoneal bleeding. Loin (low back) pain and tenderness suggests acute renal ischaemia (Russell's viper bites). Intracranial haemorrhage is suggested by lateralising neurological signs, asymmetrical pupils, convulsions or impaired consciousness (in the absence of respiratory or circulatory failure).
   f. Extent of local swelling* and necrosis
   g. ECG, blood gas analysis.
3. **Antivenom (Antivenin) therapy**:
   a. Never embark on antivenom therapy as a matter of routine. Apart from the risks and adverse effects involved (*vide infra*), such indiscriminate use is irrational because
      i. Many cases of snakebite involve non-venomous snakes.
      ii. Envenomation is not the rule even in venomous bites.
      iii. Antivenoms available are usually effective against specific species of snakes, and are of little or no benefit against other species.
      iv. Antivenom is usually in short supply, and has limited shelf-life.
   b. ***Indications***:
      i. A common early symptom of systemic envenoming is vomiting.
      ii. Bleeding persistently from the fang marks.
      iii. Discoloured urine is often indicative of haematuria. Perform urinalysis immediately.
      iv. Patients who complain of sleepiness, drooping eyelids or blurred or double vision may have neurotoxic envenoming.
      v. Important early symptoms of sea snake envenoming include generalized pain, tenderness and stiffness of muscles, and trismus.
      vi. Check other muscles innervated by the cranial nerves (facial muscles, tongue, gag reflex, etc). The muscles flexing the neck may be paralysed, giving the "**broken neck sign**" (**Fig. 11.33**).

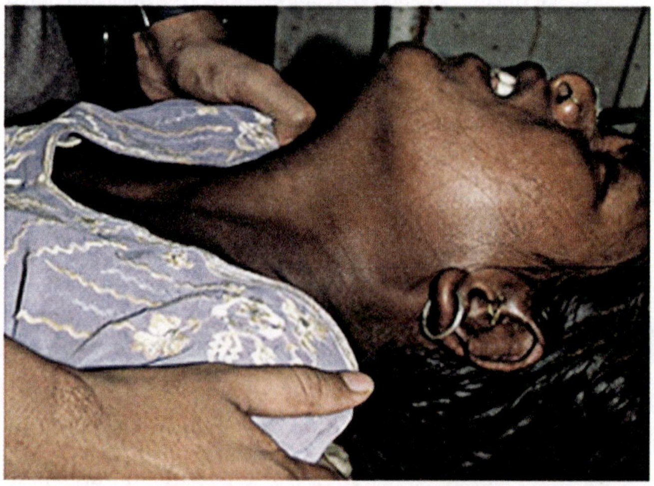

Fig. 11.33 Broken neck sign (*Courtesy*: *Dr HS Bawaskar*)

      vii. Inability of the patient to swallow, or accumulation of secretions in the pharynx, are early signs of bulbar paralysis.
      viii. "Paradoxical respiration" (abdomen expands rather than the chest on attempted inspiration) indicates that the diaphragm is still contracting but that the intercostal muscles and accessory muscles of inspiration are paralysed.
      ix. Objective measurement of ventilatory capacity is very useful. Use a peak flow meter, spirometer (FEV1 and FVC), or ask the patient to blow into the tube of a sphygmomanometer to record the maximum expiratory pressure (in mm Hg).
   c. ***Time of administration of antivenom***:
      i. Antivenom treatment should be given as soon as it is indicated.
      ii. Although antisnake venom must be administered as early as possible when signs of systemic or local envenomation develop, it is almost never too late to try antivenom therapy. Some investigators have reported beneficial effects even after a lapse of several days.

**Note*: *Mark the level of swelling on the skin every 15 min.*

d. ***Availability***:

i. In India, **polyvalent antivenom (Fig. 11.34)** is commonly available which is effective against the Big Four: Common cobra, Common krait, Russell's viper and Saw-scaled viper. It can be procured from:
   - Biological E (Evans) Limited, Hyderabad
   - VINS Bioproducts Ltd, Hyderabad
   - Bharat Serums & Vaccines, Mumbai
   - Serum Institute of India, Pune.
   - Haffkine Corporation, Parel, Mumbai

ii. The best form of antivenom is a lyophilised (freeze-dried) powder, which is produced by immunization of horses with the venom of the snakes mentioned (*vide supra*). The powder must be reconstituted in distilled water or saline just before use. If the resulting solution is opaque to any extent (**Fig. 11.35**), it has lost its efficacy and should be discarded. The antivenom must always be administered intravenously. It should not be injected into the tissues in or around the bitesite.

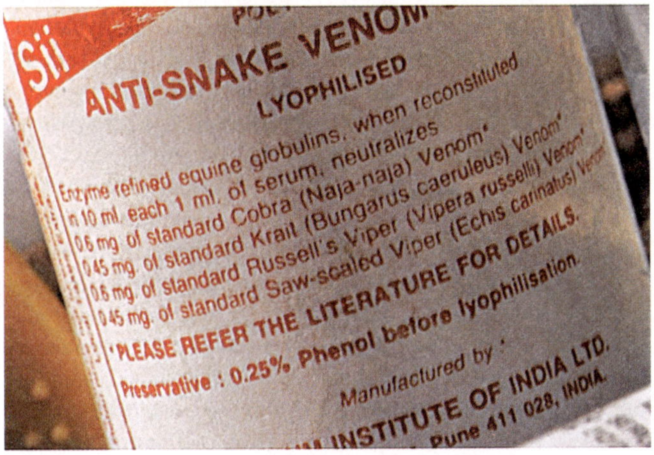

Fig. 11.34 Vial of polyvalent antivenom (*Courtesy: Ashok Captain*)

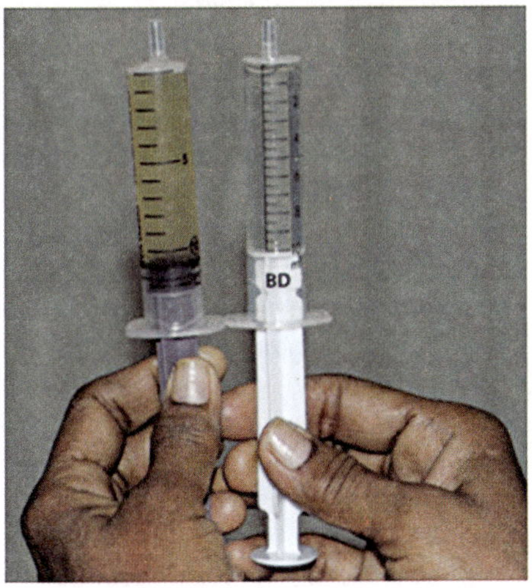

Fig. 11.35 Turbid antivenom, left (*Courtesy: Dr HS Bawaskar*)

e. ***Dose***:

i. Freeze-dried (lyophilized) antivenoms are reconstituted, usually with 10 mL of sterile water for injection per ampoule. Two methods of administration are recommended:
   - *Intravenous "push" injection:* Reconstituted freeze-dried antivenom or neat liquid antivenom is given by slow IV injection (not more than 2 mL/min). This method has the advantage that the doctor or nurse administering the antivenom must remain with the patient during the time when some early reactions may develop. It is also economical, saving the use of intravenous fluids, IV sets, cannulae, etc.
   - *Intravenous infusion*: Reconstituted freeze-dried or neat liquid antivenom is diluted in 5–10 mL of isotonic fluid per kg body weight (i.e., 250–500 mL of isotonic saline or 5% dextrose) and is infused at a constant rate over a period of 1 hr. Snakes inject the same dose of venom into children and adults. Children must therefore be given exactly the same dose of antivenom as adults.

ii. Local administration of antivenom at the site of the bite is not recommended: Although this route may seem rational, it should not be used as it is extremely painful, may increase intracompartmental pressure, and has not been shown to be effective.

iii. Intramuscular injection of antivenom: Antivenoms are large molecules which, after intramuscular injection, are absorbed slowly via lymphatics. Bioavailability is poor, especially after intragluteal injection, and blood levels of antivenom never reach those achieved rapidly by IV administration. Other disadvantages are the pain of injection of large volumes of antivenom and the risk of haematoma formation in patients with haemostatic abnormalities (**Fig. 11.36**).

The only situations in which intramuscular administration might be considered:
   - At a peripheral first aid station, before a patient with obvious envenoming is put in an ambulance for a journey to hospital that may last several hours.
   - On an expedition exploring a remote area very far from medical care.
   - When intravenous access has proved impossible.

Under these unusual circumstances, the dose of antivenom should be divided between a number of sites in the upper anterolateral region of both thighs. A maximum of 5–10 mL should be given at each site by deep intramuscular injection followed by massage to aid absorption. Local bleeding and haematoma formation is a problem in patients with incoagulable blood.

Antivenom should not be injected into the gluteal region (upper outer quadrant of the buttock) as far as possible, as absorption is exceptionally slow and unreliable, and there is always the danger of sciatic nerve damage when the injection is given by an inexperienced operator.

iv. **Recommended initial dosage of antivenom**:
- *Bungarus caeruleus*: 10–20 vials
- *Naja naja*: 10–20 vials
- *Daboia/Vipera russelli*: 10 vials
- *Echis carinatus*: 5 vials

v. **Criteria for giving more antivenom**:
- Persistence or recurrence of blood incoagulability after 6 hrs, or of bleeding after 1–2 hrs: If the blood remains incoagulable (as measured by 20WBCT) 6 hrs after the initial dose of antivenom, the same dose should be repeated. This is based on the observation that, if a large dose of antivenom (more than enough to neutralize the venom procoagulant enzymes) is given initially, the time taken for the liver to restore coagulable levels of fibrinogen and other clotting factors is 3–9 hrs. In patients who continue to bleed briskly, the dose of antivenom should be repeated within 1-2 hrs.
- Deteriorating neurotoxic or cardiovascular signs after 1–2 hrs: the initial dose of antivenom should be repeated after 1–2 hrs, and full supportive treatment must be considered.

f. ***Storage of antivenom*** – Antivenom must be stored in a refrigerator. Lyophilised antivenoms stored at below 8ºC usually retain their activity up to 5 years or more. Reconstituted solutions remain stable up to 48 hrs. Diluted solutions should be used within 12 hrs of dilution.

g. ***Reactions/Adverse effects***:

i. *Early (anaphylactic) reaction*: Usually within 10 min to 3 hrs of starting antivenom, the patient begins to itch (often over the scalp) and develops urticaria, dry cough, fever, nausea, vomiting, abdominal colic, diarrhoea and tachycardia. A minority of these patients may develop severe life-threatening anaphylaxis: hypotension, bronchospasm and angio-oedema.
- In most cases, these reactions are not truly "allergic". They are not IgE-mediated type I hypersensitivity reactions to horse or sheep proteins as there is no evidence of specific IgE, either by skin testing or radioallergosorbent tests (RAST). Complement activation by IgG aggregates or residual Fc fragments or direct stimulation of mast cells or basophils by antivenom protein are more likely mechanisms for these reactions.

ii. *Pyrogenic reaction*: Develops in 1–2 hrs of beginning the therapy. It is characterized by chills, goose fleshing, shivering, fever, sweating, hypotension. Convulsions may occur in children. These reactions are caused by pyrogen contamination during the manufacturing process.

iii. *Late (serum sickness) reaction:* Develops 1–12 days after treatment. Clinical features include fever, nausea, vomiting, diarrhoea, itching, urticaria, arthralgia, myalgia, lymphadenopathy, periarticular swellings, proteinuria and, rarely, encephalopathy.

h. ***Contraindications***:

i. There are no absolute contraindications to antivenom in life-threatening cases of snakebite.

ii. Caution may be exercised in atopic and previously sensitized individuals. These high-risk patients may be pre-treated empirically with subcutaneous adrenaline, IV antihistamines (both anti-H1, such as promethazine or chlorpheniramine; and anti-H2, such as cimetidine or ranitidine) and corticosteroid. In asthmatic patients, prophylactic use of an inhaled adrenergic beta$_2$ agonist such as salbutamol may prevent bronchospasm.

i. ***Treatment of antivenom reactions***:

i. *For anaphylactic and pyrogenic reactions*: Adrenaline is given intramuscularly (into upper lateral thigh) in an initial dose of 0.5 mg for adults and 0.01 mg/kg body weight for children. The dose can be repeated every 5–10 min, if the patient's condition is deteriorating. An antihistamine such as chlorphenamine maleate (adults 10 mg, children 0.2 mg/kg) should also be given followed by intravenous hydrocortisone (adults 100 mg, children 2 mg/kg).

ii. *For late serum sickness reaction*: A 5-day course of oral antihistamine (e.g., chlorpheniramine – 2 mg, 6 hourly). Patients who fail to respond in 24–48 hrs should be given a 5-day course of prednisolone (5 mg, 6 hourly for 5–7 days).

j. ***Prevention of antivenom reactions***:

i. *Prophylactic drugs* (adrenaline, antihistamine anti-H1 blockers, corticosteroids).

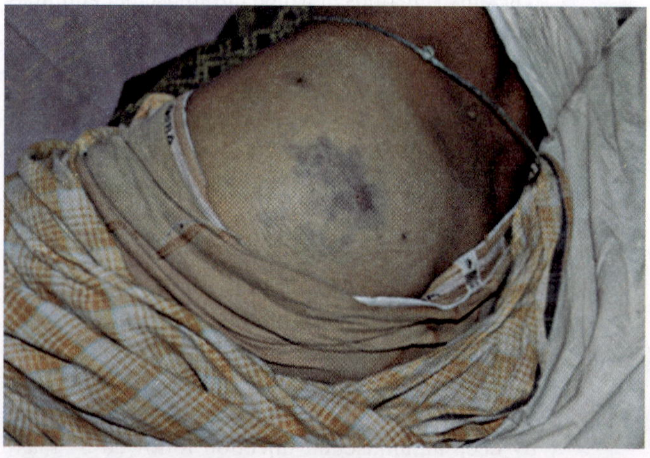

Fig. 11.36 Haematoma over gluteal region – intramuscular injection of antivenom (*Courtesy*: *Dr HS Bawaskar*)

ii. *Speed and dilution of intravenous antivenom administration*: No convincing clinical evidence has yet been published demonstrating that the strategy of slow administration of diluted antivenom reduces the risk of reactions.

4. **Additional Measures**

a. ***Treatment of bitten part***:

i. The bitten limb, which may be painful and swollen, should be nursed in the most comfortable position, but not excessively elevated as this may reduce arterial perfusion pressure in a tensely swollen limb and increase the risk of intra-compartmental ischaemia.

ii. Blisters may be large and tense, but they should be aspirated only if they seem likely to rupture (**Fig. 11.37**).

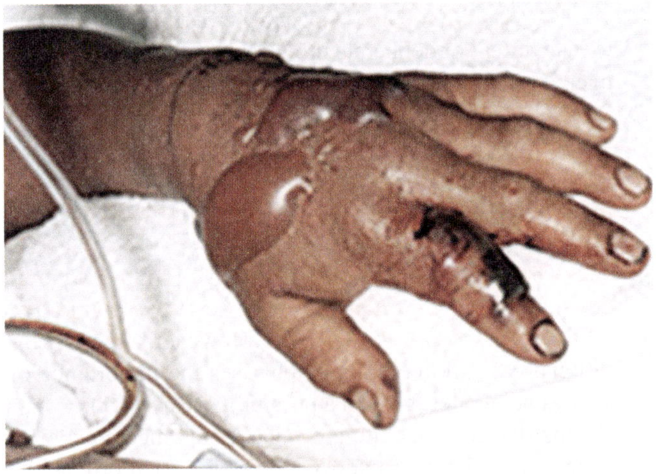

Fig. 11.37 Snakebite with blisters and swelling of limb (*Courtesy: Anders Nielsen*)

iii. Infection at the time of the bite with organisms from the snake's venom and buccal cavity is a problem with some species such as pit vipers, but prophylactic antibiotics may not be effective. Interference with the wound (incisions made with an unsterilised razor, knife, etc.) creates a risk of secondary bacterial infection and justifies the use of immediate broad spectrum antibiotics and tetanus prophylaxis.

b. ***Treatment of intracompartmental syndrome***:

i. The appearance of an immobile, tensely-swollen, cold and apparently pulseless snake-bitten limb may suggest the possibility of increased intracompartmental pressure, especially if the digital pulp spaces or the anterior tibial compartment are involved. Swelling of envenomed muscle within such tight fascial compartments could result in an increase in tissue pressure above the venous pressure, resulting in ischaemia.

ii. The most reliable test is to measure intracompartmental pressure directly through a cannula introduced into the compartment and connected to a pressure transducer or manometer (**Fig. 11.38**). Intracompartmental pressures exceeding 40 mm Hg may carry a risk of ischaemic necrosis. Fasciotomy may be required, but should not be contemplated until haemostatic abnormalities have been corrected, otherwise the patient may bleed to death.

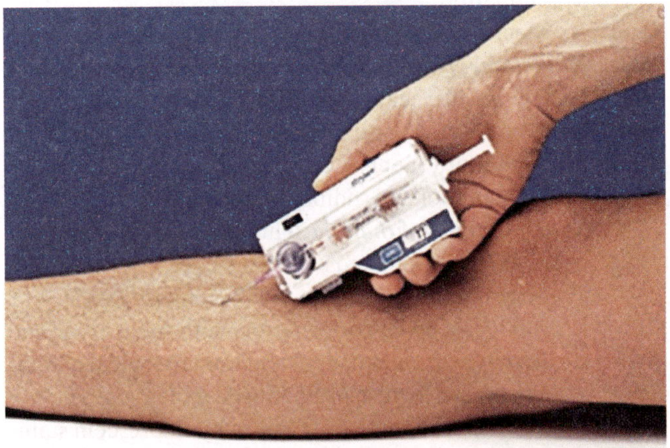

Fig. 11.38 Measuring intracompartmental pressure with Stryker pressure monitor

c. ***Treatment of coagulation abnormalities***: If coagulation abnormalities are not corrected by antivenom therapy it may be necessary to administer fresh whole blood, fresh frozen plasma, cryoprecipitates or platelet concentrates.

d. ***Hypotensive shock***: Much of the time, this can be managed by antivenom therapy. However, treatment with plasma expanders (colloid or crystalloid) may become necessary. Selective vasoconstrictors such as dopamine may be given by intravenous infusion.

e. ***Renal failure***: Most patients with acute renal failure are oliguric, defined as a urine output of less than 400 mL/day or less than 20 mL/hr. Conservative management may avoid the need for dialysis. Serum potassium, urea, creatinine, bicarbonate, etc., should be monitored frequently. Established renal failure will have to be managed by **dialysis**.

f. ***Neurotoxicity***: All patients with neurotoxic symptoms should be administered the **Tensilon test**, to judge whether anticholinesterase therapy can be beneficial. The following procedure can be adopted:

i. Atropine sulfate (0.6 mg) is given by IV injection, followed by neostigmine bromide by intramuscular injection 0.02 mg/kg. Short acting edrophonium chloride (Tensilon) is ideal for this test, but is rarely available in India. It is given by slow IV injection in an adult dose of 10 mg.

ii. The patient is observed over the next 30–60 min (neostigmine) or 10–20 min (edrophonium) for signs of improved neuromuscular transmission.

iii. Patients who respond convincingly can be maintained on neostigmine, together with atropine to block muscarinic side effects.

g. ***Respiratory failure***:
   i. Keep airway clear
   ii. Oral airway, or tracheostomy, or cuffed endotracheal intubation
   iii. Mechanical ventilation

h. ***Rhabdomyolysis and myonecrosis***: This is especially likely in the case of sea snakebites. Correct hypovolaemia and maintain saline diuresis. Myoglobinuric nephropathy can be prevented by infusing mannitol and sodium bicarbonate.

i. ***Snake venom ophthalmia***: This occurs when a spitting cobra ejects venom into a victim's eyes.
   i. Urgent decontamination by copious irrigation.
   ii. Analgesia by vasoconstrictors with weak mydriatic activity (e.g., adrenaline) and limited topical administration of local anaesthetics (e.g., tetracaine).
   iii. Exclusion of corneal abrasions by fluorescein staining with a slit lamp examination and application of prophylactic topical antibiotics.

PREVENTION OF SNAKEBITE

I. **DO's**
   a. Do wear shoes (or preferably leather boots and long trousers) when walking outdoors amid thick undergrowth or long grass.
   b. Do carry an electric torch or flashlight when walking outdoors at night.
   c. Do take care when collecting firewood, or moving logs, rocks, or debris which are likely hiding places for a snake.
   d. Do take care when climbing rocks or trees with dense foliage, or swimming in lakes or rivers with lots of weeds.
   e. Do be careful while walking under low hanging branches of trees.
   f. Do use repellents in basements, attics and storerooms to ward off rodents and snakes (e.g., DDT, naphthalene, pyrethroids, etc.).

II. **DONT's**
   a. Do not poke hand or foot into holes or crevices while walking outdoors, especially in logs of wood or among rocks or boulders.
   b. Do not hike or backpack alone in a remote area.
   c. Do not go near a snake even if it appears inactive or harmless. Slip away quietly. Do not make sudden movements.
   d. Do not handle a snake even if it appears dead. Some snakes pretend to be dead to avoid attack.
   e. Do not keep venomous snakes as pets or performing animals.
   f. Do not camp near large logs, rocky areas or tall grass, when camping outdoors. Shake out clothing, shoes and sleeping bags before use to dislodge any hidden snakes.
   g. Do not wade in the sea, especially in sand, or near coral reefs.
   h. Do not swim in muddy waters, or waters with vegetation since these are favourite hiding areas for water snakes.

SNAKES AND SNAKEBITE – FORENSIC ASPECTS

1. Snakes have been venerated and worshipped in India since ages. The mysterious power of inflicting death possessed by venomous snakes, their slithering movement, and periodic shedding of skin, inspired awe and dread among people of ancient civilizations, and led to their worship in idol form. Among all the snakes, the cobra has been the object of most attention in India. Even today, it is **worshipped by many Hindus**. Hindus generally do not kill cobras on account of such veneration. Also, there is a popular belief that he who kills a cobra will be cursed for generations.
2. Almost all cases of **snakebite** reported from around the world are **accidental** in origin, and the vast majority are due to inadvertent or deliberate provocation of a snake by a human. Snakes rarely if ever, attack human beings on their own.
3. Perhaps, the only recorded case of **suicide** accomplished with the help of a venomous snake is that of Egyptian queen **Cleopatra**, who reportedly died from the bite of an asp – likely an Egyptian cobra – after hearing of Mark Antony's death (**Fig. 11.39**).
4. While **homicides** can be accomplished by using a venomous snake as a tool, actual instances of murder committed by such an exotic method are rare. However, a recent sensational case from Kerala emphasises the importance of always being alert to such a possibility (**Box 11.1**).
5. Deaths due to snakebite are regarded as medicolegal in nature, and a forensic autopsy is mandatory. Unfortunately, clear-cut signs of envenomation may be lacking in such cases, and even fang marks may not always be discernible. Today, immunodiagnosis with the help of ELISA makes it possible to conclusively diagnose death due to snakebite by analyzing tissues around bitesite, or blister fluid, or even body fluids such as blood and urine for venom antigens.

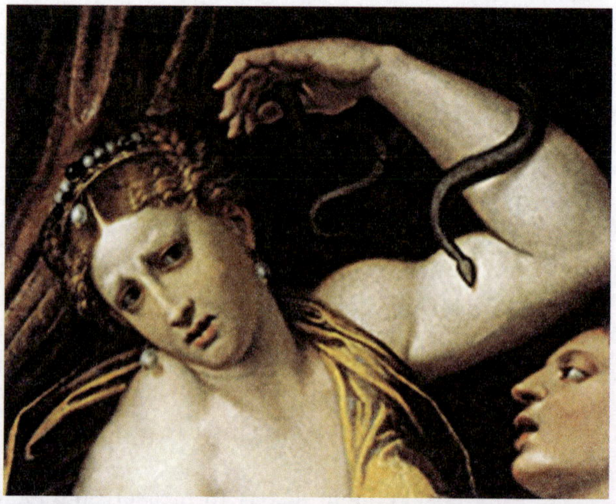

Fig. 11.39 Painting of Queen Cleopatra committing suicide by snakebite

Box 11.1—Kerala Snakebite Murder

This is a sensational case in which the victim, Uthra, a young woman, was killed by a snakebite inflicted while she was asleep on 7th May 2020. She was in her parents' home in Anchal, Kerala. Her husband, Sooraj Kumar, a bank employee, was arrested. Later, he confessed to the public media that he purchased a cobra, and introduced the snake into their bedroom, with the intention of killing his wife. Kerala Police produced strong scientific evidence that supported a charge of murder.

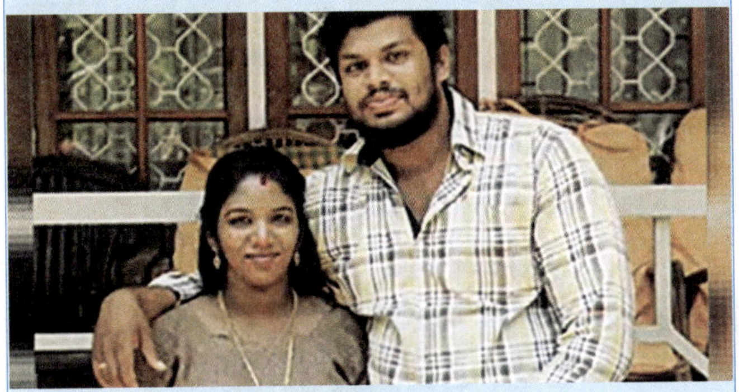

Uthra with her husband Sooraj Kumar

Uthra was a disabled young housewife who had been married for 2 years, and was the mother of a 1-year-old boy. At the time, Uthra was recovering from a previous Russell's viper bite, inflicted on 2nd March 2020, 2 months prior, at her husband's home near Adoor, and she was living in her parents' home during her recovery. The viper bite caused her to be completely bed-ridden for around 52 days, and she had to undergo plastic surgery to repair the damage. She was found unconscious in her bedroom in her parents' home, when her mother came to call her in the morning. It appeared that she had been bitten by a snake during the night of 6th May 2020. Uthra died the next day, 7th May 2020. A large Indian cobra was found in the bedroom that she shared with her husband.

According to Uthra's mother, her daughter and Sooraj went to bed after dinner. The next morning Sooraj, usually a late riser, woke up unusually early and went outside. However, Uthra did not wake up at her usual time. Her mother went into her room and found Uthra unconscious. Later, the room was searched, and the cobra was discovered and killed.

One week after his daughter's death, Uthra's father contacted the police, stating that he suspected foul play in his daughter's death. He stated that, because Uthra and her husband were sleeping in an air-conditioned room, it would have been difficult for the cobra to enter the room without being detected. Uthra had already informed her parents about Sooraj Kumar's expertise in handling venomous snakes. Approximately 2 months prior to her death from the cobra bite, Uthra had been bitten by a Russell's viper. The combination of the two incidents caused police to suspect Sooraj Kumar's involvement in this case.

The police arrested Sooraj as the prime suspect, and also a snake catcher Suresh Kumar as the second suspect in the case. On 12th July 2020, Sooraj made a public confession about the murder. He stated that he bought two snakes for Rs. 10,000 each. He admitted that he gave "sleeping pills" to his wife in order to sedate her before releasing the snake. Sooraj was booked under various sections of the Indian Penal Code for murder, attempted murder, attempted permanent injury and destruction of evidence.

During the course of the investigation, it was discovered that gold from Uthra's bank locker had been removed on 2nd March, the date of her first snakebite. In early June 2020, Uthra's father-in-law was arrested, on charges of destroying evidence and hiding 38 sovereigns of gold jewellery, which Police discovered buried in a nearby rubber plantation. Uthra's parents stated that the majority of her dowry was still missing. In August 2020, both the mother and sister of Sooraj, were arrested on charges of conspiracy, domestic violence and destruction of evidence. Although Suresh Kumar was originally one of the accused, he became a witness in the case.

Kerala Police sent the carcass of the cobra for forensic examination. It was confirmed that the cobra was 80 cm long, and capable of inflicting a fatal bite to a human.

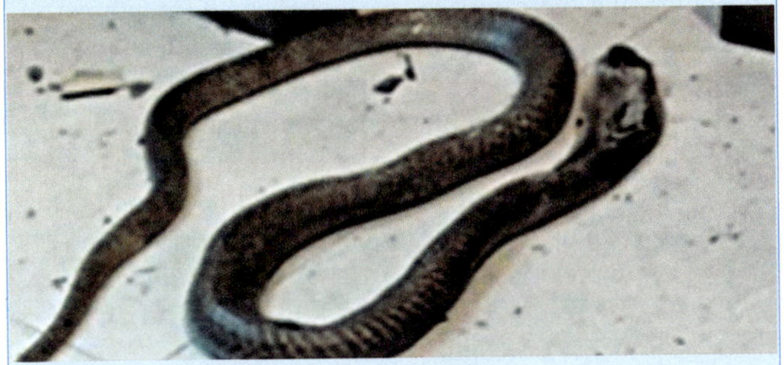

The killed cobra

Sooraj Kumar is said to have planned the murder by watching snake handling videos on the internet and receiving training to handle venomous snakes. His motive was to take ownership of his wife's dowry in gold, as well as her life insurance policy.

In December 2020, the snake catcher, Suresh Kumar, testified to the court that Sooraj contacted him and purchased a snake. Suresh learned of Uthra's death from the newspapers. Sooraj told Suresh that he no longer wished to be wed to a disabled wife and that people would attribute his wife's death to "sarpa dosha", the wrath of snakes (a popular belief). Suresh said he was distressed by Uthra's death.

In court, Sooraj was found guilty of using a live cobra to kill his wife Uthra. On 13th October 2021, Kollam Additional District and Sessions Court sentenced Sooraj to 17 years imprisonment plus two consecutive life sentences, and an additional penalty of 5 lakh rupees.

SCORPION STING

- **Arachnids** differ from insects mainly in the number of legs they possess: eight instead of six. They are further distinguished from insects by the fact they do not have antennae or wings.

- However, arachnids have two further pairs of appendages that have become adapted for feeding, defense and sensory perception.
  - The first pair, the **chelicerae**, serve in feeding and defense.
  - The next pair of appendages, the **pedipalps**, have been adapted for feeding, locomotion and/or reproductive functions.
- There are two important orders from the toxicological point of view: **Scorpiones** and **Araneae**.
- The members of **Scorpiones** comprise **scorpions**, which are capable of inflicting severe, and sometimes fatal stings, while the members of **Araneae** comprise **spiders**, which are capable of inflicting painful bites.
- **Scorpions** have eight legs and are easily recognized by the pair of grasping pedipalps, and the narrow, segmented tail, often carried in a characteristic forward curve over the back, ending with a venomous stinger. Scorpions range in size from 9 mm/0.3 inches to 23 cm/9 inches.
- The scorpion has a cephalothorax (fused head and chest) comprising the carapace, eyes, chelicerae (mouth parts), pedipalps (which have chelae, commonly called **claws** or **pincers**) and four pairs of walking legs. The six segmented tail terminates in a bulbous enlargement called **telson**. The telson contains the **stinger** and **venom apparatus**.
- Common scorpions include those of Buthidae family (**fat-tailed scorpions**) including *Hottentotta tamulus* (**Indian red scorpion**; previously known as *Mesobuthus tamulus*). It is the **commonest species seen in India** (**Fig. 11.40**). It grows up to 3 inches in length.
- Larger scorpions are found in the outdoors, e.g., *Palamneus* (*Heterometrus*) species, which grow up to 7 inches and are darker, even blackish in colour (**Fig. 11.41**).
- Scorpions are often found on the bark of trees, amidst dry firewood, piles of bricks or tiles, and in beddings, inside shoes, pockets of trousers, etc.
- Components of scorpion venom are complex and species–specific, those of the family Buthidae being the most potent. The main toxins include phospholipase, acetylcholinesterase, hyaluronidase, serotonin and neurotoxins.
- Most scorpion venoms have neurotoxins that bind reversibly to voltage gated ion channels to maintain an open state or activation, notably affecting sodium, calcium and potassium channels. Both somatic and autonomic nervous systems are affected and autonomic storm is the primary mediator of morbidity and mortality.

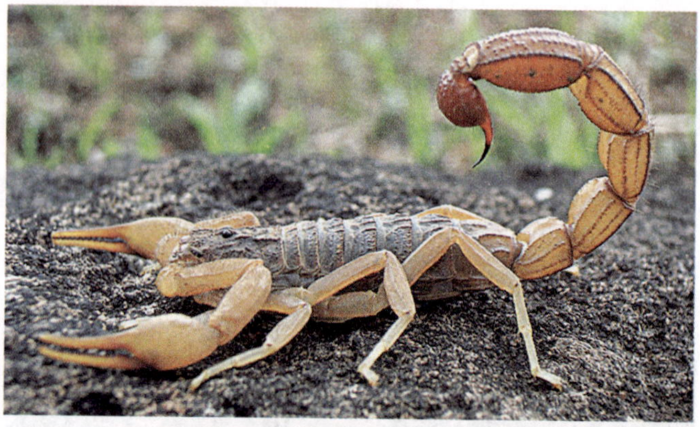

Fig. 11.40 Indian red scorpion (*Hottentotta tamulus*) (*Courtesy*: *Shantanu Kuveskar*)

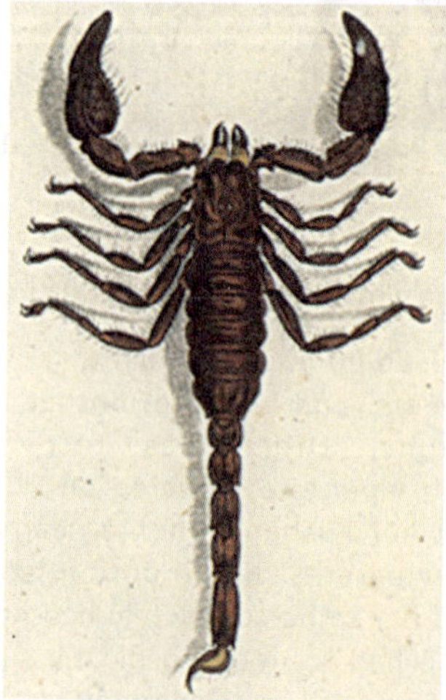

Fig. 11.41 Forest scorpion (*Heterometrus indus*)

Clinical Features

1. ***Local Features***:
   a. Pain is the main feature, along with erythema, induration and wheal.
   b. Also paraesthesia and hyperaesthesia.
2. ***Systemic Features***:
   a. **Allergic**: Urticaria, wheeze, angioedema.
   b. **Autonomic system**:
      i. *Sympathetic*: Tachycardia, hyperthermia, hypertension, tachyarrhythmias, profuse sweating (**Fig. 11.42**), urinary retention
      ii. *Parasympathetic*: Bradycardia, hypotension, urination, hypersalivation (**Fig. 11.43**), broncho-constriction, priapism (**Fig. 11.44**).
      iii. *Mixed autonomic dysfunction*.
      iv. *Cardiovascular system*:
         - Initially hypertension, tachycardia, arrhythmias, hypertensive encephalopathy, haemorrhagic stroke.
         - Later cardiovascular collapse: Cardiogenic and hypovolaemic shock, pulmonary oedema, coronary arterial spasm.
         - ECG: Tachy or brady dysrhythmias, conduction block, QT prolongation, non-specific ST and T-wave changes, ventricular ectopic activity, acute MI.
      v. *Gastrointestinal*:
         - Nausea, vomiting, diarrhoea and abdominal pain.
      vi. *Neurological*:

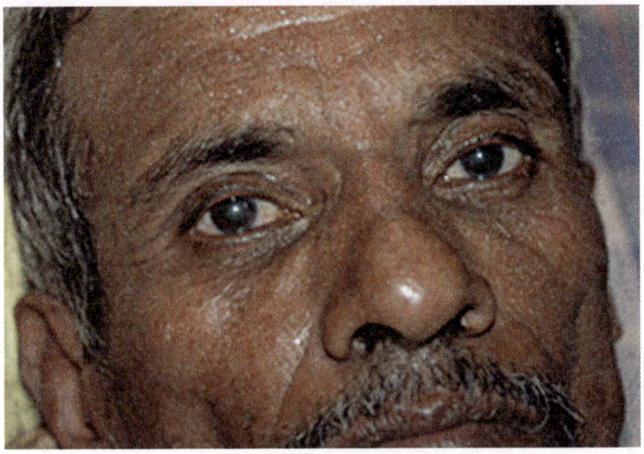

Fig. 11.42 Profuse sweating – Scorpion sting (*Courtesy*: *Dr HS Bawaskar*)

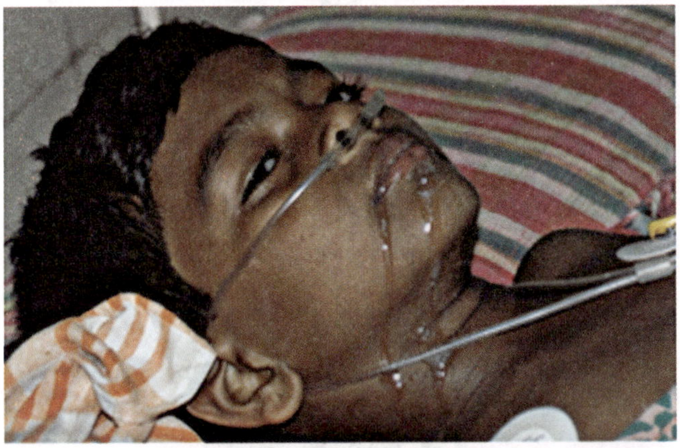

Fig. 11.43 Hypersalivation – Scorpion sting (*Courtesy*: *Dr HS Bawaskar*)

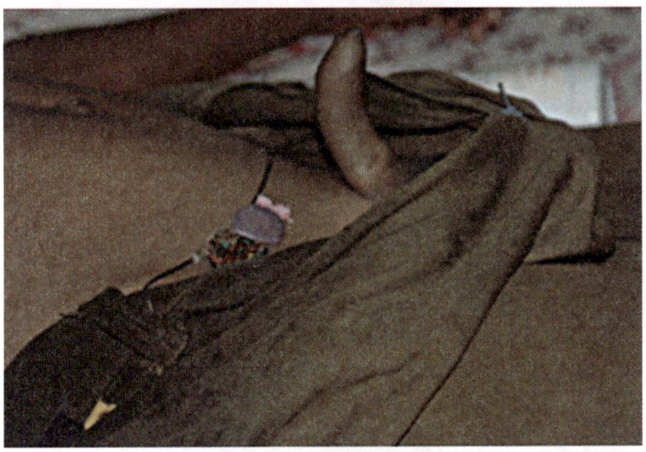

Fig. 11.44 Priapism – Scorpion sting (*Courtesy*: *Dr HS Bawaskar*)

- Cranial nerves: Nystagmus, dilated or constricted pupils, tongue fasciculation.
- Peripheral: Increased tone, spasticity, muscle jerks/clonus, brisk reflexes, ascending paralysis.
- Central effects secondary to circulatory or respiratory failure, and include coma and stroke.

vii. *Rarer complications*: Spontaneous systemic bleeding (e.g., from nose; gums; intestinal, urinary or genital tracts), disseminated intravascular coagulation, pulmonary oedema, rhabdomyolysis, renal failure.

Treatment

1. **First aid**:
   a. Reassure the patient and give paracetamol for pain.
   b. The patient, and particularly the envenomed limb, should be immobilised.
   c. All patients who have been stung should be rapidly transported to hospital, preferably in the recovery position.
   d. Maintain a clear airway and adequate ventilation in patients who are unconscious. Early anaphylaxis should be treated with adrenaline (e.g., with an auto-injector such as Epipen).
   e. Any interference with the sting site should be avoided. Do not cut into or suck from the site, nor apply tourniquets, ligatures or compression bandages.
2. **Hospital**:
   a. Maintain a clear airway and adequate ventilation in patients who are unconscious. Early intubation and ventilation may be required for respiratory compromise, coma or ascending paralysis.
   b. Assess cardiovascular status (BP, pulse and peripheral perfusion) and resuscitate the patient as required with intravenous fluids.
   c. Anaphylaxis should be managed conventionally with adrenaline, chlorpheniramine and hydrocortisone.
   d. Infiltration of the sting site with local anaesthetic or a regional nerve block may be required to relieve intense pain (this is the most useful intervention in most cases of scorpion sting).
   e. Monitor temperature, pulse, blood pressure, respiratory rate and oxygen saturation at least hourly. Monitor cardiac rhythm.
   f. Perform a 12-lead ECG in all patients who require assessment. Repeat 12-lead ECGs are recommended, especially in symptomatic patients. Check cardiac rhythm, QRS duration and QT interval.
   g. Check serum potassium, magnesium and calcium concentrations and replace as necessary to keep within the high normal range.
   h. Check ABGs and correct any hypoxia or acidosis.
   i. Check full blood count, renal and liver function, amylase and creatine kinase activities and blood glucose.
   j. Perform a chest X-ray in patients with symptoms of pulmonary oedema.
   k. All patients should be observed for at least 4 hrs in hospital. All patients with features of systemic envenoming should be observed for a minimum of 24 hrs.
   l. Antivenom may be required for systemic envenoming (or severe local envenoming). Administer antivenom by intravenous infusion of liquid or reconstituted

lyophilised antivenom diluted in 0.9% sodium chloride (adult 250–500 mL, children 10 mL/kg). Adults and children require the same dose. "Hypersensitivity" tests (intradermal or subcutaneous administration of antivenom) do not predict reactions and should not be used. Scorpion antivenom effective against *Hottentotta* (*Mesobuthus*) *tamulus* has been introduced in India. A single 30 mL dose of the monovalent antivenom is added to 100 mL of normal saline, which is infused intravenously over 30 min irrespective of patient's age.

m. Give anti-tetanus prophylaxis as required.
n. Hypotension: Correct hypotension by adequate fluid resuscitation with a crystalloid. Treat brady and tachyarrhythmias appropriately. Vasopressors and inotropes can be initiated in an emergency through peripheral venous access.
o. Agitation and delirium: Adults can be sedated with oral or IV diazepam (0.1–0.3 mg/kg). If agitation persists, consider oral (5–10 mg) or parenteral (2–10 mg) haloperidol.
p. Other measures as indicated by the patient's clinical condition.
q. **Bawaskar's Protocol**: One of India's pioneering physicians involved in treating scorpion stings (Dr HS Bawaskar) advocates a standard protocol, based on **prazocin** as add-on therapy to scorpion antivenom.

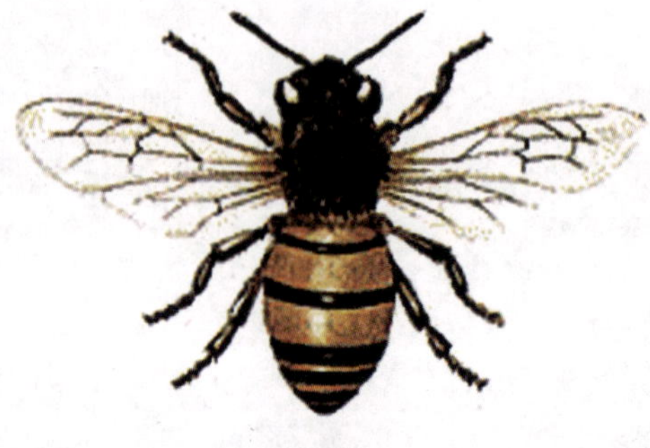

Honey Bee

Fig. 11.45 Honey bee (*Apis Mellifera*)

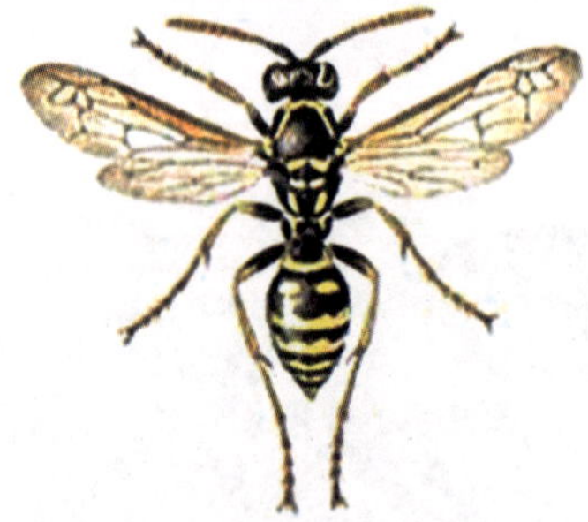

Fig. 11.46 Paper wasp (*Polistes annularis*)

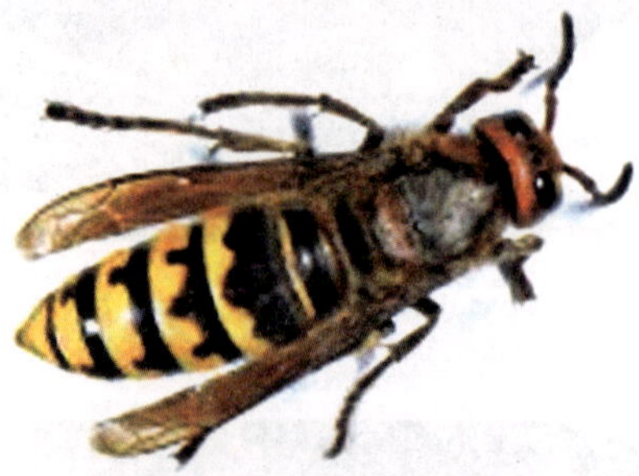

Fig. 11.47 Hornet (*Vespa crabro*)

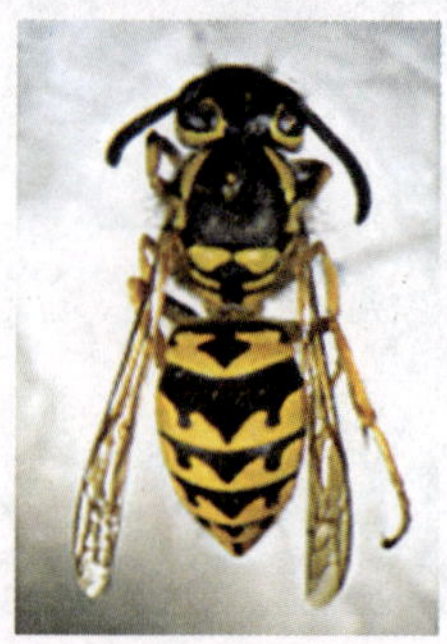

Fig. 11.48 Yellow jacket (*Vespula pensylvanica*)

BEE & WASP STINGS

- Phylum **Arthropoda** (the largest phylum of the animal kingdom) has two very important classes of venomous creatures: **Insecta** and **Arachnida**.
- **Arachnids** comprise **scorpions** and **spiders**.
- There are three orders of toxicological importance in class **Insecta**: **Hymenoptera, Lepidoptera** and **Coleoptera**.
- **Hymenoptera** comprises mainly two-winged flies and ants. The common **stinging hymenopterids** include **bees, wasps, yellow jackets, hornets** and **fire ants**. The term "hymenoptera" refers to membranous wings that characterize these insects.
- Hymenoptera stings are invariably caused by the **honey-bee*** (*Apis mellifera*) (**Fig. 11.45**), **paper wasp** (*Polistes annularis*) (**Fig. 11.46**), **hornets** (*Vespa species*) (**Fig. 11.47**) and **yellow jackets** (*Dolichovespula species*) (**Fig. 11.48**).
- Bees are attracted to sweet food and meat and can sting multiple times.
- They are found in large nests, located where shelter is available (eg, under eaves, hollows of trees, and wall cavities).
- Venom is usually injected through a sting which may be ***barbed*** (e.g., **bee**), or ***smooth*** (e.g., **wasp**) (**Fig. 11.49**).
- Bees leave behind the stings embedded in the skin, while wasps and hornets are capable of repeated stings.

Clinical Features

- **Local Reaction**:
  - In individuals not allergic to the venom, a single sting usually produces only mild effects such as local pain, redness, irritation, itching and swelling, which resolve in a few hours.
  - Local reaction becomes dangerous only if the site of the sting is in a vital location, e.g., mouth or tongue

Note*: *Different from the **bumble bee (Bombus terrestis) which is large, slow moving and stings rarely.*

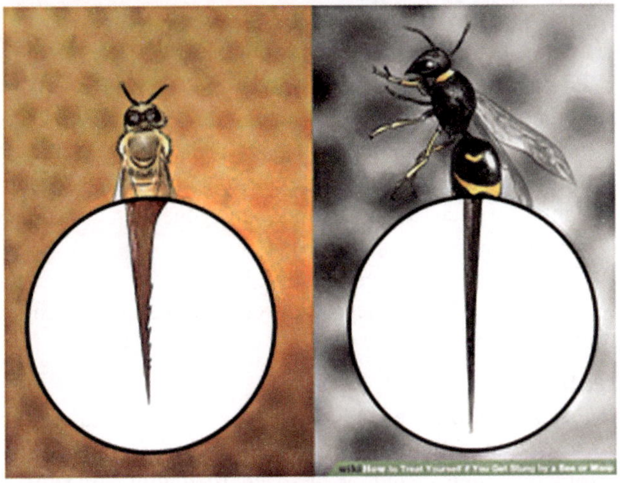

Fig. 11.49 Barbed stinger of a bee (*left*) and smooth stinger of a wasp (*right*)

(oedema leading to airway obstruction), or near the eye (cataract formation, glaucoma, etc.). External eye stings can cause pain, swelling, lacrimation, hyperaemia and conjunctival chemosis.

- Severe cutaneous infection and cellulitis have occurred after stings from yellow jackets and wasps, which may pick up virulent bacteria while foraging on decaying animal and vegetable matter.

- **Allergic Reactions**
  - ***Anaphylaxis***
    - About 4% of the human population is hypersensitive to hymenoptera venom. Yellow jackets and other wasps are the most serious offenders and cause twice as many allergic reactions as honeybees. In sensitive individuals, successive stings cause increasingly severe symptoms. Sensitization to wasp venom is said to occur much more rapidly than to bee venom.
    - Anaphylaxis is IgE-mediated, wherein the IgE antibodies attach to tissue mast cells and basophils in a previously sensitized individual. These cells are then activated, resulting in the progression of the cascade reaction of increased vasoactive substances such as leukotrienes, eosinophil chemotactic factor-A (ECF-A) and histamine.
    - Clinical features develop within a few minutes of the sting, comprising tingling sensation of scalp, flushing, dizziness, visual disturbances, syncope, abdominal cramps, vomiting, diarrhoea, dry cough, wheezing and tachycardia. In severe cases, the patient develops urticaria, angioedema, glottic oedema, profound hypotension and coma. Death may occur within minutes.
    - Individuals who have had an anaphylactic reaction to a Hymenoptera sting have a 35–60% chance of developing anaphylaxis from subsequent stings by an identical insect.
  - ***Delayed Reaction***
    - A few patients develop urticaria, skin rash, pedal oedema, and arthritis between 1 and 5 days after the sting.
    - Sometimes, a serum sickness-like syndrome occurs a week or more after the sting. This is characterized by malaise, fever, headache, urticaria, lymphadenopathy and polyarthritis. Renal failure may occur rarely.
- **Toxic Reactions**
  - Multiple stings (especially involving a swarm of bees, wasps or hornets) can cause massive envenoming characterized by vasodilation, hypotension, oedema, fatigue, vomiting, diarrhoea, headache, seizures and coma. There have been reports of acute renal failure.
  - Delayed toxic reactions can occur, characterized by normal initial laboratory results, and subsequent evidence of haemolysis, coagulopathy, thrombocytopenia, rhabdomyolysis, liver dysfunction and disseminated intravascular coagulation.

Treatment

- **Local Reaction**
  - Remove embedded stinger (common in the case of bees) by scraping with a blade or fingernail. Do not grasp the stinger with forceps which will cause further injection of venom due to squeezing.
  - Local infiltration with adrenaline 1:1000 (0.1–0.3 mL) near the sting site may help impede systemic absorption of venom.
  - Local cold compress: Local application of an ice pack at the sting site for 15 min every 30 min may decrease intensity of swelling, reduce pain and help retard absorption of venom.
  - Domestic meat tenderizer (papain) diluted 1 in 5 with tap water, is reputed to produce immediate relief of pain.
  - Antihistamines: Diphenhydramine (50 mg every 6 hrs) or chlorpheniramine (4 mg every 6 hrs).
  - Local antiseptic cream.
  - Antibiotic may be administered only if there is evidence of infection.
- **Allergic Reactions**
  - ***Anaphylaxis***:
    - 0.1% adrenaline by subcutaneous or intramuscular injection. It may be repeated in 20 min.
    - Antihistamine injection (e.g., chlorpheniramine maleate 10 mg IV or IM, or diphenhydramine 50 mg parenterally) is useful in relieving urticarial symptoms.
    - Airway management with adequate ventilation and oxygenation.
    - Bronchodilators such as salbutamol to relieve dyspnoea and wheezing.
    - Corticosteroids:
      - Methylprednisolone – 1–2 mg/kg IV every 6–8 hrs.
      - Prednisone – 40–60 mg/day.
    - Correction of hypotension and shock: Dopamine and IV fluids.

  - Continuous cardiac monitoring.
- *Delayed reaction*:
  - Antihistamines
  - Analgesics
  - Haemodialysis for renal failure
- **Toxic Reactions**
  - Parenteral antihistamines
  - Large doses of corticosteroids
  - Bronchodilators
  - Haemodialysis for renal failure

SPIDER BITE

- There are more than 40,000 species of **spiders** of which less than 300 (belonging to a single family) are non-venomous. However, only about 20 species cause serious envenoming in humans, while about 150–180 can cause significant toxicity.
- **Australian funnel web spiders** are said to be the most dangerous in the world, on clinical and venom toxicity grounds, though this claim has also been attributed to the **Brazilian wandering spider**, due to much more frequent accidents.
- The **common Indian species** that cause serious envenomation include **brown recluse, black widow, wolf spider** and **tarantula**.
- Anatomically, a spider has a cephalothorax and an abdomen with four pairs of legs fanning out from the thorax. Two claw-like fangs called **celicera** protrude from the head and are connected to **venom glands** which are under voluntary control.
- Although the venom is quite potent in many species, serious envenomation is rare because of inadequate injection mechanism, and small quantity injected with each bite.

Brown Recluse

Other Common Names

Brown fiddler, Fiddleback spider, Violin spider

Species

Loxosceles reclusa

Physical Appearance

- It is a small reddish brown or grey spider, with a brown violin shaped mark on its back (**Fig. 11.50**).
- Loxosceles spiders can be differentiated from most other "garden" brown spiders, of which there are many, by its set of six eyes (three pairs), rather than eight.

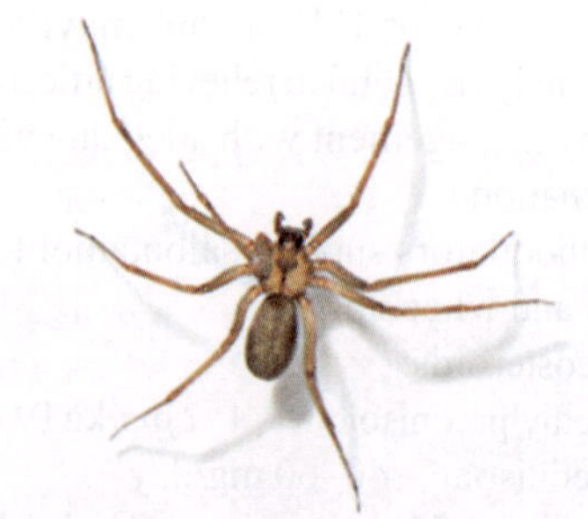

Fig. 11.50 Brown recluse

Clinical Features

1. **Loxoscelism** is the term used to describe lesions and clinical manifestations caused by bites of *Loxosceles* spp.
2. In the first 24 hrs, the area surrounding the bite becomes painful and erythematous. This is followed by skin mottling and areas of microvascular haemorrhage. Systemic symptoms such as fever, malaise and generalised erythema are common.
3. After 4–7 days, an area of painful necrosis develops at the bite site. Under the necrotic eschar, a deep slow healing ulcer may occur.

Treatment

1. Clean and dress the wound. Rest the affected area or limb.
2. Observe all patients admitted to hospital for 6 hrs. Asymptomatic patients can then be discharged with advice to return, if symptoms appear.
3. In patients with symptoms check FBC, blood film, U&Es, coagulation and LFTs.
4. Give tetanus prophylaxis, if indicated.
5. Prophylactic antibiotics are NOT indicated.
6. Apply a cold-pack. This is an effective topical analgesic and reduces the activity of spider venom.
7. Oral analgesia may be required.
8. Early surgical debridement is NOT recommended. Excision of the necrotic eschar may be appropriate if the lesion shows complications or limited and prolonged healing.

Black Widow

Species

Latrodectus erythromelas

Other Common Names

Hourglass spider

Physical Appearance

- *Latrodectus* spiders are often small-to-medium sized, and have a globular abdomen with long thin legs.
- Female widow spiders are typically dark brown or shiny black in colour (**Fig. 11.51**), usually exhibiting a red or orange hourglass on the ventral surface (underside) of the abdomen.

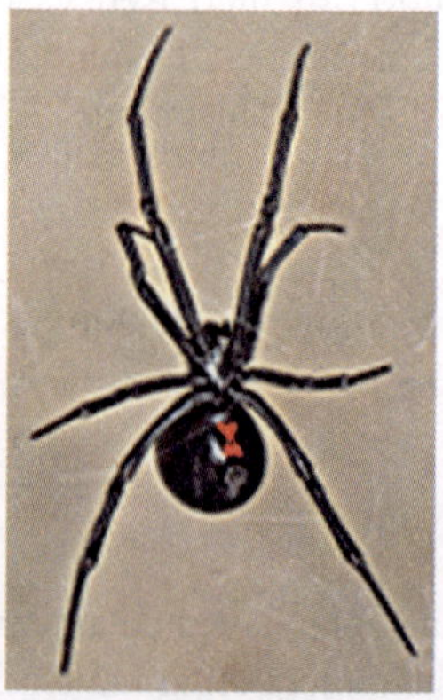

Fig. 11.51 Black widow

- Females are generally much larger than the males, and are more likely to cause human envenomation than the males.
- The prevalence of **sexual cannibalism**, a behaviour in which the female eats the male after mating, has inspired the common name "**widow spiders**". This behaviour may promote the survival odds of the offspring; however, only females of some species (rarely) show this behaviour, and much of the documented evidence for sexual cannibalism has been observed in laboratory cages where the males could not escape.

Clinical Features

Although envenomation is unlikely to be lethal, it can produce significant local and systemic effects (**Latrodectism**).

Grade 1

- Sharp pain at bitesite, with formation of a pair of red spots.
- No systemic features.

Grade 2

- Muscular pain in bitten extremity.
- Extension of pain to the trunk.
- Local diaphoresis of bitten extremity.
- No systemic features.

Grade 3

- Tender or swollen lymph nodes indicate systemic spread of envenomation.
- Generalized muscle pain.
- Generalized sweating.
- Nausea, vomiting.
- Headache.
- Tachycardia, hypertension.
- Cardiac changes include initial tachycardia followed by bradycardia and ECG abnormalities.
- Systemic lactrodectism can cause the victim to display a contorted, grimacing, sweating facial appearance, referred to as "***facies latrodectisma***."
- In severe cases, the following manifestations occur: ptosis, hyperreflexia, tremor, convulsions and respiratory compromise.

Treatment

1. Most bites require only symptomatic management. Cold packs and simple oral analgesia can be used as required.
2. Ensure tetanus immunisation is up-to-date.
3. Monitor vital signs, cardiac rhythm and measure blood sugar (BM).
4. Perform a 12-lead ECG in all patients who require assessment.
5. In all patients measure FBC, U&Es, LFTs, coagulation and CK. Observe all patients for at least 4 hrs after the bite.
6. Antivenom (if available) is considered in patients with severe pain or pronounced systemic symptoms. **There is no antivenom for the Indian species of black widow**.

Wolf Spider

- Wolf spiders belong to *Lycosa* species.
- The bite of the wolf spider is generally not associated with serious manifestations. Occasionally, it causes moderate pain, erythema, oedema or pruritis. Rarely, there is necrosis.
- Systemic manifestations may develop after 1–2 days, characterized by fever, chills, myalgia and arthralgia.
- Treatment involves supportive and symptomatic measures.

Tarantula

- The tarantula (*Lycosa tarantula*) is usually a variant of the wolf spider.
- Though all tarantulas are venomous and some bites cause serious discomfort that might persist for several days, so far there is no record of a bite causing a human fatality.
- While the bites of many species are known to be no worse than a wasp sting, accounts of bites by some species are reported to be very painful and to produce intense spasms that may recur over a period of several days.
- Tarantulas are large, hairy spiders which caused panic in Europe in the 17th century, due to a large series of bites beginning from the Italian city of Taranto and spreading to several European countries. Mass hysteria led to the development of a special dance ("**tarantella**") which was supposed to protect the envenomated victim from serious effects!
- **Tarantulas** have urticating hairs on their back legs and abdomen (**Fig. 11.52**). They range from as small as a fingernail to as large as a dinner plate when the legs are fully extended. When they feel threatened, they vibrate their hind legs together, spraying a cloud of sharp pointed hairs with numerous barbs. The hairs can also be spread to skin and eyes via direct contact when handling the spiders. The hairs are quite sharp and penetrate through many layers. Eye problems encountered include corneal and conjunctival hyperaemia, chronic granulomatous-type reactions, nodular conjunctivitis and stromal keratitis ('**spider keratouveitis**').
- Treatment involves application of ice packs, wound cleansing and antihistamines.
- If eye irritation has occurred, an ophthalmology referral should be arranged. Treatment is generally aimed at mechanical removal, topical corticosteroids and cycloplegics.

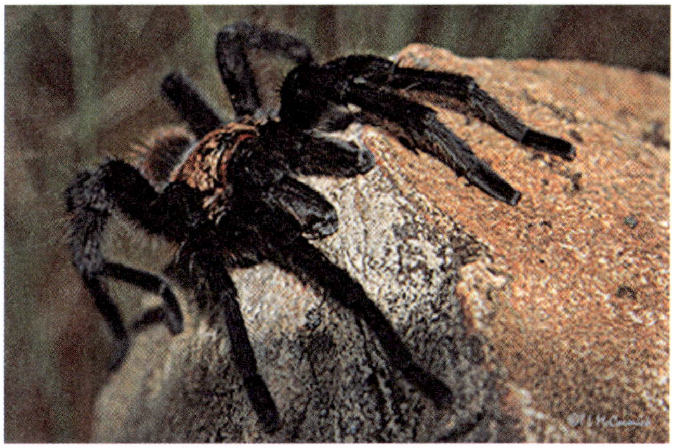

Fig. 11.52 Tarantula

Topic 12

SOCIOMEDICAL TOXICOLOGY

(Number of Competencies – 1: FM 12.1)

Teachers and students, please note:

- Topics 9–13 deal with specific categories of poisons with regard to clinical features, diagnosis and management, upon exposure to them. It is to be noted that except for Topic 13, the new curriculum does not mention medicolegal aspects at all! So, it is a moot point whether students can be assessed on these aspects.
- However, as the editor feels it is important, this book lists medicolegal aspects too (under 'Forensic Issues') for all the poisons.
- Also, there is always a possibility of a revised (corrected) curriculum being released incorporating medicolegal aspects, anytime in the future. So, it is better to be prepared!

FM 12.1: Core – Written/Viva Voce

- Describe features and management of abuse/poisoning with:
  - Tobacco
  - Cannabis
  - Amphetamines
  - Cocaine
  - Hallucinogens
  - Designer drugs
  - Solvent abuse

This topic deals with **Substance Abuse**, though this term is not mentioned explicitly in the new curriculum. However, since some preliminary information is essential before proceeding to the individual examples listed, the following prelude has been included. Kindly note that as it is not specified in the curriculum, it has been highlighted in green colour. In other words, the information falls in the "Nice to Know" area and questions cannot be asked in the University examination, but can be asked in formative assessment (internal assessment).

SUBSTANCE ABUSE

Terminology in the field of substance abuse has changed frequently leading to a great deal of confusion. Therefore, it is necessary to begin this section by defining currently used terms, and to clarify the differences between them. The nomenclature and diagnostic schemes mentioned here-in are based on the 5th **edition of *Diagnostic and Statistical Manual of Mental Disorders* (*DSM-5*)**, and the 11th **edition of *International Classification of Diseases and Related Health Problems* (*ICD-11*)**.

Definitions

- **DSM-5** categorizes **substance abuse** into two categories:
  - **Substance use disorder** refers to a cluster of cognitive, behavioural and psychological symptoms, indicating that the individual continues using the substance despite significant substance related problems.
  - **Substance-induced disorder** includes intoxication, withdrawal and other substance induced mental disorders.
- **ICD-11** categorizes **substance abuse** into four categories:
  - **Substance dependence**
  - **Harmful pattern of substance use**
  - **Episode of harmful substance use**
  - **Hazardous substance use**

Substance Dependence

- **Substance dependence** in ICD-11 is defined as a disorder of regulation of substance use arising from repeated or continuous use of that substance, and includes:
  - A strong desire to take the drug
  - Difficulties in controlling its use
  - Persisting in its use despite harmful consequences
  - A higher priority given to drug use than to other activities
  - Increased tolerance
  - A physical withdrawal state.

Addiction

- The term "**addiction**" denotes a chronic disorder characterized by compulsive use of drugs (***craving***), resulting in physical, psychological and social harm, and continued use despite evidence of that harm (***denial***).

Classification

The **10 substance classes** as mentioned in **DSM-5** are:

1. Alcohol
2. Sedative – Hypnotics and anxiolytics
3. Opioids
4. Nicotine
5. Stimulants, including cocaine, amphetamine and related substances
6. Cannabis, synthetic cannabinoids
7. Caffeine
8. Inhalants
9. Hallucinogens and other dissociative drugs
10. Emerging substances of abuse

Only those listed in the new curriculum will be discussed in this section.

TOBACCO

Sources

- **Tobacco** is the main source of **nicotine**, which is a plant alkaloid. Nicotine is usually derived from two sources:

- the large leaf tobacco plant *Nicotiana tabacum* and
- the small leaf tobacco plant *Nicotiana rustica.*

Physical Appearance

- *Nicotiana tabacum* is an annual herb, shrub or small tree; from 1 to 1.50 m tall according to the variety (**Fig. 12.1**).
- The leaves are elliptical; flowers are clustered at the end of the branches, and are long and trumpet-shaped, white-pinkish in colour (**Fig. 12.2**).
- Fruit has different forms with globular seeds.
- Every part of the plant (except the seed) contains **nicotine**, the maximum concentration of which is in the **leaves**.
- *Lobelia inflata* contains **lobeline**. It is sometimes used as a nicotine substitute.
- Nicotine is a pale yellow, hygroscopic, oily liquid with a pungent odour, and sharp, burning taste. It gradually becomes brown on exposure to air or light.

Active Principles

- *Nicotiana tabacum* and *Nicotiana rustica* contain the following alkaloids:
  - Nicotine
  - Nornicotine
  - Anabasine
  - Anabatine

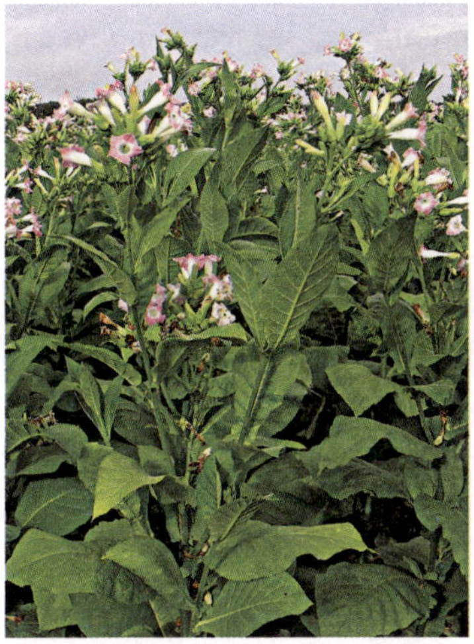

Fig. 12.1 *Nicotiana tabacum*

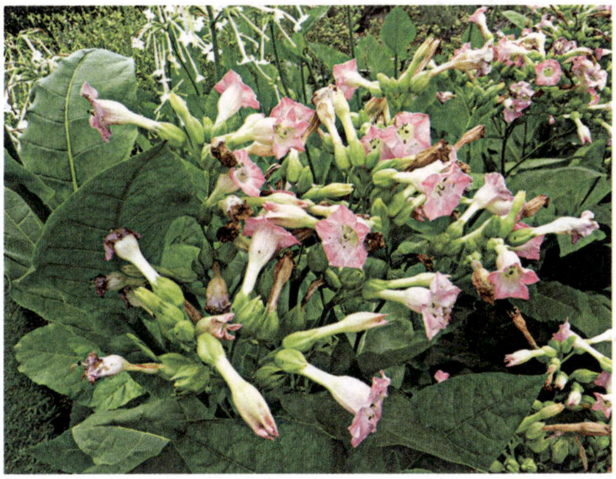

Fig. 12.2 *Nicotiana tabacum* – Flowers

Uses

- **Nicotine** is a **stimulant** of the central nervous system, and is abused widely all over the world in the form of inhalation (cigarette, cigar, pipe, beedi), nasal insufflation (snuff) or chewing.
  - By far the commonest source of nicotine poisoning (acute or chronic) results from smoking tobacco in the form of **cigarettes**. When a cigarette is lit and inhaled, the smoker is exposed to both **gaseous** and **particulate** matter.
  - **Nicotine** and **tar** are part of the particulate phase of cigarette smoke.
  - The usual nicotine content of a "regular" cigarette varies between 13 and 20 mg, while certain European and Turkish cigarettes can contain higher amounts. "Low nicotine" cigarettes contain 7–10 mg of the alkaloid. Cigars contain 15–40 mg of nicotine.
  - In India, "**bidis**" (**Fig. 12.3**) are very popular, especially among the poorer sections of society, since they are much cheaper than cigarettes. Bidis are small, brown, hand-rolled cigarettes consisting of tobacco wrapped in a ***tendu*** or ***temburni*** leaf (*Diospyros melanoxylon*) (**Fig. 12.4**). They are more harmful than cigarettes and produce higher levels of carbon monoxide, nicotine and tar. Also, because of low combustibility of tendu leaf, bidi smokers tend to inhale more often and more deeply, breathing in greater quantities of tar and other toxins than cigarette smokers.
  - After cigarettes, the next common source of nicotine toxicity results from **smokeless tobacco** which is of two kinds – **snuff** and **chewing tobacco**. Smokeless tobacco is consumed without burning the product, and is used either nasally or orally.
- Nicotine is also used as an **insecticide**.

Mode of Action

- When tobacco smoke is inhaled, nicotine enters the blood stream via the pulmonary circulation. It bypasses first pass metabolism and crosses the blood–brain barrier.

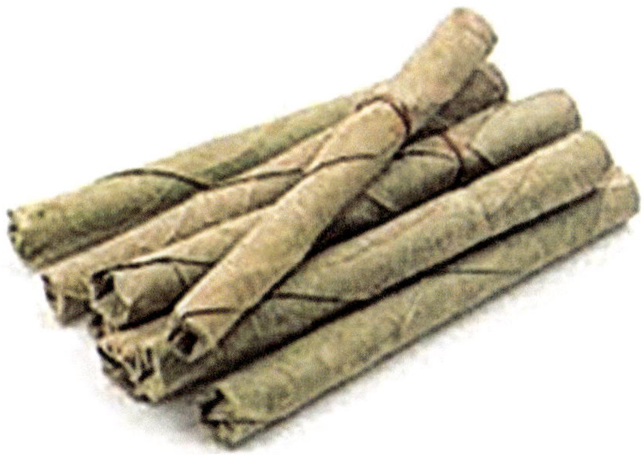

Fig. 12.3 Bidis

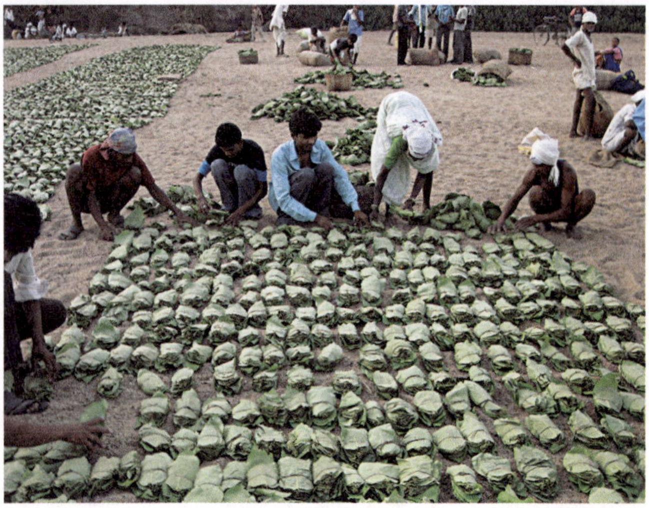

Fig. 12.4 Stacks of Tendu leaves

- Nicotine then binds stereo-specifically to select acetylcholine receptors (nicotine receptors). These receptors are present throughout the body, particularly in the autonomic ganglia, adrenal medulla, central nervous system, spinal cord and neuromuscular junctions.
- Nicotine is metabolized to **cotinine** in the liver, primarily by the enzyme CYP2A6.
- At moderate doses, nicotine stimulates the reticular activating system producing an alerting pattern on the EEG, with resultant favourable effects on memory and attention. But, higher doses cause tremor and convulsions due to a CNS disinhibition mechanism.
- Nicotine stimulation of vagal centres in the medulla induces nausea and vomiting, while the gastro-oesophagal reflux is provoked due to a lowering of sphincter pressure and increased acid secretion. Larger doses cause diarrhoea due to both central and parasympathetic excitation.
- Nicotine suppresses appetite while increasing basal energy expenditure, resulting in weight loss.
- Nicotine is sympathomimetic, and causes the release of catecholamines which increase heart rate, cardiac contractility and cause constriction of cutaneous and coronary blood vessels, while increasing blood pressure.

Clinical (Toxic) Features

1. **Acute Poisoning**:
   a. *Early Effects* (*15min-1 hour*):
      i. GIT: Nausea, salivation, vomiting, abdominal pain.
      ii. CVS: Tachycardia, hypertension.
      iii. RS: Tachypnoea, bronchorrhoea.
      iv. CNS: Agitation, anxiety, sweating, headache, blurred vision, confusion, vertigo, tremor, ataxia, muscle fasciculations, convulsions. Pupils are at first constricted, but may dilate later.

   b. *Delayed Effects (after1 hr)*:
      i. GIT: Diarrhoea.
      ii. CVS: Bradycardia, arrhythmias, hypotension, shock.
      iii. RS: Hypoventilation, apnoea.
      iv. CNS: Lethargy, weakness, hyporeflexia, hypotonia, paralysis, coma.

   Death may occur, especially in the case of ingestion of cigarettes (inadvertently) by children, or exposure to insecticidal nicotine.

   Occupational dermal exposure to wet, uncured tobacco may produce "**green tobacco sickness**" among workers, characterized by nausea, vomiting, headache, vertigo, pallor and sweating. Headache occurs frequently, especially in harvesters. Contact dermatitis can occur.
2. **Chronic Poisoning (*Addiction*)**:
   Nicotine dependence is the most widely prevalent and deadly of all substance dependencies. DSM-5 defines two nicotine-related disorders: **nicotine dependence** and **nicotine withdrawal**. The dependence-producing effects of nicotine appear to be modulated by dopamine which is increased in smokers. Nicotine also increases noradrenaline, adrenaline and serotonin levels.
   a. *Health consequences of tobacco use*:
      i. Lung cancer
      ii. Non-pulmonary cancers: Mouth, larynx, oesophagus, stomach, liver, pancreas.
      iii. Respiratory diseases: Emphysema, bronchitis, asthma, pneumonia.
      iv. Cardiovascular diseases: Coronary heart disease, hypertension, stroke.
      v. Obstetric and neonatal conditions: Abortion, abruptio placenta, placenta praevia, pre-eclampsia, growth retardation, congenital malformations, sudden infant death syndrome.
      vi. Other conditions: Peptic ulcer, osteoporosis, Alzheimer's disease.

   b. ***Nicotine withdrawal***: Manifestations of nicotine withdrawal can occur within 4–8 hrs of the last cigarette. Manifestations include changes in mood, insomnia, difficulty concentrating, restlessness, decreased heart rate and weight gain. Craving is common, and increased coughing, poor performance on vigilance tasks, etc., can occur.

Usual Fatal Dose

Nicotine is highly toxic; 2–5 mg can cause nausea, and 40–60 mg can cause death. However, survival has occurred with ingestions of 1–4 g.

Diagnosis

1. Nicotine is metabolised to **cotinine** and then to **nornicotine** which can be detected in urine and blood.
2. High-pressure liquid chromatography (HPLC) is generally utilized to assay nicotine levels. Plasma level > 40–50 ng/mL indicates serious toxicity.

Treatment

1. **Acute Poisoning**:
   a. Decontamination by stomach wash. Activated charcoal is effective and must be administered in the usual manner.

b. Since nicotine is weakly alkaline, excretion can be enhanced by acidification of urine. But, it is not recommended by most investigators.
c. Symptomatic and supportive measures:
   i. Benzodiazepines for convulsions.
   ii. Atropine for bradycardia.
   iii. IV fluids and vasopressors (dopamine or noradrenaline) for hypotension.
   iv. Respiratory compromise is managed by oxygen, intubation and positive pressure ventilation.

2. **Chronic Poisoning (Addiction)**:
   a. **Nicotine replacement therapy**:
   The rationale behind nicotine replacement is to prevent or relieve nicotine withdrawal symptoms while stopping smoking behaviour by replacing it with another behaviour. Pharmacological nicotine is of various forms and dosages.
      i. **Nicotine gum (Polacrilex)**: The first nicotine preparation that was made available for use is the nicotine gum (available as ***Nicorette*** 2 mg and 4 mg strengths). It is designed to be chewed slowly and intermittently. Approximately 50–70% of the nicotine is absorbed through the buccal mucosa, while additional amounts are absorbed through swallowed saliva.
      ii. **Nicotine transdermal patch**: The disadvantages of nicotine gum (frequent administrations, unsightly chewing, bad taste, nausea and dyspepsia) are mostly avoided by transdermal nicotine, which is available as nicotine-releasing adhesive patches of varying sizes and delivery rates. The nicotine patch is generally available in three sizes, 30 cm^2, 20 cm^2 and 10 cm^2, which deliver 21 mg, 14 mg and 7 mg of nicotine, respectively, over 16 or 24 hrs.
      iii. **Nicotine spray**: Nicotine nasal spray is an alternative to gum or patch. It is available as a metered dose inhaler containing 100 mg of nicotine at 10 mg/mL, designed to deliver 200 equivalent puffs each releasing 0.5 mg of nicotine. The recommended dose is 2 sprays (one in each nostril) every hour, subject to a maximum of 40 doses (80 puffs) in any 24-hr period.
   b. **Other therapies**:
      i. **Nicotine replacement medications**:
         - **Bupropion**: Initially marketed as an antidepressant, today it is widely used to aid smoking cessation. It inhibits the reuptake of dopamine and norepinephrine.
         - **Varenicline**: Considered to be superior to bupropion as it has shown to reduce the risk of both short-term and long-term relapse. It is a partial agonist at the alpha-4 beta-2 nicotinic acetylcholine receptors
         - **Clonidine**: Clonidine is an alpha$_2$-adrenergic agonist that has been found useful in the treatment of alcohol and opiate withdrawal. Subsequent studies on its utility in nicotine withdrawal have shown that it could be effective in promoting abstinence from cigarettes also. The usual dose recommended is 150–200 μg/day for 1 month.
      ii. **Nicotine agonists and antagonists**: These drugs have the potential to block the effect of nicotine, i.e., removing its reinforcing effect on smoking behaviour.
         - **Lobeline**, the first of these drugs to be studied in this regard, is a partial agonist that binds weakly and competitively to nicotine receptor sites. However, it has not been found to be very effective in practice, though it continues to be sold abroad as a smoking cessation aid under the brand name *CigArrest*.
         - **Mecamylamine** is a nicotine receptor antagonist that is said to reduce the craving for cigarettes, if administered for more than 6 weeks.

Forensic Issues

- Tobacco abuse has been described as being the most widespread cause of death and disability worldwide than any single disease entity. The Government of India prohibits tobacco smoking in public, and most states have begun to implement this with varying success rates.
- As far as acute nicotine poisoning is concerned, the circumstances could be accidental, suicidal or even homicidal.
  - Accidental poisoning could occur in children who play with old tobacco pipes, or who ingest cigarettes out of curiosity. Severe poisoning can result from ingestion of just 2 or 3 cigarettes. Milder poisoning can result from "experimental smoking" by adolescents. Accidental poisoning in horticulture due to the use of nicotine as a pesticide was not uncommon in the past.
  - Suicidal ingestion of nicotine pesticides used to be reported occasionally in the past, until such preparations were withdrawn from use.
  - Homicidal cases have always been rare, though a few cases do find mention in medical literature.
- Autopsy findings in death due to nicotine ingestion include characteristic odour (of stale tobacco) in gastric contents, brownish froth at the mouth and nose, congestion with brownish discolouration of oesophageal and gastric mucosa, and intense congestion of liver and kidneys.

CANNABIS

- Cannabis is among the earliest mind-altering drugs known to man and has been around for at least 4000 years. Today, it is the world's most commonly used illicit drug, with approximately 200 million cannabis users (4% of the population aged 15–64) in 2020. In terms of popularity ratings, it stands 4th among psychoactive drugs (after caffeine, nicotine and alcohol).

Sources

1. *Cannabis sativa* (**Fig. 12.5**) – A 1–4-m tall plant with coarse, rough stems and small, green flowers. The plant is loosely branched with irregularly toothed leaves that are arranged

in a pattern of 3–7 leaves per stem. Native to the Far East, the United States and Central America.

2. *Cannabis indica* (Indian Hemp) (**Fig. 12.6**) – A similar plant species to *C. sativa*, but it does not grow as tall, usually only up to 1.2 m. It is more densely branched and has broader leaves compared to *C. sativa*. Native to India.
3. *Cannabis ruderalis* (**Fig. 12.7**) – A much smaller plant than *C. sativa* and *C. indica*. Grows up to 30–60 cm when fully mature. It is unbranched or only very sparsely branched, and the leaves are very broad and short compared to the other two species. Native to Siberia and central Asia but also found in Europe and Russia.
   - *Cannabis* normally has imperfect flowers, with staminate "male" and pistillate "female" flowers occurring on separate plants (**dioecious plants**).
   - It is not unusual, however, for individual plants to bear both male and female flowers (**monoecious plants**).

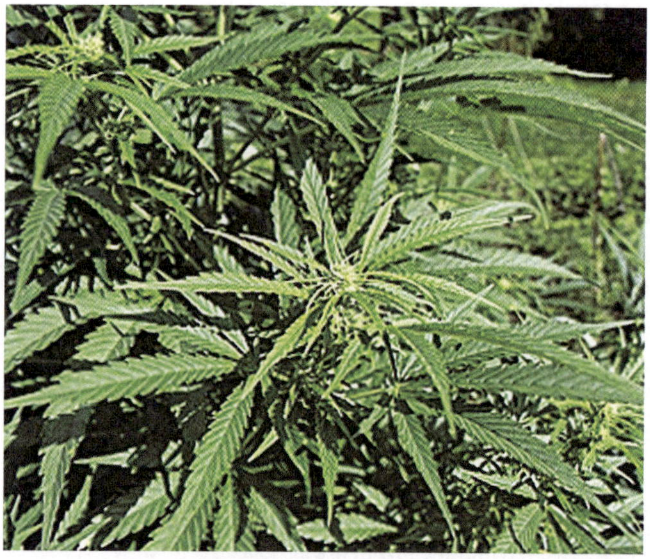

Fig. 12.5 *Cannabis sativa*

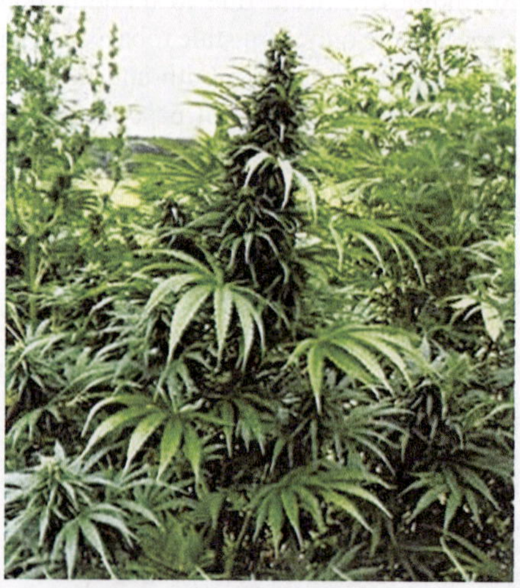

Fig. 12.6 Broad leaf of *Cannabis indica*

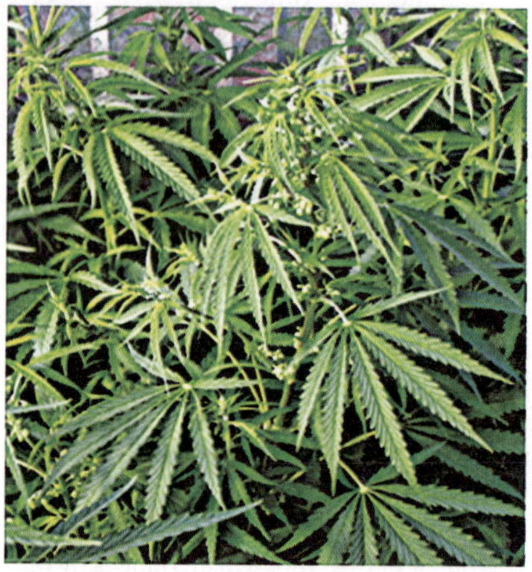

Fig. 12.7 *Cannabis ruderalis*

Active Principles

- **Cannabinoids** – primarily **delta-9-tetrahydrocannabinol (Δ9-THC)**, Δ8-THC, cannabinol and cannabidiol.
- Tetrahydrocannabinol (THC) is the main psychoactive cannabinoid. The concentration of THC is highest in the bracts, flowers, and leaves, while it is practically non-existent in the stem, root and seeds.
- Seedless (unpollinated female) plant, referred to as "**sinsemilla**" can contain high concentrations of THC (up to 5%).

Uses

- The durable fibres of the woody trunk of cannabis, referred to collectively as **Indian hemp**, has been used for centuries to produce rope and twine, as well as fine or rough cloth/fabric (**Fig. 12.8**).
- **Therapeutic uses**:
  - **Medical cannabis (medical marijuana)** refers to the use of cannabis and its constituent cannabinoids, to treat disease or improve symptoms.

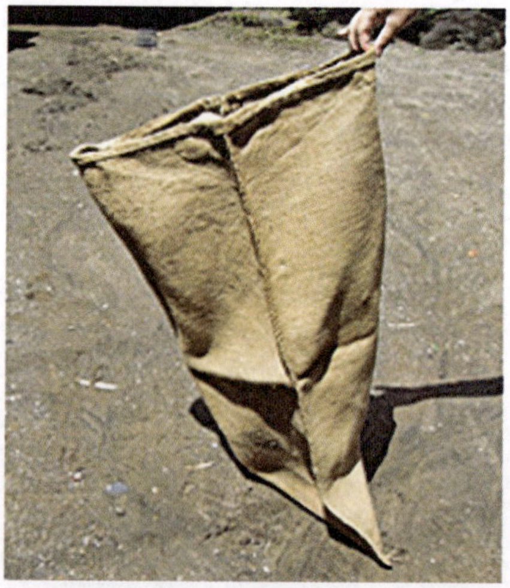

Fig. 12.8 A sack made from hemp fibre (*Courtesy: Katorisi*)

- THC in the form of a synthetic oral cannabinoid ("**dronabinol**") has been shown to be effective in controlling the nausea and diarrhoea associated with AIDS, as well as the nausea and vomiting caused by chemotherapy for cancer or AIDS. It also increases appetite and produces weight gain in both AIDS and cancer patients.
- THC possesses analgesic properties and has been tried in the treatment of pain due to cancer, and to treat chronic pain and muscle spasms.
- A cannabinoid mixture (**Sativex®**) has been licensed for the treatment of neuropathic pain associated with multiple sclerosis in various countries.

Mode of Poisoning

Toxic effects arise mainly from the abuse of various cannabis preparations for their mind-altering properties (slang terms are listed in **Table 12.1**).

1. **Marijuana**: The term "marijuana" refers to any part of the plant or its extract that is used to induce psychotomimetic or therapeutic effects.
2. **Ganja**: In India (where the term originated), the term 'Ganja' is used to refer to crushed leaves and inflorescences of female plants. It is usually smoked in a pipe ("***chillum***") or in the form of cigarettes ("***reefer***" or "***joint***") (**Fig. 12.9**). Ganja is said to contain 1–2% THC.

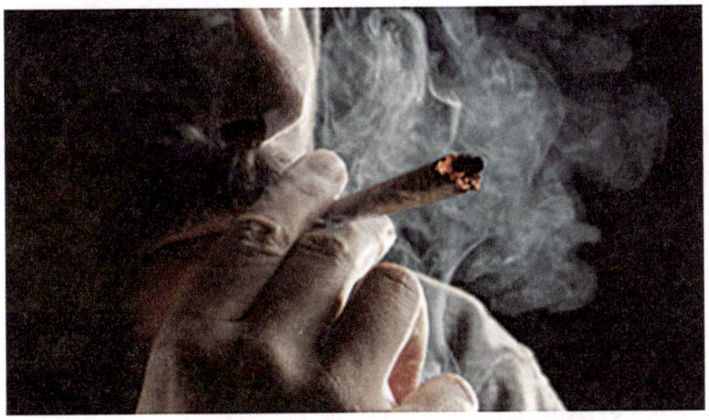

Fig. 12.9 Ganja being smoked as a 'reefer' ('*joint*')

3. **Bhang**: It is consumed by Hindus in India during festivals such as Holi and Shiv Ratri. Using mortar and pestle, the buds and leaves of cannabis are ground into a paste. To this mixture, milk, ghee, mangoes and Indian spices are added. The bhang base is now ready to be made into a thick drink, as an alternative to alcoholic beverages; this is often referred to as a "***bhang thandai***" or "***bhang lassi***".
   - Bhang is also mixed with ghee and sugar to make a purple halva, and into peppery, chewy little balls called ***golee*** (which means "bullet" as well as "pill" in Hindi).
4. **Hashish (Charas)**: This preparation is made out of dried resin (**Fig. 12.10**) collected from flower tops, and contains varying concentrations of THC up to 10%. It is popular in the Middle East and North Africa.
   - **Hashish oil** or "**liquid hashish**" is an alcohol or petrol extract which occurs as a dark green viscous liquid with the consistency of tar. It is the most potent of all cannabis preparations and contains 20–30% (or more) THC.
5. **Sinsemilla**: It is the most popular form of cannabis in the USA, and refers to seedless (unpollinated female) plant which averages 5% of THC.
6. **Marijuana "Blunts"**: This is nothing but cheap cigars sliced open, packed with cannabis and resealed. The harsh stench of the cigar masks the characteristic sweet smell of cannabis. Blunts are very popular among the youth in some parts of the USA.
7. **Cannabis Tea**: This is made by first adding a saturated fat to hot water (e.g., cream or milk) with a small amount of cannabis. It contains relatively small concentrations of THC because THC is an oil (lipophilic) and is only slightly water-soluble.

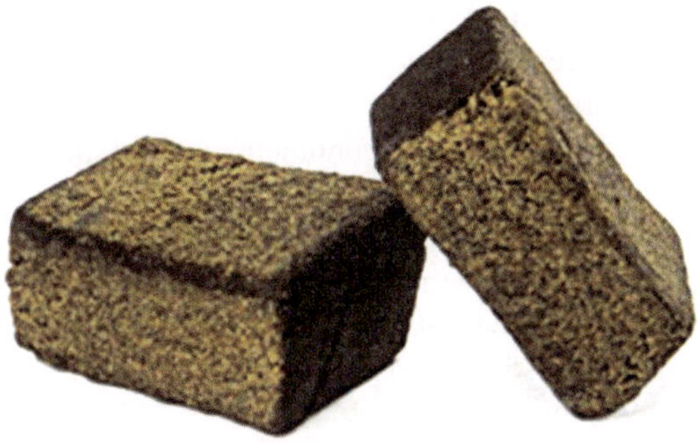

Fig. 12.10 Blocks of hashish

Table 12.1 Slang Names – Cannabis

Bhang, Bush, Dope, Ganja, Grass, Hash, Hashish, Kiff, Marihuana, Marijuana, Mary Jane, MJ, Pot, Puff, Reefer, Rope, Skunk, Tea, Torch, Weed.

Mode of Action

- A receptor site has been identified in the brain that binds reversibly and selectively with cannabinoids. Receptor binding is also present in the marginal zone of the spleen, nodular corona of Peyer's patches and cortex of lymph nodes.
- An endogenous cannabinoid-like ligand is present within the brain, named "**anandamide**"* which suggests the presence of a cannabinoid neurochemical pathway. It appears that cannabinoids exert many of their actions by influencing several neurotransmitter systems and their modulators. These include GABA, dopamine, acetylcholine, histamine, serotonin, noradrenaline and prostaglandins.
- After binding to receptors, cannabinoids also produce effects through second-messenger systems including inhibition of adenylcyclase and calcium channels, and also probably by enhancing potassium channels activity.

Drug Interactions

- Concomitant use of cannabis and ethanol produces additive effects on psychomotor performance.

***Note**: *Derived from Sanskrit "ananda" which means "bliss".*

- Concomitant use of cannabis and cocaine can greatly increase the heart rate.
- Concomitant use of cannabis and phencyclidine ("**supergrass**" or "**superweed**") produces an intensely vivid hallucinogenic experience.

Toxic Effects

I. **Acute**:

a. Euphoria with increased garrulity and hilarity, especially when smoked in a social group setting.

b. Temporal and spatial disorientation with intensification of sensation (colours become brighter, sounds become more distinct, music is heard with heightened fidelity) and increased clarity of perception.

c. At high doses, the user experiences hallucinations, sedation, and sometimes dysphoria characterized by unpleasant sensations, fear and panic.

d. Sometimes an acute toxic psychosis is precipitated with suicidal ideation, anxiety and paranoia. Occasionally, schizophrenic symptoms occur.

e. Stimulation of appetite.

f. Bloodshot eyes due to conjunctival congestion. Pupils are usually not affected.

g. Pulmonary irritation, including cough, sore throat, rhinitis and bronchitis may occur after inhalation.

h. Tachycardia, palpitations, hypotension (high doses).

i. Cannabis use has been associated with convulsions followed by cardiac arrest.

II. **Chronic Poisoning**:

a. **Amotivational Syndrome**: Chronic indulgence is said to induce an amotivational syndrome characterized by apathy, poor concentration, social withdrawal and lack of motivation to study or work. However, the actual existence of such a syndrome is being questioned by some investigators today who state that previous studies had not attempted to adequately distinguish between the effects of cannabis and pre-existing psychological status. In other words, it is difficult to determine which came first, the drug or the amotivation!

b. Heavy cannabis users demonstrate an increased tendency to develop manic, schizophreniform and confusional psychoses over a period of time.

c. **Cannabinoid hyperemesis syndrome**: Some patients with a long history (years) of cannabis abuse develop a cyclical pattern of hyperemesis occurring every few weeks or months. Patients often have a compulsion to have multiple hot showers or baths to provide symptomatic relief. Symptoms resolve with abstention from cannabis.

d. **Medical Complications**: Chronic heavy cannabis use is associated with an increased incidence of the following conditions:

i. Chronic lung disease and carcinogenesis.

ii. Cancers of mouth and larynx.

iii. Aspergillosis: Studies have shown that cannabis is often contaminated with Aspergillus spores which can cause aspergillosis in immunocompromised individuals.

Usual Fatal Dose

- There are no authentically documented cases of lethality from cannabis intoxication alone. The few cases of fatality that have been reported have not adequately ruled out the possibility of multiple-drug intoxication.
- In spite of such lack of documented fatalities, some authors have suggested that the fatal dose for IV cannabis is about 1–2 g, while it is 700 g for ingestion (of bhang).

Diagnosis

1. **Clinical**:

a. Symptomatology

b. Characteristic '**burnt rope**' odour in the breath of a recent smoker.

2. **Identification of suspected specimen**:

a. Suspend leaf or stem fragments in several drops of chloral hydrate (10%) on a microscope slide and examine under low power for characteristic "cystolith hairs." These hairs look like bear claws or elephant tusks.

b. At the base of these claws is a wart-like cluster composed of calcium carbonate deposit.

c. Add a drop of 20% HCl and note the gentle effervescent release of carbon dioxide gas in tiny bubbles.

3. **Urine levels of cannabinoids**:

a. Screening tests usually employ EMIT (Enzyme Multiplied Immunoassay Technique) or RIA (Radio Immunoassay), while confirmation is done by using GC–MS (Gas Chromatography–Mass Spectrometry).

b. THC is hydrophobic and accumulates in adipose tissue. Screening tests may be positive for up to 70 or more days, depending on the cut-off levels used and the individual's lipid stores of THC.

c. Some investigators state that after using three or more joints per day, an individual who then stops smoking cannabis completely, can still test positive for urinary THC for more than 2 months. An individual who smokes an occasional joint will test positive for 3–4 days.

Treatment

I. **Acute Poisoning**:

a. Decontamination measures in cases of ingestion.

b. Perform a 12-lead ECG in all patients who require assessment. Check cardiac rhythm, QRS duration and QT interval.

c. For agitation or delirium: Adults can be sedated with oral or IV diazepam. If agitation persists, consider oral or parenteral haloperidol. Midazolam is the most appropriate drug for managing agitation in children and young people.

d. Supportive measures.

II. **Chronic Poisoning**:

a. Psychosocial therapy consisting of attempts to promote realistic alternatives to the drug and associated life styles, along with a commitment to abstinence from psychotropic drugs.

b. A combination of interventions is recommended, including urine testing, participation in multi-step programmes, education about drug effects, drug counselling, psychotherapy and family therapy.
c. Short-term use of anxiolytic agents such as benzodiazepines may be necessary in some cases, when anxiety symptoms are severe.
d. Short-term use of antipsychotic medication may be required, if there are persistent delusional ideas or psychotic symptoms.

Medicosocial and Forensic Issues

- The mind-altering properties of cannabis probably did not receive wide attention until about 1000 BC when it became an integral part of Hindu culture in India. Cannabis is first referred to in Hindu Vedas between 2000 and 1400 BCE, in the *Atharvaveda*. Cannabis use eventually became a ritual part of the Hindu festival of Holi.
- After AD 500, cannabis began creeping westward, and references to it began appearing in Persian and Arabic literature.
- Cannabis was brought to Europe by Napoleon's soldiers returning from Egypt in the early part of 19th century.
- It made its entry into the USA at about 1920, when Mexican labourers smuggled the weed across the border into Texas. Today, in spite of all efforts at minimizing the abuse of cannabis, the drug is the most commonly used illicit substance in the USA.
- The use of cannabis among youth reached its peak in the 1960s, when the drug became associated with social protest. The **hippie generation** (**"flower people"**) (**Fig. 12.11**) was particularly fond of cannabis, to whom it was a "gateway drug" opening the doors to more potent "hard drugs" such as opiates and hallucinogens.
- In modern times, the **Rastafari movement** has embraced cannabis as a sacrament. It is a religious movement that considers cannabis to be the Eucharist, claiming it as an oral tradition from Ethiopia dating back to the time of Christ. Rastafarians tend to be among the biggest consumers of modern cannabis use (**Fig. 12.12**).
- Cannabis is frequently used among **Sufis** – the mystical interpretation of Islam that exerts strong influence over local Muslim practices in Bangladesh, India, Indonesia, Turkey and Pakistan. Cannabis preparations are frequently used at Sufi festivals in these countries.
- Recent reports of medical uses of cannabis have led to the resurgence of "**pot culture**" beginning with the 1990s. **Medical cannabis** refers to the physician-recommended use of cannabis, which is allowed in Canada, Belgium, Australia, the Netherlands, Spain and many US states.
- Several US states have **legalized** recreational use of cannabis.
- In December 2013, Uruguay became the first country to legalize growing, sale and use of cannabis. As drugs have increasingly come to be seen as a health issue instead of criminal behaviour, marijuana has also been legalized or decriminalized in Czech Republic, Colombia, Ecuador, Mexico, Portugal and Canada.

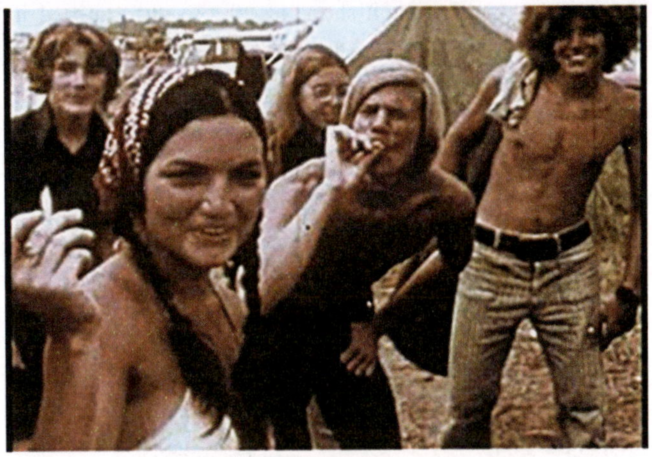

Fig. 12.11 Hippies smoking cannabis in the 1969 music festival – Woodstock (USA)

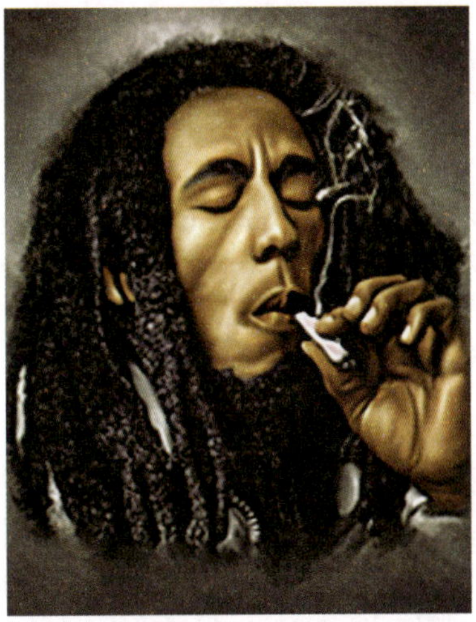

Fig. 12.12 Legendary reggae musician Bob Marley was a Rastafarian who regularly smoked cannabis

- Consumption of cannabis in various forms has always been popular in India. **Sanyasis** and **temple pujaris** use it to induce a trance-like state for the purpose of religious meditation. There are several festivals such as Holi and Shiva Ratri when widespread consumption occurs even among the general populace.
- Bhang is heavily consumed in Mathura, an ancient town of religious importance to the Hindus. But, the hub of bhang use is Varanasi (Banaras), where the bhang is prepared on its famous ghats. As bhang has served such an important role in India's culture and spiritual practices, it would be impossible to criminalize cannabis completely in the country. Cultivation of cannabis is government regulated, and illegal without a government permit. Sale of bhang is also government regulated and illegal without a permit. Those who get the permit can establish "Govt authorised" bhang

shops (**Fig. 12.13**)! Such shops are freely encountered in parts of Uttar Pradesh and Rajasthan.

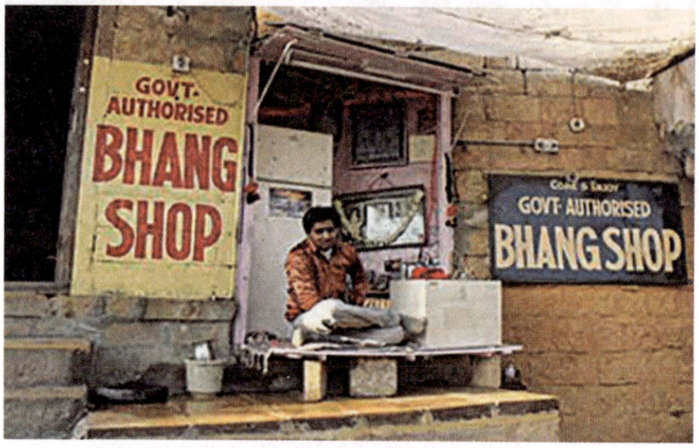

Fig. 12.13 A Govt authorised bhang shop in Jaisalmer, Rajasthan

- Bhang is no longer under the Prohibition Act in Gujarat from Feb 2017, hence its consumption has been decriminalized in Gujarat.
- While long-term cannabis use can cause serious health problems (*vide supra*), acute intoxication sometimes leads to medicolegal complications. The danger lies in the capacity of cannabis to interfere with motor skills and judgement. Operating a motor vehicle or other machinery under the influence of the drug could lead to potential loss of life or limb.
- Occasional acute psychotic reactions precipitated by long-term heavy cannabis use can cause the user to "**run amok**" in homicidal frenzy. This became well known during the Vietnam war when several American soldiers began suffering from acute toxic psychosis arising out of heavy abuse. Cannabis is also known to induce suicidal ideation brought on by anxiety and paranoia.

AMPHETAMINES

Source

- **Amphetamine** belongs to the phenethylamine family with a methyl group substitution in the alpha carbon position. It is actually the contracted form "alpha methylphenethylamine".
- **Amphetamine** is also the parent compound of its own structural class, the **substituted amphetamines**, which includes prominent substances such as bupropion, cathinone, MDMA and methamphetamine. Numerous substitutions of the phenethylamine structure are possible, resulting in several **amphetamine-like compounds**. These compounds have now collectively come to be known as "**amphetamines**." Slang terms are listed in **Table 12.2**.
- In the late 1980s, a pure preparation of **methamphetamine hydrochloride** made its appearance for the first time in Hawaii, where it was referred to as "**batu**." It quickly made its way across to the United Kingdom, Australia, Western Europe and USA, where it became popular by the slang name "**ice**" (or "**glass**") (**Fig. 12.14**).
  - While ice is produced by the ephedrine reduction method and is very pure, occurring as large translucent crystals, a variant produced by an oil-based method is called "**crystal**" (or "**crank**") (**Fig 12.15**), and is a white to yellow crystal product.
- Methamphetamine abuse began in the 1950s and reached a peak in the 1970s. It used to be referred to as "**speed**" or "**go**." The newer avatars "**ice**" and "**crystal**" are virtually the same in their pharmacological and toxic effects. Methamphetamine powder can be inhaled, smoked, ingested or injected. Ice and crystal are almost always smoked.

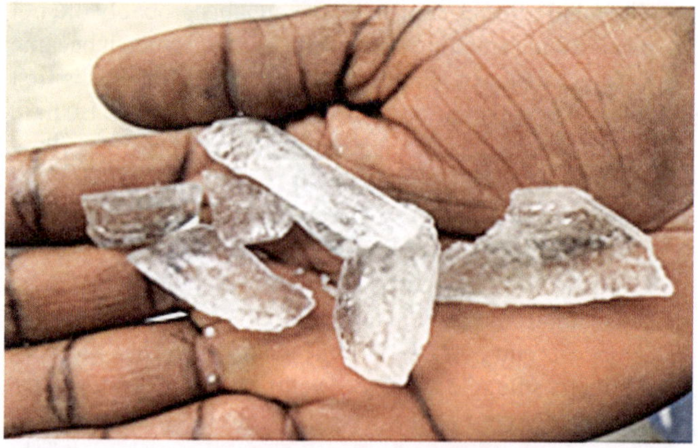

Fig. 12.14 Methamphetamine 'ice' crystals

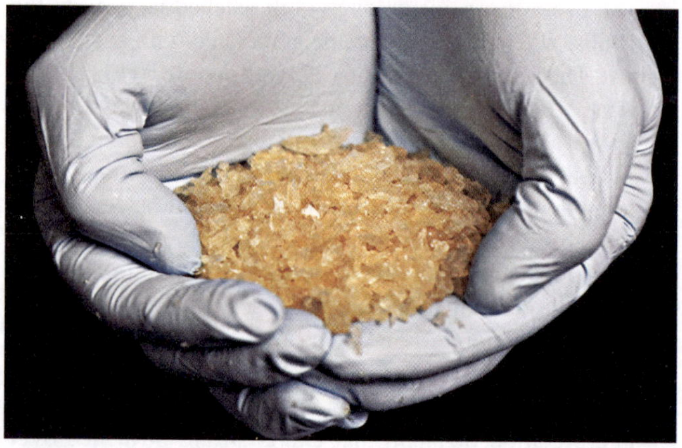

Fig. 12.15 Methamphetamine 'crank' crystals

Table 12.2 Slang names – Amphetamines

Aimies, Amphet, Bennies, Billy Whiz, Bumblebees, Clear Rocks, Crank, Croke, Glass, Ice, Mollies, Pep Pills, Pink Champagne, Rippers, Rocks, Speed, Splash, Wake Ups, Whizz

Uses

- Some amphetamines have therapeutic uses and are still available as prescription drugs in Western countries (**Table 12.3**).
- **Adderall** is a combination drug containing salts of the two enantiomers of amphetamine (levo- and dextroamphetamine). It is used in the treatment of attention deficit hyper-

activity disorder (ADHD) and narcolepsy. It is also used as an athletic performance enhancer and cognitive enhancer, and recreationally as an aphrodisiac and euphoriant.

Mode of Action

- The major mechanism of action of amphetamines involves the release of monoamines from storage sites in axon terminals, which leads to increased monoamine concentration in the synaptic cleft. The release of dopamine in the nucleus accumbens and related structures is responsible for the reinforcing and mood elevating effects of amphetamines.
- Cardiovascular effects result from the stimulation of release of noradrenaline.
- The effects of serotonin and dopamine at the mesolimbic system alter perception and induce psychotic manifestations.

Toxic Effects

I. **Acute Effects**:

a. *CNS*:
i. Euphoria
ii. Agitation
iii. Headache
iv. Paranoia
v. Anorexia
vi. Hyperthermia
vii. Hyper-reflexia
viii. Convulsions
ix. Intracerebral hemorrhage

b. *CVS:*
i. Tachycardia
ii. Hypertension
iii. Arrhythmias
iv. Myocardial ischaemia

c. *Sympathetic Effects:*
i. Mydriasis
ii. Sweating
iii. Tremor
iv. Tachypnoea

d. *Other Effects:*
i. Muscle rigidity
ii. Pulmonary oedema
iii. Rhabdomyolysis

e. *Complications:*
i. Psychosis
ii. Cerebral infarction
iii. Myocardial infarction
iv. Aortic dissection
v. Ventricular fibrillation
vi. Acute renal failure
vii. Serotonin syndrome may occur. Features of this syndrome include CNS effects (including agitation or coma), autonomic instability (including hyperpyrexia) and neuromuscular excitability (including clonus and raised serum creatine kinase).

II. **Chronic Effects**:

a. At low (therapeutic) doses, amphetamine produces modest improvements in cognition, including memory and attention. Amphetamine also improves task saliency (motivation to perform a task), and increases arousal (wakefulness), in turn promoting goal-directed behaviour.

b. Amphetamines can be taken orally, by injection, by absorption through nasal and buccal membranes; or by heating, inhalation of the vapours, and absorption through the pulmonary alveoli.

c. As with opiates, the rapid onset of effects from amphetamine injection or inhalation produces an intensely pleasurable sensation referred to as "***rush***."

d. Chronic users of amphetamines tend to fall into one or the other of the following categories:

i. *Intermittent low-dose misuse*: Some individuals (students studying for exams, military personnel on ex tended exercises, athletes, truck drivers on night trips,

Table 12.3 Therapeutic Uses of Amphetamines

Drug	Use
Amphetamine (*Benzedrine*)	Attention deficit hyperactivity disorder (ADHD), weight reduction
Dextroamphetamine (*Dexedrine*)	ADHD, narcolepsy
Methamphetamine (*Desoxyn*)	ADHD, weight reduction
Methylphenidate (*Ritalin*)	ADHD, narcolepsy
Fenfluramine (*Pondimin*)* Dexfenfluramine (*Redux*)*	Weight reduction
Phentermine (*Adipex-P, Fastin, Ionamin*) Chlorphentermine (*Pre-Sate*)*	Weight reduction
Mephentermine (*Wyamine*)	Hypotension
**Banned since 1997 in most countries.*	

etc.), consume amphetamines periodically to overcome fatigue, prolong wakefulness or elevate mood. They usually do not develop dependence.

ii. *Sustained misuse*: Some individuals who have been prescribed amphetamines for legitimate purposes, as well as some others who have been using these drugs illicitly may continue to ingest them in relatively large daily doses. Attempts to reduce the dose result in depression and lethargy.

iii. *High-dose abuse*: Individuals who relish the euphoria induced by amphetamines quickly progress to IV injections in order to enhance the "**rush**" or "**flash**." These individuals ("***speed freaks***") classically manifest the symptomatology of chronic amphetamine toxicity. They are also prone to "***speed binges***," wherein there are repeated cycles of action and reaction phases. The former is due to intake of the drug resulting in a "***high***," while the latter is due to stoppage, and is associated with acute hunger followed by intense depression or "***crash***." This provokes him to go on the action phase again, and the cycle continues until collapse or financial ruin.

e. **Manifestations of heavy chronic amphetamine use**:
   i. Hyperactivity, hyperexcitability.
   ii. Anorexia, loss of weight, emaciation.
   iii. Stereotyped behaviour (skin picking, pacing, interminable chattering).
   iv. Paranoid psychosis, unpredictable violence.
   v. Heightened sexual activity initially, followed by impotence and sexual dysfunction.
   vi. Occasionally, very rapid IV injection of a large dose produces a condition called "***overamped***," characterized by inability to speak or move even though consciousness is fully retained. Blood pressure and temperature are usually elevated.
   vii. Deterioration of *social* (family problems), *physical* (slovenly, unkempt appearance) and *economic* (loss of job, bankruptcy) status.
   viii. *Adverse psychological reactions*: Anxiety reactions, amphetamine psychosis, exhaustion syndrome, depression and hallucinosis.
   ix. *Medical complications*: Cardiomyopathy, pulmonary hypertension, neurological deficits, HIV infection, hepatitis, endocarditis, osteomyelitis.

Usual Fatal Dose

- The acute **lethal dose** of amphetamine in adults has been reported to be **20–25 mg/kg**, but individual response varies greatly due to tolerance, and toxicity correlates poorly with the amount taken.
- **Lethal blood level** is said to be around **0.2 mg per 100 ml**, though addicts can tolerate much higher levels with hardly any toxic effects.

Diagnosis

- Urine is the specimen of choice. Levels above 2 mg/100 mL indicate acute toxicity.
- Methods of analysis include TLC, RIA, HPLC and GC–MS. The last mentioned is the best.

Treatment

I. **Acute Poisoning**:

a. *Stabilization*:
   i. IV line, cardiac monitoring.
   ii. Oxygen
   iii. Monitor conscious level, pulse, blood pressure, cardiac rhythm and body temperature at least every 30 min.
   iv. Evaluate blood glucose, BUN and electrolyte levels.
   v. Perform a 12-lead ECG in all patients who require assessment. Check cardiac rhythm, QRS duration and QT interval.
   vi. Shock is a poor prognostic sign and needs to be managed effectively.
   vii. Consider oral activated charcoal (50 g for an adult, 1 g/kg for a child), if any amount of an amphetamine has been ingested within 1 hr, provided the airway can be protected.

b. *Supportive Measures*:
   i. Airway management, ventilatory support.
   ii. Rapid rehydration.
   iii. Mannitol diuresis promotes myoglobin clearance to prevent renal failure.
   iv. Assess psychological and neurological status.
   v. Gastric lavage (in cases of ingestion) with appropriate tracheal protection.

c. *Specific Measures*:
   i. For agitation or delirium: Adults can be sedated with oral or IV diazepam. If agitation persists, consider oral or parenteral haloperidol. Midazolam is the most appropriate drug for managing agitation in children and young people.
   ii. Convulsions: Control convulsions that are frequent or prolonged with IV diazepam, lorazepam or midazolam. If convulsions are unresponsive, second-line therapy is phenobarbitone sodium. An alternative is phenytoin. If convulsions persist, consider the need for referral to intensive care, general anaesthesia, intubation and ventilation. Thiopentone sodium is the preferred antiepileptic for status epilepticus not responding to the above measures.
   iii. Metabolic acidosis: If metabolic acidosis persists despite correction of hypoxia and adequate fluid resuscitation consider correction with IV sodium bicarbonate.
   iv. Hypertension:
      - Adults: Intravenous nitrates such as glyceryl trinitrate starting at 1–2 mg/hr and gradually increase the dose (max 12 mg/hr) until blood pressure is controlled. Calcium antagonists such as nifedipine, verapamil or diltiazem are an alternative as second line therapy. Sodium nitroprusside is an option for patients with hypertension

without any evidence of cardiac ischaemia, but may cause a rapid fall in blood pressure.

- Children: Consider oral/sublingual nifedipine or intravenous labetalol. Intravenous nitrates may also be used (glyceryl trinitrate 0.2 µg/kg/min).

v. Hyperthermia: Mild to moderate hyperthermia may respond to conventional cooling measures. When rising body temperature exceeds 39°C, core temperature monitoring should be considered (rectal probe) and urgent cooling measures should be employed according to local protocols.

- Cooling methods include:
    - Ice-baths.
    - Internal/invasive measures – cold fluid lavage (gastric, bladder, peritoneal), intravascular cooling techniques.
    - Ice packs to groin and axillae.
    - Mist and fan techniques.
- Dantrolene may be considered where there is muscular hyperactivity (1 mg/kg IV to a maximum of 10 mg/kg).

vi. Rhabdomyolysis: If rhabdomyolysis is present (CK activity > 5× the upper limit of the normal range), renal failure can develop particularly if the CK activity is >5000 IU/L. Give volume replacement as soon as possible and consider the need for urine alkalinization. Haemodiafiltration can effectively remove myoglobin from the circulation; haemodiafiltration combined with urine alkalinization is more effective than urine alkalinization alone.

II. **Chronic Poisoning**:

a. Cognitive behavioural treatment, making use of a combination of group and individual counselling.

b. Additionally, research suggests that daily aerobic exercise, especially endurance exercise (e.g., marathon run ning), prevents the development of drug addiction and is an effective adjunct therapy (i.e., a supplemental treatment) for amphetamine addiction.

c. A wide variety of pharmacological agents have been tried as adjuncts to the treatment of amphetamine dependence. These include imipramine and fluoxetine, but results have been disappointing.

DESIGNER DRUGS

- A **designer drug** is a structural or functional analogue of a banned substance that has been designed to mimic the pharmacological effects of the original drug, while avoiding classification as illegal, or detection in standard drug tests.
- Apart from **amphetamines**, there are several other groups of designer drugs (**Table 12.4**) which have been discussed in detail elsewhere.
- Designer drugs include psychoactive substances that have been designated by the European Union as **new psychoactive substances** (**NPS**) as well as analogues of performance-enhancing drugs such as **designer steroids**.
- Designer drugs are usually stronger and cheaper than the parent compound, and can be easily synthesized in clandestine laboratories.
- The term "designer drug" does not include new forms or new dosing routes of old drugs (e.g., cocaine used in freebase form, i.e., "crack"). It also does not include legal drugs which are abused (e.g., ephedrine, caffeine, phenylpropanolamine, etc.).
- The modern use of the term designer drug was coined in the 1980s to refer to various synthetic opioid drugs, based mostly on the fentanyl molecule (such as α-methylfentanyl). The term gained widespread popularity when MDMA ("ecstasy") experienced a popularity boom in the mid-1980s.
- The first true designer amphetamine to be developed was methylenedioxymethamphetamine (**MDMA** or **Ecstasy**), which was introduced by E Merck and Company in Germany in 1914. However, it was never marketed. It was only in the 1970s and early 1980s that it made its appearance as an "**underground drug**".* Since 1983, it has become in-

Table 12.4 Common Designer Drugs

Amphetamines	Opiate Derivatives	Methaqualone Derivatives	Arylhexyl-amines	Phenylethyl-amines
Methamphetamine (*Speed, Crystal, Ice*)	Fentanyl derivatives: α-Methylfentanyl (*China white*) Methylfentanyl	Mecloqualone	Phencyclidine	Mescaline
Methylenedioxy methamphetamine or MDMA (*Adam, Ecstasy, XTC, MDM*)	Pethidine derivatives: Methyl-phenyl-propionoxypiperidine or MPPP	Nitromethaqualone		
Methylenedioxyethamphetamine or MDA (*Love drug*)	Methyl-phenyl-tetrahydropyridine or MPTP			

***Note**: *Any drug of abuse that is not certified as having therapeutic uses by the Food and Drug Administration of USA is termed an "underground drug."*

creasingly popular among adolescents and college students as a recreational drug to be used during "**rave parties**" which are extended dance parties often lasting all night long (**Fig. 12.16**). The other designer amphetamines quickly followed and are mostly available as gelatin capsules or loose powder for ingestion. They have made their way into India in the late 1990s, and are quite openly abused by college students from affluent families.

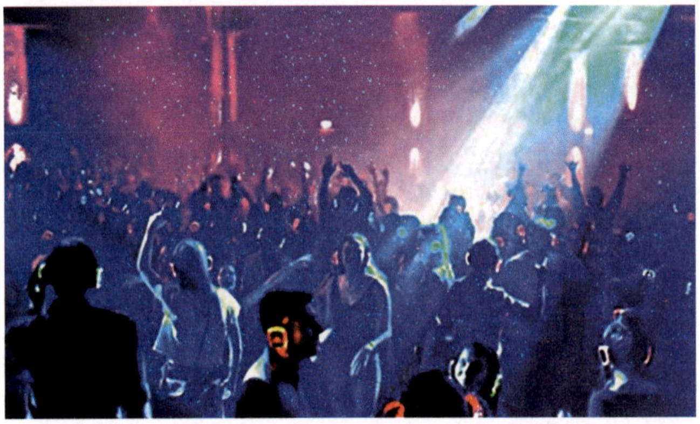

Fig. 12.16 Rave party in full swing (undisclosed location – India)

- In the late 1990s and early 2000s, there was a huge explosion in designer drugs being sold over the internet. Widespread discussion of consumptive use and the sources for the chemicals in public forums drew the attention of the media and authorities.
- The late 1990s and early 2000s also saw the first widespread use of novel **anabolic steroids** by athletes in competition. Steroids had been banned by the International Olympic Committee since 1976, but due to the large number of different anabolic agents available for human and veterinary use, the ability of laboratories to test for all available drugs had always lagged behind the ability of athletes to find new compounds to use. The introduction of increasingly formalised testing procedures, especially with the creation of the World Anti-Doping Agency in 1999, made it much more difficult for athletes to get away with using these drugs without detection, which then led to the synthesis of novel and potent anabolic steroid drugs such as **tetrahydrogestrinone (THG)**, which were not detectable by the standard tests.
- While through recent history most **designer drugs** had been either **opioids**, **hallucinogens** or **anabolic steroids**, the range of possible compounds is limited only by the scientific and patent literature, and recent years have been characterised by a broadening of the range of compounds sold as designer drugs. These have included:
  - **Designer stimulants** such as **geranamine**, **mephedrone**, **MDPV** and **desoxypipradrol**,
  - **Designer sedatives** such as **methylmethaqualone** and **premazepam** and
  - **Designer analogues** of **sildenafil** (Viagra), which have been reported as active compounds in "herbal" aphrodisiac products.
- **Designer cannabinoids** are another recent development, with two compounds JWH-018 and (C8)-CP 47,497 initially found in December 2008 as active components of "herbal smoking blends" sold as legal alternatives to marijuana, and subsequently a growing range of synthetic cannabinoid agonists have continued to appear, including by 2010 novel compounds such as RCS-4, RCS-8 and AB-001, which had never been reported in the literature, and appear to have been invented by designer drug manufacturers themselves.
- **Mephedrone** and the **cathinones** marked somewhat of a turning point for designer drugs, turning them from little known, ineffective substances to powerful substances able to compete with classical drugs on the black market. Mephedrone especially experienced a meteoric rise in popularity in 2009 and the resulting media panic resulted in its prohibition in multiple countries. Following this, there was a considerable emergence of other cathinones which attempted to mimic the effects of mephedrone, and with a newly attracted customer base, plenty of money to drive innovation.
- In the UK to avoid being controlled by the Medicines Act, designer drugs such as mephedrone have been described as "**plant food**," despite the compounds having no history of being used for these purposes. In the USA, similar descriptions ("**bath salts**" is the most common) have been used to describe mephedrone as well as methylone and methylenedioxypyrovalerone (MDPV).

This particular section will focus mainly on "designer amphetamines", while some of the other designer drugs will be discussed in subsequent sections (*see Index*).

- **Designer** or **Substituted amphetamines** are a class of compounds based upon the amphetamine structure; it includes all derivative compounds which are formed by replacing, or substituting, one or more hydrogen atoms in the amphetamine core structure with substituents.
- The compounds in this class span a variety of pharmacological subclasses, including stimulants, empathogens and hallucinogens, among others.
- Examples of substituted amphetamines include **methamphetamine**, **ephedrine**, **cathinone**, **methoxyphenamine**, **amfepramone**, **pyrovalerone**, **MDA**, **MDMA (ecstasy)**, **DOM (STP)**, etc.

Mode of Action

- While designer amphetamines share a number of properties with the original amphetamines, unlike the latter, they are potent releasers of serotonin. Chronic administration can result in permanent damage to serotonergic neurons.

Toxic Effects

- Designer amphetamines are abused by teenagers and young adults for inducing euphoria, facilitating intimacy and verbosity and heightening sexuality.

- Users of MDMA report that it "expands consciousness" without making them lose control. Sometimes these drugs are labelled "**entactogens**" for their alleged ability to increase sensitivity to touch, or "**empathicogens**," for their alleged ability to create empathy, especially before sexual encounters.
- MDMA is usually sold as 30–150 mg/dose (tablet or powder). There is current vogue for combining ecstasy with sildenafil to enhance sexual pleasure ("***sexstasy***").
- **Acute toxicity** results in nausea, anorexia, anxiety, hyperthermia, muscle rigidity, trismus, sinus tachycardia, sweating, tachypnoea, cardiac arrhythmias, metabolic acidosis, rhabdomyolysis, myoglobinuria and acute renal failure. The following have also been reported: hallucinations, paranoia, convulsions and fulminant hepatic failure.
- **Chronic use** results in anorexia, weight loss, exhaustion, jaundice, irritability, flashbacks, paranoia, depression or psychosis. However, since frequent use diminishes the pleasurable effects of these drugs, users often take them only at intervals of 2–3 weeks, and then gradually lose interest and stop intake altogether over a period of time.* There appear to be no reports of individuals who take excessive doses of these drugs frequently over an extended period of time.

Treatment

Treatment measures are essentially the same as for all amphetamine poisonings.

Medicosocial and Forensic Issues

- Amphetamines are the most widely used illicit drugs (second only to cannabis) in the United Kingdom, Australia and many parts of Europe. Significant abuse also occurs in the USA.
- After the introduction of amphetamines into clinical use in the early 1930s, they were available as prescription drugs for various indications (obesity, narcolepsy, attention deficit disorder, psychotherapy), and even sold over the counter in the form of nasal inhalers till the early 1970s. Since then their pharmaceutical use has been greatly curtailed, though many of these drugs are still available (under restriction) in Western countries. They are virtually banned in India.
- Japan experienced an epidemic of intravenous methamphetamine abuse in the years following the Second World War.
- Crystalline methamphetamine ("ice") was introduced in the 1980s in Hawaii, and quickly became popular in other countries.
- Today, designer amphetamines are a rage among adolescent party-goers, and are used extensively in the course of "**rave parties**." This fad has now gripped several metropolitan Indian cities, where tablets of Ecstasy are available freely among elite circles. Much of this popularity has to do with the copious amount of information existing on these drugs on the Internet, and the fact that unlike certain other drugs like heroin and cannabis, designer drugs are considered "hep" and "cool". Also, unlike many other hard drugs, designer drugs can be easily consumed (ingested) without the messiness of nasal insufflations, smoking or injection, and are often available as attractively shaped and coloured pills (**Fig. 12.17**).

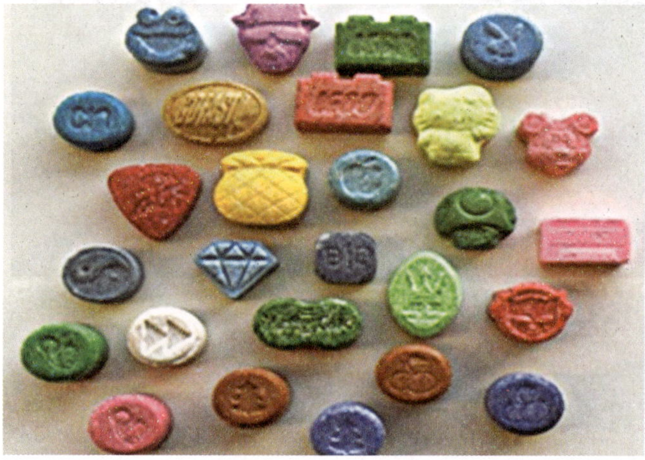

Fig. 12.17 Designer drug (Ecstasy) pills

COCAINE

Source

- Cocaine ("***coke***" or "***snow***") is a natural alkaloid present in the leaves of the coca plant, i.e., *Erythroxylum coca* or *Erythroxylum novogranatense* (**Fig. 12.18**), a shrub that grows well in South America, Mexico, Indonesia and West Indies.
- Chemically, cocaine is **benzoylmethylecgonine**, and belongs to the tropane family of natural alkaloids, other members of which include atropine and scopolamine.

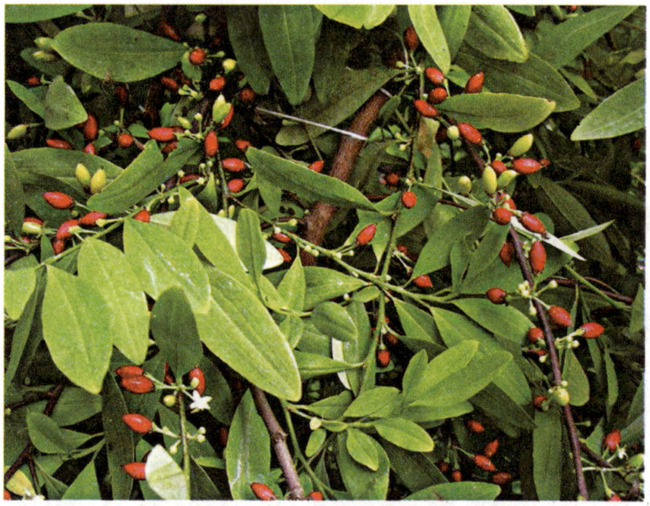

Fig. 12.18 *Erythroxylum novogranatense*

Note: *Freshmen love it, sophomores like it, juniors are ambivalent and seniors dislike it!*

- Cocaine occurs as colourless to white crystals, or white crystalline powder (**Fig. 12.19**).

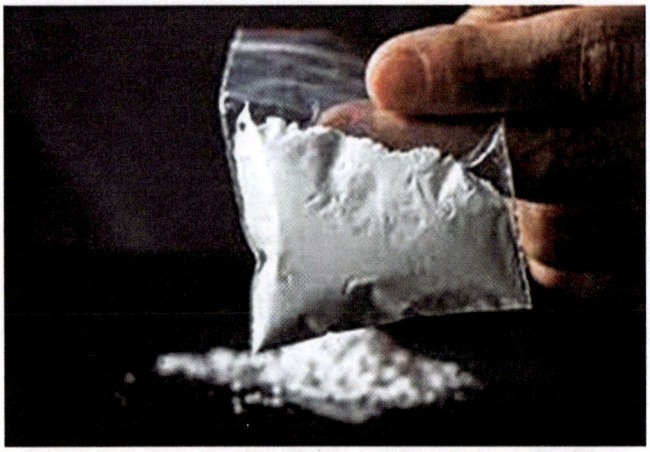

Fig. 12.19 Cocaine powder

Mode of Intake

- Cocaine is usually abused by either chewing coca leaves, smoking coca paste or "**snorting**" cocaine hydrochloride. The last mentioned is the most popular form of cocaine intake, i.e., the drug is inhaled in powder form through the nostrils (**Fig. 12.20**).
- Occasionally, cocaine hydrochloride is injected intravenously. Today, a **smokable form** of cocaine ("***crack***" or "***rock***") has virtually become a rage in the West.
- Pure alkaloidal cocaine ("***free-base***" or "***baseball***") can also be smoked.
- Occasionally, coca paste or cocaine sulphate ("***pasta***", "***bazooka***") is smoked.

  Street cocaine is often impure. The content of pure cocaine ranges from 10% to 50% (most commonly 15–20%). Cocaine which is available on the street is often adulterated with one or more of the following compounds: talc, lactose, sucrose, glucose, mannitol, inositol, caffeine, procaine, lignocaine, strychnine, amphetamine or heroin ("***speed ball***").

Uses

1. Topical anaesthetic (4–10% solution) for intranasal and bronchoscopic procedures.

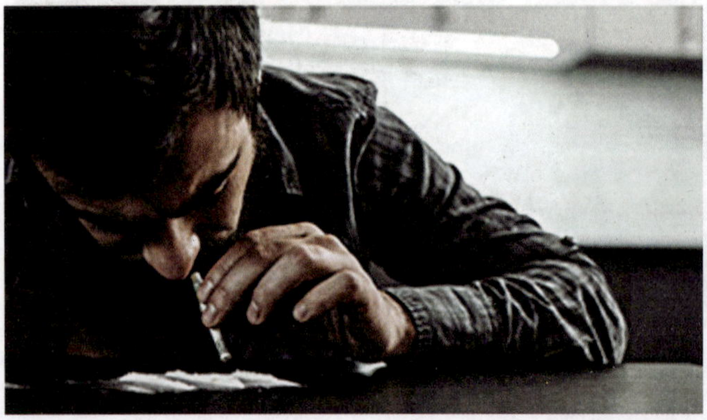

Fig. 12.20 Snorting cocaine

2. Ophthalmologic anaesthesia.
3. Relief of severe (oncologic) pain: Cocaine is one component of **Brompton's cocktail** (the others being morphine, chlorpromazine, and alcohol), which was previously popular in Europe for the control of intractable pain associated with some forms of cancer.
4. Cocaine is one of the components of **TAC** (the others being **tetracaine** and **adrenaline**) which is sometimes used as a topical anaesthetic in children with scalp and facial lacerations.

Mode of Action

1. *CNS*:
   a. **Cocaine is the most powerful (naturally derived) CNS stimulant known to man**. Stimulation of the brain occurs in a rostral-to-caudal fashion. The cortex is stimulated first resulting in excitement, restlessness and increased motor activity. Subsequent stimulation of lower motor centres produces tonic-clonic convulsions. The medulla is at first stimulated resulting in an initial increased respiratory rate, followed by depression with resultant respiratory failure.
   b. The CNS stimulant effects of cocaine are mediated through inhibition of dopamine reuptake in the nucleus accumbens.
   c. Cocaine also increases the concentrations of the excitatory amino acids, aspartate and glutamate in the nucleus accumbens. These excitatory amino acids increase the extracellular concentrations of dopamine.
   d. Cocaine also inhibits reuptake of noradrenaline and serotonin. Increase in the concentrations of the former plays an important role in the toxic effects of cocaine.
2. *Peripheral nerves*: Through direct blockade of fast sodium channels, cocaine stabilizes the axonal membrane, producing a local anaesthetic effect. Cocaine is the only local anaesthetic that interferes with the uptake of neurotransmitter by the nerve terminals and simultaneously functions as a vasoconstrictor.
3. *CVS*:
   a. Tachycardia is a prominent effect resulting from central sympathetic stimulation.
   b. The cardiostimulatory effect of cocaine is due in large part to sensitization to adrenaline and noradrenaline, preventing neuronal reuptake of these catecholamines, as well as due to increased release of noradrenaline from adrenergic nerve terminals. The increased concentrations and persistence of catecholamines near the receptors of the effecter organ lead to exaggerated sympathetic effects.

Toxicokinetics

- *Absorption*:
  - Ingestion and insufflation: Cocaine is well absorbed from oral, nasal and pulmonary routes. Onset of action on insufflation is within 1–3 min, and peak effects are seen in 20–30 min.

- Intravenous injection: Onset of action is within seconds, and peak action occurs in 3–5 min.
- Inhalation: Smoking produces effects as rapidly as IV injection.

- *Metabolism*:
  - Cocaine is metabolized by liver esterases and plasma cholinesterase to ecgonine methylester (EME), one of the major metabolites, while non-enzymatic hydrolysis results in the formation of the other major metabolite, benzoylecgonine (BE).
- *Excretion*:
  - Excretion is mainly through urine. Due to the long elimination half-life of BE, assays for its detection in urine may be successful up to 2–3 days following cocaine use.

Clinical Features

1. **Acute Poisoning**
   a. *Hyperthermia*: Body temperature often soars to 108–112°F, and does not respond to conventional antipyretics. It is often associated with rhabdomyolysis, seizures and renal failure.
   b. *CNS effects*:
      i. Headache.
      ii. Anxiety, agitation.
      iii. Hyperactivity, restlessness.
      iv. Tremor, hyperreflexia.
      v. Convulsions: Seizures may be recurrent and status epilepticus has been reported, particularly in children. Sometimes, there is lethargy and decreased level of consciousness which can persist up to 24 hrs ("***cocaine washed out syndrome***").
      vi. Cerebrovascular accidents are not uncommon, and include subarachnoid haemorrhage, intracerebral haemorrhage, cerebral infarction, etc.
   c. *Psychiatric effects*:
      i. Paranoia
      ii. Stereotypy
      iii. Hallucinations
      iv. Toxic delirium
   d. *Ophthalmologic effects*:
      i. Mydriasis.
      ii. Corneal abrasions/ulcerations due to particulate matter in smoke ("***crack eye***").
      iii. Central retinal artery occlusion and bilateral blindness due to diffuse vasospasm.
   e. *CVS effects*:
      i. Tachycardia
      ii. Hypertension
      iii. Coronary artery vasoconstriction with myocardial ischaemia and infarction.
      iv. Tachyarrhythmias of all types can occur, including sinus tachycardia, atrial fibrillation or flutter, torsades de pointes and ventricular fibrillation.
      v. Chronic cardiomyopathy can occur.
      vi. Aortic dissection and rupture.
   f. *Pulmonary effects*:
      i. Thermal injuries to the upper airway leading to epiglottitis, laryngeal injury and mucosal necrosis have been reported after smoking "crack" or free base cocaine.
      ii. Exacerbation of asthma.
      iii. Non-cardiogenic pulmonary oedema.
      iv. Pneumothorax, pneumomediastinum.
      v. Diffuse alveolar haemorrhage.
   g. *Musculoskeletal effects*: Rhabdomyolysis with hyperthermia, massive elevation of creatine phosphokinase and acute renal failure.
   h. *GI effects*:
      i. Colitis
      ii. Intestinal perforation: It is postulated that cocaine blocks the reuptake of noradrenaline leading to mesenteric vasoconstriction and focal tissue ischaemia and perforation.
      iii. Pneumoperitoneum has been reported after smoking crack cocaine.
      iv. Hepatic necrosis has been reported in overdose.
   i. *Renal effects*: Renal failure, usually secondary to myoglobinuria and rhabdomyolysis, has been reported after intravenous or intranasal cocaine use.
   j. *Uteroplacental effects*:
      i. Increased incidence of spontaneous abortion, low birthweight and abruptio placentae. Neonatal intoxication may also occur.
      ii. There are indications that cocaine may be teratogenic.
   k. *Miscellaneous effects*:
      i. Priapism has been observed after topical application of cocaine to the glans penis.
      ii. Severe metabolic acidosis has been reported due to seizures, agitation and hypotension.
   l. *Drug combination effects*:
      i. Cocaine is often combined with other drugs such as ethanol and heroin. Concurrent use of cocaine and ethanol produces additive effects on the brain. It results in the formation of the metabolite, **cocaethylene** which is more cardiotoxic, and is associated with enhanced mortality.
      ii. Combination of cocaine with heroin is referred to as "***speed ball***" and is reputed to produce a double effect of initial high "*kick*" of cocaine, followed by subsequent euphoric "*rush*" of heroin. "***Speed ball***" is usually injected.
2. **Chronic Poisoning**
   a. *Cocaine abuse*:
      i. Anorexia, emaciation.
      ii. Mydriasis.
      iii. Agitation, restlessness: A cocaine-associated ***agitated delirium syndrome*** has been identified, comprising the following in sequence: hyperthermia, delirium with agitation, respiratory arrest and death.

iv. Hallucinations, especially tactile, characterized by a crawling sensation under the skin or a feeling of ants crawling all over the skin ("***cocaine bug***" or "***formication***") (**Fig. 12.21**) with resultant excoriation, leading to irregular scratches and ulcers (***Magnan's sign***).
v. Tremor.
vi. Recurrent chest pain.
vii. Cardiomyopathy.
viii. *Psychiatric changes*: Psychosis, panic disorders, attention deficit disorders and eating disorders.
ix. Decreased libido, impotence, gynaecomastia, amenorrhoea and sexual dysfunction are common with chronic cocaine abuse.
x. "***Crack hands***": A syndrome of multiple, blackened, hyperkeratotic lesions of the fingers and palms has been described in crack cocaine smokers.

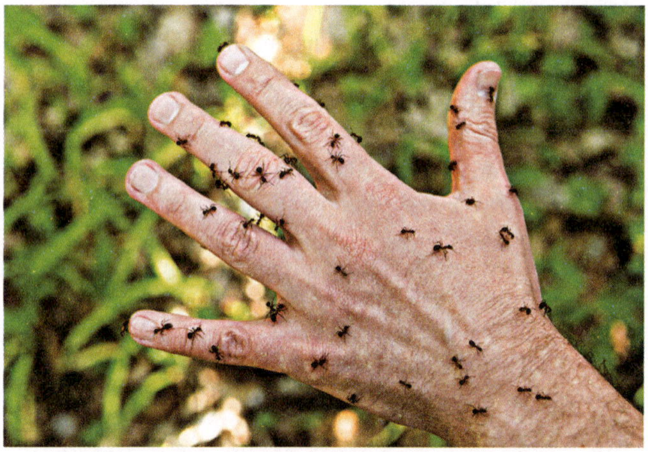

Fig. 12.21 Sensation of ants crawling over the skin ("formication") in cocaine addiction

xi. Maternal chronic cocaine use during pregnancy has been suggested as a possible factor in Sudden Infant Death Syndrome. Cocaine readily passes into breast milk and can cause adverse effects in the nursing infant.
xii. Evidence of medical complications (**Table 12.5**).

b. ***Cocaine withdrawal***: Conventionally, cocaine withdrawal is said to occur in three phases:
i. *Phase I* ("Crash"): 9 hrs to 4 days.
   - Early: Agitation, depression, anorexia, intense craving for cocaine.
   - Intermediate: Fatigue, tendency to sleep, decreased craving.
   - Late: Exhaustion, hypersomnia, hyperphagia, absence of craving.
ii. *Phase II*: Normalized sleep, improved mood, followed subsequently by return of anxiety and increased craving.
iii. *Phase III* ("Extinction"): Increased tendency to relapse.
iv. Additional points of importance:
   - Impaired colour vision (blue-yellow), which may persist for up to 2 months or more, has been reported in some patients with cocaine withdrawal.
   - Silent ischaemia has occurred upon cocaine withdrawal, and acute myocardial infarction may occur up to 2 weeks after the last cocaine use.
   - ECG changes: Increased PR intervals have been found to correlate with length of absti

Table 12.5 Medical Complications of Cocaine

CNS – Convulsions, "sympathomimetic storm," migraine headaches, cerebral infarction, intracranial haemorrhages
CVS – Hypertension, cardiac arrhythmias, myocardial infarction, cardiomyopathies, myocarditis, endocarditis, aortic rupture
RS – Alveolar haemorrhage, ARDS, pneumomediastinum, pneumothorax
GI – Mesenteric ischaemia, malnutrition
ENT – Rhinitis, nasal septal necrosis, sinusitis, laryngitis
Metabolic – Hyperthermia, hypoglycaemia, lactic acidosis, hypo/hyperkalaemia
Renal – Rhabdomyolysis-induced renal failure
Psychiatric – Paranoia, violent behaviour
Obstetric & Paediatric – Abruptio placentae, abortion, prematurity
Infections (*IV use*) – Hepatitis B, AIDS, endocarditis

nence, which is thought to reflect the remediation of a depolarization variant.
- Persistently elevated serum creatine kinase (CPK) levels have been demonstrated in abstinent cocaine abusers.

Usual Fatal Dose

- **500 mg (*oral*)**
- **100 mg (*mucosal contact*)**
- **Lethal blood level: 0.2 mg/100 mL**

Chronic users of cocaine can tolerate much higher doses.

Diagnosis

1. Blood or plasma cocaine levels are not clinically useful, although they may be advisable to be done in medicolegal cases. Qualitative urine tests using kits may be helpful in clinical diagnosis (by utilizing chromatography, radioimmunoassay, enzyme immunoassay, fluorescence polarization immunoassay and enzyme-multiplied immunoassay technique). Cocaine metabolites can be identified in the urine and provide a method for qualitatively identifying suspected cocaine poisoning or abuse.
2. Benzoylecgonine, the major metabolite of cocaine, can usually be detected in urine for 48–72 hrs after cocaine use.

Treatment

1. **Acute Poisoning**:
   Activated charcoal adsorbs cocaine in vitro under both acidic and alkaline conditions, and can be administered in cases of ingestion.
   a. *Hyperthermia*:
      i. Minimize physical activity and sedate with benzodiazepines.
      ii. Ice baths, packs, cool water with fans, etc.
      iii. Severe, intractable cases may respond to dantrolene (1 mg/kg) every 6 hrs. Alternatively, bromocriptine can be administered orally in a nasogastric tube.
   b. *Anxiety and agitation*:
      i. Diazepam 5–10 mg IV, or lorazepam 2–4 mg IV titrated to effect.
      ii. Antipsychotics such as haloperidol or droperidol, and phenothiazines are not recommended, since they can induce malignant hyperthermia and convulsions.
   c. *Convulsions*:
      i. Diazepam 5–10 mg IV, or lorazepam 2–4 mg IV titrated to effect.
      ii. Phenobarbitone 25–50 mg/min up to 10–20 mg/kg.
      iii. If seizures are not controlled by the above measures, consider continuous infusion of midazolam or propofol.
      iv. Intractable convulsions may require neuromuscular paralysis with intubation and mechanical ventilation.
   d. *Cerebrovascular accidents*: Neurosurgical consultation is mandatory.
   e. *Hypertension*:
      i. Without tachycardia:
         - Nifedipine 0.1–0.2 mg/kg IV
         - Nitroprusside 2–10 μg/kg/min IV
      ii. With tachycardia:
         - Labetolol 10–20 mg IV.
         - Nitroglycerine IV titrated to effect.
      iii. With chest pain:
         - Nitroglycerine drip.
         - If pain does not respond to nitroglycerine, use morphine (2 mg IV titrated to pain relief).
         - Obtain ECG.
         - If chest pain is strongly suggestive of a myocardial infarction, consider thrombolytic therapy.
   f. *Arrhythmias*:
      i. Sinus tachycardia: Diazepam 5–10 mg IV, or lorazepam 2–4 mg IV titrated to effect.
      ii. Supraventricular tachycardia: Diltiazem 20 mg IV, or verapamil 5 mg IV. Cardioversion (if necessary).
      iii. Ventricular arrhythmias: Obtain an ECG, institute continuous cardiac monitoring and administer oxygen.
         - Hypertonic sodium bicarbonate
         - Diazepam 5 mg IV, or lorazepam 2–4 mg IV.
         - Defibrillation (if haemodynamically unstable).
   g. *Myocardial infarction*: Acute myocardial infarction due to cocaine toxicity must be treated on the same lines as myocardial infarction in non-cocaine users, except for the use of beta blockers. Administer sublingual nitroglycerine or nifedipine 10 mg orally. For life-threatening arrhythmias, use of type IA antiarrhythmic agents may be considered. Thrombolytic therapy may be necessary if myocardial infarction is not amenable to relief by nitrates, calcium channel blockers or phentolamine.
   h. *Aortic dissection*: The hypertension that precipitated aortic dissection must be controlled immediately with nitroprusside and calcium channel blockers.
      i. Pulmonary oedema:
      i. Frusemide 20–40 mg IV.
      ii. Monitor fluids with pulmonary artery catheter.
   j. *Rhabdomyolysis*: Diuretics such as mannitol or furosemide may be needed to maintain urine output. Urinary alkalinization is not routinely recommended.
      i. Cardiac monitoring.
      ii. Serial potassium determinations.
      iii. Serial serum creatine kinase and urine myoglobin studies.
      iv. IV hydration (urine output must be maintained at 3 mL/kg/hr).
   k. *Acidosis*: Correction of acidaemia through supportive care measures such as hyperventilation, sedation, active cooling and sodium bicarbonate infusion.
   l. *Elimination enhancement measures*: Cocaine is rapidly metabolized. Forced diuresis, urine acidification, dialysis and haemoperfusion are ineffective in significantly altering elimination.
2. **Chronic Poisoning**:
   a. *Psychotherapy*: This involves cognitive-behavioural, psychodynamic and general supportive techniques.

b. *Group psychotherapy*: Interpersonal group therapy focuses on relationships, and uses the group interactions to illustrate the interpersonal causes of individual distress, and to offer alternative behaviours.

c. *Group counselling*: The most widely used form of psychosocial treatment for cocaine dependence is group counselling, in which the group is open-ended with rolling admissions; the group leaders are drug counsellors, many of whom are recovering from addiction, and the emphasis is on providing a supportive atmosphere, discussing problems in recovery and encouraging participation in multistep programmes.

d. *Pharmacotherapy*:

   i. Several drugs have been tried to help ameliorate the manifestations of cocaine withdrawal. Many of these have either not demonstrated clinical efficacy, or have produced serious side effects.

   ii. Bromocriptine has successfully reduced cocaine craving and decreased withdrawal symptoms in several studies.

   iii. Amantadine, a dopamimetic agent, increases dopaminergic transmission and has been found to be useful in the treatment of early withdrawal symptoms and short-term abstinence.

   iv. Carbamazepine has benefited some patients.

3. **Bodypacker Syndrome**:

   The practice of swallowing balloons, condoms or plastic packets filled with illegal drugs for the purpose of smuggling is called "**body packing**" (**Fig. 12.22**) and the individual who does this is referred to as a "**mule**." This must be differentiated from "**body stuffing**" in which an individual who is on the verge of being arrested for possession of illegal drugs, swallows his illicit contraband to conceal the evidence. Leaking from these poorly wrapped packets can produce cocaine toxicity. Sudden death due to massive overdose can occur in either a bodypacker or a bodystuffer, if one or more of the ingested packages burst within the gastrointestinal tract. Fatal cocaine poisoning has occurred with the rupture of just a single package.

   a. *Diagnosis*:

      i. X-ray: Plain films of the abdomen in the supine and upright positions. Radiography may not detect cellophane-wrapped packets or crack vials. Even false-negative abdominal CT scans have been reported. It is therefore advisable to perform a contrast study of the bowel with follow-up X-rays, 5 hrs after the oral ingestion of a water-soluble contrast compound such as meglumine amidotrizoate (50 mL). Daily views are performed thereafter until negative views coincide with the passage of two drug packet-free stools.

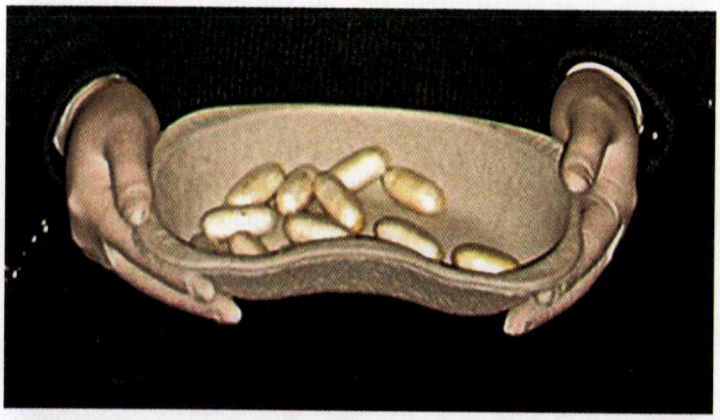

Fig. 12.22 Cocaine packets recovered from a bodypacker

   b. *Treatment*:

      i. Lavage, charcoal, as applicable.

      ii. Cathartic/whole bowel irrigation to flush the packages out of the intestines.

      iii. Symptomatic patients should be considered a medical emergency, and be evaluated for surgical removal of the packets.

      iv. Asymptomatic patients should be monitored in an intensive care unit until the cocaine packs have been eliminated. This must be confirmed by follow-up plain radiography and barium swallows.

      v. Bowel obstruction in asymptomatic patients may necessitate surgery. Endoscopic removal has been successful in some cases.

Autopsy Features

1. There are no specific findings at autopsy, except for **nasal septal ulceration and perforation**, if the deceased had been a long-term abuser of cocaine. Histological study of nasal septal mucosa in such cases may reveal characteristic changes including arteriolar thickening, increased perivascular deposition of collagen and glycoprotein and chronic inflammatory cellular infiltration.
2. Histopathology of heart may demonstrate microfocal lymphocytic infiltrates, acute coronary thrombosis, early coagulation necrosis of myocardial fibres and non-atherosclerotic coronary obstruction due to intimal proliferation.
3. Cocaine can be recovered by sampling from recent injection sites, or by **swabs from the nasal mucosa**. It can also be recovered from the liver and especially brain, where cocaine may be found not only in dopamine-rich areas such as caudate, putamen and nucleus accumbens, but also in other extra-striatal regions. Specimens obtained postmortem should be preserved with sodium fluoride, refrigerated and analyzed quickly. Tissue specimens should be frozen.

Forensic Issues

- Cocaine has been abused for centuries, but its toxic properties have been studied extensively only in the last couple of decades. In the current drug subculture, cocaine has become the "***champagne drug***" because of its cost and relative scarcity. Cocaine is a "rich man's drug" since the poorer classes cannot afford to sustain a drug habit that costs thousands of rupees every week. Therefore in India, cocaine abuse is restricted mainly to the affluent classes of society. The prevalence and extent of the problem among newer generation Indian film actors in recent times has become apparent with the arrest of several film stars for possession of cocaine. Several high-profile artists, socialites and even politicians have been caught with cocaine possession, beginning with the case of Bollywood actor **Fardeen Khan** (**Fig. 12.23**) in 2001. Khan was arrested late at night on 05 May near an ATM in Juhu, Mumbai, along with a drug peddler who had 9 g cocaine in his possession. As the actor successfully argued in court that he was in the act of purchasing only 1 g of the drug, which attracts only probation and not imprisonment, under Sec 27 of the NDPS Act, he was let off with a direction to undergo rehabilitation!

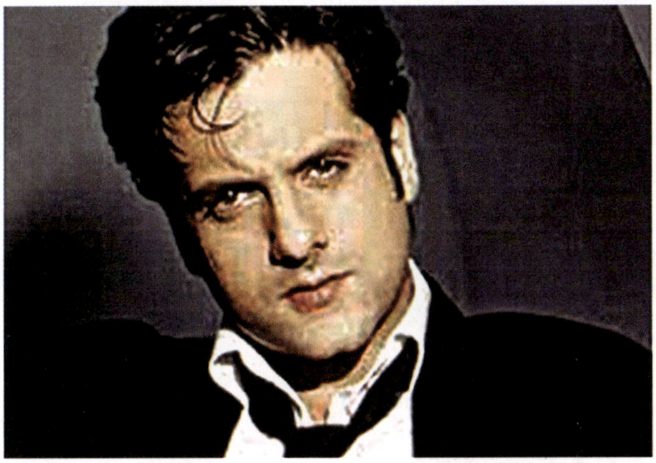

Fig. 12.23 Fardeen Khan

- Cocaine has always been popular with musicians (especially jazz and rock), other artistes and film personalities. There are innumerable rock songs eulogising the drug directly or indirectly. One of the most infamous examples is a hugely popular rock song titled "Cocaine" which was originally written and sung by JJ Cale, but was popularized by **Eric Clapton** (**Fig. 12.24**) who claimed that the song is actually against the use of cocaine, if one examined the lyrics closely!
- Today cocaine has made inroads into the general population, especially adolescents. After the cocaine epidemic of the 1970s ("***snorting seventies***") in the West, there had been a relative lull in the 1980s and early 1990s. A recent survey shows the cocaine resurgence of the 21st century has not only affected Western countries, but even poorer countries such as India. In fact a sizeable chunk of youth (including girls) from well-to-do families in metropolitan cities such as Mumbai, Delhi and Bangalore have no qualms about drug abuse, and even openly admit to using "party drugs" such as cocaine as a "cool" mode of recreation. Since cocaine has a reputation of enhancing sexual pleasure, such widespread abuse has also led to increased spread of sexually transmitted diseases such as AIDS because of high-risk sexual practices among the users.
- Cocaine abuse by pregnant mothers can lead to devastating effects on the foetus and the newborn (**Table 12.6**). There is convincing evidence that cocaine is teratogenic and can play an important role in the causation of several serious congenital anomalies (**Table 12.7**).

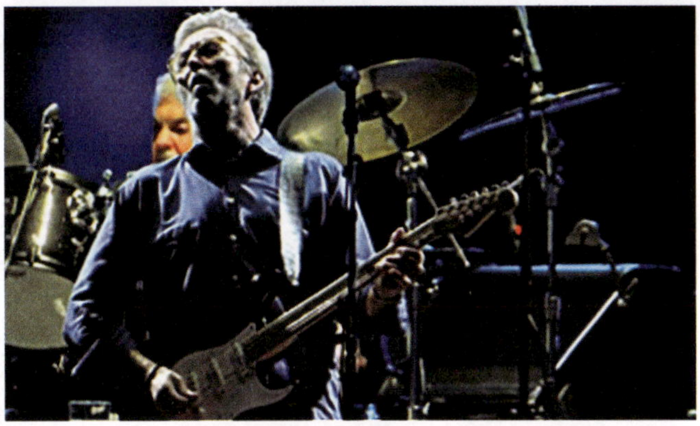

Fig. 12.24 Eric Clapton playing "Cocaine" in 2015 at Royal Albert Hall, London

- Cocaine abuse is well known for its propensity to cause sudden death not only due to its deleterious effects on health (cerebrovascular accidents, myocardial infarction, malignant hyperthermia, renal failure), but also due to its capacity to provoke the user to commit acts of aggression and violence.
- Deaths due to massive overdose are especially common among those who smuggle the drug within their bodies ("**cocaine packers**") (**Fig. 12.25**).

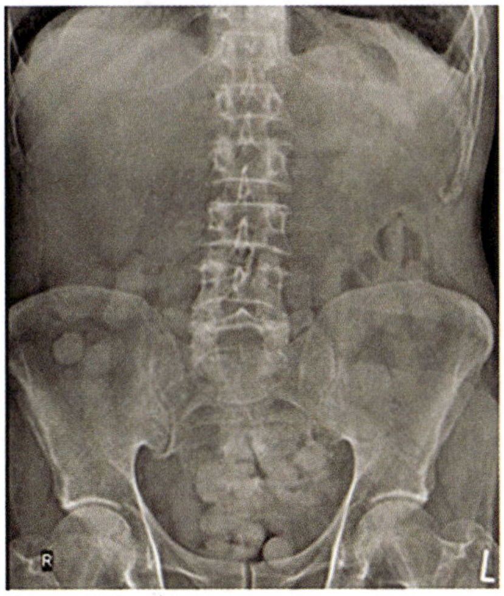

Fig. 12.25 X-ray showing multiple packets of cocaine in a "cocaine packer"

Table 12.6 Complications of Cocaine Abuse during Pregnancy

- Spontaneous abortion
- Placenta praevia
- Abruptio placentae
- Prematurity
- Placental infarction
- Intrauterine growth retardation
- Low birth weight
- Congenital anomalies
- Foetal death

Table 12.7 Some Teratogenic Effects of Cocaine

Body Area	Anomaly
Cranio-spinal	Exencephaly, hydrocephaly, encephalocoele, myelomeningocoele
Facial	Cleft lip, cleft palate, ptosis, cutis aplasia
CVS	Atrial septal defect, ventricular septal defect, transposition of great vessels, pulmonary artery stenosis, cardiomegaly
GI and GU tracts	Ileal atresia, inguinal hernia, renal agenesis, multicystic kidneys, hydronephrosis, hypospadias, hydrocoele, undescended testis
Extremities	Phocomelia, polydactyly, syndactyly

HALLUCINOGENS

Definition

- **Hallucinogens are substances that induce changes in thought, perception and mood, without causing major disturbances in the autonomic nervous system.**
- Perceptual alterations can take the form of illusions, synaesthesias or hallucinations.
  - ***Illusions*** are the result of misinterpretation of an actual experience.
  - ***Synaesthesias*** are sensory misperceptions (e.g., hearing colour or seeing sounds). Both require external stimuli for their institution.
  - ***Hallucinations**** differ from them in this important respect, since they are perceptual alterations without any external stimulation whatsoever.
  - Hallucinations may be **visual**, **auditory**, **olfactory**, **gustatory** or **tactile** in nature. Most hallucinogens induce visual or auditory hallucinations; a few cause tactile or olfactory manifestations.
  - While a number of therapeutic drugs can cause hallucinations in overdose, they are not classified as hallucinogens. A true hallucinogen is a drug that induces hallucinations in small doses (sometimes, as in the case of LSD, in microgram doses).
    - **Hollister's criteria** for establishing that a drug is hallucinogenic are as follows:
      - In proportion to other effects, changes in thought, perception and mood should predominate.
      - Intellectual or memory impairment should be minimal.
      - Stupor, narcosis or excessive stimulation should not be an integral effect.
      - Autonomic nervous system side effects should be minimal.
      - Addictive craving should be absent.
      - Most genuine hallucinogens cause vivid visual hallucinations, while the other types of hallucinations are relatively uncommon.

Classification

1. **Psychedelics**:
   a. ***5-HT receptor agonists***:
      i. *Tryptamines*:
         - Lysergic acid diethylamide (LSD)
         - Dimethyltryptamine (DMT)
         - Psilocin, psilocybin
      ii. *Phenethylamines*:
         - Methamphetamine
         - Cathinone
         - Mescaline
   b. ***Serotonin releasing agents***:
      - Methylene deoxy amphetamine (MDA)
      - Methylene deoxy methamphetamine (MDMA)
   c. ***Cannabinoids***:
      - Tetrahydrocannabinol (THC)
2. **Dissociatives**:
   a. ***NMDA receptor antagonists***:
      - Ketamine
      - Dextromethorphan (DXM)
      - Phencyclidine (PCP)
   b. ***Opioid receptor agonists***:
      - Morphine
      - Pentazocine
      - Salvinorin-A
3. **Deliriants**:
   a. ***Anticholinergics***:
      - Datura alkaloids

Lysergic Acid Diethylamide (LSD)

Source

- Lysergic acid diethylamide (LSD)** is the synthetic derivative of **ergot alkaloids**, and was originally synthesized exclusively from these alkaloids produced by the fungus *Claviceps purpurea* (**Fig. 12.26**), which is a contaminant of **rye** and certain other grains.
- Today, most LSD is synthesized entirely in the laboratory, and typically sold to addicts as liquid-impregnated blot-

****Note***: *Derived from Latin "allucinari" which means to "wander in mind."*
*****Note***: *LSD actually stands for the drug's German name: Lyserge Saure Diethylamid.*

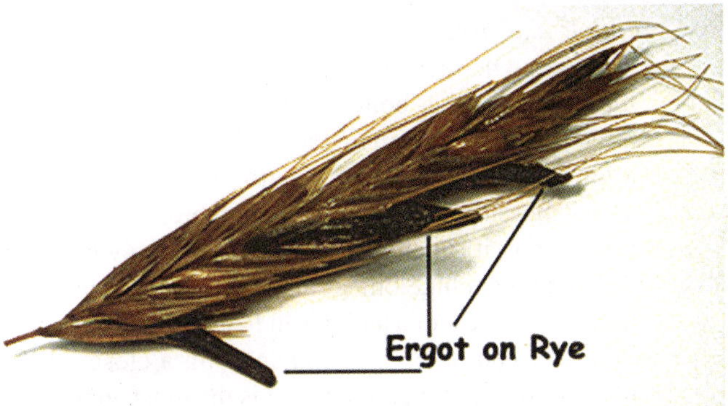

Fig. 12.26 Rye infested with *Claviceps purpurea*

ting paper or sugar cubes, tiny tablets ("*microdots*"), gelatin squares ("*window panes*"), liquid or powder.

- **Table 12.8** lists common slang names.

Table 12.8 Slang Names – LSD

LSD, Acid, Blotter Acid, Blue drops, Dome dots, Domes, Dots, LSD, Lucy, Microdot, Paper acid, Strawberry, Sunshine, White lightning, Windowpane, Yellow drops

Mode of Intake

- LSD is almost always ingested.
- Other less common routes of intake include intranasal, sublingual, smoking, conjuctival instillation and very rarely injection.
- It is not absorbed through intact skin.
- **LSD is said to be the most powerful of all hallucinogens**, and is active in doses of 50–100 µg.
- It occurs as a water-soluble, colourless, tasteless and odourless powder.
- Drugs related to LSD (lysergamides) also occur naturally in plants such as "**Morning glory**" (*Rivea corymbosa*) (**Fig. 12.27**) and "**Beach moonflower**" (*Ipomoea violacea*) (**Fig. 12.28**).

Mode of Action

- LSD is structurally related to serotonin (5-hydroxytryptamine) and is an agonist at the 5-HT_1 receptor.
  - Serotonin modulates many psychological and physiological processes including mood, personality, affect, appetite, sexual desire, motor function, temperature regulation, pain perception and sleep induction.

Toxic Effects

I. **Acute Poisoning**:

a. ***Physical***:

i. Mydriasis, hippus*
ii. Vertigo
iii. Tachycardia, hypertension
iv. Sweating, piloerection
v. Hyperthermia

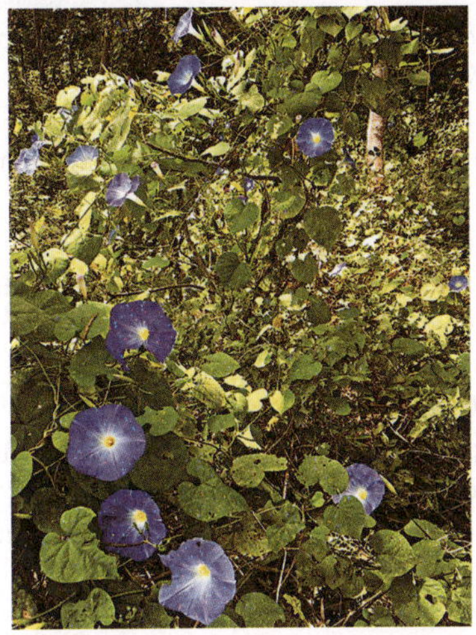

Fig. 12.27 Morning glory

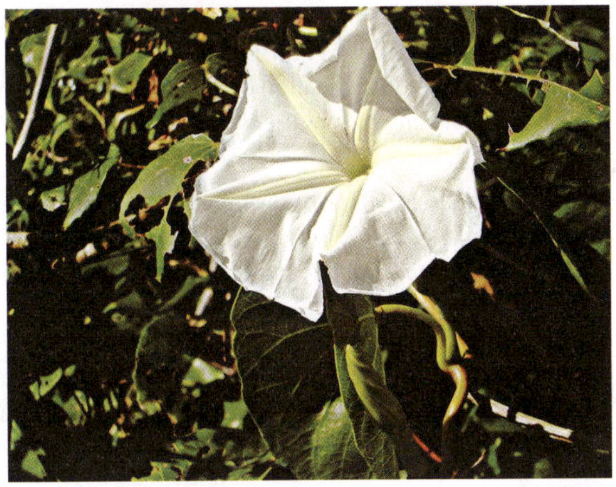

Fig. 12.28 Beach moonflower

vi. Tachypnoea
vii. Muscle weakness, ataxia
viii. Hyperactivity
ix. Coma
x. Serotonin syndrome may occur. Features of this syndrome include CNS effects (including agitation or coma), autonomic instability (including hyperpyrexia) and neuromuscular excitability (including clonus and raised serum creatine kinase).

b. ***Psychological***:

i. Euphoria or dysphoria.
ii. Vivid hallucinations, synaesthesias.
iii. *Bizare perceptual changes*: People's faces and body parts appear distorted, objects undulate, sounds may be magnified and distorted, colours seem brighter with halos around objects. Occasionally, there is depersonalisation, and the hallucinating person may feel as if he is observing an event instead of being involved in it.

**Note*: *Spasmodic contraction and dilation of pupils.*

c. ***Massive overdose***: Vomiting, coma, respiratory arrest and hyperthermia.

II. **Chronic Poisoning**:

a. Prolonged psychotic reactions which are mainly schizophrenic in nature.
b. Severe depression.
c. ***Flashback phenomena***: The person re-lives the LSD experience periodically in the absence of drug intake for months or years.
d. ***Post-hallucinogen perception disorder***: A persistent perceptual disorder often described by the person as if he is residing in a bubble under water in a "purple haze," with trailing of lights and images. Associated anxiety, panic and depression are common.
e. The following unusual phenomena have also been reported:
   i. Pareidolias – Images of faces on floor and walls, outdoors (in the foliage of trees) or floating faces hovering in space (**Fig. 12.29**).
   ii. Aeropsia – Visualization of air in the form of numerous vibrating pinpoint-sized dots ("molecules").

Diagnosis

1. Radioimmunoassay (RIA) of serum or urine: Limit of detection 0.1 ng/mL.
2. High Performance Thin Layer Chromatography (HPTLC): Limit of detection less than 1 μg/L.
3. High Performance Liquid Chromatography (HPLC): Less sensitive.
4. Gas Chromatography–Mass Spectrometry (GC–MS): Limit of detection 5 pg/mL.

Treatment

1. Avoid gut decontamination as LSD is ingested in microquantities and rapidly absorbed, rendering decontamination procedures totally redundant.
2. Do not use restraints in agitated patients; it will only exacerbate the condition.
3. Because of the short half-life and few serious medical reactions, elimination enhancement procedures such as haemodialysis, haemoperfusion, etc., are not warranted.
4. If the patient has evidence of systemic toxicity (hyperthermia, autonomic instability, diarrhoea and vomiting), monitor BP, pulse, temperature and conscious level. Check FBC, U&Es, creatinine and CK.
5. *Agitation and psychotic behaviour*:
   a. Adults can be sedated with an initial dose of oral or IV diazepam. Further boluses, given IV, may be administered if the patient remains severely agitated 10–15 min after the initial bolus. If agitation persists despite the above measure, consider oral or parenteral haloperidol.
   b. In children, it is better to manage agitation without sedation and exclude other causes (e.g., hypoxia, infection, hypoglycaemia and raised ICP). Consider nursing in a dark and quiet environment with a close relative present. If required, midazolam is the most appropriate drug for managing agitation in children and young people. Intravenous lorazepam is an alternative.
6. Treat *post-hallucinogen perception disorder* with long-lasting benzodiazepines such as clonazepam, and to a lesser extent, anticonvulsants such as valproic acid and carbamazepine. This approach must be combined with behavioural therapy. The patient must be instructed not to consume alcohol, cannabis, caffeine and other drugs which can intensify the disorder.
7. Warn patient of the risk of *flashback hallucinations* for weeks or months after the last dose of LSD. Treat flashbacks with psychotherapy, anti-anxiety agents and neuroleptics.

PHENCYCLIDINE

- Phencyclidine is commonly referred to by addicts as "**angel dust**" or "**PCP**."
  - It was developed in the 1950s as a potential general anaesthetic by Parke-Davis under the brand name Sernyl. It was termed a "**dissociative anaesthetic**" because unlike conventional anaesthetics which induced a state of relaxed sleep, PCP induced a state of catatonia with flat facies, open mouth, fixed staring, rigid posturing and waxy flexibility. Patients seemed dissociated from the environment without classical coma.
  - However, a significant proportion of patients showed severe adverse reactions during emergence, including agitation and hallucinations. Some suffered from psychosis for up to 10 days. PCP was therefore quickly withdrawn.
  - Today, **ketamine** a less potent PCP derivative is quite popular as an anaesthetic.

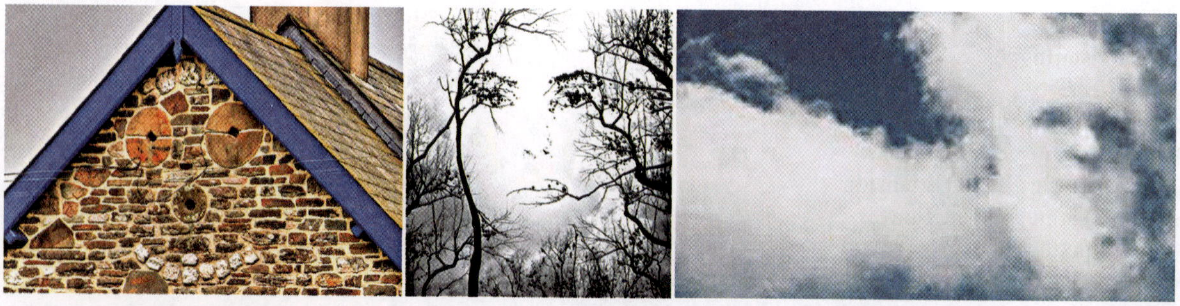

Fig. 12.29 Examples of pareidolias

Mode of Intake

- PCP is abused by smoking, insufflation, ingestion or rarely IV injection.
- It is commonly sold on the street as tablets (about 5 mg), capsules, powder (**Fig. 12.30**), aqueous or alcoholic solution, or as "***rock salt***" crystal. It is often mixed with tobacco, parsley, mint or marijuana.

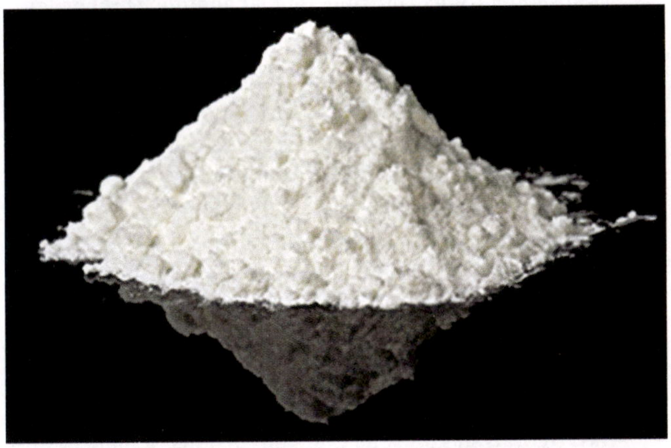

Fig. 12.30 Phencyclidine crystalline powder

Mode of Action

- Phencyclidine antagonizes the action of glutamate at the NMDA (N-methyl-d-aspartate) receptor.
- PCP also blocks presynaptic monoamine reuptake, thus directly increasing synaptic levels of dopamine and noradrenaline.
- At even higher doses, PCP blocks neuronal Na^+ and K^+ channels, as well as muscarinic cholinergic receptors. This may explain the occurrence of convulsions in PCP overdose.

Toxic Effects

- At lower doses, there may be inebriated behaviour, hallucinations, paranoia, dizziness, ataxia, nystagmus, miosis or mydriasis, slurred speech, blank staring, and tremulousness with hyperreflexia, increased muscle tone and clonic movements.
- With higher doses, features include anaesthesia and catatonic-like posturing, progressing in severe cases to myoclonic movements, dystonic reactions, convulsions and coma.
- Respiratory depression, acute lung injury and hyperthermia can rarely occur with very large doses.
- Cardiovascular features include hypertension and sinus tachycardia. Vasospasm can cause severe systemic hypertension and cerebral haemorrhage.
- Cholinergic (diaphoresis, bronchospasm, hypersalivation) and anticholinergic (urinary retention) symptoms can occur, as well as hypoglycaemia.
- Acute psychosis can occur during the recovery phase of phencyclidine anaesthesia (termed an '***emergence reaction***').

Common symptoms are summarized by the mnemonic **RED DANES**: **R**age, **E**rythema (redness of skin), **D**ilated pupils, **D**elusions, **A**mnesia, **N**ystagmus, **E**xcitation and **S**kin dryness.

Usual Fatal Dose

- **Approximately 100 mg or more.**
- Lethal blood level: 0.1 mg/100 mL.

Diagnosis

- Serum PCP levels usually do not correlate well with clinical picture. Therefore, a qualitative test (kit-based urine test) is adequate in most cases.

Treatment

1. The need for gastric lavage should be assessed carefully. Often such measures may exacerbate agitation and violence.
2. Activated charcoal may be beneficial and can be administered at a dose of 1 g/kg every 4 hrs for several doses.
3. Some authors recommend urinary acidification to enhance excretion of PCP (which is a weak base). But, only 10% of the drug is excreted in the urine, while the remaining 90% is metabolized in the liver. Hence, the practical utility of urinary acidification is negligible.
4. Haemodialysis and haemoperfusion are not beneficial.
5. As of now there is no antidote for PCP, though efforts are on to develop PCP-specific antigen binding fragmens (Fab) which can prove to be very useful.
6. For agitation and delirium:
   a. Adults can be sedated with an initial dose of oral or IV diazepam. Further boluses, given IV, may be administered if the patient remains severely agitated 10–15 min after the initial bolus. If agitation persists despite the above measure, consider oral or parenteral haloperidol.
   b. In children, it is better to manage agitation without sedation and exclude other causes (e.g., hypoxia, infection, hypoglycaemia and raised ICP). Consider nursing in a dark and quiet environment with a close relative present. If required, midazolam is the most appropriate drug for managing agitation in children and young people. Intravenous lorazepam is an alternative.
7. Reassure patients with acute dystonic reactions. These usually respond to antimuscarinic agents, e.g., procyclidine. Diazepam is an alternative. Repeat doses may be required for prolonged reactions.
8. Specific antihypertensive therapy should be instituted in patients with very high blood pressure.
9. Control convulsions that are frequent or prolonged with IV diazepam, lorazepam or midazolam. If convulsions are unresponsive to initial treatment, second-line therapy is phenobarbitone sodium. Thiopentone sodium is the preferred antiepileptic for status epilepticus not responding to the above measures.
10. Mild to moderate hyperthermia may respond to conventional cooling measures. When rising body temperature exceeds 39°C, core temperature monitoring should be con-

sidered (rectal probe) and urgent cooling measures should be employed according to local protocols.

a. Cooling methods include:
    i. Ice-baths (may achieve rapid cooling but caution in elderly/comorbidities).
    ii. Internal/invasive measures – cold fluid lavage (gastric, bladder, peritoneal), intravascular cooling techniques.
    iii. Ice packs to groin and axillae.
    iv. Mist and fan techniques.
    v. External cooling devices.
b. Dantrolene may be considered where there is muscular hyperactivity.

11. If rhabdomyolysis is present, renal failure can develop particularly if the CK activity is greater than 5000 IU/L. Give volume replacement as soon as possible and consider the need for urine alkalinization. Haemodiafiltration can effectively remove myoglobin from the circulation; haemodiafiltration combined with urine alkalinization is more effective than urine alkalinization alone.

Medicosocial & Forensic Issues

- Hallucinogen abuse has been traditionally a Western phenomenon, and drugs of abuse such as LSD and phencyclidine have always been popular only in countries such as the USA, UK, Australia and parts of Europe. The popularity of such drugs has been fuelled by their glamorous representation in films and rock music.
    - Prominent film actors who have confessed to having used hallucinogens: Cary Grant, Dennis Hopper, Jack Nicholson, Will Smith, Susan Sarandon, Kristen Bell, Frances McDormand, Sanjay Dutt.
    - Prominent Pop/Rock bands or musicians who have confessed to having used hallucinogens: The Beatles, The Beach Boys, Pink Floyd, Grateful Dead, Jimi Hendrix, Harry Styles, Nirvana, Santana.
    - Prominent films featuring hallucinogens: Apocalypse Now, Easy Rider, Natural Born Killers, Dead Man, Dev D, Jacob's Ladder, The Wall, Woodstock
- The 1960s saw an explosion of hallucinogen use almost in the form of an epidemic, and though it declined steeply in the 1970s and 1980s, there has been an alarming resurgence over the last decade. Drugs like LSD are now increasingly being abused even in India.
- The dangers of hallucinogen use do not have as much to do with acute toxicity, as with long-term psychological damage. The inevitable fallout is violent crime manifesting as assaultative behaviour, homicides and suicides. Several horrific crimes have been committed by drug-crazed individuals acting out their bizarre fantasies.

SOLVENT ABUSE

("GLUE SNIFFING", VOLATILE SUBSTANCE ABUSE, INHALANT-RELATED DISORDERS)

- **Inhalant drugs (volatile substances)** are widely available and frequently abused, especially by adolescents from poor socioeconomic background. These substances are mostly volatile hydrocarbons which are used as solvents, propellants, thinners and fuels.
    - The hydrocarbon is typically inhaled by pouring into a container for "***sniffing***," a rag or sock for "***huffing***" or a plastic/paper bag for "***bagging***." Abusers often begin with "sniffing" (lower concentrations), and progress subsequently to "huffing" and "bagging" (higher levels of exposure).
- The most commonly abused inhalants include:
    - Toluene from paints and glues
    - Petrol
    - Butane from cigarette lighter fluids
    - Halogenated hydrocarbons from typewriter correction fluids
    - Propellants
    - Dry cleaning fluids.

Toxic Effects

I. **Acute**:

a. *CNS* – Excitation, agitation, hallucinations, headache, vertigo, nystagmus, ataxia, convulsions, lethargy, stupor, respiratory depression.
b. *CVS* – **Sudden sniffing death syndrome**:
Inhaling butane gas can cause drowsiness, narcosis, asphyxia and cardiac arrhythmia. Butane is among the most commonly misused volatile solvents. Sudden death may occur by cardiac arrest.
c. Furthermore, the inhalation of any gas that is capable of displacing oxygen in the lungs (especially gases heavier than oxygen) carries the risk of hypoxia as a result of the very mechanism by which breathing is triggered.
d. *Other Effects*:
    i. Methaemoglobinaemia.
    ii. Hepatitis.
    iii. Metabolic acidosis, rhabdomyolysis, renal failure, hypokalaemia.

II. **Chronic**:

a. ***Chronic painter syndrome*** – A neurobehavioural syndrome due to solvent-induced encephalopathy, characterized by memory loss, anxiety, depression, sleep disorders, neurasthenia and personality changes. CT scan often reveals areas of atrophy, and EEG readings are usually abnormal.
b. Cerebellar dysfunction with chorea (petrol).
c. Abdominal pain, nausea, vomiting, haematemesis.
d. Cardiomyopathy
e. Hepatotoxicity
f. Pulmonary disorders – pulmonary hypertension, acute respiratory distress.
g. Dementia (petrol, toluene).
h. The main effects following chronic toluene abuse are renal tubular acidosis, resulting in hypokalaemia and muscle weakness.

Treatment

- Inhalant intoxication, like alcohol intoxication, usually requires no special treatment and resolves spontaneously. However, complications such as cardiac arrhythmias, bronchospasm, coma, etc., will require prompt treatment.
- Essentially, medical care primarily involves reassurance, quiet environment, and attention to vital signs and level of consciousness.
- Sedative drugs such as benzodiazepines are contraindicated, since they may aggravate intoxication.
- Severe agitation may require cautious control with haloperidol (5 mg for adults) intramuscularly, repeated once after 20 min, if necessary.
- Treat pulmonary oedema and/or acute lung injury with continuous positive airway pressure (CPAP) or in severe cases with IPPV and PEEP.
- Inhalant dependence requires specialized treatment by a qualified psychiatrist, and may take 3–12 months for achieving total abstinence. Relapses are not uncommon.

Medicosocial and Forensic Issues

- Volatile substances abuse (VSA) is a uniquely adolescent phenomenon, and is particularly common among lower socio-economic classes, mainly because these substances are cheap, easily available and legal to possess. Also, the mode of intake is relatively simple.
- VSA is quite common among street urchins of major Indian cities (**Fig. 12.31**), probably because these inexpensive substances offer a rare exciting experience to escape from the daily misery of poverty. Persons with adolescent conduct disorder and adult antisocial personality disorder are especially prone to VSA.
  - In India, three of the most widely abused inhalants are the Dendrite brand and other forms of contact adhesives and rubber cements manufactured in Kolkata, and toluenes in paint thinners.
  - Another very common inhalant is Erase-X, a correction fluid that contains toluene. It has become very common for school and college students to use it, because it is easily available in stationery shops in India. This fluid is also used by street and working children in Delhi.

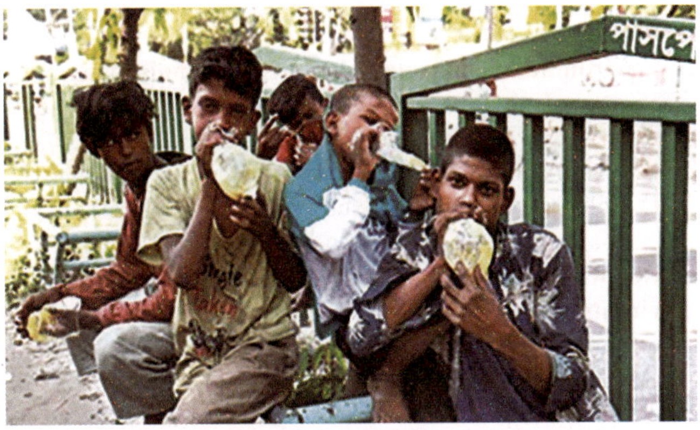

Fig. 12.31 Street children indulging in solvent abuse

Topic 13

ENVIRONMENTAL TOXICOLOGY

(Number of Competencies – 2: FM 13.1 & 13.2)

FM 13.1: Core – Written/Viva Voce
- Describe:
  - Toxic pollution of environment and its medicolegal aspects
  - Toxic hazards of occupation and industry

ENVIRONMENTAL TOXICOLOGY

Definition

- **Environmental toxicology** deals with the study of harmful effects of various chemical, biological and physical agents on living organisms.
  - **Ecotoxicology** is a sub-discipline of environmental toxicology concerned with studying the harmful effects of toxicants at the population and ecosystem levels.
- **Rachel Carson** (Fig. 13.1) is considered the mother of environmental toxicology, as she made it a distinct field within toxicology in 1962 with the publication of her book **Silent Spring**, which covered the effects of uncontrolled pesticide use. Her book was based on a series of reports on the ecological effects of the pesticide DDT.

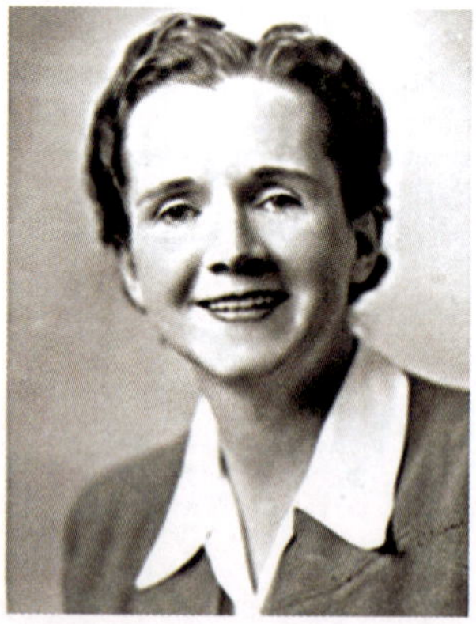

Fig. 13.1 Rachel Carson

- Organisms can be exposed to various kinds of toxicants at any life cycle stage, some of which are more sensitive than others.
- Bioaccumulation occurs when an organism stores toxicants in fatty tissues, which may eventually establish a toxic cascade and the bio-magnification of specific toxicants.
- Although legislation implemented since the early 1970s had intended to minimize harmful effects of environmental toxicants upon all species, there are serious limitations leading to progressive contamination of the environment, especially in developing countries such as India.

Sources of Toxic Pollution (Environmental Contamination)

- There are many sources of environmental toxicity that can lead to the presence of toxicants in food, water and air. These sources include heavy metals, pesticides, biological toxins and radiation, all of which can have harmful effects on living organisms.
- There can be **point sources** of pollution, for instance the drains from a specific factory, as **also non-point sources** (diffuse sources) like the rubber from car tires that contain numerous chemicals and heavy metals that are spread in the environment.

1. **Heavy Metals**:
   - The most common heavy metals involved in environmental contamination include arsenic, lead, mercury and cadmium. They are found in air, soil and water.
   - **Arsenic** is one of the most abundant elements on earth and its specific inorganic forms are very dangerous to living creatures (animals, plants and humans) and the environment. In humans, arsenic can cause cancer in the bladder, skin, lungs and liver. One of the major sources of arsenic exposure in humans is contaminated water (especially bore-well water), which is a problem in more than 30 countries in the world. In India, West Bengal faced arsenic poisoning in epidemic proportions a few decades ago (*page no. 436*).
   - Another extremely toxic metal, **lead** has been known to cause extensive environmental contamination and health problems in many parts of the world. Humans come in contact with lead through mining, fossil fuel burning and industrial use. Formerly, major sources of exposure included petrol and paint. Lead can either cause acute poisoning with headache, hypertension, abdominal pain, and renal dysfunction, or chronic poisoning with mental retardation, autism, weight loss, palsies, muscular weakness, brain damage, kidney damage, etc.
   - **Mercury** occurs either as elemental form, or inorganic salts, or organic compounds, all of which are highly toxic. Elemental mercury and inorganic salts are occupational toxicants, while organic mercury compounds are especially toxic to the marine environment. Methyl mercury came into prominence after the Minamata environmental disaster in Japan (*page no. 444*) (**Fig. 13.2**).
   - **Cadmium** is a highly cumulative heavy metal, and will accumulate inside the body throughout the life of the human/animal. It is seen mostly in rechargeable batter-

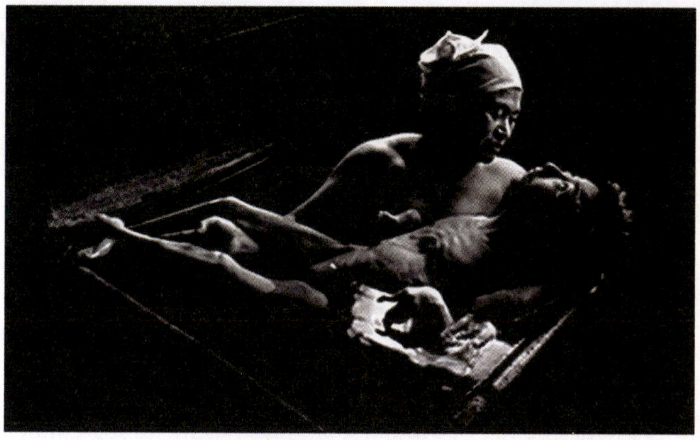

Fig. 13.2 A haunting image of a victim of Minamata disease

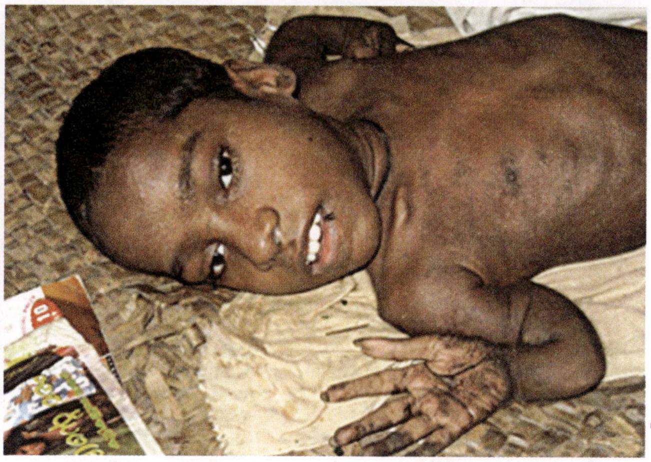

Fig. 13.3 A victim of endosulfan exposure

ies, tobacco smoke and some alloys production. Cadmium is extremely toxic to the kidneys and the bones.

2. **Pesticides**:
   - Pesticides are a major source of environmental toxicity. These chemically synthesized agents have been known to persist in the environment long after their administration. The poor biodegradability of many pesticides can result in their accumulation in various organisms with long-term deleterious effects such as carcinogenesis, teratogenesis, etc.
   - Pesticides can be categorized according to the pests they target. For example, insecticides are used to eliminate agricultural insects that attack various fruits and crops, while herbicides target unwanted weeds and other plants that reduce crop production.
   - Among the pesticides, the most notorious environmental pollutants comprise the **chlorinated hydrocarbons (organochlorines)**, which are often referred to as persistent organic pollutants (POPs) because they persist in soil and water for a very long time.
   - One of the classic examples is **dichlorodiphenyltrichloroethane (DDT)**, which is an organochlorine insecticide that has been banned due to its adverse effects on both humans and wildlife. DDT was widely used by farmers, until in 1962, the harmful effects of the widespread and uncontrolled use of DDT were detailed by Rachel Carson in her book Silent Spring. DDT has damaging effects on the liver, nervous system and reproductive system of humans.
   - By 1972, the United States Environmental Protection Agency (EPA) banned the use of DDT in the United States. Despite the regulation of this pesticide in North America and most parts of Europe, it is still unfortunately used in certain areas of the world, including India.
   - **Endosulfan** is another organochlorine insecticide with a terrible reputation. It is responsible for the Kasargod Endosulfan Tragedy in the state of Kerala (*page no. 489*) (**Fig. 13.3**).
3. **Polychlorinated biphenyls (PCBs)**:
   - **PCBs** pertain to the group of human-produced organic chemicals known as **chlorinated hydrocarbons**.
   - PCBs have certain properties (chemical stability, nonflammability) which make them useful in a number of commercial and industrial practices. Some of these include hydraulic equipment, plasticizers in paints, plastics and rubber products, and pigments, dyes, etc.
   - PCBs are organic pollutants and can persist in soil and aquatic ecosystems for a long period of time.
4. **Biotoxins**:
   - The most common examples of environmental biotoxins comprise **cyanobacteria** that produce **cyanotoxins**.
   - Cyanobacteria, or blue-green algae, are photosynthetic bacteria. They grow in many types of water. Their rapid growth ("bloom") is related to high water temperature as well as eutrophication (resulting from enrichment with minerals and nutrients often due to runoff from the land that induces excessive growth of these algae). Many genera of cyanobacteria produce biotoxins (cyanotoxins) (**Fig. 13.4**).

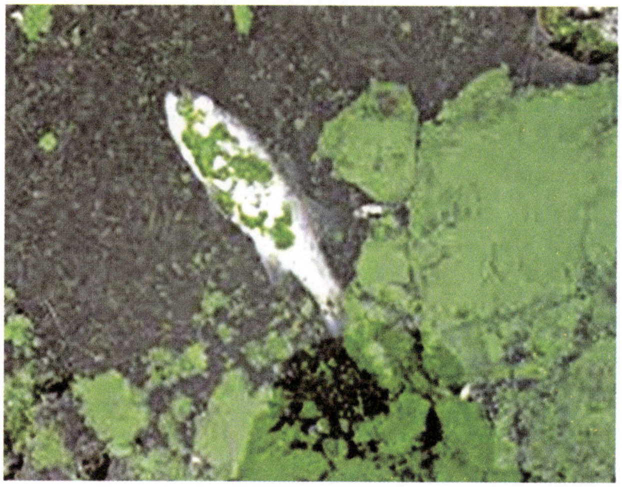

Fig. 13.3 Toxic lake water due to the presence of blue green algae

- Cyanotoxins can be dermatotoxic, neurotoxic and hepatotoxic, though death related to their exposure is rare.

5. **Radiation**:
   - Radiation is given off by matter as either rays or waves of pure energy, or high-speed particles. The former known as electromagnetic radiation, include sunlight, X-rays, radar and radio waves. Particle radiation includes alpha and beta particles and neutrons.
   - When humans and animals are exposed to high radiation levels, they can develop cancer, congenital disabilities or skin burns.

FM 13.2: Core – Written/Viva Voce
- Describe medicolegal aspects of poisoning in Workmen's Compensation Act

TOXICOLOGY & THE WORKMEN'S COMPENSATION ACT

- The **Workmen's Compensation Act (1923)**, provides for the payment of compensation by certain classes of employers to their employees for injury or accident sustained in the course of employment.
- An occupational disease contracted by a workman while in the service of an employer for a continuous period of not less than 6 months is deemed to be an injury or an accident.
- When a workman gives notice of an accident, the employer should arrange to have him examined free of charge by a qualified medical practitioner.
- If the workman refuses to be examined or treated, or after agreeing to be examined disregards instructions regarding treatment, the injury or disablement will be deemed to be of the same severity as it may have been reasonably expected to be with proper medical attention.
- In case a medical officer is asked to examine a workman and give his opinion as to whether he is partially or totally disabled from an accident or occupational disease, he should undertake the examination with great care.
- Among the list of occupational diseases mentioned under the Act, the following poisons/toxins are implicated as causative agents – arsenic, benzene, bichromates, cabon-disulphide, chromic acid, halogenated hydrocarbons, lead, manganese, mercury, nitrous fumes, organophosphates and phosphorus.
- However, the WHO has identified many more chemicals as disease-causing in the field of occupational health (**Table 13.1**).

Table 13.1 Toxic Agents Causing Occupational Diseases (WHO)

Gases	Dusts	Metals	Chemicals	Solvents
▪ Ammonia ▪ Carbon dioxide ▪ Carbon monoxide ▪ Carbon disulphide ▪ Hydrogen cyanide ▪ Hydrogen sulphide ▪ Nitrogen ▪ Sulphur dioxide	▪ *Inorganic*: - Asbestos - Coal - Iron - Silica ▪ *Organic*: - Cotton dust - Hay - Sugarcane fibre - Tobacco	▪ Arsenic ▪ Beryllium ▪ Cadmium ▪ Chromium ▪ Lead ▪ Manganese ▪ Mercury	▪ Acids ▪ Alkalis ▪ Pesticides	▪ Benzene ▪ Chloroform ▪ Trichloroethylene

Annexure I

PRE-CONCEPTION & PRE-NATAL DIAGNOSTIC TECHNIQUES (PCPNDT) ACT, 1994

- Pre-Conception & Pre-Natal Diagnostic Techniques (PCPNDT) Act, 1994 was enacted to stop female foeticides and arrest the declining sex ratio in India. It bans prenatal sex determination.
- Every genetic counselling centre, genetic laboratory or genetic clinic engaged in counselling or conducting pre-natal diagnostics techniques, like in vitro fertilisation (IVF) with the potential of sex selection before and after conception, comes under purview of the PCPNDT Act, and are banned.
- Social discrimination against women and a preference for sons have promoted female foeticide in various forms skewing the sex ratio of the country towards men.The main purpose of enacting the Act is to ban the use of sex selection techniques after conception and prevent the misuse of pre-natal diagnostic technique for sex selective abortions.

Salient Features

- Offences under this Act include
  - Conducting or helping in the conduct of prenatal diagnostic technique in unregistered units
  - Sex selection on a man or woman
  - Conducting PND test for any purpose other than the one mentioned in the Act
  - Sale, distribution, supply, renting etc. of any ultra sound machine or any other equipment capable of detecting sex of the foetus.

Main Provisions

- The Act provides for the prohibition of sex selection, before or after conception.
- It regulates the use of pre-natal diagnostic techniques, like ultrasound and amniocentesis by allowing them their use only to detect :
  - Genetic abnormalities
  - Metabolic disorders
  - Chromosomal abnormalities
  - Congenital malformations
  - Haemoglobinopathies
  - Sex linked disorders.
- No laboratory or centre or clinic will conduct any test including ultrasonography for the purpose of determining the sex of the foetus.
- No person, including the one who is conducting the procedure as per the law, will communicate the sex of the foetus to the pregnant woman or her relatives by words, signs or any other method.
- Any person who puts an advertisement for pre-natal and pre-conception sex determination facilities in the form of a notice, circular, etc., or advertises through media in electronic or print form or engages in any visible representation made by means of hoarding, wall painting, signal, etc., can be imprisoned for up to three years and fined Rs. 10,000.
- The Act mandates compulsory registration of all diagnostic laboratories, all genetic counselling centres, genetic laboratories, genetic clinics and ultrasound clinics.

Amendment in 2003

- Pre-Natal Diagnostic Techniques (Regulation and Prevention of Misuse) Act, 1994 (PNDT), was amended in 2003 to **The Pre-Conception and Pre-Natal Diagnostic Techniques (Prohibition of Sex Selection) Act (PCPNDT Act)** to improve the regulation of the technology.
- Implications of the amendment are:
  - Amendment of the Act mainly covered bringing the technique of pre-conception sex selection within the ambit of the Act
  - Bringing ultrasound within its ambit
  - Empowering the central supervisory board, constitution of state level supervisory board
  - Provision for more stringent punishments
  - Empowering appropriate authorities with the power of civil court for search, seizure and sealing the machines and equipments of the violators
  - Regulating the sale of the ultrasound machines only to registered bodies.

Annexure II

GLASGOW COMA SCALE

The Glasgow Coma Scale (**GCS**) is a neurological scale which is an objective way of recording the conscious state of a person for initial (and subsequent) assessment. A patient is assessed against specified criteria, and the resulting points provide a **score** between **3** (deep unconsciousness) and **15** (normal).

Eye response (E) - There are **4** grades starting with the most severe:

1. No eye opening.
2. Eye opening in response to pain stimulus (*a peripheral stimulus, such as squeezing the lunula area of the patient's fingernail is more effective than a central stimulus such as a trapezius squeeze*).
3. Eye opening to speech (*not to be confused with the awakening of a sleeping person; such patients receive a score of 4, not 3*).
4. Eyes opening spontaneously.

Verbal response (V) - There are **5** grades starting with the most severe:

1. No verbal response.
2. Incomprehensible sounds (*moaning, but no words*).
3. Inappropriate words (*random speech, but no conversational exchange; speaks words but no sentences*).
4. Confused (*responds to questions coherently, but there is some disorientation and confusion*).
5. Oriented (*responds coherently and appropriately to questions such as the patient's name and age, etc*).

Motor response (M) - There are **6** grades:

1. No motor response.
2. **Decerebrate posturing** accentuated by pain (*extensor response: adduction of arm, internal rotation of shoulder, pronation of forearm and extension at elbow, flexion of wrist and fingers, leg extension, plantar flexion of foot*).
3. **Decorticate posturing** accentuated by pain (*flexor response: internal rotation of shoulder, flexion of forearm and wrist with clenched fist, leg extension, plantar flexion of foot*).
4. Withdrawal from pain (*absence of abnormal posturing; unable to lift hand past chin with supraorbital pain but does pull away when nailbed is pinched*).
5. Localizes to pain (*purposeful movements towards painful stimuli; e.g., brings hand up beyond chin when supraorbital pressure applied*).
6. Obeys commands (*does simple things as asked*).

Interpretation

Individual elements as well as the sum of the score are important. Hence, the score is expressed in the following form "GCS 8 = E2 V3 M3 at 10:20 hrs".

Generally, severity is classified as:
Severe (GCS < 8);
Moderate (GCS 9–12);
Minor (GCS ≥ 13)

Glasgow Coma Scale

	1	2	3	4	5	6
Eye	Does not open eyes	Opens eyes in response to painful stimuli	Opens eyes in response to voice	Opens eyes spontaneously	N/A	N/A
Verbal	Makes no sounds	Incomprehensible sounds	Utters inappropriate words	Confused, disoriented	Oriented, converses normally	N/A
Motor	Makes no movements	Extension to painful stimuli (decerebrate response)	Abnormal flexion to painful stimuli (decorticate response)	Flexion/ Withdrawal to painful stimuli	Localizes painful stimuli	Obeys commands

Note that a motor response in any limb is acceptable. The scale is composed of three tests: eye, verbal and motor responses. The three values separately as well as their sum are considered.

Annexure III

DATURA*

Other Common Names

Angel's trumpet; Devil's apple; Devil's weed; Jamestown weed; Jimson weed; Locoweed; Stinkweed; Thorn apple

Botanical Name

Datura stramonium, D.metel (Hindu Datura), D.fastuosa

Physical Appearance

- Small coarse shrub with a strong and rather unpleasant smell, belonging to family Solanaceae which grows wild all over the Indian countryside.
- It grows to a height of 3 to 5 feet, and has a handsome foliage of dark green ovate, pointed leaves, and large tubular (trumpet-shaped) flowers which may be white (*alba*) or purple (*niger*).
- The fruit capsule is spherical with soft spines, and contains up to 200 small (2–3 mm in length) dark brown or black, reniform (kidney-shaped) seeds, which bear a superficial resemblance to chilly seeds.

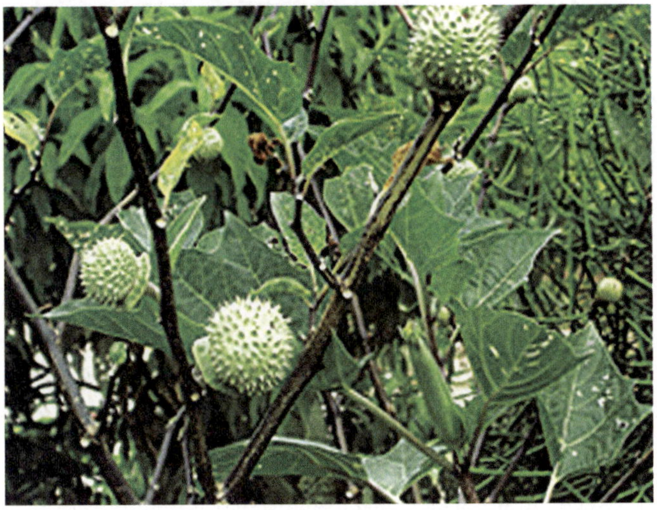

Datura fastuosa

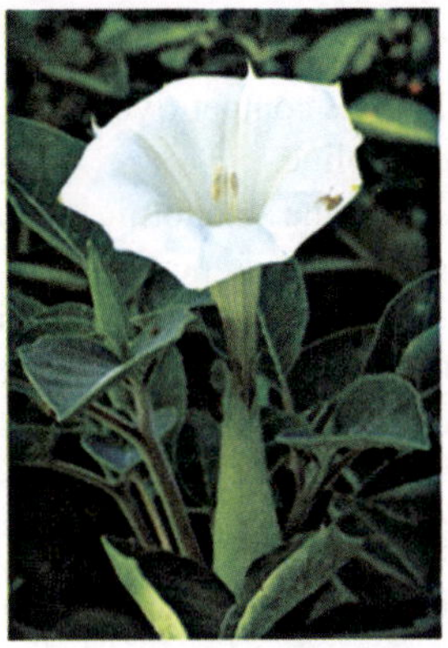

Flower of Datura

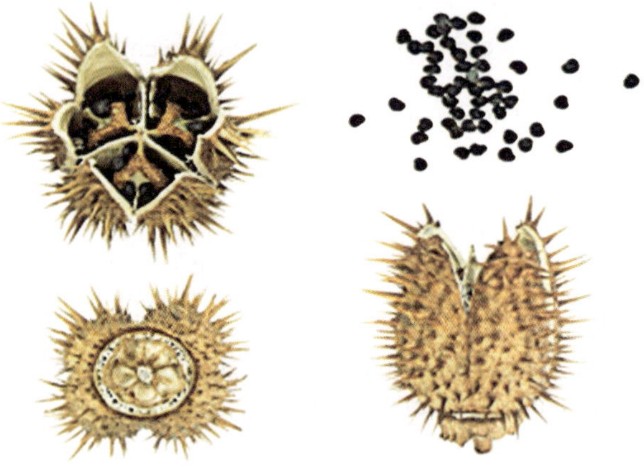

Datura fruit capsule with seeds

Uses

- Formerly, the dried leaves (usually mixed with cannabis) were used in the form of cigarettes as a remedy for asthma.
- The active principles have various uses in modern medicine (**Table**).

Toxic Part

All parts, especially seeds.

Medicinal Uses of Datura Alkaloids

Alkaloid	Uses
Atropine	1. Treatment of bradycardia, vagal syncope. 2. Preanaesthetic medication (for reducing salivation and bronchial secretions). 3. Antidote for organophosphates, carbamates, and certain mushrooms). 4. Treatment of iridocyclitis, and for facilitating refractory procedures in children (local application as eye drops or ointment).
Hyoscine	1. Antispasmodic. 2. Aid to radiological and endoscopic examination of GI tract. 3. Preanaesthetic medication. 4. Treatment of motion sickness (*transdermal patch*).

*Not mentioned as a separate entry in the new curriculum, but being discussed here because of its importance.

Toxic Principles

- Hyoscine (scopolamine), hyoscyamine, and traces of atropine, together referred to commonly as **belladonna alkaloids**.

Mode of Action

- Belladonna alkaloids competitively inhibit the muscarinic effects of acetylcholine.
- Sites of action are at the autonomic effectors innervated by postganglionic cholinergic nerves or on smooth muscles that do not contain cholinergic innervation.
- Central nervous system effects result from their central antimuscarinic actions, i.e., vagal stimulation and decrease in heart rate.

Clinical (Toxic) Features

Summarised in the classic phrase: ***blind as a bat, hot as a hare, dry as a bone, red as a beet, and mad as a wet hen***.

- The important manifestations can be better remembered as a **series of D's**:
  - **Dr**yness of mouth, thirst, slurred speech.
  - **Dy**sphagia.
  - **Di**lated pupils (with no reaction to light or accommodation).
  - **Di**plopia.
  - **Dry** hot skin, with flushing, hyperpyrexia.
  - **Drunken** gait (ataxia), hyperreflexia, convulsions.
  - **Delirium** with hallucinations, agitation, amnesia, incoherence.
  - **Dysuria**, urinary retention, bladder distension.
  - **Death**, preceded by tachycardia, arrhythmias, coma, and respiratory depression.
- Other features include cardiac conduction abnormalities and arrhythmias, paralytic ileus, hyperglycaemia, rash, and glaucoma. Abnormal liver and renal function and rhabdomyolysis have also been reported.

Usual Fatal Dose

- 50 to 100 datura seeds.
- 10 to 100 mg of atropine (usually 50 to 60 mg).

Treatment

1. **Gut decontamination**: Gastric lavage (after intubation), activated charcoal.
2. Dialysis and haemoperfusion do not appear to be effective.
3. Catheterize bladder.
4. Perform a 12-lead ECG in all patients who require assessment. Repeat 12-lead ECGs are recommended, especially in symptomatic patients. Check cardiac rhythm, QRS duration and QT interval.
5. **Agitation and delirium**: Adults can be sedated with an initial dose of oral or IV diazepam. If agitation persists, consider oral or parenteral haloperidol. In children, it is better to manage agitation without sedation and exclude other causes (e.g., hypoxia, infection, hypoglycaemia and raised ICP). Consider nursing in a dark and quiet environment with a close relative present. If required, midazolam is the most appropriate drug for managing agitation in children and young people. Intravenous lorazepam is an alternative.
6. **Hyperthermia**: Mild to moderate hyperthermia may respond to conventional cooling measures. When rising body temperature exceeds 39°C, core temperature monitoring should be considered (rectal probe) and urgent cooling measures should be employed according to local protocols. Cooling methods include ice-baths, cold fluid lavage (gastric, bladder, peritoneal), intravascular cooling techniques, ice packs to groin and axillae, etc.
7. **Antidote**: **Physostigmine** is the antidote of choice, and should be administered in serious cases. The adult dose is 2 mg IV, slowly, repeated if required, in 20 minutes. Do not give it as a continuous infusion. Continuous cardiac monitoring is mandatory. The paediatric dose is 0.5 mg IV, slowly, repeating if required, at 5 minute intervals till a maximum of 2 mg.Physostigmine is an effective but dangerous antidote, and can give rise to convulsions, asystole, hypotension, hypersalivation, and bradyarrhythmias, if administered without caution.
8. Control **convulsions** that are frequent or prolonged with IV diazepam,lorazepam, or midazolam. If convulsions are unresponsive to initial treatment, second-line therapy is phenobarbitone sodium. An alternative is phenytoin.If convulsions persist, consider the need for referral to intensive care, general anaesthesia, intubation and ventilation. Thiopentone sodium is the preferred antiepileptic for status epilepticus not responding to the above measures.
9. If **rhabdomyolysis** is present, renal failure can develop. Early volume replacement and urine alkalinization may be helpful in preventing or reducing the severity of rhabdomyolysis-induced renal failure. In an adult give 225 mmol of 8.4% sodium bicarbonate (in a child 3 - 5 mmol/kg) over one hour to increase the urine pH to greater than 7.5; further doses of bicarbonate will be required to maintain pH greater than 7.5.

Forensic Issues

- **Accidental** - Accidental poisoning may result from any one of the following ways:
  - Mistaken identity involving **capsicum seeds**.
  - Foraging children in the countryside chewing on the seeds (or other parts of the plant) out of curiosity.
  - Therapeutic misadventures.
  - Overenthusiastic use of atropine as an antidote for organophosphate or carbamate poisoning.
- **Suicidal**– Owing to easy accessibility, datura is not infrequently reported in suicidal ingestions, especially in rural parts of India.
- **Homicidal**– There have been rare instances of murder being accomplished with one or the other belladonna alkaloids.

- **Stupefaction**– The term "stupefaction" is loosely applied to the process of rendering a victim suddenly incapacitated by exposing him to a deliriant poison such as datura, in order to facilitate robbery or rape. An extract of the seeds is usually employed, which is mixed with food or drink and administered to the unsuspecting victim. Sometimes, stupefaction is induced by exposing the person to fumes of incense, by mixing datura with other constituents of an incense or joss stick (*agarbathi*). Even cigarettes may be adulterated in a similar fashion. Gullible railway or bus passengers are the usual victims who fall into the trap of accepting food, drink, or tobacco from "friendly" strangers.
- **Datura abuse** – The seeds, flowers, and leaves are ingested whole or as preparations (e.g., tea) for hallucinogenic effect. The hypnotic and hallucinogenic properties of datura have been known since ages.

Annexure IV

STRYCHNOS NUX VOMICA*

Common Names

Dog button; Poison nut

Physical Characteristics

- This is a tree belonging to family Logianaceae which grows well in South India, as well as in certain other parts of the country.
- Leaves are oval, dark or variegated green.
- Fruits are globular, and contain greyish brown disc-shaped seeds about an inch in diameter and ¼ inch thick, which are slightly concave on one side and convex on the other. The pericarp is very tough. The outer surface is satin-like due to innumerable fine, silky hairs. While the seeds are odourless, they are extremely bitter to taste.

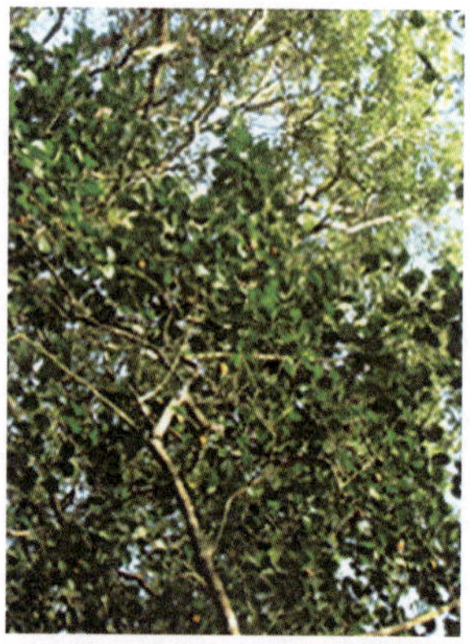

Strychnos nux vomica tree

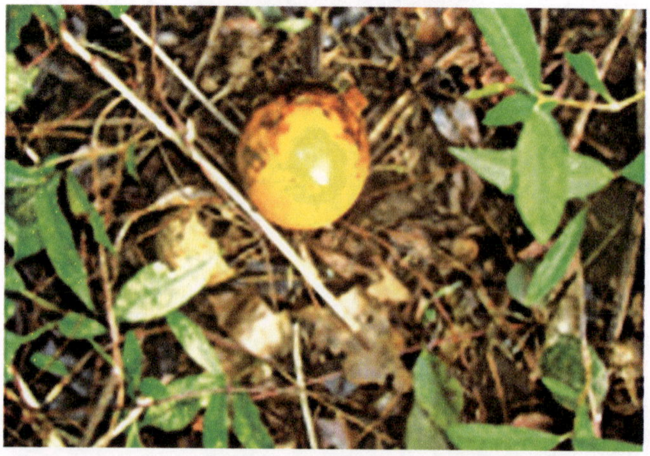

Strychnos nux vomica fruit

Uses

- The main alkaloid **strychnine** has been in use as a rodenticide since the 16th century.
- In the past, it was sometimes used for killing stray dogs (hence the name "***dog buttons***"). Killing dogs (including stray dogs) is actually illegal in India under the Prevention of Cruelty to Animals Act, 1960, and Animal Birth Control Rules 2001, besides being a criminal offence under Sections 428 and 429 of the Indian Penal Code. The punishment for such an act is rigorous imprisonment for up to 2 years, or a fine, or both
- Strychnine was first used medically in 1540, and continued to be used in many stimulants, tonics, and cathartics until as recently as the 1960s.
- Even today, strychnine is popular in folk medicine.

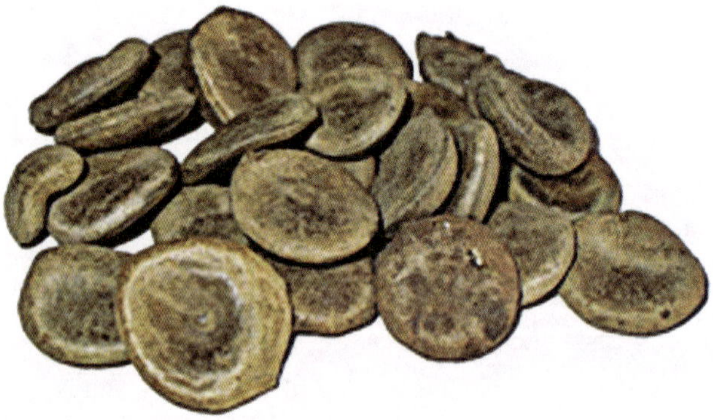

Strychnos nux vomica seeds

Toxic Part

Leaves, fruits, and seeds (in increasing order of toxicity).

Toxic Principles

Strychnine and **brucine** are the principal alkaloids, of which the former is much more powerful.

Mode of Action

- Strychnine prevents the uptake of glycine at inhibitory synapses, especially in the ventral horns (anterior horn cells) of the spinal cord.
- It results in the competitive antagonism of the inhibitory neurotransmitter at the post-synaptic spinal cord motor neurone.
- There is a net excitatory effect, and minimal sensory stimulation can set off powerful muscle contractions.

Toxic Effects

- A feeling of apprehension and anxiety is a common prodromal manifestation.
- Muscle twitching, spasms, followed by overwhelming convulsions (each lasting from 30 seconds to 2 minutes) which are precipitated by minimal external stimuli.
- **Opisthotonus** is a characteristic feature. It is due to powerful extensor spasm causing the body to be hyperextended

*Not mentioned as a separate entry in the new curriculum, but being discussed here because of its importance.

with arching of the back. Less commonly, emprosthotonus (forward bending) and pleurosthotonus (lateral bending) are seen.

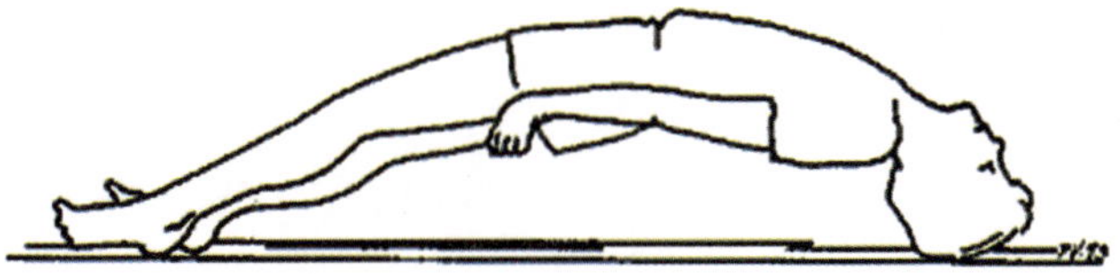

Opisthotonus

- **Trismus** (*lockjaw*), **risus sardonicus** (*sardonic smile* due to grimacing that results from facial muscle spasm). There may be frothing from the mouth.
- Mydriasis, proptosis, nystagmus, blurred vision, and loss of vision have been described.
- An important diagnostic feature is that there is complete muscle relaxation in between spasms and convulsions.
- Another feature of significance is that the patient maintains a clear sensorium during and between convulsive episodes.
- Non-specific ST and T-wave changes on ECG, and QTc and QRS prolongation secondary to hypocalcaemia have been described.

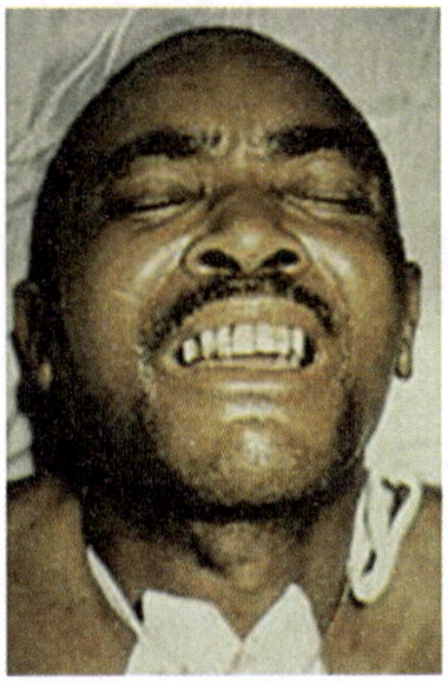

Risussardonicus

- Complications include hypoxia, hyperthermia, cardiac arrest, rhabdomyolysis, metabolic acidosis, and acute renal failure.
- The usual fatal event is respiratory failure consequent to spasm of respiratory muscles.

Usual Fatal Dose

- The minimum lethal oral dose in adults is 50–100 mg (1-2 mg/kg body weight).
- 1 to 3 gm for strychnos seeds.

Treatment

1. Cautious stomach wash with full protection of airway may be done in the absence of convulsions. However, it is better to avoid this for danger of instigating convulsions.
2. Consider activated charcoal (50 gm for adults; 1 gm/kg for children) if the patient presents within one hour of ingestion of any amount and the airway can be protected. Paralysis and administration via a nasogastric tube is likely to be required prior to administration.
3. Forced diuresis and dialysis are not advisable.
4. External stimuli should be reduced to the barest minimum. Treatment should preferably be carried out in a quiet, dark environment.
5. The key to successful management involves aggressive control of convulsions. Control **convulsions** that are frequent or prolonged with IV diazepam, lorazepam, or midazolam. If convulsions are unresponsive to initial treatment, second-line therapy is phenobarbitone sodium. An alternative is phenytoin.If convulsions persist, consider the need for referral to intensive care, general anaesthesia, intubation and ventilation. Thiopentone sodium is the preferred antiepileptic for status epilepticus not responding to the above measures. The role of newer agents such as propofol and levetiracetam in toxicological seizures is currently unclear because of a lack of clinical or animal studies.
6. If metabolic acidosis persists despite correction of hypoxia and adequate fluid resuscitation, consider correction with IV sodium bicarbonate.
7. Mild to moderate hyperthermia may respond to conventional cooling measures. When rising body temperature exceeds 39^{0}C, core temperature monitoring should be considered (rectal probe) and urgent cooling measures should be employed according to local protocols. Cooling methods include ice-baths, cold fluid lavage (gastric, bladder, peritoneal), intravascular cooling techniques, ice packs to groin and axillae, etc.
8. If **rhabdomyolysis** is present, renal failure can develop. Early volume replacement and urine alkalinization may be helpful in preventing or reducing the severity of rhabdomyolysis-induced renal failure. In an adult give 225 mmol of 8.4% sodium bicarbonate (in a child 3 - 5 mmol/kg) over one hour to increase the urine pH to greater than 7.5; further doses of bicarbonate will be required to maintain pH greater than 7.5.
9. Extracorporeal techniques will not enhance the elimination of strychnine, as it has a large volume of distribution.

Autopsy Features

- Early onset and disappearance of rigor mortis.
- Postmortem caloricity.
- Signs of asphyxia.
- Frothing at mouth.
- Dilated pupils.

Forensic Significance

- Strychnine has always had (a mostly unjustified) reputation of being the homicidal poisoner's choice for murder. In reality, strychnine has been uncommonly employed in murder owing to various obvious reasons: bitter taste, dramatic nature of symptoms (that will always arouse suspicion of foul play), and easy detectability in body fluids and tissues. However, occasional cases do get reported from time to time.

- Accidental poisoning can result in children who chew on the seeds out of curiosity while playing or foraging in the countryside.
- Previously, therapeutic misadventures used to be fairly common when strychnine was an approved constituent of various over-the-counter tonics and cathartics.
- Owing to the agonising nature of death, strychnine is rarely employed in suicide.

Index

G